INTERNAL MEDICINE

INTERNAL MEDICINE

Edited by

Clarence A. Guenter

PROFESSOR AND HEAD
DEPARTMENT OF MEDICINE
FACULTY OF MEDICINE
THE UNIVERSITY OF CALGARY
DIRECTOR, DEPARTMENT OF MEDICINE
FOOTHILLS PROVINCIAL GENERAL HOSPITAL
CALGARY, ALBERTA

With 21 Contributors

CHURCHILL LIVINGSTONE
NEW YORK, EDINBURGH, LONDON, AND MELBOURNE   1983

Acquisitions editor: *Lewis Reines*
Copy editor: *Michael Kelley*
Production editor: *Karen Goldsmith Montanez*
Production supervisor: *Nina R. West*
Compositor: *Maryland Composition Company, Inc.*
Printer/Binder: *The Maple-Vail Book Manufacturing Group*

Distributed in the United Kingdom by Churchill Livingstone,
Robert Stevenson House, 1-3 Baxter's Place, Leith Walk,
Edinburgh EH1 3AF and by associated companies, branches
and representatives throughout the world.

First published 1983

Printed in U.S.A.

ISBN 0-443-08153-0

7 6 5 4 3 2 1

Library of Congress Cataloging in Publication Data

Main entry under title:

Internal medicine.

   "With 21 contributors."
   Bibliography: p.
   Includes index.
   1. Internal medicine.   I. Guenter, Clarence A.
[DNLM: 1. Internal medicine. WB 115   I6051]
RC46.I48   1983   616   83-7514
ISBN 0-443-08153-0

CONTRIBUTORS

Werner J. Becker, M.D.
Assistant Professor of Clinical Neurosciences, The University of Calgary and Calgary General Hospital, Calgary, Alberta

Stephen K. Carter, M.D.
Professor of Medicine, School of Medicine, New York University, Vice President, Anti-Cancer Research, Pharmaceutical Research and Development Division, Bristol-Myers Co., New York, New York

Bernard Corenblum, M.D.
Associate Professor, Department of Medicine, Faculty of Medicine, The University of Calgary, Calgary, Alberta

R. Timothy Coussons, M.D.
David Ross Boyd Professor, Vice Head, Department of Medicine, The University of Oklahoma, Health Science Center, College of Medicine, Oklahoma City, Oklahoma

Thomas Enta, M.D.
Associate Professor of Medicine (Dermatology), Department of Medicine, Faculty of Medicine, The University of Calgary, Calgary, Alberta

Hugh J. Freeman, M.D.
Associate Professor of Medicine, Head of Gastroenterology, The University of British Columbia, Health Sciences Hospital, Vancouver, British Columbia

Clarence A. Guenter, M.D.
Director, Department of Medicine, Foothills Provincial General Hospital, Professor and Head, Department of Medicine, Faculty of Medicine, The University of Calgary, Calgary, Alberta

Gabriel Gregoratos, M.D.
Professor of Medicine, Director, Coronary Care Unit, Coordinator, Clinical Cardiology Services, The University of California Medical Center, San Diego, California

Jack Hirsh, M.D.
Professor and Chairman, Department of Medicine, McMaster University, Hamilton, Ontario

Alan R. Hull, M.D.
Southwestern Dialysis Center, Clinical Professor of Medicine, The University of Texas, Southwestern Medical School, Dallas, Texas

Joel S. Karliner, M.D.
Professor of Medicine, The University of California, San Francisco, Chief, Cardiology Section, Veterans Administration Hospital, San Francisco, California

T. Douglas Kinsella, M.D.
Professor of Medicine, Director, Division of Rheumatology, Department of Medicine, Faculty of Medicine, The University of Calgary, Calgary, Alberta

Robert G. Lee, M.D.
Professor and Head, Department of Clinical Neurosciences, Faculty of Medicine, The University of Calgary, and Director, Department of Clinical Neurosciences, Foothills Provincial General Hospital, Calgary, Alberta

Raymond M. Lewkonia, M.B., Ch.B.
Professor and Head, Departments of Internal Medicine and Pediatrics, Faculty of Medicine, The University of Calgary, Calgary, Alberta

R. Brian Lowry, M.D.
Professor and Head, Division of Medical Genetics, Department of Pediatrics, Faculty of Medicine, The University of Calgary, Director of Medical Genetics, Alberta Children's Hospital, Calgary, Alberta

Samuel Oleinick, M.D.
Professor of Medicine, Department of Medicine, The University of Oklahoma, Health Sciences Center, Oklahoma City, Oklahoma

John K. Ruedy, M.D.
Head, Department of Medicine, St. Paul's Hospital, Professor of Medicine, The University of British Columbia, Vancouver, British Columbia

Eldon Shaffer, M.D.
Professor of Medicine, Director, Division of Gastroenterology, Department of Medicine, Faculty of Medicine, The University of Calgary, Calgary, Alberta

Scott N. Swisher, M.D.
Professor of Medicine, Associate Dean for Research, Michigan State University, East Lansing, Michigan

Robert Volpé, M.D.
Physician-in-Chief, The Wellesley Hospital, Professor, Department of Medicine, The University of Toronto, Toronto, Ontario

Wilfred M. Weinstein, M.D.
Professor of Medicine, The University of California, Los Angeles, School of Medicine, Los Angeles, California

Ellison H. Wittels, M.D.
Clinical Assistant Professor of Medicine, The University of Oklahoma, Health Sciences Center, Oklahoma City Clinic, Oklahoma City, Oklahoma

PREFACE

The study of internal medicine is filled with intrigue and challenge. These result from the continual revision of our understanding of disease and treatment, and the immense scope of the field. This text was developed for those students and physicians who are overwhelmed by the sheer volume of material in the authoritative and encyclopedic textbooks now available. Offered in response to pleas from our students it was designed to identify themes and patterns of learning which may facilitate mastery of the essentials of this field.

The book places clear priority on selected material and less emphasis on detail which can reasonably be deferred to subsequent years of specialized training. The reader should have sound knowledge of basic medical science and a thorough background in the clinical skills of interviewing, obtaining a medical history and performing the physical examination. Certain specialized but necessary skills such as interpretation of electrocardiograms and roentgenograms are best dealt with by the fine textbooks written for those areas of laboratory diagnosis. In order to limit the contents, priorities were determined by the prevalence of disorders and the urgency of therapeutic intervention. More emphasis was placed on preventive medicine than sophisticated care of advanced disease. The priorities were clearly developed on the basis of disease in the Western World; however, the principles remain relevant for the developing countries where parasitic, diarrheal and nutritional diseases should receive greater emphasis.

Part I deals with pathophysiologic processes and therapeutic principles appropriate to multiple organ systems. The common problems of alcoholism, obesity, drug abuse, atherosclerosis, hypertension and thromboembolism are emphasized because of the potential for intervention. A clear understanding of genetics, immune mechanisms, infectious diseases, fluid and electrolyte disturbances and principles of pharmacotherapy are provided as a basis for the care of patients with disease of any organ system. The chapter on oncology outlines factors considered important in carcinogenesis, opportunities for early detection of certain types of cancer and major therapeutic advances.

Part II deals with medical problems involving the major organ systems. Emphasis is placed on the approach to understanding mechanisms, diagnosis and management. The student is urged to concentrate on synthesis of the patient problem into a cohesive formulation, scrupulously avoiding the temptation to simply list the facts. In some instances allocation of a disease to a specific organ system was arbitrary and the student may need to consult the index.

The emerging emphasis on gerontology and geriatrics would justify a separate chapter on this theme. In this text the authors were urged to integrate the emphasis on aging with the appropriate chapters, thereby conforming to the usual clinical presentation.

As a primary text, suitable to be read from cover to cover during the term of one's medical service, it is our hope that this book will cultivate the interest, understanding and clinical approach essential to the mastery of medical problems and essential to the performance of an excellent physician.

Clarence A. Guenter, M.D.

INTRODUCTION
The Approach to the Patient

THE DOCTOR-PATIENT RELATIONSHIP

Since patients' needs extend far beyond their diseases, physicians must be skilled beyond the science of medicine. The burgeoning technological and scientific advances, coupled with subspecialty based expertise, support the trend to identify each patient's problems as a disease. The sensitive clinician is often embarrassed by the lack of human interest and skill which penalizes patients in much of current medical practice. The art of medicine requires a broad commitment to the problems of the individual; this challenge was well phrased in an ancient book of healing: *bear ye one anothers burdens*. When physicians accept this involvement, patients will not be shunted indifferently from appointment to appointment or from one physician or subspecialist to another.

THE PATIENT'S ASSESSMENT OF THE DOCTOR

Every child begins a lifelong study of persons who are part of his life. Every patient brings a unique perceptive ability to assess the physician. He may come with biases regarding status, finances, personality or bedside manner. The physician refutes or confirms these by his office, car, clothes and behaviour. The die may be cast before the interview begins. If the physician survives this scrutiny, the relationship may grow. The effective physician must ultimately play a role as confidant and consultant and often as comforter and counsellor. Every encounter unfolds new dimensions in the fragile doctor-patient relationship.

Is the Doctor Interested in Me?

Undivided attention is difficult to transfer from patient to patient at short intervals. This skill is absolutely basic to development of strong relationships. Financial preoccupations, multiple commitments in a day, distractions by interruptions and interests elsewhere can paralyze the development of understanding. The ability to listen, to sense the hidden meanings, to hear beyond the expressed concerns can only be developed fully when used consistently. The patient will have enduring respect for the physician who correctly perceives an unspoken need.

Respect for a patient's comments and concerns will be demonstrated by a suitable response. Between friends each response is weighed carefully, but in the doctor-patient relationship each response is considered to be a deliberate pronouncement. Therefore a symptom ignored may be perceived as disinterest, disbelief or a medical judgement that the symptom is insignificant. The sensitive physician is attentive to each patient concern, carefully planning a suitable response. Occasionally the response is deferred, and brought to bear at a follow-up visit.

Personal interest may be off-bounds for business relationships and casual friendships, but it is central to the doctor-patient relationship. The physician who shows little interest in family, friends, work, financial status, religion, travel and life style is unlikely to assure the patient of his comprehensive knowledge of factors bearing on health and disease. Furthermore, significant factors must not be forgotten or the interest will be recognized as superficial and contrived. Good records, quickly reviewed before each visit, aid immeasurably.

The patient who has exposed himself through a doctor-patient encounter expects a special arrangement in return: opportunity to discuss concerns regarding laboratory investigation, medical problems of spouse or children, preferred consideration for appointments, and occasionally emergency services. This is not viewed as an imposition, it is part of the relationship. The physician is the patient's doctor: "*my doctor*".

Is the Doctor Honest?

Each patient is concerned that the services rendered be based on a system of trust. Evidence of credibility in all areas of behaviour will be assessed and interpreted as bearing on the medical care. Personal values are generally more apparent than we admit. Patients quickly identify double standards.

Is the Doctor Competent?

Self assurance founded on sound knowledge and clinical skills are persuasive. Arrogance, denial, superficial judgements and false confidence soon declare their folly. The patient generally warms to the physician who sincerely and humbly acknowledges that he is perplexed and needs more time for consideration or seeks the advice of a colleague. He expects understanding for his naïve enthusiasm when an alternative form of care arises, even if it is unconventional. Although not always present in the same physician, competence and humility are perceived as compatible ideals.

THE DOCTOR'S ASSESSMENT OF THE PATIENT

How Well are we Communicating?

Naïvety allows some physicians to come to firm conclusions after a single patient encounter. The skilled clinician recognizes that many unrecognized factors will only be identified with time. Just as a symptom may be irrelevant with respect to the underlying disease, the spoken communication may distract from the major patient concern. The wise clinician listens carefully to the expressed concerns and is tuned to information that may reveal problems beyond those expressed. A rapid judgement may effectively terminate the encounter, but tentative reassurance with delayed conclusions may permit additional information to be gathered. Each encounter should provide a stronger relationship, not a new diagnosis or treatment.

Is the Patient Ill?

A diagnosis and treatment rest on scientific medicine. They may prevent complications or cure disease. An early objective for each new patient encounter is to establish the presence or absence of illness. This sense of illness improves with experience but always remains imperfect. Therefore, for apparently unimportant symptoms, reassurance should be given with clear willingness to review the problems. All too often the "functional" headache becomes severe sinusitis or a brain tumour; the "smoker's" cough is later shown to be due to lung cancer.

Understanding the person with stoical or hypochondrial tendencies may be most useful. Change in living pattern, sex life and effectiveness at home or work may be more revealing than additional laboratory tests. The patient's own diagnostic preoccupations will certainly provide a clue to his anxiety and occasionally to the disease. Finally, if the patient is declared free of the disease but remains unconvinced, the problem is not resolved. Good care includes the worried well.

What is the Life Setting?

The systematic interview should include occupation, life habits and diet. All too often this information is scanty or the question is misunderstood. Stress in the working place, conflict in the home, bereavement or illness of loved ones may amplify symptoms or concerns. Frequently a visit to the home or working place will demonstrate an entirely new range of relevant data. The patient with allergic alveolitis and incapacitating asthma may never be relieved until the home visit unveils the previously denied breeding pigeons. The now abandoned house call was once a major source of clinical data.

THE ILLNESS IN CONTEXT

RELEVANT MEDICAL DATA

Every patient has a history of health or disease. Accurate records of interviews and examinations may shed new light on patient behaviour or abnormal physical findings. Previous chest roentgenograms, electrocardiograms, histological material or urinalysis may clarify the significance of a recent abnormality. Such information must always be sought and retrieved; simple recall is often in error. Telephone calls or letters to previous doctors, hospitals or laboratories will generally be richly rewarded by the improved analysis of the problem. Perseverance is essential.

THRESHOLDS FOR DISABILITY

Disability is generally experienced in relation to life tasks and recent performance. A patient with hypothyroidism may be quite oblivious to a lack of mental acuity or conversational skills but acknowledges improvement after treatment. The patient with decreased sexual drive may be unconcerned by impotence. Those who never run or climb stairs may not recognize incipient dyspnea. The physician must establish the activities and the household or community expectations of the patient. How has the activity or behaviour changed with time? What level of demand is placed on performance?

PREVALENCE AND PROBABILITY OF DISEASE

Food poisoning usually affects most participants in a shared meal. Febrile illness is predictable during a community or household outbreak of infection. Hot climates may cause heat stroke, particularly in the elderly taking parasympathetic blocking drugs. Tetanus is extremely rare in immunized persons. Pancreatitis is more likely in the alcoholic. Septicemia demands a search for the portal of entry. Coccidioidomycosis is common in California but only occurs in the Alberta resident if he travels to endemic areas. Statistical probabilities help establish diagnostic priorities but must never be given the ultimate vote.

CONSIDERATIONS FOR THE AGING

Most organ systems progressively deteriorate after age 25. The insidious decrease in function may only be apparent during intercurrent disease. After age 65 the hypoxemia and systemic toxicity of pneumonia frequently causes confusion; febrile illness may precipitate heart failure and medications may cause side effects at lower doses. By age 75–80 most organs have marginal function. Heart failure may cause severe confusion, impaired renal function and nettlesome electrolyte disturbances. Multiorgan system failure becomes commonplace. Communication may be more difficult. The relative risk of intervention is greater and the life expectancy even with a good immediate outcome may be brief.

THE PATIENT'S EXPECTATIONS OF AN ILLNESS

Benign or self-limiting disease may seem inconsequential to the physician, but the patient is only completely convinced after recovery. The wise physician recognizes this suspended conclusion by planning a follow-up. Rate of recovery, residual symptoms or concern about transmission to household or family may become major preoccupations. The physician should attempt to understand the expectations of the patient.

Chronic progressive disease and incurable malignancy are accepted in different ways. Some patients face brutal reality with courage and bouyancy while others become incapacitated by depression. The physician should assess the patient's emotional reserves and personal needs. Time and the natural history of disease may convincingly declare the prognosis when words could only alarm. Too often the physician accepts the charge to be honest and makes pronouncements of prognosis when variability in natural history defy concrete predictions. On the other hand, optimistic denial of obvious medical failure will soon be construed as incompetence. Patients may not perceive the illness in pathophysiologic terms. They do not understand the therapy as scientifically based intervention. Personal judgement, motivation and sense of well being are major determinants of compliance for each treatment or dose. This is particularly true for physicians who are patients.

The doctor and patient must identify what is expected of each other and of the illness but recognize that all three are likely to change positions in mid course.

These considerations supersede all detailed knowledge in the day to day practice of medicine. Students who learn excellent scientific medicine and understand the importance and complexity of these relationships will be distinguished by their effectiveness.

CONTENTS

Disease of Life-Style: Alcohol, Obesity, and Drug Abuse

John K. Ruedy, M.D.

The major objectives of medical care include relief of suffering, improvement of the quality of life, and prolongation of life through prevention, treatment, or cure of disease. Early in the twentieth century the life expectancy at birth was about 47 years, but it now averages 78 years. The premature deaths were predominantly due to infections, such as diphtheria, polio, tetanus, measles, smallpox, diarrheal diseases, tuberculosis, and pneumonia, and to parasitic infestations and trauma. Immunization programs, insect control, clean water, sewage management, food processing, improved nutrition, and early care for acute illness are largely responsible for the reduced mortality in early life.

These measures have influenced the developing countries to a variable degree; for example, India has an estimated life expectancy of 55 to 57 years, while Nepal continues to have a life expectancy of 42 to 47 years. In the underdeveloped countries the major hurdles relate to poverty, social customs, religions, and the lack of engineering skills and education.

Remarkably, despite the 30-year increase in life expectancy at birth in the developed countries, the life expectancy for 75-year-old persons has increased only 3 years. Considerable evidence suggests that human longevity will be limited to about 80 to 90 years, regardless of the role of acute or chronic disease. If aging and multiorgan system failure is normal, 80 to 90 years may represent the age of general demise.

The major changes in life expectancy yet to be achieved probably relate to acute and chronic disease resulting from life-style and habits. These remediable factors are intimately related to behavior and emotional status. If neonatal death due to prematurity is excluded, the most common causes of life-years lost to premature death are trauma and suicide. Half of the deaths due to trauma are alcohol and drug related; suicide has its roots in emotional and social unrest. Alcohol, obesity, and drug abuse represent three major health problems that are products of life-style. These are discussed in this chapter. Similar life-style problems such as cigarette smoking, environmental pollution, and noncompliance with medical treatment are discussed elsewhere in relation to appropriate organ systems or diseases.

ALCOHOL AND ITS MEDICAL CONSEQUENCES

In North America there are twice as many admissions to hospital for treatment of alcohol-related disorders as for myocardial infarction. In some areas the number of deaths resulting from cirrhosis secondary to alcohol approaches the number of deaths resulting from coronary artery disease. Half of all suicides, homocides, and motor vehicle accidents are alcohol related. Of every 10 patients in a general hospital, 2 to 4 can be expected to have a drinking problem. Physical symptoms are common in alcoholism, but patients are very likely to complain about such symptoms without volunteering information about a drinking problem. Thus the diagnosis of an alcohol-related symptom is frequently missed until the disorder is advanced. Often the effects of alcohol are superimposed on other medical illnesses, leading to inappropriate diagnosis and treatment. Unfortunately frustration with the frequency of diseases related to alcohol sometimes engenders physician neglect and disinterest in the patient's problems. This contrasts strikingly with the positive attitude physicians have toward other "self-inflicted" disorders such as sports injuries.

The major overt manifestations of ethanol excess are cirrhosis of the liver and central nervous system symptoms including intoxication, the alcohol withdrawal syndrome, and a variety of neurological sequelae. Ethanol overuse, however, has many other less obvious, though important consequences, which are summarized in Table 1.1. An understanding of

Table 1.1   Some of the Common Medical Consequences of an Excessive Intake of Alcohol

Intermediary metabolism
   Increased production of lactate, acetoacetate, and β-hydroxybutyrate
   Increased production of fatty acids and triglycerides
   Decreased urate excretion
   Hyperglycemia and hypoglycemia
   Induction of hepatic microsomal enzymes
Nutritional deficiency
   Reduced intake
   Malabsorption
Hematological effects
   Vacuolization of red cell precursors
   Megaloblastic pancytopenia (folate deficiency)
   Sideroblastic anemia (? pyridoxine deficiency)
   Macrocytosis, target cells, and acanthosis
   Hemolytic anemia
   Iron deficiency anemia
   Impaired phagocytic function
   Thrombocytopenia and rebound thrombocytosis
Water, electrolytes, and minerals
   Inhibition of secretion of antidiuretic hormone
   Increased osmolality
   Hypomagnesemia, hypocalcemia, hypophosphatemia, hypokalemia
Neurological consequences
   Acute inebriation
   Withdrawal reactions
   Wernicke-Korsakoff syndrome
   Alcoholic cerebellar ataxia
   Polyneuropathy
Myopathy
   Skeletal
   Cardiomyopathy
Gastrointestinal disorders
   Esophageal lacerations
   Esophageal varices
   Gastric erosions and hemorrhagic gastritis
   Atrophic gastritis
   Gastric ulcer
   Cancer of upper gastrointestinal tract
Pancreatitis
Liver disease
   Alcoholic fatty liver
   Alcoholic hepatitis
   Cirrhosis
Pulmonary disease
   Aspiration pneumonia
   Anaerobic infections
   Tuberculosis
   Rib fractures

the mechanisms of these effects is important in the management of alcoholic patients.

METABOLIC CONSEQUENCES OF ETHANOL IN THE LIVER

A variety of metabolic abnormalities are influenced by the chronicity of alcohol intake, the nutritional state of the patient, genetic factors, and the presence of congeners in the alcohol consumed. Predominant among these biochemical effects are the following:

1. Increased production of lactate, acetoacetate, and beta-hydroxybutyrate
2. Increased production of fatty acids and triglycerides
3. Decreased urate excretion
4. Hyperglycemia and hypoglycemia

Many of these changes can be explained by the products of the hepatic metabolism of ethanol. The major metabolic pathway involves the cytosolic enzyme, alcohol dehydrogenase (ADh), which catalyses the conversion of ethanol to acetaldehyde:

$$C_2H_5OH + NAD^+ \xrightarrow{ADh} CH_3CHO + NADH + H^+$$

In this reaction hydrogen is transferred from ethanol to the cofactor nicotinamide adenine dinucleotide (NAD), yielding its reduced form, NADH. Oxidation of the excessive NADH takes place in the mitochondria, but the oxidation capacity is limited. As a consequence there is an increase in the reducing equivalents in the liver with the production of acetaldehyde. The altered redox state of the liver affects many reactions that are dependent on NAD. Some of the effects are evident only within the hepatocyte and, therefore, are not amenable to direct measurement by clinical laboratory methods. Others, however, are reflected in changes in serum constituents.

Increase in Lactate and β-Hydroxybutyrate

The principal metabolic reaction that may be measured clinically is the conversion of pyruvate to lactate. The excess production of NADH enhances the production of lactate from pyruvate (Fig. 1.1), so that an increased lactate-pyruvate ratio can be measured in the peripheral blood following the intake of alcohol. Other variables, however, such as exercise, thiamine status, and carbohydrate metabolism affect this ratio, making it unreliable

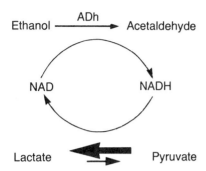

Fig. 1.1 The influence of alcohol on lactate and pyruvate.

as a clinical index of ethanol abuse. This increased production of lactate may result in significant metabolic acidosis, and this acidosis can be enhanced by another NAD-dependent reaction influenced by alcohol, the enhanced production of β-hydroxybutyric acid from acetoacetate. Neither lactate nor β-hydroxybutyrate are measured by the usual techniques for measuring ketones in serum or urine. The clinical suspicion of excess lactate or β-hydroxybutyrate is based on measurement of an increased anion gap without an important degree of ketosis in an alcoholic patient.

Lipid Metabolism

The reactions of the tricarboxylic acid cycle are depressed by the excess of NADH. Mitochondria utilize the hydrogen equivalents derived from the oxidation of ethanol in place of those ordinarily generated from oxidation of fatty acids. Ethanol replaces fatty acids as the major energy source for the liver, and fatty acids accumulate. In addition, the excess of NADH favors the generation of α-glycerophosphate from glucose, which enhances the accumulation of triglycerides in the hepatocyte. Both of these changes contribute to the development of the alcoholic fatty liver and to an increase in serum lipoproteins and triglycerides. The increase in fatty acids can serve as a source for increased production of acetoacetate, which is manifested clinically as ketoacidosis.

Hyperglycemia and Hypoglycemia

Chronic ingestion of ethanol results in two disturbances of glucose metabolism which are apparent clinically. The first is a diabetic-like moderate glucose intolerance which is not severe enough to require insulin. The mechanisms of this abnormality are probably multiple and are poorly understood. In some instances the nutritional state of the patient and the presence of hepatic or pancreatic disease secondary to ethanol use may be important. Ethanol ingestion results in an increased output of growth hormone which through its antiinsulin effect can impair the peripheral utilization of glucose. In addition, ethanol enhances the secretion of epinephrine, which induces hyperglycemia through activation of glycogen phosphorylase and enhanced breakdown of hepatic glycogen. In acute human experiments, propranolol has been shown to block the hyperglycemia produced by alcohol. The clinical importance of alcohol-induced glucose intolerance lies in the diagnostic confusion it creates, which can lead to a mistaken diagnosis of diabetes mellitus, liver disease, or chronic pancreatitis.

Alcohol-related hypoglycemia, the second abnormality of glucose metabolism, is of greater clinical importance. Hypoglycemia can occur after alcohol ingestion in the absence of any other precipitating factor, but it is particularly severe in fasting and malnourished individuals, in alcohol-naive children, and in patients receiving insulin or other hypoglycemic drugs. It is also most likely to occur in individuals who have severe hepatic disease or whose stores of hepatic glycogen are low for other reasons. Among the mechanisms responsible for ethanol-induced hypoglycemia is the increase in NADH and interference with NAD-dependent reactions. Hepatic gluconeogenesis is impaired because of the reduced hepatic levels of pyruvate and the depressed activity of the tricarboxylic acid cycle that, in turn, impairs the utilization of amino acids. Further, an enhanced production of α-glycerophosphate from glucose accentuates the hypoglycemia. Clinical recognition of hypoglycemia in the alcoholic is difficult, since the severe signs of hypoglycemia—confusion, stupor, and coma—can be easily misdiagnosed in the alcoholic patient. Even when recognized and treated, alcohol-related hypoglycemia has a mortality rate of about 10 percent.

Metabolism of Ethanol and Effects on Hepatic Enzymes

Ethanol is principally metabolized by the liver under the influence of the enzyme alcohol dehydrogenase, which consists of a mixture of isoenzymes whose pattern varies among individuals. In some groups, including individuals from Switzerland, Chile, and Japan, atypical alcohol dehydrogenase isoenzymes have been isolated that, in vitro, have 3 to 6 times the activity of normal ADh. The rate of metabolism of ethanol in vivo, however, does not increase to the same extent, because the rate-limiting step in the oxidation of ethanol is the reoxidation of reduced nicotinamide adenine dinucleotide (NADH). Ethanol is also oxidized by a microsomal ethanol oxidizing system (MEOS). Like other substances metabolized by microsomal enzymes, ethanol induces a proliferation of the microsomal fraction of the hepatic cell that comprises the smooth endoplasmic reticulum.

The rate of metabolism of ethanol approximates 120 to 150 mg/kg/hour or 200 to 240 g/day; however, the rate is highly variable among individuals. Chronic ethanol intake induces the MEOS and in the alcoholic the clearance of ethanol can be nearly twice that in normals. The heavy drinker can eliminate 360 g/day, the approximate amount contained in 700 ml (24 ounces) of whiskey or 8 liters (8½ quarts) of beer. Other drugs that induce microsomal enzymes, such as barbiturates, oral contraceptives, and phenytoin, can result in an increased ethanol clearance. Less is known about their influences on the major metabolic pathway of ethanol—the alcohol dehydrogenase system.

Changes in the rate of ethanol metabolism occur in a variety of disorders such as cirrhosis that lead to a diminution of hepatic function. ADh can also be inhibited by drugs such as chloral hydrate. If chloral hydrate is taken with alcohol, higher levels of alcohol are reached earlier—the metabolic explanation of the Mickey Finn. The patient with an alcoholic fatty liver, however, usually has a normal or enhanced clearance of alcohol.

A rise in serum γ-glutamyl transpeptidase (γGT) occurs as a result of hepatic induction of the enzyme by alcohol, and similar increases can be observed following the use of barbiturate, cocaine, narcotics, or phenytoin. In general, serum γGT concentrations in alcoholics average twice the upper limit of normal. In normal volunteers, increased levels of γGT occur acutely and return to normal within a few days after exposure to alcohol. The serum concentration of the enzyme is frequently used as the most specific marker of hepatocellular damage due to ethanol. However, it is important to consider the possibility of enzyme induction before attributing above-normal γGT concentrations to hepatic damage.

NUTRITION

Nutritional deficiencies are frequent in alcoholics because (1) they often have diets that are poor in essential nutrients; (2) ethanol alters the absorptive and digestive function of the gastrointestinal tract; and (3) malnutrition itself can alter intestinal function. Notably, the most common lethal complication of alcohol excess—hepatic cirrhosis—develops even with normal diets; its incidence correlates best with the amount of alcohol consumed and not with a history of dietary deficiency.

Each gram of alcohol provides approximately 7 Cal of energy; thus, the chronic alcoholic consuming 360 g/day of alcohol can meet his caloric needs through alcohol alone. This occurs at the expense of nutrient protein, vitamins, and minerals. Alcoholic beverages are particularly deficient in ascorbic acid and thiamine. The frequency of the deficiencies of these two vitamins in alcoholics justifies the widespread practice of administering multivitamin preparations to alcoholics admitted to hospital. Symptoms and signs of thiamine deficiency, in particular Wenicke's encephalopathy, may develop in alcoholic patients after admission to hospital during intravenous feeding with glucose. This is presumably due to the utilization of thiamine in the metabolism of the administered glucose.

Moderate malabsorption is a frequent finding in alcoholics and is often due to multiple factors. The upper small intestine is exposed to high concentrations of ethanol during drinking; the rapid improvement in absorptive capacity seen after cessation of alcohol suggests that ethanol can directly impair intestinal function. However, the mechanism of this interference is poorly understood. There is little relationship among various nutrients and the degree of malabsorption. Malabsorption of the water-soluble vitamins thiamine, folic acid, and B_{12} can be demonstrated, whereas the absorption of xylose and fat is commonly unaffected.

Steatorrhea of moderate degree, 5 to 15 g of fecal fat per day, has been described in one third of alcoholics. This is probably a result of structural changes in the intestinal epithelium due to ethanol or malnutrition, or is secondary to the accompanying chronic hepatic and pancreatic complications of alcoholism. A strong relationship has been shown between folate deficiency and malabsorption in alcoholics, and it is probable that folate deficiency plays a major role in the impaired intestinal function in alcoholics. Severe protein malnutrition can be responsible for functional and structural alterations of the small intestine and can lead to a reversible reduction of pancreatic exocrine secretion. The role of protein malnutrition in alcoholic malabsorption is unclear.

HEMATOLOGICAL EFFECTS

Alterations in hematopoiesis are common in the alcoholic patient. Vacuolization of the red cell precursors in the bone marrow is a common abnormality in intoxicated patients, although a return to normal morphology usually occurs after an abstinence of one week. The functional importance of this finding is not known, but its resemblance to the changes seen after chloramphenicol suggest that it represents toxic depression of erythrocytes. A megaloblastic pancytopenia is observed in many alcoholics secondary to the diminished intake of folate and interference by ethanol with folate absorption. Malnourished alcoholics frequently have a sideroblastic anemia. The accumulation of iron in the mitochondria, which causes this morphological change, represents an abnormality in heme production. In alcoholics, sideroblastic anemia is thought to be due to pyridoxine (vitamin B_6) deficiency, which results from both decreased pyridoxine intake and enhanced hydrolysis of the vitamin caused by acetaldehyde.

In alcoholics with liver disease, abnormalities in red cell morphology are frequently seen. These include macrocytosis, target cells, and acanthosis. Macrocytosis can be secondary to folate deficiency, in which the volume of the red cell is increased. When macrocytosis occurs with normal folate nutrition, the red cells have increased diameter only (thin macrocytes). These macrocytic cells have an increased lipid content and an increase in osmotic resistance. Target cells appear to be an exaggerated form of the thin macrocyte. Normal red cells, when transfused into subjects with thin macrocytosis and target cells, adopt similar abnormal shapes. Irregularly spiculated and contracted red blood cells, referred to as *spur cells* or *acanthocytes*, are usually seen in patients with advanced alcoholic cirrhosis and are associated with a hemolytic anemia. The mechanism responsible for this morphological change is not known.

A low-grade hemolytic anemia is frequently associated with advanced hepatic disease of alcoholics. An association has been observed between hypophosphatemia which occurs frequently in alcoholics, and hemolytic anemia. It has been postulated that diminished erythrocyte levels of ATP lead to increased red blood cell rigidity and hemolysis. Spherocytes are frequently observed in such cases. Another suggested association, that of hemolytic anemia, acute fatty liver, hypercholesterolemia, and hyperbilirubinemia—the so-called Zieve's syndrome—is less convincing, and the evidence of hemolysis or a causal relationship with the hyperlipidemia is questionable.

Bleeding esophageal varices are often responsible for iron deficiency anemia in the cirrhotic alcoholic, and an anemia of chronic disease may occur, presumably related to infection or active cirrhosis.

Ethanol administration decreases both the migration of granulocytes into a focus of inflammation and the phagocytic function of macrophages. Granulo-cytopenia, in the presence of a bacterial infection, is a common observation in alcoholics. Folate deficiency and hypersplenism may contribute to this abnormality, but the major cause remains unknown. Characteristically, the leukopenia is associated with thrombocytopenia and is transient, with "rebound" leukocytosis occurring 2 to 4 days after admission to hospital. These alterations in white cell function contribute to the increased susceptibility of alcoholics to bacterial infection.

Thrombocytopenia is a common finding in intoxicated subjects, and often accompanied by evidence of abnormal platelet function. Characteristically, a "rebound" thrombocytosis occurs in about 10 days after alcohol intake is stopped, regardless of whether there has been an initial thrombocytopenia. The mechanism of these changes in platelet numbers and function are not known. It is important to point out that thrombocytopenia in an alcoholic patient may be a manifestation of one or more of a variety of conditions, including hypersplenism, severe folate deficiency, disseminated intravascular coagulation, or septicemia.

WATER, ELECTROLYTES, AND MINERALS

Ethanol exerts a diuretic effect by inhibiting the secretion of antidiuretic hormone by the supraoptic-neurohypophyseal system. This effect is seen only during the time when alcohol concentrations in the body are rising and is lost once alcohol concentrations are stable or are decreasing. No consistent effects on the renin-angiotensin-aldosterone system have been described. The major effects of alcohol on fluid balance, however, are most often secondary to the changes in acid-base balance that accompany alcohol excess.

Serum osmolality is increased by ethanol. The measurement of serum osmolality and calculation of the osmolal gap has been suggested as a simple method for estimating the serum concentration of ethanol. (Table 1.2)

Ethanol causes a marked increase in the amount of magnesium and calcium lost in the urine. It is probable that the hypocalcemia is at least partly secondary to the hypomagnesemia. Magnesium has been shown to be necessary for the increased secretion of parathormone that normally follows hypocalcemia. In addition, tissue resistance to the influence of parathormone has been demonstrated in the presence of hypomagnesemia. The number of cases reported in which parathormone has been measured is too small to differentiate which of these two mechanisms

Table 1.2 **Estimation of Serum Ethanol Concentrations from Serum Osmolality**

$$\text{Calculated serum osmolality} \quad \text{mosm/L} = \frac{2(Na^+)}{\text{mmol/L}} + \frac{(\text{Glucose})}{\text{mmol/L}} + \frac{(\text{Urea nitrogen})}{\text{mmol/L}}$$

$$\text{Glucose (mmol/L)} = \frac{\text{mg/L}}{180} \qquad \text{Urea nitrogen (mmol/L)} = \frac{\text{mg/L}}{28}$$

$$\frac{\text{Osmolal gap}}{\text{(mosm/L)}} = \frac{\text{Measured}}{\text{osmolality}} - \frac{\text{Calculated}}{\text{osmolality}}$$

$$= \text{Approximately 10 mosm/L}$$

Osmolal gap in excess of 10 may be due to ethanol

$$\therefore \frac{\text{Ethanol concentration}}{\text{mmol/L}} = \text{Osmolal gap} - 10$$

is of more importance in the hypocalcemia of alcoholism. Spontaneous correction of the hypocalcemia ordinarily occurs after several days of hospitalization and normal nutrition. This return to normal can be hastened by correcting the accompanying hypomagnesemia, but the same result cannot be obtained predictably by administering parathormone.

The alcoholic has many other reasons for hypocalcemia besides hypomagnesemia. Frequently there is a poor dietary intake, and mild steatorrhea may lead to malabsorption of vitamin D or precipitation of calcium with fatty acids in stool. Hypocalcemia may be a manifestation of pancreatitis, which frequently accompanies alcohol abuse.

The mechanism of the hypomagnesemia of alcoholism is unclear. An increase in urinary losses of magnesium can be shown in the normal volunteer receiving ethanol while the ethanol concentrations are rising, but not when a stable concentration is reached. In alcoholics, an increased urinary loss of magnesium is frequently accompanied by an increased loss of lactate; it has been proposed that the magnesium loss is secondary to the formation of insoluble chelates of magnesium and lactate in the tubular urine, and that these chelates prevent reabsorption of magnesium.

Hypophosphatemia has been observed in as many as 50 percent of alcoholic patients admitted to hospital. Hypophosphatemia probably results from a combination of (1) decreased intake; (2) an intracellular shift of phosphate accompanying the utilization of administered glucose in the peripheral tissues of the poorly nourished, glycogen depleted alcoholic; and (3) an increased loss associated with hypomagnesemia, hypokalemia, or acidemic states associated with alcoholism. As with other conditions associated with phosphate depletion, the serum phosphate drawn in the emergency room may be considerably higher than that determined later after the administration of parenteral glucose.

Hypophosphatemia can have a number of important acute clinical consequences in the alcoholic, including neuromuscular, hepatic, and hematologic complications. Neurological symptoms including severe muscle weakness, circumoral paresthesiae, coma, convulsions, and death have been attributed to hypophosphatemia. Two mechanisms have been proposed. Hypophosphatemia may result in a decrease in brain cell ATP, resulting in neurologic dysfunction, or may be due to hypoxemia accompanying the decreased release of oxygen from red blood cells, which is associated with a reduction in red blood cell 2,3-diphosphoglycerate (2,3-DPG). Muscle contraction is known to be dependent on inorganic phosphorus compounds, and depletion of muscle phosphorus may explain the muscle weakness. A brisk hemolytic anemia has been described in occasional patients with hypophosphatemia. The red cells characteristically show a change to a microspheric shape, with increased rigidity and decreased survival. All of these changes revert quickly to normal with phosphate administration. Red blood cell ATP, which is required for maintenance of normal red blood cell membrane integrity, can be shown to be severely depleted in such patients. The chemotactic, phagocytic, and bacteriocidal activity of leukocytes and the normal function of platelets may be also profoundly affected by phosphate depletion, leading to an increase in susceptibility to infection and hemorrhage. Hypophosphatemia has been associated with more rapid hepatic decompensation than seen in cirrhotic patients with normal serum phosphate. It has been suggested that hypophosphatemia blunts the increase of erythrocyte 2,3-DPG (which occurs in cirrhosis), and that this results in hepatic hypoxemia and progressive liver injury.

NEUROLOGICAL COMPLICATIONS OF ALCOHOL

The most obvious effects of alcohol are those on the central nervous system. Excessive intake results in acute alcoholic intoxication, while subjects who drink chronically suffer withdrawal reactions when they diminish or stop their intake. Chronic alcoholism leads to a variety of irreversible neurological syndromes, and superimposed on these may be neurological symptoms of nutritional deficiencies that are common in the chronic alcoholic.

Acute Inebriation

Acute alcoholic intoxication is so common and the symptoms and signs so well known that the diagnosis is rarely missed. In contrast, other conditions such as the neurological sequelae of head injuries, behavioral disturbances, confusion and coma from a variety of causes, and meningitis may be misdiagnosed as being due to alcohol. The "odor of alcohol" on the breath is not only a misnomer, since it is due to impurities in the alcohol consumed, but is misleading as an index of the severity or presence of ethanol intoxication. Its presence should not terminate a search for other causes of altered mentation.

The inebriating effects of ethanol are due to its direct alteration of the function of membrane-associated proteins such as enzymes or receptors. However, the specific action of alcohol is not yet known. The effects are approximately related to the concentration of alcohol, but are influenced as well by the rate at which the concentration rises and by the tolerance to alcohol that develops with chronic intake. The explanation of such adaptation is also not known. Serum concentrations above approximately 20 mmol/L are associated with mild intoxication. Motor incoordination and ataxia can be demonstrated at this concentration. At concentrations of 60 mmol/L alcoholic stupor can occur, and coma is common at higher concentrations.

Alcoholic coma should be considered a medical emergency. It is often accompanied by depression of the respiratory center with resulting respiratory acidosis; the respiratory depression is not reversible by opiate antagonists. Hypotension occurs as a result of hypovolemia due to the initial diuresis that occurs with rising alcohol levels and the fluid loss of accompanying acid-base disturbances and to the direct depression of myocardial contractility and vascular smooth muscle by ethanol and its major breakdown product acetaldehyde. Further, the cardioregulatory center of the medulla is depressed at high ethanol concentrations.

Although drunkenness most often follows a benign course, alcoholic coma is frequently accompanied by metabolic complications that can be life threatening in susceptible subjects. Alcoholic hypoglycemia, due to the inhibition of gluconeogenesis in the liver during ethanol metabolism, is associated with a mortality of 10 percent. It is most frequently observed in malnourished alcoholics. It is also seen in well nourished adults and in children who accidentally drink alcohol. The symptoms often blend imperceptably with those of drunkenness, beginning several hours after drinking is stopped. Hypomagnesemia, hypocalcemia, and acid-base disturbances can dominate the clinical picture. To the extent that they are presently understood, the mechanisms of these changes have been described above.

Diagnosis of alcohol-induced stupor or coma is best made by measuring serum or exhaled ethanol concentrations. If these measurements are not readily available, an estimate of the probable concentration of alcohol present can be made by comparing calculated and measured serum osmolality. Once the contribution of glucose and urea nitrogen has been taken into account, most of the osmolal gap can be explained by the presence of alcohol (Table 1.2).

Treatment of alcoholic stupor or coma consists of careful attention to adequate respiratory function and the correction of any accompanying metabolic abnormalities. Because of the frequency of deficiencies of thiamine and ascorbic acid in the chronic alcoholic, it is prudent to administer these vitamins as a precautionary measure. Respiratory stimulants or measures that attempt to hasten the metabolism of alcohol entail more risk than benefit.

Alcohol Withdrawal Reactions

A variety of disturbances of perception and psychomotor activity occur upon reducing or stopping the intake of alcohol. The most severe symptoms occur in chronic drinkers who have developed tolerance and who cease drinking abruptly. Severe withdrawal reactions, however, are common in individuals who have imbibed heavily for as short a period as 1 to 2 months, and can appear as early as 6 to 8 hours after the last drink when alcohol is still present in the serum but concentrations are falling. The predominant manifestations of withdrawal include tremulousness, disordered perception, seizures, and delirium tremens. Symptoms can occur singly or in combination. Alcohol withdrawal symptoms may constitute the reason for hospital admission, but a common occurrence is the onset of symptoms in alcoholic individuals several days after admission to hospital for intercurrent illness. The onset may be masked and delayed if the patient has received an anesthetic for a surgical procedure.

Tremulousness

Eight to 24 hours after cessation of drinking the subject is often tremulous. This frequently occurs in drinkers after a night's sleep. They awaken with "the shakes" and frequently relieve these symptoms with a drink. This sensation of apprehensive overalertness is frequently accompanied by a coarse irregular tremor of about 6 to 8 oscillations per second. Similar to other metabolic tremors, it is aggravated by activity and anxiety. The patient may be unable to feed himself, walk, or speak. The tremor is milder at rest and can be dampened by propranolol, suggesting that it may be due in part to excess adrenergic activity. Other common accompanying symptoms of anxiety, including excessive sweating and tachycardia, support this hypothesis; these symptoms, too, can be partially ameliorated by propranolol. Myoclonic jerks may be precipitated by mild stimuli. The patient may show slight confusion and may be irritable. These symptoms usually are maximal 24 to 36 hours after stopping alcohol, but the tremulousness and apprehension can last for 10 to 14 days.

Disordered Perception

Many subjects suffering tremulousness complain of nightmares and the distortion of sights and sounds. These altered perceptions are typically unpleasant or threatening, and are difficult to separate from reality. Insomnia and an increased duration of rapid eye movement (REM) sleep is characteristic of alcohol withdrawal. Bad dreams appear to merge with disordered perception. Frank hallucinations can occur. In contrast to the schizophrenic who seems to accept hallucinations with equanimity, the alcoholic is disturbed, frequently responding in an argumentative or combative way to the hallucinations. In contrast to frank delirium tremens, the alcoholic suffering from hallucinations is at most mildly confused, retaining reasonable orientation and recent memory.

Alcoholic mania, the sudden appearance of auditory hallucinations in an alcoholic who otherwise has a clear sensorium, should be distinguished from withdrawal symptoms. Vocal hallucinations, including reproachful, disapproving, and threatening voices, may persist for days or weeks. If short lived, the patient responds to the hallucination by taking protective action such as barricading his room, or calling the police, although self-destructive action may ensue. If chronic, the symptoms merge with other symptoms more suggestive of schizophrenia. The mechanism of alcoholic mania is not understood.

Convulsions

A major complication, generalized tonic clonic seizures occurring singly or in clusters of 2 to 6 seizures over several hours may arise 6 to 48 hours after the cessation of drinking. The seizures typically accompany the tremulousness of withdrawal and are ordinarily self-limited. About 25 percent of alcoholics suffering withdrawal seizures will develop delirium tremens. It is important to distinguish withdrawal seizures from other causes of convulsive disorders. Alcoholics with epilepsy may suffer convulsions during withdrawal, although it is most common for such seizures to occur during drinking. Focal symptoms during a seizure or in the post-ictal state, status epilepticus, the onset of seizures before 6 hours or after 48 hours of stopping drinking, the presence of abnormalities on the EEG between seizures, and the occurrence of seizures following a short period of drinking, all suggest an underlying seizure disorder.

Termination of an alcohol-withdrawal seizure can be best achieved with intravenous diazepam. Metabolic abnormalities such as hypomagnesemia should be identified and treated. Phenytoin is relatively ineffective in preventing withdrawal seizures. Long-term anticonvulsant treatment is not indicated for uncomplicated alcoholic withdrawal seizures. Decreased metabolic clearance of phenytoin in an alcoholic during drinking and during withdrawal, increased clearance during dry periods, as well as the likelihood of noncompliance make dosing too uncertain to be useful.

Delirium Tremens

The most dangerous form of alcohol withdrawal is delirium tremens. This syndrome can occur abruptly or may be preceded by tremulousness, hallucinations, or withdrawal seizures. Treating nutritional deficiencies, tremulousness, withdrawal seizures, or metabolic abnormalities with vitamin supplements, propranolol, anticonvulsants, magnesium, or phosphate does not prevent progression to delirium tremens. The onset is usually more than 48 hours after the last drink but it may be delayed as long as 7 to 10 days. The mortality rate in uncomplicated delirium tremens is 15 percent.

The major feature of delirium tremens is a marked state of confusion. The patient is profoundly tremulous, markedly agitated, and disoriented with respect to time, place, and person, and frequently suffers vivid and threatening hallucinations. Often the patient must be restrained. He may be incontinent and unable to feed himself. Signs of autonomic hyperactivity are present, with dilated pupils, tachycardia, tachypnea, sweating, and fever. Shock, hypothermia, and sudden death sometimes occur. Most often however there is full recovery with little memory of the episode.

The mechanism of delerium tremens is not clear. The syndrome can be understood as a "rebound release" of neurones following chronic suppression by alcohol. This is most clearly demonstrated by the increased activity of the respiratory center, which occurs 8 to 12 hours after drinking is stopped and characteristically results in a respiratory alkalemia.

The patient with delirium tremens should be sedated so that he will not harm himself and so that adequate fluids can be administered. Fluid requirements must be carefully monitored; as much as 7 liters of fluids may be required every 24 hours. The usual choice for sedation is a benzodiazepine. The familiarity that most physicians have with diazepam and the availability of an intravenous formulation make this the drug of choice. Phenothiazines and other antipsychotics should be avoided, since some of them lower the seizure threshold and unpredictable cardiovascular effects accompany their use in the patient with delirium tremens. A careful search for intercurrent or complicating illness must be made repeatedly. Metabolic complications of alcoholism must be anticipated and treated. Glucose solutions should initially be accompanied by thiamine supplements because of the frequent borderline nutritional status of the patient.

Wernicke-Korsakoff Syndrome, Cerebellar Ataxia and Polyneuropathy

Several neurological disorders arise as a consequence of chronic alcohol abuse. The disturbances most frequently observed include the following:
1. Wernicke's disease
2. Korsakoff's psychosis
3. Alcoholic cerebellar ataxia
4. Polyneuropathy

Although these disorders may occur in isolation, they more commonly occur together in a variety of combinations. For this reason the most common neurological sequelae are now referred to as the Wernicke-Korsakoff syndrome. The global confusional state characteristic of Wernicke's disease often masks the characteristic confabulational amnesia of Korsakoff's psychosis, which only becomes obvious when the mental symptoms of Wernicke's disease disappear. The ataxia of Wernicke's disease is indistinguishable from alcoholic cerebellar ataxia, which sometimes occurs alone. Polyneuropathy is present in more than 80 percent of patients who have symptoms of Wernicke's disease and Korsakoff's psychosis. Thiamine deficiency is clearly implicated as the causal factor in the Wernicke-Korsakoff syndrome, and improvement in cerebellar ataxia follows thiamine administration. It is more difficult to attribute the polyneuropathy of alcoholism to a specific nutritional deficiency since it can be caused by deficiencies in one of a variety of vitamins, including thiamine, pyridoxine, vitamin B_{12} and folate. In alcoholic patients, these four neurological disorders are so frequently associated with one another that they can be considered to represent different facets of a single disease process. All can occur in the absence of alcoholism in nutritionally deprived subjects.

Wernicke's Disease

Wernicke's disease consists of a triad of symptoms of disturbed eye movements, a confusional state, and ataxia. The symptoms tend to develop slowly over a few days or weeks, although they may be precipitated acutely by parenteral glucose treatment of nutritionally deficient alcoholics admitted to hospital or emergency rooms.

The ocular disorder is most frequently a horizontal nystagmus on lateral gaze. This is often accompanied by a lateral rectus palsy that is characteristically bilateral. If the sixth nerve palsy is severe, there may be no nystagmus. Conjugate gaze palsies are also common, most frequently involving horizontal gaze. A sluggish pupillary response to light is sometimes seen. More rarely the disorder is accompanied by ptosis and complete opthalmoplegia.

The patient is apathetic, inattentive, and indifferent. Frequently, questions will be ignored or answers will stop in mid-sentence with the patient rolling over and going to sleep. The patient can be easily awakened and will reveal a confusional state with disorientation as to time, place, and person. Rarely a depressed level of consciousness with stupor and coma can be seen.

Wernicke's disease is accompanied by a severe ataxia of gait. Examination of the patient in the supine position is often surprisingly normal. Ataxia of the upper extremities, if present, is mild. Cerebellar speech is usually not present. Moderate to severe ataxia is usually present in heel to shin testing. The dramatic neurological signs, however, occur in the standing position. The patient may be completely unable to walk. If able, he walks with a wide-based gait, taking short, irregular, shuffling steps. Truncal instability can be demonstrated frequently by asking the patient to turn rapidly in the standing position. Falls are frequent.

Korsakoff's Psychosis

This disorder is characterized by a profound memory disturbance, the severity of which is out of keeping with other components of mentation and behavior. The patient is unable to recall past events (retrograde amnesia) and is unable to remember new information (antegrade amnesia). However, other mental functions are preserved. The patient is able to understand spoken and written commands and can solve problems, providing the information is within his limited memory span. In the acute phase of the disorder the patient often confabulates, providing factitious and fabricated accounts of recent events. The disorder is most commonly seen in poorly nourished chronic alcoholic patients but may be caused by atherothrombotic disease of the posterior cerebral arteries, trauma, basilar meningitis, seizure disorders, and degenerative diseases including the early phases of Alzheimer's disease.

Alcoholic Cerebellar Degeneration

The symptoms and signs of alcoholic cerebellar degeneration are indistinguishable from the ataxia that characterizes Wernicke's disease. Occasionally the signs occur in the absence of confusion or ocular-movement disorders. It is then appropriate to use the separate diagnostic label of alcoholic cerebellar degeneration. The symptoms occasionally are acute in onset, in which case the prognosis for recovery is better than if the disorder progresses slowly.

The pathological findings in the Wernicke-Korsakoff syndrome are closely related to the clinical manifestations of the disorder. Necrotic nerve cells and fibers with an associated glial reaction in the diencephalon explain the amnesic symptomatology, while similar lesions in the anterior lobes of the cerebellum, particularly in the vermis, explain the disturbance of gait. In alcoholic cerebellar degeneration identical lesions in the cerebellum are found. Less severe pathological changes in the third and sixth nerve nuclei and vestibular nucleus explain the eye movement disorders. The relatively mild pathological changes in these nuclei correlate with the greater likelihood of recovery from eye movement symptoms, compared with ataxia or amnesia.

These lesions all result from thiamine deficiency. However, the nature of the biochemical abnormality responsible for cell destruction is not known. Thiamine serves several functions within the central nervous system. Bound to the neural membrane, thiamine triphosphate is important for maintaining membrane excitability and for ion transport. In addition, it is a cofactor of decarboxylase and transketolase, enzymes that are important for the metabolism of pyruvate and the production of reduced nicotinamide dinucleotide phosphate (NADH).

The clinical diagnosis of the Wernicke-Korsakoff syndrome is straightforward, provided the patient can be examined and the signs are not masked by accompanying diseases or withdrawal symptoms. Thiamine deficiency can be more specifically assessed by measuring the activity of red blood cell transketolase, its activity is low in deficient patients, and is greatly enhanced by the addition of exogenous thiamine. Increased levels of pyruvate and lactate can be expected in thiamine deficiency, due to the reduced activity of pyruvate decarboxylase.

It is important to recognize and treat patients with ocular signs, since early administration of thiamine can prevent progression to the less readily reversible state accompanied by ataxia and confusion. The frequency of thiamine deficiency and the precipitation of signs of thiamine deficiency during glucose infusion in the alcoholic justify the routine administration of thiamine to chronic alcoholic patients at the time of admission to emergency rooms or hospitals. The usual initial dose of 50 mg daily until a normal diet is resumed is larger than necessary but there is no apparent risk in exceeding the required dose. Patients with overt Wernicke-Korsakoff syndrome show a variable recovery. Ocular muscle disturbances usually resolve completely within hours to several days, although horizontal nystagmus may remain a permanent feature. Ataxia improves much more slowly over days or weeks, and about 50 percent of patients are left with a disturbance of gait. The global confusional state is entirely reversible, but with clearing, the deficit in memory characteristic of Korsakoff's psychosis may become prominent. Complete recovery from Korsakoff's syndrome occurs very slowly, sometimes taking a year or more and is only achieved in a minority of patients (about 20 percent).

Peripheral Neuropathy

A variety of lesions of peripheral nerves are common in the chronic alcoholic, including the following:

1. Alcoholic polyneuropathy
2. Traction or compression mononeuropathy
3. Toxic or drug induced neuropathy

Alcoholic polyneuropathy is common in chronic alcoholics with the Wernicke-Korsakoff syndrome but has also been observed in alcoholics receiving thiamine and pyridoxine supplemented beverages. It is therefore likely that the disorder is due to factors other than vitamin deficiency. The neuropathy, however, is indistinguishable clinically and pathologically from the neuropathy of thiamine deficiency, so-called dry beriberi. There is a symmetrical impairment of sensory, motor, and reflex function more prominent in distal segments. The patient may be asymptomatic or may complain of burning feet, paresthesiae, and mild distal weakness. In severe cases the feet may be so sensitive that bed covers touching the feet are painful and wrist drop and foot drop occur. Pathologically there is a noninflammatory degeneration of the myelin sheath. Response to nutrition and vitamin supplementation is slow and often incomplete.

During acute intoxication or withdrawal, traction or traumatic mononeuropathies are common. "Saturday night palsy" due to compression of the radial nerve in the radial groove of the humerus commonly presents as a wrist drop. Ulnar and peroneal palsies and brachial plexus traction injuries are common.

Drug induced neuropathies occur with increased frequency in the alcoholic. Isoniazid causes a sensory neuropathy due to the accompanying pyridoxine deficiency. Pyridoxine should be routinely given during isoniazid treatment in the chronic alcoholic. Disulfiram and hydralazine occasionally cause a neuropathy in alcoholic subjects. Illicit alcohol (moonshine) has been associated with toxin-induced neuropathies, including lead neuropathy from drinking whisky distilled in lead-lined radiators and triorthocresylphosphate (ginger jake paralysis) from drinking contaminated ginger liquor. Triorthocresylphosphate is presently used as a plasticizer, varnish softener, and heat stabilizer in fuels and glues.

ALCOHOLIC MYOPATHY

Several disorders of skeletal and cardiac muscle occur in alcoholics. Although common, these complications are not specific and are indistinguishable from disorders seen in a variety of other diseases.

Acute and chronic forms of alcoholic myopathy have been described. Acute alcoholic myopathy is infrequent but potentially lethal. This condition occurs characteristically after an alcoholic binge which does not appear to differ from other short periods of excessive drinking. Upon arising in the morning the patient notices weakness of the limb-girdle muscles, particularly the hip flexors and quadriceps so that sitting up or getting up from bed is difficult. Cramps may occur in the affected muscles, and in severe cases the muscles become tender, swollen, and discolored by the blue-green appearance of myoglobin released from the necrotic muscle fibers. More commonly the symptoms are mild and are masked by symptoms of alcoholic withdrawal. The weakness frequently resolves over several days, although in severe cases it can last for several weeks. If myonecrosis is severe, the myoglobinuria can be associated with acute renal failure, which may be complicated by severe hyperkalemia as a consequence of the potassium released from affected muscle as well as the compromised renal function.

The mechanisms of acute alcoholic myopathy are uncertain. The characteristic occurrence following a binge of drinking suggests a direct toxic effect of alcohol on the muscle; however, electrolyte and mineral disorders are common accompaniments and may play a contributory role. Hypokalemia as well as hypophosphatemia have each been shown to be associated with acute muscle necrosis. Potassium or phosphate depletion in the alcoholic patient may be severe enough to account for acute myopathy. Hypokalemia or hypophosphatemia as a precipitating factor may be missed if the measurements are made after potassium and phosphate have been lost into the blood from the damaged muscle.

The diagnosis of acute alcoholic myopathy is obvious in severe cases but is frequently missed in mild cases. Myoglobin in the urine may be suspected if the urine Hemastix or benzidine tests are positive in the absence of hematuria or hemoglobulinuria. Serum creatinine kinase (CK), aldolase, and aminotransferase enzymes are elevated. About 50 percent of patients admitted to hospital due to recent alcohol abuse have elevated CK enzymes. Withdrawal seizures can cause elevation of CK without evidence of muscle necrosis.

The important aspect of treatment of acute alcoholic myopathy is the prevention of acute renal failure. This is accomplished by insuring adequate renal blood flow and a high tubular urine flow with osmotic diuretics. Dialysis may be required to control hyperkalemia.

Chronic myopathy in the alcoholic consists of the insidious development of weakness in proximal muscle groups, particularly of the shoulder girdle and pelvis. The weakness is usually symmetrical and associated with wasting. The muscles are painless and there are usually increases in serum CK, aldolase, and aminotransferase enzymes. After cessation of alcohol there is usually a gradual return to normal function.

Alcohol has been suspected to be related indirectly to two distinctive cardiomyopathies. Thiamine deficiency associated with the malnutrition of chronic alcoholism is responsible for beriberi that is characterized by the insidious development of high-output cardiac failure. Another peculiar syndrome restricted to heavy beer drinkers from Canada, Belgium, and the United States consists of acidemia, polycythemia, pericardial effusion, and shock with impaired myocardial contractile function. Although the condition has been attributed to cobalt added to beer as a foam-stabilizing agent, other factors are probably responsible since cobalt has been used as a therapeutic agent in certain anemias in much higher doses, without these consequences.

In addition to these two specific conditions it is evident that chronic drinking can lead to a nonspecific cardiomyopathy that is unresponsive to thiamine. The patient usually presents with biventricular cardiac failure and marked cardiomegaly due to both hypertrophy and dilatation. There are no characteristic histological findings and the diagnosis is made by exclusion of atherosclerosis, hypertension, and other cardiovascular disorders. The findings and course of alcoholic cardiomypathy are indistinguishable from those of idiopathic cardiomyopathy.

GASTROINTESTINAL DISORDERS

The drinker is subject to a variety of gastrointestinal disorders. Morning nausea and retching is a frequent complaint, and its suppression by further drinking contributes to the drinking problem. Concentrations of alcohol of 10 percent or less stimulate pepsin and hydrochloric acid but are not associated with any morphological change in the gastric mucosa. Concentrations of alcohol over 20 percent inhibit acid and pepsin secretion but enhance mucous production and delay gastric emptying. Erosions of

the gastric mucosa are commonly seen with higher concentrations, an effect that is probably due to the direct toxic effect of alcohol on the mucosa. Half of all patients admitted to many metropolitan hospitals with hemorrhagic gastritis will have ingested alcohol or acetylsalicylic acid, or both, shortly before the onset of bleeding. Atrophic gastritis and gastric ulcers are frequent. An increased incidence of cancer of the mouth, pharynx, larynx, and esophagus is observed in alcoholics. Since many are also heavy smokers, this effect may not be due solely to the drinking of alcoholic beverages.

Massive blood loss from the gastrointestinal tract in the alcoholic is most often due to erosive gastritis. However, it may be due to lacerations of the mucosa at or below the esophageal junction, which most often occur after forceful or repeated retching or vomiting. Esophageal varices secondary to the portal hypertension of cirrhosis and peptic ulcer are other common causes of hematemesis in the alcoholic.

Pancreatitis

Chronic ingestion of alcohol is damaging to the pancreas. Up to 45 percent of alcoholics at autopsy show chronic damage to the pancreas. Morphological changes in the pancreatic ducts as well as abnormalities in pancreatic secretion can be shown in many alcoholics who are asymptomatic. Overt pancreatitis tends to occur only after several years of drinking (mean 18 years in men, 11 years in women). There is no evidence that acute pancreatitis can be caused by the alcoholic binge. These observations suggest that alcoholic pancreatitis is a form of chronic (relapsing) pancreatitis, and that acute manifestations are almost always superimposed on a chronically damaged gland rather than de novo attacks of acute pancreatitis. The risk of alcoholic pancreatitis rises not only with the mean amount of alcohol imbibed each day but with the mean intake of protein as well, although the effect of protein is less marked. The effect of fat is more complex, with an increased risk seen attending both excessively low or high fat diets. The pancreatic secretion in alcoholics contains a higher concentration of protein than that in nonalcoholics, and protein precipitates can be seen frequently in chronic pancreatitis. It is possible that the precipitation of protein in pancreatic juice serves as a matrix for the formation of pancreatic calculi with secondary atrophy of adjacent ductal epithelium, fibrosis, stricture formation, and obstruction. Dilation of ducts, cyst formation, and atrophy of exocrine parenchyma served by the obstructed ductules further characterizes the development of alcoholic chronic pancreatitis. Other factors such as hyperlipidemia may play a role in the pathogenesis of pancreatitis of alcoholism.

Abstinence from alcohol usually results in a reduction of symptoms of pancreatitis to a tolerable level in 50 percent of patients. The patient should avoid an excessively high protein diet (that is, more than 110 g/day). In addition, a fat intake of about 100 g appears to be associated with the lowest risk.

Liver Disease

Altered metabolic function of the liver is universal following the ingestion of alcohol. Morphological changes in the liver are common in the alcoholic, and they consist of three distinct pathological processes:

1. Fatty metamorphosis
2. Alcohol hepatitis
3. Cirrhosis

These conditions are discussed in detail in Chapter 12, under Alcoholic Liver Disease.

LUNG DISEASE

Alcohol may predispose to lung infections through impaired granulocyte, alveolar macrophage, and mucociliary function. However, aspiration of oropharyngeal contents during bouts of inebriation, poor hygiene, and socioeconomic factors that promote crowding and cross-infection are also important factors in the alcoholic or binge drinker. Aspiration pneumonia and anaerobic pleuropulmonary infections are common. Tuberculosis is common and more difficult to treat because of poor patient compliance. Chest trauma with initially unrecognized rib fractures contributes to atelectasis and pneumonia. Lung cancer is much more common in the alcoholic, but cigarette smoking is a more major predisposing factor in most alcoholics (see Chapter 15).

ALCOHOLISM

Alcoholism is a chronic relapsing condition that fulfills three major criteria of an addictive disorder: physical dependence, tolerance, and psychological dependence. Physical dependence and tolerance occur simultaneously, beginning with the first drink and increasing as a function of the dose until a maximum level has developed. Early refractoriness to the effects of alcohol are seen in the fact that, even in the nonalcoholic, the effects of alcohol are much more pronounced as the concentration increases during drinking than at identical concentrations when concentrations are decreasing. In addition, marked attenuation of the effects of alcohol are observed with a second dose taken several days after the initial exposure. There is also convincing evidence of acute physical dependence. In animals the seizure threshold of convulsant drugs is markedly reduced 8 to 12 hours after an injection of alcohol. In man the symptoms of hangover are in a large part withdrawal symptoms. The development of chronic physical dependence and tolerance is related to both the dose and duration of alcohol exposure. It reaches a maximum beyond which no further enhancement of tolerance and dependence occurs, despite further increases in alcohol exposure. Although it is commonly thought that the disappearance of dependency and tolerance occurs rapidly, this is probably not so if sensitive measures are used to evaluate changes. Residual physical dependence and tolerance may persist for months or years.

Surprisingly little is known about the mechanism of dependence and tolerance to alcohol, and about whether the mechanisms are similar for the acute and chronic state. Enhancement of metabolism of alcohol has been suggested, since the drug can be shown to induce the microsomal ethanol oxidizing system (MEOS). The major route of metabolism, however, is catalyzed by alcohol dehydrogenase, and it appears doubtful that the minor increase in the rate of ethanol metabolism by MEOS demonstrated with chronic dosing can explain the large amount of tolerance that develops. There is no evidence that altered adsorption, distribution, or uptake in the brain of alcohol accompanies chronic drinking. Major interest has therefore focused on some cellular alteration that renders the organism refractory to the effects of alcohol. Most theories are based on the induction of protein synthesis, which applies to other addicting drugs. A prominent hypothesis is that of disuse hypersensitivity. According to this model, alcohol reduces the effects of a transmitter influencing cellular function by blocking its synthesis, release, or activity at the cellular receptor. This reduction of transmitter output or effect leads to an increase in the sensitivity of the cell to the transmitter, perhaps through the proliferation of more receptors. As the sensitivity increases, the dose of alcohol must be increased to achieve the same diminution in transmitter function, in other words, tolerance. On cessation of alcohol, a "normal" amount of transmitter can thus interact with a supersensitive cell. No specific alcohol receptor, however, has been demonstrated, and it is possible that the effects of alcohol are due to a generalized disturbance of the conformation or constituents of cell membranes. According to this hypothesis, alcohol disrupts normal membrane function, increasing the fluidity of the membrane. To compensate and maintain adequate function in the presence of alcohol, conformational or chemical changes occur to "stiffen" the membrane. Increasing doses of alcohol become necessary to interfere with cell function (tolerance develops), while cessation of alcohol results in cells with abnormal characteristics and function, resulting in withdrawal reactions. In addition to biochemical theories, a variety of behavioral mechanisms have been postulated as the basis for physical dependence and tolerance. There is little evidence to support or refute any of these theories since it is difficult to isolate behavioral from biological variables.

Much less is known about the mechanisms of psychological dependence to alcohol. Whereas tolerance and physical dependence appear to be a universal effect of alcohol, less than 10 percent of individuals who consume alcohol demonstrate the craving for alcohol and the compulsion to drink that characterize the alcoholic. This aspect of alcoholism is probably of more importance in determining the success or failure of prevention or treatment methods in alcoholism. Many factors are important in determining whether drinking alcoholic beverages will lead to alcoholism. The availability of alcohol has been shown to influence the intake as well as the frequency of complications of alcohol. Total alcohol intake has been shown to decrease during periods of economic hardship; and the number of motor vehicle accidents and the mortality rate due to cirrhosis have been shown to increase as the relative price of alcohol decreases. Genetic factors seem important. There is a much greater probability of alcoholism in adopted children having a biological parent who was alcoholic than in those having nonalcoholic biological parents. Social factors, the acceptance by peers of drinking alcohol, and psychological factors clearly contribute to the development of alcoholism. No unique or specific constitutional, environmental, or psychological configuration, however, characterizes the alcoholic.

Diagnosis

Alcoholism has been variously defined, with no general agreement on what features distinguish the disorder from merely drinking alcohol in excess of the limits accepted by the culture. It is a progressive disorder that eventually results in physical and psychological dependence, and serious damage to social relationships and health. If untreated, it ends usually in permanent mental damage, physical incapacity, and early death.

The premonitory signs and the early diagnosis of alcoholism are frequently missed. A suspicion of alcoholism should be raised in patients complaining of any of the following symptoms: heartburn, morning cough with retching, tremor in middle age, insomnia, anxiety and tension, purpura or ecchymoses, hepatic enlargement, macrocytes in peripheral blood, hyperglycemia, and sensitivity when inquiries into drinking habits are made.

Alcoholism usually occurs without the drinker's conscious knowledge. Guilt and anxiety about drinking lead to denial by the individual of his problem. This fact may be better appreciated when it is realized that as many as one out of every five adult patients seen by an average physician may be alcoholic. Alcoholism is prominently associated with many psychological and behavioral disturbances and stressful life-events, which house officers have been shown to neglect or fail to recognize in their patients. When the diagnosis is made, the patient may have difficulty accepting it because of the stigma associated with the condition and the patient's inability to face living without alcohol. It is the duty of the physician not only to convince the patient of the diagnosis but to point out the risk of the disorder as well. Since depression is a very common affective disturbance in alcoholics, with suicide a potential hazard, care must be taken in identifying the dangers of alcoholism. The physician should avoid any accusatory approach based on the conception that the disorder is one of willful self-destruction. The approach should be open, honest, and sympathetic. Comparisons with other physical illnesses that require continuous treatment and restrictions, such as diabetes or hypertension, are often helpful both with the physician's attitude and the patient's understanding. The physician should reflect on whether the relapse of an alcoholic should arouse attitudes any different from those he has toward the noncompliance of the hypertensive with dietary or drug regimens.

Treatment

The treatment of the alcoholic patient is complex. Effective treatment can rarely be provided by the physician unless he has restricted his practice to the treatment of alcoholism. Comprehensive treatment can be provided by specialized groups such as Alcoholics Anonymous, occupational programs, religious organizations, community health services, the Salvation Army, and psychiatric units specializing in the treatment of alcoholism.

Successful treatment is dependent on three factors. First, education about the harm of alcohol is essential. Second, alcohol addiction must be replaced by an activity, habit, or hobby that involves an available group of supportive and understanding persons, that is demanding in time and effort, and that increases self esteem. Third, strict control of drinking, or preferably abstinence, is basic to successful treatment. A variety of ancillary methods including psychoanalysis, behavioral modification, aversion therapy, and disulfiram have been employed, but the overall results are disappointing. In addition (if alcoholics with specific psychiatric disorders are excluded) there is no evidence that antianxiety or antipsychotic drugs are helpful. Clearly, the treatment program must be individualized. For example, unique cultural differences can influence the selection of treatment modalities. North American native people characteristically are not preoccupied with schedules, order, or competitiveness, and successful treatment must take into account the spiritual values and timelessness of such cultures, recognizing the importance of ethnic pride.

OBESITY

Obesity is a morbid condition in western society that has long been ignored, relative to other disease states. This is probably because it is often an unrewarding problem, due to its usual refractoriness to treatment. Physicians frequently have the simplistic concept that it is solely caused by dietary excess and cured by dietary moderation in a basically psychologically inadequate patient. This latter misunderstanding often leads to patient-doctor friction and patient self-recrimination.

Man's concept of obesity has changed drastically over the centuries as is attested by the idolized female figures of the ancient, plump Venus de Milo, and in this century the very slender Twiggy. These models reflect society's expectations of the ideal amount of body fat. Historically, a large amount of body fat provided visible evidence of success through abundance of foodstuffs and the ability to survive periods of starvation. Now, however, the ideal amount of body fat is defined as that associated with the minimum mortality and morbidity in the individual.

Fat itself, as well as providing insulation and padding, is the body's primary energy storage area. Triglyceride does not require water or electrolytes for storage, and when metabolized yields 9 Cal/g, almost twice the energy of carbohydrate or protein.

MEASUREMENT OF BODY FAT AND DEFINITION OF OBESITY

Obesity means an excess of body fat, and the term should be distinguished from overweight, which means an excess of weight but does not specify the tissue present in excess. The precise application of the term "obesity" is unclear because total body fat is difficult to quantitate with techniques that are widely available; and what constitutes an excess is debatable. Weight and height can be measured accurately, but they do not take into account body build, nor do they specify the tissues accounting for the weight. Clinical inspection to assess fat quantity and distribution, together with weight and height measurements, permits comparison to standards charts categorized by age, sex, and body build. A simple rule estimates fatness on the basis of height: *Ideal weight* for women is 100 pounds for the first 5 feet, plus 5 pounds for each additional inch; ideal weight for men is 106 pounds for the first 5 feet, plus 6 pounds for each additional inch.

Skin-fold measurements provide a more specific index of subcutaneous fat; measurements of biceps, triceps, and subscapular areas combined are better than a single measurement when compared to standard tables. These measurements are only reproducible when performed by an experienced person, and they become less reproducible with increased body fat. Nevertheless, they provide quantitation of small changes in subcutaneous body fat in a given individual and are therefore a useful tool. Skin-fold measurements (triceps plus subscapular areas) of 51 mm in men and 70 mm in nonpregnant women (ages 20 to 29 years) are greater than the 95th percentile for this population. Soft tissue x-rays have been used, but because skin-fold measurements have been shown to provide as reproducible an assessment, the radiological technique has been abandoned. Ultrasound may be used with great accuracy to determine the distance from skin to muscle interface. Its only drawback is its lack of availability and the error that may be introduced by different skin thickness. Density measurements employing total body immersion corrected for lung volume are accurate but tedious and are not generally available.

Dilutional techniques using the Fick principle determine the size of body compartments in which a given marker substance diffuses, and can provide a measure of body fat. Three dilutional techniques are in use: measurement of body water, measurement of cell mass, and measurement of fat mass. Antipyrine, urea, tritiated water, or dueterium oxide are used to quantitate total body water. A formula is then applied to calculate body fat, based on assumption of the proportion of body water in tissues. Cell mass can be measured by radiolabelled ^{40}K, using a total body counter. The thicker the fat layer, however, the less gamma radiation is transmitted, and therefore spuriously low estimates are observed in obese subjects. Cyclopropane and radioactive krypton are fat soluble and provide good estimates of total fat mass but require many hours for equilibration.

The idea that it is healthy to be thin is entrenched in the minds of physicians and the public. This was supported by early data that suggested that the ideal weight—the weight associated with the lowest mortality—was considerably below the average. However, more recent studies suggest that the ideal weight may be as much as 40 percent higher. Although the issue has not been settled, all still agree that large deviations from the average are associated with increased mortality and morbidity. In any individual, body fat may be considered excessive if reduction in the amount of body fat is likely to improve risk factors of disease, such as blood pressure, blood lipids or hyperglycemia, or symptoms such as angina or joint pains.

Morbid obesity is defined as an excess body fat resulting in body weight at least 100 pounds or 70 percent over the ideal. This term is used to distinguish a group of patients with greatly increased morbidity and mortality who have a very low probability of long-term weight loss through traditional medical means.

The prevalence of obesity is difficult ot quantitate since it has been defined so variably and it is influenced greatly by ethnic, social, and economic factors. It is clear, however, that obesity is a significant problem in western nations and developing countries; more common in women than in men, the incidence of significant obesity is at least 10 percent in females and 5 percent in males; about half of morbidly obese individuals gain most of their weight as adults.

ETIOLOGY AND PATHOGENESIS

Obesity always results from an excess of caloric intake over caloric expenditure. In the vast majority of obese patients there is no assignable cause other than overnutrition. This, however, may lead to an inappropriately simplistic idea of the pathogenesis of obesity.

Body weight and total body fat in most adult individuals remain steady or change very slowly. Thus, food deprivation or over-feeding will lead to transient deviations in body fat which will normalize if the individual is left to his own devices. This has led to the concept of central regulation, much the same as that for temperature. In fact, the hypothalamus has been shown to play a key role in the regulation of body fat. A feeding center as well as a satiety center has been localized in the hypothalamus. Stimulation of these centres can lead to cortical activation resulting in feeding or the inhibition of feeding respectively. Lesions produced in one or other centre can lead to a changing of the set point, with a new body fat compartment size. Significant input stimuli to these centers may include gastric and intestinal distention, absorption of food, metabolic end-products of food and hormone secretions, and may be influenced by inputs from the central nervous system itself. The recognition of these pathways and the responsible neurotransmitters is leading to a new understanding of traditional theories of obesity as well as of the effects of anorectic drugs and other therapeutic modalities.

Excessive caloric intake mediated through pathologic feeding behavior likely has a complex etiology. Social, familial, and psychological factors influence food intake. Further, in the obese, external cues to food, such as its smell, taste, and its mode and environment of presentation, affect eating behavior to a much greater extent than in normal individuals.

Body weight is also influenced by the amount of energy expended. Energy expenditure is primarily a function of basal metabolic rate. With an increase in body fat, the basal metabolic rate decreases as expressed in terms of weight, although it remains the same if expressed per surface area. With caloric restriction, the basal metabolic rate decreases. Further, obesity limits the amount of activity possible, and obese people actually perform fewer spontaneous movements. Thus, the reduced caloric expenditure of the obese contributes to the fat storage.

A major factor in determining the size of the fat cell compartment is the number of fat cells. Fat cells divide in early life, probably until the time of puberty, but it is also likely that fat cells can be induced at other times from mesenchymal cells following long-term weight gain. The fat cells so gained do not disappear with weight loss. Significantly obese patients, particularly those who gained their weight in early life, may have three to five times as many fat cells as normal individuals. This has lead to the term hyperplastic obesity—meaning an increased number of fat cells—in distinction to hypertrophic obesity, which indicates that the fat cell size is increased, accounting for the increase in total body fat. In many individuals there is both an increase in fat cell size and number.

Fat cell size may be regulated by several mechanisms. With weight loss, lipoprotein lipase levels increase, enhancing triglyceride uptake. In addition, insulin sensitivity of fat cells increases due to an increased number of functional insulin receptors and enhances glucose uptake by the fat cell. Further, a metabolic end-product of triglyceride breakdown such as glycerol may be sensed by the hypothalamus, causing altered feeding behavior aimed at normalizing what it regards to be the normal fat cell compartment size.

Genetic Causes

A number of rare genetic disorders are characterized by obesity. These include the Laurence-Moon-Biedl syndrome, characterized by mental retardation, retinitis pigmentosa, polydactyly and syndactyly, skull deformities, and hypogenitalism; Alstrom's syndrome, characterized by retinal degeneration, nerve deafness, diabetes mellitus, and obesity; Prader-Willi syndrome, characterized by hypertonia, mental retardation, short stature, and hypogenitalism; and hyperostosis frontalis interna, characterized by virilism and hyperostosis of the frontal bones, occurring in older women. It is probable that a hypothalamic disorder is fundamental to the pathogenesis of obesity in these disorders. In other obese subjects familial factors are not of simple inheritance patterns and environmental factors play a major role.

Endocrine Causes

Hyperinsulinism, either secondary to an insulinoma or exogenous in etiology, can be associated with weight gain. However, this weight gain is usually modest at most. In Cushing's syndrome, the weight gain is usually moderate in amount and associated with centripetal obesity and lessening of lean body mass, producing the typical habitus with features of moon facies, supraclavicular fat deposits, buffalo humps, buttock wasting, and thinning of the skin and abdominal striae. It is a rare cause of obesity. Twenty-four hour urine 17-hydroxycorticoid excretion may be elevated in obesity, and much less commonly plasma cortisol levels may be increased. The

levels can be suppressed with exogenous glucocorticoids, although occasionally such suppression may be somewhat incomplete (see Chapter 13). Patients with polycystic ovaries with reduced or absent menses, and hirsutism may suffer a moderate weight gain. Hypothalamic disorders due to tumor, trauma, vascular accidents or infection are rare causes of morbid weight gain. Phenothiazines, antidepressants, and estrogens are among the many drugs which can cause weight gain. The mechanisms of the drug effects have not been clearly established.

COMPLICATIONS OF OBESITY

Mortality increases in a graded fashion as body fat exceeds the ideal. This is particularly so for the young and, conversely, the association of increased risk with excess weight diminishes with age. Thus, the morbidly obese patient of age 30 to 40 years may have twelve times the risk of death that a patient of the same age and sex would have at an ideal weight. The risk is primarily related to cardiovascular disease, hepatobiliary disease, and diabetes mellitus (Table 1.3).

Obesity itself has not been clearly defined as a separate risk factor for coronary artery disease. However, since many obese patients have associated risk factors of hypertension, glucose intolerance, or hyperlipidemia, the distinction is difficult. It is important to recognize that the increased risk of coronary artery disease associated with obesity may be ame-

Table 1.3   Adverse Effects of Obesity

General
    Increased surgical and maternal risk
    Psychosocial distress
    Joint symptoms, osteoarthritis
    Increased risk of accidents
Cardiovascular
    Hypertension
    Increased angina
    Increased heart failure
    Increased venous disease of lower limbs
Respiratory
    Restrictive lung function
    Hypoxemia
    Sleep apnea syndrome
    Intermittent upper airway obstruction
    Hypoventilation
    Polycythemia
    Cor pulmonale
    Thromboembolism
Metabolic
    Hyperglycemia and glucose intolerance
    Increased circulating insulin
    Hyperlipidemia
Gastrointestinal
    Cholelithiasis

liorated by treating other risk factors present in the patient.

With increased fat cell size, a patient becomes less tolerant of glucose. This has been attributed to a decrease in the number of insulin receptors. This trend increases with time and is reversed by decreased fat cell size. Obese patients have increased circulating insulin levels and they are less prone to ketoacidosis. Reversal of the hyperglycemia associated with obesity is best accomplished by weight loss.

Hyperlipidemia is usually associated with high levels of very low density lipoprotein (VLDL) due to the hyperinsulinemia. As well, the increased free fatty acid turnover in the obese results in an increased hepatic production of VLDL. No defect in removal of VLDL from plasma has been found, and there is no major change in LDL, the major determinant of plasma cholesterol concentrations. Total body cholesterol is increased in obesity, primarily due to increased tissue cholesterol stores. Cholesterol turnover may also be increased, leading to increased cholesterol excretion in the bile and an increased incidence of gallstones.

Hypertension is more common in the obese. Blood pressure must be measured with an appropriate-sized cuff (bladder width approximately 40 percent of the circumference of the arm). Using too small a cuff leads to spuriously high blood pressure readings, but even when the appropriate pressure cuff is used there is an increased incidence of hypertension in the obese. The etiology of the hypertension is unclear. Blood volume is increased, while peripheral vascular resistance is usually normal. The hypertension is usually responsive to weight loss and volume depletion by diuretics.

Obesity can lead to reduced vital capacity and breathing at low lung volumes with ventilation-perfusion mismatch and hypoxemia. Hypoventilation may occur in severe obesity and may be typical of the Pickwickian syndrome, or more commonly associated with intermittent upper airway obstruction and sleep apnea. Frequently these patients develop polycythemia, pulmonary hypertension, and cor pulmonale. Even moderate amounts of weight loss may ameliorate the process. Progestational agents have been used to increase ventilation in the obesity-hypoventilation syndrome.

Obese patients are at an increased surgical and obstetrical risk. Although there is an increased maternal mortality rate, the perinatal mortality rate is not usually increased in obesity. The obese have impaired sexual and reproductive function as well and have an increased risk of endometrial cancer. Various mechanical disorders such as osteoarthritis and varicose veins are common in obesity.

Although there is no good evidence that obesity is secondary to any psychiatric disorder, there is impairment of self-image and increased risk of psychoneurosis, most likely secondary to the pressures of a society that discriminates against the obese socially and sexually, as well as in the business world.

TREATMENT

The obese patient should be evaluated for underlying causes, associated conditions, and complications. Treatment goals must be established at the outset, formulating an individualized regimen for the treatment of the excess fat (Table 1.4). Weight loss is frequent with most treatment regimens; however, weight maintenance is infrequent for prolonged periods of time with any treatment other than surgery. It is a fundamental principle that without a change in life-style success will be temporary. The important persons related to the family should be involved as much as possible. Such involvement will provide support and understanding and greatly increase the chances of success.

It must be understood as well by both the physician and the patient that weight loss will be generalized with all techniques aside from plastic surgery. For example, in the case of patients with centripetal obesity, the fat loss will come as much from the arms as from the trunk, and the patient will be left with the same body habitus after weight loss.

Weight loss is primarily due to loss of fat, protein, and water after an initial small weight loss due to glycogen depletion. Excess water loss seen with diuretics, the osmotic diuresis associated with ketogenic diets, and following small-bowel bypass may mislead the observer. Potential harm may ensue due to water and salt depletion and other metabolic abnormalities. As a patient loses weight, plateaus will be reached. These weight plateaus may be related to decreased basal metabolic rate, but they are often due to water retention (associated with increased levels

Table 1.4 **Major Therapeutic Modalities for Obesity**

For Modest Obesity
   Balanced hypocaloric diet
   Exercise
   Lifestyle, behavior changes
   Anorectic drugs under special circumstances
For Severe Obesity
   (More than 100 lb overweight)
   Aggressive treatment as above
   If rigorous medical treatment fails:
      Intestinal bypass surgery
      Gastroplasty with or without intestinal bypass

of reverse triiodothyroxine (T3) and decreased levels of normal T3). This is explained by the role of T3 in the regulation of the Na–K–ATP pump. Such cycles in fluid balance can be verified by following skinfold measurements, which will show fat loss despite lack of weight loss or even weight gain. Such measurements provide great reassurance to the patient who would otherwise consider the treatment to have failed.

Although obesity is associated with an increased risk of death and morbidity, radical treatment is not indicated for most patients with no other risk factors or associated conditions and who have happy lifestyles. It is important that treatment goals be realistic. Setting an unachievable goal may result in the patient abandoning lesser degrees of success achieved with small losses in weight.

Patients with the best prognosis are those with tangible secondary gains, such as reduced insulin dosage, reduced incidence of anginal attacks, controlled hypertension, and lessening of joint pain; those with only moderate obesity; and those younger patients from high socioeconomic groups.

Whatever treatment is employed, more calories must be burned than ingested. There are no magic treatments.

Diets

Diets must be hypocaloric in relation to the patient's energy expenditure and must be tailored to the individual's life-style. Ethnic background, family preferences, tastes, and working hours such as shift work may make most diets inappropriate and futile. If a short period of weight loss is needed, fasting may be appropriate, but for long-term weight loss and weight maintenance, a highly hypocaloric diet will be best tolerated.

The typical obese patient when dieting will skip meals and reduce eating to one large meal a day, usually at dinner or during the evening. This timing results in a higher percentage of the calories ingested being stored as fat, resulting at least partially from selectively increased insulin sensitivity of the adipocytes following fasting. Such patients will feel less well and when fasting will be capable of less exercise for even short periods of time during the day. It is therefore critical that at least three meals a day be ingested.

Diets should be drawn up in conjunction with a dietician. Nutritional adequacy can be checked by comparing the patient's diet with standard tables such as the Recommended Daily Dietary Allowances. Generally, any diet less than 1200 calories

(large calorie) will be deficient in some nutrients, and the patient should receive vitamin supplementation and should be followed medically. A 500 to 1000 calorie deficit per day can usually be tolerated without undue hunger and can provide a weekly weight loss of 1 to 2 pounds. Such a weight loss will discourage the patient unless he or she is forewarned that this is the expected rapidity of weight loss, and that continuing such a diet over many weeks will provide a significant loss of body fat. Dietary advice should also encourage the patient to enjoy special events, such as parties and holidays on a limited scale. This advice will help the patient to adapt, and will lessen the chance of significant noncompliance due to perceived failure.

There are no special foods that "burn" calories. Many popular diets will be low in carbohydrates, the so-called ketogenic diets that will promote a water diuresis and thereby increase weight loss. Since the increased weight loss is fluid, the patient may be temporarily more satisfied; however, diets of this kind will only lead to noncompliance as the patient regains many pounds after stopping the diet, which he or she finds intolerable for long periods of time. There is no evidence that these diets provide faster fat loss. The suggestion that they reduce appetite has not been uniformly verified. The idea of a special protein-sparing diet is unproved. Liquid protein diets should not be used. A number of deaths have been reported with these diets, often associated with myocardial damage or prolonged QT intervals, or both. The best way to spare protein is to ingest adequate calories and protein.

Fasting cannot be tolerated long because of the appetite and metabolic abnormalities that develop. Volume depletion with azotemia and postural hypotension, hyperuricemia with possible gout, and other metabolic abnormalities may result. In general, fasts should only be attempted under medical supervision, and then only if rapid weight loss (which is to a large extent water) has some tangible purpose such as preparing the patient for intensive psychological therapy.

Surgery

All medical treatments, with the exception of surgery, have limited success in reducing body fat. But because of the morbidity and mortality associated with it, surgery is reserved for a selected group of obese subjects. Several principles are of paramount importance in assessing surgery for obesity. As in any evolving field, one must be cautious of abandoning accepted practices too quickly as new procedures appear. Further, the surgery that is performed by each individual surgeon at his own institution must be judged separately, as even small differences in technique may make major differences in results. Obesity surgery is major surgery, and a continuing and significant change in life-style is necessary. For these reasons preoperative education of the patient and postoperative follow-up, preferably by a team of interested doctors, nurses and dieticians, is fundamental.

Many types of surgery have been attempted. *Jaw wiring* limits intake and often results in weight loss, but dental caries are common and the weight loss lasts only as long as the wires remain intact. It has very few advocates. *Lipectomy* has been attempted on a monumental scale by some surgeons. Results have generally been poor and unsightly unless the surgery is used either to tidy up after significant weight loss from another weight loss procedure or to treat localized adiposity. Vagotomy alone has also been performed with inconsistent results and inadequate weight loss.

The two other major types of surgery entail variations of gastric reduction and small bowel bypass.

Small Bowel Bypass

There are many types of small bowel bypass procedures. These take the majority of the small intestine out of continuity and connect it to the large intestine as a blind loop. The vascular supply remains intact, and the bowel can subsequently be reconstituted if necessary. The eating pattern becomes normal and decreased caloric intake results; these are the major factors in weight loss. Why there are such changes after the operation remains uncertain.

This procedure is the oldest of the weight loss operations. It has the longest record and the most significant weight loss and weight maintenance associated with it. Balanced against its success in weight reduction are its complications, most of which can be understood as short gut or end–blind-loop syndromes.

As the patient does have a short gut, diarrhea and deficiencies in potassium, magnesium, calcium, iron, vitamins (especially fat-soluble vitamins and vitamin B_{12}), folate, copper, zinc, and proteins can occur. Hyperoxaluria may also occur, resulting in increased incidence of oxalate renal stones. The hyperoxaluria probably occurs because of increased oxalate absorption.

The blind loop syndrome is associated with bloating, increased diarrhea, dermatitis, and arthritis. Liver disease is also seen and may be ameliorated by treating protein deficiencies. The diarrhea and its concomitant problems decrease with time as the bowel in continuity increases in size and functional capacity. Osteomalacia and cirrhosis are possible long-term, serious sequelae. Because of its effectiveness, intestinal bypass is considered the preferred procedure in some institutions for morbidly obese patients; and in contrast to the gastric procedures, intestinal bypass can result in a significant reduction in serum cholesterol, although HDL usually decreases as well.

Gastric Surgery

There are basically two types of gastric procedures: one that only limits the gastric pouch size and one that combines this with a gastrojejunostomy.

The simple gastroplasty or the gastric partitioning has been most widely adopted. Here a small proximal pouch having a volume of 40 to 60 ml is formed by stapling across the stomach, leaving a small channel of 12 mm in diameter to the distal stomach. Variations include putting the channel on the greater or lesser curvature, running staples at angles parallel to the lesser curvature, reducing the channel size to as little as 7 mm, as well as using different types of staples and sutures. After the procedure there is a marked diminution in meal size and a gradual loss of weight.

Postoperative complications include chest infections, staple-line failure, splenic laceration, and subphrenic abscesses. Deficiencies in iron, thiamine, and calcium have been reported, although rarely.

The gastric bypass, on the other hand, is a technically difficult procedure, with a higher rate of postoperative complications and a high incidence of ulceration. It has a greater associated weight loss than that of the gastroplasty, but it is performed in few institutions at the present time.

Decision as to whether a patient is a candidate for obesity surgery must be individualized and preferably agreed upon by an interested internist as well as the surgeon involved; psychiatric and other opinions may also be required. In general, the patient should be 100 pounds or 100 percent over his or her ideal weight, should have suffered repeated failures of medical attempts at weight loss, should have a relatively stable life pattern with no addictions, should be between the ages of 18 and 50 years, and should have no contraindicating medical illnesses. The low-weight limit is selected because at that weight or above the chance is very small that significant weight loss could be maintained without surgery. The lower age limit is selected because surgery too early in life can curtail growth. The upper age limit reflects the increased operative mortality and morbidity and the lower risk of obesity associated with age.

Exercise

In sedentary persons, the calories expended with planned exercise are relatively few compared to those eaten; thus it must be emphasized that exercise cannot take the place of dietary restrictions. In some subjects exercise will decrease appetite. More body fat than lean tissue is lost when diet and exercise are combined. Exercise also increases glucose tolerance, lowers blood pressure, decreases serum triglycerides, and helps to change the overall life-style of the obese. Exercise is more difficult for the obese because of mechanical limitations and social pressures, and so the program should be individualized.

Patients should be encouraged to develop a systematic, daily program that emphasizes dynamic rather than isometric exercises. Walking, swimming, skating, cross-country skiing, or cycling are all preferable to weight lifting or pushups. Exercise should be graded initially, beginning with short periods of low intensity exercise and working up to activities that increase the pulse rate at least 30 to 40 beats per minute. In addition to the planned exercise program, patients should be encouraged to routinely walk up stairs rather than ride elevators, to walk to work or to do shopping if possible, and to develop active hobbies. Competitive sports and exhaustive exercise should be avoided until initial weight reduction and physical conditioning make them safe.

Behavior Therapy

Because obese people respond less well to internal cues such as sweetness of food and gastric contractions and are affected more by external cues such as the taste and smell of food and the surroundings, techniques to change the patient's behavior regarding food acquisition and ingestion are fundamental. These techniques include keeping records to provide a data base of patient insight and to provide direction for change; control of stimuli that result in eating; physically changing eating patterns themselves; and reinforcement of the new behavior through practical and cognitive means. For example, eating from smaller plates with smaller utensils or chopsticks, removing dishes of food from the table, eating snacks

before shopping to reduce binge buying, and restructured thinking regarding food and weight are all useful.

By itself, behavior therapy lacks long-term effectiveness and must therefore be used in conjunction with dietary and exercise therapy.

Drugs

Anorectic drugs are clearly effective in augmenting fat loss. Their use is limited by the fact that they have a circumscribed (usually 4 to 6 weeks) duration of effect in increasing weight loss; the amphetamine-like drugs are addictive; they have significant side effects; and when they are discontinued, *weight gain* commonly occurs, which may even exceed the amount of weight lost. Their use lies primarily in promoting urgent weight loss, as before elective surgery, and in those in whom weight loss is necessary and all else has failed or is not possible. They should be combined with a complete exercise and diet program.

Thyroid hormone increases fat loss but also loss of lean mass; and because of its side effects it has no part in the treatment of obesity. Human chorionic gonadatropin injections have no greater effect than placebo, although they do have well-documented side effects. Other drugs developed to block various phases of the absorption of nutrients are experimental and can lead to significant nutritional deficiencies.

Unconventional Treatments

Cellulite, the dimpled appearance of skin said to result from altered tissue, is simply due to hypertrophied fat cells. It has no special significance and will disappear with reduction of total body fat. Hypnosis and acupuncture cannot be recommended, although they do provide short-term weight loss as do most treatments that provide sympathetic counseling combined with prudent advice. They do not provide a change in life-style and have not been documented to cause a sustained weight loss.

In summary, treatment for the moderately overweight is most effectively accomplished by a combination of diet, behavior therapy, and exercise modification. Anorectic drugs are useful in the occasional patient in whom no other treatment is possible or practical and in whom there is a great need for weight loss. Obesity surgery is only advisable for the morbidly obese when all else has failed.

THE ILLICIT USE OF DRUGS AND THEIR MEDICAL CONSEQUENCES

The ready availability of a variety of drugs and mood-altering substances has resulted in widespread and highly variable use. Some people decide to remain as free from such substances as possible. Others vigorously, even religiously, avoid alcohol and marijuana, but become chronic users of sedatives and analgesics. Chronic misuse of drugs may develop surreptitiously, and acute suicidal misuse may occur as a result of mental derangement produced by lesser doses. At present suicide is the second most common cause of life-years lost in North America, and drug overdose accounts for the majority of such deaths, particularly in females.

MARIJUANA

Since earliest recorded history man has used drugs to relieve his anxiety, lift his spirits, or otherwise modify his mental environment. Products of the Indian hemp plant, *Cannabis sativa*, are among the oldest known substances used for these purposes. In North America the most popular material at present is marijuana, which has about one-tenth the potency of the less widely used hashish. The overall nonmedical use of drugs seems to remain relatively constant throughout history; only the specific substances selected for use vary from time to time. It is therefore important that patients receive advice on which substances in current use are least damaging to the individual and society.

The risks to health of marijuana use remain controversial. However, they are neither serious enough to support the present penalties for possessing this drug, nor are they as innocuous as some wish to believe.

The immediate pharmacological effects of marijuana are well known, and as is true of all substances that alter mood, the effect varies depending on the dose, the environment, and individual expectations. A small dose causes an initial increase in sympathetic activity, resulting in tachycardia, whereas higher doses result in orthostatic hypotension due to centrally mediated sympathetic inhibition and parasympathetic stimulation. Memory is impaired, sensations are enhanced, and tasks dependent on learning, memory, and attention are impaired. These psychological changes are characteristically fluctuant, occurring in waves. The effects are ordinarily mild if marijuana is used in the absence of other drugs affecting the central nervous system and in doses ordinarily taken in North America. Tolerance to the acute effects of marijuana, mild withdrawal symptoms, and psychological dependence occur. These characteristics satisfy the usual criteria for an addictive drug.

Except for the tachycardia that can persist for months after stopping marijuana, there is little agreement about chronic effects. If brain damage, psychosis, or an amotivational syndrome is causally related to marijuana use, these complications are uncommon and singularly difficult to identify. It is often impossible to separate such effects from preexisting conditions and from the influence of life-style. A conjunctivitis that can persist for months after stopping smoking has been described in smokers in some countries (particularly India) but not in others. Mild hormonal changes suggesting a suppression of the hypopituitary-thalamic axis accompany chronic administration of tetrahydrocannabinol, one of the active components of marijuana. A mild reduction of sperm count occurs in men and reproductive function is impaired in experimental animals. Additional effects of heavy regular smoking include a decrease in T-lymphocyte reactivity and squamous metaplasia of the bronchial epithelium.

BENZODIAZEPINES

It is estimated that 10 to 20 percent of the adult population of the United States, Canada, and Western Europe use psychotropic drugs, of which the principal agents are the benzodiazepines. The benzodiazepines are predominantly used medically as well as by self medication for relief of anxiety. Within limits, symptoms of anxiety are normal and can be an important drive; more severe symptoms are pathological, and they impair performance. It is therefore difficult to provide an objective assessment of the level of misuse of these drugs without details of the severity of symptoms and the implications of their use or nonuse on productivity. As with marijuana, the relative risks of benzodiazepines must be weighed against the risks of alternative remedies that would probably be used in the absence of benzodiazepines.

The addictive potential of these drugs is low. Nevertheless, physical and psychological dependence and drug-seeking behavior can occur. As with alcohol and marijuana, the individual who abuses benzodiazepines seldom is forced to steal or commit other crimes to pay for his drugs. With one important exception, the addition of benzodiazepines to multiple drug use does not appear to increase the risk to the individual. The exception is the abstaining alcoholic for whom the simple act of prescribing benzodiazepines to relieve anxiety is almost a guarantee that he or she will return to alcohol. The reason for this is probably psychological: by prescribing benzodiazepines the physician makes legitimate the use of a substance to modify mental processes.

Clinical manifestations of the benzodiazepine abstinence syndrome are mild and short lived, and because of the long duration of effect of most benzodiazepines the onset of the abstinence syndrome is delayed, occuring, for example, between 3 to 6 days after stopping diazepam. The symptoms of apprehension, unease, dizziness, and insomnia are virtually impossible to distinguish from the symptoms for which the drug was initially used.

There is very low potential for producing physical dependence to the benzodiazepines compared with barbiturates and other sedative-hypnotics. Nevertheless, the medical use of these drugs should be limited to those conditions that are known to be influenced by treatment.

In order to limit the risk of physical and psychological dependence to the benzodiazepines, the following principles should be followed:

1. Benzodiazepines should only be used to relieve symptoms of anxiety if these symptoms are severe enough to impair performance, and should then be used only for a short time.

2. Benzodiazepines should be considered as suppressive and not curative agents. Other measures should be used to modify the factors causing anxiety.

3. If used for several weeks, benzodiazepines should be reduced gradually to avoid withdrawal symptoms that may be confused by the patient and physician as symptoms of recurrence of the anxiety disorder.

4. Benzodiazepines and other sedative-hypnotics should be avoided in abstaining alcoholic patients.

5. Benzodiazepines are ineffective in and probably detrimental to some patients with depression. Care should be taken to identify symptoms of depressive illness in a patient presenting with anxiety.

OPIOIDS

Opioids include drugs that in the past have been referred to as narcotics, a term originally selected because of the somnolence or sleep accompanying their use. The appellation now has a variety of nonmedical connotations. Because of the close structural chemical relationship with the principle alkaloid of opium, morphine, the drugs have also been referred to as opiates. The currently popular term opioids permits the inclusion of drugs such as propoxyphene, which has pharmacological effects similar to those of opiates even though structurally similarity may be argued.

Use of opioids is characterized by the development of tolerance and physical and psychological dependence. All drugs of this type have these characteristics, although the risk of addiction varies greatly from agent to agent. No class of opioids is entirely free from addiction liability.

Tolerance

The usual pattern of the development of tolerance is gradual shortening of the duration between doses required to provide analgesic, narcotic, or euphoric effects, and an increase in the dose required to give equivalent effects. Tolerance is seldom a problem with patients with acute pain who request increased doses of opioids at decreased intervals; the common clinical practice of prescribing analgesia in minimum effective doses when requested by the patient very often results in patients receiving doses of narcotics that are inadequate to suppress pain. The development of tolerance is related to the constancy of tissue concentration of opioids and can be lost a few days after stopping the drug. This explains the occurence of severe intoxication and death in heroin addicts who take their usual dose of heroin after a few days of abstinence.

The risk of addiction with medical use of opioids is small. The risk is undoubtedly related to the size of dose and the duration of treatment. However, the current practice in analgesic use of prescribing narcotics on an "as required" basis in relatively small doses carries the risk that it reinforces the notion that acute drug administration brings well-being. It has been repeatedly shown that smaller total doses of narcotics are required to relieve acute pain if the drugs are given continuously intravenously or by other routes in a manner that prevents the recurrence of pain.

Tolerance does not develop at the same rate or to the same degree for all of the effects of a particular narcotic. Little tolerance develops to the pupillary constriction and decreased gastric motility observed with the narcotics; thus the finding of constricted pupils in an overdosed patient remains a useful clinical clue even in the narcotic addict. There is cross-tolerance between compounds to many of the effects of opioids.

Physical Dependence and the Abstinence Syndrome

Physical dependence is characterized by the occurrence of a typical syndrome upon stopping the narcotic or upon administration of a narcotic antagonist such as naloxone. The phenomenon of physical dependence is closely related to that of tolerance. Withdrawal symptoms confirm physical dependence. The characteristics of withdrawal are similar for all opioid drugs although variable in severity.

The first clinical symptoms of morphine or heroin withdrawal occur 8 to 12 hours after the last dose and reach their peak between 36 to 48 hours, with severe symptoms disappearing by 90 hours in most patients. Symptoms occur instantly if a narcotic antagonist is administered to a narcotic addict. The onset and peak of withdrawal signs is dependent on the time course of the drug's action, with the earliest symptoms occurring 2 to 3 hours after the last dose of meperidine and dihydromorphinone, 4 to 6 hours after morphine and heroin, 8 hours after codeine, and 12 hours after methadone. The earliest symptoms include anxiety, perspiration, yawning, and a craving for drug. This progresses after several hours to include lacrimation, rhinorrhea, mydriasis, and gooseflesh, followed by muscle twitches, aching muscles and bones, hot and cold flashes, and anorexia. Still later an increase in temperature, blood pressure, pulse rate, and respiration rate and depth occurs, with vomiting, diarrhea, weight loss, and insomnia. The minimum daily dose of heroin required to produce withdrawal reactions is approximately 24 mg and the severity of the reaction is dose related. Since most street sources of heroin contain 1 to 5 mg of heroin per bag and the average street habit is three to six bags per day, psychological rather than physical dependence is typical of the street addict, and abstinence symptoms tend to be mild. Individuals using hydromorphinone tend to have more severe reactions, probably because relatively larger doses of this drug are available compared with heroin. Withdrawal symptoms from methadone tend to be less intense though more prolonged than with shorter addicting opioids. Paradoxically, methadone withdrawal precipitated by narcotic antagonists can be severe.

The diagnosis of opioid dependency is suggested by a history of daily use of an opioid for at least a month, previous withdrawal reactions, miotic pupils, and positive urine tests for opioids. Since these drugs are frequently mixed with quinine, a finding of quinine in the urine is confirmatory. Small doses of naloxone can be administered at 20 minute intervals, observing for piloerection, mydriasis, and sweating as signs of acute withdrawal.

Abstinence symptoms are frequently mild and require no treatment. Patients with objective evidence of withdrawal signs such as piloerection and mydriasis can be treated as outpatients with methadone substitution, provided they can be seen every 24 hours for repeat observation and dose administration. Usually 15 to 20 mg of methadone every 12 hours is sufficient with a progressive reduction of the drug over 7 to 10 days. Treatment must be individualized, and some patients may require methadone withdrawal treatment over 3 to 4 weeks.

Methadone withdrawal, however, is not essential; opioids can be stopped abruptly, and the symptoms of muscle and bone pain, anxiety, insomnia, and vomiting can be suppressed with clonidine.

Treatment of Opioid Dependence

Three principal methods of treatment are available in North America for treating opioid dependence. These include methadone maintenance, deconditioning with narcotic antagonists, detoxification, and group identification.

In contrast to heroin, which must be given parenterally and which produces short-lasting euphoria almost immediately, methadone is effective orally with an onset of action in 30 minutes. No euphoria or narcotic effect is obtained if methadone is used at a dose less than that to which an addict is tolerant. Duration of action is prolonged, lasting 24 to 36 hours. These characteristics of methadone make it useful in replacing other narcotics. Continuous methadone use prevents the "drug hunger" that persists after acute symptoms of narcotic withdrawal have subsided; this persistent hunger contributes to a return to the narcotic habit in many individuals. An additional advantage of methadone is that during full maintenance treatment the dose of heroin or other illicit narcotic required to produce euphoria exceeds that which is ordinarily available to the addicted individual. Unfortunately, methadone itself is subject to abuse, and administration of the drug in maintenance programs must be carefully and continuously supervised. Mental performance appears to be normal in methadone patients receiving carefully tailored doses. Successful pregnancies are possible, with one third of newborns likely to suffer moderate withdrawal symptoms. Anaesthetic and surgical treatment can be undertaken while continuing methadone as long as the precaution is taken to avoid the use of narcotic antagonists such as pentazocine, since severe withdrawal symptoms will otherwise ensue. Evaluation of the large methadone maintenance program in New York State shows that after 5 years over 60 percent of patients continue in the program and most are working.

The use of deconditioning in treating narcotic addiction is based on the belief that both the association of euphoria with narcotics and the association of relief from withdrawal symptoms with methadone greatly increase the likelihood of continued addiction or recidivism when the subject has been successfully withdrawn from narcotics over a short period of time. If relief provided by narcotics is blocked by narcotic antagonists, drug-seeking behavior and physical dependence should diminish. Narcotic antagonists such as cyclazocine that are devoid of narcotic effects and to which tolerance does not appear to develop have been used, and as with methadone the success is dependent on continued administration of the antagonist and surveillance of the individual. Group identification has been used in an attempt to resolve social and interpersonal conflicts that are believed to contribute to addiction.

Treatment of narcotic addiction should not be regarded with pessimism. The surprising number of veterans of the Vietnam conflict who were addicted to heroin and who, after returning to the United States, have been successful in abstaining from narcotic use, provides optimism that others who are addicted can successfully withdraw.

Complications of Illicit Narcotic Use

Complications of narcotic use arise from the pharmacological effects of the drugs as well as from the manner in which the drugs are prepared and administered. Coma due to the central nervous system effects of narcotics or other substances such as alcohol, and suicidal or homocidal deaths are frequent in the narcotic population. Deaths due to overdosage itself are unusual and are very frequently caused by inappropriate treatments provided by friends of the patient. The medical approach to the diagnosis and treatment of narcotic overdosage is similar to that for other central nervous system depressant drugs.

Infectious Complications

Hepatitis is the most common medical condition in narcotic addicts requiring hospitalization. The spectrum of liver disease is wide. Acute hepatitis is indistinguishable in clinical symptomatology and etiology from hepatitis in the nonaddicted young adult population. Hepatitis B antigen (HBAg) is found in 80 percent of cases within 2 weeks of the onset of symptoms, if sensitive measurement techniques are used. Almost all addicts have laboratory or biopsy evidence of hepatic dysfunction, with the most common syndrome being an asymptomatic nonprogressive hepatitis with focal portal mononuclear inflammation, so-called chronic persistent hepatitis. Since alcohol is often consumed in excess by addicts, the etiology of the chronic hepatic changes is unclear. Most often HBAg is persistently present, and it seems most likely that the chronic hepatitis is due to viral infection rather than any direct drug toxicity.

Pulmonary infections are common in addicts, probably because of the drug-induced respiratory depression and a life-style that often includes smoking and drinking. Aspiration pneumonia with necrosis of lung tissue due to bronchial obstruction and infection by a mixture of aerobic and anaerobic organisms is common. Pneumonia is most frequently due to *Streptococcus pneumoniae*. However, staphylococci and streptococci (group A) appear to be responsible for pneumonia more frequently in the addict than in the nonaddict. Tuberculosis is likewise more frequent, probably due to the fact that addicts frequently reside in areas of high population density and low income, where the disease is still common.

The intravenous injection of nonsterile material provides a ready portal of entry for a variety of bacteria that cause infectious endocarditis. This infection in the addict is more often due to organisms usually considered saprophytic, such as *Candida* organisms or *Staphylococcus epidermidis* and *Staphylococcus aureus*, and sometimes involves multiple organisms. It affects the right-sided heart valves more commonly than is the case in the nonaddict. Clinical suspicion of the complication must be high, since the principle symptoms of anemia, low-grade fever, and malaise can often be easily attributed to other causes in the narcotic addict. Septic pulmonary emboli may present as multiple lung nodules or thin-walled cavities.

Osteomyelitis, due to the hematogenous spread of *Pseudomonas aeruginosa* and less frequently to *Staphylococcus aureus* and *Candida* species, is frequently localized in the lumbar vertebrae or intervertebral discs and sacrum, although other areas may also be infected. The addict is also susceptible to rapidly progressive fascitis and myositis due to aerobic streptococci, a variety of anaerobic organisms, and *Clostridium tetani*.

Acute neurological complications of illicit narcotic use are legion. Toxic amblyopia with optic atrophy probably secondary to the quinine that narcotics and other drugs are frequently mixed with, mononeuropathy, polyneuropathy resembling the Guillain-Barré syndrome, and transverse myelitis are reported with greatly increased frequency in the narcotic addict. It remains unclear whether these disorders are a result of a direct toxic effect of the narcotic or additives, due to vascular injury secondary to a vasculitis or ischemic due to transient hypotension.

Repeated injection into veins of the forearm and hands can result in local areas of necrosis, cellulitis, tenosynovitis, and thrombosis of superficial veins (needle tracks). The characteristic puffy hands of the chronic addict, which resemble the findings in postmastectomy lymphedema, are due to obliteration of veins and lymphatics due to irritant effects of drugs or contaminants. Edema fluid becomes organized and the initial pitting edema is replaced by nonpitting brawny edema.

Acute renal failure due to acute myoglobinuria occurs in the narcotic addict probably as a result of trauma, concomitant alcohol ingestion, and metabolic causes. Nephrotic syndrome due to a focal membranous and proliferative glomerulonephritis occurs with greater frequency in addicts than in nonaddicts. The pathologic findings are similar to those seen in lupus erythematosis and renal allografts with subendothelial deposits of IgM and complement. Whether this immunological disorder is triggered by components of bacteria injected with the illicit drug or by heroin itself remains unresolved.

Overdosage with Drugs Depressing the Central Nervous System

Accidental or intentional overdosage with drugs that depress the central nervous system is one of the most common causes of coma in patients brought to emergency departments. The drugs involved are varied, determined predominantly by what is available to the patient. Often a combination of drugs is taken and alcohol often contributes to the clinical state. The most frequent drugs implicated include the benzodiazepines, barbiturates, nonbarbiturate hypnotics, antidepressant and antipsychotic drugs and narcotics.

The severity of the drug overdose state is assessed by the depth of coma and the degree of interference with normal neurological, respiratory, and cardiovascular function. Other drugs such as salicylates, acetaminophen, and lithium can have lethal consequences with little evidence of depression of the central nervous system. Care must be taken in these patients to apply different criteria and not to assume that the risk is small merely because central nervous system function is only mildly impaired.

Patients are most often semiconscious or comatose and are unable to provide a history. Acquaintances who accompany the patient can often provide reliable information regarding drugs that were likely available to the patient. The drugs most often involved vary with communities and with subcultures within communities, so knowledge of drugs involved in previous patients can be very helpful.

Physical examination must immediately focus on the respiratory system, since morbidity and mortality of coma due to drug overdose is directly related to respiratory function. The rate and depth of respiration may be helpful, but in a comatose patient alveolar hypoventilation is best assessed by measurement of arterial blood gases. Cyanosis is helpful when present, but it is a late sign of hypoxemia. If respiration is depressed, the narcotic antagonist naloxone should be employed in an attempt to reverse any narcotic-related depression of the respiratory center. This carries a risk of precipitating a withdrawal reaction in the narcotic addict. The duration of action of naloxone is short, about 2 hours, and repeated doses may be required until the longer-lasting effects of the narcotic agonist have dissipated. The severity of overdosage due to central nervous system depressant drugs is usually graded according to the depth of coma and the function of the respiratory and cardiovascular systems.

The depth of coma can be graded in a standardized manner using the Glasgow Coma Scale which is based on eye opening, verbal and motor responses as outlined in Table 1.5.

Clinical findings may suggest specific drugs (Table 1.6), but overdoses are frequently taken after drinking alcohol and often involve more than one drug. Respiratory depression should always suggest opioid drugs, particularly if the other systems are relatively spared. Dilated pupils and tachycardia suggest anticholinergic effects frequently observed with tricyclic and tetracyclic antidepressant drugs. The anticholinesterase drug, physostigmine, can reverse most of the effects of tricyclic overdosage. It should only be used in the presence of anticholinergic signs, since in the absence of cholinergic blockade physostigmine can cause marked central stimulation resulting in tachycardia and hypertension. Mixed neurological signs of unconsciousness with increased tone, restlessness, tonic convulsions, and respiratory depression are characteristic of methqualone. Barbiturates and nonbarbiturate hypnotics frequently cause hypotension which responds to volume expansion and inotropic drugs.

Gastric washings, blood, and urine should be stored for drug analysis. However, the use of screening measurements for toxins is generally not necessary since treatment is nonspecific. In selected instances when the patient fails to respond to treatment, such measurements are useful in confirming the diagnosis or, if negative, suggesting that re-

Table 1.5 **Assessment of Levels of Central Nervous System Depression**

1. Eyes	a. Open	Spontaneously	4
		To Verbal Command	3
		To Pain	2
	b. No response		1
2. Best Motor Response	a. To Verbal Command	Obeys	6
	b. To Pain	Localizes pain	5
		Flexion withdrawal	4
		Decorticate rigidity	3
		Decerebrate rigidity	2
		None	1
3. Best Verbal Response		Oriented and Converses	5
		Disoriented and Converses	4
		Inappropriate words	3
		Incomprehensible sounds	2
		None	1

The painful stimulus used is usually knuckle pressure on the sternum. A numerical grade can be assigned to each of the three categories and progress of the patient monitored.

newed attention should be given to alternative diagnosis such as intracranial vascular accidents, trauma, metabolic causes, or infection including meningitis.

Special efforts may be required to treat these patients with the necessary compassion. The natural tendency to take a judgmental or authoritarian approach is unlikely to reduce the risk of recurrence and may detract from the objectivity with which clinical decisions should be reached.

Treatment should be aimed at maintaining adequate respiratory function. Oxygen administration, endotracheal intubation, and assisted ventilation may be necesaary. Adequate intravenous fluids should be given to correct any deficit and to provide mainte-

Table 1.6 **Clinical Findings That Suggest Specific Drugs**

Clinical Findings	Drug to Consider
Central nervous depression	
Respiratory depression	Opioids
	Barbiturates
	Benzodiazapines
Dilated pupils, tachycardia, arrhythmias	Tricyclic and tetracycline antidepressants
Increased tone, seizures	Methaqualone
Chronic tachycardia, impaired memory	Marijuana
Hyperventilation, mild confusion, metabolic acidosis	Salicylates

nance requirements. Once the respiratory care is established, further absorption of the drug (if taken by mouth) should be prevented by performing gastric lavage. When performed with the head in a slightly dependent position, aspiration into the lungs is unlikely. Forced diuresis should not be used, since few drugs are appreciably reabsorbed by the renal tubules. If phenobarbital is identified as the causative drug (an unusual occurrence, since this drug is no longer used to treat anxiety disorders), osmotic diuretics can be used to enhance the rate of renal clearance. Alkalinization of the urine can further decrease tubular reabsorption of the phenobarbital because of the increased trapping of ionized drug within the tubules.

Approximately one third of patients treated for coma due to drug overdosage have received previous psychiatric treatment and one third have been treated for similar episodes at least once previously. Upon recovery, all patients should be assessed by a psychiatrist.

OVERDOSAGE WITH ACETAMINOPHEN AND SALICYLATES

Patients who have taken overdoses of acetaminophen, salicylates, and other drugs often have less dramatic presenting signs than the comatose patient. Nevertheless, in patients who receive in-hospital treatment, the lethality of acetaminophen and salicylate overdosage is, if anything, higher than that due to central nervous system depressant drugs.

Acetaminophen

Acetaminophen is metabolized in the liver by the microsomal enzymes known as mixed function oxidases, principally to sulfate and glucuronide conjugates. A small amount of a therapeutic dose (about 4 percent) is excreted unchanged in the urine and a smaller amount is converted by microsomal enzymes to a reactive N-hydroxylated metabolite. In therapeutic doses this metabolite combines preferentially with glutathione and is excreted as a conjugate of cysteine or acetylcysteine. In an overdose, however, the supply of glutathione is exceeded and the N-hydroxylated metabolite can bind covalently to portions of the hepatic cell, causing hepatic necrosis.

There are several phases to the clinical course of acetaminophen toxicity. Within a few hours of ingestion, nausea, vomiting, sweating, and palor appear. The severity of these symptoms is usually related to the size of dose taken. This phase is followed by a quiescent period of 24 to 48 hours after which symptoms and signs of hepatic damage occur, usually beginning 3 to 5 days after the drug is ingested. This phase varies in severity from asymptomatic elevation in hepatic enzymes to frank hepatic coma. If the patient recovers there is no evidence of permanent hepatic damage.

If more than 100 mg/kg of acetaminophen (7.5 g in an ordinary adult) has been ingested, the poisoning should be considered potentially severe. It is important that antidotal treatment be given as early as possible in order to prevent progression to hepatic necrosis. Serum concentration measurements provide a reasonable estimate of severity if interpreted in relation to the time of ingestion. Since absorption often continues for some time after ingestion of a large dose, single measurements before 4 hours are unreliable. Antidotal treatment with the glutathione substitute N-acetylcysteine should be initiated and continued until a serum concentration of acetaminophen is available. Nomograms relating expected toxicity to the serum concentration and serum half-life of acetaminophen are used to determine whether antidotal treatment should be continued.

Treatment should include reducing further absorption using emesis or gastric lavage. Activated charcoal should not be used if acetylcysteine will be used by mouth, since charcoal will absorb the antidotal drug.

Salicylate

Salicylate-containing drugs are widely available and overdosage remains an unfortunately common occurrence. The spectrum of cases encompasses accidental overdosage in children, whose conditions rapidly progress to a metabolic acidemia; suicidal attempts in young adults, whose conditions frequently do not progress beyond the initial phase of respiratory alkalosis; and the surreptitious development of mild confusion and malaise in patients taking salicylates chronically, who have increased the dose slightly to suppress symptoms or in whom excretory processes for salicylates have changed.

The patient with salicylate overdose is usually conscious, although mild confusion or somnolence are common in elderly patients. The clinical features are dominated by the metabolic effects of the drug, which include hypoglycemia, salt and water depletion, hypokalemia, respiratory alkalosis, metabolic acidosis, and, rarely, hypoprothrombinemia.

Salicylate rapidly produces a marked reduction of liver glycogen and brain glucose, probably because of increased peripheral utilization of glucose. This occurs secondary to salicylate interference with the transfer and storage of energy in phosphate bonds derived from the oxidation of foodstuffs (uncoupling of oxidative phosphorylation). In salicylate overdosage, particularly in infants, blood glucose can be low and brain glucose can be reduced even when blood glucose concentrations are normal. For this reason, solutions containing glucose should be given in salicylate overdosage even if blood glucose is normal.

Lethality of salicylate poisoning in animals is related more directly to the concentration of salicylate in the brain than in the blood. In acidemic states salicylate distributes more readily into tissues, including the brain, since about twice as much salicylate is in the unionized, diffusable form at pH 7.2 compared with pH 7.4 (pKa of salicylate = 3.5). A primary goal in treating salicylate poisoning should therefore be to avoid systemic acidemia. This can be achieved by the administration of sodium bicarbonate.

Salicylate has complex effects on salt, water, and acid-base balance. The uncoupling of oxidative phosphorylation leads to increased oxygen consumption and carbon dioxide production, the respiratory center responds, and ventilation is increased largely by an increase in the depth of breathing. Many salicylate preparations contain codeine and the respiratory response may be blunted, with a resulting respiratory acidosis. With increased serum concentrations of salicylate the respiratory center is directly stimulated and the rate and depth of ventilation increase, leading to respiratory alkalosis. At even higher concentrations, a metabolic acidosis occurs due to a variety of factors: if the phase of respiratory alkalosis is prolonged there is a compensatory renal loss of bicarbonate; increased glucose utilization leads to an increase in production of pyruvate, lactate, and acetoacetate; salicylate ion itself displaces 2 to 3 mmol HCO_3; and renal perfusion and function may be impaired due to fluid and electrolyte changes. The fluid and electrolyte state is complicated by the loss of sodium and water due to the hyperventilation and sweating that accompanies the increased but inefficient metabolism.

Potassium losses in salicylate poisoning can be large. Salicylate itself enhances renal potassium loss, perhaps through interference with Na-K transport mechanisms. In respiratory alkalemia intracellular potassium concentrations increase so that in the renal tubules the potassium gradient between the tubular cell and tubular urine increases, thus enhancing transfer into the urine. In acidemia, a primary buffering mechanism is the entry of hydrogen ion into cells, displacing potassium from body cells into the plasma space and from renal tubular cells into urine, leading to high renal losses.

Treatment of salicylate overdosage should include attention to the above features and to glucose, alkali, sodium (and water), and potassium (the mnemonic GASP may aid recall).

Salicylate taken in large doses for several days can cause hypoprothrombinemia due to an interference with vitamin K. Since small doses affect platelet function, bleeding complications can occasionally be seen. Vitamin K effectively reverses the hypoprothrombinemia.

Ancillary treatment of salicylate overdosage may include gastric emptying with syrup of ipecac, or lavage with the usual precaution against aspiration. Activated charcoal adsorbs salicylate and can be given by mouth. Alkalinizing the urine to a pH between 7 and 8 traps more salicylate in the ionized, nondiffusible form in tubular urine, diminishing tubular reabsorption and enhancing loss. Little increase in loss is observed by lesser increases in urine pH. It is difficult to achieve this degree of alkalinization with bicarbonate alone. The carbonic anhydrase inhibitor acetazolamide is effective in increasing the pH of urine by enhancing bicarbonate loss. Two risks of acetazolamide must be considered. The bicarbonate loss can precipitate or aggravate a metabolic acidemia—an undesirable complication in salicylate overdosage—and can lead as well to greater potassium loss since the bicarbonate must be lost with an accompanying cation. Therefore acetazolamide should not be used without bicarbonate and without correction of potassium deficits. In severe cases, particularly where renal function is impaired, salicylate can be effectively removed by hemoperfusion through a resin column.

Salicylate overdosage is sometimes recognized because of the findings of an unexplained metabolic acidemia with an increase in anion gap. Other toxins such as methyl alcohol, ethylene glycol, and ethanol should be considered in the differential diagnosis of such cases.

The usual criteria for assessing the severity of overdosage due to central nervous system depressants cannot be used in salicylate poisoning. Severity can be assessed by an estimate of dose taken, by serum concentration measurements, and by the extent of acid-base disturbance. Mild overdosage is seen with doses less than 150 mg/kg, whereas severe states are seen with doses over 400 mg/kg. Infants and elderly patients are at higher risk. Serum concentrations less than 3 mmol/L are associated with mild overdosage, whereas concentrations over 7 mmol/L are associated with severe states. Single measurements can be misleading, since continued absorption may occur for many hours after absorption in overdosage. Any degree of acidemia suggests a severe poisoning.

STIMULANTS AND HALLUCINOGENS

A variety of chemicals are used to stimulate the central nervous system or induce hallucinations. Cocaine and the amphetamines are the predominant drugs used to provide stimulation, while lysergic acid derivatives including dimethyltryptamine (DMT) and phencyclidine are the most popular hallucinogens. These substances are particularly hazardous because of the small difference between lethal doses and those which provide the desired effect. There are differences in the pharmacological effects and the chronic consequences of these substances.

Cocaine, a naturally occurring local anesthetic, stimulates the central nervous system and results in a feeling of excitement with increased perceptual awareness and euphoria. Increased motor activity may proceed to tremor and convulsions. Hypertension, tachycardia, and ventricular fibrillation are the major cardiovascular adverse effects. The local vasoconstrictor effects result in nasal septal perforation after chronic intranasal application. In high doses hallucinations occur, and with chronic high doses a psychosis marked by paranoia and proneness to violence is observed. True physical dependence is not seen.

Amphetamine results in psychic effects similar to those of cocaine. Unlike cocaine, however, tolerance to amphetamine develops quite rapidly. Chronic use causes a psychosis marked by paranoia, prolonged hallucinosis, and proneness to violent behavior. Cardiovascular effects include marked hypertension that can result in cerebral hemorrhage.

The hallucinogens such as lysergic acid characteristically produce a change in mood and perception accompanied by visual hallucinations and a distortion of body image. Depersonalization, acute panic, and schizophrenia-like reactions are observed. The autonomic effects of these drugs are largely sympathomimetic, with increased blood pressure, tachycardia, mydriasis, and piloerection. Chronic lysergic acid use can lead to severe depression and recurrent hallucinogenic effects in the absence of the drug (flashbacks).

Overdosages with amphetamines, lysergic acid, cocaine, and phencyclidine lead to similar clinical states characterized by the following:

1. Apprehension, anxiety, restlessness, and irritability
2. Adrenergic signs, including dilated pupils, tachycardia and hypertension
3. Muscle spasms and rigidity, hyperreflexia, and convulsions

Paranoia suggests amphetamine toxicity, hallucinations suggest cocaine or lysergic acid ingestion, and bizarre behavior and agitation with mild sensory stimuli suggest phencyclidine ingestion. However, substances often consist of mixtures, including such additional compounds as caffeine, strychnine, procaine, heroin, and quinine. It is therefore often impossible to identify the causative drug from the clinical picture. Knowledge of the trends of drug use in the community can be invaluable.

Treatment should consist of reducing sensory stimuli, since agitation and convulsions are often precipitated by noise, excitation, or bright lights. If the patient is unconscious the treatment is similar to that of a central nervous system depressant with attention to adequate ventilation. Severe apprehension and convulsions are best managed with diazepam. Patients who are severely agitated or psychotic can be treated with haloperidol. This drug should be used rather than phenothiazine since it does not have anticholinergic properties. Phenothiazines can interact with some street drugs such as dimethyltyramine to cause severe hypertension, increase muscle rigidity in patients with phencyclidine toxicity, and exaggerate toxic effects of anticholinergic drugs such as scopolamine.

THE PHYSICIAN'S ROLE IN RECOGNIZING AND PREVENTING DRUG ABUSE

It is estimated that about 7 million Americans and Canadians misuse prescription drugs. Some of this misuse begins inadvertently. For others it is abetted because physicians fail to appreciate the risk of long-term or repeat prescriptions of addicting drugs, and because pharmacists are reluctant to call the physician's attention to problem patients or inadvisable prescribing practices. In the United States it is estimated that at least 20 percent of the total 600 kilograms of amphetamines dispensed annually is provided directly from physicians' offices, without the benefit of the additional surveillance by pharmacists. Some of the misuse is of a criminal nature. Careless placement of prescription forms provides easy access for those who want to purchase mind-altering drugs. Physicians themselves are at particular risk of addiction because of their access to drugs.

The patient who has an actual or potential problem of addiction to alcohol or other drugs is often difficult to identify because the stigma attached to drug use causes patients to deny misuse. Information from the patient should be obtained in a diplomatic and nonjudgmental manner. The inquiry, "Many people use drugs today. What drugs have you used in the past?" followed by, "What drugs are you using now?" is more likely to provide reliable information than the more terse, "Do you drink or do you use drugs?" The adolescent who changes from long-time reliable friends to new companions who are not brought home, may have a drug problem. Deteriorating school performance and breakdown in family communication may be clues to misuse of drugs, but may also reflect normal adolescent stress. Personality changes including poor personal hygiene, increased hostility, unexplained absences from work, and withdrawal from community, family, and leisure activities should suggest alcohol or other drug misuse.

Physical examination may raise suspicion of a drug habit. Tachycardia at rest is often found in amphetamine and marijuana users. Needle puncture sites, needle tracks due to thrombosed superficial veins, hyperpigmented macules or punched out atrophic 1 to 5 cm depressions in the skin, regional lymphadenopathy, and miosis should be carefully searched for and are suggestive of intravenous and subcutaneous drug abuse. Bruxism (grinding of teeth during sleep) is observed in amphetamine abusers, and perforation of the nasal septum occurs in persistent users of cocaine snuff.

The physician can help to prevent the abuse of drugs by recognizing the individual who already has a problem and by identifying those at greatest risk. The individual who smokes and uses alcohol is more likely to misuse drugs than the nonsmoker and abstainer. The abstaining alcoholic is particularly likely to relapse if given antianxiety drugs. Ready availability of drugs is an important contributing factor to initiating a habit. In order to avoid this tragedy, physicians should scrupulously avoid prescribing self-medication with potentially addicting drugs, including benzodiazepines. Addicting drugs should only be provided to patients in small quantities for short treatment courses, and should not be dispensed directly from the physician's office unless all of the safeguards and records expected of a pharmacy outlet are meticulously maintained. Care should be taken that prescription blanks are not easily available for misuse by drug-seeking patients.

REFERENCES

1. Becker, E.C.: Medical Complications of Drug Abuse. Adv. Int. Med. 24:183, 1979.
2. Casarett, L.J., Doull, J.: Toxicology, The Basic Science of Poisons. New York, MacMillan, 1975.
3. Clark, W.D.: Alcoholism: blocks to diagnosis and treatment. Am. J. Med. 71:275, 1981.
4. Eckardt, N.J., et al: Health hazards associated with alcohol consumption. JAMA 246:648, 1981.
5. Kricka, L.J., Clark P.M.S.: Biochemestry of Alcohol and Alcoholism. New York, John Wiley and Sons, 1979.
6. Lieber, C.S.: Metabolic Aspects of Alcoholism. Baltimore, University Park Press, 1977.
7. Nahas, G.G.: Current status of marijuana research: symposium on marijuana held July 1978 in Reims, France. JAMA 242:2775, 1979.
8. Sellers, E.M., Naranjo, C.A., Peachey, J.E.: Drugs to decrease alcoholic consumption. N. Engl. J. Med. 305:1255, 1981.
9. Sherlock, S. (ed): Alcohol and disease. Br. Med. Bull. 38:1–108, 1982.
10. Stunkard A.J. (ed): Obesity. Philadelphia, W.B. Saunders, 1980.
11. Teasdale, G.: Assessment of coma and impaired consciousness. Lancet II:81, 1974.
12. Van Itallie, T.B., Kral, J.G.: The dilemma of morbid obesity. JAMA 246:999, 1981.

2

Atherosclerosis

Ellison H. Wittels, M.D.

Arteriosclerosis is a general term used to describe disease processes which lead to loss of elasticity and to thickening of the arterial wall. Atherosclerosis is the most common form of arteriosclerosis. The term comes from the Greek "athero" meaning porridge and "sclerosis" meaning hardening, the name being derived from the gruel or porridge-like material found in the center of the atherosclerotic plaque. Atherosclerosis affects the intima and the inner media of large and medium sized muscular arteries, and large elastic arteries. Atherosclerosis affects the aorta, the extra- and intracranial cerebral arteries, the coronary arteries, the visceral arteries, and the peripheral vascular bed. The vast majority of cerebrovascular, coronary artery and peripheral vascular disease is caused by atherosclerosis. Clinically, the lesion can cause symptoms in several different ways. Gradual occlusion of a vessel can cause ischemic pain such as claudication cr angina pectoris. Sudden occlusion of the vessel can lead to infarction or sudden death. The atherosclerotic lesion can ulcerate, causing distal embolization of atheromatous material or clots, with ischemia or infarction resulting. The plaque can lead to vessel wall weakening with aneurysm formation and possible rupture of the vessel. The clinical symptoms depend upon which part of the vascular system is involved, the rate of progression of the atherosclerotic lesion, and whether the lesion in the vessel is proximal, distal, or diffuse (Table 2.1).

It is most important to remember that the development of the atherosclerotic plaque takes many years. Atherosclerosis may progress at varying rates in different parts of the vascular bed in the same individual. Atherosclerosis can be present without clinical symptoms. The clinical symptoms, can, however, develop in seconds or minutes, even though the underlying lesion is long standing. The length of time it takes for the atherosclerotic lesion to develop and the variability of clinical symptoms has caused a great deal of difficulty in understanding this disease process.

Table 2.1 **Common Organ Involvement and Clinical Manifestations of Atherosclerosis**

Region Involved	Clinical Features
Cerebral blood vessels	Vascular bruit (particularly at bifurcation of carotid arteries)
	Transient ischemic attacks
	Vascular thrombosis with cerebral infarction (see Chapter 14)
Coronary blood vessels	Arrhythmias
	Ischemic pain
	Myocardial infarction (see Chapter 16)
Peripheral blood vessels	Vascular bruit (particularly over iliac and femoral vessels)
	Ischemic Pain (intermittent claudication)
	Trophic changes ranging from loss of skin appendages to gangrene
Aorta and abdominal vessels	Vascular bruit
	Vascular calcification (seen by roentgenogram)
	Abdominal aortic aneurysm
	Renal vascular hypertension
	Mesenteric insufficiency

EPIDEMIOLOGY

Atherosclerosis is the major cause of death in Western societies. In 1978, almost one million people died from cardiovascular disease, accounting for 51.3 percent of all deaths in the United States. Approximately 650,000 of the almost one million deaths were from coronary artery disease. By comparison, all forms of cancer accounted for approximately 400,000 deaths in the United States in 1978. In 1979 over 4 million Americans had clinical symptoms of coronary artery disease.

Atherosclerosis is a disease which affects men much more than women. After the menopause the incidence of vascular disease becomes more equal between the two sexes. It is a disease which affects primarily individuals from the fifth through the seventh decades of life. A man has a 37 percent chance and a woman has an 18 percent chance of developing clinically significant cardiovascular disease by the time they reach 65 years of age.

Atherosclerosis involves the expenditure of approximately 27 billion dollars a year. Of this, 6 billion dollars is in direct medical care. Another 21 billion dollars consists of indirect costs secondary to premature death and lessened productivity.

In the United States over the last several decades there has been a marked decline in the death rate from cardiovascular disease. This includes both coronary artery disease and stroke. It has occurred in both males and females, white, black, and in all age groups. The death rate from stroke has declined approximately 32 percent over the last decade. In the United States from 1969 through 1977 the death rate from coronary heart disease declined almost 23 percent. In Canada the decline was approximately 11 percent. Evidence of a decrease in mortality from cardiovascular disease has been found in other countries as well. At the same time several countries, such as France and England, have continued to show an increase in the death rate from coronary artery disease. It is not clear whether the incidence of cardiovascular disease has shown a similar decline.

Several postulates have been advanced to explain the reason for the decrease in the death rate. Part of the decreased death rate may be due to more rapid transportation of critically ill patients as well as to Coronary Care Units with better monitoring. New medication for the treatment of coronary artery disease and coronary bypass surgery also may have been beneficial. Better diagnostic testing to identify early atherosclerotic disease has also been advanced to explain some of the decrease in the death rate. In the last several decades, there has been increased emphasis on preventive medicine. Diseases associated with the development and exacerbation of atherosclerotic disease have been treated more aggressively. It is postulated that this may also have played a major role in the decrease in cardiovascular disease.

Understanding the reason for the decline of death from atherosclerotic disease is most important, since a better understanding of this decline offers hope for further improvement.

PATHOGENESIS

ANATOMY AND HISTOLOGY

The muscular artery has three layers, the intima, the media and the adventitia. The intima is bounded on the luminal side by a single endothelial cell layer. The endothelial cell layer bars the passage of substances from the vessel lumen into the vessel wall. Substances may pass from the lumen into the vessel wall through intercellular junctions (100–200 angstrom in size) or penetrate the endothelial cell through endocytotic vesicles. These allow incorporation of molecules approximately 600–1,000 angstrom in size. Also found in the intima are very small numbers of smooth muscle cells and some connective tissue. As a person ages the number of smooth muscle cells in the intima increases. The media is bounded by the internal elastic membrane on its luminal side and the adventitia. The media consists of smooth muscle cells, collagen, elastic fibers, and proteoglycans. The external elastic lamina separates the media from the adventitia. The adventitial layer is composed mostly of fibroblasts, smooth muscle cells, collagen and proteoglycans. The intima and the inner media are nourished by perfusion of substances from the lumen. The outer part of the media and the adventitia are nourished by the vasovasorum, a complex of arterioles and venules.

Atherosclerosis includes three different pathologic components. These are the fatty streak, the fibrous plaque, and the complicated lesion. In each of these three types, smooth muscle cell proliferation, connective tissue deposition, and intra- and extracellular lipid are found. The atherosclerotic lesion should be looked upon as a continuum rather than as discrete components. Also, within the same individual there can be a mixture of the three different types of atherosclerotic lesions at the same time.

The fatty streak is a pale yellow flat intimal lesion. Lipid, principally cholesterol and cholesteryl ester, is the predominant abnormality. The lipids are found in foam cells, cells with vacuolated cytoplasm. These cells have been postulated to be derived from smooth muscle cells and/or macrophages. The juvenile fatty streak begins within the first few months after birth starting first in the proximal aorta. It later progresses to the thoracic and the abdominal aorta. The amount of aortic intimal involvement increases to about 50 percent by the time an individual reaches 25. Fatty streaks also appear in the coronary arteries and later in life in the cerebral vessels. Interestingly, females have more extensive fatty streaks than do males. The progressive fatty streak consists of lesions that in many ways resemble the juvenile fatty streak. It often contains more extracellular lipid from necrosis of the lipid laden foam cells and more collagen and elastic fiber than the juvenile fatty streak.

It is uncertain whether the juvenile fatty streak is the forerunner of subsequent atherosclerotic lesions. In the aorta, there is little relationship between the juvenile fatty streak and subsequent atherosclerotic lesions. There is better correlation in the coronary arteries. It is possible that the progressive fatty streak represents a transition between the juvenile fatty streak and the fibrous plaque which is more pathognomonic of atherosclerosis.

The fibrous plaque is a white-to-gray elevated lesion that protrudes into the vessel lumen. It appears some 15–20 years later than the fatty streak. These plaques are correlated with clinical symptoms of atherosclerosis. All of these plaques have a central core of extracellular lipid and cell debris and are covered by a thick capsule of collagen and elastic tissue along with smooth muscle cells. Again, cholesterol and cholesteryl ester are present.

The hallmark of the complicated lesion of atherosclerosis is calcification. This develops in the fibrous plaque following necrosis, thrombosis, or hemorrhage. These are the most common type of atherosclerotic lesions that produce clinical symptoms.

A fourth lesion may be associated with the subsequent development of atherosclerosis. This fibroelastic lesion, or intimal cushion consists of proliferated smooth muscle cells in the subendothelium along with some connective tissue but little lipid. The intimal cushion develops especially at sites of branching in the vessels. It has been noted as early as the 34th week of fetal development and with increasing age, intimal thickening increases. It is found much more frequently in males than in females. It appears that the areas involved with intimal cushions are more susceptible to atherosclerotic plaque formation.

CELLULAR AND METABOLIC MECHANISMS

The endothelial cell, serum lipids, the coagulation system, and smooth muscle cell are of paramount importance in the initiation and development of the atherosclerotic plaque.

Endothelial Cell

The endothelial cell serves a number of important functions. It is a barrier between the lumen and the wall of the vessel. Substances may move from the lumen into the vessel wall through intercellular junctions and by pinocytosis. The endothelial cell synthesizes and secretes proteins including collagen and glycoproteins. It also secretes proteoglycan, a heparin like substance, and prostacyclin (PGI_2) and has a role in the clearance of thrombin and vasoactive amines. Thus the endothelial cell layer can be viewed as a mechanical barrier as well as a metabolically active barrier.

Injury to the endothelial cell layer can result in increased permeability or death of cells followed by multiplication of surrounding cells and re-endothelialization. Carbon monoxide, antigen-antibody complexes, elevated cholesterol, fatty acids, homocystine, hypertension, and vasoactive peptides such as angiotensin and the catecholamines, have all been shown to cause increased endothelial cell permeability or injury. While each of these substances may not induce the same injury to the endothelial cell, all will cause disruption of this cell layer. Damage to the endothelial cell has been postulated as the initiating factor in the development of atherosclerosis.

The early concept that atherogensis stems from the absence of the endothelial cell lining with increased movement of plasma protein, platelets and lipoproteins, from the lumen into the vessel wall, has been disputed by recent experimental data. Intimal thickening and lipid accumulation have been found to be more marked beneath areas of re-endothelialization than beneath areas which have been denuded of their endothelial layer. In areas which have been recently re-endothelialized, cellular activity is much increased. For example, there is increased synthesis of sulfated glycosaminoglycans which can bind plasma proteins such as LDL and may inhibit lysosomes. In addition, less cholesteryl ester hydrolase activity is found in re-endothelialized areas when compared to the de-endothelialized aortic wall. Thus it appears that altered metabolic activity, and binding of the plasma proteins rather than simple transport of proteins across the denuded endothelial wall plays a central role in the atherogenic process.

Smooth Muscle Cells

Approximately 3 to 5 days after endothelial cell injury has occurred, smooth muscle cells migrate from the media through the internal elastic lamina and into the intima where they proliferate. The smooth muscle cells are the source of collagen, elastic fiber and glycosaminoglycan in the intima. Over time, the intimal lesion may regress into a thickness of only 1 or 2 cell layers.

The intimal proliferation of smooth muscle cells

is the essential cellular response associated with the progression of atherosclerosis. Smooth muscle cells can migrate into the intima either secondary to adaptation of the wall to increased pressure or in response to injury to the endothelial cell layer. Several factors play a role in the stimulation of smooth muscle cell migration and proliferation. Disruption of the platelets at the subendothelial layer releases a glycoprotein called platelet derived growth factor. This factor plays a major role in the proliferation of the smooth muscle cells. In addition, several other factors have been found to increase smooth muscle proliferation. These include a growth factor from the LDL fraction of hyperlipidemic serum, an insulin growth factor from diabetic serum, endothelial cell growth factor and a monocyte macrophage growth factor. Accumulation of cholesteryl ester in smooth muscle cells produces a foam cell which becomes toxic and dies, releasing the cholesteryl ester into the surrounding connective tissue. The macrophage or monocyte may also function as a foam cell in the atherosclerotic plaque.

Studies of primary smooth muscle cell cultures have added more information about the metabolism of the smooth muscle cell. The smooth muscle cell is maintained in two states, the contractile state and the synthetic state. The change from a contractile to a synthetic state has been termed "modulation". In a contractile state, during the first 5 days or so in culture, the cells contract and respond to platelet derived growth factor. The smooth muscle cells can be maintained in a contractile state by keeping them at high density in culture. If the smooth muscle cells are placed in sparse culture, they lose their capacity to contract over a period of 7 to 9 days. This parallels a loss of most of their cytoplasmic myosin. The cells become responsive to platelet derived growth factor and synthesize connective tissue. Modulation provides an explanation for the delayed smooth muscle cell response following endothelial injury. It also increases the importance of platelet derived growth factor in stimulating the migration of smooth muscle cells from the high cell density media to the sparse density intima where modulation could occur.

At present, several theories are available to explain smooth muscle cell proliferation in the intima. The monoclonal theory proposes that a single cell type proliferates in the atherosclerotic plaque. The cell has been altered by chemical or viral agents, such as cigarette smoke, develops a proliferative advantage, and this single cell type multiplies. The second theory is the clonal senescence hypothesis. With age, the fibroblast and smooth muscle cells lose their capacity to multiply. This leaves only stem cells capable of division. The stem cells are inhibited by a negative feedback control via chalone which is secreted from

smooth muscle cells. As the aging smooth muscle cells decrease, the concentration of chalone decreases. As the chalone decreases the stem cells are released from feedback control and proliferate. Thus in the media where there are a large number of smooth muscle cells the loss of chalones in the aging smooth muscle cells would have a minimal effect upon smooth muscle cell proliferation. In the intima, the loss of feedback inhibition could lead to a significant increase in stem cell replication.

A third hypothesis to explain smooth muscle proliferation in the atherosclerotic process is the "response to injury hypothesis". In this hypothesis, endothelial cell injury or disruption is the initiating event. The disruption of the endothelial cell barrier exposes the underlying subendothelial connective tissue to platelets which through adherence, aggregation and release of growth factor stimulate the proliferation of smooth muscle cells from the media into the intima. Connective tissue is formed. Plasma protein such as low density lipoprotein accumulates. Eventually, the endothelial barrier is restored and the lesion regresses if the injury and the tissue response are limited. If injury to the endothelium is continuous or repeated, however, further proliferation of smooth muscle cells and accumulation of connective tissue and lipid occur. There is relatively little information to document how regression occurs. The response to injury hypothesis puts increased emphasis on risk factors and repetitive injury.

Clotting Mechanisms

As early as 1852, Rokitansky proposed that the atherosclerotic plaque resulted from the organization of mural thrombi. Since then, the relationship between atherosclerosis and coagulation has been investigated. Currently, major areas of investigation center on prostaglandin metabolism and on the role of platelets.

Arachidonic acid is the most common precursor of prostaglandins. Two oxidative pathways are available for free arachidonic acid. One pathway, found in human platelets, converts arachidonic acid to thromboxane A_2. Thromboxane A_2 has two major effects: aggregation of platelets and constriction of arteries. The second oxidative pathway leads to the production of prostacyclin (PGI_2). Prostacyclin is a powerful inhibitor of platelet aggregation and vasodilating agent. Thus the actions of thromboxane A_2 and prostacyclin are opposite. PGI_2 is produced in large amounts by the vascular endothelial cells and by vascular smooth muscle cells. One of the fundamental characteristics of the normal endothelium is its nonreactivity to platelets, leukocytes, or clotting factors. PGI_2 may play a role in this. The vascular smooth muscle cells which are actively proliferating in the intima form significantly higher PGI_2 levels than when they are in the media. This may be a protective mechanism in the face of injury to the endothelial cell wall. In early atherosclerosis, there is suppression of PGI_2 generation with normal thromboxane generation.

When the endothelial surface is injured, the adhesion of the platelets to the subendothelial connective tissue collagen is almost instantaneous. Subsequent aggregation of platelets begins in about 15–30 seconds and will persist over 48 hours. Thromboxane A_2 is released, which may promote further platelet adherence and aggregation and contribute to vasoconstriction. Platelets also release the platelet-derived growth factor which plays such a central role in chemotaxis and the proliferation of smooth muscle cells. Experimental data substantiating the role of platelets in the atherosclerotic process have come from several experiments. Swine, homozygous for von Willebrand's disease, have platelets that do not adhere to collagen. These swine are resistant to spontaneous and hypercholesterolemic atherosclerosis. They develop flat fatty lesions and endothelial damage but no intimal proliferation. If an experimental animal is made thrombocytopenic and its vascular endothelium is then damaged, development of atherosclerotic lesions is also prevented.

Thrombosis is a major complication of atherosclerosis. Examination of obstructed coronary arteries has established that the platelet thrombus which may lead to obstruction of the vessel is associated with recent hemorrhage into an underlying atherosclerotic plaque. According to the erythrocyte-hemodynamics hypothesis, the event that begins arterial thrombosis is fissuring of atherosclerotic plaques, which leads to hemorrhage into the vessel wall and release of red cell ADP into the plasma. The ADP is responsible for activating platelets and their subsequent aggregation as mural thrombi. Thrombosis may occur over an atherosclerotic plaque in the absence of rupture of the atheroma. The thrombus becomes replaced by fibrous and vascular tissue, which is called organization.

Thus the coagulation system is involved with atherosclerosis in several ways. It may play a role in the etiology of atherosclerosis through the release of platelet-derived growth factor, contribute to acute complications through mural thrombus formation, and promote or inhibit clotting through the balance of thromboxane or prostacylin generation.

RISK FACTORS

In recent years, there has been increased emphasis on identifying persons at risk to develop atheros-

clerotic disease. The presence of a risk factor in an individual means there is an increased likelihood of developing the atherosclerotic lesion and of developing it at an earlier age than if the risk factor were not present. This does not imply a cause-effect relationship between the risk factor and atherosclerotic disease. Likewise, the presence of a risk factor in an individual does not in itself mean that the person is going to develop atherosclerosis.

Three major risk factors have been identified for coronary artery disease. They include elevated cholesterol, hypertension, and cigarette smoking. Minor risk factors for coronary artery disease include diabetes mellitus, elevated triglyceride, sedentary lifestyle, type A personality, male sex, positive family history, and obesity (Table 2.2). There is some evidence that obesity is a risk factor only through its association with elevated triglyceride, diabetes, elevated blood pressure, and lack of physical activity which are often found among obese patients. It may in itself not be a risk factor (see Chapter 1).

For cerebrovascular disease and stroke, hypertension and diabetes seem to be major risk factors. Elevated triglycerides are found in a significant percentage of patients with cerebrovascular disease. For peripheral vascular disease, cigarette smoking seems to be a major risk factor.

Often, it is found that an individual will have several risk factors. For example, the patient may smoke cigarettes and have elevated serum cholesterol. Risk factors are not only additive but may well be synergistic.

Cholesterol and Lipoproteins

The lipoproteins which have been considered to be atherogenic include the low density lipoprotein (LDL), the intermediate density lipoprotein (IDL), the chylomicron remnant, and the very low density lipoprotein (VLDL). The heavy density lipoprotein (HDL) has been found to protect from the development of atherosclerotic disease. The major component of these lipoproteins with atherogenic effect

Table 2.2 **Risk Factors–Coronary Artery Atherosclerosis**

Major	Minor
Elevated cholesterol	Diabetes mellitus
Elevated blood pressure	Elevated triglyceride
Cigarette smoking	Type A personality
	Male
	Age
	Family history
	Lack of exercise
	Obesity

is probably cholesterol. (See Hyperlipidemias below.)

In 1862, Virchow suggested that the lipids in the atherosclerotic lesion were derived from plasma by "imbibition or insudation". Several lines of evidence support the critical role that cholesterol plays in the development of atherosclerotic disease, especially coronary artery disease.

In humans, the atherosclerotic plaque contains a markedly increased amount of cholesteryl ester compared to the normal artery. Lipids comprise about 60 percent of these plaques. At this time, it is felt that the cholesterol in the plaque is largely derived from plasma lipoproteins, especially LDL cholesterol. The movement of the LDL cholesterol into the atherosclerotic plaque is about ten times faster than the movement of cholesterol into a normal arterial wall. This would indicate that the formation of the atherosclerotic plaque can become more and more self-propagating in the face of elevated serum cholesterol. The presence of excess cholesteryl ester in the atherosclerotic plaque has led some investigators to hypothesize that the basic defect in atherosclerosis resides in the intracellular lysosome. According to this theory, with defective lysosomal metabolism of the LDL cholesterol, the cholesteryl ester accumulates to a level which becomes toxic. This leads to cell necrosis and release of cholesteryl ester into the surrounding extracellular space.

The Framingham study, which included over 5,000 adults followed for many years, has clearly shown a relationship between increasing serum cholesterol levels and coronary artery disease. In this study a serum cholesterol level above 180 mg/dl seemed to have increased risk of coronary disease. A person with a cholesterol of 260 mg/dl had a five times greater risk of developing coronary artery disease than a person with a cholesterol of 200 mg/dl. Most other epidemiologic studies have shown a direct relationship between increasing serum cholesterol level and the incidence of coronary artery disease.

The induction of atherosclerotic lesions by high cholesterol feeding has been demonstrated in numerous animal studies and in experimental animals. As early as 1928, Anitschkow induced regression of the atherosclerotic plaque in rabbits by decreasing their high cholesterol feedings. Subsequently, experiments in rabbits, dogs, birds, pigs and non-human primates have confirmed the reversibility of arterial lesions by discontinuing high cholesterol feedings.

Reports have also appeared in the literature demonstrating regression or lack of progression of vascular disease following surgical procedures to lower cholesterol, as well as during the use of medication and diet together. It is currently felt that the more advanced, complicated lesions will regress more slowly than the earlier lesions.

Over the last few years studies have been undertaken to prove the effectiveness of cholesterol lowering in the treatment of coronary artery disease. These trials were either primary prevention trials, among subjects who had no previous evidence of coronary disease, or secondary prevention trials in subjects who had previously diagnosed coronary artery diease. The diet trials showed no clear benefit from lowering serum cholesterol levels; the reduction was usually in the range of 10 to 12 percent. Several studies have also employed lipid lowering drugs in an attempt to prove the benefit of cholesterol lowering. The Coronary Drug Project used clofibrate, estrogen, thyroid, and nicotinic acid and reduced serum cholesterol in the range of 15–25 mg/dl. The results of this study showed some decrease in non-fatal myocardial infarction among those patients taking nicotinic acid. A second study using a bile acid-binding agent to lower serum cholesterol, achieved 37 mg/dl lowering of cholesterol. This study showed a decrease in coronary artery disease mortality.

The benefit of cholesterol lowering has been difficult to discern in some studies. There are several possible reasons for this. Atherosclerosis is a multifactorial disease; the disease is hard to quantitate, an identical baseline and rate of progression among participants are difficult to establish, and it is impossible to hold all variables but one constant in human studies.

In summary, it is agreed that elevated cholesterol is a significant risk factor in the development of coronary disease. In experimental animals the role of cholesterol in the development of the plague is established, and lowering of cholesterol can lead to regression of the disease. It is possible that in humans, benefits from cholesterol lowering will depend upon the achievement of a much greater reduction in circulating cholesterol levels. Currently the Lipid Research Clinic primary prevention trial is underway. By use of a prudent heart diet (cholesterol lowering, see Treatment below) and a bile-acid sequestering agent to lower serum cholesterol, an attempt is being made to assess more rigorous serum cholesterol lowering in the prevention of coronary artery disease.

Smoking

Smoking has been recognized as a significant risk factor for atherosclerosis, especially for coronary artery disease and peripheral vascular disease. When smoking occurs in association with other risk factors, it has a marked synergistic effect. There are several mechanisms by which smoking seems to exacerbate atherosclerotic disease. The build-up of carbon monoxide among smokers shifts the oxyhemoglobin dissociation curve to the left, with reduced oxygen release to the tissues and potential tissue hypoxia. In a person with marginal blood flow to an organ, this may cause exacerbation of ischemic disease. Hypoxia may also be harmful to the endothelial cell. Carbon monoxide from cigarette smoke has been found to injure the endothelial cell barrier, which may initiate the atherosclerotic process as described below. It is estimated that by discontinuing cigarette use, it will take up to ten years before the risk of coronary disease returns to the same baseline as that of the person who has never smoked. HDL levels rise with cessation of cigarette smoking, suggesting an important role of lipid metabolism in association with smoking.

Hypertension

Hypertension is considered a major risk factor for both cerebral vascular disease and coronary artery disease. Several mechanisms by which hypertension can play a role in the development of atherosclerosis have been postulated. It may affect lipoprotein transport by increased pinocytosis across the endothelial cell or increased size of the intercellular endothelial junctions. Angiotensin increases the interendothelial cell junctions.

The earliest lipid deposits in atherosclerosis occur at sites in the vasculature that are exposed to excess hemodynamic stresses, particularly branching points and curves in the vessel. It has been postulated that the development of atherosclerosis is a sequel to the forces of blood flow which tend to be increased in major vessels of hypertensive individuals.

Diabetes

The mechanism by which diabetes may lead to increased risk of atherosclerosis is not certain. Atherosclerosis is, however, the most common complication of diabetes. It will account for three-fourths of the deaths of diabetics in North America. Recently, hyperinsulinemia has been shown to be an independent risk factor for the development of atherosclerosis. It can alter the metabolism of the arterial wall and stimulate smooth muscle cell proliferation. Hyperinsulinemia may have the effect of increasing very low density lipoprotein (VLDL) formation and release from the liver. If this occurs, more VLDL would be available for catabolism at the endothelial cell. This may lead to release of increased VLDL remnants and LDL. (See Hyperlipidemia below.) Abnormalities of clotting function, specifically abnormal platelet function, have also been implicated in the development of atherosclerosis in diabetic patients.

Obesity

Obesity, as noted earlier, may not be an independent risk factor, but may be associated with such factors as diabetes, hyperinsulinemia, sedentary lifestyle and hyperlipidemia. High density lipoprotein (HDL) levels are decreased in obese patients. With weight reduction the HDL levels increase. Obese patients have also been shown to have elevated insulin levels associated with insulin resistance.

Triglycerides

The role of triglycerides in atherosclerosis is somewhat controversial. The Framingham study seems to downplay elevated triglyceride when not associated with elevated cholesterol or diabetes. The Stockholm prospective study found elevated triglycerides to be an independent risk factor. It has been accepted that elevated triglyceride in association with elevated cholesterol or with diabetes becomes a significant risk factor. As previously noted, HDL plays a significant role in the metabolism of VLDL triglyceride (see Hyperlipidemias below).

Sedentary Life-Style

Great controversy has surrounded the role of exercise in determining risk of developing atherosclerosis. HDL is increased with vigorous and systematic exercise such as jogging 12 miles a week. Myocardial infarction is more commonly fatal in the sedentary than in the physically active. Hypertension, obesity and smoking may be easier to treat when accompanied by an exercise conditioning program. Therefore a systematic and sustained exercise program may be useful in reducing risk factors, at least in special groups of patients.

THE HYPERLIPIDEMIAS

LIPOPROTEINS AND LIPID METABOLISM

Since the major blood lipids (cholesterol, triglycerides, and phospholipids) are insoluble and cannot circulate freely in aqueous solution, they are bound to proteins and transported through the plasma as lipid-protein complexes or lipoproteins. The major lipoprotein families are interrelated and are classified according to their density (as determined by ultracentrifugation) or by their electrophoretic mobilities. The physical properties of each plasma lipoprotein are determined by its chemical composition (Table 2.3). The major types of lipoproteins include the chylomicrons, the very low density lipoproteins (VLDL), the intermediate density lipoproteins (IDL), the low density lipoproteins (LDL) and the heavy density lipoproteins (HDL).

Dietary fat absorption begins with the formation of *chylomicra* particles and intestinal VLDL which are secreted into the intestinal lymphatics where apoprotein-C is added. Endogenous triglyceride synthesis occurs by hepatic lipogenesis, from fatty acid sources in the fasting state, or from carbohydrates and chylomicron triglyceride after meals. This hepatic synthesis is enhanced by dietary carbohydrates, alcohol ingestion, and any state which produces increased insulin levels. Apoprotein-C is added in the plasma to form VLDL. Cholesterol may be absorbed from the intestine or synthesized in the body. Almost all cells can synthesize cholesterol but the major sites are liver and intestinal mucosa. Absorption of cholesterol from the diet will reduce hepatic cholesterol synthesis. Cholesterol may be eliminated from the body by the liver where it is directly secreted into the bile or converted into bile acids. Cholesterol functions as a component of cell membranes and as a precursor of steroid hormone synthesis. It circulates in lipoprotein particles and is available for peripheral cell use. The chylomicrons carry the exogenous cholesterol and triglyceride from the intestine to the blood stream. By weight, 90 percent of the chylomicron is composed of triglyceride. The triglyceride

of the chylomicron is hydrolyzed by lipoprotein lipase, an enzyme found on the endothelial cell of peripheral tissue blood vessels. This produces glycerol and fatty acids and the chylomicron "remnant" remains, consisting of cholesteryl ester, and apoproteins. In the liver, the remnant is further catabolized. The remnant cholesterol can inhibit cholesterol synthesis by the liver by inhibiting HMG CO-A reductase, the rate limiting enzyme in cholesterol synthesis by the cell. The total circulation time for the chylomicron and the chylomicron remnant is 4.5 minutes.

Endogenous triglyceride secreted mainly by the liver, is carried by the very low density lipoprotein and serves to transfer energy to peripheral storage sites. The VLDL is produced in increasing amounts in response to increased carbohydrate and fatty acid loads to the liver. The VLDL carries triglyceride and cholesterol in about a 5:1 ratio. This cholesterol can come either from the chylomicron remnant or be synthesized de novo by the liver. There thus is a relationship between VLDL production and the person's diet.

The triglyceride is hydrolyzed by endothelial cell lipoprotein lipase, leaving the smaller IDL. Ultimately, the IDL is metabolized to LDL. The half-life of the VLDL is 1-3 hours.

Recently, data has been presented to show that the cholesterol-loaded chylomicron remnants and the VLDL remnants are taken up by arterial walls and are atherogenic. It is possible that the fatty acids released during hydrolysis of chylomicrons may cause injury to the endothelial cell layer.

The *low density lipoprotein* carries approximately 70 percent of the cholesterol found in the plasma. In unusual circumstances the LDL can be produced directly by the liver but, generally, it results from the

Table 2.3 **Characteristics of Lipoproteins**

	Chylomicron	VLDL	LDL	HDL
Size	750–12,000 Å	300–800 Å	250 Å	180–220 Å
Density (Ultracentrifuge	0.96	0.96–1.006	1.006–1.063	1.063–1.21
Electrophoretic origin	Origin	Pre Beta	Beta	Alpha
Major APO Proteins	B	B	B	AI
	CI	CI		AII
	CII	CII		E
	CIII	CIII		
Lipid Composition	Triglyceride exogenous	Triglyceride endogenous	Cholesterol	Cholesterol
Source	Small bowel	Liver and small bowel	Derived from VLDL	Liver and small bowel
Function	Transport dietary fat	Transport endogenous triglyceride	Transport cholesterol	Source of APO C, removes free cholesterol from tissue

breakdown of VLDL. The LDL attaches to receptors in the plasma membrane of cells; these receptors are called "coated pits". By the process termed "endocytosis", this area of the cell surface invaginates and the low density lipoprotein cholesterol is brought into the cell and fused with the cellular lysosomes. Within the lysosomes the protein is hydrolyzed and the cholesteryl ester of the LDL is hydrolyzed to free cholesterol and fatty acid. The free cholesterol which is released can have several fates. It can be released from the cell, it can be incorporated into the cell membranes, or can be reesterified by the enzyme acyl-CoA: cholesterol acyltransferase (ACAT). At the same time, inside the cell 3-hydroxy-3-methyl-glutaryl coenzyme A reductase (HMG-CoA reductase) is active in the production of cholesterol. The free cholesterol which has been released from the LDL cholesterol has several modifying effects upon the cell. It decreases the activity of the HMG-CoA reductase. It increases the activity of ACAT, and it decreases the LDL receptor activity. Thus, the LDL receptor mechanism is involved in the delicate feedback to regulate cellular cholesterol production and metabolism.

A second mechanism for LDL cholesterol uptake by the cell is by pinocytosis. This is independent of the LDL receptors. A third mechanism for LDL degradation is by macrophages which bind altered LDL. This method is less efficient than the primary LDL receptor system. In man, the majority of LDL degradation takes place through receptor sites and endocytosis.

Heavy density lipoprotein is produced mainly by the liver. Approximately 50 percent of the HDL mass is protein, 20 percent is cholesterol and cholesteryl esters and phospholipids make up another 30 percent. HDL apoprotein AI, activates lecithin cholesterol acyl transferase (LCAT). This enzyme permits esterification of free cholesterol. The cholesteryl ester is later transferred back from HDL to IDL. In this way, the VLDL triglyceride core is converted to a cholesteryl ester core in the IDL. This allows a reverse transport of cholesterol from the periphery back to the liver where it may be excreted. HDL is also involved in the hydrolysis of chylomicrons and VLDL, since it is a reservoir for APO C II, which activates endothelial cell lipoprotein lipase. HDL may therefore play a prominent role in preventing atherosclerosis by partially blocking the uptake of LDL in the peripheral tissues and mobilizing free cholesterol from the peripheral tissues. HDL is increased after cessation of smoking, in persons active in vigorous exercise programs and in premenopausal women. The half life of HDL is approximately 5 to 6 days. The Framingham study proved a direct correlation between LDL cholesterol levels and coronary disease. The same study also has shown an inverse relation between HDL cholesterol level and coronary artery disease. Premenopausal women who are known to have a decreased incidence of coronary artery disease have a 30-60 percent higher level of HDL than adult males. Normal HDL levels in males run from 40-50 mg/dl. Individuals with familially increased HDL levels, familial hyperalphalipoproteinemia, have HDL levels of 70 mg/dl or more. They have been found to have a decreased morbidity and mortality from coronary artery disease.

HYPERLIPOPROTEINEMIA

The hyperlipidemias by definition have cholesterol and/or triglyceride elevations above the 95 percentile of the normal population for that individual's age and sex.

Hyperlipidemia must be considered clinically important because:

1. Symptomatic disorders may be caused by the lipid excess,

2. Hyperlipidemia may result from an underlying disorder. Currently the major interest in hyperlipidemia stems from its relationship with atherogenesis (especially coronary artery disease). Other disease may result from hyperlipidemia, as in pancreatitis due to type V hyperlipoproteinemia. Identification and treatment of the underlying hyperlipidemia usually prevents recurrent episodes of abdominal pain.

The secondary hyperlipidemias result from a drug or another disease, and removal of the drug or treatment of the other disease results in normalization of lipid levels (Table 2.4).

Hyperlipidemia is usually asymptomatic and goes undetected unless routine lipid levels are measured, or the patient presents with skin manifestations of the increased lipid (Xanthomas). Measurement of the serum lipids should be carried out in the patient with a family history of premature atherogenesis or with coexisting risk factors for atherogenesis whereby hyperlipidemia would pose an added risk. Otherwise, the presenting feature of the hyperlipidemia may be with end stage vascular disease.

Table 2.4 **Secondary Hyperlipoproteinemias**

I. Endocrine: diabetes, Cushing's disease hypothyroidism, pregnancy
II. Nonendocrine: nephrotic syndrome, uremia, obstructive hepatic disease, pancreatitis, dysglobulinemia
III. Drugs: estrogens, corticosteroids, alcohol, thiazides, Dilantin

Pathogenesis of Hyperlipidemia

Hyperlipidemia may be caused by disorders of the lipoprotein transport system by four mechanisms:

1. Increased production of triglyceride containing lipoproteins:

Overproduction of VLDL results in fasting hypertriglyceridemia, and may be part of two genetic disorders, familial hypertriglyceridemia and familial combined hyperlipidemia, the latter may have family members with hypercholesterolemia. These genetic abnormalities of overproduction of VLDL may be simulated by any hyperinsulinemic state such as obesity, estrogen administration, acromegaly and possibly glucocorticoid therapy. Enhanced VLDL production also may be induced by alcohol ingestion.

2. Decreased Removal of Triglycerides:

Severe insulin deficiency will cause decreased induction of the lipoprotein lipase. This causes the decreased removal of lipids in uncontrolled diabetes. Both chronic renal failure and hypothyroidism have decreased triglyceride removal, possibly due to decreased lipoprotein lipase action. The greatly increased triglyceride concentration may produce eruptive xanthomas, abdominal pain due to acute pancreatitis, and lipemia retinalis. Usually the plasma triglyceride concentration is over 1500 mg/dl at this time. A rare genetic deficiency of lipoprotein lipase or deficiency of apo C-II will result in decreased peripheral removal of exogenous and endogenous triglyceride, resulting in increased plasma levels of chylomicrons and VLDL particles. (See Type I & V hyperlipoproteinemia below.)

3. Decreased Removal of the Remnant Lipoprotein (IDL)

This is a rare genetic disease which results in increased levels of both cholesterol and triglyceride, approximately to the same level. This is one lipoprotein disorder which cannot be diagnosed by mere measurement of fasting lipid levels and observation of the serum after being left overnight at 4°C. The abnormal lipoprotein, IDL, results in cholesterol-rich VLDL particles. A definitive diagnosis may be confirmed by ultracentrifugation or by apo E-III assay, since a deficiency of this apoprotein frequently underlies this disorder. Although some clinical features such as palmar xanthomas and tuberous xanthomas may exist, these are not specifically pathognomonic of this disorder. Ischemic heart disease and peripheral vascular disease are increased in patients afflicted with this disorder.

4. Decreased Peripheral Removal of LDL:

LDL is removed after binding by the β apoprotein to specific cell surface receptors, and patients with familial hypercholesterolemia have a genetic deficiency in the quantity or quality of these peripheral receptors. This results in decreased LDL metabolism with resultant increased plasma concentrations.

In addition to the decreased peripheral removal of LDL, cellular production of cholesterol is increased due to abnormal regulation of HMG CoA reductase. Thus, even though the membrane defect is primary, the resultant hypercholesterolemia is due to decreased removal and increased production of cholesterol.

The physical finding of xanthomas (usually in the extensor tendons at the back of the hands, and in the Achilles tendon) and the association with premature ischemic heart disease are well established. The familial form of this disease is Type II A Hyperlipoproteinemia described below.

Modest elevations of LDL may also occur from patients who ingest large amounts of animal fat. Such diet-induced hyperlipidemia responds well to dietary restriction.

Familial Hyperlipidemia

The genetic classification of lipidemias is complicated. Some of the disorders appear to be due to a single inherited factor transmitted as an autosomal dominant trait, others appear to be polygenetically transmitted, and still others seem to be primarily transmitted as a dominant trait modified by secondary factors. Even in a given kindred some subjects may have hypercholesterolemia, others hypertriglyceridemia, and the remainder a combined hyperlipidemia. Five phenotypes outlined by Frederickson have been widely used to categorize hyperlipidemia.

Type I hyperlipoproteinemia consists of elevated chylomicrons. The defect in type I hyperlipidemia is the absence of lipoprotein lipase. The triglyceride level is significantly elevated. The cholesterol may also be slightly elevated. The reason for the elevated cholesterol is that even though the chylomicrons contain 90 percent triglyceride, they also contain about 5 percent cholesterol; the marked increase in chylomicrons results in increased total cholesterol. Type I hyperlipidemia is generally a disease of infants and young children. It is inherited as an autosomal recessive trait. The children have hepatosplenomegaly secondary to lipid deposition in the reticuloendothelial system. They complain of abdominal pain and often have pancreatitis. Generally, death is in childhood or in the very early teens.

Type II hyperlipoproteinemia is divided into type II-A which has elevated LDL, cholesterol and normal triglyceride and type II-B with elevated LDL, cholesterol and elevated VLDL triglyceride. Type II disease is inherited as an autosomal dominant trait and is associated with a marked increase of premature coronary atherosclerosis. The serum cholesterol is greater than 500 mg/dl. Xanthoma develop early usually by age three, four or five. There is a strong family history of hyperlipidemia. The patient often succumbs from coronary artery disease in preadolescent or early adolescent years. Patients with heterozygote type II-A familial hypercholesterolemia comprise about one in every 500 people in a general population but about one in every 20 patients who have myocardial infarction. They have about 40 percent of normal LDL receptor sites and cholesterol values are from 300-500 mg/dl. There is a strong family history of hyperlipidemia. Xanthoma appear in adolescence. They often succumb from premature coronary artery disease in their 30's, 40's or early 50's.

The effect of the LDL receptor deficiency is loss of feedback control with elevation of the LDL cholesterol level. In patients who have heterozygous type II-A hypercholesterolemia, the elevated plasma LDL cholesterol compensates for the diminished LDL receptors. A relatively normal amount of LDL is degraded each day by the receptor mechanism. In patients with homozygous type II-A hypercholesterolemia, the LDL receptor system is functionally absent. With no feedback control the plasma LDL cholesterol is markedly elevated. While only 15 percent of the plasma cholesterol metabolized is by pinocytosis, in both Type II A and B familial hypercholesterolemia, the expanded plasma pool of LDL cholesterol leads to an increased absolute amount of cholesterol taken up by this process. With increasing levels of LDL, the scavenger cells take up larger amounts of cholesterol.

In the Western hemisphere, normal cholesterol values of 250-260 mg/dl are often found. This is 3-5 times higher than the level required for plasma LDL to deliver cholesterol to body cells. The excess cholesterol would be handled through pinocytosis. This may explain why "normal" cholesterol levels do not necessarily represent protection from atherosclerosis among Western societies.

Type III hyperlipidemia is characterized by elevations in both cholesterol and triglyceride and an increase in the VLDL and IDL. This has been termed a broad beta disease with the VLDL having both beta and prebeta mobility on electrophoresis. The VLDL cholesterol: plasma triglyceride ratios are 0.3 or greater. This compares with normal VLDL cholesterol:plasma triglyceride of approximately 0.2 or less. Patients with Type III hyperlipidemia have an increased risk of premature atherosclerosis involving the coronary arteries or peripheral vasculature. They often have elevated uric acid and glucose intolerance.

Type IV hyperlipidemia has an elevated very low density lipoprotein. In this syndrome the triglyceride is elevated and the cholesterol is either normal or slightly elevated. The elevated cholesterol reflects approximately 20 percent of the VLDL lipoprotein which contains cholesterol. With enough VLDL elevation, the cholesterol may be somewhat elevated. Patients with this type of hyperlipidemia may have obesity, diabetes, or premature atherosclerosis.

Type V hyperlipidemia is a combination of hyperchylomicronemia and elevated VLDL. In this syndrome the lipoprotein lipase activity is diminished. The triglycerides are significantly elevated. The cholesterol may also be elevated. These patients have infiltration of liver with triglyceride. They often present with pancreatitis.

TREATMENT OF ATHEROSCLEROSIS

The mainstay of therapy for atherosclerosis is symptomatic treatment (see chapters dealing with each organ system). In general these measures are directed to improve blood flow and reduce tissue metabolic demands. Antiplatelet therapy (ASA) has been recommended for people with cerebrovascular disease. It is unknown whether this will have significant benefit. Treatment of peripheral vascular disease or coronary disease through medications such as beta blockers, calcium antagonists, and nitrates may provide symptomatic relief. Vascular bypass surgery is rapidly becoming a standard treatment. It has been found that graft closure is increased among people who resume cigarette use or who have high triglycerides. Thus, in patients who have undergone bypass surgery the need for risk factor modification remains important.

The treatment and reduction of risk factors in each individual is suggested in the hope it will prevent, lessen, or delay the clinical signs and symptoms of atherosclerosis. Recently there is some support for treatment aimed at inducing regression of the atherosclerotic plaque.

At the present time more aggressive identification and earlier treatment of risk factors seems warranted; the long term objective must be prevention rather than treatment of established disease. Medication as a means to prevent or treat atherosclerosis in humans is controversial.

DIAGNOSIS AND MANAGEMENT OF HYPERLIPIDEMIA

Patients with premature coronary artery disease, a strong family history, xanthomas, recurrent pancreatitis, or other features suggesting hyperlipidemia, should have cholesterol and triglyceride blood levels measured. All lipid measurements should be obtained after an adequate fast (8 to 12 hours) and should not be performed within two weeks of an acute illness or three months of a major stress such as surgery or myocardial infarction. The patient should not be taking lipid lowering medication. The first step in diagnosis is inspection of the plasma after overnight refrigeration at 4°C; chylomicrons produce a creamy layer at the top of the serum, while turbidity within the serum indicates an increase of VLDL particles due to their ability to refract light. In addition to measurement of the cholesterol and triglyceride, it is useful to determine the HDL cholesterol level, since elevated HDL would suggest reduced risk for atherosclerosis while elevated LDL cholesterol would suggest increased risk. Assessment of total cholesterol, total triglycerides and HDL, after inspection of the serum after overnight refrigeration, usually permits establishment of a specific lipoprotein abnormality. Occasionally, particularly to diagnose Type III hyperlipidemia, more sophisticated methods such as ultracentrifugation must be used. Detailed family studies may be essential to establish the type of hyperlipidemia, and the patient risk.

If patients are asymptomatic and are not overly at risk on the basis of the lipid type, family history, or concomitant risk factors, then the only rationale for therapy is to attempt to decrease the enhanced cardiovascular risk factors. Therefore, the overall age and health of the individual as well as the state of the vascular disease in that individual must be taken into consideration. Generally, the younger and healthier the patient, especially with a family history of related disease, the greater the rationale for lipid lowering therapy.

Treatment of any primary hyperlipidemia begins with the diet. The principle of dietary treatment of hypercholesterolemia is to decrease the cholesterol intake by decreasing the percentage of calories ingested as saturated fat with concomitant increase in the percentage of calories from polyunsaturated fat. There should be a general change from consumption of animal protein to vegetable protein, and the fiber content of the diet may be increased. The intake of polyunsaturated fat, saturated fat, and dietary cholesterol must all be considered. The addition of 2 gm of unsaturated fat appears to have the same benefit on lowering cholesterol as removal of 1 gm of saturated fat. Some physicians place more emphasis on decreasing the level of cholesterol intake in order to reduce plasma cholesterol. Thus there is controversy regarding the optimal diet. The polyunsaturated to saturated fat ratio should be about 1.0. For patients with a high risk of atherosclerosis, a *prudent heart diet* can be recommended. This consists of 30 percent of calories in dietary fat, a polyunsaturated to saturated fat ratio of 1.0, and a cholesterol content of less than 300 mg/day.

The treatment of hypertriglyceridemia is usually caloric restriction to attain close to ideal body weight, some dietary restriction of carbohydrate and severe limitation on the use of alcohol. Patients with isolated hyperchylomicronemia respond to a fat restricted diet supplemented with medium chain triglycerides which are not transported as chylomicra.

When diet therapy alone fails to correct the lipid levels then lipid lowering drugs may be considered. These drugs usually should be reserved for patients with a greatly enhanced risk of developing early atherogenesis or other complications of hyperlipidemia.

Hypercholesterolemia is initially treated with bile acid sequestrants such as cholestyramine which result in net fecal excretion of bile acid which therefore promote increased hepatic conversion of cholesterol into new bile acids. This results in an absolute decrease in the circulating cholesterol levels, a decrease, however, limited by the compensatory increase in the cholesterol synthesis by the liver. These drugs also interfere with the absorption of fat soluble vitamins and other drugs, so multivitamins and drugs should be administered at times other than when the bile acid binding resin is administered. Nicotinic acid also reduces plasma cholesterol levels and is useful in combination with the bile acid binding resins. Recent preliminary results using antagonists to HMG Co-A reductase have been encouraging.

Moderate hypertriglyceridemia usually responds to clofibrate, but there has been recent concern about its safety. The mechanism of action is unclear. The drug clofibrate may be particularly helpful in Type III hyperlipidemia; anabolic or progestational agents may be useful in females with Type V hyperlipidemia.

It should be borne in mind that each of the medications has distinctive side effects and contraindications. The physician must weigh the risk versus the benefits before undertaking drug therapy of hyperlipidemia.

Even though a reduction in risk seems to have been demonstrated when the cholesterol is less than 180 mg/dl, a routine program to reduce serum cholesterol to 180 mg/dl cannot be generally recommended. Vigorous cholesterol lowering may be appropriate for selected patients with increased risk.

An isolated finding of a low HDL cholesterol appears to be associated with an increased risk for premature coronary atherosclerosis. Attempted treatments to raise the HDL cholesterol level have been of unproven benefit. HDL cholesterol has been found to increase with exercise and an exercise program in keeping with the patient's physical abilities would certainly be reasonable. While alcohol consumption in moderate amounts has also been found to elevate HDL cholesterol, the use of alcohol cannot be recommended because of its deleterious effects on other organ systems.

SMOKING CESSATION

Perhaps the clearest benefit from risk factor identification comes to subjects who stop smoking. While the risk of atherosclerotic vascular disease may only drop to non-smokers' levels in 10 years, ischemic symptoms, which result from carboxyhemoglobin, improve within hours. Furthermore, the risk of sudden death during a myocardial infarction is much higher in the smoker, and this risk is reduced to non-smokers levels within 48 hours.

TREATMENT OF HYPERTENSION

See Chapter 3

WEIGHT REDUCTION, EXERCISE

Principles for control of obesity are described in Chapter 1. Exercise is an integral part of a good weight control program. Furthermore, systematic exercise may help control systemic blood pressure, reduce sudden death during myocardial infarction, and perhaps, reduce atherogenesis. Vigorous and regular exercise appear essential, but no precise guidelines are firmly established. At present, careful assessment should precede an exercise program. Uncontrolled hypertension, ischemic heart disease, symptomatic pulmonary disease and arrhythmias must be identified and treated. Exercise prescriptions should emphasize dynamic exercise (walking, jogging, cycling, swimming), gradually increasing in workload over several weeks, till peak desired activity is reached. These must be carried out 3 to 5 times per week to ensure that conditioning is maintained.

REFERENCES

1. Armstrong, M.L.: Regression of atherosclerosis. Atherosclerosis Reviews, Vol. 1, New York, Raven Press, 1976.
2. Arteriosclerosis, Vol. 1, No. 5, September/October 1981.
3. Goldstein, J.L., Brown, M.S., Atherosclerosis: The low density lipoprotein receptor hypothesis. Metabolism, 26:1257–1275, 1977.
4. Gotto, A.M., Smith, L.C., Allen, B. (eds.): Atherosclerosis V: Proceedings of the Fifth International Symposium. New York, Springer-Verlag, 1980.
5. Havel, R.J., Kane, J.P.: Therapy of hyperlipidemic states. Ann Rev Med, 33:417, 1982.
6. Stanberry, J.B., Wyngaarden, J.B., Fredrickson, D.S., The metabolic basis of inherited disease. New York, McGraw-Hill, 1972.
7. Stein, E.A., Glueck, C.J., Morrison, J.A.: Coronary risk factors in the young. Ann Rev Med, 32:601, 1981.

3

Hypertension

John K. Ruedy, M.D.

THE PHYSIOLOGICAL DETERMINANTS OF BLOOD PRESSURE
    Control of Blood Pressure
MEASUREMENT OF BLOOD PRESSURE
DEFINITION OF ARTERIAL HYPERTENSION
CLASSIFICATION OF HYPERTENSION
ESSENTIAL HYPERTENSION
    Incidence of Hypertension
    Pathogenesis
    Consequences of Hypertension
    Manifestations of Essential Hypertension
    Assessment of the Patient with Hypertension
    Treatment of Essential Hypertension
HYPERTENSION SECONDARY TO ENDOCRINE DISEASE
    Adrenal Cortex
    Estrogen and Postgesterone-Induced Hypertension
    Adrenal Medulla
    Other Endocrine Causes
COARCTATION OF THE AORTA
RENAL CAUSES
REFERENCES

THE PHYSIOLOGICAL DETERMINANTS OF BLOOD PRESSURE

Arterial blood pressure, the pressure exerted on the walls of the arteries by the contained blood, is largely determined by two physiological variables: stroke volume of the heart and the resistance to the forward flow of blood in the arterial tree.

Maximum pressure, the *systolic pressure*, occurs at the beginning of the ejection phase of ventricular systole when blood is rapidly thrust into the aorta. The resultant sudden distension of the aorta produces a pressure wave that is partly accommodated by moving blood forward at a greater velocity but also by creating a pulse wave that progresses distally down the arterial tree much more rapidly than the blood itself. As the pulse wave moves peripherally, its velocity progressively increases until in the small arteries its velocity is 100 times greater than the velocity of the blood. Backward deflection of this first portion of the pressure wave from the periphery results in a systolic pressure in the brachial artery that is usually 20 to 40 mmHg higher than the pressure in the aorta. In addition, as the pulse wave moves peripherally, the high-pressure portion of the wave is more rapidly transmitted than are the low-pressure portions. The delayed, higher and more peaked pulse wave of the dorsalis pedis artery is compared graphically with that of the femoral artery in Figure 3.1. Systolic pressure results from the superimposition of the pressure due to the rapid ejection of blood from the left ventricle into the aorta on the minimum arterial pressure, that is, the diastolic pressure. The major determinants of systolic pressure are summarized in Table 3.1.

Minimum arterial pressure, or *diastolic pressure*, is determined by the elasticity of the aorta and the larger arteries (which forces blood against the closed aortic valve and, distally, down the arterial tree) and the resistance met by forward blood flow. Approximately 70 percent of the resistance to the forward flow of blood is due to the arterioles (*resistance vessels*), with the remainder accounted for by the large arteries, venules, and veins. Arteriolar resistance, and therefore diastolic pressure, can be increased actively by arteriolar vasoconstriction or passively by structural changes in the arteriolar wall, such as edema. Arteriolar vasoconstriction can be induced through a variety of means, including stimulation of alpha-adrenergic receptors, release of vasoactive substances such as angiotensin II, vasopressin, and prostaglandins, and physiocochemical influences such as alkalosis, decreased osmolality, and high concentrations of potassium. Factors that can increase diastolic pressure are outlined in Table 3.2.

Mean blood pressure is not simply the arithmetic average of the systolic and diastolic pressure. Rather, it is a function of the height and contour of the arterial pulse wave. In most instances, the contour of the arterial pulse is such that the mean pressure is ap-

Table 3.1 Factors Increasing Systolic Pressure

1. Increased stroke volume or rate of left ventricular emptying
   Exercise
   Stimulation of beta-adrenergic cardiac receptors
   Thyrotoxicosis
2. Decreased aortic elasticity, distensibility, or capacity
   Coarctation
   Aortic arteriosclerosis
   Atheroma, thrombi, or emboli within the aorta or major arteries.
3. Increased diastolic pressure

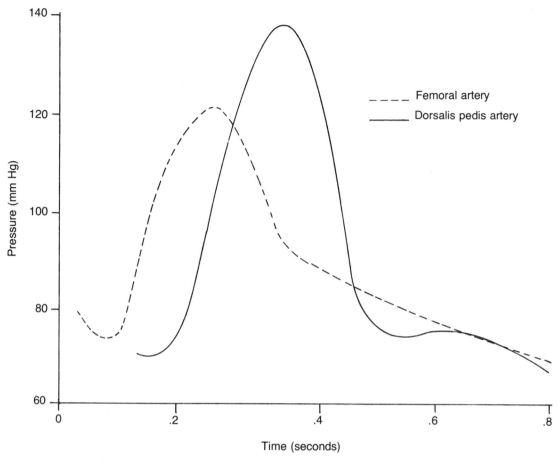

Fig. 3.1 Pressure curves in normal femoral and dorsalis pedis arteries.

proximately equal to diastolic pressure plus one third of the pulse pressure.

CONTROL OF BLOOD PRESSURE

During changes in posture, blood pressure is maintained through the autonomic nervous system. Baroreceptors in the carotid sinus, heart, and large ves-

Table 3.2 **Factors Increasing Diastolic Pressure**

1. Increased arteriolar resistance
   Active constriction
      a. cathecholamines, angiotensin II, certain prosta-
         glandins, and other vasoactive substances
      b. physicochemical changes—alkalosis, hyper-
         kalemia
   Passive
      a. edema
      b. intravascular obstruction due to thrombi or
         emboli
      c. increased blood viscosity
2. Increased systolic pressure
3. Increased heart rate

sels influence the activity of the vasomotor and cardiomodulator centers of the medulla. A drop in intravascular pressure results in decreased nerve traffic from the baroreceptors and medullary center activity. The resultant inhibition of parasympathetic fibers to the heart causes an increase in the rate and the force of contraction, and the concomitant stimulation of sympathetic fibers causes vasocontriction of resistance vessels, producing an increase in blood pressure. Baroreceptor function is often tested clinically by measuring lying and standing blood pressures and pulse rates. Unfortunately, unless these observations are made under controlled conditions, such as using a tilt table, changes are widely variable in normal individuals, particularly during the first minute after standing. Subsequent changes are more predictable. The following are useful normal ranges for adjustments to the upright posture at one minute: an increase in heart rate from 0 to 20 beats per minute, an increase in diastolic pressure from 0 to 15 mmHg, and an increase or decrease in systolic pressure of 15 mmHg (-15 to $+15$ mmHg).

Increases in blood pressure and pulse rate that accompany such intellectual exercises as mental arithmetic are also mediated by the autonomic nervous system through the medullary centers. These centers are heavily innervated by adrenergic and serotonergic fibers: the adrenergic receptors appear to respond to norepinephrine by reducing activity. Clinical testing of the blood pressure response to mental arithmetic is a useful maneuver, since the response is not dependent on afferent fibers. The antihypertensive drugs methyldopa and clonidine may owe much of their antihypertensive effects to an interaction with the central adrenergic receptors in the medulla.

Several mechanisms are responsible for more long-term control of blood pressure. These include the baroreceptor system, the renin-angiotensin-aldosterone system, and the renal blood-volume mechanism.

The renin-angiotensin-aldosterone system is summarized in Figure 3.2. Renin is released into the circulation from storage granules in the juxtaglomerular cells of the kidney in response to reduced renal artery perfusing pressure or to extracellular fluid volume depletion. This enzyme hydrolyzes renin substrate (a plasma α_2 globulin) to yield the decapeptide angiotensin I. Angiotensin I is further hydrolyzed by converting enzyme from the lung, plasma, kidney, and vascular endothelium to the octapeptide angiotensin II. The converting enzyme also destroys bradykinin, which induces vasodilatation, and therefore may influence blood pressure by more than one means. Angiotensin II, the most powerful vasoconstrictor substance known, elevates pressure as a result of interaction with specific receptors in arteriolar smooth muscle as well as through a central action. In addition, angiotensin II is the most important stimulus to the production of aldosterone by the adrenal cortex. While renin is cleared by the liver with a plasma half-life of 10 to 15 minutes, angiotensin II is destroyed enzymatically with a half-life of only 1 or 2 minutes; one breakdown product, the hectapeptide des-Asp-angiotensin II (Angiotensin III) is much less active as a pressor substance than angiotensin II but is equipotent for stimulation of aldosterone production. The physiologic role for angiotensin III is not established.

A variety of stimuli can increase renin secretion from the juxtaglomerular apparatus, including a decrease in perfusion pressure, a decrease in extracellular fluid volume, beta-adrenergic stimulation, and decreases in plasma sodium and potassium. Clinical assessment of the activity of the renin-angiotensin-aldosterone system must be made with knowledge or control of all of these variables. Assessment is further complicated by the fact that direct measurement of renin is not yet practical. Current methods depend on measuring the amount of angiotensin I that is generated in an in vitro system; plasma renin activity (PRA) depends on the amount of renin present and the supply of renin substrate. In liver disease, reduced amounts of substrate may yield low PRA levels in spite of normal amounts of renin, while in pregnancy and following oral contraceptive drug use, increased renin substrate may yield high PRA levels in spite of normal amounts of renin. This problem is obviated by adding exogenous renin substrate in excess, and results are then expressed as plasma renin concentration.

Although blood pressure can be maintained in the absence of renin and angiotensin, it is believed that the renin-angiotensin-aldosterone system normally participates in blood pressure control, particularly in situations of changing sodium and fluid balance. It appears that in most situations renin is more closely related to sodium balance than to blood pressure control. Salt and water deprivation leads to an increase in renin release, but also to a blunting of the sensitivity of the arterioles to the pressor effects of angiotensin. The increase in renin release due to sodium deprivation does not produce hypertension. In face of an excess of sodium, renin secretion diminishes but the sensitivity of the arterioles to angiotensin increases. There is ample evidence that changes in the renin-angiotensin-aldosterone system occur in hypertension. However, it is probable that in essential hypertension the changes are secondary rather than primary in etiologic importance.

An important blood pressure control mechanism

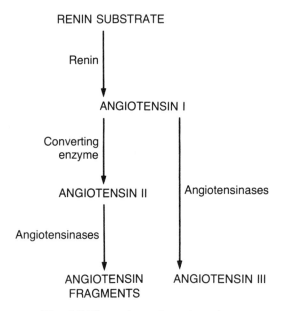

Fig. 3.2 The renin-angiotensin system.

depends on the ability of the kidney to respond to an increase in arterial pressure by increasing the output of sodium and water, that is, pressure diuresis or natriuresis. The diuresis results in decreased extracellular fluid volume, decreased venous return, and decreased cardiac output, returning blood pressure to normal. This mechanism has the ability to return the blood pressure to its previous level and to override other control mechanisms. A seven-fold increase in urine volume results from a rise in renal arterial pressure from 100 to 200 mmHg. If blood pressure is lowered, urinary output of salt and water decrease. This powerful control mechanism prevents long-term changes in the level of blood pressure, but in hypertension there is a change in the relationship between pressure and natriuresis. The resetting of this control mechanism can be caused by a variety of factors such as renal parenchymal or renal vascular disease, hyperaldosteronism, antidiuretic hormone release, renal arteriolar vasoconstriction due to sympathetic nervous system stimulation or norepinephrine release, or stimulation of salt appetite with a subsequent increased intake of sodium.

MEASUREMENT OF BLOOD PRESSURE

Indirect measurement of blood pressure using a sphygmomanometer provides a sufficiently accurate estimate of arterial pressure for clinical purposes. In comparison with direct intraarterial measurement, pressures are usually slightly underestimated; however, correlation between readings using the two methods is very high. Pressure recorded at the time that the Korotkoff sounds are muffled provides the closest estimate of diastolic pressure, but there is considerable interobserver variability using this cutoff, and diastolic pressure is generally more reliably estimated at the time when sounds disappear. Overestimates can occur in obese patients if the occluding cuff is too small, since the brachial artery is not as easily compressed because of the increased amount of intervening tissue. Overestimates also occur in the elderly when peripheral vessels are very sclerotic and difficult to compress.

Blood pressure is very variable during the day. Most individuals, be they normotensive or hypertensive, show a progressive rise in blood pressure during the day with a peak in the early evening and a marked fall during the early hours of sleep. Fluctuations tend to be greater in hypertensive subjects as well as in the elderly. Such factors as excitement or nervousness, exercise, and a full urinary bladder frequently cause increases in blood pressure. The use

of basal blood pressure recordings taken in the lying and standing position after 15 to 30 minutes of recumbency have been recommended in order to provide more accurate and reliable estimates of the average blood pressure of an individual. The Framingham study cast serious doubt on the advantages of basal blood pressures since the risk of cardiovascular complications of hypertension was related to the height of casual readings whether or not basal recordings were also elevated. This study also showed a surprising reproducibility of casual readings in individual subjects. For practical purposes blood pressure recordings should be made when the physician and the patient are calm and extraneous stimuli have been eliminated. It is common to observe a fall in blood pressure over the first few office or clinic visits of a patient who initially had elevated recordings. Mean changes between the initial and second visit casual readings average 25 mmHg systolic and 10 mm diastolic. This must be taken into account in evaluating the contribution of therapy to blood pressure control.

DEFINITION OF ARTERIAL HYPERTENSION

The definition of arterial hypertension is difficult because of several observations: (1) the distribution of pressure values in an unselected group of individuals is continuous, without cutoff levels that can be used to define normotensive and hypertensive groups. (2) The relationship between cardiovascular consequences of hypertension and the height of blood pressure is also continuous and no critical value of systolic or diastolic pressure can be identified as a threshold below which no harm is associated with the level of pressure. In fact, a gradient of increase risk of cardiovascular complications has been shown in subjects with pressures within the usually accepted normal range. (3) The definition of hypertension is complicated because men and blacks suffer cardiovascular complications of hypertension more readily than do women and whites. (4) The excess mortality relating to hypertension in the elderly is lower than in the young, presumably because the risk of death from other causes increases with age.

One approach, useful at least for epidemiologic purposes, is found in the World Health Organization definition of hypertension. Arterial hypertension is defined as a casual blood pressure greater than 160/95 (mmHg), normotension is defined by pressure below 140/90, and pressure between these readings is considered borderline. These arbitrary levels must be used clinically with careful assessment of the risk of pressure elevation in the individual. For example, in a black male under age 45, a repeated reading of 140/90 is of more prognostic concern than a similar pressure in a woman or an older individual.

CLASSIFICATION OF HYPERTENSION

All physiological factors responsible for the maintenance of normal blood pressure have been implicated in the etiology of hypertension, including the arterial baroreceptors, the integrating and controlling centers of the central nervous system, the sympathoadrenal system, and the renin-angiotensin-aldosterone system. In some hypertensive disorders a single abnormality of one of these mechanisms has been demonstrated; however, in essential hypertension the initiating and sustaining pathophysiologic factors are unknown and undoubtedly involve changes in a variety of homeostatic controls of blood pressure. For clinical purposes an etiologic classification of hypertensive disorders is the most practical (Table 3.3).

ESSENTIAL HYPERTENSION

In most subjects with elevated blood pressure, no cause can be found, and by exclusion a diagnosis of essential hypertension is made. This is a misnomer, but attempts to replace the term *essential* by "pri-

Table 3.3   Classification of Hypertension

Etiologic Classification	Most Frequent Causes
1. Essential hypertension	
2. Endocrine causes	
Adrenal cortex	Primary aldosteronism
	Cushing's syndrome
Pheochromocytoma	
Hyperparathyroidism	
3. Renal causes	
Renal artery stenosis	Atheroma
	Fibromuscular hyperplasia
Parenchymal renal	Acute glomerulonephritis
disease	Diabetic nephropathy
Trauma	Perinephric hematoma
4. Neurogenic causes	Brain-stem encephalitis or
(usually transient)	ischemia
	Increased intracranial
	pressure
5. Mechanical causes	Atherosclerosis of aorta
	Coarctation of aorta
6. Iatrogenic	Oral contraceptive
	treatment
	Sodium retaining drugs,
	particularly in patients
	with renal disease
7. Toxemia of pregnancy	

Table 3.4   Frequency of Hypertension in North America by Age and Sex

	Percentage with systolic pressure ≥160 mmHg	Percentage with diastolic pressure ≥100 mmHg
Men (age in years)		
40–49	10	4
50–59	20	7
≥60	40	12
Women (age in years)		
40–49	5	2
50–59	35	10
≥60	50	18

mary" or "cryptogenic" have not been widely accepted. Whether essential hypertension represents a single disorder or a group of independent diseases remains unresolved.

INCIDENCE OF HYPERTENSION

Whatever upper limit of blood pressure is selected above which a diagnosis of hypertension is made, there is no doubt that hypertension is common. In industrialized countries four factors have been shown to be associated with hypertension: age, race, elevated blood pressure in blood relatives, and obesity. In North America 10 percent of men and 5 percent of women under age 40 years have systolic pressures ≥ 160 mmHg. Elevated pressures become more common in women than men at age 45 or 50 years. A progressive increase in the incidence of elevated pressure with age is observed in populations with a high salt intake. A similar increase is not observed in communities with a low salt intake. In blacks the frequency of hypertension is almost twice that in whites. Hypertension is three to four times more common in brothers and sisters of subjects with hypertension than in individuals with normotensive siblings. The frequency of hypertension in North America by age and sex is shown in Table 3.4.

PATHOGENESIS

The pathogenesis of essential hypertension is not known and its discovery is frustrated by the uncertainty about whether any of the present animal models have any relevance to essential hypertension, since none mimic precisely the pathophysiology of the disease in man. It has been proposed that subsets of patients with essential hypertension, who differ in regard to plasma volume, cardiac output, or level of function of the renin-angiotensin-aldosterone system, suffer from hypertensive disorders of differing etiology. However, it is equally plausible that these pathophysiologic changes represent various stages in the development of a single disorder.

Two further precautions in interpreting the various hypotheses regarding the pathogenesis of hypertension deserve emphasis. Each successful therapeutic intervention such as the low salt rice diet, ganglionic blocking drugs, saluretic agents, adrenergic blocking drugs, inhibitors of the renin-angiotensin-aldosterone system, and inhibitors of calcium transport has given birth to new theories regarding the etiology of hypertension. The fact that blood pressure can be lowered by a pharmacologic agent is most often of no greater significance in delineating the etiology of hypertension than is the observation that fever can be lowered by antipyretic drugs in identifying the cause of a variety of febrile diseases. Further, atherosclerosis plays a very important role in the morbidity and mortality of hypertension. Studies linking such outcomes of hypertension as stroke or coronary artery disease with etiologic variables such as diet, life-style, or smoking, will be confusing unless the effects of all the factors contributing to an increased susceptibility to atherosclerosis are identified.

Sodium Intake

An association between the prevalence of hypertension and the average daily sodium intake has been shown. In Alaskan Eskimos who have an average salt intake of 4 grams the prevalence of hypertension is 4 percent, in Americans with an average intake of 10 grams the prevalence is 10 percent, while in northern Japanese, with intakes over 20 grams, the prevalence reaches 25 percent. Within populations, however, it has been difficult to demonstrate an association between salt intake and hypertension. Possible reasons for the lack of correlation within populations include narrow range of intakes within each group, the possibility that intake early in life is more important than intake during adulthood, the imprecision in identifying salt intake, particularly in industrialized societies where most processed foods are heavily salted, and the oversimplified approach in many studies of expecting a linear association in a disorder in which the pathogenesis is probably multifactorial.

Salt restriction to a level necessitating an unpalatable diet (less than 10 mmol/day of sodium) can result in a lower blood pressure in hypertensive patients. This effect, however, is not universal, and is achieved in less than 50 percent of patients with hypertension. Dahl has identified two strains of rats,

one which responds quickly to an increase in dietary salt with a severe rise in blood pressure, and the other apparently immune to this hypertensive effect of dietary salt. The salt sensitive strain has been shown to differ from the salt resistant strain in the production of about twice the amount of the adrenal corticosteroid, 18-hydroxy-11-deoxycorticosteroid (18-hydroxy-DOC), a weak mineralocorticoid under the control of ACTH. Whether similar differences in adrenal corticoid metabolism are the basis for differences in blood pressure responses to salt in man remains to be shown.

The evidence supporting the importance of salt in the etiology of hypertension is stronger than that for the variety of other putative environmental factors, including occupation, obesity, crowding, and other stressful situations. Nevertheless, high salt intake alone cannot be accepted as the sole initiating factor in essential hypertension.

Heredity

The most convincing evidence supporting the importance of genetic factors in hypertension is found in studies of twins. Monozygotic twins have a much greater risk of hypertension if the sibling is hypertensive compared with dizygotic twins. In comparing the influence of environment and heredity in twins who had been separated from birth, the genetic factor has been found to be a substantially more important determinant of hypertension than the environment. Hypertension is three to four times more common in siblings of hypertensive subjects than in siblings of normotensive individuals. However, the magnitude of the familial factor should be placed in perspective. The statistical association shows, for example, that for an increase in systolic pressure of 100 mmHg above normal in the hypertensive subjects an increase of only 25 mmHg in systolic pressure can be anticipated in blood relatives. Studies in man, in contrast with other animal experience, suggest that the genetic susceptibility to hypertension is graded and probably polygenic.

Autoregulation Theory

It has been proposed that sodium retention occurs at an early stage of hypertension, expanding plasma volume and increasing cardiac output. In order to protect tissues from over perfusion, autoregulatory vasoconstriction occurs with a subsequent increase in peripheral resistance and a fall in cardiac output. Support for this hypothesis derives largely from unsubstantiated animal and computer models, and the factor leading to the initial sodium retention remains unexplained by this hypothesis.

Cardiac Output

Some young patients with elevated pressure have an elevated cardiac output, and a proportion of such subjects show increases in plasma catecholamines and renin activity. The initially increased cardiac output may be followed by a progressive rise in peripheral resistance (through autoregulation or vascular hypertrophy) and a fall in cardiac output. However, in the majority of patients with essential hypertension, a preliminary phase during which cardiac output is increased has not been recognized, and many young patients with borderline hypertension and raised cardiac outputs do not go on to develop sustained hypertension.

Neurogenic Causes

The pressor effects of norepinephrine have attracted interest to the sympathetic nervous system as the source of the dysfunction in essential hypertension.

Some young patients with a hyperkinetic circulatory state have symptoms suggestive of sympathetic hyperactivity including palpitations, sweating, tachycardia, systolic hypertension, and increased plasma renin activity. Some have been shown to have increased responsiveness to the beta-adrenergic stimulant isoproterenol. However, in most patients with sustained essential hypertension, it has been difficult to demonstrate an abnormality in the functioning of the sympathetic nervous system.

Baroreceptor function has been shown to be altered in some patients with essential hypertension, with a "resetting" so that higher pressures are required to trigger a decrease in stimulating influences from medullary centers. However, the evidence in support of a causal relationship between the decreased sensitivity of baroreceptors and the elevated pressure in hypertension is scant, and it appears that with aging there is a loss of baroreceptor sensitivity that is independent of hypertension.

Changes in central control of blood pressure are important in the hypertension associated with such conditions as encephalitis and ischemia of the medullary centers, and hypertension in animals can be induced by destruction of specific tracts. However only very indirect methods are available for assessing the function of medullary modulating centers in man, so that there is no present evidence that essential hypertension results from an altered function of medullary controlling centers.

Humoral Causes

A variety of humoral causes in addition to the catecholamines have been studied as possible etiologic factors in essential hypertension. A variety of vascular and central nervous system sites contain prostaglandins, histamines and serotonin, kallikreins and bradykinin, and tissue enzymes capable of forming angiotensin I in the presence of renin substrate (so-called tissue iso-renins). The role of these local humoral substances in controlling peripheral vascular resistance as well as in hypertension remains unknown.

Renin-Angiotensin-Aldosterone System

Angiotensin II, in doses just sufficient to increase the plasma concentrations out of the normal range, immediately increases arterial pressure. Further, in animals, doses insufficient to acutely increase arterial pressure result in elevated pressure after several days. This delayed effect is possibly due to the sodium retention that occurs as a result of the direct effects of angiotensin II, and to the increased release of aldosterone. In some patients with hypertension of renal origin, renin is elevated and blood pressure can be lowered with drugs that inhibit renin release or that interfere with the renin-angiotensin-aldosterone system in other ways. Although one of the most potent stimuli for renin release is the reduction of extracellular fluid volume through salt restriction, changes in renin secretion over the normal range of salt intake in industrialized countries (100 to 250 mmol Na per day) are small, and salt may play little role in maintaining normal blood pressure. Values for renin activity can only be interpreted in relation to sodium balance, which may be estimated from knowledge of the 24 hour urine output of sodium. It must be emphasized that urinary losses of sodium are not an accurate reflection of sodium balance if the kidney is not handling sodium normally, as in a variety of forms of renal disease. Renin and aldosterone measurements related to sodium balance in patients with essential hypertension have revealed very heterogeneous results (Table 3.5). Most subjects have normal plasma renin activity and aldosterone secretion rates.

The identification of groups of patients with essential hypertension and low plasma renin activity and normal or low aldosterone secretion rates has led

Table 3.5 Most Common Findings of Renin-Aldosterone System in Essential Hypertension

	Percentage of subjects
Normal renin	
Normal aldosterone	45
Low renin	
Normal aldosterone	20
Low aldosterone	8
High renin	
Normal aldosterone	10
High aldosterone	7
Other combinations	10

to the hypothesis that these patients have expanded extracellular fluid volume and normally suppressed renin activity. Attempts to confirm extracellular fluid volume expansion in such patients have not been universally successful, and search for a factor, possibly an abnormal mineralocorticoid, responsible for such volume expansion has been unrewarding. Interpretation of the meaning of low renin and aldosterone results is further complicated by the fact that there is a progressive decline in both of these values with age. Aldosterone secretion rates on a normal sodium diet decrease 50 percent from age 20 to age 50 years, and plasma renin activity after one hour of ambulation (on a normal sodium intake) decreases to 85 percent from age 20 to age 50 years. It is likely that most patients with low renin represent a different stage of hypertension. The patients tend to be older, have more stable blood pressure, and tend to respond more dramatically to diuretics than do subjects with normal renin.

Present evidence suggests that alterations in the functioning of renin-angiotensin-aldosterone are the exception rather than the rule in essential hypertension, and that changes are secondary to changes in intravascular volume or other disturbances such as altered sympathetic nervous system activity, rather than primary etiologic factors of the disease. In contrast, the renin-angiotensin-aldosterone system has a causative role in malignant hypertension, renovascular hypertension, and hypertension associated with rare renin-secreting tumors.

CONSEQUENCES OF HYPERTENSION

Indirect Vascular Consequences

In North America more than half of all deaths are attributable to cardiovascular disease, with coronary artery disease, atherothrombotic stroke, and congestive heart failure constituting the most common disorders (Table 3.6). Elevated blood pressure is the most common and most important presently recognized precursor of these lethal conditions. In addition to these atherosclerotic sequelae of elevated arterial pressure, hypertension is complicated by more direct vascular damage, including the necrotizing vasculitis of malignant hypertension, hypertensive encephalopathy, intracerebral hemorrhage, hypertensive retinopathy, nephrosclerosis, and dissecting aortic aneurysm.

Most of the information on the consequences of hypertension arises from the Framingham study. This study, initiated in 1949, includes careful clinical cardiovascular observations on more than 5,000 men and women aged 30 to 62 years at the time of entry. In order to ascertain the rate of development of cardiovascular complications, subjects have been followed at intervals of two years. This study, along with actuarial studies performed by a number of insurance companies, has established that the risk of death and of cardiovascular disease is closely related to blood pressure: the risk increases with increases in diastolic or systolic pressure and, further, the risk diminishes progressively with lower blood pressures (Table 3.7). There is no apparent cutoff level below which the risk does not continue to decrease; this is so whether the raised systolic pressure occurs in a young subject when the underlying fault may be an increased cardiac output due to increased sympathetic activity, or in the elderly when the systolic pressure is influenced by the loss of distensibility of the aorta.

The influence of hypertension on life expectancy is striking. A 45-year-old man has the following life expectancies, depending on casual blood pressure readings: with a blood pressure less than 140/95, 32 years; with a pressure of 140/95 to 140/100, 26 years; and with a pressure over 140/100, 20 years.

The morbidity and mortality of hypertension is dominated by the increased susceptibility of hypertensive patients to atherosclerosis. However, the mechanisms of atherogenesis are not established (see Chapter 2).

Table 3.6 Causes of Death in Hypertension

	Approximate percentage of deaths in patients with hypertension	
	Without Treatment	With Treatment
Stroke	40	20
Congestive heart failure	20	8
Myocardial infarction	20	42
Uremia	10	3
Unrelated to hypertension	10	27
	100	100

Table 3.7   **Increased Incidence of Vascular Disease Associated with Hypertension**

| | Incidence rate compared with normotensive group | | | |
	Coronary Artery Disease	Stroke	Intermittent Claudication	Congestive Heart Failure
Hypertensive status				
Men				
Borderline	1.6	2.9	1.4	2.6
Hypertensive	2.5	8.2	2.1	6.7
Women				
Borderline	1.8	2.8	1.9	2.2
Hypertensive	3.4	7.6	3.6	4.6

Direct Vascular Consequences

Hypertension directly affects the cardiovascular system in several different ways (Table 3.8). Necrosis of the arteriolar wall, or fibrinoid necrosis, is the hallmark of malignant hypertension. (See following discussion of Malignant Hypertension.)

Hypertensive encephalopathy is thought to be due to a direct effect of hypertension, occurring when the blood pressure exceeds that to which the cerebral arterioles can respond by constricting to prevent excessive cerebral perfusion. Failure of autoregulation results in focal arteriolar dilatation, edema, and ischemia, and, if untreated, frank ischemic infarction. If treated aggressively before permanent damage occurs hypertensive encephalopathy is completely reversible. (See following section on Hypertensive Encephalopathy).

Small cystic infarctions are another vascular effect of hypertension peculiar to small arteries of the brain, most particularly those in the basal ganglia, the thalamus, the cerebellum, and the internal capsule. These lacunar infarctions are almost exclusively found in patients with hypertension. It is unclear whether they represent direct vascular damage or whether they are due to disseminated thrombotic occlusions of small arterioles. Clinical distinction between lacunar infarcts, small intraparenchymal hemorrhages, and atherosclerotic ischemic infarcts can be extremely difficult. Prior to the availability of antihypertensive drugs, stroke accounted for about 40 percent of the

Table 3.8   **Direct Vascular Consequences of Hypertension**

Malignant hyptertension (fibrinoid necrosis of arterioles)
Hypertensive encephalopathy (arteriolar spasm)
Lacunar infarctions of basal ganglia, cerebellum, subcortical areas
Intraparenchymal intracranial hemorrhages
Left ventricular hypertrophy and congestive heart failure
Nephrosclerosis
Dissecting aortic aneurysm

mortality associated with hypertension. There has been a progressive decline in the prevalence of stroke, and currently this complication accounts for less than 20 percent of the mortality associated with hypertension.

With left ventricular hypertrophy and congestive heart failure it may be clinically impossible to separate the influence of hypertension from that of superimposed coronary artery disease. Congestive cardiac failure in a hypertensive patient is an ominous complication with a 5-year survival rate of 40 percent in men and 60 percent in women. There is little difference between the prognosis of subjects with and subjects without overt ischemic heart disease, and there is no evidence that diastolic pressure is a more important determinant of this complication than systolic pressure. There has been a progressive decline in the prevalence of congestive heart failure as a cause of mortality in hypertensive patients. Prior to presently available drug therapy, 20 percent of hypertensive patients succumbed to congestive heart failure. Now less than 10 percent of the deaths among hypertensives are associated with this complication.

Progressively decreasing renal function culminating in azotemia is most often seen in patients with rapidly progressing hypertension, who often show other evidence of severe vascular damage such as hypertensive retinopathy and the pathologic changes of fibrinoid necrosis of renal arterioles. This process can be halted by control of blood pressure, and some improvement in renal function can be anticipated. The frequency of this complication as a terminal event in hypertension has decreased with the advent of drug treatment of hypertension. Another pathologic change, so-called benign nephrosclerosis, consisting of hyaline degeneration, particularly of the afferent arterioles of the kidney but found in other organs, is a nonspecific change that accompanies increasing age. Hypertension and diabetes appear to enhance the development of this lesion. Its clinical significance is unclear. The major effect is probably a result of the decrease in distensibility of affected vessels. Arteriolar responses to changes in posture, mediated by the baroreceptor reflexes, may be blunted, contributing to postural hypotension. It is conceivable that a decrease in the stretchability of the arterioles of the juxtaglomerular apparatus, due to this hyaline degeneration, could explain the progressive decrease in renin activity observed with age.

Dissecting aortic aneurysms are rare in the absence of hypertension. However, their occurrence almost always depends as well on an indirect vascular effect of hypertension such as atherosclerosis, or on unrelated conditions such as destructive diseases of the vascular media, for example, cystic medial necrosis.

MANIFESTATIONS OF ESSENTIAL HYPERTENSION

Blood Pressure Levels

Since there is no threshold cutoff pressure that determines the presence or absence of cardiovascular risk and since many other factors determine the risk, hypertension is defined arbitrarily (see preceding section, Definition of Hypertension). Two pragmatic approaches in determining a diagnosis of hypertension are to identify the pressures that considerably exceed the mean for groups of similar age and sex and to identify the pressures above which there is at least a 50 percent increase in mortality. Unfortunately, such information is not yet available for all age groups (Table 3.9).

No universally accepted term has been adopted to describe individuals who do not fall clearly into a normotensive or hypertensive category. Some have applied the term *borderline hypertension* to such individuals. Others have defined it more specifically to include subjects with systolic pressures between 140 and 160 mmHg and diastolic pressures between 90 and 95 mmHg. The term has also been used to describe subjects with intermittently elevated pressures who at other times are normotensive. Further semantic confusion has arisen because the term *labile hypertension* has been used to refer to individuals with intermittently elevated pressures as well as to individuals who remain in the hypertensive range but show wide fluctuations in pressure from one reading to the next. Since terms are used interchangeably, readers must be wary in evaluating reports that refer to groups of individuals or individual subjects whose pressures fall in the "gray" zone between normotension and hypertension and subjects who have fluctuating pressures.

Some subjects have elevations of systolic pressure with no increase in diastolic pressure; the term *systolic hypertension* is appropriate for such individuals. Others, particularly the elderly, have greater increases in systolic than diastolic pressure, with both in the abnormal range. Some young patients have elevated blood pressure, predominantly systolic, with an accompanying tachycardia. They often have other symptoms suggesting excess sympathetic activity including flushing or pallor, palpitations, and dermographism. Vigorous cardiac action and functional systolic murmurs are often present, and the condition has been labeled the *hyperdynamic* or *hyperkinetic circulatory state*. Some of these individuals have high renin responsiveness and increased circulating catecholamines. It is uncertain whether the tachycardia, increased cardiac output, and elevated systolic pressure are due to increased beta-receptor sensitivity or increased sympathetic activity. However, small doses of beta-blocking drugs usually ameliorate all of the symptoms and signs in these subjects. Many of these subjects do not develop fixed essential hypertension, and the relationship of the hyperdynamic circulatory state to hypertension remains unclear.

Most patients with essential hypertension have a blood pressure that is chronically elevated and readings that are reasonably stable and reproducible from one examination to the next after the initial one or two office visits. Such elevated pressure is referred to variably as *fixed, sustained, established, or chronic hypertension*.

Children

Essential hypertension is rare in children, and 90 percent of children with hypertension have elevated pressure due to kidney disease or other causes. The natural history essential hypertension in children has been inadequately studied and the outcome is unknown. There is no reason to suspect that the benefits of therapy of essential hypertension are any less than

Table 3.9 **Blood Pressure Levels that Are "Abnormal"**

	Male	Female
Children ≤ age 10 years above 95th percentile of blood pressure		115/80
Adolescents, pressure greater than one standard deviation above mean	130/85	125/80
Arterial pressures above which there is at least a 50 percent mortality:		
Adults ≤ age 45	130/90	160/95
Adults > age 45	140/95	

those in the adult, although in children the threshold level defining an increased risk has not been well established.

The Elderly

Elderly patients tend to have greater increases of systolic than diastolic pressure. The significance of this systolic elevation, which is mostly due to decreased aortic distensibility, is unclear. Some studies have shown an increased risk of stroke and coronary artery disease in subjects over age 65 years who have only systolic hypertension. Frequently excessive elevation of systolic pressure only reflects the severity of hypertension, per se. The benefits of lowering pressure in the elderly are not known. Further, treatment is difficult since it is often limited by postural hypotension.

Pregnancy

Normally the diastolic pressure can be expected to fall by 10 mmHg during the first trimester and to slowly rise back to the usual pressures in the third trimester. In pregnancy, diastolic pressure greater than 110 mmHg represents severe hypertension and requires urgent treatment.

Symptoms and Signs

Essential hypertension is most often asymptomatic until complicated by direct or indirect vascular complications. Under ordinary circumstances these ensue after years of pressure elevation. In the earlier stage several symptoms have been ascribed to hypertension, including headache, epistaxis, and dizziness.

Headache is a frequent symptom in patients who know about their blood pressure elevation but is unusual in subjects who are unaware of their disease. In patients with diastolic pressures greater than 120 mmHg who are unaware of the elevation, headache can be expected as a spontaneous complaint in 5 percent, while another 15 percent will admit to headache on direct questioning. In patients knowing their diagnosis, headache will be volunteered by more than 50 percent. This suggests that psychological factors play a role in the generation of headache in many patients. One type of headache is particularly characteristic of hypertension. This consists of an occipital stiffness, or ache, worst on awakening and re-

lieved after being ambulant for an hour or more. The headache is sometimes a "weekend headache," occurring on a Saturday or Sunday morning, and is presumably due to transient rises in intracranial pressure that occur in hypertensive subjects during sleep. A minimum of 6 hours of sleep is usually required to produce symptoms, thus explaining the occurrence on weekends when patients are more likely to remain in bed longer. The headache of depressive illness can be distinguished from the classic headache of hypertension because headaches associated with depression tend invariably to occur morning after morning, irrespective of the length of sleep, and they are poorly localized. The headache of hypertension is unusual if the diastolic pressure is less than 120 mmHg. Migraine has been associated with hypertension, but if migraine is more prevalent in hypertensive patients this increase is not striking. The headache of hypertension cannot be distinguished from headaches due to other conditions leading to raised intracranial pressure such as intracranial tumors. An occipital, morning headache is most frequent in patients with pressures that are rapidly rising and therefore is an important warning that the need for blood pressure control is urgent.

Epistaxis has been popularly ascribed to hypertension. Many of the studies supporting an association neglect the fact that only 10 percent of patients with nosebleed seek medical care. Epistaxis does not appear to be more frequent in hypertensive subjects. However, if epistaxis occurs in a hypertensive patient it tends to be more severe.

A variety of symptoms, including fatigue, insomnia, dizziness, depression, palpitations, and breathlessness have been ascribed to hypertension. There is no convincing evidence that any of these symptoms are related to hypertension that has not yet been complicated by direct or indirect vascular damage.

Nocturia is a common symptom of hypertension, particularly during a period when the pressure is rising. If the elevated pressure becomes fixed, nocturia tends to disappear.

The severity of symptoms of hypertension as well as of the direct vascular complications are related not only to the degree of elevation of pressure but to the length of time over which the pressure has increased. This is most evident in pressure elevations during pregnancy. A rapid rise in pressure with florid direct vascular consequences is also seen in some nonpregnant patients with essential hypertension. This has been termed *accelerated hypertension*. Accelerated hypertension is often accompanied by early morning headache, diastolic pressures over 120 mmHg, and retinal hemorrhages and exudates.

Malignant Hypertension

The clinical term *malignant hypertension* is reserved for those patients with hypertension with pressures usually above 180/130 mmHg and retinal changes that include papilledema. Malignant hypertension should not be diagnosed in the absence of papilledema. If the papilledema is not associated with hemorrhages or exudates, or if the fundal changes are strikingly different in severity in one eye, other reasons for the fundal changes, such as subarachnoid hemorrhage, should be considered. The patient with malignant hypertension may be asymptomatic, but more frequently he or she suffers from headache and symptoms attributed to heart failure or renal insufficiency. Malignant hypertension can occur in essential hypertension or secondary hypertension, but it is distinctly unusual in primary aldosteronism and in coarctation of the aorta. It is much less common in patients with long established moderate blood pressure elevation than in subjects whose pressures have increased to a similar moderate level over a short period of time—suggesting that the vascular hypertrophy of chronic hypertension may protect the vasculature against direct vascular damage due to high pressure.

Two different morphological lesions are observed in arteries in malignant hypertension, but neither are pathognomonic of the disorder. The predominant lesion is that of *necrotizing arteriolitis* involving the small arteries and arterioles of most organs. Fibrin, other plasma proteins, collagen matrix, and necrotic cell debris are deposited in the media of vessels, giving a homogeneous eosinophilic appearance on light microscopy that is referred to as *fibrinoid necrosis*. The factor responsible for this lesion is unclear. One attractive hypothesis is that arterioles constrict in response to rapidly rising arterial pressures. This process is not maintained throughout the arteriole, and it becomes patchy with scattered dilated arteriolar segments. In these areas the endothelium is disrupted, and the vessel wall becomes permeable to plasma proteins and larger molecular weight substances.

The second lesion seen in malignant hypertension is that of *intimal proliferation*, particularly of the interlobular arteries of the kidney. Microscopically, this proliferative endoarteritis consists of circumferentially located smooth-muscle cells, acid mucopolysaccharides, and collagen, and is often associated with intravascular platelet thrombi. The renal cortex distal to the affected arteries undergoes ischemic atrophy; however, hypertrophy of the juxtaglomerular apparatus may be observed, presumably in response

to the decrease in pulsatile blood flow. The subsequent excess in renin production may be responsible for a further rise in pressure through activation of the renin-angiotensin-aldosterone system. Renin is characteristically elevated in patients with malignant hypertension.

Patients with malignant hypertension often prove to have hemolytic anemia with deformed red blood cells ("burr" cells) on blood smears. In addition, some patients show evidence of intravascular coagulation with increased fibrin split products, thrombocytopenia, and reduced fibrinogen. These effects are probably secondary to vascular damage with platelet and fibrin deposition in smaller arterioles. Red blood cells are damaged as they pass through the fibrin mesh. It has been postulated that these microangiopathic changes represent the fundamental pathophysiological event that distinguishes benign from malignant hypertension. However, this theory, too, fails to provide an explanation for the initial vascular damage needed to trigger intravascular coagulation. Malignant hypertension is accompanied by a very poor prognosis: 80 percent of untreated patients die within a year. This complication of hypertension is fortunately now seen rarely. The process of fibrinoid necrosis is rapidly halted by lowering of blood pressure, although there is not necessarily a complete reversal of the damage that has occurred. If malignant hypertension is treated the prognosis improves, with a 60 percent 5-year survival rate in patients without azotemia and a 25 percent 5-year survival if azotemia is present. Malignant hypertension is entirely preventable with present methods of treatment.

Hypertensive Encephalopathy

Hypertensive encephalopathy is believed to be due to an elevation in pressure that exceeds the capacity of the cerebral arterioles to constrict and autoregulate cerebral blood flow. Cerebral edema ensues. This complication develops over several days and is usually heralded by fluctuating neurological symptoms, including confusion, somnolence, blurred vision, headache, nausea, and vomiting, which in later stages progress to seizures, stupor or coma, and focal neurological deficits. Focal neurological deficits rarely occur until late in the course of hypertensive encephalopathy. Blood pressure is usually more than 180/130 (mmHg) and retinal changes usually include hemorrhages or papilledema, or both. The distinction between hypertensive encephalopathy and malignant hypertension is made by the predominance of symptoms of severe neurological dysfunction in encephalopathy. The distinction between encephalopathy and stroke can be more difficult, particularly since blood pressure can be transiently increased in many patients with stroke, and stroke can complicate the course of encephalopathy. Focal deficits, particularly if they are persistent, do not occur in hypertensive encephalopathy until late in the course of this disorder; if they are found, the physician should be alert to the likelihood of a cerebrovascular accident. The distinction is important clinically, since prompt reduction of pressure is essential in the successful treatment of patients with hypertensive encephalopathy but can seriously compromise adequate brain perfusion in stroke.

Small Vessel Occlusive Disease: Lacunar Infarction

The most common cerebrovascular lesion found at autopsy in elderly patients with hypertension consists of small lacunar infarctions chiefly in the basal ganglia, thalamus, cerebellum, and the internal capsule. These lesions may have no clinical manifestations, or they may cause mild focal neurological deficits that are often heralded by a few days of transient symptomatology. Symptoms can include a pure motor hemiplegia, unilateral ataxia, dysarthria and upper limb ataxia, or unilateral sensory loss. Occasionally, more diffuse lesions induce syndromes consisting of bilateral motor-system involvement and organic dementia. There is often complete clinical recovery.

Intraparenchymal Cerebral Hemorrhage

Hypertension easily outranks other etiologic factors such as blood dyscrasias, rupture of arteriovenous malformations, or neoplasms as the cause of intraparenchymal hemorrhages. The most frequent sites for such hemorrhages are:

1. The cerebral hemispheres, with clinical symptoms including a profound hemiparesis and sensory loss, often with conjugate deviation of the eyes in the direction of the affected hemisphere.

2. The thalamus, with contralateral sensory loss and often hemiparesis due to involvement of the adjacent internal capsule.

3. The pons, with deep unconsciousness, decerebrate posturing, and quadriparesis.

4. And the cerebellum, with ataxia, vomiting, and progression to stupor and coma.

Symptoms due to intraparenchymal hemorrhage are typically of sudden, onset with headache and rapid progression of neurological signs. Most hemorrhages are not contained within the parenchyma and extend into the ventricles or subarachnoid space. Death, which occurs in 85 percent of patients within 1 month, often is due to brain herniation with compression and hemorrhagic infarction of the pons and midbrain.

The heart not only suffers from the consequences of high blood pressure but may play a primary role in hypertension. Some patients with borderline hypertension and others with longstanding essential hypertension and widely fluctuating arterial pressures have increased myocardial contractility, heart rate, and stroke volume. Often such subjects have other symptoms that suggest an increase in sympathetic activity, including palpitations, flushing, and sweating. In longstanding hypertension with stable elevations of blood pressure, however, subtle signs of diminished cardiac function can be demonstrated by analysing systolic time intervals. Later, electrocardiographic signs of left ventricular hypertrophy ensue as the left ventricle hypertrophies as a compensatory mechanism for the increased arterial pressure. The hypertrophy consists of an increase in myocardial cell size as well as a proliferation of the collagen-supporting tissue. This type of ventricular hypertrophy occurring in response to an increase in pressure load is ordinarily associated with diminished cardiac function that accompanies the ventricle's inability to eject the same stroke volume as the normal heart at the same end-diastolic pressure. Clinical symptoms of left heart failure are ominous symptoms in the hypertensive subject. Even mild reduction of blood pressure, however, can provide dramatic relief of these symptoms and signs of heart failure. Occasionally patients with hypertension can have symptoms and signs that are predominantly those of right heart failure. Why these patients are spared from clinical manifestations of pulmonary edema is unclear.

Most often the cardiac manifestations of hypertension are not due to the direct vascular effects of hypertension alone but are combined with and frequently dominated by the symptoms and signs of coronary atherosclerosis and ischemic heart disease.

Impairment of vision due to thrombosis of a branch of the retinal vein or of the central retinal vein itself, and scotoma due to occlusions of small arterial branches, occur commonly in hypertension. Striking changes in retinal vasculature are often found on fundoscopic examination in hypertensive patients who have no visual complaints.

ASSESSMENT OF THE PATIENT WITH HYPERTENSION

History

Assessment of the patient with hypertension must take into account the circumstance under which the elevated blood pressure was discovered. This usually entails one of the following situations:

1. During routine or screening examinations
2. At a time when the patient is being seen for some unrelated condition
3. When the patient presents with symptoms of hypertension or of the atherosclerotic vascular damage associated with hypertension
4. In a hypertensive emergency

It is often helpful to ask the question, "When was your blood pressure last measured as being normal." Dating the onset can be assisted also by seeking information from the patient in regard to insurance, school, or employment examinations. Since the rate of rise of pressure as well as the level of pressure determines the likelihood of vascular damage, knowing the duration of elevated pressures is important. In addition, the sudden onset or exacerbation of hypertension can be an important clinical clue to renal causes of the disorder.

In addition to the setting in which elevated pressures are found, other purposes of the history in a hypertensive patient must be kept in mind. Among these is the collection of information to assist in the assessment of:

1. Etiologic factors and the probability of secondary rather than essential hypertension
2. Severity of the hypertension and of the direct and indirect vascular damage to heart, kidney, brain, and optic fundi
3. Other risk factors of atherosclerosis
4. Factors that affect the method of treatment

There are two difficulties in approaching the management of a patient with elevated arterial pressure. First is the fact that knowledge of elevated pressure produces or accentuates symptoms that were not previously noticed by the patient and also contributes to absenteeism from work. It is therefore often necessary to allay anxiety by reassuring the patient of the lack of immediate harm from the elevated pressures. Further difficulty may arise if the patient attributes symptoms unrelated to elevated pressure to hypertension, and subsequently varies treatment according to the severity of these symptoms. This results in unsatisfactory blood pressure control, and

can be avoided if the physician carefully avoids erroneously reinforcing the patient's belief that his other symptoms are related to the hypertensive process.

A positive family history of hypertension or atherosclerosis in the absence of polycystic kidney, hyperparathyroidism, or rarely endocrine tumors, strongly supports the diagnosis of essential hypertension. A negative family history is less convincing, since many patients in the past suffered undiagnosed hypertension. In the young patient with an elevation of pressure that is predominantly systolic, other symptoms suggestive of sympathetic overactivity may be present, including flushing, pallor, palpitations, and sweating, suggesting a hyperkinetic circulatory state. Palpitations, sweating, and paroxysmal headache comprise the typical triad of symptoms of pheochromocytoma, but other symptoms such as weight loss are also important clues to this catabolic state. Muscle weakness, polyuria, and cramps are characteristic of aldosteronism, although this disorder is usually discovered by biochemical tests in patients without symptoms. The history should include inquiry into the possibility of renal injuries in contact sports, and back injuries. A history of hematuria or loin pain following the injury suggests a perirenal hematoma or an intrarenal hemorrhage.

A complete drug history may reveal oral contraceptives or estrogens as contributing to the elevated blood pressure. Other drugs such as carbenoxolone or foods such as licorice can cause hypertension. Often the patient has been previously treated for hypertension; it is important to ascertain previous responses to drugs as well as to make an estimate of the likelihood of compliance in following a treatment regimen.

Careful inquiry should be made of symptoms of ischemic heart disease or left ventricular failure. Nocturia is a frequent complaint during the time when blood pressure is rising, although it tends to disappear when pressure is stable. Impairment of vision in a portion of the visual field of one eye suggests retinal venous thrombosis, and scotomata suggest thrombosis of small retinal arterioles.

Physical Examination

Physical examination of the subject with elevated blood pressure is aimed at assessing the severity of the hypertensive disease, looking for evidence of direct and indirect vascular consequences of hypertension, and searching for clues that suggest that the patient has hypertension secondary to a remedial disorder. Emphasis is placed on examination of the cardiovascular system, the optic fundi, the kidneys, and the neurological system.

Cardiovascular Examination

For accuracy blood pressure should be recorded in a reasonably quiet environment using a proper sized cuff (width equal to 40 percent of the circumference of the arm) and with the arm in a position so that the antecubital fossa is at the level of the heart. If the usual size of cuff is used on an obese arm, blood pressure will be overestimated since the relatively narrow cuff is less able to compress the tissue between it and the brachial artery. If the antecubital fossa is 10 to 15 cm below the heart, as is the case with the arm hanging down, both systolic and diastolic pressures will be approximately 10 mmHg higher than if the arm is extended. Except in cases of urgency, conclusions regarding the blood pressure level should be based on two readings taken on different visits.

In children, adolescents, and young adults with elevated brachial artery pressures, blood pressure should be measured in the legs using an appropriately wide cuff in order to identify coarctation of the aorta. Examination of pulses should be routine in the assessment of all subjects with elevated pressures. Other physical signs that suggest coarctation include an ejection systolic murmur that is heard best between the left scapula and spine, or pulsating collateral vessels around the scapulae and in the intercostal spaces, particularly when the patient is sitting forward. Patients with an untreated coarctation rarely live to age 60. Thus there is little likelihood that this would be the cause of hypertension in an older patient.

Elevated pressures with a narrow pulse pressure are characteristic of hypertension due to advanced parenchymal renal disease. Predominantly systolic elevations with wide pulse pressure suggest loss of distensibility of the aorta due to arteriosclerosis in the older patient or the hyperkinetic circulatory state in young patients. In this disorder a tachycardia usually accompanies the elevated pressure. Bradycardia from any cause may be associated with a systolic elevation of blood pressure due to the increased stroke volume.

Peripheral pulses and the characteristics of the peripheral circulation should be recorded. A delayed, dampened femoral pulse in the young patient suggests coarctation of the aorta. Diminished or absent pulses are also found if large vessels are occluded by arteriosclerosis. The walls of the radial artery should not normally be palpable when the vessel is pressed against the radius. The thickened walls of arteriosclerosis may be felt, and further evidence of arteriosclerosis can be found in a tortuous brachial artery that moves like a spring with each pulse wave. Auscultation of the vessels should be carried out to discover bruits of stenotic channels. A high-pitched unilateral bruit, in the epigastrium radiating into the flank, or in the renal angle posteriorly, suggests renal artery stenosis.

Left ventricular hypertrophy may be identified at bedside examination if the apex beat is displaced laterally and there is a well localized thrust. The forceful cardiac action associated with anxiety may produce a similar apex beat although usually not lateral to the midclavicular line. Thick chest wall structures can dampen the palpable and visible evidence of left ventricular hypertrophy, accurate assessment depends on radiologic, electrocardiographic, or echocardiographic investigations. A fourth heart sound (presystolic or left atrial gallop) is commonly heard in hypertensive patients and disappears with lowering of pressure. The second sound at the aortic area is often increased. A soft ejection aortic systolic murmur is frequently heard, and is of no importance. Mitral systolic and early diastolic murmurs at the left sternal border are manifestations of valvular insufficiency and can mean severe cardiac involvement.

Fundoscopy

The examination of the optic fundi can be critical in assessing the severity of hypertensive disease. For clarity it is important that fundal changes be described to avoid confusion regarding different grading systems. Some difficulty has arisen over the meaning of fundoscopic findings, because in most hypertensive patients they represent a composite of changes directly due to hypertension and changes due to the commonly superimposed arteriosclerotic process. Two fundamental differences distinguish the retinal arterioles from vessels of similar caliber elsewhere in the body. Adjacent endothelial cells of retinal vessels abut one another tightly, without any intercellular space. Factors such as histamine that modify capillary and arteriolar permeability with resultant edema do not affect these tight junctions of the retinal arterioles. Only if functional or structural damage has occurred in these arterioles will substances diffuse out of the vessels. Sodium fluorescein, which escapes from damaged retinal arterioles, has been very useful in the study of retinal vascular disease. The second difference is that there is no autonomic innervation of the retinal arterioles, and their caliber is therefore a result of circulating or local factors, with the latter being of predominant importance.

The usual response of the retinal arterioles to an increase in pressure is vasoconstriction. Normally the retinal arterioles are seen as gently curving vessels gracefully bifurcating toward the periphery of the retina with a caliber about 2/3 that of the veins. The arterioles have a marked central stripe on their surface due to the reflection of light. In hypertension, particularly in the absence of superimposed arteriolar structural changes, and in conditions in which the rise in blood pressure has occurred quickly as in eclampsia or malignant hypertension, the arterioles show diffuse narrowing, a change that is completely reversible with effective treatment. Another early change is focal narrowing of retinal arterioles separated by intervening portions that appear normal in caliber. This irregular segmental narrowing is due largely to hypertrophy of the muscle of the media.

Other changes in the retinal arterioles of hypertensive patients represent the hypertrophy of vascular smooth muscle and hyaline degeneration of the arteriolar wall (arteriosclerosis). The vessel wall not only thickens but becomes more opaque so that the central white stripe of reflected light widens. Because of the copper color sometimes associated with such changes, some observers have used the term "copper wiring" to describe the affected vessels. Further hyaline degeneration and fibrosis leads to a homogenous "silver wiring" of the arterioles. There is generally poor agreement between observers regarding these findings. If the patient is more than 60 years of age the changes may be seen in the absence of hypertension. The younger the patient the more important these changes become in assessing the severity of hypertension.

In the normal fundus the arteriolar wall is thin enough to permit the dark color of the vein to show at arteriovenous crossings. With thickening of the arteriolar wall associated with age or hypertension, the vein appears to taper and disappear from view before it is actually crossed by the arteriole. Such AV nipping or nicking is partially due to the increased opacity of the arterioles but is also due to backward displacement of the vein by the more rigid arteriole. This displacement provides an end-on view of the vein as it dips behind the arteriole, accounting for the heaped up appearance of the vein on either side of the crossing. Again, these changes are seen in older patients in the absence of hypertension. About 10 percent of normotensive individuals under age 45 years show such changes, while 40 percent of normotensive subjects over age 50 years have identical changes.

Retinal hemorrhages, exudates, and papilledema are more readily recognized than are the arteriolar changes of hypertension. Their presence is most frequently due to hypertension, although similar changes may be seen in diabetes, bleeding disorders such as thrombocytopenia, systemic lupus erythematosis, leukemia, and severe anemia. The presence of retinal hemorrhages is usually the first fundoscopic evidence that hypertension is in a rapidly progressing phase. Flame-shaped hemorrhages around the disc are most common. This location is due to the greater pressure in the capillaries near the disc, and the shape represents spread in the nerve fiber layer. Hemorrhages due to hypertension are rarely found lateral to the macula. Other hemorrhages appearing as dots or blots occur deep to the nerve layer.

Swelling of the optic disc, or papilledema, is only seen in rapidly advancing severe hypertension. Characteristically there is little loss of visual acuity or visual fields. The earliest premonitory sign of papilledema is engorgement of the veins on the disc, supporting the theory that the papilledema is secondary to venous outflow obstruction caused by raised intracranial pressure. In those patients in whom raised intracranial pressure is not present the edema may be due to ischemic injury of the optic nerve fibers.

Fundoscopic changes of hypertension and the prognosis associated with retinopathy are summarized in Table 3.10.

Abdominal Examination

Careful auscultation of the abdomen may reveal bruits suggesting renal artery stenosis or may disclose enlarged kidneys suggesting polycystic disease.

Neurologic Examination

The neurologic examination may serve to identify evidence of hypertensive or arteriosclerotic cerebrovascular disease, and may provide an important baseline against which to compare future neurologic signs.

Investigations

Characteristically in essential hypertension there are no abnormalities in serum or urine electrolytes, in measurements of the renin-angiotensin-aldosterone system, or in plasma or urinary catecholamines. Investigational procedures are helpful in a number of

Table 3.10   **Prognosis: Approximate Percentage of Untreated Patients Surviving 10 Years**

		Men	Women	Comments
Grade I	Generalized or focal arteriolar narrowing, increased width of light reflex	75	85	Similar changes occur with aging. Little agreement between observers on those changes.
Grade II	As Grade I with further increase in width of light reflex. Arteriovenous nipping	35	70	Generalized and focal narrowing may be masked by sclerotic changes
Grade III	Grade II changes with hemorrhages, cotton wool spots, and/or hard exudates	15	25	Hemorrhages and cotton wool patches may be seen alone or together, and indicate severe disease
Grade IV	Grade III changes with papilledema	5	15	Loss of visual fields or acuity are unusual symptoms until changes are very advanced.

other ways, including the following:

1. Assessment of extent of hypertensive or atherothrombotic damage to heart and kidneys
2. Recognition of the presence of other risk factors of cardiovascular disease
3. Diagnosis of remediable causes of hypertension other than essential hypertension
4. Recognition of coincident disorders that modify the selection of drugs because of the likelihood of adverse effects

Subjects with borderline hypertension or those with modestly elevated blood pressure require little investigation beyond a complete urinalysis, whereas patients with rapidly progressive hypertension may require extensive investigations (Table 3.11). It has been estimated that reversible causes of hypertension can be found in only 2 of every 100 subjects with elevated pressures on screening examination, and that surgery is only useful in the management of 3 out of every 1,000 hypertensive patients each year. Although these figures vary depending on the nature

Table 3.11   **Screening Laboratory Tests Recommended in Patients with Hypertension**

All patients
    Urinalysis including microscopic examination
    Serum creatinine
    Blood sugar
    Cholesterol, triglycerides, high-density lipoproteins
    Chest x-ray
    ECG
+ If mineralocorticoid hypertension suspected
    Serum Na, K, Cl, HCO_3
    Plasma renin activity
+ If severe hypertension or if pheochromocytoma suspected
    Urine metanephrine or
    Urine VMA
+ If renovascular hypertension suspected
    Isotopic renal scan or
    Intravenous pyelogram and renal arteriogram
+ Before diuretic-antihypertensive therapy
    Serum Na, K
    Serum Ca, PO_4

of a physician's practice, they emphasize the rarity of presently recognized remediable causes of hypertension.

Assessment of Extent of Cardiovascular Disease

A chest x-ray may be useful in assessing the size of the left ventricle, but a more sensitive assessment is provided by the electrocardiogram. Left ventricular hypertrophy is suggested if the deepest S wave in lead V_1 or V_2 and/or the tallest R wave in lead V_5 or V_6 is equal to or greater than 30 mm. These changes are usually accompanied by ST segment deviation in a direction opposite to the main QRS direction, a QRS duration of 0.09 seconds or more, and left axis deviation of -30 degrees or more. The electrocardiogram may also show changes due to ischemic heart disease.

In slowly progressing essential hypertension the kidney is relatively spared from damage, compared with the heart. It is unusual for such patients to have proteinuria greater than $1+$ or more than an occasional red or white blood cell. If the urinalysis shows more than $2+$ proteinuria with a fixed low specific gravity or with more cells or casts, parenchymal kidney disease must be suspected as a primary cause of hypertension. In rapidly progressing malignant hypertension, marked proteinuria usually accompanied by microscopic hematuria is characteristic. Screening measurements of renal function such as serum creatinine and blood urea nitrogen are usually normal in essential hypertension. If mildly elevated, a creatinine clearance should be performed to provide a more accurate assessment of renal function. Reduction of creatinine clearance suggests either that essential hypertension has been present and inadequately treated for many years or that parenchymal renal disease is the cause of the hypertension. In addition, progressive deterioration of renal function is seen in rapidly progressing and malignant hypertension.

Other Risk Factors

It is illogical to embark on antihypertensive treatment aimed at preventing the progression of atherothrombotic and hypertensive cardiovascular disease without attempting to modify other risk factors such as obesity and smoking. Further, modest elevations of blood pressure in an individual with another important risk factor such as diabetes may merit antihypertensive treatment, while in a patient with no other cardiovascular risk factors such increases might only require observation, since synergistic effects of a combination of several risk factors has been shown. A sizeable increase in susceptibility to atherosclerotic vascular disease has been associated with hypercholesterolemia, hypertriglyceridemia, low plasma HDL, hypertension, cigarette smoking, diabetes mellitus, gout, and obesity, among other factors. Unfortunately the evidence of benefit accruing from modification of some of these factors is not (yet) available. In order to identify risk factors, measurement of blood sugar, plasma lipids, and uric acid is justified in most patients with essential hypertension.

Diagnosis of Remedial Causes of Hypertension

A careful history and physical examination is all that is required to rule out remediable causes of hypertension in most subjects with elevated arterial pressures (Table 3.3). The search for remediable causes of hypertension through laboratory investigation is more important in young hypertensive patients and in severe hypertension. Selection of investigation in each individual is based on the likelihood of finding specific causes and the likelihood that the patient will benefit from specific treatment if a remediable cause is found.

Factors which suggest a renal parenchymal or renovascular cause of hypertension include the following:

1. Age less than 30 years
2. History of renal trauma or hematuria
3. Sudden onset of or increase in diastolic hypertension
4. Rapidly progressing hypertension with evidence of direct vascular sequelae
5. Palpable kidney(s)

6. Biphasic or continuous bruit in the epigastrium and radiating to one flank
7. Hypertension that is not controlled by medical therapy

Coarctation of the aorta should be suspected in the presence of diminished and delayed femoral pulses in a subject under age 60 with elevated pressures in the arms.

Hypertension related to oral contraceptives may be the most common cause of secondary hypertension.

Hypertension resulting from aldosterone usually does not have distinctive symptomatology or physical signs. However, the following findings are suggestive:

1. Generalized muscle weakness, tetany, cramps, and polyuria
2. Hypokalemia (serum potassium less than 3.5 mmol/L) associated with a urine potassium of more than 30 mmol/24 hours in the absence of diuretic therapy for the preceding 7 days. A serum sodium toward the upper limit of normal and metabolic alkalosis are usually present. Additional causes of hypertension associated with hypokalemia are listed in Chapter 9 under hypokalemia. Other endocrine causes of hypertension should be suspected if there are symptoms or signs suggestive of Cushing's syndrome or acromegaly (see Hypertension Secondary to Endocrine Disease).

Pheochromocytoma is a rare cause of hypertension. Investigation should be pursued in patients with hypertension who also have the following:

1. Unexplained weight loss or hyperglycemia
2. Paroxysms of hypertension, sweats, headache, palpitations
3. Personality changes, anxiety
4. Hypertension precipitated or aggravated by antihypertensive drugs or anesthesia
5. Postural hypotension

Very few asymptomatic patients with hypertension and a normal urinalysis, normal serum potassium, and normal blood sugar turn out to have a remediable cause of hypertension.

Recognition of Coincident Disorders

The use of the antihypertensive diuretic drugs may be complicated by an elevation of blood sugar due to interference with insulin secretion by the pancreatic islet cells. This is more common in patients with a preexisting abnormal glucose tolerance, but at times hyperglycemia is precipitated in subjects with previously normal blood sugar control. These drugs may also be complicated by an elevation of uric acid due to inhibition of tubular secretion. Although the hyperuricemia is of no apparent consequence in the normal individual, the manifestations of gout may be worsened in the patient with gout. The benzothiadiazines and related diuretics increase the urinary loss of potassium and may cause hypokalemia, whereas the use of spironolactone and related drugs may be followed by hyperkalemia. The benzothiadiazines also reduce the urinary excretion of calcium, and a transient mild hypercalcemia may occur with their use. This may lead to difficulty in the diagnosis of hyperparathyroidism. Because of these effects, pretreatment measurements of blood sugar, uric acid, serum potassium, and calcium are helpful (Table 3.11).

TREATMENT OF ESSENTIAL HYPERTENSION

The aim of treatment of essential hypertension is to prevent the direct vascular complications of the disease and to retard the development of atherothrombotic disease.

Benefits of treating elevated pressure are beyond question in the malignant phase of hypertension as outlined above. In less severe essential hypertension treatment results in a marked reduction of the incidence of malignant hypertension, congestive heart failure, and renal failure (Table 3.6). The incidence of stroke as well as the recurrence of stroke is reduced by treatment of hypertension, and this effect is most marked in men under age 60 with a diastolic pressure over 104 mmHg. There is no evidence at present that myocardial infarction is prevented by antihypertensive treatment. Since the introduction of effective antihypertensive treatment, myocardial infarction has replaced stroke as the most common cause of death in the patient with hypertension.

No long-term studies are available that permit evaluation of benefits of treatment of hypertension in individuals with lower risks of cardiovascular complications, as in women, older patients (over age 60), subjects with isolated systolic pressure elevation, and patients with diastolic pressures less than 105 mmHg. Justification for treating such patients is based on the demonstration of the graded risk of elevated systolic pressure, no matter the level, the age, or the sex, and on extrapolation of results of studies that have concentrated largely on middle-aged men. It is probably beneficial to reduce blood pressure in

men age 45 years or less with pressures over 130/90 (mmHg), in men over age 45 years with pressures over 140/95, and in women of any age with pressures over 160/95. In the absence of increased diastolic pressure benefit is likely in individuals under age 60 if the systolic pressure is over 150 mmHg, and over age 60 if the systolic pressure is over 180 mmHg (see Tables 3.9 and 3.12). Pressures above these thresholds have been shown to be associated with at least a 50 percent increase in the risk of death. These threshold pressures for treatment are probably conservative.

Salt Restriction

Restriction of the intake of sodium results in a reduction of blood pressure in almost all patients with hypertension. The restriction of sodium intake, however, must be severe. The Kempner rice-fruit diet, for example, has a content of less than 10 mmol/day and its unpalatability and the consequent poor compliance probably explains why less than 50 percent of patients achieved a reduction in blood pressure when this treatment was used. If sodium intake is reduced to 75 mmol/day many hypertensives will achieve a reduction in blood pressure equivalent to that with a diuretic-antihypertensive drug. If the intake exceeds 150 mmol/day, there is no lowering of blood pressure. An intake of less than 75 mmol/day is difficult to achieve since popular North American foods such as meat and eggs have a high sodium content, and sodium is also contained in the widely used preservatives sodium benzoate and sodium glutamate. In spite of these difficulties subjects with mild hypertension should be informed that a diet containing less than 75 mmol Na/day may obviate the need for drug treatment. In patients with diastolic pressures over 105 mmHg, an intake of sodium over 150 mmol/day will reduce the effectiveness of diuretic as well as nondiuretic antihypertensive drugs. In practice, compliance with salt restriction to 75 mmol/day is poor.

Table 3.12 Recommended Threshold Pressures above which Treatment Should be Instituted

	Men	Women
Systolic and diastolic elevations		
Age ≤45 years	130/90	
		160/95
Age >45 years	140/95	
Predominant systolic elevations	(Men and Women)	
Age ≤60 years	150	
Age >60 years	180	

Weight

The patient should be encouraged to reduce weight to that considered ideal. Weight reduction of 10 kg or more in the overweight hypertensive patient is followed by a lowering of blood pressure. This effect is independent of the reduction of sodium intake that usually accompanies dietary approaches to the treatment of obesity. Obesity is an independent risk factor for cardiovascular morbidity and mortality so that maintenance of ideal weight may benefit the obese hypertensive patient in more than one way.

Compliance

The major difficulty in achieving blood pressure control in hypertensive patients is failure of the patient to adhere to dietary restrictions or drug regimens. Many factors contribute to poor compliance with therapy, particularly when regimens require behavioral change, are complex or of long duration, or are associated with side effects. The asymptomatic nature of essential hypertension is also important, since clinical improvement is not apparent to the patient.

Drug Therapy

In spite of the attractiveness of selecting drugs based on a consideration of the pathophysiologic factors causing the elevated pressure, the pathogenesis in most patients with essential hypertension remains obscure and therapy remains aimed empirically at the lowering of the increased arterial pressure. Since the aim of treatment is primarily to prevent the cardiovascular complication of hypertension and since many of these complications are a consequence of atherosclerosis, other contributing factors including obesity, hyperlipidemia, and smoking should not be neglected.

If two or more drugs are used concomitantly in treatment, the antihypertensive effects are approximately additive. Concurrent therapy permits the use of smaller doses of each drug and reduces the severity of dose-related side effects. Nevertheless, since the variety of possible side effects increases with the number of different agents employed and since compliance decreases with increasing complexity of therapy, treatment is more likely to be successful if a single drug can be used. Treatment should generally be instituted with a single drug, and the dose should be increased until adequate control is achieved, or until the ceiling dose of the drug is reached (that is,

until no further blood pressure lowering can be anticipated, or intolerable side effects occur). If blood pressure control is inadequate, an alternative drug can be tried or a second drug can be added, depending on the amount of blood pressure reduction achieved with the initial agent.

The side effects of the primary treatment should be avoided if possible by selecting an alternative antihypertensive drug rather than adding another drug. The addition of a potassium-sparing diuretic or a potassium supplement to antihypertensive diuretic treatment complicated by hypokalemia should only be contemplated if there are reasons for not replacing the diuretic with an alternative drug such as a beta-adrenergic antagonist. Compliance will be best if the drug regimen is simple.

The drugs presently available to treat essential hypertension include principally the following:

1. The diuretic-antihypertensive group
2. Drugs interacting with the adrenergic system, including adrenergic receptor antagonists, centrally acting drugs, and adrenergic neurone antagonists
3. Arterial vasodilators

The main consideration in selecting a drug is that it effectively lowers blood pressure with a minimum of side effects. In general the less potent drugs are associated with milder side effects; however, it is clearly not to the patient's benefit to use an ineffective but well-tolerated drug. The choice of drug is frequently influenced by the risk of side effects. It may be necessary, for example, to avoid the use of diuretics in subjects with gout or hyperuricemia, and the use of kaliuretic diuretics in individuls with greater risk of hypokalemia, such as patients receiving digitalis glycosides. Beta-adrenergic antagonists, on the other hand, increase the likelihood of bronchospasm in predisposed subjects, can worsen cardiac failure by reducing adrenergic drive to the heart, and can aggravate intermittent claudication because of the reduction of cardiac output and peripheral blood flow. Further, the manner in which a drug is used is frequently as important as the particular drug selected. The use of two or more drugs at an ineffective dose level, is all too frequent and erroneously results in patients being considered refractory to treatment by their physicians.

The *drugs of first choice* in treatment are the antihypertensive-diuretic drugs, hydrochlorothiazide or the closely related chlorthalidone. These drugs are identical in all known effects, but chlorthalidone has the advantage of acting for longer than 24 hours, making the occasional missed daily dose of less importance. Blood-pressure lowering reaches a maximum after three weeks of treatment, and it may take at least this length of time before blood pressure returns to its pretreatment level after stopping the drug. The initial hemodynamic change is a reduction in stroke volume and cardiac output with a rise in total peripheral resistance. However, after several weeks of treatment, cardiac output returns to normal and peripheral resistance falls. These effects are probably secondary to circulatory adjustments to the loss of sodium as well as to the drugs' relaxing of vascular smooth muscle. The ceiling dose of hydrochlorothiazide beyond which no further saluresis or antihypertensive effects can be anticipated is about 150 mg/day, while that of chlorthalidone is about 100 mg/day. If doses near this ceiling are employed, almost all patients will show a reduction in serum potassium to the lower limit of normal or slightly below. This mild hypokalemia is rarely symptomatic and of no proven risk to the patient, and it can be helpful as a measure of compliance. Other unwanted biochemical effects are increases in uric acid, which are of no apparent consequence except in the patient with coexistent gout and hyperglycemia. Spironolactone, a competitive aldosterone antagonist, provides blood-pressure lowering similar to equivalent doses of hydrochlorothiazide. However, the drug is tolerated less well because of digestive complaints and gynecomastia. Occasional patients may show further lowering of pressure up to a ceiling dose of 400 mg. Triamterene has little antihypertensive effect. In the patient with normal renal function, furosemide must be given several times daily to achieve blood-pressure reduction similar to that of chlorthalidone. Its use in hypertension should be limited to those patients with renal failure who require a diuretic because of sodium retention but who are resistant to the less potent diuretics.

The advantage of selecting a diuretic as the initial drug to treat hypertension is that all patients with normal renal function can be expected to achieve some lowering of blood pressure, with the average reduction in mean arterial pressure being 15 percent. Patients with low renin responsiveness generally show a greater reduction of about 25 percent; and those with high renin responsiveness show a smaller reduction of about 5 percent. A further advantage of initial diuretic antihypertensive drugs is that the other drugs, with the exception of the beta-adrenergic antagonists, lead to sodium retention and usually must be used concomitantly with a saluretic drug.

The beta-adrenergic receptor antagonist drugs comprise a useful alternative initial drug in the treatment of essential hypertension. The drug of choice is propranolol. The hemodynamic effects are very similar to those seen with the diuretics, with an initial reduction in cardiac output and rise in peripheral resistance, and a subsequent reduction in peripheral resistance. The sites of action responsible for these effects remain unclear, and as with many antihypertensive drugs more than one site of action is probably important. The most likely actions include an antagonistic action at beta-adrenergic receptors of the adrenergic nerve endings, accompanied by a reduction of norepinephrine release. A central site of action resulting in a reduction of efferent sympathetic activity also appears likely. The direct effects of the drugs in reducing cardiac output and renin release are probably less important in their antihypertensive effectiveness in essential hypertension. A practical ceiling dose of propranolol is 240 mg/day. This dose can be given once daily with control of blood pressure equivalent to more frequent doses. The additional blood-pressure lowering achieved with higher doses is ordinarily small, and larger doses are not well tolerated if given once a day. Beta-adrenergic responsiveness may be necessary in cardiac failure, bronchospastic conditions, and bradyarrhythmias. If such conditions coexist with or complicate the use of propranolol, all beta-adrenergic antagonist drugs are best avoided. Minor pharmacologic or pharmacokinetic advantages of the present variety of beta-adrenergic antagonists are unimportant, and because of its long and widespread use, propranolol remains the beta-adrenergic antagonist of first choice. An occasional patient may tolerate one beta-adrenergic antagonist better than another for no apparent pharmacologic reason.

The advantage of selecting a beta-adrenergic antagonist drug as the initial drug is their unique control of blood pressure in the face of emotional excitement and exercise. These drugs are also very useful in ameliorating the hyperkinetic circulatory state characterised by a predominant increase in systolic pressure and sinus tachycardia. Blood-pressure reduction is not universal: about 25 percent of patients with essential hypertension do not achieve any blood-pressure reduction with propranolol alone and some actually experience an increase in pressure. In those who respond, an average reduction of 15 percent in mean arterial pressure can be expected—very similar to that achieved with diuretics.

Most patients can be controlled with antihypertensive diuretic drugs or beta-adrenergic antagonist drugs used alone or together, provided that drugs can be increased to their ceiling doses and that patients are compliant.

It is difficult to maintain blood-pressure control of hypertensive patients in the low normotensive range and it is not known whether the benefits of such aggressive therapy outweigh the risks. At present a reasonable aim is to attempt to reduce pressures to pressures considered in the borderline range or lower: less than 130/85 (mmHg) in male adolescents; less than 130/90 in adult males up to age 45; less than 140/95 in males over age 45; less than 125/80 in female adolescents; and less than 160/95 in adult women.

A variety of other drugs are available for use in patients not controlled with diuretics and beta-adrenergic antagonist drugs. With chronic use, all of these agents induce salt and water retention, so these drugs must be used with attention to salt restriction and most often must be used with a diuretic. Methyldopa is equivalent in potency to the beta-adrenergic antagonist drugs but is associated with more frequent adverse effects of fatigue, difficulty in concentrating, and other mental symptoms. The drug lowers blood pressure largely through its breakdown product α-methylnorepinephrine, which acts as a false transmitter at central sites, thereby reducing the sympathetic outflow under the control of the medullary cardiovascular modulating center. Hydralazine lowers blood pressure through arterial vasodilation. Unfortunately an increase in force of cardiac contraction and tachycardia often accompany its use. This may be detrimental to patients with coexistant ischemic heart disease. These effects can be prevented with the concomitant use of propranolol. Minoxidil, clonidine, and guanethedine are more potent antihypertensive drugs. Unfortunately, in doses that provide more blood-pressure lowering than diuretics, propranolol and hydralazine side effects are very common and often limit the size of doses that can be given.

Two new drugs appear promising but their role in the treatment of hypertension remains to be established. Captopril, an angiotensin-converting enzyme inhibitor has strong mechanistic attraction. Nifedipine, an arteriolar vasodilator and calcium blocking drug also shows promise.

Treatment of Hypertension in the Elderly

Decisions regarding treatment of hypertension in the elderly cannot be based on the results of comparative trials since such trials have not yet been reported. Tolerance of antihypertensive medications declines with age. Nevertheless, patients over age 65 years with diastolic pressures equal to or greater than 95 mmHg or with systolic pressures equal to or greater than 180 mmHg should receive treatment. Lower threshold pressures may be applicable to patients with concomitant cardiac failure since reduction of afterload may markedly improve the cardiac function of the failing heart.

Treatment of Hypertensive Emergencies

In patients with accelerated hypertension it is urgent to lower blood pressure to halt the acute vascular damage due to the raised pressure. The drugs used are similar to those employed in long-term therapy; however, it may be necessary to use more than one drug from the outset to achieve an effective lowering of blood pressure. Once control of the acute situation has been attained, it may be possible to simplify the drugs required for long-term therapy.

Even more unusual are hypertensive emergencies in which it may be important to lower blood pressure in a matter of minutes or hours rather than days. Conditions of this kind include the following:

1. Hypertensive encephalopathy and malignant hypertension
2. Hypertension and dissecting aneurysm
3. Hypertension and acute pulmonary edema
4. Preeclampsia and eclampsia

In these conditions the acute damage is directly related to the elevated pressure, and reduction of pressure must be prompt. Many agents are available but two appear to be most useful because of their potency and predictability. Nitroprusside given intravenously with careful regulation of the rate of infusion is probably the most useful drug, provided there are adequate facilities for continuous monitoring of the patient. The onset of effect is instantaneous, and the effect is evanescent so that pressure returns to its previous level within 2 minutes of stopping the infusion. The second useful drug is diazoxide. This drug can be given by intermittent intravenous injections in increasing amounts at 5 to 10 minute intervals until the desired effect is achieved or until a dose of 300 mg is reached. The maximum effect is usually achieved in 3 to 5 minutes and there is a slow rise in pressure to previous levels within 6 to 12 hours. The initial dose should be small (50 to 100 mg) to identify those individuals who are very sensitive to the drug. In the initial phase of treatment combinations of drugs should be avoided to reduce the risk of an excessive lowering of blood pressure, which can occur due to unpredictable interactions. If diazoxide is continued for more than 24 hours, a saluretic will be required to overcome the sodium-retaining effects of the drug.

If a predominant manifestation of the hypertensive emergency is pulmonary edema, reducing venous return to the heart may result in a reduction of blood pressure. Furosemide is a useful agent. If antihypertensive therapy is also required, nitroprusside, diazoxide, or alternative drugs should be used with extra caution because of the possibility of combined effects with furosemide.

Hypertensive emergencies requiring immediate blood-pressure lowering are rare relative to the number of patients with diastolic pressures of 130 mmHg or greater seen in emergency departments. In hypertensive patients who have suffered a stroke it is not unusual to observe a transient increase in blood pressure. Except in cases of intracranial bleeding, rapid reduction of blood pressure may compromise blood flow and further ischemic damage may occur. Such patients usually respond to bedrest and continuation of their usual antihypertensive medications.

HYPERTENSION SECONDARY TO ENDOCRINE DISEASE

ADRENAL CORTEX

The adrenal cortex produces three hormones that enhance sodium-potassium exchange across a variety of cell membranes including the distal tubular cells of the kidney. These are aldosterone, corticosterone, and deoxycorticosterone (DOC). This effect at distal tubular sites in the kidney results in sodium retention, extracellular fluid volume expansion, and suppression of renin secretion by the kidney. Since sodium is retained in an amount slightly in excess of water, the serum sodium in patients with mineralocorticoid hypertension tends to be at the upper limit of normal. Continued accumulation of sodium, however, does not occur, since a variety of ill-defined volume control mechanisms permit the kidney to escape from the full effects of the increased mineralocorticoids. Edema, therefore, is unusual. Disorders characterized by an increased secretion of mineralocorticoids are characterized by elevated arterial pressures, although the hypertension is rarely severe. Although the hypertension is related to the retention of sodium, the mechanisms by which blood pressure is increased are not clear. Initially, volume expansion may be important, but if the condition persists an increase in the peripheral resistance is observed. Potassium loss occurs in exchange for the sodium retained by the distal tubular cells, and probably as well through the same escape mechanism that reduces sodium reabsorption in the proximal tubule. This potassium loss is responsible for most of the clinical features of mineralocorticoid excess: loss of concentrating ability of the kidney, with polyuria and polydipsia; hypokalemic metabolic alkalosis; muscle fatigue and weakness; and electrocardiographic signs of hypokalemia, such as prominent U waves or ectopic rhythms. The alkalosis may predispose to signs of tetany.

Mineralocorticoid hypertension occurs in the following situations (see Chapter 13):

1. Primary hyperaldosteronism
2. Cushing's syndrome
3. Congenital adrenal hyperplasia with (a) corticosterone excess due to 17-α-hydroxylase deficiency, or (b) deoxycorticosterone excess due to 11-β-hydroxylase deficiency
4. Exogenous administration of corticosteroids, carbenoxolone, or excess intake of licorice

In the absence of iatrogenic causes, the most common form of mineralocorticoid hypertension is primary hyperaldosteronism due to a unilateral adrenal adenoma or, more rarely, to bilateral cortical nodular hyperplasia. Primary hyperaldosteronism is found in less than 1 percent of patients with hypertension. The possibility of hyperaldosteronism should be considered in all hypertensive subjects having unexplained hypokalemia, which can be precipitated easily by another factor such as moderate diarrhea, diuretic agents, or sodium loading. Additional support for the possibility is the finding of a high urinary potassium loss (greater than 60 mmol/24 hours) in the face of hypokalemia and the absence of other kaliuretic influences. In light of these findings, estimation of plasma renin activity can be very useful. If plasma renin is normal or high, or if it rises after intravascular volume reduction or ambulation, primary hyperaldosteronism is ruled out. Low renin activity or low renin responsiveness is suggestive but not diagnostic of hyperaldosteronism, since about 20 percent of patients with essential hypertension show these changes. Primary hyperaldosteronism is distinguished from secondary hyperaldosteronism by the finding of a normal or high circulatory renin activity in the secondary form. In the face of the finding of low renin activity, the diagnosis of primary hyperaldosteronism can only be confirmed by measurement of aldosterone secretion and the response to suppression of secretion by saline loading, or other maneuvers. Localization of an adenoma causing hyperaldosteronism can be achieved by computerized axial tomography or adrenal venography. The latter technique also permits collection of effluent blood from the adrenal gland so that measurements of aldosterone can be made. If there are no lateralizing signs, primary hyperaldosteronism is probably due to bilateral cortical hyperplasia. The treatment of choice for an adrenal adenoma is surgical removal, while hyperplasia is best treated medically with salt restriction and the aldosterone antagonist spironolactone.

Other forms of mineralocorticoid hypertension are rare. In some patients with Cushing's syndrome, increased amounts of deoxycorticosterone are secreted; however, in many patients no excess of mineralocorticoids can be demonstrated, and renin activity is usually normal. Further, glucocorticoid-induced hypertension occurs when salt retention is prevented. Therefore some factor other than sodium retention is instrumental in the pathogenesis of the hypertension of Cushing's syndrome. ACTH infusions can result in the secretion of unusual steroids, including dihydroxyprogesterone, which can produce blood pressure elevation without sodium retention. It appears likely that dihydroxyprogesterone or other unusual steroids are responsible for the elevated pressures observed in Cushing's syndrome.

ESTROGEN AND PROGESTERONE-INDUCED HYPERTENSION

A small increase in blood pressure occurs in most women receiving estrogens, and a few women show marked rises in pressures and even malignant hypertension. Less is known about the influence of progesterone, but synthetic progesterone can be shown to have a sodium-retaining effect that could unmask or aggravate hypertension. Hypertension induced by oral contraceptive medications is said to be the most common secondary cause of hypertension discovered in general practice. The mechanism of the elevation of blood pressure is not known, nor is the importance known of the increase in plasma renin substrate induced by estrogens. The effect of estrogen and progesterone on blood pressure may take several months to become evident and several months to dissipate following cessation of the drugs.

ADRENAL MEDULLA

The catecholamines, adrenaline, and noradrenaline are secreted by the adrenal medulla. Normally, the adrenal medulla is the only source of adrenaline, whereas the predominant source of noradrenaline is the sympathetic nerve endings. Noradrenaline is a potent pressor substance causing hypertension by vasoconstriction of skin and splanchnic arterioles (and veins) secondary to alpha-adrenergic stimulation as well as by an increase in cardiac stroke volume due to beta-adrenergic cardiac stimulation. Adrenaline, alone, induces a rise in systolic pressure due to cardiac stimulation, although at low concentrations diastolic pressure may fall secondary to dilatation of skeletal muscle arterioles (beta-adrenergic stimulation). At higher doses the peripheral alpha-adrenergic effect of adrenaline may supervene, causing an increase in total peripheral resistance. The catecholamines have important metabolic effects, including glycogenolysis and acceleration of breakdown of triglycerides to form free fatty acids. In addition the catecholamines cause changes in mental function and sweating. Tumors of the adrenal medulla or of the neuroectodermal tissue (located usually at sites of sympathetic ganglia) secrete excessive amounts of adrenaline and noradrenaline. Neuroblastomas and more primitive types of tumor often secrete, in addition, large quantities of the precursors dopa, dopamine, and their metabolites. Pheochromocytomas are the most frequently offending tumors, with 85 percent located in the adrenal medulla. The remaining pheochromocytomas are located chiefly near the abdominal aorta, with rare tumors arising in the urinary bladder, near the aortic arch, or in the central nervous system. Fifteen percent of tumors are multiple and 10 percent are malignant.

Most pheochromocytomas result in the intermittent secretion of both adrenaline and noradrenaline, producing characteristic paroxysms of adrenergic symptoms of sweating, palpitations, throbbing headache, and pallor, with systolic and diastolic hypertension. The release of adrenaline results in a catabolic state, so that characteristically the patient when directly questioned will admit having had weight loss. Central nervous system symptoms of anxiety and tremulousness may be prominent. Blood sugar is usually elevated. An associated cholelithiasis has been recognized in 25 percent of cases; however, the explanation of this association is not clear.

Unfortunately, some tumors do not produce the characteristic intermittent symptoms but instead induce sustained hypertension. If the principal secretory product is noradrenaline, as may be the case in tumors located outside the adrenal medulla, metabolic symptoms may be absent, and if dopamine and other precursors are present in large amounts, postural hypotension may be the presenting complaint. Other patients without measurable dopa or dopamine may suffer postural hypotension, presumably due to the relative intravascular volume depletion that sometimes accompanies the hypertension of pheochromocytoma. Pheochromocytoma may be seen in association with neurofibromatosis and multiple endocrine neoplasms.

All patients with hypertension who have any symptoms suggestive of paroxysmal attacks of adrenergic symptoms, such as weight loss, excessive sweats, anxiety, tremulousness, or changes in mood or affect, should be screened for pheochromocytoma. The most useful screening tests are measurements of catecholamines or their breakdown products in the urine. Urine vanillylmandelic acid measurements will be falsely negative in 30 percent of cases. Methyldopa, monoamine oxidase inhibitors, clofibrate, and nalidixic acid can interfere with the test, producing false negative results, while stress and exogenous catecholamines (nose drops)can cause false positives. Measurements of urinary metanephrines are associated with 5 percent false negatives, but false positive results can be due to stress, exogenous catecholamines, methyldopa, monoamine oxidase inhibitors, and chlorpromazine. Methylglucamine, an ingredient of many x-ray contrast materials, may cause a false negative result. Pharmacologic tests are now very rarely necessary to provide confirmation of a pheochromocytoma. Computerized axial tomography has provided a very useful means of anatomically localizing the tumor.

Although pheochromocytoma probably causes hypertension in less than 0.4 percent of subjects with elevated pressures, the cost to the individual of a missed diagnosis is very high. This justifies the use of urinary vanillylmandelic acid and/or urinary metanephrine screening measurements in all hypertensive individuals with severe hypertension, as well as in those who have any symptoms conceivably related to excess catecholamines.

OTHER ENDOCRINE CAUSES

Hypercalcemia due to vitamin D excess or hyperparathyroidism is associated with systolic and diastolic hypertension that does not always resolve with correction of the hypercalcemia. The mechanism is unknown. Multiple endocrine neoplasms (MEN) can include parathyroid, pituitary, and pancreatic islet-cell tumors (type 1), or hyperparathyroidism, medullary carcinoma of the thyroid, and pheochromocytoma (type 2). Patients with these rare conditions may present with hypertension.

COARCTATION OF THE AORTA

Narrowing of the aorta due to a coarctation results in a reduction in the size of the chamber that is immediately available to receive the stroke output of the heart. This probably explains the systolic and diastolic hypertension observed in coarctation, as well as rarer conditions reducing the aortic lumen such as Takayasu's disease. Renin activity has been variably reported as normal or increased in subjects with aortic coarctation, and in some patients a reduction in pulsatile blood flow to the kidney result-

ing in increased renin release may contribute to the hypertension. In longstanding coarctation, total peripheral resistance is increased, but the mechanism responsible for this change is unclear.

The diagnosis of coarctation must be considered in all young hypertensive patients, and the diagnosis should be made clinically. Careful assessment should be made for the characteristic radial-femoral pulse delay, pulsating collateral vessels around the scapulae and posterior intercostal spaces, and a bruit heard over the left scapula. Chest x-ray will show notching of the inferior margin of the ribs due to collateral vessels and sometimes left ventricular hypertrophy or pre- and post-stenotic aortic dilatation.

RENAL CAUSES

The kidney can be responsible for hypertension in two major ways. Renal parenchymal disease is one of the most common causes of secondary hypertension. In most instances the disease is bilateral and the most important hemodynamic abnormality responsible for the elevated pressure is sodium retention due to the inability of the kidney to excrete a "normal" intake of salt at "normal" levels of pressure. In many instances levels of renin activity are excessive, relative to the increased extracellular fluid volume. Blood pressure can usually be controlled by salt restriction and diuretics, although often the more potent loop diuretics such as furosemide must be used to obtain a diuresis. In chronic renal failure, hemodialysis or peritoneal dialysis most frequently corrects the elevated pressures, although in a few instances such volume-reducing maneuvers result in an increase in pressure. In such patients the elevated pressures are largely determined by an inappropriately high renin activity. The most frequent causes of hypertension due to renal parenchymal disease include the following (see Chapter 11):

1. Acute post-streptococcal glomerulonephritis
2. Chronic glomerulonephritis or pyelonephritis—the "end-stage" kidney
3. Diabetic glomerulonephritis
4. Polycystic kidney disease

Unilateral renal disease has been associated with hypertension, although the association is less definite and the mechanisms less well understood than with bilateral disease. A unilateral shrunken kidney in most instances represents the end result of an acquired disease such as unilateral pyelonephritis; in some cases unilateral nephrectomy has resulted in control of hypertension. Such a therapeutic approach should only be considered if medical therapy has failed. If the contralateral kidney is of normal rather than increased size, bilateral renal disease is probably present. Unilateral hydronephrosis has occasionally been associated with hypertension, and amelioration of the hypertension has been achieved in some patients through relieving the obstruction. In some cases of unilateral shrunken kidney and unilateral obstructive disease, high renin activity can be demonstrated, but this is not a universal finding. Cysts can compress renal vessels or renal tissue, causing ischemia with ensuing renin release. Vascular tumors (hemangiopericytomata) and very rarely Wilm's tumors can cause hypertension through production of renin by the tumor. Such patients usually have hypokalemic alkalosis and high aldosterone levels.

The second major renal cause of hypertension is renovascular hypertension. The mechanisms of hypertension following narrowing of a renal artery have been intensively studied. Upon constriction, renal perfusion on the affected side is reduced, and even before there is a fall in glomerular filtration rate there is an increase in tubular reabsorption of salt and water. Urine from the affected kidney is reduced in volume and has a lower salt content than that from the normal side. At the same time, renin content of the renal vein of the affected kidney rises. Blood pressure increases largely because of the increased release of renin.

These functional abnormalities have given rise to a variety of tests for determining the presence of renovascular hypertension. Since most depend on comparison with the contralateral kidney they are most helpful if the disorder is unilateral. These observations, or tests, include the following findings:

1. A more dense and persistent appearance of contrast material on the affected side during intravenous pyelogram
2. A slowed rise in isotopic activity on the affected side during isotope renography, and a slower fall because of the lower flow rate
3. Increased concentration of renin in the renal vein of the affected side
4. Decreased concentration of sodium relative to creatinine in the urine from the affected side

The first two tests are useful noninvasive tests applicable in screening hypertensive subjects in whom a renovascular cause is suspected. The latter two tests are more predictive, but are subject to a variety of technical errors. If a functional abnormality is confirmed the diagnosis is not complete without demonstration of an anatomic lesion, usually with a renal arteriogram.

Since the mechanism responsible for elevated pressures in renovascular hypertension is almost always related to an increased release in renin, attempts have been made to use angiotensin antagonists to assess whether or not the hypertension is renin dependent, and therefore more likely to be renal in origin. Saralasin, a competitive antagonist of angiotensin II, has been studied extensively, but at present it is unreliable in screening patients for possible renovascular causes of hypertension.

A variety of disorders causing renal artery narrowing are responsible for renovascular hypertension. These include the following:

1. Atherosclerosis
2. Fibromuscular hyperplasia
3. Congenital stenosis
4. Extrinsic pressure by tumor, or fibromuscular bands
5. Thrombi or emboli

Atherosclerotic narrowing is the most common lesion causing hypertension in the elderly. Overall, the results of surgical correction of such lesions do not differ from the results of medical therapy, so that a conservative approach to searching for renovascular hypertension in the elderly is appropriate. A mortality rate in surgically treated elderly patients of 9 percent can be expected. In younger patients the most common lesions are dysplasias of fibrous or muscular tissue of the renal arteries. Although the adventitia and intima may be selectively involved, the most common site affected is the media, and the most common change consists of thickened fibromuscular ridges that create a "string of beads" appearance, particularly in the distal 2/3 of the main renal artery and often progressing into the major branches. This medial fibromuscular dysplasia is most common in women under the age of 40 years, and lesions are frequently bilateral. In contrast with the outcome seen with atherosclerotic lesions, the results of surgery for these lesions are good, with a cure rate in selected patients of over 90 percent.

The high cost of diagnosing renovascular causes of hypertension and the disappointing results of surgery in the atherosclerotic group have led, correctly, to limiting the use of screening investigations for renovascular hypertension to a small group of patients. Screening of this kind is generally now reserved for younger patients with severe hypertension or with a recent acceleration of their hypertension.

REFERENCES

1. Esler, M., Julius, S., Zweiffer, A., et al: Mild high-renin essential hypertension: neurogenic human hypertension? N. Engl. J. Med. 296:405, 1977. Haber, E.:

The role of renin in normal and pathological cardiovascular homeostasis. Circulation 54:849, 1976.

2. Fries, E.D., Arias, L.A., Armstrong, M.L. et al: Veterans administration cooperative study group on antihypertensive agents: effects of treatment on morbidity in hypertension: results in patients with diastolic blood pressures averaging 115 through 129 mmHg. JAMA 202:1028, 1967.

3. Genest, J., Koiv, E., Kuchel, O. (eds): Hypertension, Physiopathology and Treatment. New York, McGraw-Hill, 1977.

4. Hypertension Detection and Follow-Up Program Cooperative Group: Five-year findings of the hypertension detection and follow-up program. I. Reduction in mortality of persons with high blood pressure, including mild hypertension. JAMA 242:2562, 1979.

5. Hypertension Detection and Follow-up Program Cooperative Group: The effect of treatment on mortality in "mild" hypertension. N. Engl. J. Med. 307:976, 1982.

6. Swales, J.D.: Clinical Hypertension. Chicago, Year Book Medical Publishers, 1979.

4

Clotting and Bleeding Disorders

Jack Hirsh, M.D.

Part 1: Thrombosis and Embolism

A thrombus is an intravascular deposit composed of fibrin and formed blood elements. The relative proportion of the formed elements in thrombi differs from that in blood because their accumulation is partly selective. Thrombosis occurs in four major sites: the veins, the arteries, the microcirculation, and the heart. The pathogenesis, the structure, and the complications of thrombi in each of these sites differ considerably. In part 1 of this chapter, the pathogenesis, epidemiology, clinical manifestations, and management of venous thromboembolism will be discussed in detail, but thrombi occurring at the other three sites will be mentioned only briefly, since their clinical manifestations and complications are discussed elsewhere in this book.

VENOUS THROMBOEMBOLISM

Venous thromboembolism (venous thrombosis resulting in pulmonary embolism) is a serious disorder that usually complicates the course of sick, hospitalized patients but occasionally affects ambulant and otherwise healthy individuals. Pulmonary embolism has been estimated to account for 200,000 deaths each year in the United States. An even larger number of patients suffer from nonfatal venous thromboembolic disease, which causes considerable

morbidity and prolongs hospital stay in its acute phase, and is responsible for the postphlebitic syndrome, which is a long-term complication of extensive acute venous thrombosis.

VENOUS THROMBOSIS

Pathogenesis

The formation, growth, and dissolution of venous thrombi and pulmonary emboli represents a balance between the various thrombogenic stimuli that an individual is exposed to and a number of protective mechanisms. The factors that predispose to venous thrombosis are activation of blood coagulation, vascular damage, and stasis (Table 4.1). The protective mechanisms include the inactivation of activated coagulation factors by circulating inhibitors, clearance of activated coagulation factors by the reticuloendothelial cells of the liver, and dissolution of fibrin by a variety of fibrinolytic enzymes derived from plasma, endothelial cells, and circulating leukocytes.

Thrombogenic Factors

Activation of blood coagulation The process of blood coagulation follows a series of complex steps that terminate in the formation of a fibrin clot. (These are described in Hemostasis, part 2 of this chapter.)

Tissue thromboplastin is released into the blood stream during surgery and following tissue injury, and is probably made available locally by vessel-wall

Table 4.1 **Causes of Venous Stasis**

1. Immobilization
2. Raised central venous pressure
3. Extrinsic venous pressure
4. Intraluminal obstruction due to old venous thrombosis
5. Venous dilatation

cells at sites of vascular damage and by activated leukocytes that migrate to areas of vascular damage. Factor XII is activated on contact with subendothelial tissues exposed to circulating blood as a result of vascular injury.

Vessel damage The normal intact endothelium is nonthrombogenic and neither reacts with platelets nor with blood coagulation proteins.

When a vessel is damaged, there is endothelial loss and exposure of subendothelium that reacts with both platelets and the blood coagulation system. Platelets and leukocytes rapidly accumulate in the subendothelium at sites of endothelial loss, and the blood coagulation mechanism is activated. Platelets adhere to a number of components of the subendothelium, including collagen and basement membrane. These adhering platelets release adenosine diphosphate and thromboxane A_2 (which is a product of platelet prostaglandin synthesis), and aggregate under the influence of these two agents. This process of platelet aggregation is associated with a change in the platelet membrane that facilitates blood coagulation on the membrane's surface and so accelerates thrombin generation and fibrin formation.

Vascular damage produced by mechanical trauma is important in the pathogenesis of venous thrombosis that occurs in patients who have major orthopedic surgery to the lower limbs. Venous damage almost invariably results when patients suffer trauma to a lower limb. It is also possible that calf veins are subjected to external pressure and subtle injury in patients who lie in bed for prolonged periods and so may contribute to the calf vein thrombosis in some immobilized patients.

Stasis Stasis predisposes to venous thrombosis by preventing clearance of activated coagulation factors by the liver. Venous return from the limbs is greatly enhanced by contraction of calf muscles, which act as a peripheral venous pump that propels blood from the deep veins of the calf in the direction of the heart. During recumbancy, the soleal sinuses are dependent and dilated with blood, particularly if drainage into the deep veins of the calf is sluggish. Venous stasis also occurs as a result of interference of venous return (in patients with heart failure), or as a consequence of venous obstruction caused by extrinsic compression by a pregnant uterus or a pelvic mass, by the iliac artery crossing the left iliac vein, or by an intraluminal obstruction due to previous venous thrombosis. Stasis also occurs in patients with venous dilatation due to varicose veins, particularly in elderly patients if they are bedridden, in pregnant women, and in individuals who are taking pills containing estrogen.

Reduced Inhibitory or Clearance Mechanisms

Inactivation of activated coagulation factors by circulating inhibitors Activated coagulation factors are proteolytic enzymes with the amino acid serine at their active site. These serine proteases are inhibited by a number of naturally occurring protease inhibitors. Of these, antithrombin III is the most important, since it inhibits a number of activated coagulation factors and is responsible for most of the antithrombin activity in plasma. The rate of inhibition of activated coagulation factors by antithrombin III is markedly accelerated by heparin.

Hepatic inactivation and clearance of activated clotting factors The liver removes activated coagulation factors from the blood. Thrombosis has been reported following infusion of concentrates of Factors II, VII, IX, and X in patients with liver disease. These concentrates contain a small amount of activated coagulation factors that, in patients with liver disease, may not be adequately cleared and so may lead to thrombosis.

Fibrinolytic system Clot lyses takes place actively by enzymatic action (see Part 2 Hemostasis.)

Risk Factors in Thromboembolism

A number of clinical conditions are associated with venous thrombosis, including surgical and nonsurgical trauma, increasing age, malignant disease, immobilization, heart failure, previous venous thrombosis, myocardial infarction, paralysis of the lower limbs, varicose veins, obesity, the use of oral contraceptive pills, and parturition (Table 4.2). Relatively uncommon disorders that may be complicated by venous thrombosis include systemic lupus erythematosus, polycythemia vera, and homocystinemia.

A number of laboratory abnormalities have also been identified that predispose patients to venous thrombosis. Some of these are longstanding abnormalities that may be inherited and others are transient acute changes that occur in response to tissue injury or intravascular coagulation.

Longstanding Abnormalities

Decreased antithrombin III activity Antithrombin III is an important coagulation inhibitor. It inhibits activated Factors XII, XI, IX, X, and thrombin, and the rate of its inhibition of these enzymes is markedly increased by heparin. Approximately 75 percent of the plasma antithrombin activity is derived from antithrombin III, which is the only inhibitor that is diminished during blood coagulation.

There have been a number of reports of idiopathic and secondary venous thrombosis occurring in families with a deficiency of antithrombin III. The trait is inherited in an autosomal dominant manner, and affected patients have antithrombin III levels at 40 to 60 percent of normal. Although it is difficult to obtain exact figures on the risk of thrombosis in affected individuals, review of the literature indicates that over 50 percent of affected individuals develop thromboembolic events before the age of 50 years. The thromboembolic events may be spontaneous, may occur during pregnancy, or may arise when the patient is exposed to high-risk states such as surgery, trauma, or an acute medical illness.

Thrombocytosis There are anecdotal reports indicating that patients with persistent thrombocytosis associated with either myeloproliferative disorders or postsplenectomy have an increased risk of thromboembolic events. This risk appears to be limited to patients who have an unsuccessful splenectomy for hemolytic anemia or an inappropriate splenectomy for sideroblastic anemia or myelofibrosis.

Polycythemia Patients with polycythemia rubra vera have an increased risk of arterial and venous thromboembolic events. It is likely that both the increased blood viscosity associated with the high hematocrit and the thrombocytosis that frequently occurs in this disorder contribute to the thrombotic tendency. Erythrocytosis per se associated with cyanotic congenital heart disease has also been reported

to predispose patients to pulmonary arterial thrombosis, but the evidence for this association is more tenuous.

Reduced fibrinolytic activity A number of clinical studies have reported a possible association between defective fibrinolysis and thrombosis. Decreased fibrinolytic activity has been reported to occur in patients taking oral contraceptives, in women in the last trimester of pregnancy, in patients with malignant disease, and in obese individuals. A proportion of patients with recurrent superficial and deep venous thrombosis have reduced fibrinolytic activity, measured either as a vessel-wall plasminogen activator from biopsy of superficial veins or as circulating plasminogen activator. In uncontrolled studies, treatment of some of these patients with anabolic steroids has been reported to both increase fibrinolytic activity and reduce the frequency of episodes of recurrent venous thrombosis.

Pathology

Venous thrombi usually form in regions of slow or disturbed flow, and begin as small deposits that frequently occur in the large venous sinuses in the calf, in valve cusp pockets in either the deep veins of the calf or the thigh, or in venous segments that have been exposed to direct trauma.

These initial deposits may be composed either of masses of platelet aggregates (white thrombi) or of fibrin with interspersed red cells that have only a small platelet component (red thrombi). Their composition is influenced by the nature of the throm-

Table 4.2 **Clinical Conditions with High Risk of Thromboembolism**

	Risk of Thrombosis	Recommended Prophylaxis
Genito-urinary		
Surgery		
Transurethral	7–10%	External pneumatic compression*
Abdominal	5–25%	
Neurosurgery	20–25%	External pneumatic compression*
Orthopedic		
Elective hip	40–60%	Oral anticoagulants commencing postoperatively or Dextran
Fractured hip	40–60%	Oral anticoagulants commencing postoperatively
Major knee surgery	60–70%	External pneumatic compression*
Major trauma to lower limbs	50%	External pneumatic compression or Dextran or Oral anticoagulants after patient has stabilized
Myocardial Infarction	20–40%	Low dose heparin* or full dose heparin or oral anticoagulants
Stroke	60%	Intermittent pneumatic compression or low dose heparin
Other high risk medical groups		Low dose heparin

* Efficacy demonstrated by clinical trial.

bogenic stimulus; fibrin–red-cell thrombi form in areas of stasis, while platelet thrombi form at sites of vessel damage.

When the nidus of the thrombus grows out of the valve pockets, it propogates in the direction of flow. A nidus of this kind is composed of a mixture of platelets and fibrin. If the thrombus occludes the lumen, further propogation occurs in the form of a red coagulation thrombus composed of red cells and interspersed fibrin.

The underlying vein wall varies considerably in its reaction to thrombosis. In some instances there is only minimal vessel involvement with focal elevation of underlying endothelium and occasional clumps of granulocytes, while in others there is a marked inflammatory change with edema of the vessel wall, infiltration with granulocytes, and massive loss of endothelium. In some circumstances, this marked inflammatory reaction may be the cause of venous thrombosis, but it is likely that this reaction occurs as a consequence of thrombosis in most instances. A number of mediators of the inflammatory reaction are generated by the various blood components incorporated in the thrombus, and may contribute to its development and clinical manifestations.

The pain, tenderness, and swelling that occur in acute deep-vein thrombosis can be explained by the local inflammation at the site of thrombosis and by the venous distension and raised venous pressure that occur as a result of proximal obstruction.

Natural History

The fate of venous thrombi is determined by the balance between factors that promote further deposition and factors that lead to removal (Table 4.3). Thrombi may extend, undergo lysis, become organized, or embolize. Complete spontaneous lysis of large thrombi is a relatively uncommon event; even when patients with venous thrombosis are treated with heparin to prevent further deposition, complete lysis occurs in less than 20 percent of cases.

***Table 4.3* Factors Influencing Natural History of Venous Thrombosis**

Extension	Removal
1. Persisting thrombogenic stimulus.	1. Fibrinolysis (by plasma or cellular fibrinolytic system).
2. Severe endothelial damage.	2. Organization.
3. Stasis due to venous obstruction by the thrombus.	3. Embolization.

Pulmonary embolism is commonly associated with venous thrombosis. If the thrombus that becomes embolized is small (which is frequently the case when it arises in the calf), it usually produces no clinical manifestations. But if the embolized thrombus is large, it frequently produces clinical symptoms.

Most clinically significant emboli arise from thrombi in the proximal veins of the leg (popliteal, femoral, or iliac veins), although large thrombi of the calf vein may also produce clinically symptomatic emboli occasionally. Fatal pulmonary emboli usually arise from large thrombi in the proximal veins, but even relatively small emboli may prove fatal in patients whose cardiopulmonary function is already compromised.

Thrombi that do not embolize or that undergo slow dissolution tend to organize and may recanalize, thereby predisposing patients to the postphlebitic syndrome or to recurrent acute venous thrombosis.

Clinical Manifestations

The majority of patients who develop venous thrombi have no clinical manifestations. When symptoms or signs of venous thrombosis occur, they are caused by obstruction of venous outflow, by inflammation of the vessel wall or perivascular tissue, by a combination of these two factors, or by embolization of the thrombus into the pulmonary circulation. The more common clinical symptoms and signs of venous thrombosis are discussed below. None are specific for venous thrombosis because all can be caused by other pathological processes involving the lower limbs or pelvis.

Pain and Tenderness

Pain and tenderness are the most common clinical manifestations of venous thrombosis, and are probably caused by local inflammation of the vein wall or perivascular tissue or by venous distension. Typically, these symptoms improve after a few days of bedrest and treatment, particularly with elevation of the leg, but may recur during early mobilization.

Swelling

Swelling is due to edema that may be caused either by obstruction of large proximal veins or by inflammation of perivascular tissues. The swelling may be marked, and may be associated with obvious pitting edema; or it may be mild, and may be detected only as increased tissue turgor of the calf muscles, most readily appreciated by careful palpation of the relaxed calf.

Venous Distension, Prominence of Subcutaneous Vessels

Venous distension and prominence of subcutaneous vessels is a relatively uncommon manifestation of acute venous thrombosis.

Discoloration

Discoloration is a relatively uncommon and nonspecific manifestation of venous thrombosis. The leg may be pale, cyanosed, or a reddish purple in color. Marked palor may occur in the early stages of acute iliofemoral vein thrombosis, and is thought to be caused by arterial spasm. Cyanosis is caused by impaired venous return and stagnant anoxia, occuring in patients with obstructive iliofemoral vein thrombosis. Rarely, the leg may be diffusely red, hot, and inflamed due to marked perivascular inflammation, and when this occurs venous thrombosis may be difficult to differentiate from cellulitis.

Phlegmasia cerula dolens is the term used to describe the marked swelling and cyanosis that occurs with obstructive iliofemoral vein thrombosis. The obstruction to flow may impair arterial inflow and so produce marked tissue ischemia. The leg is very painful, swollen, cyanosed, and may be covered with multiple petechial hemorrhages. The patient may be hypotensive due to marked pooling of blood in the affected leg, and there may be a mild thrombocytopenia due, probably, to platelet consumption. These features usually subside gradually when the patient is treated with heparin and confined to bed with the leg elevated. Occasionally, however, the cyanosis may progress to venous gangrene if the obstruction is not removed immediately by thrombectomy.

Palpable Cord

When a vessel that is easily palpable becomes thrombosed, it may be felt as an obvious cord. This is not a common sign, and it does not differentiate acute venous thrombosis from longstanding disease.

Diagnosis

Clinical Diagnosis

The clinical diagnosis of venous thrombosis is both insensitive and nonspecific. It is now well recognized that patients without symptoms or with relatively minor symptoms and signs can have extensive venous thrombosis, while those with overt clinical features suggestive of deep vein thrombosis frequently have no objective evidence of thrombosis.

Clinical diagnosis is insensitive because many dangerous thrombi do not cause complete obstruction to venous outflow and are not associated with vessel wall inflammation. The clinical diagnosis is nonspecific because many other disorders produce pain and swelling in the leg that simulate venous thrombosis.

Because the clinical manifestations of venous thrombosis are not specific, the diagnosis should be confirmed by tests that clearly establish whether venous thrombosis is present.

Diagnosis Using Objective Tests

The objective diagnostic tests that have been adequately evaluated are venography, plethysmography, Doppler ultrasound, and ^{125}I-fibrinogen leg scanning.

Venography   is the most definitive method currently available, and, if adequately performed and interpreted, it can be used to reliably confirm or exclude the diagnosis in patients with clinically suspected venous thrombosis. The external iliac veins and common iliac veins are not always well visualized by ascending venography and so femoral venography may be required occasionally to exclude isolated iliac vein thrombosis.

Venography has a number of disadvantages. It is invasive, it produces pain, it may induce clinically significant phlebitis in a small percentage of patients, and it is expensive and time consuming. For these reasons, venography has been replaced or supplemented in many centers by noninvasive testing in patients with clinically suspected venous thrombosis.

Impedance plethysmography (IPG)   is sensitive and specific for proximal vein thrombosis in symptomatic patients but is insensitive for calf vein thrombosis. In patients with clinically suspected venous thrombosis, a positive IPG result can be used to make therapeutic decisions in the absence of clinical conditions known to produce false-positive results. A normal result essentially excludes a diagnosis of proximal vein thrombosis but does not exclude calf vein thrombosis. False-positive results may occur with disorders that interfere with arterial inflow or venous outflow. These include severe congestive cardiac failure, constrictive pericarditis, severe arterial insufficiency, hypotension, and external compression of veins. Most of these disorders are readily recognized on clinical grounds. False-positive results may also occur if the technician performs the test incorrectly or if the patient is not relaxed. The test cannot be performed in some patients, for example, those who are in a plaster cast or who cannot be adequately positioned because of immobilization or pain

Doppler ultrasound is sensitive for symptomatic proximal vein thrombosis but relatively insensitive for calf vein thrombosis. Its major drawback is that its interpretation is subjective and requires considerable skill and experience. However, in skilled hands, it is almost as sensitive for symptomatic proximal vein thrombosis as is IPG. Doppler ultrasound is more specific than IPG in patients with raised venous pressure or arterial insufficiency, and it can be used in patients who have their legs in plaster or who are in traction.

^{125}**I-fibrinogen leg scanning** detects calf vein thrombi and thrombi in the distal half of the thigh that are actively accumulating fibrin. False-positive results occur if scanning is performed over a hematoma or a large wound, over an area of inflammation, or if there is very extensive edema, but in the absence of these conditions leg scanning is both sensitive and specific for acute calf and lower thigh vein thrombosis. Leg scanning should not be used as the only diagnostic test in patients with clinically suspected venous thrombosis because it fails to detect thrombi in approximately 30 percent of patients (many of which are thrombi in the iliac vein), and because there may be a delay before a sufficient amount of fibrinogen accumulates in the thrombus to make the test positive; a delay of this kind is unacceptable in patients with proximal vein thrombosis. However, leg scanning is a valuable diagnostic test when used to complement IPG in patients with clinically suspected venous thrombosis. In the majority of patients with acute venous thrombosis, the leg scan becomes positive within 24 hours of injection of ^{125}I-fibrinogen, but in some patients with symptomatic acute venous thrombosis it may take 48 or even 72 hours for enough radioactivity to accumulate in the thrombus to permit making a positive diagnosis.

A Practical Approach to Diagnosis

If venography is the only objective test available, it should be performed on all patients with leg symptoms or signs compatible with venous thrombosis. If noninvasive tests are available and applied in an appropriate way, they can be used as a substitute for venography in the majority of these patients. IPG detects over 95 percent of all proximal vein thrombi but it fails to detect 70 to 80 percent of calf vein thrombi. If the IPG is positive in the absence of conditions known to produce false-positive results, a diagnosis of venous thrombosis can be confidently made and the patient can be treated appropriately. If it is negative, however, the patient can be followed up with repeated IPG examinations over the next 6 or 7 days to detect extending calf vein thrombosis, or can be followed by ^{125}I-fibrinogen leg scanning used in the same way as the IPG if the operator is very skilled in its use.

Differential Diagnosis of Symptoms and Signs

Pain and/or Tenderness

Muscle strain or trauma Muscle ache may occur when the leg muscles have been subjected to unusual types or amounts of activity.

Muscle tear Fibers of the gastrocnemius or, less commonly, plantaris muscle may be torn as a result of sudden strong stretching of contracting calf muscles during plantar flexion. When this occurs, the patient experiences a sudden severe pain in the back of the leg, which may simulate a direct blow to the calf muscles. Examination reveals local tenderness, and it may be possible to palpate the localized swelling caused by hematoma.

After a number of days, an ecchymosis may appear either in the posterior aspect of the medial malleolus or in the anteromedial part of the leg, but this is not an invariable finding.

Direct muscle trauma sustained during a vigorous sporting activity or during an accident may produce delayed pain and swelling due to hematoma and inflammation.

Spontaneous muscle hematoma Occasionally, patients who are treated with anticoagulants develop pain and swelling of the leg without obvious trauma or following mild trauma.

Neurogenic pain Compression of the sciatic nerve or lateral cutaneous nerve of the thigh produces leg pain that is easily differentiated from venous thrombosis because of its characteristic distribution.

Ruptured Baker's cyst When a Baker's cyst (popliteal cyst) ruptures, the fluid contents track down the planes between the muscle tissues of the calf and produce an inflammatory response with pain, tenderness, heat, and swelling, which may simulate the clinical features of acute venous thrombosis. In most cases, but not always, there is a history of arthritis of the knee or of traumatic or operative injury to the knee. The diagnosis can be readily established by arthrography, but since venous thrombosis and ruptured Baker's cyst may occur in the same patient, it is necessary to specifically exclude venous thrombosis before attributing the acute clinical features to a ruptured Baker's cyst.

Inflammation of other tissues in the lower limb Lower limb cellulitis, lymphangitis, vasculitis, myositis, and panniculitis may each produce pain and tenderness of the lower limb. These conditions can usually be differentiated from venous thrombosis on clinical grounds alone when they are fully developed, but may occasionally be confused with venous thrombosis in their early stages or if they are atypical.

Varicose veins Patients with varicose veins frequently have pain and tenderness in the calf when they have been standing for a period of time. Occasionally, an obvious superficial varicose vein becomes inflamed and thrombosed and the pain is more severe. When these clinical features occur in association with more diffuse pain in the calf or with edema of the leg, it may be difficult to exclude an associated deep vein thrombosis without performing objective diagnostic tests.

Pregnancy and patients taking oral contraceptives Pain and tenderness in the leg may occur in pregnancy or in individuals taking an oral contraceptive pill containing estrogen. Occasionally, the pain and tenderness in pregnant patients is associated with marked swelling of the calf or the thigh, which may be unilateral. In many cases, these symptoms and signs are not due to venous thrombosis. The cause of pain and tenderness is uncertain but may be due to venous dilatation caused by estrogens, to inflammation of the vein wall without associated thrombosis, or to muscle cramps in pregnant patients. Compression of the iliac vein by the enlarged uterus may contribute to unilateral leg swelling in pregnancy.

Swelling without Associated Pain and Tenderness

A number of conditions other than venous thrombosis can produce edema or swelling of the leg with or without associated pain and tenderness.

Compression of the iliac vein External compression of the iliac vein by tumor, hematoma, or abscess may be impossible to differentiate from acute iliofemoral vein thrombosis on clinical grounds alone. Definitive differentiation between acute venous thrombosis and external compression can be made when the venogram shows either smooth symmetrical indentation characteristic of the external compression, or an intraluminal filling defect characteristic of acute thrombosis.

Compression of the left common iliac vein may produce chronic swelling that is usually painless, or it may produce acute exacerbations of swelling that last for hours or days and then subside. The leg swelling is thought to be due to impaired venous return, which occurs as a result of fibrosis and narrowing of the left common iliac vein where it is crossed by the right iliac artery.

The post phlebitic syndrome Typically, patients with the postphlebitic syndrome have longstanding symptoms of swelling associated with an ache in the calf that occurs on standing or leg exercise. Some of these patients present with repeated episodes of more severe swelling and pain, which may be associated with calf tenderness, and in these patients it may be difficult to exclude a complicating acute venous thrombosis as the cause of the symptoms.

Leg immobilization Swelling not caused by venous thrombosis frequently occurs in patients whose leg has been immobilized soon after removal of the plaster cast or after limb paralysis caused by stroke or spinal cord injury. Many of these episodes of swelling are not caused by venous thrombosis, although it is well recognized that thrombosis frequently complicates leg immobilization. The mechanism of swelling is uncertain but may be due to alterations in venous tone or capillary permeability.

Leg inflammation Inflammatory conditions of the leg such as cellulitis, panniculitis, erythema nodosum, and severe myositis may cause diffuse swelling, but these can usually be differentiated from venous thrombosis because of other associated characteristic features.

Lymphedema Leg swelling is a characteristic feature of impaired lymphatic drainage. In its severest form, lymphedema is nonpitting and brawny, but milder forms of lymphedema may be pitting. When lymphedema occurs as a result of a congenital defect in the lymphatic channels, it is rarely difficult to differentiate from venous thrombosis, but when it is acquired as a result of trauma to the lymphatic vessels, which may occur after hip surgery, leg fracture, or as a consequence of compression of major lymphatic channels by leg plaster, it may be impossible to distinguish it from edema caused by venous obstruction without performing objective tests.

Lipedema   occurs in females and often becomes obvious in adult life. The leg swelling is due to accumulation of subcutaneous fat and is, therefore, chronic and not associated with pitting or signs of inflammation. On examination of the leg it is readily distinguished from edema caused by venous thrombosis.

Self-induced edema   Occasionally, factitious syndromes may simulate venous thrombosis. Pain, tenderness, and swelling may be produced by self-inflicted injury to the legs by application of a venous tourniquet or by other bizarre methods.

Prophylaxis

Two approaches can be used to prevent clinically significant venous thromboembolism: primary prophylaxis, and early detection and treatment of subclinical venous thrombosis. Primary prophylaxis is more effective and less expensive, and is the method of choice in most clinical circumstances.

A number of prophylactic methods have been shown effective in preventing venous thrombosis and pulmonary embolism in well-designed clinical trials (Table 4.4).

Low-Dose Heparin

Low-dose heparin is given subcutaneously in a dose of 5,000 units 2 hours preoperatively and then either every 8 or 12 hours postoperatively. It is important to continue prophylaxis for the entire high-risk period, that is, until the patient is fully ambulant. Low dose heparin is of limited effectiveness in patients who have had hip surgery.

External Pneumatic Compression

External pneumatic compression is a highly effective form of prophylaxis. The intermittent compression device may be applied preoperatively, at operation, or in the early postoperative period, and it should be worn while the patient is in bed for the entire postoperative period.

It is effective in preventing thrombosis in general surgical and neurosurgical patients and in patients having major knee surgery, but it does not appear to be effective in patients with hip surgery. This approach has the advantage that it is not associated with bleeding and can be used with other forms of prophylaxis.

Oral Anticoagulants

Oral anticoagulants given in doses that double the prothrombin time are very effective in preventing both the occurrence of venous thrombi and their extension. This approach is most effective when commenced preoperatively so that there is an anticoagulant effect at the time of operation. However, when used in this way, oral anticoagulant prophylaxis produces an increased risk of bleeding, and most surgeons find this unacceptable. An increased risk of bleeding also occurs when oral anticoagulants are commenced at the time of operation, but this may be reduced to acceptable levels if treatment is commenced 2 or 3 days postoperatively in a dose that prolongs the prothrombin time to 1.5 to 2 times control value on the 5th to 6th postoperative day.

Dextran

Dextran given in volumes of at least 500 ml over a 4 to 6 hour period at the time of operation, and then daily for 2 to 5 days, is an effective form of prophylaxis. The use of dextran is associated with a slight risk of bleeding when commenced at the time of surgery, and may produce circulatory overload, particularly in elderly patients. It is an effective and acceptable form of prophylaxis in patients undergoing general surgical procedures or elective hip surgery.

Choice of Prophylaxis in Various High-Risk Groups

The applicability of different forms of prophylaxis varies among the different high-risk groups. From a practical point of view, the choice of prophylactic agent in any group depends on its efficacy, safety, and feasibility when administered to the group under consideration.

Table 4.4   **Prevention of Venous Thrombosis**

Proven effective prophylactic methods
1. Low dose heparin.
2. Intermittent pneumatic compression.
3. Oral anticoagulant.
4. Dextran.

Promising prophylactic methods which require further study
1. Graduated compression stockings.
2. Electrical stimulation of calf muscles.
3. Aspirin (for orthopedic surgery).
4. Low dose heparin plus dihydroergotamine.

Elective abdominal or thoracic surgery   The risk of venous thromboembolism in patients undergoing elective abdominal or thoracic surgical procedures can be subdivided into three categories depending on the patient's age, the nature and the extent of the operative procedure, and whether there is a history of previous venous thromboembolism. Although there is considerable overlap between these groups, the proposed division is clinically useful (Table 4.5).

In low-risk patients, it would be reasonable to use physical methods, such as graduated compression stockings or early ambulation, as the only form of prophylaxis, unless they develop a complication which requires their continued confinement to bed.

Moderate-risk patients should be treated prophylactically with low-dose heparin or with intermittent pneumatic compression.

Patients in the high-risk group can be treated with a combination of external pneumatic compression and low-dose subcutaneous heparin commencing in the early postoperative period and continuing until the patient is fully ambulant.

Orthopedic surgery and leg and pelvic trauma

Elective hip surgery   Between 40 and 60 percent of patients who have elective hip surgery develop venous thrombosis; 20 percent develop proximal vein thrombosis, and 1 to 2 percent have a fatal pulmonary embolus. Two forms of prophylaxis, oral anticoagulants and dextran, are effective in preventing venous thromboembolism in patients undergoing elective hip replacement. Results with both low-dose heparin and aspirin have been inconsistent.

Fractured hip   Prophylaxis in patients who sustain a fracture of the neck of the femur is even more difficult than in patients having elective hip surgery. The frequency of venous thrombosis in this group of patients is similar to that in patients undergoing elective hip surgery, but fatal pulmonary embolism

poses a greater risk, occurring in about 5 percent of these patients. Many of these patients are elderly and, therefore, are particularly, at risk for bleeding when given anticoagulant therapy, and are considerably at risk for volume overload if treated prophylactically with dextran.

At present, it would be reasonable to use oral anticoagulants commencing 48 to 72 hours after surgery in a dose that prolongs the prothrombin time to 1 to 1.5 times control value at 5 to 6 days after surgery.

High-risk medical patients   *Myocardial infarction*   Between 20 and 40 percent of patients who sustain acute myocardial infarction develop calf vein thrombodis. Low-dose heparin is effective in reducing the frequency of venous thrombosis detected by leg scan in these patients, but there is no evidence that this approach is effective in preventing systemic embolism. Patients with extensive acute myocardial infarction are at high risk for developing systemic embolism, and they should be treated with a combination of full doses of heparin and oral anticoagulants commencing at the time that they are admitted to the hospital. Heparin therapy can then be stopped after 3 to 5 days, and oral anticoagulants can be continued for 3 to 4 weeks. Alternative approaches that are likely to be as effective include (1) oral anticoagulants (used alone) administered at the time of admission to the hospital and then daily with the aim of increasing the prothrombin time to 1.5 times control value after 4 or 5 days; (2) subcutaneous heparin in doses of 7,000 to 10,000 units 3 times daily while the patient remains in the hospital; and (3) subcutaneous heparin for the first 3 or 4 days in combination with oral anticoagulants that are continued until the patient is discharged from the hospital. The moderate dose subcutaneous heparin regimen is particularly useful if facilities for laboratory monitoring are not available. Patients with subendocardial my-

Table 4.5   Categories of Risk and Suggested Prophylaxis in Elective Abdominal and Thoracic Surgical Patients

	Low Risk	Moderate Risk	High Risk
Risk of Thromboembolism	Age under 40 and uncomplicated or minor surgery	Age over 40. Abdominal, pelvic or thoracic surgery.	Age over 40. Recent venous thrombosis. Extensive surgery for malignant disease.
Calf vein thrombosis	Less than 3%	10 to 40%	30 to 60%
Proximal vein thrombosis	Less than 1%	2 to 8%	6 to 12%
Fatal pulmonary embolism	Less than 0.01%	0.1 to 0.7%	1 to 2%
Prophylaxis of choice	Early ambulation Graduated compression	Low dose heparin or intermittent pneumatic compression	Continuous low to moderate dose heparin or intermittent pneumatic compression plus low dose heparin or oral anticoagulants

ocardial infarction have a lower risk of systemic embolism, and in these it is reasonable to limit prophylaxis to low-dose heparin while they remain in the hospital.

THE POSTPHLEBITIC SYNDROME

Pathophysiology and Clinical Manifestations

The postphlebitic syndrome is caused by venous hypertension that occurs as a consequence of either valve destruction and venous reflux or persistent outflow obstruction. Recanalization and valve destruction produce an increase in venous pressure, which ultimately destroys the valves of the perforating veins of the calf that normally direct flow from the superficial to the deep system. When this occurs, flow is directed from the deep into the superficial system during muscular contraction, and this leads to impaired viability of the subcutaneous tissues and ultimately to venous ulceration.

The initial symptoms of the postphlebitic syndrome are swelling of the ankle and the leg, and a heavy aching pain in the calf and the ankle that is most marked after the patient has been standing or walking and that is relieved by rest and leg elevation. Pigmentation, induration, and prominent venules develop with time around the ankle and the lower third of the leg, and, in the most severe form of this disease, ulceration develops around the region of the medial malleolus. Venous claudication is another possible symptom, which is a bursting calf pain occurring on exercise usually in patients with persistent proximal obstruction.

Relationship of the Postphlebitic Syndrome to the Site and Extent of Thrombosis

In patients with marked iliofemoral vein thrombosis, the swelling may never disappear, while in patients with less severe proximal vein thrombosis, the swelling may subside after initial treatment but recur months or years after the initial event. Other symptoms of the postphlebitic syndrome may be delayed for 5 to 10 years.

The postphlebitic syndrome usually occurs as a complication of proximal vein thrombosis, and the severe symptoms of bursting pain and leg ulceration occur mainly with iliofemoral vein thrombosis. Calf vein thrombosis is generally not considered a predisposing cause of the postphlebitic syndrome; but this view may be erroneous, because it is based on retrospective studies that have used clinical features to differentiate between calf vein thrombosis and proximal vein thrombosis.

Management of the Postphlebitic Syndrome

Prevention of postphlebitic syndrome

A number of approaches can be used to prevent the postphlebitic syndrome. These include (1) prevention of venous thrombosis in high risk patients, (2) treatment of calf vein thrombosis with heparin to prevent extension into the more proximal veins, and (3) treatment of proximal vein thrombosis with thrombolytic therapy or thrombectomy. The true benefits of the latter forms of therapy are not established.

Treatment of the postphlebitic syndrome

The initial management of postphlebitic leg ulcers is conservative, since the majority of these heal with bed rest and leg elevation. Swelling can be controlled by well-fitting compression stockings, which also appear to reduce the frequency of leg ulceration, even when ankle pigmentation and induration are already present. These stockings compress superficial veins and so control reflux.

Various medications have been used to treat leg ulceration in the postphlebitic syndrome. The most effective appear to be the hydrophilic powders that absorb moisture and necrotic debris. Postphlebitic ulcers that recur despite conservative treatment are difficult to manage. Various surgical procedures have been attempted, including skin grafting, varicose vein stripping, and ligation of the recanalized popliteal or femoral veins.

PULMONARY EMBOLISM

Pathophysiology

Most clinically detectable pulmonary emboli are associated with, and probably arise from, thrombi in the deep venous system of the legs.

The pathophysiological consequences of pulmonary embolism are caused by its effect on lung tissue, gas exchange, and right heart function.

Effects on Lung Tissue

The lung derives its oxygen from the bronchial circulation, the pulmonary arterial circulation, and from alveolar oxygen. Because oxygen is provided from multiple sources, impairment of pulmonary arterial flow does not usually produce ischemia of pulmonary parenchyma. However, the oxygen supply to the distal lung tissue may be impaired in (1) patients with chronic lung disease, because they frequently have abnormalities of their bronchial circulation; (2) patients with chronic heart disease, because of pulmonary venous congestion; or (3) patients in whom the embolus reaches a critical length and is located in a distal pulmonary vessel. There are two consequences of impaired oxygenation of lung parenchyma. These are ischemic atelectasis and pulmonary infarction. Atelectasis may result from loss of surfactant, and pulmonary infarction occurs when there is death of parenchymal tissue. The pulmonary infarct is characteristically hemorrhagic due to blood that enters the infarcted area via the bronchial circulation. Since the terminal branches of the pulmonary arteries perfuse conical regions of the lung, the infarct characteristically appears wedge-shaped, with the base of the wedge on the pleural surface. Both atelectasis and pulmonary infarction may be associated with pleural effusion.

The Effects of Gas Exchange

Pulmonary embolism creates areas of dead space in regions of the lung that are ventilated but not perfused. This results in a local decrease in carbon dioxide tension that in turn leads to constriction of the terminal airways of the involved lung. In addition, shunting occurs because hypoxia and thromboxane A_2 (a prostaglandin product) released from platelets and lung tissue at the site of embolism produce airway constriction in regions of the lung that are normally perfused.

Hypoxemia is a frequent but not invariable accompaniment of pulmonary embolism. Its precise mechanism is uncertain, and the severity of hypoxemia may not always bear a close relationship with the size of the embolus. Factors that may be important include (1) constriction of the terminal airways and alveolar ducts of parts of the lung, causing reduced ventilation/perfusion ratios, (2) hyperperfusion and pulmonary edema of nonembolized parts of the lung; and (3) regional hypoventilation caused by chest pain from pleurisy or decreased compliance of parts of the lung that are affected by pulmonary embolism.

The Effect on Right Heart Function

Pulmonary embolism produces pulmonary hypertension as a result of the combined effect of mechanical obstruction and pulmonary arterial vasoconstriction. The degree of mechanical obstruction produced is closely related to the size of the embolus and its location in the pulmonary circulation. The mechanism of pulmonary arterial vasoconstriction is not known, but probably includes reflex neural factors and humoral agents such as prostaglandins that are released locally from either platelets or pulmonary vascular tissue. The combination of mechanical obstruction and vasoconstriction leads to an increase in pulmonary vascular resistance that, if sufficiently severe, results in right ventricular failure and, if cardiac output is sufficiently impaired, in peripheral circulatory failure or shock.

Factors that Influence Clinical Manifestations of Pulmonary Embolism

Size of Embolus

Small emboli (which obstruct lobular or smaller branches) only produce clinical symptoms or signs if they are multiple or recurrent, if the patient's cardiorespiratory system is compromised by other disease, or if they obstruct a peripheral pulmonary artery and produce atelectasis or pulmonary infarction. Larger pulmonary emboli may also be asymptomatic; they produce clinical manifestations because they produce hemodynamic changes that interfere with right heart function, because they compromise gas exchange, or because they are associated with pulmonary infarction or atelectasis. In patients with normal cardiopulmonary reserve, approximately 60 percent or more of the pulmonary vasculature must be obstructed before significant hemodynamic changes are produced.

Previous Cardiorespiratory Status of the Patient

If the cardiorespiratory status of the patient is compromised, even relatively small pulmonary emboli may produce a critical rise in pulmonary vascular resistance and result in right heart failure and peripheral circulatory failure. In addition, these patients are more likely to develop atelectasis or pulmonary infarction, because the oxygen supply to their pulmonary parenchyma may already be compromised.

*The Rate of Lysis of the Pulmonary
Embolism*

The embolus may undergo complete lysis; it may
extend or migrate distally into the pulmonary circulation; or it may shrink and undergo organization
leaving residual webs. In most cases, pulmonary emboli undergo fairly rapid lysis so that they either disappear or become greatly reduced in size, weeks to
months after the embolic event.

Impaired resolution is most common in patients
who have very large emboli or who have chronic
heart or lung disease. Most patients, including those
with impaired resolution, suffer no clinically important long-term consequences or pulmonary embolism; however, a minority of patients with impaired resolution and chronic pulmonary arterial
obstruction develop chronic thromboembolic pulmonary hypertension.

Pathophysiology of Clinical Manifestations (Table 4.6)

Dyspnea and Tachypnea

These occur commonly, but their mechanisms are
not defined. Possible contributing factors include:
anxiety, hypoxemia, splinting of the chest wall
caused by pleuritic chest pain, stimulation of intrapulmonary receptors, and changes in inspiratory
work as a result of atelectasis, lung edema, or infarction.

Pain

Two types of chest pain occur in patients with pulmonary embolism. The most common and characteristic is the pleuritic pain caused by inflammation
of the pleura overlying areas of pulmonary infarction
or atelectasis. The pleuritic pain is typically sudden
in onset, aggravated by breathing, and may be associated with mild chest wall tenderness. It may remain localized to a small area of the chest wall or
may gradually spread from its original location over
a larger area.

The less common type is a central anterior chest
pain that occurs in patients with massive pulmonary
embolism and is indistinguishable from ischemic
heart pain. It is usually of brief duration. The cause
of the pain is uncertain but may include dilatation of
the main pulmonary artery, or right ventricular ischemia as a result of acute pulmonary hypertension.

**Table 4.6 Pathophysiology of Clinical
Manifestations of Pulmonary Embolism**

Clinical Features	Possible Mechanisms
1. Dyspnea and Tachypnea	a) Hypoxemia
	b) Splinting of chest because of pleural inflammation
	c) Decreased lung compliance
	d) Stimulation of intrapulmonary receptors
	e) Anxiety
2. Pain	a) Pleural inflammation
	b) Dilatation of main pulmonary artery
3. Hemoptysis	a) Pulmonary infarction
	b) Congestive atelectasis
4. Syncope	a) Reduced cardiac output and hypotension
	b) Arrhythmia
	c) Hypoxemia
5. Cyanosis	a) Hypoxemia
	b) Stagnant anoxia associated with poor tissue perfusion
6. Apprehension and Anxiety	a) Catacholamine release
7. Impaired Consciousness	a) Hypoxemia
	b) Hypotension
8. Hypotension	a) Reduced cardiac output
9. Cardiac Manifestations	a) Acute pulmonary hypertension
10. Chest Findings	a) Pleural inflammation
	b) Pulmonary consolidation or collapse
	c) Bronchoconstriction

Hemoptysis

Hemoptysis is a relatively infrequent feature of
pulmonary embolism. Its presence indicates that pulmonary injury has occurred and has produced alveolar hemorrhage. Clear evidence of infarction is
commonly but not always present in patients with
hemoptysis.

Syncope

Syncope may occasionally be the first and most
prominent manifestation of pulmonary embolism. It
usually occurs only in massive pulmonary embolism
and is caused by a reduction in cardiac output, which
in turn results in hypotension and transient impairment of cerebral blood flow; it is usually associated

with dyspnea and right heart failure. Occasionally, syncope may be caused by an arrhythmia that complicates pulmonary embolism.

Cyanosis

Central cyanosis only occurs in patients with major pulmonary embolism and is caused by hypoxemia. Peripheral cyanosis may also occur as a result of reduced tissue perfusion in patients who are hypotensive.

Apprehension, Anxiety, and Tachycardia

Apprehension, anxiety, and tachycardia may be prominent features of major pulmonary embolism. The mechanism is not clearly understood but the occurrence of these symptoms is likely to be mediated by stimulation of the sympathetic autonomic nervous system and release of catecholamines.

Hypotension

Hypotension occurs in patients with massive pulmonary embolism and is caused by a reduced cardiac output due to increased pulmonary vascular resistance.

Cardiac and Lung Abnormalities

The clinical manifestations resulting from pulmonary hypertension and lung injury are discussed later in this chapter in the section Diagnosis of Pulmonary Embolism.

Diagnosis

The clinical diagnosis of pulmonary embolism is nonspecific and insensitive. It is nonspecific because many conditions may produce similar clinical manifestations and it is insensitive because many, if not most, pulmonary emboli are clinically silent.

The clinical manifestations of pulmonary embolism are characterized by a number of syndromes among which there is often considerable overlap. These include (1) transient dyspnea and tachypnea with no other associated clinical manifestations; (2) the syndrome of pulmonary infarction or ischemic pneumonitis, which includes pleuritic chest pain, cough, hemoptysis, pleural effusion, and pulmonary infiltrates on chest roentgenograms; (3) right sided heart failure associated with severe dyspnea and tach-

ypnea; (4) cardiovascular collapse with hypotension, syncope, and coma; and (5) various less common and less specific symptom complexes, including confusion, fever, wheezing, resistant heart failure, and unexplained arrhythmias.

Physical Signs

The physical signs of pulmonary embolism are nonspecific and varied, and often do not reliably indicate the severity of the pulmonary vascular obstruction. Although venography shows that patients with pulmonary embolism usually have leg vein thrombosis at the time of clinical presentation, these thrombi often produce no detectable signs or symptoms, and only 30 percent of patients with pulmonary embolism have clinical evidence of venous thrombosis.

The physical findings in patients with submassive pulmonary embolism may be limited to tachypnea and tachycardia, or there may be some of the cardiac or respiratory manifestations of massive embolism.

Massive pulmonary embolism is associated with tachypnea, tachycardia, cyanosis, and an altered mental and conscious state that varies from anxiety to frank coma. The patient may be hypotensive and may have pulsus parodoxus. The jugular venous pressure is elevated, often with a prominent *a* wave that may sometimes be difficult to appreciate by clinical examination. A loud pulmonary second sound may occur due to increased pulmonary vascular pressure, and a gallop rhythm (S3 and S4) may be present due to right ventricular failure. A systolic murmur may be heard; this may be an ejection murmur due to embolic obstruction of the main pulmonary artery or, rarely, a pan-systolic murmur due to tricuspid incompetence. The electrocardiogram may be normal or may reveal a right axis shift, a right bundle branch block, or inversion of inferior or anteroseptal t waves.

The chest findings are nonspecific. Patients with pulmonary infarction characteristically have reduced movement of the affected portion of the chest, and there may be signs of pulmonary consolidation, atelectasis, pleural friction rub, crackles, or a pleural effusion.

Fever may occur in pulmonary embolism even in the absence of pulmonary infarction, and when it does the patient's temperature is usually less than 38.5°C. Mild polymorphonuclear leucocytosis is common.

Because of the nonspecificity of the clinical manifestations in pulmonary embolism, clinical suspicion should always be confirmed by objective tests. The most useful tests are the chest roentgenogram, the perfusion and ventilation lung scan, the pulmonary angiogram, and objective tests for venous thrombosis.

Diagnostic Tests

Chest roentgenogram   The chest radiograph may be normal or more frequently may show non-specific abnormalities including regions of hypoperfusion, patchy infiltrates, nonsegmental basilar atelectasis, unilateral or bilateral pleural effusions, or the uncommon but typical wedge-shaped densities. A chest roentgenogram is necessary for the proper interpretation of the perfusion lung scan and may demonstrate conditions that simulate pulmonary embolism (for example, pneumothorax or pulmonary edema).

Perfusion lung scan   The perfusion lung scan detects areas of reduced blood flow. A normal lung scan virtually excludes a diagnosis of pulmonary embolism. However, an abnormal scan cannot be taken as evidence of pulmonary embolism, since many pulmonary disorders are associated with impaired pulmonary vascular perfusion.

Ventilation scan   The ventilation scan, when used in conjunction with the perfusion scan, increases the specificity of the perfusion lung scan by identifying regions of reduced pulmonary perfusion that result from impaired ventilation. Perfusion defects that are associated with matching ventilation abnormalities and a normal chest x-ray are unlikely to be caused by pulmonary embolism, while multiple large perfusion defects in regions that ventilate normally, are likely to be caused by pulmonary embolism.

Pulmonary angiography   is the most definitive diagnostic test for pulmonary embolism. The accuracy of this technique has been improved in recent years by selective pulmonary arterial catheterization and magnification techniques.

Objective tests for venous thrombosis   Venography or impedance plethysmography can detect venous thrombosis in patients with clinically suspected pulmonary embolism, and in the appropriate clinical setting this can be used as an indication to treat patients with anticoagulants.

A Practical Approach to the Diagnosis of Pulmonary Embolism

If the clinical manifestations suggest pulmonary embolism, further investigation is required. Conditions that may simulate pulmonary embolism, such as pneumothorax, fractured rib, lobar pneumonia,

carcinoma of the lung, mitral stenosis, pericardial effusion, and left ventricular failure, may be apparent on chest roentgenograms. The ECG may be diagnostic of myocardial infarction or pericarditis (Table 4.7). If the chest film is normal or nondiagnostic, a six-view perfusion lung scan should be performed. If the perfusion lung scan is technically adequate and normal, a diagnosis of pulmonary embolism can be excluded, and no further investigations are required. However, an abnormal perfusion lung scan requires further investigation. This occurs most commonly in obstructive lung diseases.

Three approaches can be used. These are to perform ventilation scanning, venography, or a pulmonary angiogram, and the choice between these approaches is influenced by the clinical circumstances and the availability of the test procedure. If facilities are available, a ventilation scan should be performed first, since the results obtained can be used to either confirm or exclude a diagnosis of pulmonary embolism in some patients. If a ventilation scan cannot be performed, either a venogram or a pulmonary angiogram should be performed. If the venogram or pulmonary angiogram show filling defects characteristic of venous thrombosis or pulmonary embolism, the patient should be considered for treatment. A negative pulmonary angiogram excludes pulmonary embolism, but a negative venogram does not exclude the possibility that the patient's symptoms are due to pulmonary embolism. In these patients, the management decisions may have to be based on other clinical factors, but a pulmonary angiography should be performed if possible.

Differential Diagnosis of Clinical Manifestations

Dyspnea, Pleuritic Chest Pain, and Hemoptysis

Dyspnea, pleuritic chest pain, and hemoptysis are common features of numerous diseases discussed in detail in Chapter 15.

Table 4.7   Conditions which May Simulate Pulmonary Embolism Clinically but which Can Be Excluded by the Result of Chest Roentgenogram or ECG

Submassive Pulmonary Embolism	Massive Pulmonary Embolism
Pneumothorax	Left Ventricular Failure
Fractured Rib	Mitral Stenosis
Lobar Pneumonia	Tension Pneumothorax
Carcinoma of Lung	Pericardial Tamponade
Mitral Stenosis	Dissecting Aneurysm of
Left Heart Failure	Ascending Aorta
Pericarditis	Acute Myocardial Infarction

Acute Right Heart Failure

If acute right heart failure complicates pulmonary embolism, it is almost always associated with severe dyspnea and tachypnea. Dyspnea and heart failure also occur in any condition with biventricular failure, and may occur in patients with mitral valve disease. Patients with chronic obstructive lung disease may develop acute respiratory failure with pulmonary hypertension, severe dyspnea, and right heart failure.

The nonthrombotic causes of pulmonary embolism include fat embolism, amniotic fluid embolism, and tumor emboli. Fat embolism is almost always a complication of long bone fractures, and it occurs within a short time of trauma. Dyspnea may be a prominent feature, and it is often associated with other features, including petechiae, confusion, thrombocytopenia, and fever. Amniotic fluid embolism almost always occurs as a complication of difficult labor, and it is associated with features of disseminated intravascular coagulation. The chest roentgenogram shows diffuse bilateral infiltrates in fat or amniotic fluid embolism.

Cardiovascular Collapse

The conditions that may be confused with massive embolism and peripheral circulatory failure include myocardial infarction with cardiogenic shock, acute pericardial tamponade, acute massive blood loss, gram-negative septicemia and, occasionally, spontaneous pneumothorax (see Table 4.7).

Treatment of Venous Thromboembolism

Objectives of Treatment

The main objectives of treating venous thromboembolism are (1) to prevent death from pulmonary embolism, (2) to prevent the postphlebitic syndrome, (3) to reduce morbidity resulting from the acute event, and (4) to achieve these objectives with a minimum of side effects and cost.

The therapeutic approaches available are either directed at removing the obstruction by mechanical or enzymatic means, preventing its extension by inhibiting blood coagulation, or preventing pulmonary embolism from leg vein thrombosis by interrupting the inferior vena cava (Table 4.8). Although removing the thromboembolic obstruction is clearly the most desirable on theoretical grounds, this is not usually indicated nor is it often possible, and, in practice,

most patients are treated with anticoagulants. Anticoagulant therapy is highly effective and prevents death from pulmonary embolism in over 95 percent of patients who present with venous thrombosis or pulmonary embolism. Heparin may also prevent the postphlebitic syndrome in patients with calf vein thrombosis by limiting propagation of thrombi into the proximal veins, but it is less effective in preventing the postphlebitic syndrome in patients who present with proximal vein thrombosis. Total lysis is infrequent with heparin therapy. Instead, the thrombus usually becomes organized and eventually produces valvular incompetence, which in turn leads to venous hypertension and to the postphlebitic syndrome.

In theory, the most effective way of preventing the postphlebitic syndrome in patients with proximal vein thrombosis would be to remove the thrombus either by surgical or enzymatic means. However, thrombectomy is usually complicated by nearly recurrence and is, therefore, rarely performed. Thrombolytic therapy is associated with a higher risk of bleeding than is heparin therapy, and it is contraindicated in patients who have had major surgery or trauma within 10 days of the thrombotic event. Further, thrombolytic therapy may not prevent the postphlebitic syndrome if the valves are damaged and become incompetent. Complete lysis with thrombolytic agents is uncommon if the thrombus has been present for 96 hours or longer, because thrombi become resistant to lysis as they age; in many patients who have symptomatic venous thrombosis, the thrombus has been present for a number of days at the time of presentation.

Most patients with pulmonary embolism including those with major pulmonary embolism recover completely if treated with heparin. A small number of these patients remain unresponsive to conservative measures and die during the dirst few days after the embolic event unless the obstruction can be rapidly removed either by pulmonary embolectomy or thrombolytic therapy. The indications for these approaches are controversial, and their correct application requires considerable experience and clinical judgement (see section which follows on Drug Treatment of Thrombosis).

The Use of Anticoagulants in the Treatment of Venous Thrombosis and Pulmonary Embolism

Heparin is the treatment of choice in patients with venous thromboembolic disease because it is relatively safe and is effective in preventing extension of

Table 4.8 Approaches to the Treatment of Venous Thromboembolism

Treatment	Principle	Effectiveness in Preventing			Side Effects	Cost	Availability	Comment
		Recurrence	Death	Post-Phlebitic Syndrome				
Heparin	Prevents Extension	+++	+++	+ (Calf vein thrombosis)	+	+	+++	Very Effective Therapy
Thrombolytic Therapy	Removes Obstruction	+++	+++	++	+++	+++	+	Limited to Special Cases
Thrombectomy	Removes Obstruction	±	±	±	++	++	++	Not Effective
Pulmonary Embolectomy	Removes Obstruction	N/A	+	N/A	+++	+++	+	Rarely Indicated
Vena Caval Interruption	Prevents Pulmonary Embolism	+++	+++	–	++	++	++	Only Indicated in Special Circumstances

venous thrombosis and pulmonary embolism. The standard approach to anticoagulant therapy is to administer heparin intravenously in full doses for a period of 7 to 10 days. In most patients, heparin therapy is followed by treatment with oral anticoagulants which are then continued for a period of 6 to 12 weeks. Ideally, oral anticoagulant treatment should be started 4 to 5 days before heparin is stopped, since there may be a delay before the antithrombotic effect of oral anticoagulants is achieved. In patients who have an increased risk of bleeding or when anticoagulant control is difficult or inconvenient, moderate doses of subcutaneous heparin (8,000 units) can be used instead of oral anticoagulants. This can usually be administered by the patient. Moderate dose subcutaneous heparin is as effective as oral anticoagulants and is associated with less bleeding, but is more expensive.

Acute iliofemoral vein thrombosis   If there are no contraindications, thrombolytic therapy should be considered in patients with isolated proximal vein thrombosis.

Major pulmonary embolism (massive and submassive)   Thrombolytic therapy produces accelerated lysis of pulmonary embolism over the first 24 to 48 hours and should be considered in patients who have a major life-threatening pulmonary embolism.

Patients who are likely to benefit most from thrombolytic therapy are those with associated cardiopulmonary disease. Spontaneous resolution is frequently impaired or delayed in these patients and they are clinically unstable; they are prone to sudden episodes of arrhythmia or cardiopulmonary arrest. Further, these patients are more likely to die if they develop recurrent pulmonary embolism.

Pulmonary embolectomy may be life-saving if immediate relief from pulmonary vascular obstruction is required. This approach is indicated in patients who have massive pulmonary embolism, who have cardiac arrest, or whose conditions have deteriorated despite conservative treatment with heparin or a thrombolytic agent. It is important to emphasize that clinical deterioration in these patients may be caused by complications such as arrhythmias, acidosis, hemorrhage, or severe hypoxemia, and these complications should be identified and treated aggressively before pulmonary embolectomy is considered.

Treatment of Patients Who Have a Relative Contraindication to Anticoagulant Therapy

The contraindications to anticoagulant therapy are listed in Table 4.9. Three approaches can be used for the management of patients with venous thrombosis

Table 4.9   Contraindications to Anticoagulant Therapy

Relative Contraindications:
Severe hypertension
Major recent surgical operation
Recent major trauma
Recent stroke
Active gastrointestinal hemorrhage
Bacterial endocarditis
Severe renal failure
Severe hepatic failure
Hemorrhagic diathesis

Absolute Contraindications:
Malignant hypertension
Serious active bleeding (either postoperative, spontaneous or associated with trauma)
Recent brain, eye or spinal cord surgery
Subarachnoid or cerebral hemorrhage

when there are relative contraindications to anticoagulant therapy:

1. Treat patients with heparin by continuous infusion but monitor the effect carefully so that the anticoagulant level is maintained in the low therapeutic range (the equivalent of 0.1 to 0.2 units of heparin per ml or 1.2 to 1.5 times prolongation of the patient's own baseline Activated Partial Thromboplastin Time).

2. Perform a caval interruption procedure to prevent pulmonary embolism or recurrent embolism.

3. Withhold treatment until the period of hemorrhagic risk subsides. (This approach can only be used if the patient has calf vein thrombosis, if surveillance with ^{125}I-fibrinogen leg scanning is available to detect extension, and if risk of bleeding is transient). See Table 4.10.

Treatment of Patients Who Have an Absolute Contraindication to Anticoagulant Therapy

If there is an absolute contraindication to anticoagulant therapy in patients with proven venous thromboembolism who are not terminally ill, then

Table 4.10   Treatment of Patients with Contraindications to Anticoagulant Therapy

Relative Contraindications:
Carefully controlled moderate dose heparin.
Caval interruption.
If calf vein thrombosis and facilities available, screen with leg scanning and IPG until relative contraindications no longer present.

Absolute Contraindications:
Caval interruption.
If calf vein thrombosis screen and only use caval interruption if thrombosis extends.

either a caval interruption procedure should be performed or, if the patient has calf vein thrombosis and facilities are available for surveillance, the patient can be managed by monitoring for extension with twice daily ^{125}I-fibrinogen leg scanning and IPG.

General Measures for the Treatment of Deep-Vein Thrombosis

Although pain is a common feature of deep vein thrombosis (DVT), analgesics are not often required because symptoms tend to subside with rest, leg elevation, and heparin therapy. Heparin may relieve pain through an ill-defined and hypothetical anti-inflammatory effect. If analgesics are required, aspirin-containing drugs should be avoided, since they affect hemostasis, and when used in combination with heparin, they increase the risk of bleeding. Drugs such as acetaminophen are appropriate; narcotics such as meperidine (pethadine) or morphine are rarely required to treat the pain of venous thrombosis. Drugs should not be administered by intramuscular injection, since this may cause serious bleeding in patients treated with anticoagulants.

If symptoms of pain and/or swelling are severe, the patient should be confined to bed until they subside. During this time, the foot of the bed should be elevated to encourage venous return and reduce leg edema. Symptoms subside in most patients in 2 or 3 days, and these patients should then be encouraged to gradually resume normal activity; however, patients with severe iliofemoral vein thrombosis may need to remain in bed for a week or longer. If symptoms are not severe, the patient can be treated with anticoagulants while he or she is ambulant. There is a theoretical risk that pulmonary embolism may be induced by movement; however, there is no evidence that this occurs, and therefore a diagnosis of venous thrombosis should not in itself be an indication for bed rest. In some patients, edema persists, while in others it recurs when normal activity is resumed. This can be controlled by using well-fitted compression stockings. These should be worn indefinitely in patients with persistent leg swelling to prevent the development of a more severe postphlebitic syndrome. Antibiotics should not be used in patients with venous thrombosis who are febrile unless indicated, because of associated infection.

General Measures for the Treatment of Pulmonary Embolism

In patients with pulmonary embolism and pleurisy, the pain may be very severe, and analgesia is frequently required. If pain cannot be controlled by simple analgesics, narcotics such as pethadine or morphine may be required.

Oxygen therapy is indicated in all patients with hypoxemia. This can be given either by face mask or intranasally, and its effect can be monitored by ear oximetry. Arterial blood gas analysis may be associated with arterial bleeding during heparin therapy; for this reason, radial punctures should be performed cautiously, with prolonged arterial compression.

Pleural effusions may complicate pulmonary embolism, but they are usually small and therapeutic aspiration is rarely, if ever, required. If diagnostic thoracentesis is necessary, it should be performed before heparin therapy is commenced or when the level of circulating heparin is low. A narrow gauge needle should be used, and care should be taken to avoid hepatic or splenic puncture.

Occasionally, differentiation between pulmonary infarction and pulmonary infection may prove difficult, and a decision may be made to treat with both anticoagulants and antibiotics until these two conditions can be more clearly differentiated. Once a diagnosis of pulmonary embolism is established, antibiotics should be withdrawn.

Hemoptysis complicating pulmonary infarction is not a contraindication to anticoagulant therapy, since in most cases it is minor, and even though it may be accentuated with anticoagulants, it is rarely life-threatening. Very rarely, massive pulmonary hemorrhage does complicate pulmonary infarction and anticoagulant therapy must be stopped and alternative methods must be used to treat pulmonary embolism. Increased pulmonary vascular resistance may be relieved to some extent by correction of hypoxemia, and by isoproterenol, which is a powerful pulmonary arterial vasodilator.

ARTERIAL THROMBOSIS

Arterial thrombi occur in regions of disturbed flow, distal to bifurcations or stenoses, or within aneurysmal dilatations. Arterial thrombi invariably occur at sites of endothelial damage when subendothelial structures are exposed to the flowing blood. The most common lesion predisposing to arterial thrombosis is atherosclerosis.

The pathogenesis of arterial thrombosis and atherosclerosis are closely related (see Chapter 2). Platelets contribute to the formation of atherosclerosis by releasing lysosomal enzymes that damage vascular endothelium and a platelet growth factor that stimulates the migration of smooth muscle cells from the media into the subendothelial layer to form the smooth muscle plaque (also known as the *fibrous pla-*

que), which is the forerunner to atherosclerosis. In its early stage, the atherosclerotic plaque is covered with endothelium, and it leads to flow disturbances and narrowing of the lumen. As the plaque grows, the overlying endothelium becomes ulcerated and platelets adhere to the connective tissue. Because of rapid flow, the platelet thrombi are usually not totally occlusive but remain as mural thrombi and become incorporated into the vessel wall, increasing the size of the atherosclerotic plaque. The mural thrombus may embolize into the microcirculation and produce complications by obstructing end arteries or by releasing vasoactive agents that produce spasm of distal vessels. Most emboli are asymptomatic or unrecognized, but when embolization occurs in the cerebral circulation, the patient may suffer transient attacks of cerebral ischemia or stroke, and when embolization occurs in the coronary circulation, it may lead to rhythm disturbances or sudden death.

THROMBOSIS OF THE MICROCIRCULATION

Disseminated thrombosis of the microcirculation can be caused by activation of blood coagulation, by diffuse endothelial damage, or by disseminated platelet aggregation. Activation of blood coagulation leading to disseminated thrombosis classically occurs in patients with malignancy or following obstetrical accidents. Diffuse endothelial damage occurs in the vasculitides, and septicemia following extensive burns. Disseminated platelet aggregation occurs in a condition known as thrombotic thrombocytopenic purpura. Most microcirculatory thrombi are of the mixed variety containing fibrin and platelets, but in thrombotic thrombocytopenic purpura the thrombi are almost entirely composed of platelet aggregates. The clinical manifestations of *disseminated intravascular thrombosis* are related to organ ischemia, such as in the brain, the heart, or the kidney, and to hemorrhagic phenomena caused by consumption of blood coagulation factors and platelets.

CARDIAC THROMBOEMBOLISM

Thrombosis of the cardiac chambers occurs in disorders of the endocardium, myocardium, valve structures, and as a result of the insertion of vascular prostheses. Thrombotic deposits frequently occur at sites of inflammation of the cardiac valves in patients with endocarditis. These thrombi are small and composed of a mixture of platelets and fibrin. Systemic arterial embolism to the brain, the kidneys, the splanchnic circulation, and occasionally to the coronary arteries is an important complication of endocarditis.

Myocardial damage caused by myocardial infarction, myocarditis, or cardiomyopathies is frequently complicated by mural thrombosis. These cardiac thrombi vary in size and consist of fibrin enmeshed in ventricular trabeculations. Systemic embolization is an important complication of intracardiac thrombi.

Rheumatic heart disease, particularly when it involves the mitral valve and is complicated by atrial fibrillation, is frequently associated with thrombosis and systemic embolism. Thrombi that consist mainly of fibrin and red cells occur in the dilated left atrium.

The incidence of thromboembolism in patients who have prosthetic heart valves appears to be decreasing with improvement in valve design, but it remains a common problem, particularly with mitral valve replacement. These red thrombi contain fibrin and red cells with only a minor platelet component, and they frequently embolize.

DRUG TREATMENT OF THROMBOSIS

Three classes of antithrombotic agents are available for clinical use. These are anticoagulant drugs, drugs that suppress platelet function, and thrombolytic drugs.

Anticoagulant Drugs

Anticoagulant drugs have been used clinically for almost 40 years and have an established place in the treatment of venous thromboembolic disease and systemic embolism, but their value in arterial thrombosis is less well established. There are two types of anticoagulant drugs in clinical use: heparin and the vitamin K antagonists.

Heparin

Heparin acts as an immediate anticoagulant by binding to antithrombin III. Antithrombin III inactivates the activated clotting Factors XIIa, XIa, IXa, Xa, and thrombin, all of which are enzymes with a serine active site. In the absence of heparin, antithrombin III is a slowly progressive inactivator of these coagulation enzymes, but the rate of inactivation is markedly accelerated in the presence of heparin. When heparin binds to the antithrombin III molecule, it produces a conformational change that greatly increases the affinity of the antithrombin III for these clotting factor enzymes.

Administration of heparin   Heparin can be administered by intravenous or subcutaneous injection. It should not be administered by intramuscular injection, because of the danger of local hemorrhage from a punctured intramuscular vessel. When administered intravenously, it can be given by continuous or intermittent infusion. All three methods—continuous or intermittent infusion or subcutaneous injection—are acceptable, but administration by continuous infusion is associated with a lower frequency of bleeding and is, therefore, preferable to the intermittent route, provided that laboratory facilities are available for monitoring the rate of infusion. Most experience with subcutaneous heparin has been limited to its use as a prophylactic agent in high-risk patients, but subcutaneous heparin can also be used if there is difficulty in maintaining an intravenous line.

The response to a single intravenous dose of heparin varies considerably between patients. In some, a dose of 70 units/kg given by intravenous injection produces a marked anticoagulant effect that lasts for 2 to 3 hours, while in others the anticoagulant effect wears off within one half to one hour. Heparin is cleared more rapidly in pulmonary embolism than in venous thrombosis.

The optimal therapeutic dose of heparin is that which prevents extension of thrombosis with a minimal risk of bleeding. Experimentally, the dose that prevents extension of established thrombosis when heparin is given by continuous infusion is one that prolongs the partial thromboplastin time (PTT) to approximately twice the preheparin level; this corresponds to a heparin level (using heparin assay) of approximately 0.3 units/ml. Less well controlled studies in man are consistent with these experimental observations.

When heparin is administered by continuous intravenous infusion it should be given in an initial loading dose of 5,000 units and then as a continuous infusion in a dose of 24,000 units administered over 24 hours. This dosage regimen will provide an adequate therapeutic level (heparin level of 0.2 to 0.4 units/ml, PTT of 1.5 to 2 times control) in 70 to 80 percent of patients. In the other 20 to 30 percent, the dose will either have to be increased or decreased to reach this level of anticoagulant effect. The activated partial thromboplastin time or heparin level should be measured in approximately 6 hours and again within 24 hours after commencing heparin treatment, and then daily. In patients who are at serious risk of bleeding, (for example, patients in the early postoperative period or patients with an associated hemostatic defect), the dosage of heparin may have to be modified as follows: an initial bolus dose of 3,000 units and an initial infusion rate of 18,000 to 20,000 units/24 hours with more frequent monitoring to maintain levels at the lower limit of the anticoagulated range.

Intermittent intravenous heparin is usually administered every 4 hours with the aim of maintaining some heparin in the circulation at all times. To achieve this, the patient must be exposed to periods of marked hypocoagulability because of the relatively short half-life. Monitoring should be performed to ascertain that the heparin effect is being obtained and that it is not cumulative. Heparin is usually administered in a dose of 5,000 to 7,000 units every 4 hours with the aim of elevating the PTT to approximately 1.2 to 1.5 the control value 3 hours after injection.

The subcutaneous route of heparin administration is particularly useful when long-term treatment with heparin is indicated or when it is used on an outpatient basis. The risk of local bleeding can be minimized by injecting the heparin through a narrow gauge needle, using a concentrated solution of heparin so that only a small volume is required, and by applying pressure for at least 5 minutes after injection. The most convenient site is the anterior abdominal wall because of the subcutaneous fat. When subcutaneous heparin is used therapeutically (rather than prophylactically), it is given in a dose of 10,000 to 15,000 units every 12 hours with the aim of maintaining the minimum heparin concentration above 0.2 units/ml.

The Vitamin K Antagonists

The vitamin K antagonists are readily absorbed when administered by the oral route. The oral anticoagulants in common use are coumarin derivatives. These drugs act by interfering with a vitamin K-dependent postribosomal step in the hepatic synthesis of clotting Factors II, VII, IX, and X.

Drugs including aspirin, phenylbutazone, sulfonamides, oral antibiotics, sulfinpyrazone and anabolic steroids augment the effect of vitamin K antagonists. Many of these drugs act by displacing the oral anticoagulant from its carrier protein, thereby making more anticoagulant available. Dangerous bleeding may result if patients taking oral anticoagulants also take prescribed drugs that augment the effects of oral anticoagulants, unless careful laboratory monitoring is performed. Some of these drugs, particularly aspirin, also suppress platelet function and may contribute to bleeding through this effect. Other factors that potentiate the effect of oral anticoagulants include excessive alcohol intake, because of interference with liver function; diarrhea, because of interference with vitamin K absorption; a decrease in vitamin K intake; and liver disease.

Barbiturates are the most important class of drugs that inhibit the action of vitamin K antagonists. They achieve this effect by inducing the synthesis of hepatic enzymes that increase the rate of catabolism of the coumarin derivatives.

Other factors that inhibit vitamin K antagonists include an increased vitamin K content in the diet, oral contraceptives (because they increase the synthesis of blood coagulation factors), and hereditary resistance to the vitamin K antagonists.

Bleeding During Anticoagulant Therapy, and its Control

Bleeding during oral anticoagulant therapy is relatively uncommon in the hemostatically competent individual, provided that anticoagulation is monitored and maintained within the therapeutic range. However, bleeding becomes a more common complication in patients who are treated with anticoagulants in the early postoperative period, who are hemostatically impaired, or who have a local lesion such as a peptic ulcer or malignancy—even when the monitoring tests show that anticoagulation is maintained within the defined therapeutic range.

When bleeding is mild, there is rarely an indication to reverse the effect of the anticoagulant drug, but when serious bleeding occurs, particularly if it is life-threatening, prompt reversal of the anticoagulant effect is necessary. Serious bleeding during heparin therapy should be treated with the antidote protamine sulphate, which combines with and inactivates heparin immediately. Approximately 1 mg of protamine sulphate neutralizes approximately 100 units of heparin. Serious bleeding during treatment with the oral anticoagulants or overdose of oral anticoagulants should be treated with vitamin K_1 given by injection in a dose of 5 to 25 mg. If bleeding is life-threatening, the patient should be treated with Factor II, VII, IX, or X concentrates.

Antiplatelet Drugs

A great many compounds inhibit platelet function in vitro, and a number of these have been shown to inhibit thrombosis in experimental animals. Three that have been widely tested clinically are aspirin, dipyridamole, and sulfinpyrazone. The antithrombotic effect of aspirin is thought to be mediated through its inhibitory effect on the synthesis of thromboxane A_2 by platelets. The antithrombotic effect of dipyridamole is thought to be related to its ability to elevate platelet cyclic AMP levels by inhibiting the enzyme phosphodiesterase. The antithrombotic effect of sulfinpyrazone is poorly understood, and may be due in part to its ability to reversibly inhibit platelet prostaglandin synthesis and, therefore, to inhibit thromboxane A_2 production by the platelet. All three of these agents have been shown effective in the management of certain thromboembolic states in man. Aspirin is effective in relieving symptoms in patients with thrombocytosis and spontaneous platelet aggregation; in preventing systemic embolism in patients with prosthetic heart valve replacement when combined with oral anticoagulants; in reducing the frequency of transient cerebral ischemic attacks, stroke, and death in males with transient cerebral ischemia; and possibly in reducing recurrent myocardial ischemic complications in patients who have suffered a myocardial infarction.

Dipyridamole is effective in reducing systemic embolism when combined with oral anticoagulants in patients with prosthetic heart valves. Sulfinpyrazone is effective in reducing the frequency of thrombi that occur in arteriovenous shunts in patients undergoing chronic renal dialysis.

Thrombolytic Agents

Two thrombolytic agents in current use are streptokinase and urokinase. Both are plasminogen activators and produce thrombolysis by converting plasminogen to plasmin, which in turn lyses fibrin. Both of these drugs accelerate lysis of major pulmonary emboli and venous thrombi in man. They are associated with a higher frequency of bleeding than heparin, and therefore the decision regarding their use must always be weighed against the risks of therapy.

Part 2: Hemostasis and Bleeding

The normal hemostatic mechanism prevents blood loss from intact vessels and stops excessive bleeding from severed vessels. Prevention of blood loss from intact vessels is influenced by the structural integrity of the vessels and by the presence of a normal number of functional platelets. The arrest of bleeding from severed vessels is achieved through interaction between the blood vessel wall, blood platelets, and plasma proteins.

When a vessel is severed, it constricts, blood is shed, and the processes of platelet adhesion, aggregation, and blood coagulation are initiated. Vascular constriction is transient, lasting less than a minute, and is contributed to by local contraction of vascular wall cells in response to injury and, possibly, by vasoactive substances.

Platelets adhere to the subendothelial connective tissue and to the basement membrane, release adenosine diphosphate, and synthesize and release thromboxane A_2, an end product of platelet prostaglandin synthesis. Both of these agents stimulate platelets to aggregate to form an unstable platelet plug at the site of injury. All of these events occur within less than a minute of vessel injury, and then the unstable platelet plug is gradually stabilized over the next few minutes by fibrin, which is the final product of the blood coagulation process. The fibrin component of the hemostatic plug gradually increases in amount as the platelets undergo autolysis, and after 24 to 48 hours the hemostatic plug is transformed into fibrin. The fibrin is then digested by enzymes derived from the plasma (plasma fibrinolytic system) and from leukocytes and other cells (cellular fibrinolytic system), and the defect in the vessel wall is covered with endothelium.

The processes of platelet adhesion, platelet aggregation, blood coagulation, vessel constriction, and fibrinolysis are linked by a complex series of interactions. The initial vessel wall contraction that occurs in response to injury is contributed to by thromboxane A_2 synthesized by and released from platelets when they come in contact with the damaged vessel. Thrombin, an enzyme produced during blood coagulation, activates vascular wall cells to synthesize Prostanlahdia I_2 (PGI_2) and may contribute to the subsequent vasodilatation. Platelets activated by collagen, adenosine diphosphate, thromboxane, or thrombin undergo changes in their surface membranes that facilitate the alignment of blood coagu-

lation proteins in optimal proportions and so accelerate the blood coagulation process on the platelet surface. Thrombin is a powerful platelet-aggregating agent in its own right and causes platelets to release adenosine diphosphate and to synthesize and release thromboxane A_2.

THE BLOOD COAGULATION PROCESS

The process of blood coagulation follows a series of complexes that terminate in the formation of a fibrin clot. The coagulation proteins circulate as proenzymes, or zymogens, which are sequentially converted to active enzymes. The blood coagulation process can be activated either through the intrinsic or extrinsic pathways.

Activation of the intrinsic pathway is initiated by conversion of the proenzyme Factor XII to its enzyme when blood comes in contact with a nonendothelialized surface such as a damaged vessel wall or prosthetic device. In vitro, Factor XII is activated by contact with the wall of the test tube. The activated Factor XII, in turn, converts the zymogen Factor XI to the enzyme Factor XIa, a reaction that is calcium-independent; all subsequent blood coagulation reactions require calcium. Factor XIa activates Factor IX, and Factor IXa in the presence of Factor VIII, and phospholipid activates Factor X. The rate of this reaction is greatly increased by the presence of phospholipid and by the prior exposure of Factor VIII to thrombin or Factor Xa. The extrinsic pathway is activated in vitro by exposing blood to phospholipoprotein extracts from various tissues (such as brain or lung), which are known as tissue thromboplastins. Tissue thromboplastins combine with and activate Factor VII, and this Factor VII tissue-thromboplastin complex in turn activates Factor X, bypassing a number of time consuming steps in the intrinsic clotting pathway.

The extrinsic pathway is probably stimulated in vivo by exposure of blood to damaged endothelium or to extravascular tissues, both of which have tissue thromboplastin activity. The intrinsic and extrinsic pathways meet at a common point at the activation of Factor X, and beyond this point blood coagulation continues along a common pathway. Activated Factor X in the presence of calcium, phospholipid, and

Factor V converts prothrombin to thrombin. This reaction is also markedly accelerated by the prior exposure of Factor V to thrombin. The enzyme thrombin interacts with fibrinogen, splitting it into a large fibrin monomer fragment and into small polypeptide fragments known as fibrinopeptides A and B. The fibrin monomer fragments copolymerize to form fibrin polymers that precipitate as insoluble fibrin when a critical concentration of fibrin monomer is reached. The fibrin polymers are initially linked by noncovalent bonds but become covalently bound under the influence of activated Factor XIII.

Blood coagulation is modified by a number of positive and negative feedback loops and by interaction between the intrinsic and extrinsic pathways.

The coagulation system may be activated in vivo by tissue thromboplastin at the level of Factor VII, by contact activation at the level of Factor XII, by activated platelets at the level of Factor XI, or by enzymes derived from malignant cells at the level of Factor X. Tissue thromboplastin is released into the bloodstream during surgery and following tissue injury, and is probably made available locally by vascular wall cells when they are damaged and by activated leucocytes that migrate to the area of vascular damage. Factor XII is activated on contact with subendothelial tissues that are exposed to circulating blood as a result of vascular injury or when blood comes in contact with prosthetic devices. The observations that mucin, including mucin produced by mucin-secreting adenocarcinoma and other extracts of malignant cells, are able to activate Factor X directly, suggests the possibility that this may be one of the mechanisms by which thrombosis is induced in patients with cancer. The ability of stimulated platelets to activate Factor XI directly probably explains the lack of a hemorrhagic diathesis in patients with Factor XII deficiency.

FIBRINOLYSIS

There are two components of the blood fibrinolytic system: a plasma component and a cellular component (Fig. 4.1). The basic reaction of the plasma fibrinolytic system is the conversion of a beta globulin, plasminogen, to an active proteolytic enzyme, plasmin. Plasminogen activation occurs by two different pathways; a pathway linked with the activation of Factor XII and a pathway in which the activator originates from endothelial cells. The plasminogen activators exert their fibrinolytic action by hydrolysing a specific bond in plasminogen, converting it to plasmin. When plasmin is formed in plasma, it rapidly binds to α-2-antiplasmin so that fibrinogen and other circulating plasma proteins are protected from its proteolytic effect. When plasmin is produced in excess, the α-2-antiplasmin binding site becomes saturated, plasmin binds to α-2-macroglobulin and interacts with fibrinogen, which is

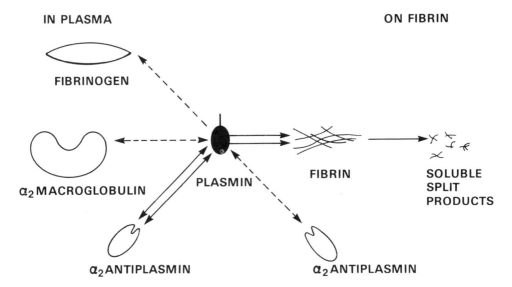

Fig. 4.1 When plasmin is formed in plasma, it is rapidly inactivated by a_2 antiplasmin. Excess plasmin combines with a_2 macroglobulin or is available for proteolysis of fibrinogen and other blood coagulation factors. When plasmin is formed on fibrin, it is protected from the effect of a_2 antiplasmin and is, therefore, available for fibrinolysis.

rapidly degraded. In contrast, plasmin that is formed within the interstices of a fibrin clot is protected from inactivation by α-2-antiplasmin, since its binding to fibrin protects it from the inhibitor. Both tissue plasminogen activator and plasminogen are adsorbed to fibrin. This is an important mechanism for localising fibrinolytic activity on the fibrin surface. Plasminogen activator is constantly present in blood in normal healthy individuals but very little, if any, plasminogen activation occurs under normal circumstances. On the other hand, when intravascular coagulation occurs, there is evidence of activation of the fibrinolytic system, presumably because the circulating plasminogen activator is adsorbed to fibrin along with plasminogen and so induces local fibrinolysis. Although it has been suggested that the fibrinolytic system is in dynamic equilibrium with the coagulation system, turnover studies with labeled components of the coagulation and fibrinolytic system in healthy human subjects indicate that this process of continuous activation is either minute or nonexistant.

FIBRINOLYTIC BLEEDING

Abnormal bleeding caused by increased fibrinolytic activity has been described in association with a congenital deficiency of α-2-antiplasmin, and as an acquired abnormality in patients with liver disease who are exposed to trauma. The mechanism of acquired fibrinolytic bleeding is thought to be due to impaired hepatic clearance of plasminogen activator released from damaged vascular wall cells.

A number of factors contribute to the hemostatic defect in pathological fibrinolytic states. These include digestion of fibrin in wounds and hemostatic plugs, interference of normal fibrin clot formation by plasmin proteolysis products of fibrin and fibrinogen, and by hypofibrinogenemia and decreased levels of other coagulation factors induced by plasmin-induced proteolysis.

DEFECTIVE HEMOSTASIS

Abnormal bleeding can be caused by defects in any of the components in the hemostatic system, including blood vessels, platelets, blood coagulation proteins, or excessive fibrinolytic activity (Table 4.11).

These abnormalities may be inherited or acquired, may occur as isolated or mixed deficiencies, and may be associated with minimal or no pathological bleeding, or may produce life-threatening bleeding.

The clinical problems produced by abnormal

Table 4.11 **Bleeding Disorders**

Vascular Disorders
  Purpura simplex
  Senile purpura
  Purpura associated with infection and drugs
  Vasculitis (Henoch-Schoenlein purpura)
  Scurvy
  Hypercortisolism and rheumatoid arthritis
  Amyloid disease
Platelet Disorders
  Thrombocytopenia
  Platelet function disorders
Coagulation Factor Disorders
Pathological Fibrinolysis

bleeding include acute anemia and hypovolemic circulatory failure; compression of vital structures such as pharynx, brain, or blood vessels produced by internal bleeding; chronic iron deficiency anemia due to chronic or recurrent blood loss; and bleeding into joints or muscles that may lead to contractures and deformities.

DIAGNOSIS OF BLEEDING DISORDERS

Abnormal bleeding, either overt or hidden, is a common manifestation of a variety of disorders. The physician must determine whether the patient is bleeding as a result of local factors such as a peptic ulcer, dysfunctional uterine bleeding, or hemorrhoids, or whether the patient has a generalized hemostatic defect. Patients with a mild hemostatic defect can present difficult diagnostic problems because the abnormality may only declare itself when it is unmasked by local factors or by trauma. In contrast, patients with severe hemostatic defects do not present diagnostic difficulties because the bleeding manifestations are usually readily apparent.

The diagnosis of a clinically suspected bleeding disorder is made by taking a careful history, performing a complete physical examination, performing screening tests, and, if indicated, performing special tests of hemostasis.

The clinical history is the most important single factor in the diagnostic process. It is usually possible to determine from the history whether the patient has a generalized hemostatic defect and whether the defect is inherited or acquired, and it may be possible to determine whether the defect is likely to be a vascular or platelet abnormality, a coagulation abnormality, or a mixture of the two. Specific investigations are required to determine the precise nature of the abnormality.

The patient is likely to be suffering from a generalized hemostatic defect if bleeding occurs from multiple sites, if it is spontaneous, or if it takes the form of petechiae, hematomas, very large bruises, or hemarthrosis. In contrast, nose bleeding, uterine bleeding, and gastrointestinal bleeding are much more frequently caused by local factors, and even when they occur in combination (for example, uterine bleeding and gastrointestinal bleeding) they are more likely to be manifestations of two local abnormalities rather than of a generalized bleeding abnormality.

Patients with severe inherited disorders usually present in infancy or childhood, may have a family history of bleeding, and often give a history of bleeding in response to previous operations or trauma. On the other hand, patients with mild inherited hemostatic defects may present for the first time in adult life, often after exposure to trauma or surgery, and in these patients it may be difficult to determine whether the hemorrhagic disorder is inherited or acquired.

Inherited bleeding disorders may be transmitted as either an autosomal or a sex-linked recessive trait. By obtaining a careful family history it may be possible to establish the hereditary nature of the condition and therefore narrow down the number of diagnostic possibilities. Every effort should be made to interview as many of the patient's relatives as possible and to obtain a detailed history from these relatives. Histories obtained about relatives from either the patient or the patient's parents are frequently unreliable. A positive family history of bleeding is of great value in establishing a diagnosis of an inherited bleeding disorder but a negative history does not exclude this possibility, particularly if the family history is only obtained from the patient, or if the number of family members is small. In obtaining a history of previous response to surgery or trauma, specific enquiries should be made about bleeding from the umbilical cord at birth, bleeding after circumcision, tooth extraction, tonsillectomy, and abdominal operations. If tonsillectomy or major abdominal operations have been tolerated without excessive blood loss, it is unlikely that the patient is suffering from a severe or even moderately severe inherited bleeding disorder.

Many acquired hemostatic defects are associated with an obvious underlying disorder such as liver disease and kidney disease, but occasionally careful enquiry may be necessary to obtain a history of drug ingestion.

Differentiation between a vascular, platelet, or coagulation defect is frequently possible. In the typical case, a patient with a vascular or platelet disorder has spontaneous skin and mucous membrane bleeding, petechiae and superficial bruising, and bleeding that starts within seconds of injury and is prolonged, but does not usually recur once stopped. In contrast, patients with coagulation defects typically develop deep spreading hematomas, bleeding into joints, hematuria, and retroperitoneal bleeding. In these patients, post-traumatic bleeding may be delayed sometimes for hours after the traumatic episode and then may recur at a later date for up to 4 to 5 days.

LABORATORY DIAGNOSIS OF BLEEDING DISORDERS

Laboratory investigations are required to determine the precise nature of the underlying bleeding disorder. Initially, screening tests are performed for vascular, platelet, and coagulation disorders, and based on the results of these and the patient's history, additional, more complex, time consuming and expensive tests may be performed.

Screening Tests for Vascular and Platelet Disorders

The two most important screening tests in patients with suspected vascular or platelet disorders are the bleeding time and the platelet count. The tourniquet test for vascular fragility is less useful because it has both limited sensitivity and specificity for platelet and vascular disorders. The template bleeding time is used to determine the time required for bleeding to stop from incised small subcutaneous vessels. A blood pressure cuff is applied to the upper arm and inflated to 40 mm Hg, either 2 or 3 standard incisions 1 mm deep and 5 mm long are made in the skin of the anterior aspect of the forearm, and the time taken for bleeding to stop is measured. The bleeding time is an index of the initial stages of the hemostatic plug formation. The upper limit of normal for the template bleeding time is 6 minutes. It is prolonged in patients who have abnormalities of vascular contraction, thrombocytopenia, or in those with platelet functional disorders characterised by abnormal adhesion of platelets to the damaged vessel, abnormal release of adenosine diphosphate or thromboxane A_2, or abnormal aggregation with adenosine diphosphate. The bleeding time is usually normal in patients with coagulation disorders, presumably because fibrin formation is not required for primary arrest of bleeding from the small vessels that are severed in the subcutaneous tissues.

The platelet count can be assessed by direct counting using either a hemocytometer or particle counter—or by careful inspection of the blood film, which provides a semiquantitative assessment. Inspection of the blood film may also reveal large platelets, which are seen in patients with thrombocytopenia and associated rapid platelet turnover, with myeloproliferative disorders, and with a rare inherited platelet function abnormality known as Bernard-Soulier syndrome.

The normal range for the platelet count is 150,000 to 400,000/mm^3. Although there is no absolute relationship between the platelet count and the incidence or severity of bleeding, spontaneous bleeding is uncommon if the platelet count is above 40,000/mm^3 but is frequent and often severe when the platelet count is less than 10,000/mm^3. If spontaneous bleeding does occur in patients with platelet counts above 40,000/mm^3, the possibility of an associated platelet functional disorder or coagulation defect should be considered.

Screening Tests for Coagulation Disorders

The thrombin time, prothrombin time, and partial thromboplastin time, are tests designed to detect a significant coagulation abnormality in either the intrinsic or extrinsic pathway, or in the final step of coagulation—the coversion of fibrinogen to fibrin.

Partial Thromboplastin Time

The partial thromboplastin time is a screening test for the intrinsic coagulation pathway. The principle of the test is to activate Factor XII with a surface activator such as kaolin or celite, and then, after a period of incubation, to add phospholipid and calcium to the plasma. Phospholipid substitutes for platelets, and calcium is required since the plasma used for these tests is collected in a chelating anticoagulant. Factor VII is not required for this reaction, and therefore the partial thromboplastin time becomes normal in patients with a Factor VII deficiency.

The partial thromboplastin time is abnormal in patients with deficiencies of Factors XII, XI, IX, VIII, X, V, prothrombin, or fibrinogen. The test is relatively insensitive to deficiencies of Factor V, prothrombin, and fibrinogen. In addition, prolongation of the partial thromboplastin time is seen in patients with disorders of prekallekrein and kininogen, both of which are required for the activation of Factor XI by Factor XII.

Prothrombin Time

The prothrombin time test is performed by adding tissue extract and calcium to citrated platelet-poor plasma. Tissue thromboplastin combines with and activates Factor VII, which in turn activates Factor X. Activated Factor X in the presence of Factor V and phospholipid converts prothrombin to thrombin, and the thrombin then converts fibrinogen to fibrin. The prothrombin time bypasses the intrinsic clotting pathway and is normal in patients with deficiencies of Factors XII, XI, IX, and VIII. It is abnormal in patients with deficiencies of Factors VII, X, V, prothrombin, or fibrinogen.

Thrombin Clotting Time

The thrombin clotting time test is performed by adding thrombin to platelet-poor plasma. Thrombin converts fibrinogen to fibrin, and this test bypasses all other steps in the coagulation sequence. Therefore, the thrombin time is normal in patients with deficiencies of Factors XII, XI, IX, VIII, X, V, VII, and II. The thrombin time is also normal in patients with any condition that interferes with the conversion of fibrinogen to fibrin. These include hypofibrinogenemia, inhibitors of thrombin such as heparin, and inhibitors of fibrin polymerization such as the proteolysis products of fibrin.

Thus, by performing these three screening tests, it is possible to localize the coagulation factor defect and assign it to either the intrinsic pathway (abnormal partial thromboplastin time), the extrinsic pathway (abnormal prothrombin time), abnormalities of the common pathway (prolonged partial thromboplastin time and prothrombin time), and abnormalities of the final step in blood coagulation (prolonged thrombin time). Combined abnormalities of the prothrombin and partial thromboplastin time also occur in the presence of multiple defects, while an abnormality of all three screening tests occurs in severe hypofibrinogenemia or in patients with multiple defects.

Special Tests

The special tests that may be required after the patient's history, physical examination, and screening tests are evaluated include (1) specific coagulation factor assays; (2) platelet function tests to measure the platelet release reaction and platelet aggregation; (3) assay for von Willebrand's factor (see below), which is performed by testing the ability of platelets to aggregate, with a substance known as ristocetin; (4) tests for circulating inhibitor; (5) tests for disseminated intravascular coagulation; and (6) tests for pathological fibrinolysis.

VASCULAR DISORDERS

It may be difficult to differentiate vascular disorders from platelet disorders on clinical grounds and the diagnosis of a vascular defect is usually made after thrombocytopenia and a platelet functional defect have been excluded. The vascular bleeding disorders are a heterogeneous group of conditions caused by a variety of abnormalities involving either the vessels themselves or the perivascular connective tissue. Clinically, these disorders are characterized by easy bruising and spontaneous bleeding from small vessels. The vascular wall defects may be caused by inflammatory or immune processes or by congenital weaknesses in the vessel wall, while the perivascular disorders are usually degenerative in nature and associated with loss of perivascular supporting connective tissue.

Most cases of bleeding due to vascular disorders alone are not severe and rarely are life-threatening. The bleeding is usually into the skin causing petechiae or ecchymoses, or both, but in some conditions there is also excessive bleeding from mucous membranes. In many of these conditions, the standard screening tests used for the investigation of patients with a bleeding disorder show little or no abnormality. The bleeding time is usually normal, but the tourniquet test might be positive.

The vascular defects may be inherited or acquired. The most common inherited hemorrhagic disorder caused by a vascular abnormality is *hereditary hemorrhagic telangiectasia*. This relatively uncommon disorder is transmitted as an autosomal dominant trait and therefore affects both sexes equally. Telangiectases begin to appear in the skin and mucous membranes usually during early adult life. The basic underlying abnormality is a defect in the subendothelial connective tissue, which results in multiple dilatations of capillaries and arterioles. Because of their thinness, the vascular dilatations bleed easily. The most common symptom is epistaxis, but bleeding may occur from the gastrointestinal tract and rarely in other organs. Anemia may occur due to chronic blood loss and iron deficiency. The tourniquet test and bleeding time are normal, and although there have been isolated reports of abnormalities of platelet function in patients with hereditary hemorrhagic telangiectasia, these are probably chance associations

and are unlikely to contribute to the mechanism of hemorrhage. The lesions in the skin are mainly seen on the face, on the tips of the fingers, and on the feet, while the mucous membrane lesions are seen in the mouth and on the lips, tongue, cheeks, and palate. The lesions blanche on pressure and tend to become more numerous and larger with advancing age.

Other inherited vascular and perivascular defects are very rare. They include a number of connective tissue disorders due to defects in collagen or elastin. These include Ehlers-Danlos syndrome, osteogenesis imperfecta, and pseudoxanthoma elasticum. In all three of these disorders there is an inherited abnormality of connective tissue that leads to extreme vascular fragility and to abnormalities of the skin and skeletal system.

ACQUIRED VASCULAR DEFECTS

The more common acquired vascular defects are purpura simplex (simple easy bruising), senile purpura, purpura associated with infections and drugs, Henoch-Schönlein syndrome, scurvy, corticosteroid administration, rheumatoid arthritis, and amyloid disease.

Purpura Simplex

Purpura simplex is a common, benign disorder that usually first presents in adolescence or early adult life and occurs predominantly in women who are otherwise healthy. The disorder is characterized by recurrent bruising, either spontaneous or following minor trauma, that is most often seen on the legs, arms, and trunk. The bruises are occasionally preceeded by pain, which is probably caused by rupture of small blood vessels. The cause of the disorder is unknown. The diagnosis is made on the basis of characteristic clinical manifestations and by excluding other causes of easy bruising, the most common of which are platelet functional disorders, particularly the acquired disorder associated with aspirin ingestion and the disorder associated with mild von Willebrand's disease. In purpura simplex, all tests of hemostasis are normal. The disorder does not cause excessive bleeding at operation, and there is sometimes a family history in the female members of the family.

Senile Purpura

Senile purpura is the term used to describe the purpura and the ecchymoses that occur mainly on the extensor aspect of the forearm and the hand in elderly subjects. The skin in the affected parts is inelastic and thin, and histological section shows atrophy of subcutaneous connective tissue, which results in the skin being freely moveable over the deep tissues. The purpuric lesions are thought to be caused by the excessive mobility of the skin and subcutaneous tissue, which results in tearing of the small subcutaneous vessels.

Purpura Associated with Infections and Drugs

Purpura associated with bacterial, rickettsial, or viral infections may be caused by direct vascular toxic damage or may be contributed to by thrombocytopenia with or without disseminated intravascular thrombosis. Viruses and bacteria may directly invade vascular endothelium, may release toxins, or vascular damage may be caused by microthrombi induced by the direct interaction of viruses or bacterial products with blood platelets.

A number of drugs have also been reported to cause purpura without associated thrombocytopenia, although frequently drug-induced purpura is thrombocytopenic.

Henoch-Schönlein Syndrome

The Henoch-Schönlein syndrome is a hypersensitivity reaction characterized by widespread inflammation of capillaries and other small blood vessels. This results in increased vascular permeability, perivascular edema, and perivascular hemorrhage.

The condition occurs most commonly in children but may occur in adults, and usually presents in an acute form with a macular rash, purpura, arthalgia, gastrointestinal pain, and hematuria. In most cases, there is no obvious preceeding event but the condition may follow upper respiratory tract infection or drug ingestion.

The distribution of the purpuric rash is fairly characteristic, occurring on the buttocks, on the backs of the elbow, on extensor surface of the arms, on the extensor surface of the lower leg, on the ankle, and on the foot. It is usually bilateral and symmetrical. The purpuric lesions may occur in crops and be associated with a macular papular rash and subcutaneous edema, and occasionally may be frankly hemorrhagic.

Scurvy

Scurvy, which is caused by vitamin C deficiency, is associated with increased vascular fragility, which results in defective formation of vascular connective tissue. Hemorrhage commonly occurs in the skin and is manifested both by petechiae and ecchymoses. The legs are a common site of hemorrhage, and the petechiae are frequently perifolicular. The bleeding time is often prolonged, and the tourniquet test is usually positive.

Cushing's Disease and Rheumatoid Arthritis

Bruising is a common feature of Cushing's disease and of patients treated with large doses of corticosteroids for a prolonged period of time. These patients lose subcutaneous tissue that supports blood vessels coursing between muscle and skin, so that the vessels readily bleed even with mild trauma. Bleeding is fairly severe, and takes the form of bruising or multiple petechial hemorrhages and purpuric spots. Patients with rheumatoid arthritis also lose subcutaneous tissue and frequently develop lesions similar to those seen in senile purpura.

Amyloid Disease

Amyloid deposits in the perivascular tissue cause increased vascular fragility that frequently leads to purpura and hemorrhage. Characteristically, the blood vessels that have been infiltrated with amyloid tissue are very fragile, so that even mild trauma such as simple stroking may cause hemorrhage in the skin. The cutaneous areas most frequently affected include the eyelids, the mucous membranes, and the intertrigenous folds. Amyloid disease of the lungs or liver may cause fatal hemorrhage after needle biopsy.

PLATELET DISORDERS

Hemostasis may be impaired by either a quantitative defect (thrombocytopenia) or a qualitative defect (platelet functional abnormality). Platelets are derived from megakaryocytes, which are multinucleated cells found in the bone marrow. Megakaryocytes arise from mononuclear precursors that undergo nuclear replication without cytoplasmic replication so that they become multinucleate. Cytoplasmic maturation also occurs, and membranes form that set apart the cytoplasm into platelet subunits, which eventually are released into the bloodstream as mature platelets. In the normal marrow, about 25 percent of the megakaryocytes are immature and contain no apparent granules, and 75 percent show varying degrees of granulation.

Platelet production is under the control of thrombopoietin, a humoral agent, which acts both to increase the number of megakaryocytes formed from precursor cells and to increase the rate of cytoplasmic maturation and platelet release. Thrombopoietin blood levels rise in thrombocytopenic states, but its site of synthesis is unknown.

After their release from megakaryocytes, platelets circulate for approximately 10 days as cytoplasmic discs in a concentration of approximately 250,000 platelets/mm^3 of blood. Young platelets recently released from the marrow are larger than platelets that have been in the circulation for a number of days. Approximately 20 to 30 percent of the platelets are pooled in the spleen, while the remaining 70 to 80 percent circulate in equilibrium with a splenic platelet pool. Splenic enlargement is associated with a marked increase in splenic pooling so that up to 80 to 90 percent of the total body platelets may be pooled in the spleen in patients with marked splenic enlargement. When there is an increase in platelet turnover, for example, when an accelerated rate of platelet destruction is taking place, platelets are released prematurely from the marrow and so the proportion of large platelets in the circulation increases.

ETIOLOGY OF THROMBOCYTOPENIA

Thrombocytopenia may be caused by disorders that decrease the rate of platelet production, increase the rate of platelet destruction, or result in an increase in splenic platelet pooling. A reduction in the rate of platelet production may be associated with a reduced number of megakaryocytes in the marrow or may result from ineffective platelet production from normal numbers of megakaryocytes. Amegakaryocytic or hypomegakaryocytic thrombocytopenia may be caused by a variety of agents that produce marrow damage, including radiation, chemicals, and drugs, and may be caused by intrinsic bone marrow abnormalities such as leukemia or when bone marrow is replaced with malignant cells or fibrous tissue. Ineffective thrombopoiesis associated with normal numbers of marrow megakaryocytes is seen in megaloblastic anemia and occasionally in myeloproliferative disorders.

Thrombocytopenia Associated with Increased Platelet Destruction

There are three basic mechanisms responsible for the premature removal of platelets from the circu-

lation. These are immune-mediated platelet destruction, thrombin-induced platelet aggregation, and platelet damage due to interaction with other stimuli. In all cases, thrombocytopenia stimulates the marrow so that megakaryocyte and platelet production are increased. If the stimulus to platelet destruction is relatively mild, the platelet count may be compensated to near normal.

Immune Thrombocytopenia

Three types of immune thrombocytopenia are recognized clinically: chronic immune thrombocytopenia, acute immune thrombocytopenia, and drug-induced thrombocytopenia.

Chronic immune thrombocytopenia Chronic immune thrombocytopenia may be primary, or may occur in association with other immune disorders, such as disseminated lupus erythematosus or lymphoproliferative disorders such as chronic lymphocytic leukemia and Hodgkin's disease. In this disorder, the platelets are coated with autoantibodies that sensitize the platelets so that they are phagocytosed by cells in the reticuloendothelial tissues. There is some evidence that lightly sensitized platelets are mainly destroyed in the spleen, while very heavily sensitized platelets are destroyed in the liver and in other reticuloendothelial tissues throughout the body.

Treatment of chronic immune thrombocytopenia is directed toward reducing the level of circulating autoantibody and reducing the rate at which sensitized platelets are destroyed by the reticuloendothelial system. Various immunosuppressive agents such as cyclophosphamide and vincristine decrease the titer of circulating autoantibodies, while splenectomy relieves thrombocytopenia in a large percentage of these patients mainly by removing a principle site of platelet destruction. Corticosteroids act at both levels. They decrease production of autoantibodies and also decrease the rate at which sensitized platelets are removed or destroyed by phagocytic cells.

Acute immune thrombocytopenia Acute immune thrombocytopenia is a self-limiting condition that is probably caused by immune complexes that adhere to platelets and lead to their premature destruction. The antigenic component of the immune complex may be a virus or bacterial product or, frequently, it remains unidentified. Clinically, patients with acute immune thrombocytopenia develop thrombocytopenia with an increase in platelet associated IgG, 7 to 14 days after acute viral infection or in the acute stages of a bacterial infection. Thrombocytopenia usually persists for approximately a week and occasionally may last up to 3 or 4 weeks.

Drug-induced immune thrombocytopenia Most cases of drug-induced immune thrombocytopenia are thought to be caused by immune complexes formed between the drug-plasma protein (the antigen), and an antibody-directed against this antigen. Immune complexes are absorbed onto the platelet's surface, leading either to premature destruction in the reticuloendothelial system or to intravascular lysis, a complement-mediated mechanism.

Nonimmune Destructive Thrombocytopenia

Thrombocytopenia is a common feature of disseminated intravascular coagulation and is caused by the interaction of platelets with thrombin. Other less well-defined mechanisms of accelerated destruction include prosthetic heart valves, large hemangiomas, and thrombotic thrombocytopenic purpura. The likely mechanism of premature platelet destruction in patients with prosthetic heart valves and giant hemangioma is interaction of platelets with a nonendothelialized surface, which results in platelet damage and premature destruction. The mechanism of thrombocytopenia in the condition, known as thrombotic thrombocytopenic purpura, is a matter for debate. There is evidence that thrombocytopenia is associated with an increase in the concentration of platelet-bound IgG, and it is likely that in many of these cases the thrombocytopenia is immune-complex induced. However, the clinical manifestations of this disorder differ from those of drug-induced immune complex thrombocytopenia in one important respect: the disseminated intravascular platelet aggregation associated with thrombotic thrombocytopenic purpura produces serious focal organ ischemia.

Thrombocytopenia Due to Splenic Pooling

Thrombocytopenia is associated with increased splenic pooling in patients with marked splenic enlargement. Thrombocytopenia due to increased splenic pooling is seen in portal hypertension. In splenomegaly associated with lymphoproliferative and myeloproliferative disorders, the thrombocytopenia is contributed to both by splenic pooling and impaired platelet production.

Platelet Functional Disorders

These disorders may be primary or may occur in association with recognized disorders. The primary disorders may be inherited or acquired. Patients present with abnormal skin and mucous membrane bleeding, and in some patients the bleeding time is prolonged and mucous membrane bleeding may be severe and even life-threatening.

Failure of Platelets to Adhere to Subendothelium

Failure of platelets to adhere to subendothelial connective tissue is seen in von Willebrand's disease and the Bernard-Soulier syndrome. In von Willebrand's disease, there is either a quantitative or a qualitative abnormality in the Factor VII molecule. The Factor VIII molecule can be considered to subserve two major functions in hemostasis: to act as a cofactor in the intrinsic pathway of blood coagulation (the coagulant portion of the molecule) and to act as a bridge between endothelium and platelets (the von Willebrand portion of the factor molecule). In the Bernard-Soulier syndrome the platelets have a membrane abnormality associated with a lack of one of the membrane glycoproteins that is a receptor for the von Willebrand portion of the Factor VIII molecule. Patients with the Bernard-Soulier syndrome have giant platelets which are also relatively ineffective in supporting blood coagulation. Abnormalities of platelet adherence to subendothelium have also been described in hypergammaglobulinemia, possibly because the gammaglobulin coats the platelets and interferes with their adhesion to subendothelial structures.

Failure of Platelets to Release Adenosine Diphosphate

There are two types of release defects. One is associated with reduced levels of adenosine diphosphate in the platelet-dense granules, called *storage pool disease*, and the other is associated with an abnormality of the platelet release mechanism. In patients with storage pool disease, there is a family history of the defect, the skin bleeding time is prolonged, and the bleeding manifestations vary from mild to severe. In the second type of release defect, patients have normal amounts of ADP in their granules but do not release the ADP in response to collagen, thrombin, and adrenalin. This type of abnormality is seen in patients with myeloproliferative syndromes, and following cardiac bypass surgery in which a pump oxygenator has been used.

Defective Platelet Prostaglandin Synthesis

When platelets are exposed to various stimuli including collagen, thrombin, and adrenalin, the platelet surface enzyme phospholipase A_2 is activated, and this in turn cleaves arachidonic acid from membrane phospholipid. The arachidonic acid is then oxidized by cyclo-oxygenase to the endoperoxides PGG_2 and PGH_2; PGH_2 is converted to thromboxane A_2 under the influence of the enzyme thromboxane synthetase. Thromboxane A_2 stimulates platelets to release adenosine diphosphate (ADP) and causes platelet aggregation.

Aspirin and some other anti-inflammatory drugs block thromboxane A_2 formation by inhibiting the enzyme platelet cyclo-oxygenase. The effect of aspirin on platelets is of considerable interest because of its possible therapeutic applications. Although aspirin is cleared from the bloodstream rapidly (within 30 minutes of ingestion), the platelet function defect produced by aspirin lasts for up to 4 to 7 days. This is because aspirin irreversibly acetylates the enzyme cyclo-oxygenase and so inhibits platelet function for the life span of the circulating platelets. Primary deficiencies in cyclo-oxygenase and thromboxane synthetase have also been described, and these patients have an aspirin-like release defect.

Failure of Platelets to Aggregate with Adenosine Diphosphate

Failure of platelets to aggregate with ADP occurs in a rare inherited platelet disorder known as *thrombasthenia*. Thrombasthenic platelets lack a membrane glycoprotein that is thought to be a receptor for ADP. The platelets do not aggregate with ADP, thrombin, or collagen, and the patients may have a severe bleeding abnormality with bruising, petechiae, and purpura.

Failure of Platelets to Accelerate Blood Coagulation on their Surface

Platelet phospholipid is normally made available for blood coagulation on the platelet surface when platelets aggregate. Therefore, a failure of availability and impaired blood coagulation arises in any disorder that interferes with platelet aggregation. A qualitative defect of platelet phospholipid has been described in a number of families with bleeding disorders and is also a feature of the Bernard-Soulier syndrome.

Mixed Defects that Are Less Well Characterized

Abnormalities of platelet aggregation and release occur in patients with renal failure, myeloproliferative disorders, and hypergammaglobulinemia. Platelet functional abnormality in renal failure is reversible by dialysis, and is caused by a retained metabolite, guanidinosuccinic acid, which interferes with platelet function.

COAGULATION DISORDERS

Abnormalities of blood coagulation can arise because (1) there is a defect in synthesis of the coagulation molecule, (2) the coagulation molecule synthesized is functionally defective, (3) the plasma clearance of the coagulation factors is increased (due to its participation in intravascular coagulation, destruction by proteolytic enzyme, or abnormal renal clearance), and (4) by the inactivation of coagulation factors by circulating antibodies.

The coagulation factors fibrinogen, prothrombin, Factors V, VII, IX, X, XI, XII, and XIII are synthesized in the liver. Synthesis of Factors VII, IX, X, and prothrombin is vitamin K-dependent. Factor VIII is synthesized in the endothelial cells and it then acquires coagulant activity by an unknown process.

HEREDITARY DISORDERS

The most common pure coagulation disorder is hemophilia A, or Factor VIII deficiency. In hemophilia A, Factor VIII antigen and von Willebrand factor is present in normal amounts, but the molecule is defective in coagulant activity. The other inherited disorders of coagulation factors have not been as well characterized; in some there is evidence of synthesis of a defective molecule, while in others there appears to be a reduced synthesis of the coagulation factor, but the factor retains normal function. In the very severe form of von Willebrand's disease there is a marked decrease in the level of Factor VIII antigen, which is paralleled by a marked coagulation defect. In the milder forms, Factor VIII antigen is moderately depressed and this is usually paralleled by a decrease in Factor VIII coagulant activity, although in some of the variants there are considerable discrepancies between the levels of Factor VIII antigen (assayed immunologically), von Willebrand factor activity (assayed by the ristocetin platelet aggregation test), and the Factor VIII coagulant activity. In these variants, the Factor VIII coagulant activity tends to be proportionately higher than the other measurements.

Both hemophilia A (Factor VIII deficiency) and hemophilia B (Christmas disease, Factor IX deficiency) are transmitted as sex-linked recessive traits. Von Willebrand's disease is transmitted as an autosomal dominant trait, often with incomplete penetrance, while all of the other inherited coagulation disorders are thought to be transmitted as autosomal recessive traits. As a general rule, there is a good correlation between the severity of the patient's symptoms and the severity of coagulation deficiency in patients with hemophilia A and hemophilia B. For patients with hemophilia A or hemophilia B, levels of coagulation factor activity of less than 1 percent of normal are associated with severe bleeding symptoms, levels of 1 to 5 percent are associated with moderate bleeding symptoms, while patients with levels between 5 and 20 percent of normal usually only have a mild hemorrhagic defect. In contrast, Factor XII deficiency and deficiencies of the other contact activation factors prekallekrein and kininogen may produce a marked laboratory-detected defect but no clinical bleeding. Factor XI deficiency may also produce a marked laboratory-detected defect but the clinical symptoms are disproportionately mild. In Factor VII deficiency, the clinical effects also tend to be disproportionately less than the defects detected by laboratory tests, although some patients with Factor VII deficiency have severe bleeding. Both Factor V and Factor X deficiencies are very uncommon; clinical bleeding occurs, but the relationship between the laboratory defect and the severity of bleeding is not well characterized. Severe Factor XIII deficiency produces clinical bleeding, but all screening tests for coagulation disorders are normal. This deficiency is diagnosed by demonstrating increased solubility of a fibrin clot in solvents such as 5 mol/L urea.

Hemophilia A

Hemophilia A is due to a Factor VIII abnormality and is transmitted as a sex-linked recessive trait. The clinical disorder is seen almost exclusively in affected males. Females carry the trait but, with rare exceptions, do not have a significant coagulation deficiency.

Various grades of severity of hemophilia are recognized, and the severity of the clinical manifestations closely parallel the concentration of Factor VIII in the patient's plasma. Bleeding manifestations in severely affected patients are usually obvious in early childhood and tend to be both severe and spontaneous. The first manifestation in patients with severe hemophilia may be bleeding at the time of circumcision, but many severely affected hemophiliacs do not bleed abnormally until they reach the stage of toddling. Moderately affected patients do not bleed spontaneously unless they have a local lesion, and these patients may have their first episode of abnormal bleeding in adult life following operative trauma. Severe hemophiliacs have bleeding into muscles and joints, which may lead to permanent crippling unless treated promptly and adequately. Posttraumatic bleeding characteristically occurs in deep wounds, and it continues for days. Any large hematomas that form may compress nerves and occasionally even produce severe vascular occlusion leading to gangrene. Oral-pharyngial bleeding is one of the most dangerous complications of hemophiliac hemorrhage, because it may produce severe respiratory obstruction.

Principles of Treatment

The physician caring for patients with lifelong bleeding disorders must be prepared not only to manage episodes of bleeding but is also required to make a strong commitment to manage the social and psychological problems encountered by both the patient and parents. Patients with lifelong bleeding disorders should, if at all possible, be managed by a group of medical and paramedical specialists in the field. In advising parents on their children's upbringing, a balance must be struck between protecting the child from injury and bringing him or her up as normally as safety will permit. The child should be encouraged to participate in noncontact sports and to develop interests that will not expose him or her to hazards in later life.

Bleeding episodes are managed using both local measures and replacement therapy. The outlook for the hemophiliac has improved considerably because of the availability of Factor VIII concentrates that can be used at the first sign of bleeding. This is important, both because it becomes more difficult to treat hemorrhage once a large hematoma has developed than to prevent it in early stages, and because early treatment minimizes joint deformities and muscle contractures in later life.

Spontaneous bleeding usually can be controlled if the patient's Factor VIII level is increased to over 20 percent of normal. If, however, major surgery is contemplated, or if there is serious posttraumatic bleeding, or if bleeding has occurred into a vital organ, the level of Factor VIII should be increased to approximately 60 percent of normal. Factor VIII has a biological half-life of approximately 10 to 15 hours. It is not stable when stored in blood and is usually administered as Factor VIII concentrate prepared from fresh plasma. Two forms of Factor VIII concentrates are available: cryoprecipitate, in which the Factor VIII is concentrated approximately 12-fold, and more highly purified Factor VIII concentrates that are available commercially as freeze-dried preparations.

In the past, fresh frozen plasma was used, but this practice has essentially been replaced by the use of Factor VIII concentrates. The increased availability of purified Factor VIII concentrates has revolutionized the life of the hemophiliac. It is now possible to teach the hemophiliac child self-treatment at home at the earliest suspicion of a bleed. The Factor VIII concentrate is stored in an ordinary refrigerator, the patient dissolves the freeze-dried concentrate, and injects the solution intravenously. This has greatly increased the mobility of families and made them far less dependent on the medical profession. It has reduced the frustration and inconvenience of frequent visits to emergency departments of hospitals and hospital admission, and has virtually abolished crippling hemarthroses.

The local measures used in treating hemophilia include resting the affected part and protecting it from further trauma. If the bleeding site is obscured by a large blood clot, as often occurs with mouth bleeding, particularly after tooth extraction, the clot should be gently removed after replacement therapy with Factor VIII concentrate has been given, and a protective dressing should be placed over the area.

Hemophilia B, or Christmas disease

Hemophilia B is due to a deficiency of Factor IX. Like hemophilia A, it is transmitted as a sex-linked recessive trait. Factor IX is much more stable in vitro and has a longer survival in the circulation. Because of its stability in vitro, stored plasma can be used to replace Factor IX, and because of its longer half-life infusions do not have to be given as frequently. A Factor IX concentrate is now available, and this has greatly facilitated the management of these patients.

Von Willebrand's Disease

Von Willebrand's disease is characterized by a prolonged bleeding time, which is due to defective interaction of platelets with subendothelial connective tissue and a low Factor VIII level. The platelet function defect can be demonstrated by measuring platelet aggregation produced by the antibiotic ristocetin. Unlike hemophilia A and hemophilia B, the severity of von Willebrand's disease varies considerably within a given family. Bleeding is usually mild and of the skin and mucous membrane variety, but occasionally, particularly in patients who are severely affected, it may be catastrophic and even fatal. Fresh plasma and cryoprecipitate is effective in controlling bleeding because it both increases the level of circulating von Willebrand factor and induces a rise in the plasma level of Factor VIII coagulant activity in the patient. Thus, following transfusion of plasma or cyroprecipitate, there is an immediate rise in Factor VIII equivalent to the amount infused, followed by a slow rise in Factor VIII coagulant activity that reaches a maximum in 6 to 12 hours and falls to pretreatment levels in approximately 48 hours. The bleeding time also is often shortened, but the effect is transient and lasts for only 2 or 3 hours after infusion.

When patients with von Willebrand's disease require surgery, attempts should be made to shorten the bleeding time as well as to increase the Factor VIII level. This can best be done by frequent cryoprecipitate infusion, that is, every 3 hours. Factor VIII concentrates are not as effective as cryoprecipitate in shortening the bleeding time, probably because there is loss of von Willebrand factor activity during their preparation.

ACQUIRED DISORDERS

Acquired coagulation disorders occur much more commonly than inherited coagulation disorders. Often there are multiple coagulation deficiencies, and in some of these there is an associated qualitative and/or quantitative platelet abnormality. The three most common acquired coagulation disorders are vitamin K deficiency, liver disease, and disseminated intravascular coagulation.

Vitamin K Deficiency

Vitamin K is required for a postribosomal modification of the coagulation proteins Factors II, VII, IX, and X. Vitamin K is obtained from various food sources, particularly green vegetables. It is fat soluble and therefore is poorly absorbed by patients having any of the various malabsorption states. Vitamin K deficiency occurs in adults usually in conditions that produce fat malabsorption, including biliary obstruction, small-bowel disease, and chronic pancreatic disease. Mild forms of vitamin K deficiency are common in hospitalized patients who are not receiving vitamin K supplements and who are being treated with antibiotics and intravenous fluids. Patients with vitamin K deficiency promptly respond to parenteral vitamin K therapy.

Vitamin K deficiency occurs in neonates, producing a condition known as *hemorrhagic disease of the newborn*. It has also been described following the administration of certain drugs to the mother, including oral anticoagulants, anticonvulsant drugs such as phenobarbitone and phenyntoin, and aspirin given in very large doses.

Vitamin K is required for the carboxylation of terminal glutamic acid residues on the coagulation Factors II, VII, IX, and X. In the absence of this carboxylation reaction, the coagulation factors do not bind to the platelet's surface (a reaction that is calcium dependent), and therefore coagulation is defective.

Liver Disease

Abnormalities of the coagulation tests are frequently seen in patients with liver disease. Bleeding, when it occurs, is usually only of mild or moderate degree. Troublesome and even life-threatening bleeding, although relatively uncommon, occurs following trauma or, particularly, if there is a local lesion or lesions such as esophageal varices or peptic ulcer. Severe bleeding also occurs in patients with fulminant hepatitis or chronic liver disease in the terminal stage.

A number of factors contribute to the hemostatic defect associated with liver disease. These include defective synthesis of the vitamin K–dependent clotting factors, defective synthesis of Factor V, and, in very severe liver disease, defective synthesis of fibrinogen. Patients may also have thrombocytopenia (particularly those with chronic liver disease), portal hypertension, and congestive splenomegaly. In addition, fibrinolytic activity is increased in patients with chronic liver disease because the liver is a site of synthesis of antiplasmin and the site of clearance of plasminogen activator, which is released into the bloodstream following surgery or trauma. Defective synthesis of coagulation factors is probably the most important mechanism responsible for the hemostatic defect in liver disease.

Consumption Coagulopathy or Disseminated Intravascular Coagulation

Consumption coagulopathy is a disorder in which diffuse intravascular coagulation causes a hemostatic defect which is due to the reduction of clotting factors and platelets because they are utilized or consumed in the thrombotic process. Consumption coagulopathy can complicate a variety of clinical conditions; it is usually acute but occasionally may be subacute or chronic.

Intravascular coagulation is frequently activated by relatively trivial stimuli, but the process is usually self-limiting because the activated clotting factors are rapidly inhibited and cleared. However, when a stimulus is extensive or when there is a breakdown in the protective mechanisms, disseminated intravascular coagulation with or without microthrombosis and thrombocytopenia may occur and lead to severe bleeding. The factors that stimulate blood coagulation include trauma, either surgical or spontaneous, amniotic fluid embolism, immune complexes, viruses and bacteria, products of malignant tissue, or extensive endothelial damage as is seen in burns or endotoxemia. When these stimuli activate the clotting process, the blood gradually becomes incoagulable because platelets, fibrinogen, prothrombin, Factors V and VIII, and occasionally some of the vitamin K dependent clotting factors are altered and either lose their activity or are cleared from the circulation. The fibrin that is formed is deposited diffusely throughout the small vessels in the body and is eventually digested by the fibrinolytic system. This secondary increase in fibrinolytic activity is usually localized to the site of intravascular thrombosis and does not result in an increase in systemic fibrinolytic activity. However, the breakdown products of fibrin, known as fibrin split products or fibrin degradation products, circulate and may contribute to the hemostatic defect by interfering with both fibrin formation and platelet function.

The clinical manifestations of consumption coagulopathy or disseminated intravascular coagulation are quite varied. In the majority of patients, no symptoms are apparent but evidence of a hemostatic defect is detected on laboratory testing. Bleeding is more likely to occur if the patient has been exposed to surgical trauma or childbirth, but when the degree of consumption is severe, bleeding may be spontaneous. Consumption coagulopathy can also lead to organ damage as the result of ischemia, which occurs secondary to diffuse intravascular thrombosis. The organs most severely affected are the kidneys, the heart, the lungs, and the brain. The red cells may

Table 4.12 **Labortory Features of Disseminated Intravascular Coagulation**

Thrombocytopenia
Fragmented red blood cells
Reduced Factor V, VIII, fibrinogen, prothrombin
Circulating fibrin complexes
Increased plasmin
Fibrin degradation products

also be damaged as they pass through vessels that are partly blocked by thrombus or fibrin material. This leads to marked distortion of the red cells and produces a hemolytic anemia that has been called *microangiopathic hemolytic anemia*. The diagnosis of disseminated intravascular thrombosis is suspected by finding prolongation of the thrombin clotting time, the prothrombin time, and the activated partial thromboplastin time in association with thrombocytopenia (Table 4.12). The more specific tests that point to a diagnosis of disseminated intravascular coagulation are increased levels of circulating fibrin complexes in the plasma and increased concentrations of fibrin split products in the serum. The principles of treatment of consumption coagulopathy include elimination of the precipitating factor (for example, septicemia by antibiotic treatment), replacement of depleted coagulation factors and platelets, and inhibition of the coagulation process by heparin. In practice heparin is rarely required, since elimination of the precipitating factor and replacement are sufficient to reverse the process.

Pathologic Fibrinolysis

Pathologic fibrinolysis is a rare cause of acquired bleeding (except if fibrinolytic therapy is used) and is limited to patients with liver disease who are exposed to surgical or nonsurgical trauma.

REFERENCES

1. Adar, R., Salzman, E.W.: Treatment of thrombosis of veins of the lower extremities. N. Engl. J. Med. 292:348, 1975.
2. Barnes, R.W., Wu, K.K., Hoak, J.C.: Fallibility of the clinical diagnosis of venous thrombosis. JAMA 234:605, 1975.
3. Browse, N.L., Clemenson, G., Lea, Thomas, M.: Is the postphlebitic leg always postphlebitic? Relation between phlebographic appearances of deep-vein thrombosis and late sequelae. Br. Med. J. 281:1167, 1980.
4. Clayton, J.K., Anderson, J.A., McNicol, G.P.: Preoperative prediction of postoperative deep vein thrombosis. Br. Med. J. 2:910, 1976.
5. Coon, W.W., Coller, F.A.: Some epidemiologic considerations of thromboembolism. Surg. Gynecol. Obstet. 109:487, 1959.
6. Dalen, J.E., Alpert, J.S.: Natural history of pulmonary embolism. Prog. Cardiovasc. Dis. 17:259, 1975.
7. Davies, G.S., Salzman, E.W.: The pathogenesis of deep vein thrombosis. In: Joist, H.J., Sherman, L.A. (eds), Venous and Arterial Thrombosis. New York, Grune & Stratton, 1979, p 1.
8. Gallus, A.S., Hirsh, J., Hull, R.: Diagnosis of venous thromboembolism. Semin. Thromb. Hemost. 2:203, 1976.
9. Gallus, A.S., Hirsh, J.: Treatment of venous thromboembolic disease. Semin. Thromb. Hemost. 2:291, 1976.
10. Gallus, A.S., Hirsh, J.: Prevention of venous thromboembolism. Semin. Thromb. Hemost. 2:232, 1976.
11. Hirsh, J.: Hypercoagulability. Semin. Hematol. 14:409, 1977.
12. Hirsh, J., Genton, E.: Thrombogenesis. In: Root, W.S., Berlin, N.I. (eds), Physiological Pharmacology. New York, Academic Press, 1974. p 99.
13. Hull, R., Hirsh, J., Sackett, D.: Clinical validity of negative venogram. Circulation 64:622, 1981.
14. Hull, R., Hirsh, J., Sackett, D.L., Powers, P., et al: Combined use of leg scanning and impedance plethysmography in suspected venous thrombosis: an alternative to venography. N. Engl. J. Med. 296:1497, 1977.
15. Hull, R., Hirsh, J., Sackett, D.L., Stoddart, G.: Cost effectiveness of clinical diagnosis, venography and noninvasive testing in patients with symptomatic deep vein thrombosis. N. Engl. J. Med. 304:1561, 1981.
16. Hull, R., Hirsh, J.: Prevention of venous thrombosis and pulmonary embolism with particular reference to the surgical patient. In: Joist, J.H., Sherman, L.A. (eds), Venous and Arterial Thrombosis. New York, Grune and Stratton, 1979. p 93.
17. Kakkar, V.V., Stamatakis, J.D., Bentley, P.G., et al: Prophylaxis for postoperative deep-vein thrombosis. JAMA 241:39, 1979.
18. McNeil, B.J.: Ventilation-perfusion studies and the diagnosis of pulmonary embolism: concise communications. J. Nucl. Med. 21:319, 1980.
19. Moser, K.: Pulmonary embolism: state of the art. Am. Rev. Respir. Dis. 115:829, 1977.
20. Robin, E.D.: Overdiagnosis and overtreatment of pulmonary embolism: the emperor may have no clothes. Am. Intern. Med. 87:775, 1977.
21. Salzman, E.W., Davies, G.C.: Prophylaxis of venous thromboembolism: analysis of cost-effectiveness. Ann. Surg. 191:207, 1980.

5

Neoplasia

Stephen K. Carter, M.D.

WHAT IS CANCER?

Defining cancer is not easy. Both scientists and laypeople have used *cancer, neoplasm, tumor,* and *malignancy* as if the terms were synonymous. *Cancer* today has become a layperson's term that is used almost exclusively to indicate a process having the biological characteristics of a malignant neoplasm.

A *neoplasm* has been defined as a relatively autonomous growth of tissue. It is autonomous in the sense that it is not subject to the factors that govern the individual cells and the overall cellular interactions of the functional organism, but because a neoplasm is not completely autonomous, it is described as relatively autonomous. Further, a neoplasm is described as a growth, which implies a progressive increase in its size. The rate of growth may be rapid or slow in comparison with normal host tissues. Neoplasms commonly grow more rapidly than their normal host tissue of origin, but this is not universally true.

A neoplasm can be either benign or malignant. The principle behavioral characteristics of benign and malignant neoplasms are outlined in Table 5.1. The majority of these differences are relative. The most critically important difference is that benign tumors do not metastasize, whereas a malignant neoplasm has this ability. A *metastasis* is defined as a secondary growth of a neoplasm, originating from the primary tumor and growing within the host organism in a location distant from the initial site of the neoplastic growth.

Metastases can occur through several pathways. The most obvious one is through the blood stream. Tumor cells are carried by the blood to new sites where they initiate a new growth. It has been shown that cancer cells in the circulation are a common occurrence, and that the number of cells that enter the bloodstream is far greater than the number that ever give rise to metastatic lesions. Another common route for metastases is via the lymphatic system. Some tumors may become implanted in other sites by mere physical movement from one site to another. This is commonly seen in ovarian and gastrointestinal neoplasms when cancer cells from one side of the peritoneal activity become implanted in the other side.

Metastases are usually found in the draining regional lymph nodes of the primary site or in lung, liver, and bone tissues. Certain tumors have a predisposition to metastasize to certain organs. Cancer of the prostate commonly metastasizes to bone, sarcomas tend to metastasize to the lung, while colorectal cancers predominantly metastasize to the liver.

Metastasis involves a complex series of sequential steps whereby malignant tumor cells invade adjacent tissues and penetrate into lymphatic and circulatory systems, detach from the primary tumor mass, spread to near and distant sites, come to rest and invade at these secondary sites, and finally proliferate to form new tumor foci. This last part usually involves only a small percentage of the cells that actually get into the circulation. The invasion that begins the process is thought to occur by mechanical extension or by enzymatic destruction of the extracellular tissue matrix, or both.

After implantation of blood-borne tumor cells in the microcirculation, the next step is usually extravasation or secondary invasion of the endothelium and its underlying basement membrane. This process can involve deposition and dissolution of a fiber matrix around the arrested tumor cells. This arrest in

Table 5.1 **Behavioral Characteristics of Benign versus Malignant Neoplasms**

Benign	Malignant
1. Encapsulated	Nonencapsulated
2. Noninvasive	Invasive
3. Highly differentiated	Poorly differentiated
4. Rare mitoses	Mitoses relatively common
5. Slow growth	Rapid growth
6. Little or no anaplasia	Anaplastic to varying degrees
7. No metastases	Metastases

(Adapted with permission from Pitot HC: Fundamentals of Oncology. New York, Marcel Dekker, 1978.)

capillaries is a nonrandom phenomenon, and therefore it is unlikely that mechanical considerations are the only ones at play. It has been postulated that circulating malignant cells may recognize unique capillary vascular endothelial cell surface determinants in some way.

Penetration of the vascular endothelium probably occurs at points of endothelial cell retraction, although diapedesis or intracellular penetration may also occur. The retraction of vascular endothelial cells caused by interactions between tumor cells and endothelial cells results in net movement of malignant cells to the basement membrane surface of higher adhesive potential. Subsequent invasion may then be due to tumor enzymes secreted by cell surfaces, and secretion of tumor angiogenesis factors may then be responsible for vascularization of the secondary colony, leading to rapid growth.

Metastasis constitutes one of the primary challenges to the oncologist. Although we know much about the clinical manifestations of the metastatic process, little is understood yet about the biochemical, immunologic, genetic, and hormonal mechanisms involved in tumor cell separation, survival during circulation, adhesion to and penetration through the endothelial walls, establishment of secondary tumors in the perivascular tissues, and eventual further metastasis to still more distant sites. Tumors are composed of a heterogeneous population of cells. Different histologic types of tumors differ in their ability to metastasize as do different clonogenic foci within a single tumor. Numerous factors influence the metastatic potential of a tumor. These include the growth characteristics, the blood supply, the host-tumor immunologic interactions, and the nutritional status of the patient, including metabolic factors that are largely undefined. The essential factors that determine the establishment of secondary lesions are the structure of the plasma membrane, the separation of the cell cluster from the primary lesion, the arrest in and infiltration through the lymphatic

or vascular vessel, and, finally, the growth of the micrometastasis.

After the behavioristic dichotomy of benign versus malignant has been distinguished, neoplasms are then classified histogenetically in terms of the type of tissue from which the neoplasm has arisen. This breaks down into six broad classifications outlined in Table 5.2.

Some basic facts about cancer that are important to keep in mind are the following: (1) Neoplasms can only develop from cells that have the ability to proliferate. (2) Tumor cells can resemble their tissue of origin but usually are not as mature and are therefore spoken of as being undifferentiated, poorly differentiated, or anaplastic. (3) Regardless of the stimuli that may cause neoplastic transformation, neoplasms arise usually after a prolonged latent period. (4) Hyperplasia and dysplasia often precede the development of neoplasia by months or years. (5) Neoplastic cells may lie dormant for long periods of time. (6) Spontaneous regression of malignant neoplasms has been known to occur. (7) No completely distinctive ultrastructural or biochemical difference between a cancer cell and a normal cell has yet been identified.

Cancer is not exclusively a problem of cell proliferation but rather is a problem combining the processes of proliferation and differentiation. Differentiation is the result of a genetic program that is able to make an organ as adaptive as possible to the range of environmental variations in which it evolved. Cancer tissues differ from normal tissues insofar as they are unable to recapitulate the total program that develops during normal differentiation and leads to an orchestrated collection of organism-serving cells.

One characteristic of neoplastic cells is the loss of contact inhibition. When normal cells are placed on a glass surface they will grow and migrate until they touch each other, and then they will stop. This phenomenon is known as contact inhibition. When cancer cells are placed in a similar situation they will continue to grow when they make contact and will grow into a multilayered mass.

EPIDEMIOLOGY

The American Cancer Society estimates that almost 56 million people now living will eventually have cancer, which is one person in four according to present rates. There are over 3 million Americans alive today who have a history of cancer. Of these, 2 million had the diagnosis made more than 5 years ago. In 1981 it was estimated that about 805,000 people will be diagnosed as having cancer in the United

Table 5.2 **Examples of Neoplasms Based on the Histogenetic Classification**

Tissue of Origin	Benign	Malignant
1. Epithelial neoplasms		
Epidermis	Epidermal papilloma	Epidermal carcinoma
Stomach	Gastric polyp	Gastric carcinoma
Biliary tree	Cholangioma	Cholangiocarcinoma
Adrenal Cortex	Adrenocortical adenoma	Adrenocortical carcinoma
2. Connective tissue neoplasms		
Fibrous tissue	Fibroma	Fibrosarcoma
Cartilage	Chondroma	Chondrosarcoma
Bone	Osteoma	Osteogenic sarcoma
Fat	Lipoma	Liposarcoma
Smooth muscle	Leiomyoma	Leiomyosarcoma
Skeletal muscle	Rhabdomyoma	Rhabdomyosarcoma
3. Neoplasms of the hemopoietic and immune systems		
Lymphoid tissue	Brill-Symmer's disease	Lymphosarcoma (lymphoma)
		Lymphatic leukemia
		Reticulum cell sarcoma
		Hodgkin's disease
Thymus	Thymoma	Thymoma
Granulocytes		Myelogenous leukemia
Erythrocytes	Polycythemia vera	Erythroleukemia
Plasma cells		Multiple myeloma
4. Neoplasms of the nervous system		
Glia	Astrocytoma	Glioblastoma multiforme
	Oligodendroglioma	
Meninges	Meningioma	Meningeal sarcoma
Neurons	Ganglioneuroma	Neuroblastoma
Adrenal medulla	Pheochromocytoma	
5. Neoplasms of multiple tissues		
Breast	Fibroadenoma	Cystosarcoma phylloces
Kidney		Wilms' tumor
Ovary, testis, etc.	Dermoid (benign teratoma)	Malignant teratoma
6. Miscellaneous neoplasms		
Melanocytes	Nevus	Melanoma
Placenta	Hydatidiform mole	Chorionepithelioma
Ovary	Granulosa cell tumor	Granulosa cell tumor
	Cystadenoma	Cystadenocarcinoma
Testis		Seminoma

(Adapted with permission from Ritchie, A.C.: The classification, morphology and behavior of tumors. In: Florey H. (ed), General Pathology, 4th ed. Philadelphia, W.B. Saunders, 1970. p 675.)

States. Of these, about 268,000 or, around one third, will be alive at least 5 years after treatment. This figure rises to 41 percent when normal life expectancy and the risk of dying from other causes is taken into consideration.

Cancer can occur at any age and it is the leading cause of death from disease in children 3 to 14 years of age. The incidence and mortality of individual cancers varies with both sex and age. The mortality for the five leading cancer sites in major age groups by sex, in the United States, in 1977, is given in Table 5.3. In children under age 15 years, leukemia is the leading cause of cancer death for both sexes. Above age 15 years the number one killer differs for each of the sexes. Breast cancer dominates among women until above age 75 years, when large bowel takes over as number one. In males, lung cancer is the leader after the age of 35 years.

When age-adjusted national death rates for cancer in the United States are studied it is seen that there has been a steady rise since 1930. In 1930 the number of cancer deaths per 100,000 population was 143. In 1940 it was 152. By 1950 it had risen to 158, and in 1977 to 175. This has been mainly due to an increasing incidence of, and mostly due to, lung cancer. As for other sites, it has either remained steady, or in a few cases (for example, stomach and cervical cancer) has actually declined (Table 5.4).

Table 5.3 Mortality for the Five Leading Cancer Sites in Major Age Groups by Sex, United States, 1977

Under 15 years		15–34 years		35–54 years		55–74 years		75+ years	
Male	Female	Male	Female	Male	Female	Male	Female	Male	Female
Leukemia 633	Leukemia 422	Leukemia 755	Breast 623	Lung 10,110	Breast 8,348	Lung 44,112	Breast 17,341	Lung 14,060	Colon & rectum 11,953
Brain and nervous system 414	Brain and nervous system 302	Brain and nervous system 474	Leukemia 553	Colon & rectum 2,434	Lung 4,528	Colon & rectum 13,504	Lung 13,045	Prostate 11,645	Breast 8,166
Bone 58	Bone 47	Testis 423	Brain and nervous system 316	Pancreas 1,307	Colon & rectum 2,283	Prostate 8,851	Colon & rectum 12,190	Colon & rectum 8,811	Lung 4,341
Connective tissue 50	Connective tissue 46	Hodgkin's disease 352	Uterus 303	Brain & nervous system 1,200	Uterus 2,093	Pancreas 6,378	Ovary 6,000	Pancreas 3,205	Pancreas 3,778
Lympho- and reticulo-sarcoma 49	Lympho- and reticulo-sarcoma 35	Skin 254	Hodgkin's disease 235	Leukemia 1,046	Ovary 2,063	Stomach 4,652	Uterus 5,573	Bladder 3,121	Uterus 2,970

Table 5.4   **Twenty-five–year Trends in Age-adjusted Cancer Death Rates per 100,000 Population, 1950–52 Compared to 1975–77**

Sex	Sites	1950–52	1975–77	Percentage Changes	Comments
Male	All sites	169.8	213.3	+ 25.6	Steady increase mainly due to lung cancer.
Female	All sites	146.7	135.0	− 8.0	Slight decrease.
Male	Bladder	7.2	7.2	a	Slight fluctuations; overall no change.
Female	Bladder	3.1	2.1	− 32.3	Some fluctuations; noticeable decrease.
Male	Breast	0.3	0.3	a	Constant rate.
Female	Breast	25.9	27.0	+ 4.2	Slight fluctuations; overall no change.
Male	Colon & rectum	25.9	26.1	a	Slight fluctuations; overall no change.
Female	Colon & rectum	25.5	20.0	− 21.6	Slight fluctuations; noticeable decrease.
Male	Esophagus	4.7	5.4	+ 14.9	Some fluctuations; slight increase.
Female	Esophagus	1.2	1.5	a	Slight fluctuations; overall no change in females.
Male	Kidney	3.3	4.7	+ 42.4	Steady slight increase.
Female	Kidney	2.0	2.2	a	Slight fluctuations; overall no change.
Male	Leukemia	7.7	8.8	+ 14.3	Early increase, later leveling off.
Female	Leukemia	5.3	4.9	− 7.5	Slight early increase, later leveling off.
Male	Liver	6.7	4.8	− 38.4	Some fluctuations. Steady decrease in both sexes.
Female	Liver	7.7	3.6	− 53.2	
Male	Lung	23.7	67.5	+ 184.8	Steady increase in both sexes due to cigarette
Female	Lung			+ 238.8	smoking.
Male	Oral	6.1	5.9	a	Slight fluctuations; overall no change in both sexes.
Female	Oral	1.5	2.0	a	
Female	Ovary	7.9	8.6	+ 8.9	Steady increase, later leveling off.
Male	Pancreas	8.4	11.2	+ 33.3	Steady increase in both sexes, then leveling off.
Female	Pancreas	5.5	7.0	+ 27.3	Reasons unknown.
Male	Prostate	20.7	22.2	+ 7.2	Fluctuations throughout period; overall no change.
Male	Skin	3.2	3.4	a	Slight fluctuations; overall no change in both sexes.
Female	Skin	2.0	1.9	a	
Male	Stomach	23.6	9.3	− 60.6	Steady decrease in both sexes; reasons unknown.
Female	Stomach	12.8	4.4	− 65.6	
Female	Uterus	20.7	8.9	− 57.0	Steady decrease.

[a] Percent changes not listed because they are not meaningful.

ETIOLOGY

CHEMICAL AGENTS

Agents that are able to induce tumors are called carcinogens. A wide variety of agents have been demonstrated to be carcinogenic in humans as a result of either industrial exposures, medical exposures, or societal exposures. The formation of tumors by chemical agents is now recognized as being a complex process involving several stages (Fig. 5.1). The first stage of the process is called initiation. A cell exposed to an initiating agent does not become a tumor cell until it has become exposed to the stage of promotion that causes the actual development of tumor cells capable of replicating to yield gross tumors. Promotion requires a prolonged period of time

and may well consist of more than one process. In the experimental systems where carcinogenesis has been studied, tumors do not develop when only the initiating agent or only the promoting agent is administered in appropriate doses. In addition, if the promoting agent is given prior to the initiating agent, tumors will not form. Once initiation has occurred, however, the application of the promoting agent can be delayed by many months and still cause tumor formation. This indicates that initiation, once it occurs, is irreversible. On the other hand, the promotion step seems to be at least partially reversible. When doses of a promoter are either too low or too widely spaced, it becomes less effective, despite the fact that total dose would be adequate with other dosage schedules.

The chemical structures that are carcinogenic are highly varied. These groups include alkylating agents and acylating agents, which act directly and

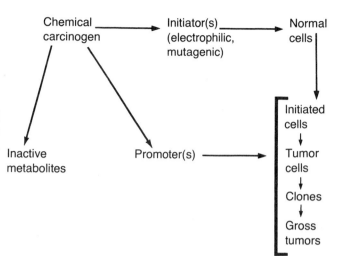

Fig. 5.1 A simplified scheme for chemical carcinogensis. (Miller, EC and Miller JA: Mechanisms of chemical carcinogenesis. Cancer 47:1055, 1981, with permission.)

can induce tumors at sites of application. There are many polycyclic aromatic hydrocarbons, aromatic amides, and amines that can induce tumors in a wide range of tissues. In addition, there are 30 known chemical carcinogens that are products of plants and microorganisms.

A chemical that is a carcinogen can be metabolized to many products. Some of these are inactive, while others have the actual structures that induce the tumors ("ultimate carcinogens"). A balance exists, with any chemical, between activation and inactivation as a result of the metabolic process. This balance is critically important in determining the carcinogenic properties of the agent.

A chemical acting as an initiator must be able to bind with nucleophilic sites in the target cells, such as DNA, RNA, or proteins. Agents that can do this are electrophilic and contain uncharged or positively charged electron-deficient atoms. The electrophiles react nonenzymatically to form covalent bonds through the sharing of electron pairs from nucleophilic atoms. The actual initiation occurs when the linked carcinogen–DNA adduct, which results from the reaction of the electrophilic carcinogen and DNA, leads to mutations within the cell. These mutations lead to the persistence of altered bases in DNA and the fixation of errors by erroneous base-pairing during replication of the DNA. Thus it seems that the initiation of carcinogenesis is a genetic event, although epigenetic processes cannot be totally excluded from consideration, and research in this area is active.

The properties of tumor promoter are less well understood in comparison with the initiating agents. Promotion differs from initiation insofar as it is par-

tially reversible and occurs over a prolonged period of time.

Apparently not all of the promoting agents require activation to electrophilic or mutagenic intermediates for activity. A chemical that has both initiating and promoting activities is called a complete carcinogen.

OCCUPATIONAL AGENTS

The fact that cancer can be caused by exposures in the work place is one of the oldest observations in cancer epidemiology. Over the years there have been a number of chemical agents in occupational settings that are either known or suspected to be important in causing cancer.

One of the most dramatic examples of occupational chemical exposure causing cancer is vinyl chloride. This chemical causes hepatic angiosarcomas, which are otherwise extremely uncommon. The rarity of these tumors made the detection within the occupational setting relatively easy based on epidemiologic observation. With chemicals that cause more common malignancies, for example, lung and bladder tumors, the epidemiologic linkage is less easy to prove. In addition to chemicals, physical factors can also be important factors in occupational cancer. Examples are ionizing radiation and ultraviolet light.

DRUGS

One of the medications associated with a cancer risk involves the administration of diethylstilbestrol (DES) during pregnancy. In 1971 a cluster of a rare form of clear cell adenocarcinoma of the vagina and cervix was reported in females aged 14 to 22 years and was linked to DES given to their mothers during pregnancy. A registry has been set up for these rare tumors, which now totals over 350 cases. Among these cases with an available maternal pregnancy history, about two thirds of the cases indicated an in utero exposure to DES or similar compounds. The follow-up on the large number of women previously exposed to DES in utero is still relatively short. As these women move into the older age ranges they should be observed to see if there are increases in cancers of the breast and cervix. Whether the males so exposed are at an increased risk of testicular cancer is now under vigorous epidemiologic study.

Another example of medical drug exposure and cancer risk involves the use of menopausal estrogens. A common medical practice that developed in the 1960s and 1970s was the administration of conjugated estrogens to menopausal women to ameliorate the sometimes difficult symptomatology associated with menopause. Starting in 1975 a series of studies has established that the use of these estrogens is associated with a significant increase in the incidence of endometrial cancer. When the use of estrogens is stopped the increased risk is quickly lost to a major degree.

RADIATION

Ionizing radiation is perhaps the most thoroughly studied human carcinogen. Despite the extensive study there is still considerable controversy concerning the magnitude of the biologic effects of low doses of sparsely ionizing radiation, such as x- and gamma rays. A variety of populations have been uncovered who received medical irradiation found to be associated with increased cancer risks. These have included patients treated for ankylosing spondylitis, tinea capitis, enlarged thymus glands, tuberculosis, postpartum mastitis, and cervical cancer; and persons receiving radioactive compounds such as thorotrast, radium, iodine, and phosphorous. In Great Britain 52 persons developed leukemia among 14,558 individuals treated by irradiation for ankylosing spondylitis. The normally expected number of cases would be only 5.5. The risk in this population appeared to be proportional to the dose observed over the entire bone marrow. In Israel among 10,842 children irradiated for ringworm of the scalp (tinea capitis) 23 developed thyroid cancer, while only 5 cases could normally be expected.

Thorium dioxide (Thorotrast) containing thorium 232 was used between 1928 and 1955 as a contrast agent for radiographic procedures. This material deposited in body tissues and resulted in continuous alpha particle exposure throughout life at a low dose rate. Three surveys of patients in Denmark, Portugal, and Germany show excesses of liver cancer, including angiosarcoma and cholangiosarcoma, and acute myeloid leukemia.

The data correlating radiation exposure and the risk of human malignancy comes predominantly from observations at moderate to high doses of radiation. Because of this the carcinogenic risks of low level radiation can be estimated only by extrapolation from observations at higher doses and dose rates, based on unproven assumptions about the nature of the dose-incidence relation and the mechanism of carcinogenesis. An important question that cannot be definitively answered is whether there exists a threshold phenomonon in the radiation carcinogenic risk. According to Upton, the growing body of information from observations of irradiated human populations, experimental animals, and cultured cells argues increasingly against the existence of a threshold. Upton suggests, however, that a linear quadratic model for estimating risk may be more appropriate than a linear model. This is based on the laboratory observations that the biological effectiveness of low linear energy transfer radiation generally decreases with decreasing dose and dose rate for carcinogenic effect. This is still a controversial area, particularly in attempting to assess risk in relation to public policy.

Significant increases in leukemia have been observed in Hiroshima and Nagasaki as a result of the atomic bomb explosions at the end of World War II. Among the most heavily irradiated atomic bomb survivors, the cumulative incidence during the first 28 years after irradiation was 10 to 20 times higher than normal, with the largest excess in those who were either children or elderly adults at the time of the explosion. The Hiroshima blast emitted a large component of fast neutrons, while the one at Nagasaki was composed almost entirely of gamma rays. The excess incidence rates rise more steeply in Hiroshima than in Nagasaki, reflecting the higher relative biological effectiveness of fast neutrons for leukemic induction.

VIRUSES AND CANCER

The study of viruses in relation to cancer has been extensive, and for many years it was hoped that a direct viral cause of cancer could be elucidated, which would lend itself to a preventive strategy. Unfortunately this goal has been elusive, and to date there is no definitively established virus known to cause human cancer.

One of the most studied viruses, in relation to human cancer, has been the Epstein-Barr virus (EBV). Burkitt discovered the lymphoma that bears his name and made the observation that the distribution of the tumor in Africa was determined by geographic features affecting climate. A climate-dependent arthropod vector was suggested by the temperature and rainfall similarities in the regions of high incidence. Cultured Burkitt lymphoma cells contained herpesvirus, and a link was established between the EBV virus and infectious mononucleosis. People who were seropositive for the virus were resistant to the disease, while those seronegative were susceptible. When studies for EBV antibody titers in patients with tumors were undertaken it was observed that they were elevated in patients with either nasopharyngeal carcinoma or Burkitt's lymphoma. Molecular hybridization has demonstrated the EBV genome in nasopharyngeal cancer cells as well as in the transformed cells obtained from Burkitt's lymphoma biopsies. Exactly how the presence of EBV inside the cell is associated with the occurrence of the chromosomal changes associated with Burkitt's lymphoma is not yet clear.

Another virus-malignancy association has been found linking hepatitis B virus and primary hepatocellular carcinoma. Hepatoma is one of the most common malignancies throughout the world, even though it is relatively uncommon in the United States. In patients with hepatoma, the frequency of chronic hepatitis B virus infection is greater than in an appropriate control population. Those regions of the world where the incidence of primary liver tumors is highest are also regions endemic for a high incidence of chronic carriers of hepatitis B virus infection. Prospective studies in Japan and Taiwan comparing chronic carriers to noninfected controls have shown a higher incidence of hepatocellular carcinoma in the infected group.

The oncogenic viruses in animals may be divided into three types. The DNA oncogenic viruses include 3 taxonomic groups: the papovaviruses, the adenoviruses, and the herpesviruses. The oncogenic RNA viruses are called oncornaviruses. Extensive experimental work has clarified many aspects of the viral-cellular interactions in avian leukosis, murine leukemia, mouse sarcoma, and mammary tumors. However, the relationship to human cancer is not clear.

A new and important discovery is that malignant transformation may be mediated by a relatively slight genetic change. These modified genes are called oncogenes. These oncogenes appear to be able to elicit the entire neoplastic phenotype. The characterization of proteins encased by oncogenes offers a powerful strategy by which the mechanisms of oncogenes might be revealed.

ASSESSING ENVIRONMENTAL CARCINOGENS

It is essential that we have reliable methods for determining specific carcinogens and their various cofactors in our environment if we are to develop a meaningful prevention strategy. Ideally, these assays would follow from knowledge of basic mechanisms of carcinogenesis. Since gaps still exist in this knowledge, the assays developed to date are less than perfect. It is estimated that at least 4 million synthetics and chemicals exist currently. Over 60,000 synthetic chemicals are in widespread use. In addition over 1,000 new chemicals enter our environment annually. Only the development of rapid short-term assays will enable us to make any significant dent in the testing of this assemblage for carcinogenic potential. A listing of the methods for detecting environmental carcinogens is given in Table 5.5.

The most reliable laboratory assay currently available to detect carcinogens is the long-term administration of an agent to rodents with pathologic determination of the increased tumor incidence. With the exception of benzene and arsenic, all of the known human carcinogens have been proven carcinogenic in rodents.

These tests are expensive and time consuming. The standard National Cancer Institute rodent assay

Table 5.5 **Current Methods for Detecting Carcinogens in our Environment**

Short-term Tests	In Vivo Approaches
Mutagenic assays	Clinical observations
Bacteria (Ames Test)	Epidemiologic studies
Mammalian cell culture	Experimental animal
Other eukaryotes, e.g.,	bioassays
yeast, drosophilla,	Rodents
mice	Larger animals
Cell transformation assays	
Assays for DNA binding,	
damage and repair or	
binding to other	
macromolecules	
Assays for chromosomal	
abnormalities and sister	
chromatid exchange	
Provision for metabolic	
activation	

of a single compound requires about 600 animals, takes over two years to compute, and costs over $400,000. This assay uses only two dose levels and often requires a high dose to achieve significant results. These doses are beyond any expected exposure that could occur in humans. How to do accurate risk extrapolations for doses expected in humans from results obtained at these high doses, is still under study. Whether a threshold dose exists for carcinogens has still not been established. Another problem with rodent bioassays is that there can be marked variations between strains and species of rodents in terms of their response to specific carcinogens.

The ability of many carcinogens to generate electrophiles that bind to cellular DNA has provided the rationale for utilizing mutagenesis in bacterial or mammalian cells as screening tests. The Ames test is the most commonly used of these, and involves mutagenesis of *Salmonella typhimurium.*

In extensive studies the Ames test has correctly predicted 90 percent of known carcinogens placed into the system. It has also predicted as negative about 90 percent of known noncarcinogens tested. Thus there is both a 10 percent false positive and false negative rate, which indicates that the best use of the Ames test will probably be as part of a panel of screening tests.

Another assay system is the malignant transformation of mammalian cells in culture, sometimes supplemented with tissue preparations for the metabolic activation of test chemicals. In contradistinction to mutagenicity assays, these systems have the formation of cancer cells as the endpoint of the assay. These tests can be performed within one to a few weeks. When injected into appropriate hosts the transformed cells can often generate tumors indicating that the in vitro endpoint correlates with the neoplastic process. There are not a large number of studies on the validation of the cell transformation systems as screens for chemical carcinogenesis.

Epidemiologic and clinical observations have uncovered many of our major environmental causes of cancers, such as tobacco, asbestos, and DES. A potent clinical tool is the *case control study* in which patients who have developed a type of cancer can be compared with controls matched with regard to environmental and occupational exposures. These studies are retrospective in nature and depend on the actual development of the cancer in question. They provide evidence for an association and must be linked to laboratory approaches if definitive cause is to be established.

The most established and studied example of human environmental carcinogenesis is the relationship between cigarette smoking and the development of lung cancer. While lung cancer was unusual in 1920, by 1950 it had risen in incidence to become the number one cause of cancer deaths in adult males in the United States. With the rise in female smoking the lung cancer incidence is now on the increase among women and may soon pass breast cancer as their number one cause of cancer death.

The major carcinogenic agents in tobacco smoke condensate are the polycyclic aromatic hydrocarbons (PAHs) such as benzopyrene and benzaanthracene. These PAHs are converted to active electropholic forms after their entry into the body tissues. One enzyme system that is responsible for the conversion of these compounds to their active metabolic form is aryl hydrocarbon hydroxylase. This membrane-bound, oxygen dependent enzyme system is found in many body tissues and is capable of converting components of cigarette smoke to potent intermediates with enhanced mutagenic and carcinogenic potential.

The process of pulmonary carcinogenesis is a multifactorial one that is highly complicated (Fig. 5.2). It probably begins with activation of polycyclic aromatic hydrocarbons in cigarette smoke or air pollution by the aryl hydrocarbon hydroxylase enzyme system. Reactive intermediate metabolites are formed, which may undergo detoxification through conjugation or other enzymatic reactions and then be excreted. Conversely, if these electrophilic metabolites are not detoxified, they may bind to cellular macromolecules such as DNA, thereby initiating mutagensis. This mutagenic damage may be reversed by DNA repair mechanisms, which return the cell to normal function. If the DNA repair mechanisms fail or are overwhelmed, then the formed mutations persist and ultimately lead to malignant transformation. This step of malignant transformation may be influenced by environmental factors such as viruses, cocarcinogens such as asbestos, promoters such as phorbol esters (which are found in cigarette smoke), or other undefined factors.

TUMOR IMMUNOLOGY

All cells on their surface contain a complex array of molecular markers consisting primarily of protein, with a small amount of carbohydrate. These molecular markers differ from one cell to another. When cells from one species are transplanted into another species, these molecular markers act as antigens and elicit an antibody response. Cancer immunology has been predicated on the concept that tumor cells are

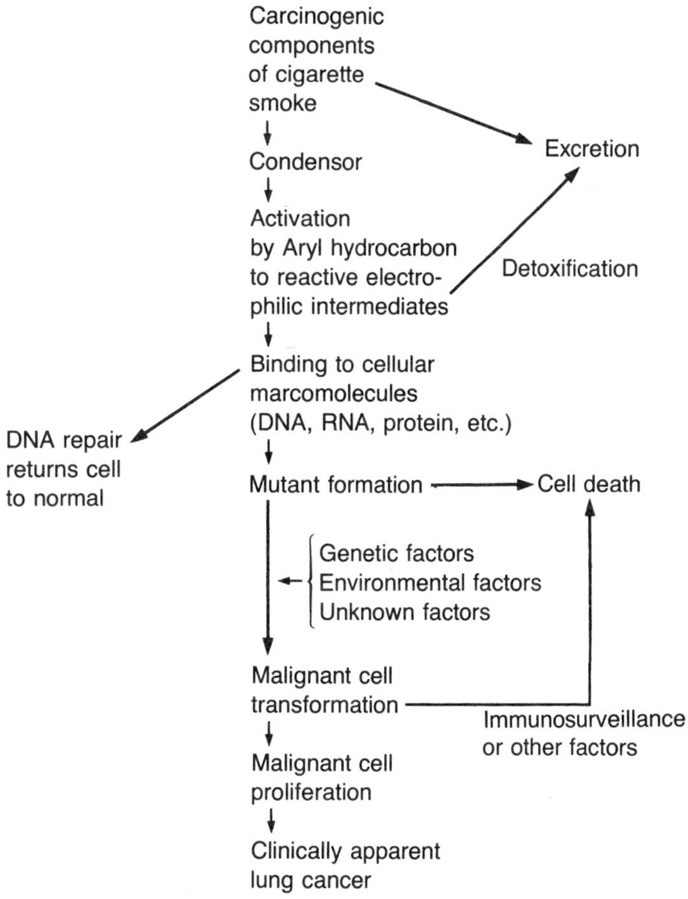

Carcinogenic
components
of cigarette
smoke

↓

Condensor

↓

Activation
by Aryl hydrocarbon
to reactive electro-
philic intermediates

→ Excretion

Detoxification

↓

Binding to cellular
marcomolecules
(DNA, RNA, protein, etc.)

DNA repair
returns cell
to normal

↓

Mutant formation ────────→ Cell death

{ Genetic factors
←{ Environmental factors
{ Unknown factors

↓

Malignant cell
transformation ──────── Immunosurveillance
or other factors

↓

Malignant cell
proliferation

↓

Clinically apparent
lung cancer

Fig. *5.2* Pulmonary carcinogenesis—Theoretical pathways. (Mc Lemore, TL and Martin RR: Pulmonary carcinogenesis: Aryl hydrocarbon hydroxylase. In: Livingston RB (Ed.). Lung Cancer I. Martinus Nijhoff, The Hague, 1981. pp 1–35, with permission.)

antigenic within their host and that they elicit some kind of immunologic host response. The initial demonstration of cancer-specific antigens came from observations in highly inbred strains of mice, possessing identical transplantation antigens on their cells. A tumor arising from one strain of mice implanted into another strain will grow initially and then regress. This is due to the effect of strain-specific transplantation antigens and not to the fact that tumors contain tumor-specific antigens. Studies with chemically induced tumors in inbred mice have proven that tumor-specific antigens exist independent of transplantation antigens. A consistent and remarkable feature of chemically induced tumors is that each tumor elicits immunity to itself but not to any other tumor. This may be due to either (1) genes that mutate as a direct result of interaction with the cancer-causing chemical; or (2) the activation genes that are ordinarily silent in the adult situation but that may be active in a fetal situation. With virus-induced tumors in mice, all tumors induced by a given virus have the same virus-specified cell-surface antigen, so

that immunization with any specific virus-induced tumor, such as polyoma virus, confers resistance to any other.

In mice, experimentally induced tumors vary greatly in their immunizing capacity. Tumor-specific antigens are described as either "strong" or "weak." This description depends on how effectively they render mice immune to subsequent challenge with the same tumor.

The rejection of tumors, like the rejection of grafted tissues from a nonrelated donor, is primarily mediated by lymphocytes. The B type cells interact with antigen and subsequently synthesize and secrete antitumor antibodies. The T cells appear to synthesize antibody-like molecules at their surface with which they recognize the antigen on subsequent challenge, enabling them to destroy antigen containing cells. T cells also release factors that mediate complex interactions between T cells, B cells, and macrophages. (see Chapter 6)

The use of antibody as an analytical probe (serologic method) for tumor-specific antigens has been given a great deal of emphasis in basic tumor immunologic research. For example, an antigen from the blood of mice with hepatic tumors is the same antigenic component found in the blood of a normal mouse fetus. This antigen, called α-*fetoprotein*, belongs to a class of substances that are manufactured in fetal life but then fall to undetectable levels shortly after birth. This occurs because the genes controlling production of these antigens are inactivated. These genes may become reactivated as a result of malignant transformation, and the antigen reappears.

Hybridomas involve the fusion of myeloma cells with lymphocytes immunized against a specific antigen. The resulting hybrid myeloma cells, or hybridoma cells, express both the lymphocyte's property of specific antibody production and the immortal character of the myeloma cells. A tumor is itself an immortal clone of cells descended from a single progenitor, and so myeloma cells can be cultured indefinitely.

In a *hybridoma* there is a technologic coupling of the immortality of a secretory cancer cell (myeloma) with the genetic mechanisms of normal antibody producing cells. The resulting hybrid cell is immortal and can produce large quantities of chemically and immunologically uniform antibodies. What usually occurs in the laboratory is the fusion of spleen cells from a mouse, stimulated with the antigen one wants to recognize with a mouse myeloma cell. The antibodies produced are mouse proteins against which humans would react immunologically. Human hybridomas can make specific human immunoglobulins.

The availability of human hybridomas opens the way to the use of their antibody products in clinical diagnosis and treatment. It would be exciting if human hybridoma antibodies could be generated against tumor-specific antigens found in the membranes of tumor cells. These antibodies, when developed, could be radiolabeled with various radionuclides for use in diagnostic imaging. These could then be used to detect micrometastases. If the antibodies were linked to radiation emitting compounds, chemotherapeutic agents, or toxins, then selective destruction of micrometastases could take place.

Whether human tumors carry antigens that can be specifically recognized by the primary host is a question that has not been resolved conclusively. There is good evidence, however, that at least some human tumors carry tumor-restricted cell-surface antigens that elicit an immune response in the patient. A variety of different types of immune mediators and effectors have been described in animals and identified, to some extent, in humans. The possibility of augmenting the host response through selective modification of various components of the response has been demonstrated in animals using a variety of chemicals, natural products, or physiologic factors. Most well-designed trials fail to demonstrate any benefit for immune modulation. Areas where positive results have been reported in well-designed trials for nonspecific stimulation of the immune response with materials such as bacillus calmette-guerin (BCG) include intrapleural BCG for stage I non–oat cell lung cancer, intravesical BCG for stage O–A bladder cancer, and BCG combined with chemotherapy in advanced ovarian cancer and non-Hodgkin's lymphoma. Further investigation in these areas continues, but immune modulation cannot as yet be routinely recommended.

THE CANCER CARE CONTINUUM

In the effort to control cancer, the research and care approaches move through a series of sequential steps that can be described as the Cancer Care Continuum (CCC) (Fig. 5.3). The CCC begins with the potential for preventing the development of cancer, which would be an ideal way to control cancer if possible. Failing the ability to prevent the development of malignant neoplasia, the next step is to attempt to detect it at a stage of development that will make it amenable to successful therapy with minimal morbidity. This early detection approach begins with the possibility of diagnosis in asymptomatic individuals, which some call screening and others call secondary prevention. This can involve mass populations or specific populations deemed to be at high risk based on epidemiologic observations. The next part of early detection involves prompt diagnosis in indi-

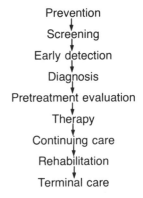

Fig. 5.3 The cancer care continuum.

viduals who are either symptomatic or who demonstrate a physical and/or laboratory sign that would be presumptively diagnostic. This will involve both public and professional education to alert the public and professionals about the early warning signs and the benefits of early detection.

The next step in the CCC is the diagnosis of malignant neoplasia itself and the immediate subsequent step of pretreatment evaluation. Pretreatment evaluation involves classifying the patient according to histology, extent of disease (staging), and functional ability. Based on pretreatment evaluation, an appropriate initial therapeutic prescription is developed for the patient within a multidisciplinary framework.

Pretreatment evaluation is followed by therapy itself, which will involve varying combinations and sequences of surgery, irradiation, chemotherapy, and hormonal manipulation, depending on the disease site and its various classifications. Treatment is followed by continuing care, which includes the appropriate continued evaluation for potential recurrence requiring further therapeutic intervention as well as the important concepts of physical and psychosocial rehabilitation. The rehabilitation of the cancer patient begins with the functional classification that precedes treatment, and should be a part of the therapeutic decision.

The final part of the CCC will be rehabilitation if the patient is cured by therapy, or terminal care if cure has not been achieved. Terminal care has received increasing emphasis with the development of the hospice concept and its varied applications.

Decision-making about the CCC must relate to two major factors: (1) What priority should be given to research activities geared toward improving the current standard of knowledge within the CCC; and (2) at best, what can be accomplished by the delivery to every individual of the current baseline of knowledge with the CCC.

Understanding the impact of the CCC within any defined population requires an epidemiologic data base. This consists of three major components. The first component is the *incidence* of cancer site by site. This incidence data is broken down by factors such as age, sex, race, socioeconomic class, and occupation. A successful approach to prevention will ultimately manifest itself as a diminished incidence rate. The second component is the *stage* at diagnosis, which in most tumor registries is broken down as local, regional, or disseminated disease. For any tumor, local disease is the most highly curable form. Because of this, the success of any screening or early detection program would manifest itself as a higher percentage of local disease at diagnosis and be re-

flected in more successful therapy data. The third component is cancer *mortality* site by site, again relating to age, sex, race, and so forth as well as to stage at diagnosis. Success in therapy will manifest itself as a diminished cancer mortality within a framework of the incidence data. A diminished cancer mortality can be due to one of two reasons: (1) an increased incidence of early stage disease allowing standard therapy to have a greater overall impact, despite the fact that the cure potential of therapy within stage is unchanged; or (2) improvements in therapy that increase the cure potential within stage and are therefore independent of any change in stage breakdowns at diagnosis.

PREVENTION

A strategy of prevention is dependent on knowledge of the causes of cancer that allow for an intervention. Since the exact cause and mechanism of malignant transformation is not clear, prevention strategy is based on environmental factors that are associated epidemiologically with increased incidence of cancer. The most dramatic example is the association of cigarette smoking and lung cancer.

The *environment*, as it relates to cancer causation, has been defined as all exogenous factors that impinge on humans, that is, the physical, dietary, behavioral, and cultural environment. Higginson has divided cancers into those caused by defined exogenous factors and those of probable environmental origin. In the first group are tumors in adults arising in the skin, respiratory tract (larynx and lung), upper digestive tract (nasopharynx and esophagus), liver, pancreas, and bladder. Also included in this group are some tumors of the endometrium and blood-forming organs.

Tobacco is a major environmental cause in this first group of tumors. One third of all cancers in males in the United States result from cigarette smoking. Among the tumors documented as related to tobacco are those of lung, pharynx, larynx, esophagus, bladder, and probably pancreas. In women, lung cancer rates are increasing due to their more recent increased cigarette smoking rate. It is estimated that within 5 years, the lung cancer death rate in women will become higher than that for breast cancer.

Alcoholism increases the risk of cancer of mouth, pharynx, larynx, esophagus, and liver. When incidence rates for these tumors are studied in alcoholics they are found to be higher than average. There is no evidence that moderate or small amounts of alcohol are associated with an increased cancer risk.

About 7 percent of cancer deaths in men and 2 percent in women are related to alcoholism. There is a common association between alcoholism and smoking that may cause a synergistic interaction in cancer causation.

The cancers of probable environmental origin are made up predominantly of tumors of the gastrointestinal tract, stomach, large intestine, endocrine-related organs (prostate, ovary and breast, uterus, cervix) and some tumors of the genitourinary tract. This group forms approximately 40 percent of cancers in males and 60 percent to 70 percent in females. Epidemiologic studies in support of this concept are those that show significant geographical variations in cancer incidence and those that show shifts in cancer incidence with migration. Examples of geographic variations include cancer of the nasopharynx, which is roughly 40 times more common among the Chinese population in San Francisco than among the white population of New York State, and cancer of the liver, which is about 30 times more common in certain parts of Africa.

Additional epidemiologic support for the role of environment in cancer causation has come from migrant studies. A classic example concerns Japanese persons who migrate to California. In Japan the incidence of stomach cancer is high, while that of colon cancer is low. When Japanese persons migrate to California they rapidly (in the next generation) develop a lower stomach cancer rate and a higher colon cancer rate, which are more typical of the white population of the state.

Socioeconomic differences in cancer incidence also support the important role of the environment. For example, in poor populations the incidence of cervical and stomach cancers are higher than average, while in higher-income groups there is a higher than average frequency of breast, brain, and prostate cancer and leukemia.

At present most of the potential approaches to preventing cancer involve taking something away from people that they either find pleasurable or that they at least are used to in their everyday existence. Tobacco, alcohol, and diet all involve behavior modification. Since these factors do not lead to cancer in all exposed individuals, it is easy for any one person to assume that he or she will not be the one to develop cancer.

SCREENING AND EARLY DETECTION

Screening is defined as the use of simple tests or examinations to differentiate those persons who have disease from those who probably do not. Put another way, screening is a technique of secondary prevention—a strategy for reducing morbidity and mortality in a population through early detection and treatment of asymptomatic patients. Screening requires a change in thinking from that used when approaching symptomatic patients. In symptomatic patients there is an acceptance of morbidity and considerable cost in the diagnosis and evaluation of disease for the purposes of appropriate treatment. Screening approaches a large number of asymptomatic individuals in whom adverse effects of the screening will weigh heavily compared with the low probability of having a relatively rare disease. The program must evaluate the gains of early diagnosis and therapy through screening in light of the adverse effects and the cost of screening.

Screening for a given cancer has three major assumptions: (1) The cancer is an important cause of neoplastic mortality and morbidity. (2) There exists a screening test that is acceptable to patients with a sufficient sensitivity and specificity. (3) The results of treating the cancer at the stage detected by screening are superior to treatment at later stages.

An appropriate cancer for screening has to be a neoplasm that causes a high mortality rate when diagnosed in the symptomatic patient. The screening approach must make the diagnosis at a lower stage (lesser extent of disease) that will enable mortality to be significantly reduced by appropriate therapy. Figure 5.4 illustrates the concept of the detectable preclinical phase (DPCP) of a neoplasm. The DPCP is the time from when the disease can first be detected by a test to the time when it is symptomatic. The prevalence of the DPCP in a population must be high enough to make screening feasible and cost-effective. This prevalence depends on disease incidence, the point at which a test can detect the preclinical phase, the rate of progression to clinical disease, and the frequency of previous screening. The higher the risk for population chosen, the higher will be prevalence of the DPCP.

The evaluation of screening programs is plagued by three difficulties: selection bias, lead time bias, and length bias. Selection bias involves those peculiar aspects of a population subset that determine participation in a cancer screening program. If these selection factors are linked in any way to disease prevalance, than a bias will exist between screened and unscreened groups. Lead time bias reflects the fact that by diagnosing a tumor earlier through screening the interval between diagnosis and death is lengthened in comparison to individuals diagnosed

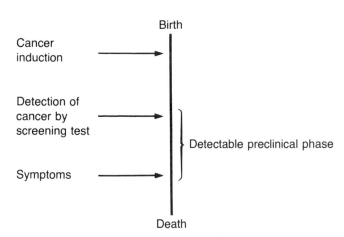

Fig. 5.4 The detectable preclinical phase. (Higgenson, H: Epidemiology for clues to etiology. In: Burchenal JH and Oettgen HF (Eds.). Cancer—Achievements, challenges and prospects for the 1980's. New York, Grune & Stratton, 1981. pp 7–25, with permission.)

when symptomatic. Thus, though death occurs at the same point in time, a screened population will live longer from the point of diagnosis than does an unscreened population. Length bias relates to the concept that cancers with long preclinical phases generally have long clinical phases, while those with short preclinical phases generally have short clinical phases. Given a population of unscreened people, a single screening is likely to lead to the diagnosis of select cases with long preclinical and clinical phases. These cases will have an improved survival because they have a long natural history.

The cost-benefit analysis of a screening program must reckon with the varying side effects of screening. These include (1) the psychologic cost of a false-positive test; (2) unnecessary work-ups of persons with false-positive tests; (3) the morbidity associated with diagnostic tests performed on persons with false-positive tests; and (4) the psychologic and physical cost of early diagnosis on those for whom early diagnosis does not prolong survival, that is, those who live longer with cancer.

The effectiveness of a screening test is determined using the concepts of sensitivity and specificity. Sensitivity asks the question, If cancer is present, what is the likelihood the screening test will be positive? Specificity asks the question, If cancer is not present what is the likelihood the screening test will be normal? The sensitivity of the test is determined by identifying the proportion of patients with disease in whom the test is positive. Similarly, the specificity of the test is determined by identifying the proportion of patients without disease in whom the test is negative.

The ideal test is one in which there is no overlap of results among patients with and without cancer. In this situation, all patients without cancer would

have test values lower than those observed among patients with cancer. In other words, there are no false positives and no false negatives. Unfortunately no such laboratory test exists at this time.

There are 12 common forms of cancer that cause 85 percent of the cancer mortality. The long-term survival rates after therapy for patients diagnosed with localized disease is significantly superior to that achieved for patients diagnosed with nonlocalized disease (Table 5.6).

The early detection of breast cancer involves three techniques: breast self-examination (BSE), physical examination, and low-dose mammography. The American Cancer Society recommends the monthly practice of BSE by women of all ages, beginning in

Table 5.6 **Twelve Common Tumors Accounting for 85 Percent of Cancer Mortality and the Percentage Diagnosed in a Localized Stage**

Tumor	Percentage Localized at Time of Diagnosis
Bladder	68
Larynx	58
Cervix-uterus	53
Prostate	48
Kidney	44
Rectum	43
Breast	41
Colon	40
Oropharynx	34
Ovary	27
Lung	16
Stomach	15

(Adapted with permission from Miller, D.G.: If you look for early cancer you will find it! Your Patient and Cancer 1(6):25–31, July 1981.)

the high-school years. There have been two major studies in this area. The screening procedures detect tumors at an earlier stage. Table 5.7 lists the sensitivity and specificity of the three procedures based on two large-scale studies.

DIAGNOSIS

The diagnosis of cancer requires two critical steps. The first step is the establishment of the diagnostic hypothesis that cancer may exist in a patient. This is followed by the second step, which involves a series of tests geared toward either definitely making or excluding the diagnosis of cancer. In the beginning, there is a need for sensitive tests that when normal permit a confident exclusion of malignancies. The process ultimately requires a very specific test that when abnormal confirms the presence of malignancy. In most cases this is a biopsy followed by pathologic examination, or at least pathologic study of some tissue, for example, cytologic material.

The diagnosis of cancer in a patient is one of the most serious that can be made. This diagnosis can only be firmly established when a trained pathologist recognizes a pattern of cellular growth in tissue or cells that he judges to be neoplastic. The process of determining whether a very thin slice of tissue magnified many times is benign or malignant, is not an exact science. Pathologists can make mistakes, and therefore the clinician and the pathologist should work together as a team to make the diagnosis, and, ideally, pathologists should be physicians first and histopathologic experts second.

It should be kept in mind that a piece of tissue removed from a patient has to go through a series of preparatory steps before it can be "read" by the pathologist. This may involve freezing the specimen or coagulating it with chemicals, producing a variety of artifacts. It is essential that a department of pathology employ the best possible staff of histotechnologists, and they should be directed to work together closely

to develop the best possible sections for microscopic interpretation. Another critical part of this process is the adequacy of the biopsy specimen that is received.

The diagnosis of lung cancer can be made by fiberoptic bronchoscopy, bronchial brush biopsy, percutaneous needle biopsy, cytologic evaluation, and thoracotomy. Of these, the easiest is the collecting of sputum for cytologic examination, and it is relatively inexpensive. This procedure, using the papanicolaou staining technique, will be positive in 40 to 60 percent of patients with bronchogenic carcinoma. The sensitivity of sputum cytology depends on the location and size of the primary tumor. More positives are found with centrally located lesions than with peripheral tumors. The larger the primary tumor the more cytologic positives are observed. If the sputum cytology is positive, then the presence of a malignant neoplasm can be definitively assumed. False positives with cytology are rare. Unfortunately the diagnosis of histologic subtypes of bronchogenic carcinoma are not perfect with this technique, particularly in the diagnosis of squamous cell lesions. To the extent that therapy will be dependent on histology, this needs to be kept in mind.

Fiberoptic bronchoscopy is a relatively noninvasive technique with a sensitivity of greater than 80 percent in detecting lung cancer. If the tumor is centrally located, the sensitivity is 94 to 100 percent, but it falls to 61 to 71 percent in peripheral lesions. As with sputum cytology a positive biopsy is definitive in making the diagnosis.

A diagnostic technique that is now being used more commonly is percutaneous aspiration needle biopsy. The overall sensitivity is greater than 80 percent but the risk of morbidity is greater than with bronchoscopy. With this technique the sensitivity is greater for peripheral lesions, where it is about 87 percent, compared with central lesions, where its sensitivity drops to 66 percent.

The final diagnostic approach that has total sensitivity and specificity is thorocotomy, but this is the diagnostic procedure with the greatest risk of morbidity and mortality.

It would thus appear that a logical initial approach to making the diagnosis of a suspected lung cancer would be cytologic analysis of the sputum. More invasive diagnostic procedures should be reserved for those individuals who have at least three sputum samples showing no evidence of malignant cells.

In suspected central lesions, the next technique should be fiberoptic bronchoscopy with brush or forceps biopsy. In suspected peripheral lesions, percutaneous needle biopsy would be more sensitive. Since the risk of needle biopsy is higher, bronchos-

Table 5.7 **Sensitivity and Specificity of Procedures Used in Breast Cancer Screening**

Screening Technique	Percentage Sensitivity		Percentage Specificity
	BCDDP[a]	HIP[b]	
Breast self-examination	25	56	
Physical examination	24	29	95
Mammography	62	24	97

[a] Breast Cancer Detection Demonstration Project
[b] Health Insurance Plan of New York Project

copy might still be preferable in selected patients with compromised lung function.

Similar principles should determine the approaches to other suspected tumors.

TREATMENT

"Although cancer remains the number one health concern of the American people, it is also one of the most curable chronic diseases in the United States today," states Dr. Vincent T. DeVita, Jr., in his preface to the 1980 Directors Report and Annual Plan for the National Cancer Program. He points out that 41 percent of newly diagnosed serious cancers are curable using surgery, radiotherapy, and chemotherapy, either singly or in combination.

Great strides have been made in the treatment of cancer in the last 30 years. For many years, cancer was a disease that could only be cured if the tumor was found at a localized stage and was amenable to complete surgical excision. The ability to cure localized tumor was enhanced by the development of modern megavoltage irradiation techniques, as well as by refinements in surgical techniques, anesthesiology, and control of infectious complications. By the end of the 1950s, a plateau had been reached in the ability to cure cancer by local control modalities at the stages being found at the time of routine diagnosis.

In the last twenty years, the full flowering of cancer chemotherapy and the subspecialty of medical oncology have added a new dimension to the curative potential of cancer treatment. Unlike surgery or irradiation, chemotherapy has the potential to kill tumor cells anywhere in the body, and so can be used to treat metastatic disease. In its early years, chemotherapy was restricted in its use to two broad clinical situations within oncology. The first was the treatment of malignancies disseminated intrinsically at diagnosis, such as leukemias, advanced stage lymphomas, and other hematologic malignancies. The second situation was in solid tumors with clinical evidence of metastasis. These were mostly after curative attempts had been made with surgery and/or irradiation. The traditonal concept was to use the therapeutic modalities in sequence, with chemotherapy as the last resort for palliation.

In the 1950s, it was recognized that some tumors were remarkably sensitive to cytotoxic chemicals. These included acute leukemia of childhood, the malignant lymphomas (especially Hodgkin's disease), choriocarcinoma in women, and testicular cancers in men. An armamentarium of drugs was developed, and it was recognized that each drug had its own individual spectrum of clinical efficacy and organ-related toxicities. Cancer was clearly understood to be a multitude of different diseases, each with its own natural history, pattern of spread, and responsiveness to surgery, irradiation, and drugs.

As the 1960s began, two major developments in clinical oncology began to coalesce from the earlier data base of clinical research. One development was the aggressive use of combinations of drugs, with a curative intent, within the context of the cell kill hypothesis of cancer chemotherapy (see Clinical Research).

The implications of the cell kill hypothesis were to treat as aggressively as possible (using maximally tolerated dosages) to achieve zero tumor cells before resistance occurred. Combinations of drugs offered the potential of increased tumor-cell kill through differing mechanisms of action, as well as a lessened potential for early resistance for the same reason. Empirically, it was discovered that combining active drugs, led to more effective combinations. The curative triumphs of childhood leukemia and Hodgkin's disease evolved from daring oncologists combining active drugs in an aggressive manner designed to achieve total tumor-cell eradication.

The second development was the concept of combined modality treatment utilizing chemotherapy immediately after local control therapy. This evolved out of the understanding that many tumors, after local control was accomplished, would relapse with a metastatic pattern. The reason for this was that microscopic foci of metastatic disease existed at the time of initial diagnosis but were not identified by current diagnostic techniques. Certain clinical situations were discovered to be highly predictive of metastatic failure. An example was breast cancer with tumor found in axillary lymph nodes. For tumors where cancer chemotherapy has been shown capable of shrinking clinically evident metastatic disease, the cell kill hypothesis predicted even greater cell destruction against microscopic foci of metastasis.

Cure is defined as a disease-free survival curve that parallels that of a comparable population without malignancy. The biological requirement for cure is total eradication of all malignant cells, regardless of the treatment modality. This may be accomplished by surgical excision, radiation ablation, cytotoxic drug destruction, or any other effective means.

Treatment of cancer can be either curative or palliative in its intent. The aggressiveness of the treatment prescription is determined to a great degree by whether cure is deemed possible or not. The aggressiveness of any therapeutic plan has to be balanced against the toxic risk, combined with the expected course of the disease if no treatment at all is given. Other considerations include the age of the patient, comorbidity factors, and a range of psychosocial or socioeconomic nuances.

Cure requires a blend of local and systemic control based on the individual tumors and how they evolve, along with their patterns of spread. Solid tumors tend to be conceptually divided into compartments for the purpose of classification and the elucidation of appropriate therapy (Table 5.8). These compartments involve the primary tumor (T) and the regional lymph nodes (N), which become lumped under the therapeutic concept of local control. The metastases (M) are the aspect that are addressed under the rubric of systemic control (see Tumor Staging).

While local control and systemic control are often conceptually separated, they are in fact interrelated in a variety of ways. Failure to achieve initial local control may lead to secondary systemic spread. Systemic therapy can kill tumor cells in the primary local and regional areas as well as those that are disseminated, thus having an impact on local control. Local control therapy, particularly irradiation, may compromise the ability to deliver optimal systemic therapy. Systemic therapy given concomitantly or prior to surgery and/or x-ray may compromise the ability to achieve local control. In addition, the elucidation of successful systemic adjuvant therapy may change the strategic approach to local control.

The greatest opportunity for cure for any cancer occurs with the primary therapeutic approach. In general, the smaller the tumor burden and the more localized the tumor, the greater chance there is for cure. If a tumor is diagnosed prior to its regional and/or disseminated extension, then the cure potential is usually high. With regional spread cure is still possible, but the percentage of patients in whom this is accomplished falls. When cancer is disseminated, then the cure potential is very low to nil, with a few exceptions.

Tumor Staging

The first step after making the diagnosis of a malignant neoplasm is to classify the tumor with the specific intent of treatment planning (Fig. 5.5). This classification of the malignancy involves three broad approaches. The first approach is histologic classification. Histologic classification elucidates the cell type involved and characteristics that relate to biologic aggressiveness. It is not enough to know that a malignant lymphoma exists within a patient. It is essential to differentiate between Hodgkin's disease and non-Hodgkin's lymphoma. Within non-Hodgkin's lymphoma, it is critical to separate out the good risk (predominantly nodular) lesions from the poor risk (predominately diffuse) lesions. In bronchogenic carcinoma, it is of paramount importance to separate the oat cell cancers from the squamous cell, adenocarcinomas, and large cell tumors, since the patterns of spread and responsiveness to therapy differ so greatly between oat cell and non–oat cell lung cancers.

The second type of classification involves determination of the extent of tumor spread. This is commonly called staging, and usually relates to a local, regional, and metastatic component that is broken down into the shorthand of TNM discussed previously. Accurate quantitation of tumor is beneficial for the following reasons:

1. It aids to communication among the various groups that treat cancer and report their end-results.
2. It aids in the selection of the most appropriate therapy for a given individual patient.
3. It assists in determining the prognosis of individual patients and groups of patients.
4. It helps in evaluating cancer-control measures (clinical trials).

These classifications are generalizations that have to be applied to the circumstances of individual pa-

Table 5.8 **Generalization for Solid Tumors Regarding Primary Curative Intent Therapy Based on Extent of Disease Spread**

Tumor Compartment	Predominant Primary Curative Modality	Potential Adjuvant Mode
Local (T)	Surgery	⟶ Radiation or Chemotherapy
	or X-ray	⟶ Surgery or Chemotherapy and/or
Regional (N) (lymph nodes)	Surgery	⟶ Radiation or Chemotherapy
	X-ray	⟶ Surgery and/or Chemotherapy
Metastases (M)	Chemotherapy	⟶ Surgery or X-ray

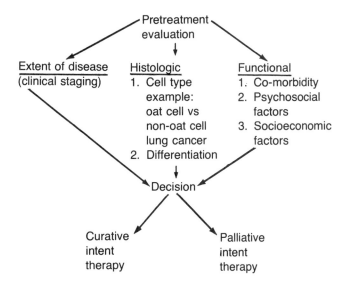

Fig. 5.5 Pretreatment evaluation and the initial decision in treatment planning.

tients, all of whom are unique individuals. It needs to be recognized that statistics do not apply to the individual. All systems of classification are manmade and impose human concepts of order on witnessed phenomena and accumulated behavior. There is no law that demands that a particular cancer should conform to our concepts of its methods of spread.

Proper staging of any tumor requires information obtained by careful physical examination, specific diagnostic procedures, and ultimately surgical exploration. A preliminary classification can be made at any point in the work-up, but a final staging requires completion of all of these procedures.

The TNM Classification

Staging divides tumor spread into three compartments (Table 5.9). The first compartment is the primary tumor itself (designated T). Staging within this compartment details the size and/or the extent of local spread of the primary tumor. In some tumors, such as breast and head and neck cancers, tumor size is the critical variable in determining the stage within the T compartment. In other tumor sites, such as large bowel and bladder, it is depth of tumor penetration in the organ that determines the stage. Determining the T stage can be accomplished clinically for some tumors, for example, head and neck cancer; but for others, this determination can only be made pathologically, for example, large bowel cancer.

The second compartment involves the draining regional lymph nodes (designated N). The determi-

nation of lymph node involvement has been deemed critically important because lymph nodes are believed to provide an initial barrier to widespread tumor dissemination. Therefore therapy that can control all tumor in the lymph nodes has a curative potential. It has also been recognized that involvement of the regional lymph nodes constitutes, for many tumors, the most potent prognostic variable for ultimate cure or relapse. Staging within the N compartment involves either the number of lymph nodes involved, the size of the involved nodes, the number of lymph node changes involved, or some combination of these. However, the most critical determination remains whether the nodes are involved ($N+$) or are tumor free (N_0). The ability to determine nodal involvement can be through either clinical examination (head and neck) or tissue examinations. For the great majority of cancers tissue

Table 5.9   TNM System for Classification of Cancer

T = Primary tumor
T_0: No evidence of primary tumor
T_{IS}: Carcinoma in situ
T_{1-4}: Progressive increase in tumor size and involvement
N = Regional lymph nodes
N_0: Regional lymph nodes not demonstrably involved with tumor
N_{1-3}: Increasing degree of demonstrable abnormality of regional lymph nodes
N_x: Involvement of regional lymph nodes cannot be assessed
M = Distant metastases
M_0: No evidence of distant metastases
M_{1-3}: Ascending degrees of distant metastases

examination is necessary to determine whether the lymph nodes are involved. For some tumors radiographic assessment, such as lymphangiography, can give a strong clinical impression of whether the nodes are involved or not.

The last conceptual compartment of tumor spread is the metastatic compartment (designated M). In most staging classifications, merely the presence of metastatic disease ($M+$) or its absence (M_0 or $M-$) is determined (Table 5.10).

Staging is a complex interaction of clinical staging, surgical evaluative staging, and pathologic staging (Fig. 5.6). The relative importance of these three approaches to staging differs from tumor to tumor. Clinical staging has as its major function the determination of whether a surgical approach to cure is feasible. This is the foremost immediate role of clinical staging in lung cancer, colon cancer, stomach cancer, prostate cancer, and most, if not all, of the solid tumors. Surgical evaluative staging is done by the surgeon on the operating table and leads to a decision to attempt a curative resection, perform a palliative resection, or merely "open and close." Pathologic staging has as its main function prognostic subsetting, which enables a rational decision to be made about the appropriateness of adjuvant therapies.

Cure or Palliation

The crucial early decision in pretreatment planning for any tumor is whether cure is feasible. If cure is a reasonable possibility, then aggressive therapy is indicated along with certain calculated risks of treatment-related morbidity and mortality. The psychosocial impact of amputation, mastectomy, laryngectomy, colostomy, or cystectomy are worth facing if cure may possibly be gained. Where cure is not considered possible, palliation becomes the goal. This is

Table 5.10   Generalized Approach to Staging Using TNM Classification

Stage I: No extension beyond tumor		
T_1	N_0	M_0
T_1	N_x	M_0
Stage II: Tumor has extended to regional lymph nodes		
T_1	N_1	M_0
T_1	N_2	M_0
T_2	N_0	M_0
T_2	N_1	M_0
T_2	N_2	M_0
T_2	N_x	M_0
Stage III: Tumor has spread beyond the walls of the organ and to distant areas of the body		

defined as prolongation of survival, relief of symptoms, and maintenance of function as near normal as possible. The aggressiveness of treatment acceptable for palliation is dependent on the potential benefit that can be expected and the natural history predicted if no therapy is undertaken.

The potential therapeutic decisions that can be made within a given cancer are numerous. Each tumor has three or four stages and multiple subsets within each stage. Each of these stages, and their subsets, has various possible combinations of surgery, radiation, drugs, and hormonal manipulations as primary, secondary, or even tertiary therapy. Into this mix psychosocial, economic, and travel factors must be added. Therefore, therapeutic decision-making is a highly complex process.

Clinical Research

The decision-making process of treatment planning can be viewed as occurring in two contexts. The first context is individual patient care, and the second context is clinical research. Well-conducted clinical research gives to all participating patients the benefit of optimal application of what is known to be currently achievable. Clinical cancer research is an interactive process with four major inputs (Fig. 5.7): the disease, the modality, the strategy, and the design. Each of the manifold diseases called cancer are different in terms of their natural history, patterns of spread, response to treatment, and patterns of relapse after therapy. Each disease has its own clinical research strategy that utilizes the various modalities in differing sequences and/or combinations, depending on stage, histology, and functional abilities. This disease-oriented strategy can be viewed as being in conflict with, to some degree, the modality-oriented strategy. A new drug has a fixed generalized strategy of phase I→phase II→phase III. These phases of study for a new drug must take place in patients with cancer, and therefore must relate to the disease-oriented strategy. In what instances is it appropriate to perform a phase I or II study of a new drug in breast cancer as against colon cancer as against leukemia? Those investigators solely concerned with drug development might have an opinion that differs from that held by an investigator who specializes in breast cancer or leukemia. Therefore, the clinical oncologist must balance a large number of specific disease-oriented strategies with modality-oriented strategies for new drugs, radiation therapy approaches, surgical techniques, immunologic modulation concepts, and new combined modality strategies.

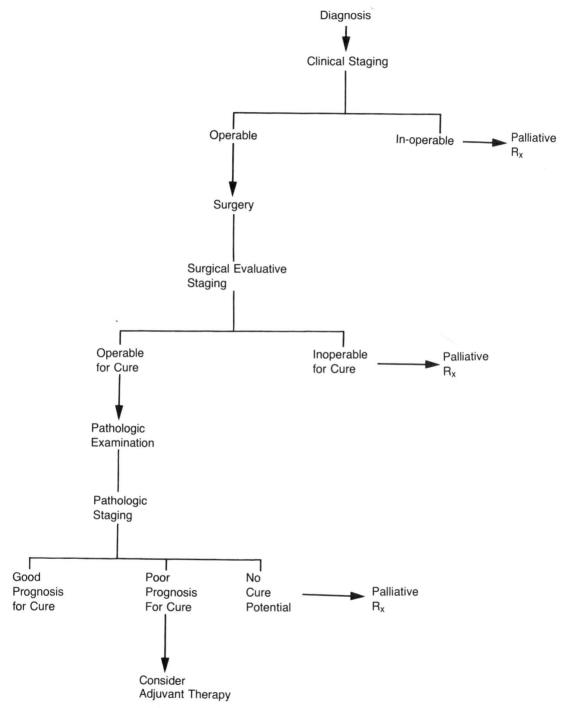

Fig. 5.6 Generalized flow for an operable solid tumor encompassing the three types of disease staging.

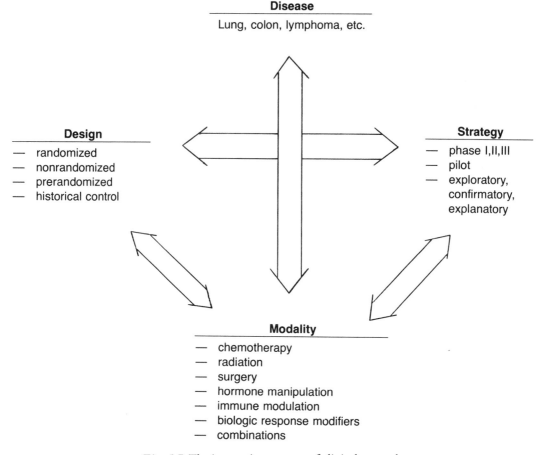

Disease

Lung, colon, lymphoma, etc.

Design

— randomized
— nonrandomized
— prerandomized
— historical control

Strategy

— phase I,II,III
— pilot
— exploratory,
  confirmatory,
  explanatory

Modality

— chemotherapy
— radiation
— surgery
— hormone manipulation
— immune modulation
— biologic response modifiers
— combinations

Fig. 5.7 The interactive process of clinical research.

The essence of good clinical research is having ideas worthy of testing. The organization of clinical research should be geared toward optimizing the ability of an innovative idea to reach clinical evaluation. The testing of a new idea or approach is an exploratory study, and it usually falls under the rubric of a *pilot study*. If the approach involves a new drug, the first study is labeled *phase I*. The phase I aspect involves developing the appropriate dose level and schedule for the drug or combination. The *phase II* aspect involves an early efficacy evaluation to decide if further studies are indicated.

After the completion of an exploratory study, the critical decision that has to be made is whether further studies are indicated. With a new combination of drugs, the phase I study may assess the tolerability of the combination as determined by the achievable dose level of the individual drugs. If some responses are observed in this exploratory study, then enthusiasm may be great for further study; and if no responses have been observed, the opposite may occur. With a single new drug, failure to see responses in a phase I study does not preclude the phase II approach. With a combination, a lack of activity may be a more important observation.

Clinical research must be organized to optimize and facilitate the knowledge flow from exploratory to confirmatory studies, and then on to explanatory studies. The exploratory study is best performed within a single institution or a small number of collaborating institutions. The confirmatory and explanatory studies require larger patient numbers, and, in most instances, will require the collaboration of multiple institutions.

Surgical Treatment

Surgery is the oldest modality available for treating patients with cancer. Since the turn of the last century, surgeons have defined the safe limits of resections, improved the techniques of reconstruction, and learned how to operate with limited morbidity.

By the 1950s most of these advances had been made, and the outcomes following surgery have changed little since.

The classical principles of surgical oncology can be outlined as follows:

1. In excising a tumor a certain amount of normal tissue surrounding the cancer also has to be removed.

2. Many cases spread initially to the regional lymph nodes, and so removal of the tumor-bearing organ along with its adjacent nodes should be attempted when feasible.

3. Some tumors tend to metastasize late, and so even when locally advanced these tumors can be cured by aggressive surgery involving resection of multiple organs.

4. The first surgical procedure has the greatest chance of success, and so the initial approach should be as aggressive as possible if cure is a possibility. This precept led to the adage "big operations for small cancers," a concept that may have been excessively applied, in light of current understanding.

It is now recognized that many tumors have microscopically disseminated by the time of diagnosis, when they appear clinically localized. Radical procedures involving extensive node dissection may not necessarily improve results over less disfiguring procedures. The role of the host's immune response to the tumor has become one of the major areas of research interest for the surgical oncologist, and some hypothesize that total eradication of the last cell by the surgical knife may not be required for cure. Some have gone as far as to postulate that removal of the regional lymph nodes draining a tumor may remove a natural immunologic barrier.

The surgeon has to be familiar with the patterns of spread associated with each individual type of cancer and the potential relapse patterns as he attempts to determine the optimal surgical approach to achieve tumor control. Tumors have various patterns of local invasion. Some tumors excite a desmoplastic reaction and cause a hardness in the invaded tissues that helps the surgeon distinguish surgical margins. The surgeon commonly determines the margin around a cancer by visible and tactile changes and then attempts to remove enough surrounding tissue to account for microscopic invasion. The surgical margins are also dictated by natural anatomic boundaries, by cosmetic factors, and by experience.

Once the diagnosis is established the surgeon works as part of a multidisciplinary team to stage each patient. Rigorous attempts are made to determine whether the cancer has spread, and to which sites, before proper treatment can be decided.

The prognosis for a given patient with cancer is predicted on the basis of a complex of factors that Patterson describes as tumor-related factors, host-related factors, and physician-related factors.

Tumor-related factors include the size and location of the tumor, its cellular characteristics, its invasiveness, and, after pathologic staging, the lymph node involvement or the lack thereof. Size is usually inversely proportional to the prognosis for cure. Large tumors are not only more difficult to remove but have a greater chance of having microscopically metastasized. Undifferentiated neoplasms with a high mitotic rate and rapid doubling time generally have a poor prognosis compared with well-differentiated tumors with low mitotic rates and slow doubling times. Squamous cell lesions of the head and neck area are a location where this is a particularly potent prognostic variable.

Host-related factors include the patient's general condition and age and the stage of his or her immunologic system. Many patients have concomitant morbid conditions that can affect whether adequate treatment can be administered. These include other physical conditions and the psychological status of the patient. It takes a reasonably strong patient, both physically and emotionally, to handle the full effects of aggressive therapy, which may cause discomfort, pain, and physical deformity. Immunity to cancer is expressed through humoral factors (tumor-specific antibodies) and cellular factors (activated lymphocytes and macrophages). Many studies have shown that patients whose immune system is intact, especially with regard to delayed hypersensitivity, have a better prognosis than those who are anergic when tested with a battery of skin tests.

Physician-related prognostic factors include the appropriateness of therapy, the adequacy of the therapeutic application, and the adequacy of the follow-up. The appropriateness of the treatment depends on an adequate diagnostic work-up, accurate staging, and thorough pretreatment evaluation by all of the disciplines that can have a meaningful input. The therapy, once decided on, needs to be carried out by qualified personnel with access to an adequate laboratory and competent nursing support. Effective follow-up is essential to the care of cancer patients so that recurrence can be detected early and cure provided when possible.

Radiation Therapy

Radiation therapy exerts a selective effect on the tumor. Ideally, radiation therapy should completely eradicate a tumor without damaging in any way the surrounding normal tissue. Unfortunately, this ideal is rarely achieved with current approaches. The effectiveness of radiation for a given tumor depends on a combination of the following factors:

1. The difference between the radiosensitivity of the neoplastic cells and that of the normal cells.

2. The difference between the intracellular repair capacity of the neoplastic cells and that of the normal cells. The accumulated radiation injury in the tumor cells may become so great that they die, while normal cells will tend to survive because of a greater rate of recovery.

3. The ability of normal tissues and organs to repair themselves if they are regionally damaged.

All ionizing radiations deposit their energy in matter through charged particle interactions, that is, through collisions between high-velocity charged particles and the orbital electrons of the medium. These high-velocity charged particles deposit their energy in discrete and randomly distributed energy-deposition events along their paths. Each charged-particle energy-deposition event liberates an average of 60 electron volts of energy into a sphere of 3 nm in diameter. This results in the sphere containing excited and ionized molecules that rapidly transform into free radicals that can interact with biological molecules in their vicinity. These free radicals can interact with DNA in a manner lethal to the cell unless metabolic repair processes remove the damaged moiety. In terms of eradicating neoplastic cells with irradiation, more than one energy deposition event must occur within a small volume. This may involve (1) a single target requiring several hits, (2) several close targets each needing one hit, or (3) additive sublesions.

Linear Energy Transfer (LET) is defined as the energy imparted to matter by one charged particle traversing some specified length. LET is a complex function of velocity and charge of the ionizing particle. Standard irradiation, with 250 KV, cobalt 60, or 10 MEV linac machines are described as low LET since they are sparsely ionizing. High LET irradiation, utilizing heavy ions on pl-mesons, is described as densely ionizing. Fast neutrons are intermediate density radiations, but are usually also described as high LET.

New types of therapeutic radiation are compared in terms of relative biologic effectiveness (RBE). RBE is defined as follows:

$$RBE = \frac{\text{Dose of standard radiation required to produce a given effect}}{\text{Dose of test radiation required for the same effect}}$$

The standard radiation is usually taken as 200 to 500 KVP orthovoltage x-rays. Numbers greater than 1.0 means greater efficiency, since a lower dose of the test radiation is therefore required to achieve the comparable effect. High LET radiations can reach an RBE of 8.0 experimentally.

The RBE depends on at least eight interactive factors, such as (1) linear energy transfer of radiation, (2) radiation dose, (3) fractionation pattern, (4) dose rate, (5) biological test system, (6) endpoint under study, (7) oxygenation status, and (8) presence or absence of a sensitizer or protector.

The concept of radiosensitivity addresses the susceptibility of cancer cells to irradiation and how effectively and efficiently they are killed by it. The clinician tends to view this as an inherent biologic characteristic of the tumor or tissue. Among the most highly radiosensitive tumors are the malignant lymphomas, testicular seminoma, dysgerminomas, granulosa cell carcinomas, and leukemia. Squamous cells lesions of the head and neck and tumors of the uterus, the cervix, the skin, the esophagus, and the bladder are generally considered to have fairly high radiosensitivity.

The choice of radiation therapy depends on the therapeutic ratio, the anatomic extent of the tumor, and the condition of the host. The relationship between normal tissue tolerance dose and the tumor lethal dose determines the therapeutic ratio. The normal tissue tolerance dose is a measure reflecting an attempt to express the minimal and maximal injurious dose of radiation acceptable to the clinician. This requires the assignment of an arbitrary but useful percentage for the risk of complications. The minimal tolerance dose is defined as the dose to which a given population of patients is exposed under a standard set of treatment conditions resulting in no more than a 5 percent severe complication rate within 5 years after treatment ($TD_{5/5}$). The maximal tolerance dose is defined similarly, but here it entails 50 percent severe complications in 5 years under the same conditions ($TD_{50/5}$). Low tolerance tissues have a TD_{50} of 500 to 4,500 rads and include the gonadal tissues of the testes and ovaries, and fetus, the developing breast, and whole bone marrow. For these tissues the TD_{50} is 500 to 1,000 rads. If the whole lung and kidneys are treated with 2,500 rads or more, fatal radiation pneumonitis or nephritis will develop. The whole liver is at risk at 3,000 to 3,500 rads, and the heart is vulnerable if its entire volume is exposed to doses greater than 4,500 rads. Moderate tolerance tissues have a TD_{50} of 5,000 to 7,000 rads, which approaches the highest levels of exposure in clinical radiation therapy. Tissues having this degree of radioresistance are the ureters, the vagina, the adult breast, the adult muscle, the bile ducts, and the articular cartilage.

When approaching the tumor tissue the radiation oncologist speaks about the tumor lethal dose, which is defined as the dose that achieves 95 percent tumor control (cure) probability (TCD_{95}). The dose that will actually be prescribed for a given tumor will not be a fixed dose but will vary with tumor size and extent, tumor type, pathologic grade and differentiation, and the tumor's response to radiation.

The highly radiocurable tumors have a TCD_{95} range of 3,500 to 6,000 rads. Seminomas, lymphosarcomas, Hodgkin's disease, neuroblastomas, Wilms' tumor, histiocytic lymphomas, medulloblastomas, retinoblastomas, dysgerminomas, and Ewing's sarcoma all fall within this range.

Tumors with a TCD_{95} range of 6,000 to 7,000 rads, such as moderate to large tumors of the oral cavity, pharynx, bladder, cervix, uterus, ovary, and lung require a risk of exceeding normal tissue tolerance to achieve cure.

Radioresistant tumors have a TCD_{95} of 8,000 rads and higher, and include large (T_3, T_4) tumors of the head and neck and breast, melanomas, osteogenic sarcomas, soft-tissue sarcomas, gliomas, and thyroid cancer.

Complications include an acute inflammatory reaction consisting of vasculitis, small vessel injury, tissue edema, and subsequent scarring with fibrosis. Hepatitis, pericarditis, transverse myelitis, esophagitis, pneumonitis, myocarditis, or nephritis may be major life-threatening complications.

The choice of a dose depends on the potential for cure weighed against the probability of complications. Dose must be individualized for each patient, weighing the host-related factors such as comcomitant morbid conditions, psychologic conditions, age, and ability to return for treatment and follow-up.

Chemotherapy

Cancer chemotherapy has a relatively brief history, in contrast to surgery and irradiation, as a modality of cancer treatment. Modern cytotoxic chemotherapy of cancer began in the late 1940s with the initial trials of nitrogen mustard at Memorial Hospital in New York. This drug was soon followed by actinomycin D and methotrexate, and by the recognition that various drugs could selectively skill neoplastic cells. As a result of this, drug development programs were born, and in 1954 the Cancer Chemotherapy National Service Center at the National Cancer Institute was born by mandate of Congress. In the subsequent 25 years, a wide range of anticancer drugs have been discovered.

Successful chemotherapy, for the most part, has meant combination chemotherapy. For a given type of cancer, the essential first step leading to chemotherapy success has been the elucidation of active single agents. Active single agents are the requisite building blocks for a successful combination chemotherapy strategy.

Wherever possible, complete remission should be the goal of cancer chemotherapy. Complete remission is defined as the disappearance of all evidence of tumor. The rapid relapse that occurs in most diseases, when therapy is discontinued after complete remission is apparently achieved, indicates that residual tumor still remains. The concept of *pathologic complete remission* is gaining credibility. To ascertain whether it has been achieved involves extensive laboratory, radiologic, and invasive examination to attempt to document the presence of residual cancer. In tumors such as the malignant lymphomas and ovarian cancer, this increased stringency has lead to a much stronger correlation of complete remission with major survival benefit.

The rationale for the use of drugs in the treatment of cancer is to achieve the selective killing of tumor cells. Underlying this rationale are the principles of the *cell kill hypothesis*. The principles are as follows:

1. The survival of an animal (with transplantable leukemia) is inversely related to either the number of leukemic cells inoculated or the number remaining after treatment.

2. A single leukemic cell is capable of multiplying and eventually killing the host.

3. For most drugs, a clear relationship exists between the dose of drug and its ability to eradicate tumor cells.

4. A given dose of a drug kills a constant fraction of cells, not a constant number, regardless of the cell numbers present at the time of therapy.

This fourth principle means that cell destruction by drugs follows first-order kinetics. For example, treatment reducing a cell population from 1,000,000 to 10 cells should reduce a population of 100,000 to 1 cell. The clinical implications of first-order cell destruction are the following: For eradication, the dose of drug or drugs should be elevated to the maximum limits tolerated by the host; or treatment should be started when the number of cells is small enough to allow the destruction of tumor at drug doses that are reasonably well tolerated.

The logical conclusion derived from the above hypothesis is that the best opportunity for achieving cure exists during the early disease stage. It is more difficult to eradicate disseminated than localized cancer, and much easier to control small tumors than large ones.

It must be recognized that the first-order kinetics of neoplastic cell kill is valid only when all tumor cells are similarly exposed and both the growth fraction and the ratio of sensitive cancer cells to permanently drug-resistant cancer cells are the same. Since large tumor masses have variable blood supplies with mixtures of hypoxic and oxic cells, and since pharmocologic tissue sanctuaries are known to exist for many drugs, it is obvious that the concept can only be generally applied to most therapeutic situations.

Cell Kinetics

All replicating cells that are synthesizing DNA go through a series of phases known as the cell cycle (Fig. 5.8). At the completion of mitosis (M) the cell spends a variable period of time in a "resting" phase (G_1), during which the synthesis of DNA for cell replication is apparently absent while the synthesis of RNA and protein continues normally. In late G_1 (the G_1-S conversion), an unknown signal initiates a burst of RNA synthesis and shortly thereafter the period of DNA synthesis (S phase) begins, and the cell is committed to undergo division or remain polyploid. Next, the cell ceases DNA synthesis during the G_2 phase before entry into mitosis, although RNA and protein synthesis continue. In mitosis, the rates of protein and RNA synthesis diminish abruptly while the genetic material is segregated into daughter cells. An additional resting phase (G_0) of the cell cycle has also been described. G_0 cells are not in cycle but are capable of proliferation; they constitute the cells that for the most part are refractory to cancer chemotherapeutic agents.

Tumor growth is dependent on the proliferating pool (growth fraction) of cells in the tumor. The rate of growth and the doubling time of small tumors depends largely, but not entirely, on the percentage of cells in the mitotic cycle. The cell types in any individual tumor can be represented in four compartments (Fig. 5.9). Tumor cell populations probably resemble a renewing population of normal cells. Some cell differentiation may be associated with inability to divide beyond one or two cell divisions, but tumor cells could be continually renewed from the tumor stem cell or clonogenic pool. Such a model would explain current cytokinetic information and would suggest that cancer cells are not totally unresponsive to growth control mechanisms. Cell population kinetics provide one approach to understanding drug susceptibility in some tumors.

Pharmacokinetics

Another reason for the success or failure of chemotherapy may be related to the pharmacologic disposition of drugs in patients. A drug cannot influence the tumor in a favorable way unless it reaches the

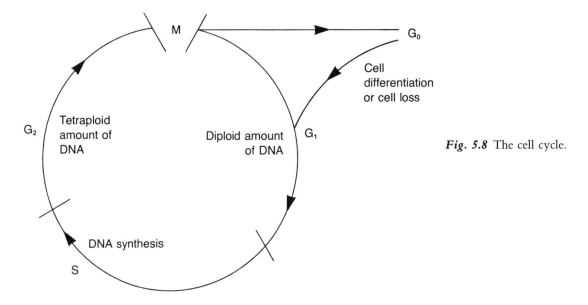

Fig. 5.8 The cell cycle.

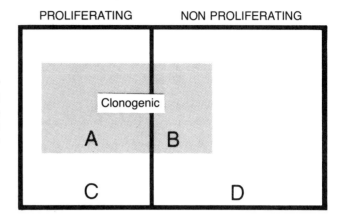

PROLIFERATING   **NON PROLIFERATING**

Clonogenic

A   B

C   D

Fig. 5.9 Types of cell in a tumor. (A) Clonogenic proliferating cells (drug sensitive); (B), clonogenic nonproliferating cells (G_0 cells); (C) nonclonogenic proliferating cells (doomed cells); (D) nonclonogenic nonproliferating cells (end cells).

tumor site and remains there in a tumoricidal concentration for a sufficient period of time to kill the tumor cells. In general, the purpose of pharmacologic studies is to tell the physician how to get an effective concentration (C) of drug to the target site for a long enough time (T) to bring out the desired effect. First, the optimal C × T for the tumor must be estimated for the real target—the tumor cells that are susceptible to killing by the drug. Second, the calculation of optimal C × T for the safety of the patient must reckon with the percentage of normal cells (such as bone marrow cells) that are at risk by being in DNA synthesis, mitosis, or any other susceptible phase of the cell cycle. Third, the cell population kinetics of both tumor cells and normal cells are perturbed as a result of drug administration, so that after the perturbation the size of the growth fraction and therefore the potential for drug effect are altered. The optimum C × T should kill the maximum number of tumor cells with minimum lethality in cells of normal tissue.

Resistance

Resistance to cancer chemotherapy may be either natural (innate) or acquired. Natural resistance means that the tumor is resistant from the outset of treatment. Acquired resistance occurs after therapy has begun, as a result of epigenetic or genetic phenomena. Both kinds of resistance may be brought to clinical attention as a result of the selective pressure exerted by the therapy: treatment selectively destroys the sensitive population of cells with subsequent overgrowth of the resistant population. In advanced tumors, where cell burden is high, heterogeneity of sensitivity is likely.

Spontaneous mutations have been shown to arise with resistance to various antimetabolites in mammalian cells. Other factors that contribute to natural drug resistance include a low growth fraction and long generation time of the tumor and the failure of drugs to enter pharmacologic sanctuaries.

Clinical resistance involves host as well as tumor factors. The toxicity to normal tissues, such as bone marrow, limits the doses of drugs that can be administered. Many drugs are highly active in vitro at concentrations that could never be achieved in man because of normal tissue dose restrictions. In order to fully understand clinical resistance, comparisons should be made between drug effects on tumor and on normal host systems, and of the different responses of sensitive and resistant tumor.

Some factors at the cellular level may explain why certain tumors' cells are resistant and while others are sensitive. These include (1) transmembrane transport of drug into the cell; (2) extent of phosphorylation of purine and pyrimidine analogs; (3) extent of catabolism, for example, deamination, decarboxylation, phosphorolysis, hydrolysis, reduction, oxidation, or esterfication of drug to inactive forms; (4) altered affinity of target enzymes for inhibiting drugs; (5) different pathways of precursor utilization for DNA synthesis by tumor cells; (6) extent of repair of drug-induced damage; (7) drug induction of enzymatic activity in tumor or normal tissue; (8) distribution of drug receptors in cell surfaces, cytoplasm, or nucleus; (9) immune inactivation of antigenic drugs; (10) fraction of cell population in drug-sensitive phases of the mitotic cycle.

In any given case of acquired resistance, more than one of these factors may be involved. With a few exceptions, for example, hair follicles, normal tissue resistance is constant, and strategies to predict sensitivity can concentrate on the tumor cells.

Factors Affecting Choice of Chemotherapy

Factors that affect the choice of chemotherapy include (1) general sensitivity of the tumor to chemotherapy, (2) specific sensitivity of an individual's tumor to individual agents, (3) the likelihood of response and clinical improvement versus serious toxicity (assessment of therapeutic index), (4) whether chemotherapy is to be used in the setting of advanced disease as a single modality, in a combined modality (such as with radiation therapy for regional disease), or in the adjuvant setting after potentially curative surgery.

Since acute leukemia, lymphomas, pediatric solid tumors, breast and ovarian cancer, and small cell lung cancer are generally sensitive to chemotherapy, the choice of antineoplastic drug treatment is generally an appropriate one, even if the patient is bedfast from his disease. Conversely, the relative chemoinsensitivity of renal, pancreatic, esophageal, colorectal, non–small cell lung cancer, and melanoma, coupled with the negative effect of adverse performance status on the likelihood of a response—together, these lead most medical oncologists to avoid the toxicity of presently available chemotherapy in nonambulatory patients having these diagnoses. Whether to treat the ambulatory patient who has dissemination of one of these cancers depends on several factors, including the patient's own informed desire for treatment, the availability of adequate facilities, and the possibility that the patient's participation in a therapeutic research protocol could yield long-range benefits.

To be able to determine the specific sensitivity (or lack thereof) of an individual patient's tumor to chemotherapeutic agents, is a long sought but frustratingly distant goal. The importance of the hormone receptor content of a mammary tumor, in determining whether endocrine therapy should be employed, represents the most significant advance as of this writing.

Recent work with effects of chemotherapeutic agents on colony formation by human tumor cells in vitro is promising. Briefly, it appears that use of a two-layer agar culture system may selectively promote the growth of tumor stem cells on a short-term basis, making it possible to assay drug effects on this population in vitro: the incidence of false negatives (no effect in vitro, effect seen in vivo) is practically zero, while that of false positives (effect in vitro, no effect in vivo) is about 30 percent. Problems with this "clonogenic" assay system are still major, including time and expense of the procedure, inability

to grow some tumors, and interobserver reproducibility.

DRUGS IN CURRENT USE

A total of 39 drugs, including hormonal agents, are now commercially available in the United States. Many of these are listed in Table 5.11 along with their major indications and toxicity patterns. In addition, there are 13 agents that are still under investigation but that have demonstrated evidence of meaningful anticancer activity.

At present, chemotherapy is involved in curative-intent therapy for selected tumor types (Table 5.12). The drugs are used alone or in a combined modality setting. In addition, combined modality studies are going on involving several other tumor types. Tumors in which chemotherapy achieves a significant complete remission rate with resultant prolongation of survival and occasional long-term disease-free survival are listed in Table 5.13.

COMPLICATIONS

Cancer can cause life-threatening emergencies that every physician needs to be familiar with. These oncologic emergencies can be broken down into three categories (Table 5.14).

Spinal Cord Compression

Spinal cord compression is one of the most devastating complications of cancer. The most common tumors associated with spinal cord compression are lung and breast cancer. Anatomically there are two types of compression, extradural compression and intramedullary compression from metastasis within the spinal cord. Extradural compression is the most common type. Hematogenous metastasis implants in the vertebral body, from which point the tumor moves out to compress the dura, thereby compressing the cord directly. Another mechanism is retroneural growth from the paraspinal areas through the intervertebral foramina with the development of secondary compression by direct impingement on the cord.

The primary symptom associated with spinal cord compression is pain, which may be insidious and is most often attributed to a low-back pain syndrome. The pain often becomes radicular. Pain is followed in sequence by paresis and paralysis of the lower extremities. Sensory loss in the extremities occurs after motor weakening. The final problem is autonomic dysfunction with bowel and bladder incontinence.

Clinical awareness is an important factor in making the diagnosis. Confirmation of the diagnosis is achieved by myelography or CT scanning. This not only makes the diagnosis but delineates the level of the cord compression and establishes the amount and distribution of tumor. In terms of therapy, surgical decompression is the primary modality for most tumors. This is accomplished by posterior laminectomy to allow for expansion of the edematous cord within a confined space, thus relieving the pressure on the neurologic tissue. Radiation therapy is the treatment of choice for spinal cord compression secondary to radioresponsive tumors such as multiple myeloma and lymphoma. Radiation therapy is invariably indicated after laminectomy, even for patients with radioresistant tumors, to attack residual disease. Corticosteroids are usually given prophylactically along with the radiation to diminish edema. The two primary determinants of prognosis in spinal cord compression are the duration of the neurologic deficit and the density, or severity, of the neurologic deficit.

Superior Vena Cava Syndrome

The superior vena cava syndrome (SVC) is caused by compression of the vena cava, usually by lymph nodes. It is usually caused by malignancy, although in earlier times syphilitic aneurisms and mediastinal infection were common. The two most common oncologic causes are bronchogenic carcinoma, accounting for nearly 75 percent of all cases, and malignant lymphomas. In bronchogenic carcinoma the SVC syndrome is more common with right-sided lesions by a ratio of 4 to 1. Impingement on the vein leads to a decreased flow rate and subsequent stasis. Eventually caval thrombosis can develop, and is found in one third of patients at autopsy with SVC syndrome.

The most common physical signs of the acute SVC syndrome are venous distension of the neck and upper thorax (75 percent), facial edema (50 percent), thoracic or upper extremity edema (40 percent) and conjunctival edema (25 percent). The symptoms include headache, cough, dyspnea, and visual disturbances. The chest x-ray may demonstrate a large mass in the mediastinum, but with metastatic mediastinal tumor the lesion may be quite small.

The SVC syndrome is a clinical diagnosis and the primary treatment is radiation because of the local lesion and the responsiveness of mediastinal tumors to radiation therapy. High dose intermittent radiation is most commonly used. In highly responsive tumors, chemotherapy can also be used and is the treatment of choice if prior mediastinal radiation precludes the further use of this modality.

Hypercalcemia

Hypercalcemia develops in as many as 10 percent of patients with advanced malignancy. It may be directly related to the tumor (secretion of parathyroid hormone or osseous metastases), or, rarely, it may be related to another morbid process, such as primary hyperparathyroidism. If it is due to osseous metastases, the breast and multiple myeloma are the most common tumors. In patients without bone metastases, most cases of hypercalcemia are due to lung cancer and renal cell carcinoma.

Clinical signs, symptoms, and management are discussed in Chapter 13.

The most important approach to the patient with hypercalcemia is to gain control of the underlying tumor. If the tumor burden is reduced this may be enough to return the serum calcium to normal levels. The cytotoxic drug mithramycin inhibits bone resorption and is useful in all cases of hypercalcemia of cancer, regardless of the pathophysiologic mechanism.

REHABILITATION

The goal of rehabilitation is to return the patient to his or her optimal functioning level, including physical restoration, social functioning, and emotional well-being. This intervention includes inpatient and outpatient care, home care, discharge planning, pastoral care, and hospice and skilled nursing facilities. It often includes pain control and nutrition therapy. Rehabilitation is not limited to the person with cancer—it includes the patient's family as well.

Prevention of disability is the ideal, and, therefore, rehabilitation begins at the time of diagnosis, with efforts aimed at maximum restoration of lost function. Continued support may be required throughout the period of patient care. Yet, many patients fail to take part in rehabilitation programs, and many health professionals fail to provide effective and comprehensive rehabilitation.

The responses evoked by diagnosis, treatment, and

(Text continues on p. 146.)

Table 5.11 Commercially Available Cancer Chemotherapy Drugs*

Drug	Formulation	Major Indications	Acute Toxicity	Delayed Toxicity
Alkylating Agents				
Busulfan (Myleran—Burroughs Wellcome)	Oral	1. Chronic granulocytic leukemia 2. Polycythemia vera	Nausea and vomiting; rare diarrhea	*Bone marrow depression;* pulmonary fibrosis; hyperpigmentation; cutaneous reactions; alopecia; gynecomastia; amenorrhea; menopausal symptoms; sterility; azoospermia; leukemia; chromosome aberrations; cataracts; hyperuricemia
Chlorambucil (Leukeran—Burroughs Wellcome)	Oral	1. Chronic lymphocytic leukemia 2. Hodgkin's disease 3. Non-Hodgkin's lymphoma 4. Ovarian carcinoma		*Bone marrow depression;* pulmonary fibrosis; leukemia
Cyclophosphamide (Cytoxan—Mead Johnson)	Oral and Intravenous	1. Acute and chronic lymphocytic leukemia 2. Breast carcinoma 3. Bronchogenic carcinoma 4. Hodgkin's disease 5. Non-Hodgkin's lymphoma 6. Multiple myeloma 7. Ovarian carcinoma 8. Uterine cervix carcinoma	*Nausea and vomiting;* anaphylaxis	*Bone marrow depression; alopecia;* hemorrhagic cystitis; sterility (may be temporary); pulmonary fibrosis; hyperpigmentation; secondary malignancies; nonspecific dermatitis
Mechlorethamine (nitrogen mustard; HN2; Mustargen—Merck)	Intravenous	1. Bronchogenic carcinoma 2. Hodgkin's disease 3. Non-Hodgkin's lymphoma	*Nausea and vomiting;* local reaction and phlebitis	*Bone marrow depression;* alopecia; diarrhea; oral ulcers
Melphalan (1-phenylalanine mustard; Alkeran—Burroughs Wellcome)	Oral	1. Breast carcinoma 2. Malignant melanoma 3. Multiple myeloma 4. Ovarian carcinoma 5. Testicular seminoma	Mild nausea; hypersensitivity reactions	*Bone marrow depression* (especially platelets); possible pulmonary fibrosis; interstitial pneumonitis; leukemia
Thiotepa (triethylenethiophosphoramide; Thiotepa—Lederle)	Intravenous	1. Bladder cancer (intravesically) 2. Breast carcinoma 3. Hodgkin's disease 4. Ovarian cancer	*Nausea and vomiting;* local pain	*Bone marrow depression;* alopecia (one case)
Antimetabolites				
Cytarabine HCl (cytosine arabinoside; Cytosar-U—Upjohn)	Intravenous	1. Acute granulocytic leukemia 2. Acute lymphocytic leukemia	*Nausea and vomiting;* diarrhea; anaphylaxis	*Bone marrow depression;* megaloblastosis; oral ulceration; hepatic damage

140

Drug	Route	Indications		Toxicity
Floxuridine (FUDR—Roche)	Intraarterial	1. Liver metastases from gastrointestinal malignancies	*Nausea and vomiting;* diarrhea	*Oral and gastrointestinal ulceration;* bone marrow depression; neurological defects, usually cerebellar; pigmentation; alopecia; dermatitis
Fluorouracil (5-FU; Fluorouracil—Roche; Adrucil—Adria)	Intravenous	1. Bladder carcinoma 2. Breast carcinoma 3. Colorectal carcinoma 4. Gastric adenocarcinoma 5. Hepatoma 6. Ovarian carcinoma 7. Pancreatic adenocarcinoma 8. Uterine cervix carcinoma 9. Basal cell and squamous cell skin carcinoma (topically)	*Nausea and vomiting;* diarrhea	*Oral and gastrointestinal ulcers; bone marrow depression;* increased lacrimation; neurological defects, usually cerebellar; pigmentation; alopecia; dermatitis
Mercaptopurine (6-MP; Purinethol—Burroughs Wellcome)	Oral	1. Acute granulocytic leukemia 2. Acute lymphocytic leukemia 3. Chronic granulocytic leukemia	*Nausea and vomiting;* diarrhea	*Bone marrow depression;* cholestasis and rarely hepatic necrosis; *oral and intestinal ulcers;* chromosomal aberrations; anorexia; hyperuricemia
Methotrexate (MTX; Methotrexate—Lederle; Mexate—Bristol)	Oral Intravenous	1. Acute lymphocytic leukemia 2. Breast carcinoma 3. Bronchogenic carcinoma 4. Choriocarcinoma 5. Osteogenic sarcoma 6. Squamous cell carcinoma of head and neck 7. Testicular carcinoma 8. Uterine cervix carcinoma	*Nausea and vomiting;* diarrhea; fever; anaphylaxis	*Oral and gastrointestinal ulceration,* perforation may occur; *bone marrow depression;* hepatic toxicity including cirrhosis and acute hepatic necrosis; renal toxicity; pulmonary infiltrates; osteoporosis; chills, fever; alopecia; depigmentation; cutaneous reactions; infertility; menstrual dysfunction; aphasia; paresis; convulsions
Thioguanine (6-TG; Thioguanine—Burroughs Wellcome)	Oral	1. Acute granulocytic leukemia 2. Acute lymphocytic leukemia	Occasional *nausea and vomiting*	*Bone marrow depression;* possible hepatic damage; stomatitis
Natural Products Asparaginase (Elspar—Merck) Source: Enzyme	Intravenous	1. Acute lymphocytic leukemia	*Nausea and vomiting; fever,* chills; headache; *hypersensitivity;* hyperglycemia	CNS depression or hyperexcitability; acute hemorrhagic pancreatitis; coagulation defects; renal damage; hepatic damage
Bleomycin (Blenoxane—Bristol) Source: Antibiotic	Intravenous	1. Hodgkin's disease 2. Non-Hodgkin's lymphoma 3. Squamous cell carcinoma of head and neck 4. Testicular carcinoma 5. Uterine cervix carcinoma	*Nausea and vomiting; fever;* anaphylaxis and other allergic reactions	*Pneumonitis and pulmonary fibrosis; cutaneous reactions;* stomatitis; alopecia; hyperpigmentation; Raynaud's phenomenon

Table 5.11 (Continued)

Drug	Formulation	Major Indications	Acute Toxicity	Delayed Toxicity
Dactinomycin (actinomycin D; Cosmegen—Merck) Source: Antibiotic	Intravenous	1. Choriocarcinoma 2. Osteogenic sarcoma 3. Sarcomas (general) 4. Testicular carcinoma	*Nausea and vomiting;* diarrhea; local reaction and phlebitis	*Stomatitis; oral ulceration; bone marrow depression;* alopecia; folliculitis
Daunorubicin (Daunomycin; Cerubidine—Ives) Source: Antibiotic	Intravenous	1. Acute granulocytic leukemia 2. Acute lymphocytic leukemia	*Nausea and vomiting;* red urine (not hematuria); severe tissue damage on extravasation; transient EKG changes	*Bone marrow depression; cardiotoxicity; alopecia;* stomatitis; cutaneous toxicity; hyperuricemia; anorexia; diarrhea;
Doxorubicin (Adriamycin—Adria) Source: Antibiotic	Intravenous	1. Acute granulocytic leukemia 2. Acute lymphocytic leukemia 3. Bladder carcinoma 4. Breast carcinoma 5. Bronchogenic carcinoma 6. Endometrial carcinoma 7. Hodgkin's disease 8. Neuroblastoma 9. Non-Hodgkin's lymphoma 10. Prostate carcinoma 11. Sarcomas (general) 12. Squamous cell carcinoma of the head and neck 13. Testicular carcinoma 14. Thyroid carcinoma	*Nausea and vomiting;* red urine (not hematuria); severe local tissue damage and necrosis on extravasation; diarrhea; transient EKG changes; ventricular arrhythmia; hypertensive encephalopathy; angioneurotic edema	*Bone marrow depression; cardiotoxicity* (may be irreversible); alopecia; stomatitis; cutaneous toxicity; hyperuricemia; anorexia; diarrhea; fever, chills; urticaria; anaphylaxis; conjunctivitis; lacrimation
Mithramycin (Mithracin—Dome) Source: Antibiotic	Intravenous	1. Testicular carcinoma	*Nausea and vomiting;* diarrhea; fever	*Hemorrhagic diathesis; bone marrow depression* (thrombocytopenia); hepatic damage; hypocalcemia and hypokalemia; stomatitis; cutaneous reactions
Mitomycin (Mutamycin—Bristol) Source: Antibiotic	Intravenous	1. Breast carcinoma 2. Colorectal carcinoma 3. Gastric carcinoma 4. Lung carcinoma 5. Pancreatic carcinoma	*Nausea and vomiting;* local reaction if extravasation; fever	*Bone marrow depression* (cumulative); stomatitis; renal toxicity; alopecia; pulmonary fibrosis; hepatotoxicity at high doses
Vinblastine sulfate (Velban—Lilly) Source: Plant	Intravenous	1. Breast carcinoma 2. Choriocarcinoma 3. Hodgkin's disease 4. Non-Hodgkin's lymphoma 5. Testicular carcinoma	*Nausea and vomiting;* local reaction and phlebitis if extravasation	*Bone marrow depression;* alopecia; stomatitis; loss of deep tendon reflexes; jaw pain; paralytic ileus

142

Drug	Route	Indications	Acute Toxicity	Delayed Toxicity
Vincristine sulfate (Oncovin—Lilly) Source: Plant	Intravenous	1. Acute lymphocytic leukemia 2. Breast carcinoma 3. Hodgkin's disease 4. Neuroblastoma 5. Non-Hodgkin's lymphoma 6. Sarcomas (general)	Local reaction if extravasation	*Peripheral neuropathy* (loss of deep tendon reflexes, numbness, tingling and muscle weakness); neuritic pain; *alopecia*; mild bone marrow depression; constipation leading to paralytic ileus
Miscellaneous Drugs Carmustine (BCNU; BiCNU—Bristol)	Intravenous	1. Brain tumors 2. Colorectal carcinoma 3. Gastric carcinoma 4. Hepatoma 5. Hodgkin's disease 6. Multiple myeloma 7. Non-Hodgkin's lymphoma	Nausea and vomiting; local phlebitis	*Delayed leukopenia and thrombocytopenia* (may be prolonged); pulmonary fibrosis (may be irreversible); delayed renal damage; gynecomastia
Cisplatin – Cis-Diamminedichloro-platinum; Cis-DDP; Platinol—Bristol)	Intravenous	1. Bladder carcinoma 2. Osteogenic sarcoma 3. Ovarian cancer 4. Squamous cell carcinoma of the head and neck 5. Testicular carcinoma 6. Uterine cervix carcinoma	Nausea and vomiting; anaphylactic–like reactions; fever	*Renal damage*; bone marrow depression; ototoxicity; hemolysis; hypomagnesemia; hyperuricemia; peripheral neuropathy; hypocalcemia; hypokalemia
Hydroxyurea (Hydrea—Squibb–	Oral	1. Chronic granulocytic leukemia	Nausea and vomiting; allergic reactions to tartrazine dye	*Bone marrow depression*; hyperkeratosis and hyperpigmentation; stomatitis; dysuria, alopecia
Lomustine (CCNU; CeeNU—Bristol)	Oral	1. Brain tumors 2. Bronchogenic carcinoma 3. Colorectal carcinoma 4. Hodgkin's disease	Nausea and vomiting	*Delayed leukopenia and thrombocytopenia*; stomatitis; alopecia; transient elevation of transaminase activity; neurological reactions
Procarbazine HCl (Matulane—Roche)	Oral	1. Brain tumors 2. Hodgkin's disease 3. Non-Hodgkin's lymphoma	Nausea and vomiting; CNS depression	*Bone marrow depression*; stomatitis; dermatitis; peripheral neuropathy; pneumonitis
Hormones **Corticosteroids** Prednisone or prednisolone	Oral	1. Acute lymphocytic leukemia 2. Chronic lymphocytic leukemia 3. Breast carcinoma 4. Multiple myeloma 5. Hodkin's disease 6. Non-Hodgkin's lymphoma		Mental aberrations; gastric ulcers; glucose intolerance; osteoporosis; hypertension; cataract formation

143

Table 5.11 (Continued)

Drug	Formulation	Major Indications	Acute Toxicity	Delayed Toxicity
Estrogens Diesthylstilbestrol (DES)	Oral	1. Breast carcinoma 2. Prostate carcinoma	*Nausea and vomiting;* cramps	*Fluid retention; hypercalcemia; feminization;* uterine bleeding; if given during pregnancy, may cause vaginal carcinoma in offspring; increased frequency of vascular accidents
Ethinyl estradiol (Estinyl—Schering; others)	Oral	1. Breast carcinoma 2. Prostate carcinoma		Same as DES above
Androgens Fluoxymesterone (Halotestin—Upjohn)	Oral	1. Breast carcinoma		*Fluid retention; masculinization;* cholestatic jaundice; hypercalcemia; painful hypertrophy of clitoris; hirsutism
Testosterone propionate (Oreton—Schering; others)	IM	1. Breast carcinoma		*Fluid retention;* masculinization; hypercalcemia
Progestins Hydroxyprogesterone caproate (Delalutin—Squibb)	IM	1. Endometrial carcinoma	Local abscess, pain	Hypercalcemia; cholestatic jaundice
Medroxyprogesterone acetate (Provera—Upjohn; others)	Oral	1. Breast carcinoma 2. Endometrial carcinoma 3. Renal cell carcinoma	Orally: nausea (rare) IM: local pain, abscess at injection site	Fluid retention; hypercalcemia
Antiestrogen Tamoxifen citrate (Nolvadex—Stuart)	Oral	1. Breast carcinoma	Nausea and vomiting; hot flashes; transient increased bone or tumor pain	Vaginal bleeding and discharge; rash; hypercalcemia; retinopathy; corneal changes; decreased visual acuity; peripheral edema; depression; dizziness; headache

* Numerous other drugs are available or under active study.

Table 5.12 **The Varying Curative Roles of Cancer Chemotherapy**

A. Tumors in Which Chemotherapy Used Alone Has a Curative Potential

Tumor	Stage	Representative Regimens	Comments
Acute lyphocytic leukemia	NA	*Induction:* Vincristine + Prednisone ± Daunorubicin *CNS prophylaxis:* Intrathecal Methotrexate ± Craniospinal Irradiation *Maintenance:* Methotrexate and 6-Mercaptopurine with periodic reinduction	Curative potential in children under age 15. Complete remission induction about 90 percent but long-term maintenance required.
Hodgkin's Disease	III–IV	"MOPP": Nitrogen mustard Oncovin (Vincristine) Procarbazine Prednisone	Complete remission induction 65–80 percent. Maintenance of no proven value. Important to pathologically restage complete remissions.
Diffuse Histiocytic Lymphomas	III–IV	"CHOP": Cyclophosphamide Doxorubicin Oncovin (Vincristine) Prednisone *or* "BACOP": Bleomycin Doxorubicin Cyclophosphamide Oncovin Prednisone	Complete remission induction 50–60 percent. Maintenance of no proven value. Important to pathologically restage complete remissions.
Testicular Carcinoma	III (disseminated disease)	"PVB": Cisplatin Vinblastine Bleomycin	Complete remission in about 75 percent. Can use surgery in patients with partial response to further induce complete remission. Long-term maintenance of no proven value. Data predominantly in nonseminomatous histologies.
Burkitt's Tumor	IV	Cyclophosphamide	
Uterine Choriocarcinoma	Metastatic	Single-agent Methotrexate *or* Actinomycin D + Methotrexate + Alkylating Agent	Single agents give 95 percent cure in low-risk patients while combinations give 70–80 percent complete remission in high-risk patients.

B. Tumors in Which Chemotherapy Increases the Cure Rates When Used as Adjuvant to Surgery and/or X-ray Therapy

Tumor	Stage	Local Control Therapy	Representative Regimens	Comments
Breast Cancer	II	Surgery ± x-ray	"CMF" Cyclophosphamide Methotrexate 5-Fluorouracil "CMFVP" Above 3 drugs + Vincristine and Prednisone	Data most persuasive for premenopausal women and suggestive for postmenopausal women.
Osteogenic Sarcoma	Clinically localized	Radical amputation	High-dose Methotrexate + Vincristine ± Doxorubicin	Data suggestive from historically controlled studies but not proven in prospectively randomized studies.

Table 5.12   (Continued)

B. Tumors in Which Chemotherapy Increases the Cure Rates When Used as Adjuvant to Surgery and/or X-ray Therapy

Tumor	Stage	Local Control Therapy	Representative Regimens	Comments
Wilms' Tumor	Local or regional spread	Surgery and x-ray	Actinomycin D + Vincristine	

Embryonal Rhabdomyosarcoma	Local or regional spread	Surgery and x-ray	Cyclophosphamide
			  + Actinomycin D
			  + Vincristine	

Ewing's Sarcoma	Localized disease	x-ray	Cyclophosphamide
			  + Vincristine
			  + Actinomycin D	

side effects vary among individuals, but the range of response is extremely broad. Depression, fear, anger, guilt, avoidance, denial, and so on affect the person's self-esteem, sense of worthiness, and sense of competence at home and at work.

The medical care system rewards those patients who do well; the emphasis is on improving one's health at the time one enters the health care system. It encourages patients to do certain exercises, observe special diets, and follow other specific medical recommendations. Cancer care tends to remove the patient from normal activity and to place him or her totally in the hands of the physician and the often intolerable treatment regimen, thus making the patient passive, with feelings of loss of control and inadequacy to deal with the situation.

Table 5.13   Tumors in Which Chemotherapy Can Achieve Complete Remission in More Than One Fourth of Patients Treated with Resultant Significant Prolongation of Survival and Occasional Long-term Disease-free Survival

Tumor	Representative Regimens	Comments

Small Cell Anaplastic Lung Cancer	Cyclophosphamide
	  + Doxorubicin
	  + Vincristine
	or
	Lomustine (CCNU)
	  + Cyclophosphamide
	  + Methotrexate
	or
	"POCC":
	Procarbazine
	Oncovin
	Cyclophosphamide
	Lomustine (CCNU)
		In "limited" disease, combination chemotherapy plus irradiation gives complete response in >50 percent with 2-year disease-free survival of about 20 percent.

Ovarian Cancer	Doxorubicin
	  + Cyclophosphamide
	  ± Cisplatin
		High complete response rate in patients with minimal residul cancer after surgery. Cytoreductive surgery may be helpful. Pathologic determination of complete response with surgery indicates those with long-term survival benefit.

Nodular Lymphomas	"CVP": Cyclophosphamide Vincristine Prednisone *or* Single-agent Chlorambucil or Cyclophosphamide	Aggressive chemotherapy may have curative potential in nodular mixed lymphomas. In nodular lymphocytic, conservative therapy with single agents may be preferable.

Acute Non-lymphocytic Leukemia	Arabinosyl Cytosine
	  + either Daunorubicin or Doxorubicin
	  ± Thioguanine or Vincristine + Prednisone
		Complete remissions in more than half the patients treated. Bone marrow transplantation in remission may offer curative potential.

Table 5.14 Life-threatening Situations Secondary to Malignancy

Neurologic lesions
    Spinal cord compression
    Cerebral metastases
Mediastinum or midline structure lesions
    Superior vena cava obstruction
    Laryngotracheal obstruction
    Pericardial invasion
Endocrinologic or metabolic effects
    Hypercalcemia
    Paraneoplastic syndrome, for example, inappropriate
       ADH secretion
    Endocrine organ tumors

To help determine the response and support service required, evaluation by psychosocial personnel can be invaluable in defining the management issue. Identifying the functional problems of the person with cancer at the time of diagnosis or as soon as they arise is vital, if appropriate support and intervention are to be provided.

For those patients fortunate in having a remission, there is always fear of recurrence or metastases. The subsequent course can bring up new psychologic and social issues for the patient, the family, and the health professional. Professional support can help to determine other losses in the patient's life, and the support services needed and ways to mobilize them.

Much has been written regarding the health professional's own difficulty in discussing the diagnosis and providing support. Patients react differently to their diagnosis and prognosis. They are influenced by their own psychologic status as well as by the skill and tact of the physician providing the information. The physician and other team members must keep in mind that the effects of cancer are neither physiologically nor psychosocially uniform.

An area receiving special attention is sexuality. Patients experiencing mastectomy and ostomy are often singled out immediately for sexual counseling. In addition, the effect of chemotherapy on fertility and ovarian function, indications of treatable menopause in patients with Hodgkin's disease, the need for effective hormonal replacement, and patient counseling are receiving greater attention. The consequences to personal and family relationships with resultant emotional distress and sexual dysfunction emphasize the need for a combined medical and rehabilitation approach.

The therapeutic environment itself can create special problems, for example, isolation of some leukemic patients, and it raises the issue of lack of physical contact by family members, friends, and physicians. Physical barriers prohibit hugging, touching, and thus comforting the patient.

Vocational Rehabilitation

A common concern among cancer patients is their ability to maintain economic and vocational independence in the way they were accustomed to prior to their illness.

Cancer is one of the life-threatening diseases that usually leaves a person quite capable of working. Yet, discussion with vocational counselors, patients, and health professionals reveals confusion and concern about possible discrimination in employment of individuals with a history of cancer and a misunderstanding of their ability to continue employment. Such discrimination is illegal and it is very difficult to prove or study. Reasons given for job discrimination against cancer patients include fear of endless sick periods, fear of contagion, concern for increased insurance cost and workman's compensation claims, and concern for pensions and other fringe benefits paid by the employer.

Physical Rehabilitation

Many therapies for cancer cause functional defects in patients, which can hinder their return to normal, everyday activities. Ideally, any potential functional defects from therapy should be identified at the time initial treatment is planned. At this time the patient's rehabilitation needs should be identified and built into the planning process.

The primary goals of rehabilitation should be (1) *restoration* of the patient to a normal functioning capacity; (2) *support* of the patient to minimize the physical, psychosocial, and vocational problems of functional deficits that cannot be restored; and (3) *palliation* when survival is not expected to be prolonged.

Communication Deficits

The communication deficit that has received the greatest attention is the one caused by laryngectomy. The alaryngeal deficit can be relieved by training in esophageal speech, the use of an artificial electric larynx, or the surgical creation of air tunnels. Such procedures allow the patient to communicate with others.

Communication deficits also exist in patients who have undergone surgical procedures for tumor in the nasal, oral, or pharyngeal areas. They may also occur after ligation of the common carotid artery or following cerebrovascular accidents in elderly cancer patients.

Speech therapists should be called upon wherever they may be helpful.

Intestinal Stomas

Surgical treatment of gastrointestinal, gynecologic, and genitourinary malignancies can result in both psychic and psychosocial problems for the patients. Essential to minimizing these problems is proper placement of the stoma. An optimal placement based on a pretherapeutic evaluation, the abdominal contours, and the type of collection device to be utilized can do much to achieve full acceptance with minimal morbidity. Conversely, poor placement can result in seepage of the intestinal contents with skin irritation and even skin breakdown.

Several physiologic problems must be kept in mind. One of these is excessive gas and odor. An oral medication such as charcoal and bismuth subcarbonate may help as a deodorizer. More important is the combination of proper diet and irrigation. The role of irrigation, as against natural evacuation, is still under some debate, as is the constitution of an optimal diet.

Another critical factor is careful selection of the collecting appliance. The application site should be observed closely in the early postoperative period to evaluate whether the patient is sensitive to the rubber ring or adhesive used to fix the ring to the abdominal skin.

A difficult transition can exist when an ostomy patient leaves the hospital to go home. Attention to the home care facilities is of paramount importance. This transition can be facilitated by a home visit by a trained enterostomal therapist or an ostomy volunteer visitor, and adequate follow-up is essential.

Cancer Amputation

Amputation of an extremity in a cancer patient does not differ greatly from amputation for other reasons. Many times the cancer amputee is at a relative advantage, since the site is elective and can be chosen where vascularity and tissue trauma are not a major problem. In addition, cancer amputations often occur in young, vigorous individuals. However, cancer amputations generally are more radical than those performed for vascular deficiencies and trauma. The entire bone often has to be removed and, therefore, below-knee or below-elbow amputations are often not possible.

The rehabilitation process should begin as soon as the decision for amputation is made. Both the patient and family must be made aware of what rehabilitation program is planned, when a prosthesis can be fitted, and what the costs will be. Psychologic counseling, particularly in teenage patients, will often be needed. Exercise programs to strengthen important muscles can be initiated immediately. Vocational counseling for the working individual is also very important.

In the immediate postoperative period the lower-extremity amputee needs to be instructed in crutch walking. In addition, evaluation and training in transfer activities and the activities of daily living should be given. Of great benefit to cancer amputees has been the use of an immediate postoperative prosthesis, which requires the services of a prosthetist in the operating room.

As Enelow states, "Emotional support is provided by any action on the part of a help-giving person, such as a physician or other health professional that communicates his interest in, liking for, or understanding of the patient and that helps give the patient a feeling of security in this relation. It is the major element in psychotherapy, but should be part of every doctor-patient relationship."

REFERENCES

1. American Cancer Society: Cancer Facts and Figures. 1981.
2. Boice, J.D.: Cancer following medical irradiation. Cancer 47:1095–1108, 1981.
3. Carter, S.K., Bakowski, M., Hellmann, K.: Chemotherapy of cancer. 2nd ed. New York, John Wiley & Sons, 1981.
4. Chapman, R.M., Sutcliffe, S.B., Malpas, J.S.: Effects on sexual function. JAMA 242:1881, 1979.
5. Healy, J.E.: Rehabilitation of the patients with cancer. In: Management of the Patient with Cancer. Philadelphia, W.B. Saunders, Philadelphia, pp. 61–80, 1976.
6. Higgenson, H.: Epidemiology for clues to etiology. In: Burchenal J.H., Oettgen, H.F. (eds), Cancer—Achievements, Challenges and Prospects for the 1980s. New York, Grune & Stratton, 1981. pp 7–25.
7. Hoover, R., Fraumeni J.F.: Drug-induced cancer. Cancer 47:1071–1080, 1981.
8. Klein, G.: Viruses and cancer. In: Burchenal J.H., Oettgen H.F. (eds), Cancer—Achievements, Challenges and Prospects for the 1980's. New York, Grune & Stratton, 1981. pp 81–101.
9. Love, R.R., Camilli, A.E.: The value of screening. Cancer 48:489–949, 1981.
10. McLemore, T.L., Martin, R.R.: Pulmonary carcinogenesis: Aryl hydrocarbon hydroxylase. In: Livingston R.B. (ed), Lung Cancer I. Boston, Martinus Nijhoff, 1981. pp 1–35.
11. Miller, D.G.: Prevention and detection in primary practice. Your Patient and Cancer 1(6):25–31, 1981.

12. Miller, E.C., Miller, J.A.: Mechanisms of chemical carcinogenesis. Cancer 47:1055–1064, 1981.
13. Nelson, N.: Cancer prevention. Cancer 47:1065–1070, 1981.
14. Patterson, W.B.: Principles of surgical oncology. In: Rubin P. (ed), Clinical Oncology—A Multidisciplinary Approach. University of Rochester School of Medicine, 1974.
15. Payne, E.D., Krant, M.J.: The psychosocial aspects of advanced cancer. JAMA 201:1238, 1969.
16. Pitot, H.C.: Fundamentals of Oncology. New York, Marcel Dekker, 1978.
17. Ritchie, A.C.: The classification, morphology and behavior of tumors. In: Florey H. (ed), General Pathology. Philadelphia, W.B. Saunders, 1962. pp 551.
18. Rubin, P. and Poulter, C.A.: Principles of radiation oncology and cancer radiotherapy. In: Rubin P. (ed), Clinical Oncology—A Multidisciplinary Approach. Unive.rsity of Rochester School of Medicine, 1974.
19. Shottenfeld, D.: Epidemiology of cancer: An overview. Cancer 47:1095–1108, 1981.
20. Wienstein IB: The scientific basis for carcinogen detection and primary cancer prevention. Cancer 47:1133–1141, 1981.

6

Disorders of Immunity

Samuel Oleinick, M.D.

PRINCIPLES OF IMMUNOBIOLOGY

The immune system, assisted by the accessory systems of host resistance, functions to preserve a specific form of homeostasis: the preservation of "self". Invasive microorganisms which might produce harm are isolated, inactivated, or eliminated. Mutated cells which are potentially malignant are destroyed. Biological or chemical toxins are *neutralized*.

All vertebrates possess an immune system, and the complexity of the system increases as the phylogenetic scale is ascended. Chordates and some of the subvertebrate animals including annelids and crustaceans also possess elements of the immune system.

The essential quality of the immune system resides in the cells of the lymphocyte series. Certain of these lymphocytes are capable of *memory*. The lymphocytes themselves or antibodies secreted by lymphocytes manifest *specificity*. The latter quality of *specificity* is not unique to the immune system; hormones show specificity for hormone receptors on cell membranes, enzymes show specificity for their substrates, and lectins show specificity for particular oligosaccharides, but the binding energies of immune reactants (e.g. antibodies) for their specified antigens are perhaps higher than any other biologic system of interaction.

The generation of specificity is genetically determined. A species may possess lymphocytes capable of recognizing and responding to a particular antigenic molecular configuration, or the species may lack this capability. Also, within a species of animals, certain individuals or certain experimental strains may lack the ability to respond to an antigen. The genetic regulation of responsiveness has been as-signed to a set of genes designated "immune response genes". Examples of genes associated with responses to specific antigens are listed in Table 6.1.

While immune response genes are implicated in the ultimate generation of immune responsiveness, the biology of the system is much more complicated. Ability to recognize and respond to a particular antigen may also depend on the complexity, configuration and number of antigenic sites on the antigenic molecule. Certain molecules directly appeal to B lymphocytes which can respond by synthesizing antibodies (thymus independent antigens). Other antigens require the interaction of several classes of lymphocytes for recognition and response. The latter antigens (thymus dependent antigens) invoke the cooperation of helper/inducer T cells with the responder B cells. This collaborative effort is especially important in secondary (anamnestic) responses. Collaboration is also an important component of T lymphocyte responsiveness to antigens (T helper interacting with T responder cells), eventuating in cell-mediated immunity.

The manner of presentation of antigens to the immune system has significant implications for immune responsiveness. The antigen may be bound to the macrophage surface, macrophages may degrade ingested molecules rendering those molecules more or less capable of invoking an immune response, or complexing of antigens with cellular molecules (especially plasma membrane molecules) may modify the role of the antigen for the responding lymphocyte.

Unresponsiveness to a particular antigen may be attributed to the absence of a particular immune response gene or to the elimination of reactive lymphocytes which bear the necessary receptor for the

Table 6.1   Genetic Control of Human Immune Responses

Antigen	Association with genes of the major histocompatibility complex (HLA), if known
Ra3 (Ragweed allergen)	A2; A28
Ra5 (Ragweed allergen)	Dw2; B7
Ra6 (Ragweed allergen)	Bw35
Rye I (Rye grass allergen)	B8; Dw3; A1
Rye II (Rye grass allergen)	Dw3; B8
Ag3 (Timothy grass allergen)	B7
Trichophytin	B8
Gluten	B8
Insulins:	
Bovine A-chain	A26; Cw2
Bovine C-peptide	B13

particular antigen. The latter can occur in the prenatal period or in certain species in the very early postnatal period. Antigens presented during these restricted periods trigger elimination of the specific responding lymphocytes rather than a state of immunity. To preserve this unresponsiveness, the antigen may have to persist chronically or this form of tolerance may not endure. A natural example of this mechanism is the chimerism seen in mammalian bovine twins and perhaps in certain human non-identical twins.

Unresponsiveness is more commonly explained by the mechanism of immune suppression; specific suppressor T lymphocytes regulate the immune response to these autoantigens. In many patients, autoantibodies can be demonstrated in low titers; however, in most instances this type of immune response is restricted to a very low level. Only in isolated cases, perhaps triggered by aging, tissue trauma or ischemia, infections, or exposure to exogenous cross-reacting antigens, does the suppressor system fail and significant levels of auto-immunity eventuate. Examples of this form of invoked auto-immunity are listed in Table 6.2.

Finally, the immune system is notable for the complex sequence of responses that are generated. Certain antigens only generate IgM antibodies. Other antigens generate the early wave of IgM antibodies, followed by IgG antibodies. Indeed, the switchover

Table 6.2   Examples of Human Autoimmunity Most Likely Invoked by Dysfunction of Suppressor Lymphocytes

1. Autoantibodies in systemic lupus erythematosus
2. Anti-cardiac muscle antibodies following myocardial infarction
3. Anti-brain antibodies following cerebrovascular accidents
4. Anti-thyroglobulin and anti-thyroid microsomal antibodies in thyroiditis

mechanism is poorly understood, but it is known that IgG antibodies to a particular antigen can turn off the IgM synthesizing cells probably by binding with, and activating suppressor cells (which contain receptors for IgG). The generation of cell-mediated immunity is also a complicated phenomenon which involves cell-cell interaction between T cell subclasses and macrophages.

The complexity of immune responses can be illustrated by observing the various forms of penicillin sensitivity. Certain persons, fortunately few in number, develop anaphylaxis, shock, and even death, mediated via IgE antibodies. Others develop less abrupt symptoms of "serum sickness" with urticaria, fever, and arthritis. Occasionally hemolytic anemia develops because of antibodies to penicillin which interact with penicillin absorbed to autologous red blood cells. Still others develop contact allergies (skin rashes) which are attributed to cell-mediated immunity, but most people have no identifiable adverse response.

LYMPHOCYTE CLASSES AND FUNCTIONS

Lymphocytes differentiate from lymphoid stem cells, which in post-natal life are generated in the bone marrow.

Cells of the lymphoid stem cell series differentiate into various lineages. The major populations of lymphocytes are the B cells, the T cells and the "third compartment" (third population) cells.

B Cells

In birds a lymphoepithelial organ adjacent to the cloaca called the bursa of Fabricius programs lymphoid stem cells to differentiate into B cells. In mammals the bone marrow "organ" itself is believed to play the role of the inducing organ for B cell differentiation, although earlier work suggested such a function was reserved for the appendix, the intestinal sacculus rotundus (as presented in rabbits), and the faucial tonsils.

The earliest form of B cells, called "pre-B" cells, possess the capability of reproducing and maintaining a population of cells committed to the B-cell lineage. The pre-B cell can be identified by IgM present in the cytoplasm but not on the cell surface.

Further differentiation in a step-wise fashion occurs in the B cell line. When surface IgM is present, maturation can be judged to be occurring. At subsequent stages, receptors for complement components and low affinity receptors for IgG present in antibody-antigen complexes appear on the cells. Some cells generate IgD on their surfaces; these IgD positive cells appear to resist being made tolerant ("tolerized") to specific antigens. Further differentiation is accompanied by loss of surface IgM (except for a subpopulation of cells) and IgD, synthesis of IgG, IgA or IgE, appearance of these immunoglobulins on the lymphocyte surfaces, and the appearance of the capability for these B cells to interact with T cells and macrophages. The decision as to which immunoglobulin heavy chain (IgG_1, IgG_2, IgG_3, IgG_4, IgM, IgA, IgE, or IgD) or which light chain (kappa or lambda) will ultimately be produced by the differentiated B lymphocyte is probably dependent upon a signal from a *helper T lymphocyte*. Thus, primary B lymphocytes bearing IgM or IgG on their surfaces can give rise to B lymphocytes secreting IgM or IgG as well as lymphocytes secreting IgA or IgE.

Plasma cells represent cells derived from the B lymphocyte lineage which possess the organelles for efficient synthesis of immunoglobulin (antibody) molecules.

T Cells

The T cell population of lymphocytes consists of several subpopulations which can be discriminated by various surface markers or by functional assays. Originally these cells were identified as the cells responsible for delayed type hypersensitivity (DTH) or "cell-mediated immunity." Examples of this reaction are the PPD skin test reaction (tuberculin reaction) as well as delayed hypersensitivity reactions to other bacterial, fungal, and viral extracts. In addition, T cells were noted to be of major importance in the rejection of tissue and organ transplants and in immune rejection of tumor tissue (especially solid tumors). Another compartment of T cells is that of memory T cells, important for the anamnestic response.

Further subsets of T lymphocytes include: (1) helper/inducer T cells, (2) suppressor/cytotoxic T cells, and (3) feedback regulator T cells. A family of monoclonal antibodies (OKT) currently provide the most widely used system of identifying human T cell subpopulations.

Bone marrow stem cells committed to the T lymphocyte lineage generate prothymocytes which migrate to the thymus. There, under the influence of thymic epithelial cells and thymic hormones, an early stage of thymocyte differentiation occurs. These Stage I, immunologically incompetent early thymocytes make up about 10 percent of thymus lymphocytes. The next stage of differentiation generates the Stage II "common" thymocyte which is partially immunocompetent. Approximately 70 percent of thymic lymphocytes are in this stage of differentiation. The final stage of thymocyte differentiation involves the partitioning of the cells into two lineages. One lineage is destined to be the helper/inducer T cell line, the other is the suppressor/cytotoxic cell. These two subpopulations of mature thymocytes make up 10 to 20 percent of the thymic lymphocytes.

When T lymphocytes are released from the thymus and migrate to the secondary lymphoid organs (nodes, spleen, Peyer's patches, tonsils, etc.) or circulate in the blood they loose early surface markers but preserve the markers of their helper or suppressor cell lineage. The helper/inducer cell makes up 60 percent of peripheral blood T lymphocytes. The suppressor/cytotoxic cell comprises 20 percent of peripheral blood T cells and is found in considerable concentration in the spleen.

As yet it is not well understood in which manner the third lineage of T lymphocytes differentiates. This cell, the feedback regulator T cell, interacts with helper and suppressor T cells to regulate their functioning.

Lymphocyte Markers

Three major groups of markers are in common use: (1) surface molecular markers, (2) receptors on lymphocyte membranes, and (3) in vitro functional studies.

The surface immunoglobulins on B cells and T lymphocyte differentiation markers are among the class of surface molecular markers. In addition, specific human transplantation antigens occur on certain lymphocytes. Immune response associated ("Ia") antigens, which are also known as B lymphocyte antigens or D and DR antigens, occur in mature B lymphocytes (as well as numerous other cell systems).

Various receptors occur on lymphocytes and may also be found on other hemic cells. The most widely exploited receptor is that for sheep red blood cells which is found on T lymphocytes as well as on thymocytes. The receptor is not due to sensitization to sheep red blood cells, but exists on all T cells without prior immunization. If sheep red blood cells are pretreated with the enzyme neuraminidase they will also bind to some non-T cells. The sheep red blood cell receptor assay is commonly known as the E rosette test and identifies 70 percent of peripheral blood lymphocytes which represents the circulating T cell population.

Another important receptor is that for the Fc portion of immunoglobulins. Various B lymphocytes have receptors for the heavy chain (Fc) portion of IgG as well as for IgM, IgA, and IgE. Certain T cells also have receptors for Fc portions of immunoglobulins. T lymphocytes which have receptors for IgM-Fc appear to have helper/inducer function; those with receptors for IgG-Fc act as suppressor cells for immunoglobulin synthesis, and others with receptors for IgA may play a regulatory function for synthesis of IgA by B cells.

Third population cells (see below) have receptors for various immunoglobulins. In vitro functional studies may also be performed with lymphocytes and third compartment cells. These assays are listed in Table 6.3.

Clinical Use of Lymphocyte Markers

Lymphocyte markers have contributed significantly to the basic understanding of immunologic phenomena. As will be seen in subsequent discussions, various abnormal lymphocyte mechanisms have been described in human congenital and acquired immunodeficiency disorders as well as in autoimmune diseases (especially systemic lupus erythematosus and Sjogren's syndrome). In addition, malignancies of lymphocytes (lymphomas and leukemias) are being dissected to identify their cells of origin, a characteristic which strongly influences prognosis (see Chapter 17).

Recently studies of T cell populations have been employed to monitor rejection of kidney grafts. Investigators have noted that a high ratio of T_4 to T_8 cells (helper to suppressor cells) was predictive of rejection; treatment of the patients with specific anti-T3 monoclonal antibody (to eliminate T cells from the circulation) effectively reversed episodes of rejection.

Table 6.3   In Vitro Functional Studies of Lymphocytes

1. Proliferation with mitogen stimulation (concanavalin A, phytohemagglutinin, pokeweed mitogen)
2. Proliferation in mixed lymphocyte cultures
3. Helper function for antibody synthesizing cells
4. Suppressor function for antibody synthesizing cells
5. Cytotoxic function of sensitized T cells
6. K cell cytolytic activity in antibody-dependent cell mediated cytotoxicity
7. Release of lymphokines (macrophage migration inhibitory factor, macrophage activating factor, chemotactic factors for mononuclear cells, neutrophils and eosinophils, skin reactive factor, lymphotoxin, blastogenic factor, cloning inhibitory factor, lymph node permeability factor, interferon, transfer factor)
8. Natural killer cell activity against tumor cell lines and virus infected cells

Third Compartment Cells

Cells given this designation are believed to be in the lymphocyte lineage, although a monocyte origin has also been considered. The major subpopulations of cells in this "third compartment" are:

1. null cells
2. NK or natural killer cells
3. K cells or ADCC cells.

Null cells are so designated because they lack the usual lymphocyte markers, although certain of these cells have been noted to develop specific T cell markers following treatment with thymus hormones.

Natural killer cells (NK) represent an early host defense mechanism against tumor cells and infectious microorganisms such as herpes simplex virus, brucella, malaria, and cryptococcus. There are numerous forms of natural killer cells, among which are the true NK cells, NC (natural cytotoxic cells which are probably distinct from NK cells and may be of importance in defense against solid tumors), monocytes and macrophages, granulocytes, and K cells or macrophages which mediate antibody-dependent cell mediated cytotoxicity by interacting with naturally developed antibodies.

NK cells react strongly with antibodies to certain immunoglobulin surface markers and immune antigens. NK cells can be shown to lyse certain leukemia and carcinoma cells. Other tumor cells are resistant to NK action. The lytic process does not require immunization for generation of the NK cells. However, NK activity can be augmented by interferon, antibody to NK cells, lectins such as PHA and con A, and enzymes such as neuraminidase, trypsin, chymotrypsin, and phospholipase A2. Activity of NK cells can be inhibited by prostaglandins (PGE1 and PGE2), phorbol ester, certain toxins and macrophage and T suppressor cells.

Finally, NK cells may be noted to produce interferon following stimulation by tumor cells and bacterial products such as BCG and C. parvum.

Clinically, NK cells appear to be important in tumor surveillance. In the Chediak-Higashi syndrome where there is a selective NK deficiency as well as other cell deficiencies, a high incidence of tumors is noted. In X-linked lymphoproliferative disorders, low NK activity is also seen. In active systemic lupus erythematosus, low NK activity is seen which normalizes during remission. Also, in renal transplant patients receiving immunosuppression, NK activity is decreased and may partially explain the increased incidence of malignancies in these persons.

K cells or killer cells bear a receptor for the Fc

portion of IgG, and are capable of lysing cells (especially red blood cells and lymphocytes) coated with IgG antibody. Complement is not involved in this ADCC phenomenon.

The role of macrophages and monocytes in early phenomena in the immune response and as components of immunoregulatory networks has already been described. The role of these cells in acute and chronic inflammatory responses, in granuloma formation, and in delayed hypersensitivity skin test reactions is well recognized.

Neutrophils and eosinophils are important phagocytic cells in acute inflammation and immediate hypersensitivity reactions. They provide defense against infective microorganisms and parasitic infections. The role of eosinophils as well as that of basophils and mast cells will be described in the subsequent discussion of immediate hypersensitivity.

Complement

The complement system consists of fourteen plasma proteins which interact in a sequential fashion. Six proteins are involved in the sequence known as the classic pathway (antigen-antibody pathway) and three are involved in the alternative or properdin pathway. These early pathways as well as the late common pathway are illustrated in Figure 6.1. Although activation of complement components can occur in fluid phase, the most efficient activation occurs when components interact on a membrane such as the plasma membrane of cells, basement membrane in tissues, or surfaces of microorganisms. Late component complement activation (C_8, with augmentation by C_9) eventuates in lysis of erythrocytes and susceptible nucleated cells and microorganisms. Thus, complement is an accessory system in host defense mechanisms by virtue of its ability to attack infecting organisms which have interacted with antibody or which have membrane components capable of activating the alternative pathway. In addition, complement is of primary importance in the acute inflammatory response, which operates to increase the local concentration of phagocytic leukocytes and to localize pathogens and prevent their dissemination.

Activated components of C_3 and C_5 display significant biologic actions: C_3a and C_5a are responsible for anaphylatoxic activity (vascular dilatation and permeability and bronchial smooth muscle constric-tion); C_3b and C_5b are responsible for opsonization and immune adherence. In addition other components of the complement sequence display biologic activity which may be protective against infecting microorganisms or may be deleterious to the host.

The major activators of the classic pathway are immune complexes of antigen and antibody. However, aggregated gamma globulins, cell wall lipopolysaccharides of gram negative bacteria, and complexes of C-reactive protein and type C pneumococcal polysaccharide can also achieve classic pathway activation. The alternative pathway is activatd by microbial products such as zymosan, inulin, and bacterial lipopolysaccharides, but also by aggregated immunoglobulins, and certain immune globulin fractions.

Complement is classified among the components known as acute phase reactants. These also include fibrinogen and C-reactive protein (as well as $\alpha1$ antitrypsin, ceruloplasmin, haptoglobin, $\alpha1$ acid glycoprotein, and serum amyloid A protein). Increased levels of acute phase reactant plasma proteins cause elevation of the erythrocyte sedimentation rate. Acute phase reactants, including complement, are elevated in acute inflammation and in tissue necrosis. Complement components are decreased in the plasma only when extensive circulatory and tissue fixed immune complexes widely activate the system, when aggregated gamma globulin is inadvertently introduced into the intravascular compartment, when regulatory factors (inhibitors) of complement components are decreased or absent, when unusual activators of the alternative pathway, such as the immunoglobulin known as C_3 nephritic factor (C_3NeF, an antibody to C_3 convertase, C_3bB) are present, or when individual complement components are directly activated by bacterial components (e.g., pseudomonas elastase can activate C_3 and C_5) or by proteinases such as plasmin.

Primary and secondary deficiencies of complement components have been noted in human health and disease. With the exception of C_2 deficiency and deficiency of C_1 esterase inhibitor, these deficiencies are rare.

C_1 deficiency occurs secondary to hypogammaglobulinemia. While certain complement components have been deficient with no apparent clinical consequences, most patients have developed a systemic lupus erythematosus-like picture, rheumatoid arthritis or other evidence of vasculitis. The rare deficiency of C_3 and C_5 to C_8 has been associated with severe infection.

In patients with deficiency of the inhibitor of C_1 the clinical picture of hereditary angioedema is seen. These patients also have an increased susceptibility

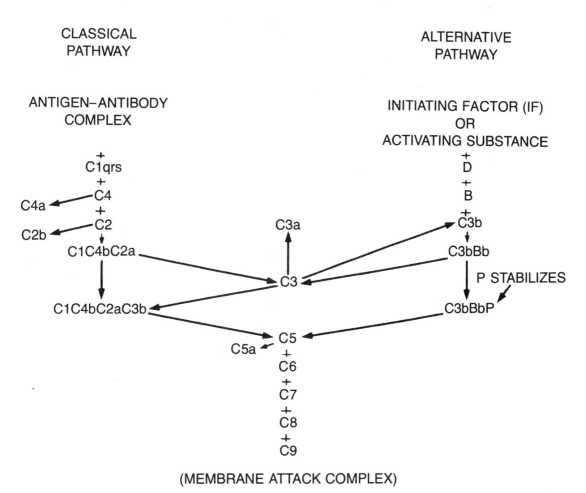

Fig. 6.1 Pathways of complement activation.

to SLE, glomerulonephritis, and other immune complex disorders. Although most deficiencies of C_1 esterase inhibitors are hereditary, fifteen instances of acquired deficiency have been reported. Most of these patients had lymphoproliferative disorders or autoimmune disease, and auto-antibodies, paraproteins, or cryoglobulins were present.

Monocytes and Macrophages

These cells, well known for their phagocytic functions, operate at multiple levels of the immune response. Precursor cells for these phagocytic cells are found in the bone marrow in the colony forming unit for granulocytes and monocytes. Upon release from the bone marrow, they circulate as monocytes and in tissues undergo conversion to macrophages and specialized cells such as microglial cells.

On the afferent arc of the immune response, macrophages (dendritic macrophages) fix particulate antigens on their surfaces and present them to responding lymphocytes. Macrophages also ingest soluble antigens and process them, subsequently presenting them complexed to soluble macrophage products to appropriate lymphocytes. Macrophage interaction with lymphocytes may occur as direct cell-cell contact, as is required for macrophage-directed T lymphocyte proliferation, or via a complex of antigen and soluble macrophage products which provide a form of helper T cell activity specific for the antigen in the complex.

On the efferent arc of the immune response, macrophages participate in inflammatory reactions, both acute and chronic. Macrophages are found in granulomas and are the precursors of epithelioid cells. They respond to secretory products of activated effector lymphocytes such as macrophage attracting factor and macrophage migration inhibitory factor. Macrophages efficiently phagocytize and degrade particulate antigens and microorganisms. In addi-

tion, these cells release numerous secretory products which play roles in inflammation and hypersensitivity reactions (Table 6.4).

IMMUNE REGULATION

Regulation of the immune response involves cellular and humoral events proceeding from the introduction of the antigen into the patient, through antigen processing and presentation, to stimulation of responding T and B lymphocytes. Along the way various regulation networks interact to ensure an immune response which is modulated to be adequate for the inciting antigen. This response is then returned to a "steady state" level of function.

Antigen-presenting and antigen-processing macrophages interact with populations of inducer T lymphocytes via cell to cell contact. The point of recognition of these two interacting cells is probably via Ia antigens (in the human D/DR antigens) on the macrophage and surface molecules complementary to Ia on the T cell. There is evidence that dendritic cells, Langerhans cells of the epidermis, endothelial cells and B lymphocytes, all of which bear Ia mark-

Table 6.4 **Secretory Products of Monocytes and Macrophages**
(The spectrum of secretory products varies with the tissue source of the mononuclear cells and their environments).

Secretory Substance	Comments
A. Hydrolytic enzymes	
1. Acid hydrolases	Rapid release effected by immune complexes, zymosan and other microbial cell wall components and mineral particles. Slow release produced by C_3b, dextran sulfates, phorbol esters and products of lymphocyte activation.
2. Lysozyme	
3. Neutral Proteinases	Very sensitive to inhibition by glucocorticoids.
(plasminogen activator, collagenase, elastase, proteoglycan degrading enzyme)	
B. Prostaglandins (PGE_2, PGI_2, $PGF_2\alpha$, and thromboxane A_2)	Products of the cyclooxygenase conversion of arachidonic acid. No products of the lipoxygenase pathway such as the leukotrienes are secreted.
C. Complement components	C_1, C_2, C_3, C_4, Bf, and factor D
D. Modulators of cellular function	
1. Lymphocyte activating factors for B and T cells	
2. Thymic maturation factor	
3. Inhibitors of proliferation of lymphocytes and fibroblasts	
4. Stimulators of collagen synthesis	
5. Stimulators of proliferation of bone marrow stem cells	
6. Endothelial cell stimulating substance (angiogenic factors)	
E. Miscellaneous	
1. Active oxygen radicals	Superoxide, hydrogen peroxide, hydroxyl radicals
2. Interferon	
3. Pyrogen	
4. Listericidal substance	
5. B12 binding protein	
6. Alpha 2 macroglobulin	Inhibits proteinases
7. Cyclic nucleotides	

ers, can also present antigen for recognition. Macrophages may also interact with T and B lymphocytes by other mechanisms.

Inducer T lymphocytes function to survey the cells of the body to insure that the surface markers of the somatic cells conform to a pre-established pattern of what is "self." Variations from this pattern (as might occur with mutational events leading to malignant cells, modification of cells by viral antigens or virus-induced antigens, or chemical and drug modification of cells) will trigger the inducer T lymphocyte to respond. The response can be the generation of cy-totoxic T lymphocytes directed against the cell bearing the foreign antigen as is illustrated in Figure 6.2.

Perhaps more importantly, the inducer T cell activated by non-self antigens interacts with precursor cells to generate effector cells. These effector cells are:

1. B lymphocytes which will then synthesize antibodies
2. effector T cells responsible for delayed type hypersensitivity reactions
3. suppressor T cells.

Although interactions of these inducer cells with pre-

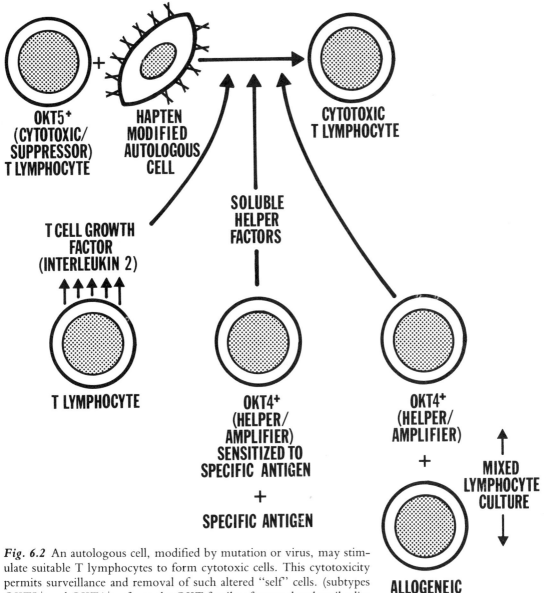

Fig. 6.2 An autologous cell, modified by mutation or virus, may stimulate suitable T lymphocytes to form cytotoxic cells. This cytotoxicity permits surveillance and removal of such altered "self" cells. (subtypes OKT5⁺ and OKT4⁺ refer to the OKT family of monoclonal antibodies used in identifying lymphocyte subsets).

cursor cells may involve cell to cell recognition on the basis of histocompatibility antigens (Ia or D/DR), in many cases the inducer T cells operate via secretion of soluble helper or suppressor factors.

Genetic control of responsiveness, or failure of responsiveness to an antigen is partially established at the level of whether the helper T cell or the suppressor T cell phenomenon is paramount. Along with generating an immune response, a parallel suppressor phenomenon is activated which will eventually damp down the antibody production. Such a response is seen in viral infection (Fig. 12.5) to turn off an IgM response when IgG antibodies to the antigen begin to accumulate.

Anti-Idiotype Network of Regulation

A second complicated regulatory system for the immune response exists. This is known as the idiotype/anti-idiotype network of regulation. Antibodies produced by a single clone of lymphocytes against a single antigen react with the antigen via the variable region of the antibodies heavy and light chains. These variable regions, because of their unique sequence of amino acids, are immunogenic in other individuals of the species and, when present in sufficient concentration, are immunogenic in the individual himself. The population of antibodies which are derived from the single clone of lymphocytes (and thus all have the same molecular structure in their variable regions) are called idiotypes or "idiotypic antibodies", and the unique variable region is the idiotypic determinant.

The lymphocytes which produce the idiotype possess that idiotype on their surface as the receptor for the antigen. T lymphocytes of the helper and suppressor populations also have specific receptors for antigen. Although these receptors are not complete antibody molecules, they do contain variable region structures and these act as idiotypes towards which specific immune responses can be generated. Soluble T cell helper and suppressor factors also contain idiotype determinants.

When sufficient cells in the lymphocyte clone synthesize idiotypic antibodies, the stage is set for activation of the anti-idiotype network of regulation. Populations of helper T cells specific for the idiotype interact with B cells which are also specific for the idiotype. The consequence of activation of the anti-idiotype helper T cell and the anti-idiotype B cell is an anti-idiotype antibody. This antibody will feed back into the system to interfere with any T or B cell bearing the idiotype as a receptor or result in the destruction of the idiotype-bearing cell. It may bind

to and block soluble helper or suppressor factors which bear the idiotype. Finally, the anti-idiotype antibody may even interact with the helper T cells which are idiotype specific, activate them, and thereby perpetuate the generation of anti-idiotype antibodies.

While the anti-idiotype network provides insight into an elegant mechanism of regulation of immune responsiveness, it also offers hope for eventual clinical manipulation of the immune system so as to achieve highly specific immune suppression. Theoretically, temporary or permanent elimination of the clone of lymphocytes producing a particular idiotype would eliminate those cells capable of making an antibody to that particular antigen or eliminate those cells responsible for the cell-mediated immunity to that antigen. This would be of great benefit in clinical transplantation and also in the treatment of autoimmune disorders.

IMMUNODEFICIENCY

Clinical conditions associated with immunodeficiency most commonly present because of impaired response to infection. Chronic or recurrent infection, incomplete clearing between episodes of infection, or infection by unusual organisms should all raise suspicion regarding the competence of the major immune systems. In general the severity of the disease correlates with the degree of deficiency and specific infections tend to occur with the particular system that is deficient. Table 6.5 is a summary classification identifying the systems that may be deficient. An enormous variety of individual deficiencies have been reported in small numbers of patients and very detailed analysis are possible, to identify the mechanisms whereby the immune systems failed. For clin-

Table 6.5 **Classification of Immunodeficiency States**

Antibody (B cell) Deficiency
    Congenital hypogammaglobulinemia
    Acquired hypogammaglobulinemia
        Idiopathic
        Secondary to immunosuppressive drugs
        Associated with protein losing conditions
    Selective immunoglobulin deficiencies e.g. IgA deficiency
Cellular (T cell) Deficiency
    Congenital thymic aplasia
    Chronic mucocutaneous candidiasis
Combined Immune Deficiency
Phagocytic Dysfunction
    Chronic granulomatous disease
    Glucose-6-phosphate dehydrogenase deficiency
Complement Deficiency

Table 6.6   **Screening Tests for Immunodeficiency**

B Cell Function	—*Quantitation of IgG, IgH, IgM and IgG subclasses
	—*Assays of antibody to common viruses
	— Antibody response to vaccines
	— Quantitative assays of B cells in blood
T Cell Function	—*Skin tests for delayed hypersensitivity to common antigens (mumps, PPD)
	— Chest radiograph to assess thymic site
	—*Skin test response to induced hypersensitivity (dimitrochlorobenzene)
	— Lymphocyte function assays (see Table 6.3, No. 7)
Phagocytic Function	—*Number and morphology of circulating polymorphonuclear leucocytes
	— Tests for chemotaxis, phagocytosis, microbial killing functions
Complement Function	—*Complement assays, particularly C_3, C_5

* Indicates generally available tests for most common abnormalities.

ical purposes it is initially important to recognize the problem and if possible categorize the system of dysfunction. Table 6.6 tabulates the screening tests most useful in recognizing common immunodeficiency disorders.

Many other conditions may result in impaired host defense to infection and cause a clinical state commonly referred to as a "compromised host." These are listed in Table 15.9. Of particular interest from an immunological perspective are the hematological malignancies which may result in impaired B or T cell function, and the use of immunosuppressive drugs (cytoxic drugs, corticosteroids, etc.) which result in altered function of both the B and T cell systems to a variable degree.

Acquired immune deficiency has become particularly important with recent recognition of an acquired immune deficiency syndrome (AIDS) in homosexual men. These men may present with clinical evidence of opportunistic infection (particularly pneumonia due to cytomegalovirus or *Pneumocystis carinii*) or an otherwise rare tumor, Caposi's sarcoma. The syndrome may result from infection, since it also occurs after blood transfusion.

The specific clinical disorders associated with immunodeficiency in the adult are dealt with in the chapters dealing with each organ system.

AUTOIMMUNITY

Autoimmune disorders result from a state in which natural unresponsiveness to self is lost. The immune system then generates a response to self-constituents causing injury or destruction. Such autoimmune phenomena may be highly specific and directed at receptors, cells, or membranes of individual organs or tissues, or they may be more generalized affecting multiple organs or tissues.

Three mechanisms are commonly suggested for this immune dysfunction (see Table 6.7, Type 2, 3, 4).

1. The action of autoantibodies on intracellular structures or cell surfaces. Such structures may be normal or modified by disease or injury. Occasionally autoantibodies directed against receptors stimulate or inhibit specialized cell functions.

2. Self antigens and autoantibodies may form immune complexes which may be deposited in vulnerable tissues. Usually injury results from associated complement deposition, granulocyte and monocyte attraction to the region, and their contribution to local cell death.

3. Sensitized T-lymphocytes may be activated to release destructive lymphokines, or cause tissue destruction through attraction of other destructive inflammatory cells.

It is frequently not clear whether a disorder is primarily a result of autoimmune mechanisms, or whether autoimmune mechanisms become a part of an underlying disease. Table 6.8 illustrates some common, better understood autoimmune conditions.

An ever increasing list of disorders is being identified as associated with autoimmune phenomena. The regulation of hormone production and the end organ response to hormones appears to be unusually vulnerable to receptor related mechanisms. Primary endocrine failure in Addison's disease, hypoparathyroidism, diabetes, hypothyroidism, and infertility have all been attributed to autoimmune mechanisms in at least some patients. Diffuse organ damage in idiopathic interstitial pneumonia or primary biliary cirrhosis may be on an autoimmune basis. Since our understanding of the triggering and potentiating fac-

Table 6.7   Immune Mechanisms that May Produce Tissue Damage (Gel and Coombs)

	Mediators:
TYPE 1: Anaphylactic (Immediate Hypersensitivity)	
—IgE antibodies bind to antigen	—Histamine, leukotriene D,
—Antigen-antibody complex on surface of	serotonin, heparin, kinins and
basophil or mast cell causes release of mediators	others
Clinical Examples: Allergic Rhinitis,	
Asthma	
Anaphylaxis	
TYPE 2: Cytotoxic	
—IgM or IgG antibodies bind to antigenic	—complement-dependent
determinants on cell surface	antibody induced cell lysis
—Complement fixation commonly occurs, leading	—antibody-dependent cell-
to cell damage	mediated toxicity
Clinical Examples: Goodpasture's Syndrome	
Idiopathic Thrombocytopenic	
Purpura	
Autoimmune hemolytic	
Anemia	
TYPE 3: Antigen-Antibody Complex	
—Circulating antibody and local or circulating	—chemotactic factors
antigens form complexes and are deposited in	
tissues	—vasoactive amines, lysosomal
—Complement fixation results in chemotaxis,	enzymes from platelets and
inflammatory reaction	macrophages
Clinical Examples: Serum sickness	
SLE	
TYPE 4: Cell-mediated (delayed hypersensitivity)	
—Actively sensitized T lymphocytes react to	—lymphokines
specific antigens	—cell lysosomes
—Lymphokines affect macrophages, PMN	
leucocytes, lymphocytes	
Clinical Examples: Skin test for delayed	
hypersensitivity	
Sarcoidosis	

tors in this group of disorders remains so elementary, definitive therapeutic intervention is not yet possible. Therapeutic approaches directed at reducing measurable antibody levels or suppressing presumed overactivity of cellular immunity are discussed where appropriate in relation to each disease throughout this book.

The impressive disease association with certain human lymphocyte antigens (particularly groups DR_2, DR_3, DR_4, and DR_5), suggests a strong pre-

Table 6.8   Autoimmune Disorders

Disease/Condition	Organ or Tissue Involved	Autoantibody
Myasthenia gravis	Acetylcholine receptors of neuromuscular junctions	Antiacetylcholine receptor antibodies
Idiopathic thrombocytopenia purpura	Platelets	Antiplatelet antibodies
Autoimmune hemolytic anemia	Red blood cells	Anti-red blood cell antibodies
Diffuse toxic goiter (Graves Disease)	Thyroid. TSH receptors	Thyroid stimulating immunoglobulins
Pernicious anemia	Gastric parietal cells	Anti-Vitamin B_{12} and anti-parietal cell antibodies
Diabetes Mellitus	Insulin receptors (peripheral)	Insulin receptor antibodies Islet cell antibodies
SYSTEMIC DISEASES		
Goodpasture's Syndrome	Lung, kidney capillaries	Anti-basement membrane antibodies
Rheumatoid Arthritis	Joints, skin, lungs	Antigammaglobulin antibodies
Systemic Lupus Erythematosus	Multiple tissues	Multiple antibodies (See Chapter 18).

Table 6.9 **Association of HLA—DR Antigens with Certain Autoimmune Diseases**

Disease	Antigen	Relative Risk
Goodpasture's Syndrome	DR 2	15 X
Juvenile Diabetes	DR 3,4	6 X
Systemic Lupus Erythematosus	DR 3	6 X
Idiopathic Membranous Nephropathy	DR 3	12 X
Pemphigus	DR 4	14 X

dilection in genetically determined subjects for certain diseases. Table 6.9 itemizes several examples where the risk of disease appears to be increased 6 to 15 times.

ALLERGY AND ALLERGIC DISEASE

In allergy, disease results from the deleterious effect of an inflammatory reaction to environmental allergens (antigens). The environmental agents are generally not intrinsically harmful. Such agents may be introduced to the body as inhalants, (pollens, fungal spores, animal dander), by ingestion (foods, food additives or drugs) or by direct skin contact. Allergy involving the nasal passages results in *allergic rhinitis*. This is probably the most common human allergy, affecting up to 10 percent of the population. The symptoms consist of attacks of profuse watery rhinorrhea, paroxysmal sneezing, nasal obstruction, and frequently itchy conjunctivitis. Such individuals commonly develop eosinophilia in the peripheral blood. Seasonal inhalants are frequently responsible and the history of seasonal symptoms may help to pinpoint the particular organic dusts (e.g., ragweed pollen during the ragweed season). The treatment of allergic rhinitis requires avoidance of the allergen if possible, and rather unsatisfactory symptomatic drug treatment. The antihistaminics reduce mucosal edema and nasal discharge, but cause anticholinergic side effects as well as central nervous system depression. Topical corticosteroids such as Beclomethasone, or inhibitors of mediator release such as Cromolyn may be helpful. This is the one group of conditions where specific *immunotherapy* with repetitive innoculations of the offending antigen has been helpful in reducing clinical symptoms. The precise mechanism by which immunotherapy is effective remains controversial.

Bronchial asthma is a poorly understood condition characterized by smooth muscle hyperreactivity in the bronchial walls. Many of these patients also have allergic rhinitis. The complex inciting factors for bronchospasm and bronchial asthma are discussed in Chapter 15. At least one major mechanism relates to the production of immunoglobulins (IgE) produced as antibodies to the inhaled antigens. On subsequent exposure the antigen antibody complex becomes attached to mast cells in the bronchial mucosa with the release of mediators. (Table 6.7, Type 1.) This release of mediators results in smooth muscle contraction (bronchoconstriction) stimulation of bronchial mucous glands to cause increased mucous secretion, increased permeability of bronchial mucosal capillaries, and perhaps secondarily results in impaired mucociliary clearance.

This process is most commonly triggered by the type 1 reaction, but is also seen in association with the type 3 and type 4 reactions. Allergies associated with the skin are discussed in Chapter 19 under atopic dermatitis.

The most florid and life-threatening form of immediate hypersensitivity is seen in generalized *anaphylaxis*. This may occur after exposure to an antigen with an exceptionally vigorous release of mediators. The reaction is rare but the most common sources of allergins responsible for anaphylaxis are outlined in Table 6.10.

Patients with anaphylaxis generally demonstrate sudden collapse within seconds or minutes after exposure to the allergen. Generally several target organs are involved causing hypotension, severe peripheral vasodilation, bronchospasm or pulmonary edema, crampy abdominal pain and diarrhea. There is generally not sufficient time to perform any diagnostic laboratory tests. In the appropriate clinical setting, this represents an extreme medical emergency. Immediate treatment should include intramuscular administration of epinephrine (1:1000 aqueous solution, 0.2 − 0.5 ml), it should be repeated every 30 minutes if necessary. Vasodilation with relative hypovolemia must be treated by intravenous volume expansion (physiologic saline) and

Table 6.10

Allergens Most Commonly Associated with Anaphylaxis

Drugs:	Foods:
Penicillin	Peanuts (other nuts)
Sulfonamides	Sea Foods
Local Anesthetics	Egg Protein
Salicylates	
Other Medications:	Stinging Insects:
Foreign serum, enzymes	Bees
Vaccines	Wasps
Allergen Extracts	

occasionally supportive vasopressor drugs. Bronchospasm may benefit from administration of intravenous Theophylline and laryngeal edema may require endotracheal intubation. Adrenal corticosteroids are generally given parenterally. Most patients require supplemental oxygen. Such urgent intervention results in frequent salvage of patients with a potentially lethal condition.

HUMORAL SYSTEMS COMMONLY ACTIVATED DURING IMMUNE MEDIATED DISEASE

It is important to recognize that many patients demonstrate more than one immune mechanism of tissue damage. Furthermore, once immune dysfunction occurs other humoral systems may develop inappropriate activity. For example, the coagulation or fibrinolytic systems may be activated (see Chapter 4), the complement system may be activated as outlined above, or the kinin system may be activated with production of bradykinin and resultant chemotaxis, smooth muscle contraction, dilatation of peripheral arterioles, and increased capillary permeability.

Unfortunately, from a clinical view point, it is rarely possible to identify a precise quantitative balance in these systems. Only when full blown disseminated intravascular coagulation becomes clinically important, when fibrinolysis results in bleeding disorders, or when complement is measureably depleted can the impact on these humoral mechanisms be identified with confidence.

REFERENCES

Immunobiology

1. Agnello, V: Complement deficiency states. Medicine 57:1–23, 1978.
2. Colten, H.R., Alper, C.A., Rosen, F.S.: Current concepts in immunology: genetics and biosynthesis of complement proteins. N. Engl. J. Med. 304:653–6, 1981.
3. Gupta, S., Good, R.A.: Markers of human lymphocyte subpopulations in primary immunodeficiency and lymphoproliferative disorders. Sem. in Hematol. 17:1–29, 1980.
4. Marsh, D.G., Meyers, D.A., Bias, W.B.: The epidemiology and genetics of atopic allergy. N. Engl. J. Med. 305:1551–9, 1981.
5. Middleton, E. Jr., Reed, C.E., Ellis, E.F., eds.: Allergy: Principles and Practice. St. Louis, C.V. Mosby Co., 1978.
6. Mullarkey, M.F.: Clinical approach to rhinitis Med Clin N Am 65:977–86, 1981.
7. Polmar, S.H.: Metabolic aspects of immunodeficiency disease. Sem. in Hematol. 17:30–43, 1980.
8. Reinherz, E.L., Rosen, F.S.: New concepts of immunodeficiency. Am. J. Med. 71:511–2, 1981.
9. Rosenthal, A.S.: Regulation of the immune response: role of the macrophage. N. Engl. J. Med. 303:1153–6, 1980.
10. Smith, P.H., Kagey-Sobotka, A., Bleecke, E.R. et al.: Physiologic manifestations of human anaphylaxis Journal of Clinical Investigations 1980:66:1072–80.

7

Infectious Disease

R. Timothy Coussons, M.D.

Part 1: Principles of Infectious Disease

This chapter deals with general principles of infectious disease and with several infectious processes that are not clearly focused on the organ systems. Since patients generally present to physicians with symptoms in one or several organ systems, most specific infections are discussed in the chapters dealing with organ systems in part II of this volume. It is assumed that the student has mastered the microbiologic classification and characteristics of organisms, or has that information readily available.

HOST-MICROORGANISM INTERACTIONS

HOST DEFENSE MECHANISMS

As we live surrounded by microorganisms, it is amazing that we are not overwhelmed by the multiplicity of bacteria, viruses, fungi, and other organisms. Familiarity with this remarkable host-parasite relationship provides a starting point for approaching infectious diseases in a systematic and rational fashion. This chapter will consider clinically important elements of the host defense mechanisms, as well as some of the factors involved in microbial virulence.

External Defense Elements

The external physical barriers met by an invading organism function as the first line of host defense. These are part of the natural resistance mechanism of the body, and include the normal microbial flora and certain external secretions that have antimicrobial action. These natural resistance elements are not specific, and therefore do not require previous exposure to a given pathogen as do the elements of acquired immunity.

The skin and mucosa are the first surface elements usually met by invading organisms, and they represent a formidable physical barrier. External secretions present on the skin's surface, including unsaturated fatty acids and lactic acid, have antibacterial properties. While the mucous membranes are somewhat less hostile to the invading organism, they also have antimicrobial actions. The pulmonary tract, for example, has a gelatinous mucous layer that entraps invading microorganisms. This mucous film is constantly swept out of the lung by ciliated epithelium lining the respiratory tract. The alveolar macrophage, which is also a part of the mucosal surface mechanism, engulfs and destroys inhaled particles. Other "external" surfaces that exist in the gastrointestinal and genitourinary tracts have different but comparable mechanisms for resisting invading organisms, in addition to their physical surface barriers. The normal flora that are an integral part of many skin and mucosal surfaces help retard multiplication of potential pathogens by bacterial interference. While bacterial interference is a complicated mechanism, it is known that antibiotic-like by-products of some normal flora inhibit proliferation of potentially pathogenic organisms. Disruption of the normal flora by extensive broad spectrum antibiotic use reduces the efficacy of bacterial interference.

Potential pathogens usually enter the body through a breach in a surface barrier produced by a scratch or a wound, or by the mechanism of attachment to and penetration of an epithelial cell surface. Our knowledge of bacterial attachment is expanding rapidly, and may well provide an important area for therapeutic intervention in the future. Epithelial cell surface attachment by an invading microorganism represents an interaction between elements on the microbial surface and receptor sites on the cell wall. Hair-like pili, called fimbriae, allow gonococci to attach to the urethral surface and resist flushing out by the urinary stream. While most infectious diseases involve penetration by the organism through the surface of the cell into the body, some do not. The enterotoxigenic *E. coli*, for example, which causes "traveler's diarrhea," does not actually penetrate the cell surface. The organism attaches itself, secretes a toxin that is absorbed, and produces symptoms without ever invading the body.

Internal Defense Mechanisms

Following invasion of a pathogen into the body, an additional series of defense mechanisms must be overcome before a disease results. The most formidable of these, at least for bacteria, is phagocytosis. The polymorphonuclear (PMN) leukocyte and the mononuclear (MN) phagocyte are the two major types of phagocytic cells involved in host defense. The PMN defends primarily against extracellular pathogens that tend to cause disease (typified by the pneumococcus). The PMN engulfs and destroys its prey. Mononuclear phagocytes are more important in the control of chronic infections caused by *Mycobacterium tuberculosis*, salmonella, and other primarily intracellular pathogens. Antigen-activated T lymphocytes and MN phagocytes produce "activated" macrophages possessing increased phagocytic and antimicrobial activity. It appears that while lymphocytes are activated specifically by certain antigens, the "activated" macrophage performs nonspecifically, attacking a wide range of potential invaders (see Chapter 6).

The humoral system of acquired immunity has a major role in adding specificity and improving the effectiveness of PMN phagocytosis. Neutrophilic phagocytosis consists of four recognized phases: chemotaxis, opsonization, ingestion, and killing. To be effective, phagocytic neutrophils must be present in adequate numbers and must be drawn to the area of invasion by a process called chemotaxis. Some chemotactic factors are released by invading organisms, but activation of the classic complement system provides additional factors instrumental in the attraction of leukocytes. Leukocytes themselves, as well as some sensitized lymphocytes, add chemotactic factors. Some invading organisms have mechanisms to inhibit chemotaxis, highlighting the complexity of the host-parasite interaction.

Opsonins react with microorganisms to enhance the success of phagocytosis. Opsonization may not require specific antibody, since it occurs through activation of the alternate complement pathway. Pneumococcal polysaccharide may result in fixation of C3, allowing opsonization of the organism to occur prior to the development of specific immunity. However, specific antibody alone, or the activation of the classic complement sequence (C1, C4, C2), plays the major role in facilitating phagocytosis as part of acquired immunity. Following opsonization, the polymorphonuclear leukocyte encloses the invader in a phagocytic pouch, called a phagosome. Neutrophilic granules fuse with the phagosome and the cell "degranulates." Granules are rich in myeloperoxidase (MPO) enzymes, among other substances that are important in bacterial killing. The mechanisms of polymorphonuclear leukocyte action are complex, including both oxygen-dependent and oxygen-independent mechanisms.

MICROBIAL VIRULENCE FACTORS AND OPPORTUNISTIC INFECTIONS

In addition to an understanding of host defense mechanisms, insight into the factors determining the microorganism's ability to cause disease is appropriate. Pathogenicity defines the microorganism's capacity to produce disease, while virulence refers to the degree of pathogenicity. It has long been recognized that there are significant differences in virulence between various strains of a given bacteria (for example, staphylococcus). One strain may colonize the majority of patients in an intensive care unit and cause little disease, while another strain may cause disease in the majority of patients colonized. Factors determining virulence are not well understood. Data from outbreaks in closed population groups suggest that rapid transmission from host to host increases virulence, probably by a process that selects out the more pathogenic organisms.

For an organism to have a high degree of virulence, it must successfully establish itself on a body surface or within the body, be able to multiply and evade the body's host defense mechanisms, and finally must produce disease by damaging the host. The penetration of the physical barriers of the skin and mucous membranes and subsequent proliferation in tissue depends on properties of the organism, some of which are genetically determined. Many organisms possess factors that directly inhibit host defense mechanisms and correlate with the degree of virulence for a given strain. The K antigens of *E. coli*, for example, inhibit phagocytosis and complement-dependent bacterial killing, thus allowing strains with high levels of K antigen to circumvent some aspects of host defense. Damage to the host is effected by multiple mechanisms; the actions of exotoxins and endotoxins are among the mechanisms best understood. Generally, exotoxins are proteins, while endotoxins are lipoprotein-polysaccharide complexes derived from bacterial cell walls. Much is known about the biochemical basis for individual exotoxin and endotoxin action that is of assistance in understanding the pathogenicity of individual disease-causing bacteria.

In recent years, our concepts of pathogenic and nonpathogenic organisms have changed as many previously "nonpathogenic" organisms have been found to cause disease in compromised patients. These so-called opportunistic infections seem to be nonpathogenic for hosts with normal, intact defense mechanisms, but are able to do considerable harm when host defense mechanisms are altered. As will be seen later, knowledge of host defense alterations often gives clinically important clues about the likely pathogens causing disease in compromised hosts (see section entitled Infection in the Compromised Host, later in this chapter).

INFECTION CONTROL, IMMUNIZATION, AND CHEMOPROPHYLAXIS

INFECTION CONTROL WITHIN THE HOSPITAL

Nosocomial infections, or hospital-acquired infections, are generally defined as infections occurring after admission that were not incubating at the time of the patient's hospitalization. Nosocomial infections are increasingly recognized as major causes of morbidity and mortality, currently accounting for 3 to 10 percent of hospital days. The cost of additional hospitalization resulting from infection exceeds one billion dollars each year in the United States.

While the hospital environment must certainly contribute to the acquisition of nosocomial infections, the severe illness of the hospitalized patient, with increased susceptibility resulting from altered host defense mechanisms, is probably more important. Hospital-acquired infections most frequently involve the urinary tract, and somewhat less frequently involve the respiratory tract, open surgical wounds, decubitus ulcers, and the sites of indwelling intravenous catheters. The organisms most commonly involved are gram-negative bacilli, but *Staph-*

ylococcus aureus continues to be a major problem. The inappropriate use of antibiotics in the hospital setting has contributed to the emergence of antibiotic-resistant bacteria. In addition, antibiotics may alter normal flora, allowing colonization by potentially pathogenic antibiotic-resistant organisms.

The prevention and control of nosocomial infections has become a major task, particularly in referral hospitals where immunosuppressed patients tend to be concentrated. The essential elements of an effective infection-control program include:

1. An effective continuing infection surveillance program, which usually involves an infection-control committee and a trained infection-control nurse. These persons have the responsibility for seeing to it that the sites of infections, the organisms involved, the antibiotic susceptibility and use patterns, and the other epidemiologic data are recorded, tabulated, and distributed to hospital physicians and personnel for review.

2. An aggressive education program that emphasizes the proper use and care of medical devices, including urinary catheters, respiratory therapy equipment, and indwelling intravenous devices, to reduce the risk of introducing infection.

3. A strictly enforced policy that requires handwashing by hospital personnel and physicians between patient contacts. This relatively simple, effective control mechanism is often neglected and needs constant reinforcement.

4. Isolation techniques. Although widely practiced, isolation techniques lack convincing data supporting their effectiveness, and the potentially negative aspects of isolation, such as reduced interaction with hospital personnel, family, and friends should also be considered. Patient isolation is most appropriate for highly contagious diseases with airborne transmission, when nonimmune personnel are involved. Hygienic or aseptic techniques for handling secretions or body fluids often permit isolation of specimens without isolation of the patient.

IMMUNIZATION IN ADULTS

Active Immunization

In the developed countries, many severe communicable diseases have been controlled as a result of vigorous and systematic immunization programs. Viral vaccines for poliomyelitis, measles, mumps, rubella, and influenza, as well as bacterial vaccines for pertussis, diptheria, tetanus, and pneumococcus

Table 7.1 Antimicrobial Prophylaxis: Prevention

Clinical Situation	Expected Organisms	Drugs
I. Rheumatic fever (established diagnosis and under 35 years of age).	*Streptococcus pyogenes*	Benzathine penicillin G, 1.2 million units IM monthly, or oral penicillin G, 200,000 units twice daily or oral sulfadiazine 1 g daily.
II. Bacterial endocarditis Known congenital or acquired valvular disease; prosthetic valve with: 1. Dental procedures associated with gingival bleeding, or surgery; and instrumentation of the upper respiratory tract.	*Streptococcus viridans*	Aqueous crystalline penicillin G, 1.0 million units, IM mixed with procaine penicillin G, 600,000 units IM, plus streptomycin 1 g IM given 30 minutes prior to procedure, followed by penicillin V 500 mg orally every 6 hours, for 8 doses.
2. Gastrointestinal and genitourinary procedures	Enterococcus	Ampicillin 1 g (IM or IV) and gentamicin (IM or IV) 1.5 mg/kg (not to exceed 80 mg) 30 minutes before procedure and repeat both every 8 hours for two more doses.
3. Cardiac surgery	*S. aureus, S. epidermidis,* Gram-negative bacilli	Cefazolin 2.0 g (IM or IV) plus gentamicin (IM or IV) 1.5 mg/kg (not to exceed 80 mg) 30 minutes before procedure; repeat both every 8 hours, for 5 more doses.
III. Meningococcal meningitis (intimate contact with proven case).	*Neisseria meningitidis*	Rifampin 600 mg orally, every 12 hours for 4 doses.

should be routinely considered. Most adults will have had the childhood programs for diptheria, pertussis, tetanus, polio, measles, mumps, and rubella, and so the major tasks, regarding adults, are to provide booster vaccines, consider special cases, and protect populations at increased risk for respiratory infection.

When immunizations have been initiated in childhood they should be continued, and in the case of diptheria and tetanus, a booster dose of the adult-type preparation every 10 years is adequate. If reliable information documenting primary immunization cannot be obtained, an initial dose followed by a booster at 1 to 2 months and a second booster at 6 to 12 months are needed. Live rubella virus vaccine is indicated in adults only for (1) males, as part of an effort to prevent or control an outbreak in a population group, or (2) nonpregnant females shown to be susceptible by rubella hemagglutination inhibition testing (titer less than 1–8) who agree not to become pregnant for three months. Live mumps vaccine should be considered for adolescent and adult males who have no history or serologic evidence of immunity, and who have not had previous live mumps vaccine. The combined measles-mumps-rubella (MMR) vaccine is recommended except for pregnant women.

The killed virus influenza vaccine is reformulated yearly in an effort to anticipate the active strains of influenza, and this should be considered for selected patients. It is indicated annually in the early fall for patients over 65 years of age, and for those of all age groups who have chronic debilitating illnesses, including heart disease, bronchopulmonary disease, renal failure, diabetes, or adrenal insufficiency. Initial immunization requires two doses at 4 to 6 week intervals, with a yearly booster to maintain reasonable protection.

Hepatitis B virus vaccine is now available for health workers at risk and active male homosexuals.

The polyvalent pneumococcal vaccine composed of purified capsular material is indicated, for the same categories of patients mentioned above, for influenza vaccine, and for individuals with sickle cell disease, asplenia, chronic alcoholism, multiple myeloma, and agammaglobulinemia. Its efficacy has been well demonstrated and its protection lasts at least 5 years.

A wide range of bacterial vaccines are under active study for patients with high risk of overwhelming bacterial infections due to pseudomonas or other gram-negative organisms that produce septic shock. These show considerable promise but remain experimental.

Passive Immunization

Patients without previous immunity may be provided temporary, complete or partial immunity to certain severe infections, by parenteral administration of hyperimmune human serum globulins. Protection of this kind should be considered for persons exposed to hepatitis A or B virus and pregnant females exposed to varicella or herpes zoster.

CHEMOPROPHYLAXIS IN ADULTS

Chemoprophylaxis is the administration of a drug prior to, during, or immediately after exposure to an infectious agent, in an attempt to prevent the development of an infectious disease. In general, "prophylactic" antibiotics are grossly overused, and contribute significantly to antibiotic abuse (see section, Problems with Antimicrobial Use, later in this chapter). To be successful, chemoprophylaxis needs to be focused on a single organism or a well-defined group of potential organisms with a known or accurately anticipated sensitivity. The chemoprophylaxis needs to be administered in a quantity sufficient and at a time interval appropriate to provide an effective blood level during the period of exposure. Considerable controversy continues about the use of prophylactic antibiotics in specific situations, and individual decisions must be made based on knowledge of each patient. The small number of usually accepted indications for prophylaxis in medical patients are outlined in Table 7.1. In addition, effectiveness is commonly agreed on for prosthetic heart valve surgery, selected bowel procedures (including colon resection), urologic surgery in patients with bacteriuria, hip prosthesis replacement, hip fractures, and selected high-risk gallbladder surgery. Benefits for surgical patients include a lower incidence of wound infection, and, in some studies, a shorter hospital stay. Prophylaxis is effective when given just prior to and during a procedure, with continuation through only the first 24 to 48 hours postoperatively.

DIAGNOSTIC METHODS IN INFECTIOUS DISEASE

HISTORY AND PHYSICAL EXAMINATION

The approach to the patient suspected of having an infectious disease has a single purpose: to precisely identify the infecting organism or organisms. This usually requires knowledge of the organ systems involved, and indicates why a thorough history and complete physical examination is the starting point of the evaluation. The history should focus on details of the onset of symptoms and their development over time. An in-depth review of systems will identify complaints that may indicate particular organ involvement. Inquiry should include home and work environment exposure, animal and bird contact, travel history, previous infectious diseases, and recognized exposure to infection. The physical examination should include a diligent search for lesions or petechiae on the skin, the mucous membranes, the nail beds, and the optic fundi. Size of nodes and presence of tenderness are noted for all lymph node areas. Abdominal examination should document liver and spleen size, as well as any detectable mass. A careful cardiac examination for murmurs is important. Genital and rectal examination in men, and pelvic and rectal examination in women should be performed routinely. Initial laboratory evaluation usually includes hemoglobin, white blood count with differential, urinalysis, chemistry screening (including liver enzymes), and a chest roentgenogram.

IDENTIFICATION OF THE ORGANISM

Specimen Collection

With a history, a physical examination, and initial laboratory data as guides, additional tests may be necessary. Ideally, testing should recover or identify the appropriate organism and document the body's reaction to it. Frequently both goals are not met. Specimens for direct examination and culture must represent the microenvironment at the infected site and must be obtained without major contamination, to be of maximum value. The physician should assume responsibility for proper collection and specimen handling. Obtaining an adequate specimen is simple from normally sterile areas such as the blood stream, pleural or peritoneal cavities, cerebrospinal fluid, and joint spaces, while obtaining it from other potentially infected areas such as the lung or open wounds is difficult and sometimes not practical.

Microscopic Examination

The direct examination of specimens (exudates and tissue samples) by appropriate microscopic techniques can often provide a rapid diagnostic clue. The gram stain continues to be the most useful technique for examining specimens for bacterial infection (Table 7.2), although methods using the specificity

Table 7.2 Gram Stain, Rapid Method

1. Prepare thin smear of the most purulent sputum on glass slide with sterile loop or swab.
2. Air-dry sputum smear.
3. Heat-fix slide to a temperature just tolerable to the skin on back of hand.
4. Cover with crystal violet for 10 sec.
5. Rinse with water.
6. Cover with Lugol's iodine for 10 sec.
7. Rinse with water.
8. Cover with 95 percent ethyl alcohol for 10 sec.
9. Rinse with water.
10. Cover with safranin for 10 sec.
11. Rinse with water.
12. Blot and dry.
13. Examine for bacterial organisms. Particularly note polymorphonuclear cells and intracellular organisms.

of immunofluorescent microscopy are becoming more available clinically. Histopathologic examination utilizing appropriate special stains to aid in recognizing organisms in tissue biopsies is useful. Close interaction between the clinician and the laboratory personnel will ensure best results.

Culture and Isolation

Culture of the organism from the appropriate specimen continues to be the standard against which newer diagnostic methods are measured. Isolation and identification of bacteria or fungi by culture on artificial media is complex and time consuming for laboratory personnel. Close coordination between the clinician and the laboratory will ensure optimal handling of specimens from sampling to incubation, including consideration of special media or environment (such as for anaerobic cultures and the like). Viral isolation, while increasingly available, should only be attempted in carefully selected patients, since the therapeutic implications are limited.

Microbiologic reports, like other data, must be interpreted in light of an individual patient's clinical situation, and not blindly accepted as representing the "diagnosis." The laboratory classification of organisms into the categories *pathogenic*, therefore meriting physician concern, and *nonpathogenic*, therefore not meriting physician concern, is of limited value as increasing numbers of *nonpathogenic* organisms are demonstrated to cause disease in compromised hosts.

Antigen Identification

In recent years, a number of techniques allowing identification of microorganisms by detection of their antigens have been introduced. These techniques are generally more rapid than cultures (hours, not days), and are quite specific. Countercurrent immunoelectrophoresis (CIE) and latex agglutination are the most widely used, with the former finding more acceptability. CIE has been of most value in the detection of bacterial antigens, particularly pneumococcal or meningococcal, in the cerebrospinal fluid of meningitis patients, or pneumococcal in blood or pleural fluid of patients with pneumonia. Less usefulness has been found for antigen identification in sputum. Levels of antigen persist for hours to days after specimens become sterile due to initial drug therapy; this feature is a major advantage of this method. Radioimmunoassay techniques have become widely used to detect hepatitis B surface antigen in blood and blood products (see Chapter 12). Clinically useful radioimmunoassay for detecting other antigens is a likely expansion of this technique.

MEASURES OF IMMUNE RESPONSE

Antibody Tests

Evidence of host-parasite interaction is sought by measurement of antibody response or by the demonstration of changes in immunity. Multiple serologic techniques (complement fixation, precipitin reactions, latex agglutination, neutralization testing, and others) are widely available to detect antibodies that have developed in response to many viral, bacterial, fungal, and some protozoan agents. A single antibody titer is rarely of value, and at least a two-fold rise in titer over time must be demonstrated to support a serologic diagnosis of active infection. "Acute" and "convalescent" sera are generally collected at 10 to 14 day intervals, to permit time for antibody production.

Skin Tests

Many viral, bacterial, fungal, and parasitic infecting agents cause the development of delayed hypersensitivity in the host. This hypersensitive or allergic state can be detected by skin testing with appropriate antigens. Since most delayed hypersensitivity persists for decades, a positive skin test in the acute situation is of limited diagnostic value in an individual patient unless a documented "conversion" from negative to positive is demonstrated. A negative test does not eliminate the possibility of infection, since conversion may require weeks to months to develop. Further, intercurrent illness or drugs may suppress delayed hypersensitivity, and not all patients having

a positive reaction will retain their reactivity over time. Tuberculosis, histoplasmosis, and coccidioidomycosis are diseases for which skin-test reactions are commonly helpful for diagnosis.

ANTIINFECTIVE THERAPY

PRINCIPLES OF ANTIMICROBIAL SELECTION

Specific therapy for infectious disease requires selection of the appropriate antibiotic for an organism known to be causing the infection (Table 7.3). In many cases the severity of the patient's illness forces the selection of antibiotic therapy when infection is suspected but the diagnosis is not yet established. The clinician should follow a logical process leading to antibiotic selection best suited to each individual patient's problem. This process should include consideration of probable infectious agents, collection of specimens, appropriate processing, initiation of antibiotic therapy selected empirically, and reevaluation of that choice on the basis of culture results and the patient's course.

A conscious decision regarding whether specimens for microscopic examination and culture are to be obtained should precede antibiotic therapy in all cases. For most hospitalized patients, specimen collection is indicated. The specimen must represent the microenvironment in the infected area, and must be free of significant contamination. If properly performed and interpreted, gram stain may be quite helpful. It is important to communicate with laboratory personnel regarding special techniques for collecting or culturing specimens. Anaerobic specimens may be obtained from collections of fluid using a needle and syringe, as for arterial punctures.

Infectious agents that are typically isolated in a particular clinical situation, including their antibiotic sensitivities, are published in the literature (Table 7.4), but this information should be supplemented and updated by data reflecting local experience with bacterial isolation and sensitivity tests. With knowledge of the most likely bacterial pathogens for a given clinical presentation, supplemented by clues from gram stains or other available specimen data, antibiotic selection can be made in a reasonable manner. Many clinical situations will warrant initiation of empirical antibiotic therapy based on this type of information prior to the availability of culture results.

Since the effective dose range for many antibiotics is narrow, consideration of body weight and renal and hepatic function may be essential. Blood levels of antibiotics should be measured during therapy in critically ill patients and patients with known renal or hepatic disease, to ensure effective levels and to reduce toxicity. After initial therapy has been started, an active review should take place, considering results of cultures and the patient's course. A change to an equally effective, less toxic antibiotic may be indicated.

INDIVIDUAL ANTIBIOTICS

While many of the antimicrobial agents available for current use have been with us a long time, a significant number of "new" agents continue to be introduced (Table 7.5). Many of the so-called new antibiotics are, in fact, refinements that may or may not represent improvements over previously available agents. The cost of the newer drugs is often great in comparison with older alternatives, and the toxicity of new agents is often poorly documented. The newer agents should be used with caution, and only accepted as replacements for existing drugs when clear-cut advantages are demonstrated.

The penicillins, the most widely used antimicrobial agents, are effective, inexpensive, and have a very wide margin of safety. Ampicillin, amoxicillin, carbenicillin, and ticarcillin represent penicillins with expanded spectrums and are useful in properly selected circumstances. Some of the penicillins recently released (piperacillin, mezlocillin) promise a further expanded gram-negative spectrum.

The cephalosoprins are clinically attractive because they are bactericidal against many gram-positive as well as a significant number of gram-negative bacilli. They may be useful for staphylococcal infections in patients who are allergic to penicillins. As a group they are relatively safe in a wide range of clinical situations, but they are seldom the drug of first choice. They are generally overprescribed since less expensive, equally effective drugs are often available. They should not be used as a routine substitute for penicillin, which is considerably cheaper and equally effective in many situations. New cephalosporins with expanded spectrums, designated as "third generation" drugs, are rapidly being marketed; the cost is high and their use is only justified in selected situations. Vancomycin is a potent bactericidal antistaphylococcal antibiotic that is used as an alternative to penicillin or cephalosporin for serious staphylococcal infections.

Erythromycin has a low incidence of significant toxicity and is effective in a wide range of gram-positive infections, particularly as an alternative to penicillin. It is particularly useful in pneumonia due to mycoplasma and Legionnaires' disease.

Clindamycin is useful as an alternative to penicillin and cephalosporin in selected situations, but its primary indication is in serious anaerobic infection where *Bacteroides fragilis* is a likely pathogen. Its association with pseudomembranous colitis (which may also occur with other antimicrobials) represents an important toxic side effect.

The aminoglycosides most commonly represented by gentamicin, tobramycin, and amikacin have bactericidal activity against a broad spectrum of gram-negative organisms. Gentamicin and tobramycin are quite comparable and should be used for serious gram-negative aerobic infections unless resistance to gentamicin and tobramycin is strongly suspected, and then amikacin is the drug of choice. Nephrotoxicity represents the clinically most important potential side effect of the aminoglycosides, and close monitoring of renal function and antibiotic levels in selected patients is required.

The sulfonamides, including the combination of trimethoprim-sulfamethoxazole, are drugs commonly used for initial treatment of uncomplicated urinary tract infections and bacterial bronchitis. They have the advantage of many years of experience and relatively low cost.

Adverse effects of antibiotics are often characteristic of the drug and must be carefully assessed before prescription or when the patient taking antibiotics presents with unexpected clinical problems.

PROBLEMS WITH ANTIMICROBIAL USE

Misuse of antimicrobial drugs has recently received considerable attention. Multiple studies have documented inappropriate prescribing practices for as many as 50 percent of patients. In addition to the high cost (approximately 25 percent of hospital drug costs), adverse effects of antibiotics include the promotion of antibiotic resistant bacteria, disturbance of the protective normal flora in the host, and unnecessary toxic and allergic reactions. The most common inappropriate antibiotic administration is for prophylactic use. While selected situations warrant short-term prophylaxis (Table 7.1), the routine administration of antibiotics in usually sterile surgical procedures or in the medical patient without proven or clinically probable infection is without merit. The routine use of combinations of two, three, or four antibiotics is another common drug misuse. The use of multiple drug combinations in selected high-risk

(Text continues on p. 180.)

Table 7.3 Properties of Selected Antibiotics

Agent	Major Antimicrobial Spectrum[a]	Routes of Administration[b]	Major Adverse Effects
Penicillins			
Penicillin G	Broad gram +, also spirochetes, *Neisseria*, *Listeria*, *Actinomyces*, clostridia, *Proteus mirabilis*, *H. influenzae*	PO IV IM	Allergy (rash or anaphylaxis—latter rare); drug fever; Coombs-positive hemolytic anemia; convulsions (high doses in renal failure)

Penicillinase-resistant penicillins
  Methicillin
  Nafcillin
  Oxacillin
  Cloxacillin
  Dicloxacillin
	Gram + especially penicillinase-producing staph (PPS)	PO
		IM
		IV
			Similar to penicillin G—plus nephrotoxicity (methicillin)

Ampicillin Amoxicillin	Gram + (not PPS), expanded gram – (*E. coli*, *H. influenzae*, *Proteus mirabilis*, *Shigella*, *Salmonella*)	PO IM IV	Similar to penicillin G but ↑ skin rash
Carbenicillin Ticarcillin	Gram + (not PPS), further expanded gram – (*E. coli*, *Proteus*, *Pseudomonas*, *Enterobacter*, *Bacteroides*, *H. influenzae*)		Similar to Penicillin G—occasional coagulopathy; high Na load (108–120 mg Na⁺/g)
Cephalosporins			

First generation
  Cephalothin
  Cefazolin
  Cephradine
  Cephapirin
  Cephalexin
  Cefaclor
	Gram + (includes PPS), moderate gram – (*E. coli*, *Klebsiella*, *Salmonella*, *Shigella*, *Proteus mirabilis*)	PO
		IV
		IM
			Similar to penicillin (may cross react with penicillin); phlebitis at IV site; positive Coombs' test; ↑ SGOT; false-positive "clinitest" pain on IM injection

Second generation
  Cefamandole
  Cefoxitin
	Similar to first but expanded gram – and anaerobic spectrum (not *Pseudomonas*)		Similar to above but limited use to date

Third Generation Cefotaxime and others	Similar to second but further expanded gram spectrum; includes some *Pseudomonas* organisms		Similar to above but limited use to date

Agent	Spectrum of activity[a]	Route[b]	Toxicity
Erythromycin	Gram + (many staph), also *Mycoplasma pneumoniae, Legionella* species, *Chlamydia trachomatis*	PO	GI intolerance PO; hepatotoxicity with estolate salt
Clindamycin	Gram + (includes PPS), *Actinomyces, Bacteroides fragilis*	IV IM PO IM IV	5 percent diarrhea; pseudomembranous colitis much less common; rash
Vancomycin	Gram + (particularly PPS) *Clostridia,* enterococci		Phlebitis; rash; fever; nephrotoxicity and deafness (dose related)
Chloramphenicol	Gram + (includes PPS), and gram –, rickettsiae, chlamydiae	PO, IV	Fatal aplastic anemia (rare); reversible ↓ RBC, ↓ WBC, ↓ platelets more common; "gray-baby" syndrome in prematures
Tetracyclines	Gram +, gram –, *Mycoplasma,* rickettsiae, chlamydiae	PO, IV	Photosensitivity; stains developing in teeth; GI irritation, negative nitrogen balance; skin rash
Sulfonamides	Gram +, gram –, *Nocardia, H. influenzae, E. coli, Shigella* and chlamydiae	PO	Hemolytic anemia (G-6-PD deficient) vasculitis; rash; fever; nausea; hematologic
Trimethoprim–Sulfamethoxazole Combination	Gram +, gram –, *Pneumocystis carinii, Mycobacterium marinum*	PO IV	Similar to above
Aminoglycosides Gentamicin Tobramycin Amikacin Kanamycin	Limited gram +, (staph, limited strept, pneumococci) broad gram –, (*E. coli, Pseudomonas, Klebsiella, Serratia, Enterobacter, Proteus, Providencia*)	IM IV	Nephrotoxicity; ototoxicity; fever; rash; neuromuscular blockade (rare)
	Gram + (staph, limited strept, pneumococci) gram – (*E. coli, Enterobacter, Proteus*)	IM IV	As above
Sodium Colistimethate Polymyxin E and Polymyxin B (similar drugs)	Most gram –, (not *Proteus, Bacteroides,* or *Serratia*)	IM	Nephrotoxicity; neurotoxicity; neuromuscular blockade
Metronidazole	Broad anaerobic spectrum (includes *B. fragilis*)	PO IV	Nausea; peripheral neuropathy; convulsions

[a] Sensitivity testing is indicated when resistance is suspected.
[b] Appropriate route of administration may vary with preparation and indication.

Table 7.4 Antibiotic Selection

Expected Organisms and Recommended Initial Antibiotics for Selected Clinical Situations
(To be reassessed after definitive identification of organisms)

Clinical Situation	Probable Organism(s)	Recommended Antibiotic	
		Primary	Alternative
Meningitis (adult	*Pneumococcus* *Meningococcus* *Streptococcus*	Penicillin (20 million units/day)	Chloramphenicol
If Postneurosurgical	Also *Pseudomonas* and *Staphylococcus*	Methicillin or equivalent and aminoglycoside[a]; if gram-negative consider moxalactam	
Pneumonitis No Underlying Disease	*Pneumococcus* or *Mycoplasma pneumonia*	Penicillin G (2.4 million units/day) Erythromycin or Tetracycline (0.5 g, 4 times daily)	
Underlying Disease (alcoholism, diabetes, chronic obstructive pulmonary disease, or immunodeficient)	Also coliforms, *Hemophilus* *Klebsiella* *S. aureus*	Methicillin or equivalent and aminoglycoside[a]	Cephalosporin and aminoglycoside[a]
	Pseudomonas organisms	Ticarcillin and aminoglycoside[a]	Cefamandole and aminoglycoside[a]
Pyelonephritis (seriously ill) Initial	Coliforms	Ampicillin	Cephalosporin, tetracycline or sulfonamide
Recurrent	Also *Proteus* and *Pseudomonas*	Aminoglycoside[a]	Colistimethate or carbenicillin

Bacterial Endocarditis			
Adult			
Classic SBE	*Streptococcus viridans* *Enterococci* (group D)	Penicillin (20 million units/day) and Streptomycin	Vancomycin
Parenteral Drug Abuse	*S. aureus* *Enterococci* (group D) *Pseudomonas* organisms	Methicillin or equivalent and aminoglycoside[a]	Vancomycin
Prosthetic Valve Endocarditis			
Early (within 6 months of surgery)	*S. aureus, S. epidermidis*, gram-negative rods, diptheroids	Methicillin or equivalent and aminoglycoside[a]	Vancomycin and aminoglycoside[a]
Late (greater than 6 months postoperative)	*Streptococcus viridans* *Enterococci* (group D) gram-negative rods	Penicillin (20 million units/day) and aminoglycoside[a]	Vancomycin and aminoglycoside[a]
Bacterial Sepsis, Adult	*S. aureus* Coliforms, other gram-negative and some gram-positive bacteria	Methicillin or equivalent Methicillin or equivalent, and aminoglycoside[a]	
Immunodeficient or Acquired in Hospital	Also *Pseudomonas*	Ticarcillin and aminoglycoside[a]	Cephalosporin and aminoglycoside[a]
Intraabdominal Infection	Coliforms Enterococci *Proteus* *Bacteroides*	Penicillin, clindamycin and aminoglycoside[a]	
Lung Abscess	*Bacteroides* *Peptostreptococcus*	Penicillin (5–10 million units/day)	Cefoxitin or clindamycin

[a] Aminoglycoside: gentamycin (1.5 mg/kg IM or IV q 8 hours) or tobramycin (1.5 mg/kg IM or IV q 8 hours) unless resistance is likely—then amikacin 7.5 mg/kg IM or slow IV q 12 hours; monitor blood levels and adjust dose.
(Modified from Coussons RT: Medical Times 107:45–53, 1979, with permission.)

Table 7.5   Antimicrobial Drugs of Choice for Selected Pathogens

Organism	First Choice	Alternative Drugs
Gram-Positive Cocci		
Staphylococcus aureus (Assume penicillinase-producing organism until susceptibilities available)	Penicillinase-resistant penicillin (PRP)	Cephalosporin; vancomycin; clindamycin
Streptococcus pyogenes	Penicillin G	Erythromycin
Streptococcus viridans group	Penicillin G and streptomycin	Vancomycin and streptomycin
Streptococcus Enterococcal endocarditis or other severe infections	Penicillin G and gentamicin or streptomycin	Vancomycin and gentamicin or streptomycin
Streptococcus pneumoniae	Penicillin G	Erythromycin; cephalosporin
Streptococcus, anaerobic	Penicillin G	Clindamycin; cephalosporin (2nd generation); chloramphenicol
Gram-Negative Cocci		
Neisseria gonorrhoeae	Tetracycline or penicillin or amoxicillin	Spectinomycin; cefoxitin
Neisseria meningitidis	Penicillin G	Chloramphenicol; cephalosporin
Gram-Positive Bacilli		
Clostridium perfringens or *tetani*	Penicillin G	Chloramphenicol; cephalosporin; tetracycline
Listeria monocytogenes	Ampicillin and gentamicin	Tetracycline; erythromycin
Enteric Gram-Negative Bacilli		
Bacteroides organisms including *fragilis*	Clindamycin	Chloramphenicol; cefoxitin; metronidazole; carbenicillin or ticarcillin
Enterobacter	Gentamicin or tobramycin	Carbenicillin or ticarcillin; cefamandole
Escherichia coli	Gentamicin or tobramycin	Ampicillin; carbenicillin or ticarcillin; cephalosporin; tetracycline; trimethoprim-sulfamethoxazole; chloramphenicol
Klebsiella pneumoniae	Gentamicin or tobramycin	Cephalosporin; kanamycin; tetracycline; trimethoprim-sulfamethoxazole
Proteus mirabilis	Ampicillin	Cephalosporin; gentamicin or tobramycin; carbenicillin or ticarcillin; trimethoprim-sulfamethoxazole
Other *Proteus*	Gentamicin or tobramycin	Carbenicillin or ticarcillin; tetracycline; trimethoprim-sulfamethoxazole
Providencia	Amikacin	Gentamicin or tobramycin cefoxitin or cefamandole
Salmonella typhi	Chloramphenicol	Ampicillin or amoxicillin; trimethoprim-sulfamethoxazole
Other *Salmonella*	Ampicillin or amoxicillin	Chloramphenicol; trimethoprim-sulfamethoxazole
Serratia	Gentamicin	Amikacin; cefoxitin; carbenicillin or ticarcillin
Shigella	Trimethoprim-sulfamethoxazole	Ampicillin; tetracycline
Other Gram-Negative Bacilli		
Acinetobacter (*mima, herellea*)	Gentamicin or tobramycin	Amikacin; trimethoprim-sulfamethoxazole
Brucella (Brucellosis)	Tetracycline	Streptomycin or chloramphenicol
Campylobacter (*vibrio*) *fetus*	Erythromycin	Tetracycline; gentamicin
Francisella tularensis (Tularemia)	Streptomycin	Tetracycline; chloramphenicol

178

	First Choice	Alternative
Other Gram–Negative Bacilli (*continued*)		
Haemophilus influenzae (Life-threatening infections)	Chloramphenicol	Ampicillin; cefamandole trimethoprim-sulfamethoxazole
Legionella pneumophila	Erythromycin	Rifampin
Pittsburgh pneumonia agent	Erythromycin	Trimethoprim-sulfamethoxazole; rifampin
Pseudomonas aeruginosa		
Urinary tract infection	Carbenicillin or ticarcillin	Tobramycin; gentamicin; amikacin
Life-threatened immunosuppressed patient	Tobramycin with ticarcillin	Amikacin with carbenicillin or ticarcillin
Acid-Fast Bacilli		
Mycobacterium tuberculosis	Isoniazid with rifampin and ethambutol	Streptomycin, paraaminosalicylic acid (PAS);
Actinomycetes		
Actinomyces Israelii (Actinomycosis)	Penicillin G	Tetracycline; clindamycin
Nocardia	Sulfonamides	Trimethoprim-sulfamethoxazole; minocycline; cycloserine
Chlamydia		
Chlamydia psittaci (Psittacosis; ornithosis)	Tetracycline	Chloramphenicol
Chlamydia trachomatis	Tetracycline	Erythromycin
Fungi		
Aspergillus	Amphotericin B	No dependable alternative
Candida species (serious deep infection)	Amphotericin B	Ketoconazole
Coccidioides immitis	Amphotericin B	Ketoconazole
Cryptococcus neoformans	Amphotericin B with flucytosine	No dependable alternative
Dermatophytes (Tinea)	Clotrimazole (topical) or miconazole (topical)	Tolnaftate (topical); haloprogin (topical); griseofulvin
Histoplasma capsulatum	Amphotericin B	Ketoconazole
Mucor	Amphotericin B	No dependable alternative
Sporothrix schenckii	An iodide	Amphotericin B
Mycoplasma		
Mycoplasma pneumoniae	Erythromycin	Tetracycline
Pneumocystis carinii	Trimethoprim-sulfamethoxazole	Pentamidine
Rickettsia		
Rocky Mountain spotted fever; endemic typhus (murine); tick bite fever; typhus; scrub typhus; Q fever	Tetracycline	Chloramphenicol
Spirochetes		
Leptospira	Penicillin G	Tetracycline
Treponema pallidum (Syphilis)	Penicillin G	Tetracycline; erythromycin
Viruses		
Herpes simplex (keratitis)	Trifluridine (topical)	Vidarabine (topical); idoxuridine (topical)
Herpes simplex (encephalitis)	Vidarabine	Acyclovir
Influenza A	Amantadine	No alternative

(Modified from: The choice of antimicrobial drugs. Medical Letter, 24:21–28, 1982, with permission.)

patients (such as immunosuppressed and granulocytopenic patients) while culture data are awaited is justified, but many combinations are prescribed without adequate clinical reason. Every physician must cultivate improved prescribing habits. An aggressive program of monitoring antibiotic use with an educational program directed at prescribers has been shown to reduce abuse, and can often be provided by the infection-control committee and nurse epidemiologist.

Part 2: Selected Topics in Infectious Disease

THE EVALUATION OF THE FEBRILE PATIENT

The evaluation of the febrile patient starts with documentation of the fever. A temperature diary with several readings daily, kept by a reliable patient, often helps define the problem in an outpatient setting. "Normal" temperature varies among individuals, as well as with the time of day and activity. For clinical purposes, an oral temperature of over 99° F (37.2° C) is considered abnormal, usually reflecting a disease state. The physiologic diurnal variation, ranging from 97° F (36.1° C) on awakening in the morning to 99° F (37.2° C) in the late afternoon, should not be misinterpreted as an afternoon fever.

Fever is a physical sign requiring an explanation, and should not be treated as a "disease." Fever most commonly indicates an infectious disease, but has multiple other possible etiologies in a given patient. The clinical setting should dictate the workup; no single diagnostic approach can be applied to all febrile patients. The otherwise healthy young adult presenting with fever lasting less than 10 days, without clinical evidence of major organ involvement, will usually have a viral syndrome and require minimal evaluation. These self-limiting illnesses are most commonly due to respiratory or intestinal viral infections. However, the older patient presenting with fever of over 2 weeks duration and with no diagnosis established after initial evaluation (history, physical examination, hemoglobin, white blood count with differential, urinalysis, chemistry screening, and chest roentgenogram) may well have a fever of unknown origin (FUO) and require extensive hospital evaluation. Diagnostic possibilities would include localized or systemic infection, malignancy, collagen-vascular disease, drug reaction, inflammatory bowel disease, or factitious fever (patient-induced), and a thoughtful planned approach is required to identify the cause. A diagnosis can be made in approximately 90 percent of patients presenting with an FUO. A careful well-executed history and physical examination is the basis for directing the evaluation of the febrile patient (see previous section, Diagnostic Methods in Infectious Disease). In addition to appropriate specimens for culture and serologic evaluation, biopsy of involved tissue and bone marrow examination may be useful. Occasionally radiographic surveys to assess kidneys, retroperitoneal lymph nodes, and the pancreas may be indicated. Clues from the history, physical examination, and initial laboratory evaluation should guide the selection of tests and specimen collection. Therapeutic trials (such as antituberculosis drugs for suspected tuberculosis) are generally not indicated and should be undertaken with caution; once they are begun they tend to reduce diligent efforts to establish a firm diagnosis. Frequent refinement of the history and repetitive physical examination are important as the workup of the FUO patient proceeds (Table 7.6). In some patients fever will be associated with disease of an organ but no definitive infectious cause, for example, lung infiltrates in patients receiving cytotoxic or immunosuppressive drugs. Management of these patients is discussed in relation to each organ system elsewhere in this volume.

Table 7.6 Major Diagnostic Considerations in Patients with Fever of Unknown Origin

Disease Process	Approximate Percentage of Patients
Infection	20–35
Tuberculosis	5–10
Abdominal abscess	5–10
Hepatobiliary infection	5
Endocarditis	5
Pyelonephritis	0–5
Other (brucellosis, infectious mononucleosis, etc.)	5
Neoplasm	10–30
Lymphoma	5–20
Carcinoma	
Renal	0–5
Pancreatic	0–5
Hepatobiliary	0–5
Other Unknown	0–5
Connective Tissue Disorder	10–25
Systemic vasculitis	5–15
Lupus erythematosus	0–5
Rheumatic fever	0–5
Other	0–5
Miscellaneous	10–25
Inflammatory bowel disease	0–5
Pulmonary emboli	0–5
Drug fever	0–5
Factitious fever	0–5
Other	5–10

RECOGNITION AND MANAGEMENT OF BACTERIAL SEPSIS

Knowledge of the clinical setting in which bacterial sepsis is common is a powerful tool in its early recognition. Patients that are recovering following gastrointestinal surgery (gall-bladder and colon surgery, particularly), patients undergoing urinary tract manipulation, patients with severe diabetes or advanced liver disease, and immunosuppressed patients with malignancy are particularly predisposed to bacterial sepsis and shock. The onset of sepsis often includes a chill, followed by fever, with subtle mental confusion, and hyperventilation associated with respiratory alkalosis, or, in more severe cases, metabolic acidosis, shock, and multiple organ failure (see Table 7.7).

With strong clinical suspicion of bacterial sepsis, three blood cultures should be promptly drawn and a urine and a sputum culture obtained. Prompt attention to any underlying focus of infection that can be surgically drained is appropriate. Broad antibiotic coverage is initially indicated, and specific antibiotic choice is influenced by the clinical situation. As an example, the patient who develops fever and a septic presentation following urinary tract manipulation will probably have a common urinary tract pathogen as the etiology of his sepsis. In the absence of a previous culture, a cephalosporin and an aminoglycoside (gentamicin or tobramycin unless resistance is likely) in high intravenous doses, constitute appropriate initial therapy. In patients where *Pseudomonas aeruginosa* infection is likely (a leukemic patient with agranulocytosis), ticarcillin or carbenicillin should be added. If anaerobic infection is probable, clindamycin should be considered as a replacement for cephalosporin. Antibiotic therapy should be re-

Table 7.7 **Clinical Features of Septicemia**

Usual (better prognosis)	Less Common (worse prognosis)
Fever	Hypothermia (<15%)
Leucocytosis	Leucopenia (<10%)
Hemodynamic Abnormalities	
Tachycardia	Hypotension
Vasodilation	Vasoconstriction
Increased cardiac output	Reduced cardiac output
Respiratory Abnormalities	
Tachypnea	Adult respiratory distress syndrome with severe hypoxemic respiratory failure (10–20%)
Respiratory alkalosis	
Mild hypoxemia	
Coagulation Abnormalities	
Thrombocytopenia	Disseminated intravascular coagulation (<10%)

viewed and monitored daily and altered if appropriate when cultures become available. It is important to include the course of the patient in any decision based on laboratory reports.

Supportive measures may be lifesaving in these severely ill patients. Vigorous fluid therapy with venous pressure monitoring, oxygen administration if hypoxemia is present, and vasoactive drugs such as dopamine in hypotensive patients may be useful. High dose steroid therapy (30 mg/kg of methylprednisolone) given as an IV bolus and repeated once 4 hours later may be helpful, although this remains controversial.

Patients with septicemia may have a mortality rate of 10 to 30 percent, which increases to 80 percent with shock. The severity of the associated or underlying disease also increases the death rate.

SEXUALLY TRANSMITTED DISEASES

Sexually transmitted diseases require intimate personal contact for their spread and propagation. These diseases have flourished as sexual practices have changed and frequent casual sexual partners replace stable, monogamous relationships. While many other diseases have aspects of sexual transmission, gonorrhea, syphilis, nonspecific urethritis, genital herpes, and trichomoniasis will be discussed here.

GONORRHEA

Gonorrhea is the most frequent "reportable" disease in the United States. It is caused by *Neisseria gonorrhoeae*, a fastidious gram-negative diplococcus whose only host is man. In males the "clap" (urethritis with dysuria and purulent urethral discharge), the most common manifestation, occurs 2 to 7 days after exposure. The incidence of infected but asymptomatic males varies, but is around 10 percent. Most gonorrhea is in fact spread by asymptomatic carriers (both male and female), since most symptomatic patients tend to seek medical treatment. Pharyngeal and anorectal gonorrhea are common in homosexual men. Pharyngeal gonorrhea can produce tonsilar exudate but is often asymptomatic and may also occur in women who practice fellatio with infected males. Anorectal gonorrhea may produce little symptomatology, although pruritis, tenesmus, and bloody purulent rectal discharge may be seen.

In females, the symptoms of uncomplicated gonorrhea are nonspecific with dysuria, frequency, and vaginal discharge often suggesting a urinary tract infection or vaginitis. Urine culture, pelvic exam, and endocervical culture on appropriate media are mandatory. In some 15 to 20 percent of women with gonorrhea, spread beyond the endocervix to the fallopian tubes occurs, producing acute salpingitis, its major complication. Gonococcemia produces distant gonococcal spread in both men and women with frequent skin and joint involvement. The diagnosis of gonorrhea is established by the demonstration of typical gram-negative diplococci seen within leukocytes from urethral or endocervical exudate. Extracellular organisms are suggestive but not diagnostic of infection. The sensitivity and specificity of the gram stain diagnosis varies considerably with observer skill, so culture confirmation is desirable. Thayer-Martin media (containing antibiotics to inhibit other organisms) with incubation in a carbon-dioxide (CO_2) enriched atmosphere should be used to culture exudates. Standard blood culture broth incubated in CO_2 enriched atmosphere is adequate for blood culture isolation. All patients with gonorrhea should have a serologic test for syphilis.

While gonococcal resistance to penicillin occurs, uncomplicated gonococcal infection in both men and women can still be adequately treated in most instances with aqueous procaine penicillin G (4.8 million units IM) in two separate sites, with 1 g probenecid given orally. Tetracycline in a total dose of 10 g over 5 days orally, or 3.5 g of ampicillin in a single oral dose with 1 g of probenecid are alternatives. Ambulatory females with acute gonococcal salpingitis should receive aqueous procaine penicillin G as above, followed by 500 mg of ampicillin, orally, 4 times daily, for a total of 10 days. Tetracycline 500 mg orally 4 times daily for 10 days is an acceptable alternative. Patients with salpingitis requiring hospitalization should receive aqueous penicillin G 20 million units daily intravenously until clinically improved and ampicillin given orally to complete a 10 day course. A follow-up culture as test of cure is desirable one to two weeks after completion of therapy.

Penicillin resistant gonococcal infection should be treated with single dose spectinomycin, 2 g intramuscularly.

ual practices. Its clinical stages can be divided as outlined in Table 7.8.

Primary syphilis, typified by the usually painless chancre that appears during the third week after exposure, continues as a common presentation. Chancres occur most frequently in the genital area, but now the mouth, the rectum, and other sites are not unusual. The lesion begins as a painless papule changing into a clean-based ulcer with an elevated, heaped up border. Lesions may be multiple, and regional lymph nodes are commonly enlarged but not tender. Dark field examination usually demonstrates the etiologic agent, the *Treponema pallidum* recognized by its corkscrew movement and coiled appearance in scrapings from these infectious lesions. Serologic confirmation is possible in over 75 percent of cases by the third or fourth week after the chancre appears. The Venereal Disease Research Laboratory test (VDRL) or its equivalent is usually adequate, and the Fluorescent Treponema Antibody Absorbent test (FTA-ABS) while more specific, is required only for confirmation in most cases. All patients with syphilis should be reported to the local public health department for follow-up of primary and secondary cases and contacts to control this highly infectious disease.

The secondary stage of syphilis is characterized by widespread macular and papular skin and mucous membrane lesions that are also highly infectious. The primary and secondary stages coincide in about one third of the patients, and secondary lesions may appear without clinical recognition of the primary stage. Systemic symptoms including fever, conjunctivitis, arthralgia, and headache may occur with generalized lymphadenopathy. Immune-complex nephropathy and hepatitis may occur. Latent and tertiary stages are summarized in Table 7.8.

Treatment for syphilis is recommended in Table 7.9. Patients under treatment for syphilis should be warned about the possibility of a Jarisch-Herxheimer reaction, with chills, fever, and malaise occurring several hours after penicillin administration. The Jarisch-Herxheimer reaction probably reflects the body's reaction to the lysis of organisms and the release of antigens. Aspirin is usually adequate for symptomatic control of the chills and fever.

SYPHILIS

Numerically, syphilis is only about 2 to 3 percent as common as gonorrhea, but its recognition and treatment are extremely important because of its potential for serious damage. During the last decade, syphilis has increased in incidence and changed its manifestations probably as a result of changes in sex-

NONSPECIFIC URETHRITIS (NSU)

NSU, or nongonococcal urethritis, is more frequent in males than gonorrhea, and is characterized by thin, mucoid, urethral discharge, usually accompanied by dysuria. It is recognized almost exclusively in males, although a counterpart probably exists in females. Diagnosis is generally by the exclusion of

Table 7.8 Clinical Stages of Syphilis

Stage	Findings	Time Since Exposure	Duration Untreated	Treponemes Present (Dark field)	Serology Percentage Positive VDRL/FTA-ABS
Primary	Chancre—not universal, penis, labia, pelvis, vagina, rectum, mouth	10–90 days (21 average)	2–6 weeks	Yes	78/85
Secondary	Maculo-papular rash, condyloma latum	6 weeks to 6 months	1–6 weeks	Yes	97/99
Latent	None	After 1° + 2°	Life-long—1/3 develop tertiary	No	74/95
Tertiary (late)					
Benign	Gumma	2–10 years	Life	No	77/95
Cardiovascular	Aortic aneurysm insufficiency	10–30 years	Life—may be fatal	Aorta +	77/95
Neurosyphilis	Asymptomatic, meningovascular, paresis, tabes dorsalis—CSF cell count and protein vary with process	5–35 years	Life—may be fatal	CSF and Brain may be +	77/95
Congenital					
Early	Rash, mucous patches, rhinitis	2 years	Neonatal	Yes	77/95
Late	Deafness, interstitial keratitis, periostitis	after 2 years	Life	No	77/95

(Modified from: Dans, P. E.: Treatment of gonorrhea or syphillis. Southern Medical Journal 68:1297, 1975, with permission.)

Table 7.9 **Recommended Treatment for Syphilis**

Stage of Infection	Benzathine Penicillin G	Aqueous Penicillin G or Procaine Penicillin G
Primary, Secondary and Latent	2 injections of 1.2 million units IM in one session	600,000 units IM daily for 8 consecutive days
Tertiary	2 injections of 1.2 million units IM on each of three sessions at 7-day intervals. Total dose 7.2 million units	600,000 units IM daily for 15 days

gonorrhea as an etiology. The gram stain shows no gonococci, but polymorphonuclear leukocytes are present. While the name suggests no etiologic factor, recent studies indicate that *Chlamydia trachomatis* may cause up to 40 to 50 percent of cases with T strain mycoplasma (*Ureaplasma urealyticum*) accounting for another 25 percent of cases. Herpes simplex and *Trichomonas hominis* are also occasionally implicated. Tetracycline, 500 mg orally, 4 times daily for 7 days is usually effective. Reinfection or relapse is common, so treatment of a regular sexual partner may be advisable.

GENITAL HERPES

Genital herpes is increasing among sexually active partners and may be the most frequent cause of genital sores. It is caused by the herpes simplex virus type II (rarely, by type I which is the cause of the common cold sore), and it manifests multiple painful vesicles at the site of infection within one week of exposure. The vesicles typically break open, revealing shallow nonindurated ulcers. Satellite lesions are common. The primary infection is often accompanied by systemic symptoms, including chills, fever, myalgia, headache, and regional adenopathy. Urination may be very painful, and urinary retention may result. A Giemsa stain of vesicular fluid reveals multinucleated giant cells with intracellular inclusions, strongly supporting the diagnosis. Confirmation by tissue culture isolation, or acute and concvalescent serum (complement fixation titers) is not usually needed. The primary infection lasts several weeks, and recurrences are common. Genital herpes may be extremely discouraging and painful to the patient. In the past, specific therapy has been discouraging, but acyclovir as a topical ointment currently appears promising. Sexual contact should be avoided until lesions are healed. Infected females should obtain at least annual pap smears because of the suggested relationship between carcinoma of the cervix and herpes simplex virus type II infections.

TRICHOMONAS

Trichomonas vaginitis is an extremely common cause of sexually transmitted vaginitis. Most infected females note itching and vaginal discharge with menses. A gray-green to yellow malodorous discharge of a profuse, frothy nature is common. Motile, flagellated organisms are seen if wet preps are examined microscopically. Metronidazole in a single 2 g oral dose is effective. Simultaneous treatment of regular sexual partners is advised to reduce recurrence.

RICKETTSIAL DISEASE—ROCKY MOUNTAIN SPOTTED FEVER

The diseases caused by organisms of the family Rickettsiaceae have in the past been among the most feared by mankind. Epidemic typhus ravaged parts of Europe and Russia in the early 1900s, producing millions of deaths and infecting 20 to 30 million people. With the development of methods to interrupt the insect vectors and animal reservoirs common to most rickettsioses, Rocky Mountain spotted fever (RMSF) remains the most prominent of these diseases in the western hemisphere. RMSF is caused by *Rickettsia rickettsii*, which, like all rickettsiae, is an obligate intracellular parasite. RMSF is an acute febrile illness heralded by the rapid onset of chills, fever, and headache, accompanied by a characteristic rash that normally appears 2 to 7 days after fever starts. Early lesions are punctate, pink, and irregular, and are usually small (2 to 5 mm), beginning on the extremities, particularly the palms, soles, wrists, and ankles. Centripetal spread to the trunk, buttocks, face, and neck occurs in the first 24 hours. The rash progresses to a macular eruption by the 3rd day, and later becomes petechial or even hemorrhagic and ecchymotic as coalescence occurs between lesions. Fever may be high (39 to 40° C) and prolonged if untreated. Severe headache, myalgia, arthralgia, and vomiting occur. Shock and renal failure occur in the seriously ill. Mortality has been reported near 20 percent in untreated patients, with most fatalities occurring in older age groups. The disease is transmitted in humans in endemic areas by tick bites (*Dermacentor andersoni* and *Dermacentor variabilis*), with transmission likely only if the tick remains attached to the host for several hours. A history of a known tick bite is present in about three fourths of the patients. The diagnosis is suspected on clinical grounds and supported by a positive Weil-Felix reaction (OX-19, OX-2 titer rises) or by more specific complement-fixation testing. Early treatment with either chloramphenicol (50 mg/kg/day) or tetracycline (25 mg/kg/day) is effective. Supportive care is also important with emphasis on nutrition and adequate fluid replacement. Tick control and daily personal inspection for ticks in exposed individuals are the keys to prevention.

COMMON SYSTEMIC FUNGAL INFECTIONS

Systemic fungal infections have become more frequently recognized in the last several decades, and with the increasing longevity of immunosuppressed patients they will probably continue in importance as pathogens. These fungi are widespread in the environment, and *Candida*, for example, is a normal inhabitant of the mouth, the gastrointestinal tract, and the vagina. *Histoplasma capsulatum, Blastomyces dermatitidis*, and *Coccidiodes immitis* cause disease in normal hosts, while *Candida* and others usually affect only the compromised host.

Cryptococcosis is caused by the yeast-like fungus *Cryptococcus neoformans*, which has a worldwide distribution and is commonly found in the soil, as well as in pigeon droppings. Patients are usually unaware of exposure, and the fungus is acquired by the airborne route, often producing an asymptomatic pulmonary infection. Most symptomatic patients present with a meningoencephalitis manifesting as headache, confusion, dementia, and gait disturbances. Pulmonary and cutaneous manifestations may also occur, but are less common. Many patients have a predisposing disease, such as lymphoma or leukemia, or have been on prolonged steroid therapy. The diagnosis is generally based on cerebrospinal fluid findings of a low glucose, elevated protein, and predominantly lymphocytic cellular response. India ink preparation may reveal encapsulated yeast, but culture or detection of capsular antigen in cerebral spinal fluid or serum by latex agglutination are required for definitive diagnosis. Treatment is complicated, requiring usually both oral flucytosine and intravenous amphotericin.

Coccidioidomycosis, like cryptococcosis, is initially a pulmonary infection and is symptomatic in less than 50 percent of cases. The fungus is a soil saprophyte found in arid regions of the western hemisphere, particularly the southwestern United States where the disease is endemic. Most primary pulmonary infections present a flu-like syndrome and elicit a granulomatous reaction followed by complete healing. Complications include progressive fibronodular cavitary pulmonary disease, or disseminated disease that tends to be particularly frequent in blacks, Mexican-Americans, American Indians, and immunosuppressed patients. Chronic meningitis, with frequent relapse is the most serious of the disseminated forms. Diagnosis is usually established by antigen detection in spinal fluid by latex agglutination or agar-gel diffusion, or by demonstration of circulating antibodies. Culture may be risky for laboratory personnel because of infectivity, and should be attempted only by laboratories with appropriate facilities. Skin-test antigen material is available but is of limited value in a given patient, since it may be positive from previous conversion in patients with disseminated disease. Primary pulmonary coccidioidomycosis needs no therapy, but in progressive lung disease or disseminated forms, amphotericin B is often effective. Surgical removal of appropriate lung or bone lesions should be considered.

Blastomycosis is also acquired by inhalation, although the reservoir for the fungus, thought to be the soil, is not confirmed. While not a frequently encountered disease, most cases occur in the Southeast and mid-Atlantic United States and in South America. Patients are usually asymptomatic; clinically recognized cases most commonly involve the lung and skin. The verrucous or ulcerated skin lesions can be multiple, and tend to be painless. Bone, joint, and prostatic involvement are not rare. Skin tests and serologic testing are not useful and diagnosis rests on recovery of the organism by culture. Amphotericin B is the drug of choice, and most patients should be treated.

Candidiasis is primarily caused by *Candida albicans*, although other *Candida* species may be pathogenic. *Candida albicans* is usually present in the mouth, gastrointestinal tract, and vagina, and invasion with dissemination tends to occur only in the compromised host. Debilitated patients, patients with diabetes or malignancy and patients receiving treatment with broad spectrum antibiotics or high-dose steroids, are at particular risk. Infections are often acquired in the hospital where indwelling intravenous catheters, GI intubation, or urinary catheters are predisposing factors. Mucocutaneous involvement is frequent. With oral candidiasis, or thrush, confluent white plaques on pharyngeal or oral mucosa are typical. Pulmonary involvement is not frequent, but may occur. Blood stream invasion may be transient and may resolve when the predisposing factor such as an IV catheter is removed. If persistence of *Candida* in the blood stream continues after removal of all indwelling intravenous catheters and other predisposing factors, and the fungus is also found in a fresh urine specimen, dissemination is probable. Meningitis and endocarditis have been reported. The diagnosis rests on the demonstration of the organism (which grows readily on routine culture media) on multiple cultures. Serologic and skin tests are not helpful.

Mucocutaneous candidiasis is treated with ketoconazole. Intravenous amphotericin B remains the most effective drug for disseminated disease. Ketoconazole may be useful in addition to amphotericin B.

Sporothrix schenckii is distributed worldwide and lives on plants, so that infection results when forest laborers or gardeners innoculate themselves by minor skin trauma. The disease is usually cutaneous with a painless red papule forming at the innoculation site. Lymphatic spread with additional papules and pustules, resulting over a matter of weeks, is common. Lymph node involvement and skin ulceration are frequent. Dissemination is fortunately not common but may involve bones, joints, lungs, and the central nervous system. Culture is the only reliable diagnostic tool. Cutaneous sporotrichosis is usually successfully treated with a saturated solution of potassium iodide. Disseminated disease requires amphotericin B, which achieves only limited success.

Histoplasmosis is discussed in the section dealing with pulmonary infections (see Chapter 15).

SELECTED PROTOZOAL DISEASES

MALARIA

Malaria remains a major health problem in certain areas despite the effectiveness of World Health Organization (WHO) efforts to eradicate it. In the United States, Europe, and Canada it is generally limited to imported cases brought in by travelers from endemic areas. Malaria is caused by four species of *Plasmodium* (*P. vivax, P. ovale, P. milariae,* and *P. falciparum*), all of which are natural human parasites. The perpetuation of malaria in endemic areas requires a sizable anopheline mosquito population in contact with an infected human population. Control measures focus on both, and have been quite effective. The malaria cycle in man is well described, and var-

iations within the different species account for the clinical findings. The incubation period ranges from 10 days for *P. vivax* up to 6 weeks for *P. milariae,* and in travellers the onset may occur months after they have returned home; the interval is influenced by the species involved. Symptoms are not specific, with headache, fever and myalgia often preceding the recurrent fever. The chills and fever may be profound with temperatures up to 40 or 41° C. Sweating and prostration are common. The fever periodicity may offer a diagnostic clue. *P ovale* and *P. vivax* cause alternate day (tertian) fever, and *P. malariae* produces fever every third day (quartian). This periodicity depends on synchronization of the parasitic cycle, and is often less apparent clinically than descriptions would suggest. With disease progression, anemia, hepatosplenomegaly, and jaundice appear. Diagnosis is confirmed by the demonstration of the parasite on peripheral blood smear. Repeat smears are often required as the parasitemia is not continuous.

Treatment of the acute phases of all but chloroquine-resistant *P. falciparum* can be accomplished with oral chloroquine phosphate base, with 0.6 g by mouth, followed by 0.3 g in 6 hours, and then 0.3 g daily for 2 additional days. Combination therapy is required for resistant *P. falciparum. P. vivax* and *P. ovale* are not eradicated by chloroquine because of their persistance in the liver, and they require primaquine base 15 mg by mouth daily for 2 weeks to avoid late relapse. For personal protection, travelers to endemic areas should obtain and follow WHO recommendations applicable to their area of travel. Adults travelling to endemic areas with chloroquine-sensitive malaria should take 300 mg chloroquine phosphate base weekly, starting 1 week before arrival and continuing 6 weeks after departure from the endemic region.

TOXOPLASMOSIS

Toxoplasmosis is an extremely common infection involving birds and mammals, but the great majority of infections in humans by *toxoplasma gondii* are subclinical and go unrecognized unless identified by serologic screening. Humans are usually infected by ingesting inadequately cooked meat or through close association with cats who excrete infective oocysts in their stool. Following invasion through the gut of humans, parasitemia occurs with multiple organs becoming infected. The acute inflammatory response may result in tissue necrosis, especially in the lymph nodes, myocardium, and muscle, or on resolution of the acute infection the cyst may remain viable for the life of the host. Clinical disease is usually divided into acute toxoplasmosis, congenital toxoplasmosis, ocular toxoplasmosis, and toxoplasmosis in the immunosuppressed host.

Acute toxoplasmosis in the normal host presents primarily with generalized lymphadenopathy, fever, and fatigue. Fever is usually low but may be prolonged. Sore throat, a rash, and headache may also be reported. This illness is often described as an infectious mononucleosis-like syndrome. Other organs involved include the lungs, the skeletal muscle, the myocardium, the brain, and less commonly the eye and the liver. Laboratory findings are not specific, and the diagnosis will be missed unless antibody levels are measured.

If toxoplasmosis is acquired by a pregnant woman, transplacental infection of the fetus can occur with congenital toxoplasmosis resulting. Many cases of congenital toxoplasmosis are mild, but severe cases may cause fetal death, neurologic damage, chorioretinitis, and hepatosplenomegaly. Prevention is the key, and avoidance of potential infection should be stressed for pregnant women.

Ocular toxoplasmosis in the form of chorioretinitis may be a reactivation of congenital disease, or may occur in the acquired form. Recurrent eye pain and progressive visual loss (usually unilateral) are common. Systemic signs are few.

In the immunosuppressed patient toxoplasmosis may present as an aggressive disseminated disease, with central nervous system involvement being most prominent. Fever, pulmonary infiltrates, myocarditis, and hepatosplenomegaly are common. Aggressive diagnosis and treatment is indicated. Antibody titers are usually elevated, but the definitive diagnosis rests on demonstration of an increase in antibody levels by approximately 4 times. The indirect immunofluorescent antibody test, the Sabin-Feldman dye test, and the indirect hemagglutination test are most widely used. Demonstration of the organism in tissue by special stains establishes the diagnosis, but techniques for isolating the organism are not readily available, and they require special interest and skill. Most patients with acquired toxoplasmosis do not require treatment, but patients with active ocular disease or immunosuppressed patients with disseminated disease, particularly with central nervous system involvement, should be treated. Combined treatment with pyrimethamine and sulfonamides is recommended.

AMEBIASIS

Entamoeba histolytica is a protozoan present in about 10 percent of the world population. While present in 2 to 5 percent of North Americans, it is much more prevalent and more commonly causes disease in the tropical countries where poverty and malnutrition may be contributing factors. The organisms are injested with contaminated food or water. In the gastrointestinal tract they may invade the gut wall, causing typical amebic ulcers, and be carried to the liver to produce hepatic abscesses. Occasionally hepatic abscesses rupture through the diaphragm to produce a hepatic-pleural-bronchial fistula. Patients present with abdominal symptoms and bloody diarrhea, right upper quadrant pain, right pleural pain, or copious brownish sputum. Fever, anemia, and weight loss are characteristic. The diagnosis is made by microscopic examination of stool, pleural fluid, sputum, or hepatic abscess pus. Serologic tests are available.

Metronidazole is a potent and safe oral agent for treatment of amebic infections.

GIARDIASIS

See Causes of Diarrhea, Chapter 12.

TRICHOMONIASIS

See previous section entitled Sexually Transmitted Diseases.

ANIMAL BITES AND RABIES PROPHYLAXIS

Animal bites are common and require prompt attention to ensure the best outcome. Human bites are fortunately infrequent but also may be very serious. A brief history and an adequate physical examination to establish the nature of the injury is important. Prompt cleansing is indicated, and initial debridement should be carried out. Patients presenting 1 to 2 days after an initial injury are likely to have established infection. Surgical closure of wounds is controversial, but is deferred if infection is suspected. Tetanus toxoid should be given as a booster to those with a documented history of primary immunization, but who have not had a booster in 5 years. Patients without a convincing history of primary immunization should receive human tetanus immune globulin and should be started on a course of primary tetanus immunization. Phenoxymethylpenicillin, 250 mg by mouth 4 times a day, is indicated in fresh but not clinically infected bites. It is effective against *Pasteurella multocida*, found in the oral cavity of many animals, as well as against streptococci, some staphylococci, and anaerobes that may also be involved.

Table 7.10 Common Parasitic Infections

Parasite	Distribution	Source	Infection Rate	Major Clinical Features
Protozoan Diseases				
Malaria	Tropical and subtropical	Anopheline mosquito	Very common	Fever, anemia, splenomegaly
Trypanosomiasis	Africa, Central and South America	Cattle through insect vectors	Common locally	Fever, lymphadenopathy, hepatosplenomegaly, encephalopathy
Leishmaniasis	Tropical and subtropical, localized	Rodents and dogs through insect vectors	Very common locally	Fever, lymphadenopathy, splenomegaly, skin lesions
Amebiasis	Worldwide	Food, water, human feces[a]	Very common	Diarrhea, fever, abdominal pain, hepatic abscess, pleuropulmonary disease
Toxoplasmosis	Worldwide	Cat feces, meat[a]	Very common	Fever, lymphadenopathy, chorioretinitis
Giardiasis	Worldwide	Food, water[a]	Very common	Diarrhea, abdominal pain
Trichomoniasis	Worldwide	Human flora	Common	Vaginitis
Helminthic Infestations[b]				
Tapeworms				
Fish tapeworm	Arctic and far North	Fish[a]	Occasional	Megaloblastic (vitamin B_{12} deficiency) anemia
Beef tapeworm	Worldwide	Beef[a]	Occasional	Commonly asymptomatic
Pork tapeworm	Worldwide	Pork[a]	Occasional	Fever, muscle aches, later epilepsy, confusion
Echinococcosis (Hydatid disease)	Worldwide	Sheep, deer meat, dog feces[a]	Occasional	Liver abscess, lung mass, pleural effusion, fever
Trematodes (Flukes)				
Schistosomiasis				
S. japonicum	Far East	Water through skin	Very common locally	Early fever, rash, Later portal hypertension, cor pulmonale
S. haematobium	Africa, Middle East	Water through skin	Common locally	Fever, rash, portal hypertension, cor pulmonale, genitourinary disease
S. mansoni	Africa, S. America, Carribean	Water through skin	Common locally	Fever, rash, portal hypertension, cor pulmonale
Nematodes (Round Worms)				
Intestinal Round Worms				
Hookworms	Worldwide	Human feces[a] through skin	Very common	Anemia, fatigue, upper abdominal pain
Strongyloidiasis	Worldwide	Human feces[a] through skin	Common	Abdominal pain, diarrhea, pulmonary infiltrates, hemoptysis
Ascariasis	Worldwide	Human feces[a] through skin	Very common	Abdominal pain, bowel or biliary tract obstruction
Trichuriasis	Worldwide	Human feces[a]	Common	Asymptomatic or abdominal pain
Enterobiasis	Worldwide	Human feces[a]	Very common	Pruritis of anal mucosa
Tissue Round Worms				
Trichinosis	Worldwide	Pork[a]	Common	Fever, muscle aches
Filariasis	Africa, S. America, S. Asia	Mosquitos	Common	Fever, headache, lymphadenopathy, lymphatic obstruction, wheezing

[a] Can generally be prevented by clean water supplies, rigorous cooking of foods. Avoidance of open ponds and wearing shoes are important with those transmitted through the skin.
[b] Peripheral blood eosinophilia is a prominent feature of most helminthic infestations.

Table 7.11 **Infection in the Compromised Host**

Defect	Common Clinical Situation	Expected Pathogens
Phagocytic Function	Drug-induced granulocytopenia, acute leukemia, chronic granulomatous disease, aplastic anemia, rheumatoid arthritis, diabetes mellitus	*S. aureus, Pseudomonas,* enteric gram-negative rods, *Candida, Aspergillus, Serratia*
Antibody Deficiency	Myeloma, Waldenstrom's macroglobulinemia, chronic lymphocytic leukemia, hypogammaglobulinemias, drug-induced	*S. pneumoniae, H. influenzae Pseudomonas,* group A and B streptococci
Cellular Defects	Hodgkin's disease, sarcoid, corticosteroid therapy, drug-induced	*Mycobacteria, Candida, Cryptococcus, Herpes zoster, Toxoplasma, Pneumocystis*

Most authorities favor treating human bites initially and animal bites that present late with clinical infection, with high-dose penicillin as well as penicillinase-resistant semisynthetic penicillin.

Rabies is a fatal central nervous system infection transmitted by infected animals through their saliva. Although rabies is a rare disease in the Western hemisphere, it requires consideration with all animal bites. In the Western world, wild animals are the major source, since legislation commonly requires vaccination of pets. With the availability of human rabies vaccine, prophylaxis is easier and much safer. The recommendations of the communicable disease center or the local health department should be followed, with careful attention to animal quarantine until the presence or absence of rabies in the animal is established.

PARASITIC INFECTIONS

Countries without adequate water purification and sewage disposal systems have exceptionally high rates of parasitic infections. Although infections are rare in the developed countries, various estimates suggest 60 to 95 percent infection rates by one or more of the parasites listed in Table 7.10. When caring for patients who have travelled to these regions, the physician should consult a textbook emphasizing parasitic infections.

Malaria, trypanosomiasis, leishmaniasis, and filariasis are transmitted by insects. Schistosomiasis, hookworms, and strongyloidiasis may penetrate the skin from infested waters or soil. Most other parasites are transmitted in infected meat or feces. Clearly insect control programs, safe water supplies, avoidance of skin exposure to infected water or soil, and vigorous cooking of foods as appropriate, provide a high level of protection.

INFECTION IN THE COMPROMISED HOST

Infection due to organisms that do not typically produce disease, or overwhelming, recurrent or otherwise atypical infection due to common pathogens, should raise suspicion that the patient has altered defense mechanisms. Altered host defense mechanisms are an increasing problem as our population ages, with increased prevalence of malignant diseases, and as immunosuppressive drugs are used more widely in the treatment of malignant and collagen vascular diseases. The assessment of the immune mechanisms is discussed in Chapter 6. Infection in the compromised host may be caused by the organisms that are typically considered pathogenic, but particular attention must be given to possible opportunistic or unusual organisms. The clinical situation may suggest organisms that are known to occur in a patient with a particular type of defect, and may guide initial therapy (Table 7.11). Presentation of infection in the altered host may be subtle, with less fever, fewer constitutional symptoms, and reduced leukocytosis or antibody response. Prompt diagnostic studies with judicious cultures, biopsies, and serologic investigations are required to establish a diagnosis. The lung is most frequently involved; a detailed discussion is included in Chapter 15.

Little specific therapy is available to reconstitute the host defects, although leukocyte transfusions may be indicated in some circumstances. Any procedure that further compromises the host, such as an intravenous indwelling catheter, an indwelling urinary catheter, or an unnecessary diagnostic procedure, should be avoided unless absolutely necessary for providing information useful in the management of the patient. A treatment decision is usually required before a specific agent is recovered, and the choice must consider the clinical situation, any known host defects, and the probable pathogens. Particularly diligent efforts at specific etiologic diagnosis are required in these patients, since the clinical clues are often inadequate.

REFERENCES

1. Antimicrobial prophylaxis for surgery. Medical Letter. 23:77–80, 1981.
2. Dinarello, C.A., Wolff, S.M.: Pathogenesis of fever in man. N. Engl. J. Med. 298:607–612, 1978.

3. Stites, D.P. et al: Basic and Clinical Immunology. 4th ed. Los Altos, Calif., Lange Med Pub, 1982.

4. Goodman, R.A., Orenstein, W.A., Hinman, A.R.: Vaccination and disease prevention for adults. J. A. M. A. 248:1607–1610, 1982.

5. Grieco, M.H. (ed): Infections in the Abnormal Host. New York, Yorke Med Books, 1980.

6. Kunin, C.M., Edelman, R. (eds): The impact of infections on medical care in the United States. Ann. Int. Med. 89(5, part II):739–866, 1978.

7. Mandell, G.L., Douglas, R.G., Bennett, J.E.: Principles and Practice of Infectious Diseases. New York, John Wiley & Sons, 1979.

8. Treatment of Sexually Transmitted Diseases. Medical Letter. 24:29, 1982.

8

Inherited Diseases

R. Brian Lowry, M.D.

The frequency of genetic disease in the population is considerable, and is relatively higher in developed countries where malnutrition and infections are under control, than in undeveloped countries. It is difficult to quote a precise figure of the frequency, but a minimal estimate in British Columbia, Canada, shows that 10 percent of the population is likely to have a disease that is either totally or partially determined by genetic factors. Although genetic disease is more prevalent in the pediatric age group, nevertheless, there is an increasing awareness of genetic factors in disease in the adult population, particularly as more genetic diseases become treatable.

In terms of etiology, disease may be considered genetic or environmental, or both when there is a gene-environment interaction. This latter category is often referred to as *multifactorial inheritance*, and accounts for a large number of the common diseases that affect humans, such as diabetes mellitus, essential hypertension, and schizophrenia, as well as many congenital malformations such as cleft lip with or without cleft palate, neural tube disorders (spina bifida and anencephaly), and many forms of congenital heart disease.

The group that is totally (or almost completely) genetic in origin may be divided into *chromosomal errors* and *single-gene (Mendelian) disorders*. This latter category is further subdivided into autosomal dominant, autosomal recessive, X-linked dominant, and X-linked recessive traits. In both major categories, it is primarily the mutant chromosome or gene (*genotype*) that determines the external characteristics (*phenotype*), although it should be appreciated that there is often some variability in the expression (clinical severity) of the gene. The reason why one gene causes more severe disease in one person than in another is unknown, although it may be related to modifying factors in other genes. A gene that causes an effect in more than one system is said to be *pleiotropic*.

FAMILY HISTORY

The importance of taking a good family history cannot be overemphasized, because it is the best screening test that is available. Physicians frequently feel that it is of less importance or significance if a five- or six-generation history cannot be obtained, but such is not the case. Very useful information can be obtained by a three-generation pedigree, which is generally obtainable in every case. For example, where the index patient (also called *proband* or *propositus*) is an adult, information should be obtained on his (or her) siblings and their offspring, his children, and his parents. If one section of the family history appears to lead to pertinent information, then it may be expanded in the appropriate direction. It is necessary to be specific and to ask first of all about the disorder in question or symptoms of the disorder if there is no precise diagnosis. Second, the physician should find out if there is any specific disorder that seems to occur frequently in the family even if it is not present in the index patient. Third, the physician should ascertain whether there is any disorder present that is known to be genetically determined. Vague questions, such as inquiries about a family history of tuberculosis, allergies, or cancer should be avoided. The physician should also ask about consanguinity, particularly in the case of the parents of the index patient, and if there are any other instances of consanguinity or possible consanguinity. Consanguinity

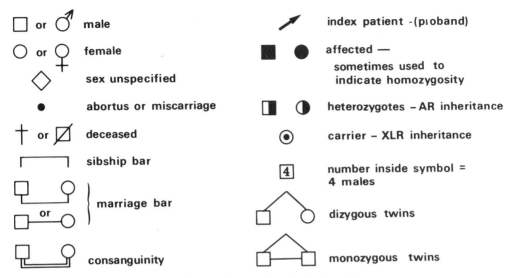

Fig. 8.1 Commonly used symbols for pedigrees.

may be suspected if the antecedents on both sides of the family come from a long settled, small, isolated community, for example, an island such as Tristan da Cunha.

The family history will be more reliable if the patient is asked to give actual names, dates of birth and death (or ages at death), and causes of death. Ethnic origins can be helpful, since there are some single-gene disorders that are more frequently found in certain groups, for example, Tay-Sachs disease in Ashkenazi Jews, hemoglobinopathies in blacks of African descent, Beta-thalassemia in Mediterranean peoples (Italians, Greeks, and others). It is useful to record the family history in pedigree form, using the symbols in Figure 8.1.

THE CONCEPT OF THE GENE

The human *genome* consists of 23 pairs of chromosomes, which in turn consist of strands of deoxyribonucleic acid (DNA) in the form of a double helix consisting of two sugar-phosphate strands connected by bases through hydrogen bonds. The bases consist of two purines, adenine (A) and guanine (G), and two pyrimidines, thymine (T) and cytosine (C). In the double-stranded DNA, adenine pairs with thymine and guanine with cytosine.

One of the properties of DNA is replication, which is accomplished by the parent strand of DNA opening up as the base pairs separate, rather like a zipper unzipping. Each single-strand DNA then attracts complementary bases according to the rule: A pairing with T, and G with C, so that ultimately two double strands of DNA are formed from one.

The production of proteins is another important function of DNA. Indeed, all gene products are proteins, either structural, such as muscle, or enzyme, such as amylase. The sequence of bases on the DNA forms the code that transcribes into messenger ribonucleic acid (mRNA), which takes the message from the nucleus into the cytoplasm and is there translated into protein (Fig. 8.2).

The mRNA bases are complementary to the DNA bases, except that A pairs with uracil (U) instead of T. A sequence of three bases constitutes a *codon*, which is a message either to code a specific amino acid or to code for a stop.

The *ribosomes* are the sites of assembly in the cytoplasm, and another RNA, known as transfer RNA (tRNA), brings a specific amino acid to the site in accordance with the code of the mRNA. The four nucleic acids are read in triplets and, theoretically, can code for 64 amino acids. The fact that there are only 20 amino acids means that some can be coded by different triplet codons. For example, phenylalanine may be coded by the sequence UUU or UUC, and there are six different codons for leucine. Some codons are responsible for the termination of transcription.

The term *gene* is used to denote a unit of heredity, and is a segment of a DNA molecule coding for a single polypeptide. Each *chromosome* is a linear array of thousands of genes. Sometimes a gene will undergo a permanent, heritable change, which is termed a *mutation*. This can occur in different ways, such as substitution, deletion, or insertion of base pairs. Most mutations are stable and constitute a permanent alteration in DNA. The causes are largely unknown, but events such as exposures to radiation, chemicals, or viruses can be responsible. The "spontaneous" rate of mutation ranges from 10^{-4} to 10^{-6} per gene per generation. Mutations can have very serious consequences. For example, the change from glutamic acid to valine in the beta chain of hemoglobin produces hemoglobin S, that is, the sickle hemoglobin; or if the change is from glutamic acid to lysine, hemoglobin C is produced. Both have resulted from a change at the sixth position of the polypeptide chain.

Other mutations can cause the polypeptide chain of a protein to end prematurely, thus resulting in a deletion of genetic information. Deletion of a base, if it occurs, may cause the remainder of the message to shift, that is, a frame-shift mutation, again resulting in a different message with functional consequences.

Structural gene mutations, such as the hemoglobinopathies, account for many of the Mendelian disorders in humans. Jacob and Monod proposed additional genes that control or regulate the structural gene and thus the amount of the product. Regulatory mechanisms in humans are less well understood than are those in bacteria, but it is known that these mechanisms can be influenced by a number of factors such as hormones and histones (protein components of

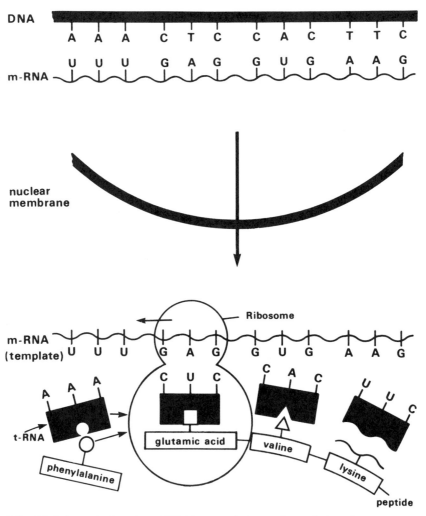

Fig. 8.2 Schematic drawing of DNA transcription and translation. (From Emery AEH: Elements of Medical Genetics. 4th ed. Edinburgh, Churchill Livingstone, 1975, with permission.)

chromosomes). In one form of beta thalassemia (β + thal) there is reduced synthesis of the beta chain mRNA, which is probably an example of a mutation in a controller gene.

CHROMOSOMAL DISORDERS

In somatic cells the normal number of chromosomes in man is 46 (diploid number), composed of 23 pairs. Twenty-two of the pairs are known as *autosomes* and the remaining pair are the *sex chromosomes*. These are designated XX in the female and XY in the male. In gametes there are only 23 chromosomes (the haploid number), and the diploid number is restored at fertilization in most instances. Each pair of chromosomes can be identified by the overall size, the location of the major constriction known as the *centromere,* and the unique pattern of banding after staining. When chromosomes of a metaphase spread are arranged in their pairs, the array is known as a *karyotype*, and by convention the short arm of a chromosome is designated by the letter *p* (petit) and the long arm by the letter *q*. Prior to the development of the special staining preparations, it was impossible to distinguish some of the chromosomes into exact pairs, and consequently one of the early classifications designated groups A through G. With the advent of better methods that produce dark and light (or bright and dull) bands, the chromosomes are now referred to by number (Fig. 8.3). Many different banding methods are employed, and these enable each individual chromosome to be identified, if there are abnormalities in chromosome structure, then precise breakpoints can be defined. The different regions of the chromosomes have been divided by a numerical system as is seen in Figure 8.5, which also shows the number of gene loci that have been actually mapped to specific regions of the chromosome.

To understand the reports on the results of chromosome analysis, it is necessary to refer to the terminology made on human cytogenetic nomenclature at two international conferences (Chicago 1966, and Paris 1971), some of which are detailed below and in Table 8.1. The total number of chromosomes in the karyotype is given first, followed by the sex chromosomes, for example, 46,XY means a normal male karyotype. A plus or a minus sign (+ or −) before a number or letter means additional or missing chromosomes; for example, 47,XX + 21 means a female with an extra chromosome 21, in other words, Down syndrome or trisomy 21.

Mosaicism is designated by a slant; for example,

Table 8.1 **Some Chromosome Nomenclature Symbols (Chicago and Paris Conferences)**

A–G	chromosome groups—Patau classification
1–22	autosome number—Paris Conference
X,Y	sex chromosomes
/	mosaicism, e.g., 46/47
+	additional chromosome
−	missing chromosome
cen	centromere
del	deletion
der	derivative
dic	dicentric
dup	duplication
i	isochromosome
ins	insertion
inv	inversion
p	short arm of chromosome
q	long arm of chromosome
r	ring chromosome
s	satellite
t	translocation
ter	terminal, for example, pter = terminal portion of the short arm of a chromosome

45,X/46,XX indicates mosaic Turner syndrome. Structural alterations of the short (p) or long (q) arms of a chromosome will be followed by a plus or minus sign if there is an excess or a deficiency; for example, 5p− indicates a deficiency or deletion of part of the short arm of chromosome 5. The terminology for translocations becomes complicated; however, a simple example of a person carrying a balanced translocation is 45,XY,t(DqGq), indicating that the long arm of a D group and a G group chromosome have been united in a translocation, and hence there is a reduction in the total number of chromosomes to 45.

Chromosomes are usually studied after a short-term culture using lymphocytes that are stimulated with phytohemagglutinin, a mitogen. After 72 hours, Colcemid is added to the culture to prevent further cell division and to accumulate metaphases. Cells are suspended in a hypotonic salt solution to make them swell for chromosome spreading, and they are examined after fixing. Cultures can also be done using fibroblasts from a skin biopsy or from other organs using necropsy material. Fibroblast cultures are especially helpful in the study of mosaicism. Marrow cells can be examined without culture, since a sufficient number of cells in mitosis may be seen. This technique is helpful where a rapid chromosome diagnosis is needed, for example, in a critically ill newborn infant suspected of having a chromosomal syndrome where heroic measures are being contemplated.

It should be recalled that *mitosis* is the division of somatic cells after its DNA synthesis has been completed. Each cell has 46 duplicated chromosomes,

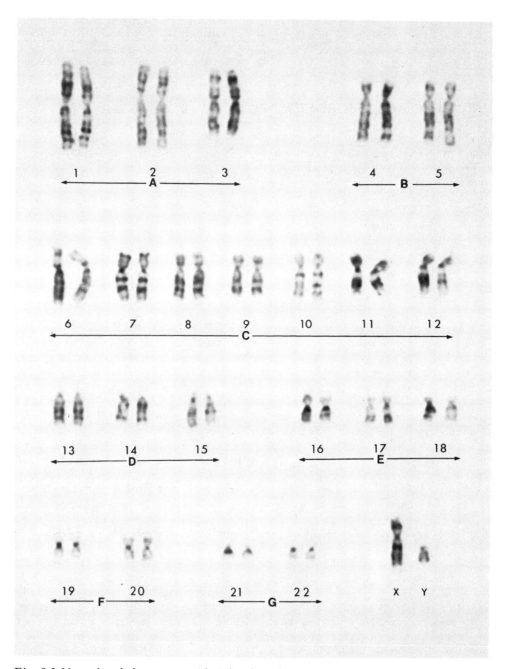

Fig. 8.3 Normal male karyotype with G-banding (by treating with trypsin and staining with Giemsa). The homologous chromosome pairs are labeled, and the seven groups A to G are indicated (2,200×). (Courtesy of Lin CC: University of Calgary.)

and after division forms two daughter cells, each having 46 chromosomes. Postzygotic errors in cell division can result in mosaicism where there is more then one cell line, as in the example quoted previously, 45,X/46,XX. *Meiosis,* on the other hand, is the reduction division that takes place in the germ cells or gametes, whereby 46 chromosomes are reduced to 23. If this fails to occur properly, the gamete may have an incorrect number of chromosomes.

The frequency of chromosome abnormalities depends on the stage of life at which they are sought. For example, about 0.5 percent of newborns have a chromosomal error, whereas the frequency in spontaneous abortuses is about 50 percent. Chromosome abnormalities may involve either the number or the structure of chromosomes.

AUTOSOMAL DISORDERS

Trisomies

In the most common type of abnormality there are three copies of a chromosome instead of two, and these are known as trisomies. The one most frequently seen in clinical practice is Down syndrome, previously known as Mongolism. Because it involves the chromosome 21, it is often referred to as trisomy 21 (Fig. 8.4). The origin of the extra chro-

mosome is a failure of separation, that is, nondisjunction at either the first or second meiotic division of oogenesis or spermatogenesis. Previously it was thought that the error always took place in oogenesis, but recent studies have indicated that the extra chromosome can be of paternal origin in approximately one fourth of cases. About 95 percent of Down syndrome infants have a trisomy 21 karyotype.

Down syndrome occurs with a frequency of approximately 1 in 600 live births. The cause of meiotic nondisjunction is unknown, although there is a well-known maternal age effect (Table 8.2). The clinical features include marked hypotonia at birth, brachycephalic skull with flattened face, epicanthic folds, upward slanting palpebral fissures, Brushfield spots in the iris, small dysmorphic ears, brachydactyly, fifth-finger clinodactyly, single palmar creases, and mental retardation. Mental retardation is usually in the moderate range, but individuals can be found

(*Text continued on p. 203.*)

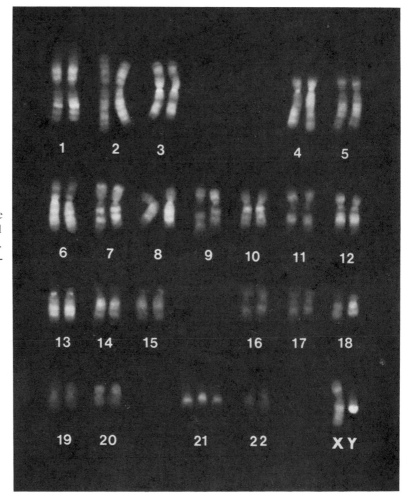

Fig. 8.4 Q-banded karyotype of a boy with trisomy 21 (Down syndrome) (2,100×). (Courtesy of Lin CC, University of Calgary.)

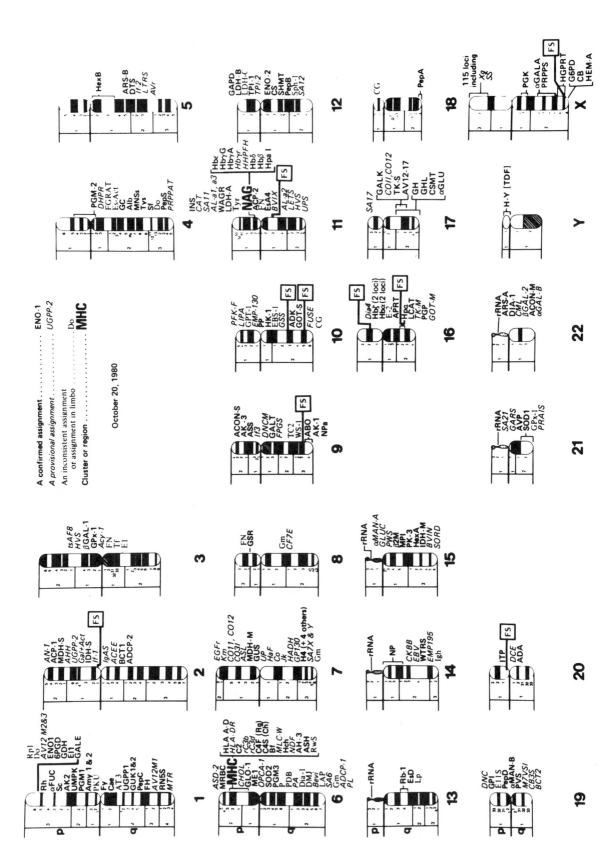

A confirmed assignment ENO-1
A provisional assignment UGPP-2
An inconsistent assignment
  or assignment in limbo .... Do
Cluster or region .... MHC

October 20, 1980

200

are those given in the International System for Human Cytogenetics Nomenclature 1978. An assignment is considered confirmed if found in two laboratories or several families; it is considered provisional if based on evidence from only one laboratory. Inconsistent assignments based on conflicting evidence and assignments for which the evidence is weaker than that for provisional assignment are separately indicated (also termed *tentative* or *in limbo*). In the Key for gene locus symbols, the chromosomal location, and in some instances the regional location, of the gene is given. Those chromosomal or regional locations indicated in parentheses represent assignments by indirect means, for example, linkage to a locus directly assigned. Also indicated are methods of assignment: F = family linkage studies; S = somatic cell hybrid studies; A = in situ annealing ("hybridization"); H-S = molecular hybridization in solution; RE = restriction endonuclease mapping; D = deletion mapping or dosage effects; AAS = deduction for amino acid sequence (Lepore phenomenon); LD = linkage disequilibrium; V = virus effects; Ch = chromosome change; OT = ovarian teratoma; EM = exclusion mapping; H = homology; R = radiation-induced gene segregation. (From McKusick VA: The Anatomy of the Human Genome. J Hered 71:370–391, 1980, with permission. Copyright 1980 by the American Genetic Association.)

KEY

ABO	ABO blood group—9q34 (F)
ACEE	Acetylcholinesterase expression—chr. 2 (D)
ACON-M	Aconitase, mitochondrial—22q11-qter (S)
ACON-S	Aconitase, soluble—9pter-p13 (S)
ACP1	Acid phosphatase-1—2p23 (D,S)
ACP2	Acid phosphatase-2—11p12-cen (S)
ACY1	Aminoacylase-1—3pter-q13 (S)
ADA	Adenosine deaminase—20q13-qter (S,D)
ADCP1	Adenosine deaminase complexing protein-1—chr. 6 (S)
ADCP2	Adenosine deaminase complexing protein-2—chr. 2 (S)
ADK	Adenosine kinase—10q11-q24 (S,D-EM)
AH3	Adrenal hyperplasia III (21-hydroxylase deficiency) (6p2105-6p23) (F)
AHH	Aryl hydrocarbon hydroxylase—2p (S)
AK1	Adenylate kinase-1 (soluble)—9q34 (F,S,D)
AK2	Adenylate kinase-2 (mitochondrial)—1p32-p34 (S,F,R)
AK3	Adenylate kinase-3 (mitochondrial)—9pter-p13 (S)
AL	Lethal antigen: 3 loci—a1, a3 on 11p13-pter; a2 on 11q13-qter (S)
Alb	Albumin—4q11-q13 (F)
AMY1	Amylase, salivary—1p1 (F-F)
AMY2	Amylase, pancreatic—1p1 (F-F)
An1	Aniridia, type 1 (chr. 2; linked to ACP1) (F)
APRT	Adenine phosphoribosyltransferase—16q (S,D)
ARS-A	Arylsulfatase A—chr. 22 (S)
ARS-B	Arylsulfatase B—chr. 5 (S)
ASD2	Atrial septal defect, secundum type (chr. 6: linked to HLA) (F)
ASH	Asymmetric septal hypertrophy (chr. 6; linked to HLA) (F)
ASL	Argininosuccinate lyase—7pter-q22 (S)
ASS	Argininosuccinate synthetase—chr. 9 (S,D)
AT3	Antithrombin III (chr. 1) (F)
AV12M1	Adenovirus-12 chromosome modification site-1—1q42-43 (V)
AV12M2	Adenovirus-12 chromosome modification site-2—1p36 (V)
AV12M3	Adenovirus-12 chromosome modification site-3—1q21 (V)
AV12-17	Adenovirus-12 chromosome modification site-17—17q21 q22 (V)
AVP	Antiviral protein—21q21-qter (S,D)
AVr	Antiviral state regulator—chr. 5 (D)

β2M (B2M)	Beta-2-microglobulin—15q14-q21 (S)
BCT-1	Branched chain amino acid transferase-1—chr. 12 (S)
BCT-2	Branched chain amino acid transferase-2—chr. 19 (S)
BEVI	Baboon M7 virus infection—chr. 6 (S)
BF	Properdin factor B—chr. 6 (in MHC) (F)
BVIN	BALB virus induction, N-tropic—chr. 15 (S)
BVIX	BALB virus induction, xenotropic—chr. 11 (S)
C2	Complement component-2—chr. 6 (in MHC) (F)
C4F	Complement component-4 fast—chr. 6 (in MHC) (F)
C4S	Complement component-4 slow—chr. 6 (in MHC) (F)
Cae	Cataract, zonular pulverulent (chr. 1: linked to Fy) (F)
CAT	Catalase—11p (S)
CB	Colorblindness (deutan and protan) (Xq28) (F)
CB3S	Coxsackie B3 virus susceptibility—chr. 19 (S)
CF7E	Clotting factor VII expression (chr. 8) (D)
CG	Chorionic gonadotropin (chr. 10 and 18; chr. 5 or 6) (S,REb)
Ch	Chido blood group—same as C4S (F)
CHOL	Hereditary hypercholesterolemia—chr. 6 (?linked to HLA) (F)
CKBB	Creatine kinase, brain type—chr. 14 (S)
CML	Chronic myeloid leukemia—22q12 (Ch)
Co	Colton blood group (chr. 7) (D,F)
COI1	Collagen I alpha-1 chain—chr. 7 and 17 (S,M)
COI2	Collagen I alpha-2 chain—chr. 7 and 17 (S,M)
COI31	Collagen III alpha-1 chain—chr. 7 (S)
CS	Citrate synthase, mitochondrial—(chr. 12 (S)
CSMT (or CSH)	Chorionic somatomammotropin—(chr. 17) (S)
DCE	Desmosteral-to-cholesterol enzyme—chr. 20 (F)
DHPR	Quinoid dihydropteridine reductase—chr. 4 (S)
Dia-1	NADH-diaphorase—chr. 22 (S)
DIA-4	Diaphorase-4—chr. 16 (S)
DMJ	Juvenile diabetes mellitus (chr. 6: ?linked to HLA) (F,LD)
DNC	Lysosomal DNA-ase—chr. 19 (S)
DNCM	Cytoplasmic membrane DNA—9qh (H-A)
Do	Dombrock blood group (?chr. 1 or 4) (F)
DTS	Diphtheria toxin sensitivity—5q15-qter (S)
E1	Pseudocholinesterase-1 (?chr. 3; linked to Tf) (F)
E2	Pseudocholinesterase-2—16cen-q22 (F)

E11S	Echo 11 sensitivity—19q (S)
EBS1	Epidermolysis bullosa, Ogna type (chr. 10) (F)
EBV	Epstein-Barr virus integration site—chr. 14 (S)
EGFR	Epidermal growth factor, receptor for—chr. 7 (S)
EII	Elliptocytosis-1—(1p; linked to Rh) (F)
EMPI30	External membrane protein-130—chr. 10 (S)
EMPI95	External membrane protein-195—chr. 14 (S)
ENO1	Enolase-1—1p36-1pter (S.F,R)
ENO2	Enolase-2—chr. 12 (S)
Es-Act	Esterase activator—chr. 4 or 5 (S)
EsA4	Esterase-A4—11cen-q22 (S)
EsD	Esterase D—13q14 (S,F,D)
FGRAT	Formylglycinamide riboside amidotransferase—chr. 4 or 5 (S)
FH	Fumarate hydratase—1q42-qter (S.R)
FN	Fibronectin—chr. 8, 11 (S)
FPGS	Folypolyglutamate synthetase—chr. 9 (S)
FS	Fragile site, observed in cultured cells, with or without folate deficient medium, or BrdU—2q11; 10q23; 10q25; 11q13; 16q124; 16q22; 20p11; Xq27 (F,S)
αFUC (FUCA)	Alpha-L-fucosidase—1p32-p34 (S.F,R)
FUSE	Polykaryocyosis inducer—chr. 10 (S)
Fy	Duffy blood group—1q13 (F,Fc)
Gal+Act	Galactose + activator—chr. 2 (S)
αGALA	Alpha-galactosidase A (Fabry disease)—Xq22-q24 (F,S,R)
αGALB	Alpha-galactosidase B—22q13-qter (S)
βGAL-1	Beta-galactosidase-1—3pter-q13 (S)
βGAL-2	Beta-galactosidase-2—22q13-qter
GALE	Galactose-4-epimerase—1p21-pter (S.LD)
GALK	Galactokinase—17q21-q22 (S.C.R)
GALT	Galactose-1-phosphate uridylytransferase—9p13 or 9p22 (S)
GAPD	Glyceraldehyde-3-phosphate dehydrogenase—12p122-pter (S.D)
GARS	Glycinamide ribonucleotide synthetase—chr. 21 (S)
GC	Group-specific component—4q11-q13 (F,Fc)
GDH	Glucose dehydrogenase—1p21-pter (1p32-pter) (S)
GH	Growth hormone—chr. 17 (S)
GHL	Growth hormone like—chr. 17 (S.RE)
αGLU (GLUA)	Alpha-glucosidase—chr. 17 (S)
GLUC	Neutral alpha-glucosidase C—chr. 15 (S)
GLO1	Glyoxylase I—6p21-6p22 (F,S)
	(continued next page)

Fig. 8.5 (continued)

GOT-M	Glutamate oxaloacetic transaminase, mitochondrial—chr. 16 (S)
GOT-S	Glutamate oxaloacetate transaminase, soluble—10q24-q26 (S,D)
G6PD	Glucose-6-phosphate dehydrogenase—Xq28 (F,S,R)
GP1.30	Granulocyte glycoprotein—7q22-qter (D)
GPI	Glucosphosphate isomerase—chr. 19 (S,D)
GPT1	Glutamate pyruvate transaminase, soluble—chr. 10 (F)
GP1	Glutathione peroxidase1—3p13-q12 (S)
GSR	Glutathione reductase—8p21 (S,D)
GSS	Glutamate-gamma-semialdehyde synthetase—chr. 10 (S)
Gm	Immunoglobulin heavy chain—chr. 6, 7, 8 (see Igh) (S,F,c,S,S)
GUK1 & 2	Guanylate kinase-1 & 2—1q32-q42 (S)
GUS	Beta-glucuronidase—chr. 7 (S)
H4	Histone H4 and 4 other histone genes—chr. 7 (A)
HADH	Hydroxyacyl-CoA dehydrogenase—chr. 7 (S)
HaF	Hageman factor—7q35 (D)
Hbα(HBA)	Hemoglobin alpha chain—chr. 16 (S-HS)
Hbβ(HBB)	Hemoglobin beta chain—11p1205-p1208 (LD,AAS,F,RE,S)
Hbδ(HBD)	Hemoglobin delta chain—11p1205-p1208 (LD,AAS,F,RE,S)
Hbγr	Hemoglobin gamma regulator—11p1205-p1208 (RE)
Hbγ(HBG)	Hemoglobin gamma chains—11p1205-p1208 (AAS,RE)
Hbε(HBE)	Hemoglobin epsilon chain—11p1205-p1208 (AAS,RE)
HBζ(HBZ)	Hemoglobin zeta chain—chr. 16 (RE)
Hch	Hemochromatosis (chr. 6; linked to HLA) (LD,F)
HEM-A	Classic hemophilia—Xq28 (F)
HexA	Hexosaminidase A—1q22-15qter (S)
HexB	Hexosaminidase B—5cen-q13 (S)
HGPRT	Hypoxanthine-guanine phosphoribosyltransferase—Xq26-qter (F,S,R)
HHPFH	Heterocellular hereditary persistence of fetal hemoglobin—11p1205-p1208 (F)
HK1	Hexokinase-1—10pter-q24 (S)
HLA(A-D)	Human leukocyte antigens—6p2105-p23 (F)
HLA-DR	Human leukocyte antigen, D-related—6p2105-p23 (F)
Hpα	Haptoglobin, alpha—chr. 16 (Fc)
Hpa1	Hpa I restriction endonuclease polymorphism—11p1205-p1208 (RE)
HVS	Herpes virus sensitivity (chr. 3 and 11) (S)
H-Y	Y histocompatibility antigen (Y chr.) (F)
IDH-M	Isocitrate dehydrogenase, mitochondrial—15q21-qter (S)
IDH-S	Isocitrate dehydrogenase, soluble—2q11 or 2q32-qter (S)
If1	Interferon-1—2p23-qter (S)
If2	Interferon-2 (chr. 5) (S)
If3	Interferon-3 (chr. 9) (S)
IgAS	Immunoglobulin heavy chains attachment site—chr. 2 (S)
Igh	Immunoglobulin heavy chains (mu, gamma, alpha)—chr. 14 (see Gm) (S)
Ins	Insulin—11p (S)
ITP	Inosine triphosphatase—20p (S)
Jk	Kidd blood group—7q (Fc)
Km	Kappa immunoglobulin light chains, Inv (chr. 7) (F-Fc)
LAP	Laryngeal adductor paralysis—(chr. 6: linked to HLA) (F)
LCAT	Lecithin-cholesterol acyltransferase—(16q22; linked to Hp alpha) (F,LD)
LDH-A	Lactate dehydrogenase A—11p1203-p1208 (S)
LDH-B	Lactate dehydrogenase B—12p121-p122 (S,D)
LDH-C	Lactate dehydrogenase C—(12p: linked to LDH-B in pigeon) (H)
LIPA	Lysosomal acid lipase-A—chr. 10 (S)
Lp	Lipoprotein-Lp—chr. 13 (F)
LTRS	Leucyl-tRNA synthetase—chr. 5 (S)
β2M (B2M)	Beta-2-microglobulin—15q22-15qter (15q12-q21) (S)
M7VSI	Baboon M7 virus sensitivity-1—chr. 19 (S)
αMAN-A	Cytoplasmic alpha-D-mannosidase—15q11-qter (S)
αMAN-B	Lysosomal alpha-D-mannosidase—19pter-q13 (S)
MDH-M	Malate dehydrogenase, mitochondrial—7p22-q22 (S)
MDH-S	Malate dehydrogenase, soluble—2p23 (S)
MEI	Malic enzyme, soluble—6p21-q16 (S)
MHC	Major histocompatibility complex—6p2105-p23 (F,S)
MLC-W	Mixed lymphocyte culture, weak (chr. 6) (F)
MNSs	MNSs blood group—4q (F,Fc)
MPI	Mannosephosphate isomerase—15q22-qter (S)
MRBC	Monkey red blood cell receptor—chr. 6 (S)
MTR	5-Methyltetrahydrofolate: L-homocysteine S-methyltransferase, or tetrahydropteroyl-glutamate methyltransferase—chr. 1 (S)
NAG	Non-alpha globin region—12p1205-1208 (S,RE)
NDF	Neutrophil differentiation factor (chr. 6) (LD)
NP	Nucleoside phosphorylase—14q13 (S,D)
NPa	Nail-patella syndrome—(9q3; linked to ABO) (F)
OPCA1	Olivopontocerebellar atrophy l—(chr. 6; linked to HLA) (F)
P	P blood group (chr. 6) (S,F)
PA	Pasminogen activator (chr. 6) (S)
PDB	Paget disease of bone—(chr. 6; ?linked to HLA) (F)
PepA	Peptidase A—18q23-18qter (S,D)
PepB	Peptidase B—12q21 (S)
PepC	Peptidase C—1q25. or 1q42 (S,R)
PepD	Peptidase D—(chr. 19) (S)
PepS	Peptidase S—4pter-q12 (S)
6PGD	6-phosphogluconate dehydrogenase—1p34-pter (S)
PGK	Phosphoglycerate kinase—Xq13 (F,S)
PGM1	Phosphoglucomutase-1—1p32; 1p221-p311; 1p33-p34 (F,S,R)
PGM2	Phosphoglucomutase-2—4p14-q12 (S)
PGM3	Phosphoglucomutase-3—6q (S,F,OT)
PGP	Phosphoglycolate phosphatase—16p (S)
PK3	Pyruvate kinase-3—15q14-qter (S)
PKU	Phenylketonuria (1p; linked to AMY) (F)
PL	Prolactin—chr. 6 (S)
PP	Inorganic pyrophosphatase—10pter-q24 (S)
PRPPAT	Phosphoribosylpyrophosphate amidotransferase—4pter-q21 (S)
PRPPS	Phosphoribosylpyrophosphate synthetase—X chr. (F,S)
PRAIS	Phosphoribosylaminoimidazole synthetase—chr. 21 (S)
PVS	Polio virus sensitivity—19q (S)
PWS	Prader-Willi syndrome—15q11-q12 (Ch)
RBI	Retinoblastoma-1—13q12-q14; 13q21-22 (Ch)
rC3b	Receptor for C3b—chr. 6 (in MHC) (S)
rC3d	Receptor for C3d—chr. 6 (in MHC) (S)
Rg	Rodgers blood group—same as C4F (F)
Rh	Rhesus blood group (1p32-pter) (F,S,D)
RN5S	5S RNA gene(s)—1q42-q43 (A)
RP1	Retinitis pigmentosa-1 (chr. 1) (F)
rRNA	Ribosomal RNA—13p12, 14p12, 15p12, 21p12, 22p12 (A)
RwS	Ragweed sensitivity—(chr. 6; ?linked to HLA) (F)
SA6	Surface antigen 6—chr. 6 (S)
SA7	Surface antigen 7—7p12-pter (S)
SA11	Surface antigen 11—11p (S)
SA12	Surface antigen 12—chr. 12 (S)
SA17	Surface antigen 17—chr. 17 (S)
SA21	Surface antigen 21—chr. 21 (S)
Sc	Scianna blood group—(1p32-p34) (F)
SHMT	Serine hydroxymethyltransferase—chr. 12 (S)
SOD1	Superoxide dismutase, soluble—21q211 (S,D)
SOD2	Superoxide dismutase, mitochondrial—6q21 (S)
SORD	Sorbitol dehydrogenase—15pter-q21 (S)
Sph1	Spherocytosis, Denver type (8p1 or chr. 12) (Fc)
SS	Steroid sulfatase (?Xp22-pter) (F,S)
TC2	Transcobalamin II—9q (?linked to ABO) (F)
TDF	Testis determining factor—prob. same as H-Y (F)
Tf	Transferrin—?chr. 3 (H)
TK-M	Thymidine kinase, mitochondrial—chr. 16 (S)
TK-S	Thymidine kinase, soluble—17q21-q22 (S,C,R)
TPI-1 & 2	Triosephosphate isomerase-1 & 2—TPI-1 on 12p12.2-pter (S)
tsAF8	Temperature-sensitive (AF8) complement—chr. 3 (S)
Tyr	Tyrosinase—(?11p) (H)
Tys	Scleroblastosis—(4q; linked to MNSs) (F)
UGPP1	Uridyl diphosphate glucose pyrophosphorylase-1—1q21-q23 (S,R)
UGPP2	Uridyl diphosphate glucose pyrophosphorylase-2—chr. 2 (S)
UMPK	Uridine monophosphate kinase—1p32 (S,R)
UP	Uridine phosphorylase—chr. 7 (S)
UPS	Uroporphyrinogen I synthase—chr. 11 (S)
WAGR	Wilms tumor—aniridia/ambiguous genitalia/mental retardation—11p13 (Ch)
WTRS	Tryptophanyl-tRNA synthetase—chr. 14 (S)
WS1	Waardenburg syndrome-1—(chr. 9; ?linked to ABO) (F)
Xg	Xg blood group (X chr., ?Xp2) (F)

Table 8.2 **Approximate Maternal Age-Specific Risks for Down Syndrome**

Age in Years	Fractional Rate
≤17–14	1/1,200
25–29	1/1,200
30–34	1/850
35–37	1/370
38–40	1/150
41–43	1/70
44–46 +	1/30

(Adapted with permission from Trimble BK, Baird PA: Maternal age and Down-syndrome: Age-specific incidence rates by single-year intervals. Am J Med Genet 2:1–5, 1978.)

who are severely retarded while others are in the milder range. About 30 percent have a congenital heart defect, often an atrial septal defect of the ostium primum type, and there is an increased frequency of leukemia. Life tables now indicate that with prompt treatment of infections, and surgery for the congenital heart defect, the life span of individuals with Down syndrome is not too different from that of the normal population.

The other autosomal trisomies that are occasionally seen are trisomy 13 and trisomy 18. Each of these show marked mental retardation with many congenital malformations and a markedly reduced life span, with few of them surviving beyond 2 years. While many autosomal trisomies are found in spontaneous abortuses, there are few if any other examples of autosomal trisomies in live births except in cases of mosaicism, for example, in trisomy 8 mosaicism. In these individuals there is mental retardation and some striking flexion deformities of the fingers and toes, with marked creasing of the sole of the foot.

Most trisomies are sporadic events. However, there are a few families in whom nondisjunction has occurred more than once, and from these, empiric recurrence risk figures have been developed. For Down syndrome, it has been shown that once a couple has had one affected child, there is a nonspecific risk of a repeat occurrence, which is about 1 percent. Such pregnancies can be monitored by means of amniocentesis, which will be dealt with in a later section.

Translocation

When nonhomologous chromosomes exchange portions, the result is known as a *translocation*. An example of this is shown in Figure 8.6, where there has been exchange of material between a chromo-some 21 and a chromosome 14. If a person carries a 14/21 translocation in balanced form, theoretically six types of gametes can be produced, only three of which are viable. Hence, the risk of such a parent having a Down syndrome infant is 30 percent. In fact, due to prenatal loss and/or gametic selection, the risks are less than that. The risks also vary with the sex of the carrier parent. Thus, the empiric risk of such a translocation parent having an affected child is generally in the 5 to 10 percent range. About 4 percent of Down syndrome cases involve a translocation, and in about one half of the cases the translocation is inherited. In another type of translocation, two of the smaller acrocentric chromosomes fuse together so that the two long arms are preserved. This may involve two chromosome 21s or a chromosome 21 and a chromosome 22. Clearly, in the case of a 21/21 translocation, a carrier parent will transmit the translocation or no chromosome 21 at all into the gamete. In the first instance the result will be a Down syndrome child, and in the second it will be a nonviable pregnancy; thus, the recurrence risk for Down syndrome is virtually 100 percent. Where the 21/22 translocation occurs in a carrier parent, there is an increased recurrence risk of Down syndrome, but as with the 14/21 example, the actual risk is less than the theoretical one, and is in the 5 to 15 percent range.

Mosaicism

Mosaicism involves an abnormality occurring after the formation of the zygote, resulting in two or more cell lines, each having a different chromosome constitution. This can occur in Down syndrome and, in fact, mosaicism accounts for about 1 percent of Down syndrome infants, many of whom are diagnosed immediately because they are no different from the usual Down syndrome infant. However, in others the diagnosis is delayed because they appear more mildly affected than the usual Down syndrome infant. Mosaicism is extremely common in the sex-chromosome disorders, particularly Turner syndrome.

Deletions and Inversions

The production of deletions and inversions involves breakage of a chromosome, usually with complete loss of a part, as in a deletion, or involves two or more breakages with resultant rearrangement of the chromosome, as in an inversion. The deletions

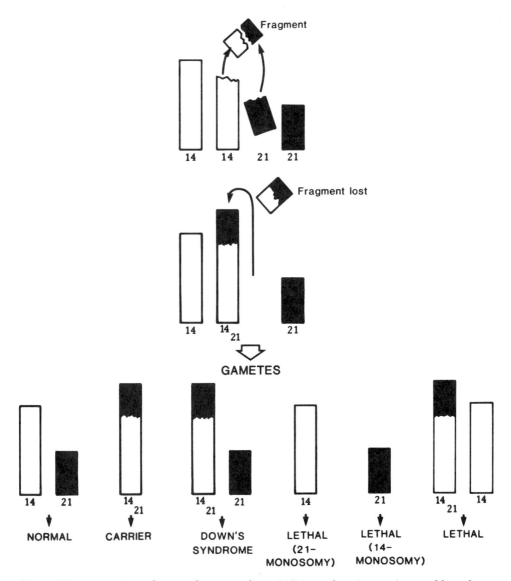

Fig. 8.6 Representation of types of gametes that a 14/21 translocation carrier would produce. The theoretical risk of Down syndrome is 30 percent. The actual risk is less. (Adapted with permission from Emery AEH: Elements of Medical Genetics. 4th ed. Edinburgh, Churchill Livingstone, 1975.)

almost always cause mental retardation, as do the trisomies, and there are several well-known examples of deletion syndromes that can be recognized by clinical characteristics.

There are two types of inversions, pericentric and paracentric. In pericentric inversions, the breaks occur on either side of the centromere, and the fragment turns upside down, thus altering the linear sequence of the genes on the chromosome and the shape of the chromosome. In a paracentric inversion, both breaks occur on the same side of the centromere,

again changing the linear sequence of the genes but not changing the shape of the chromosome. Most inversions are not associated with any specific pathology and are often found by chance.

Ring chromosomes are formed by a double breakage at each end of the chromosome, and the ends are thought to unite in the form of a ring because they are "sticky." Since they usually involve some form of deletion, they are invariably accompanied by the effects of a deletion, namely, mental retardation plus a varying array of malformations.

Chromosomal Breakage Syndromes

Three autosomal recessive conditions, ataxia telangiectasia, Fanconi's anemia syndrome, and Bloom's syndrome, are known to be associated with many different cytogenetic abnormalities such as deletions, rearrangements, and other abnormalities. All three syndromes are associated with an increased frequency of malignancies.

SEX CHROMOSOMES

If nondisjunction of the X chromosome occurs, the ovum may end up with two X chromosomes or more. If two Xs are in the egg and it is fertilized by a Y-bearing sperm, the result is an XXY karyotype (Klinefelter syndrome). If the XX ovum is fertilized by an X bearing sperm the result will be a female infant with the triple X syndrome. If the ovum contains no sex chromosome, the result will be either a conceptus 45,X (Turner syndrome) or a nonviable conceptus with a YO sex chromosome complement. In the same manner, nondisjunction in the first meiotic division of spermatogenesis may lead to a sperm with either XY or no sex chromosome complement at all, and the result of fertilization will be either a Klinefelter (XXY) or a Turner syndrome (XO). If nondisjunction takes place in a second meiosis, resulting in a sperm with two Xs or two Ys, or no sex chromosome, the result can be a XXX female, an XYY, or a Turner syndrome. Nondisjunction may take place at both first and second meiosis, resulting in a fetus with five sex chromosomes, for example, 49,XXXXY or 49,XXXXX.

Turner Syndrome

The syndrome that was originally described by Turner involved sexual infantilism in females, with short stature and certain somatic signs, such as webbed neck, congenital lymphedema, increased carrying angle of the elbow, and an increased frequency of coarctation of the aorta. Since then the concept of Turner syndrome has been greatly expanded, and the term is often used to include any disorder of the X chromosome involving a female. The overwhelming majority of XO conceptuses are lost spontaneously as abortions, so that only a very small number go to term. There is no ambiguity about the external genitalia, and such persons are unequivocally assigned as females. The diagnosis may be made at birth by the presence of congenital lymphedema and the webbed neck, but if it is not

evident at that time, then the next event that brings the patient to medical attention is likely to be growth failure during childhood, and, thus, a female with unexplained growth failure (<3 percent) should have a chromosome analysis. Others are not ascertained until the teenage years, when primary amenorrhea and lack of sexual development draws attention to the abnormality. Many of the patients who are categorized as Turner syndrome do not in fact have a 45X karyotype but rather some form of mosaicism, indicating that the nondisjunctional event has occurred after zygote formation. This results in a karyotype of 45,X/46,XX, although there are many combinations involving mosaicism. Signs and symptoms of Turner syndrome in other patients may involve deletions of the X chromosome. Usually a deletion of the short arm (Xp−) will give rise to short stature and amenorrhea, whereas deletions of the long arm (Xq−) may only yield primary amenorrhea. Another karyotype that is found in patients with signs of the Turner syndrome is that involving an isochromosome. The latter is formed by horizontal division, rather than vertical division, of the centromere, with the result that the daughter chromosomes involve both duplication and deficiency; in other words, an isochromosome of the short arm means there is no long arm, and vice versa. Many of the chromosomes involve duplication of long arms with loss of the short arm genes, and hence the patients are very similar to the classic 45,X patients. Figure 8.7 illustrates the formation of an isochromosome.

Most patients with abnormalities of the X chromosome involving Turner syndrome or a similar picture have normal intelligence, although there may be problems in space-form perception and certain learning difficulties. Most Turner-syndrome-like patients are totally infertile, but there are a few examples of patients becoming pregnant, with considerable risk of fetal abnormalities. These patients require psychological management for their short stature (most will end up in the 140 cm range), and appropriate vocational counselling, since many jobs that are traditionally available to females may not be available to females with short stature. Such counselling is a continuous and ongoing process, first for the parents of such a patient and then for the patient herself.

Kleinfelter Syndrome

Klinefelter syndrome refers to a male with an extra X chromosome, that is, 47,XXY. The genitalia are generally unambiguous, and hence the assignment at

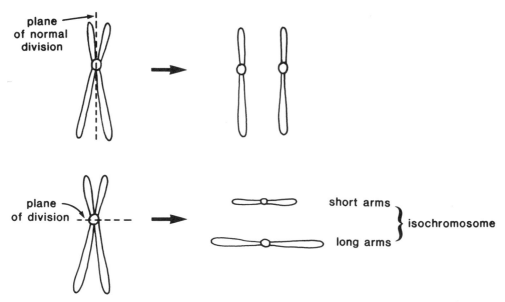

Fig. 8.7 Isochromosome formation. (Adapted with permission from Emery AEH: Elements of Medical Genetics. 4th ed. Edinburgh, Churchill Livingstone, 1975.)

birth is male. Newborn surveys have revealed that the disorder is common, about 1 in 400 male births. Diagnosis may be delayed for many years because many have normal intelligence, although there is mild mental retardation in a significant proportion of patients. At adolescence, these patients usually have insufficient masculinization; their voices are more highly pitched than normal for males, their testes are small, they lack body and facial hair, and they develop significant gynecomastia. Body build may be eunuchoid. Infertility is usually due to seminal tubule dysgenesis, with resulting azoospermia. Mosaicism is also seen in Klinefelter syndrome. Endocrine, educational, and psychologic management are generally required.

XYY Syndrome

The XYY syndrome refers to those males who have two Y chromosomes (Fig. 8.8). This may result in a male with significantly increased stature and behavioral changes, although the percentage of XYY men who do have behavioral problems is somewhat uncertain.

Triple X Syndrome

Triple X syndrome females with 47,XXX karyotype may be completely normal, or in some instances may have associated mild mental retardation.

Intersex States

In true hermaphroditism, chromosome analysis is likely to yield an unequivocal 46,XX karyotype in most cases. The next largest group show mosaicism as 46,XX/46,XY or 46,XX/46,XXY, and a very small number are 46,XY.

Individuals with an XO/XY form of intersex, also known as mixed gonadal dysgenesis, have a variable phenotype. Many appear similar to Turner syndrome patients and possess female external genitalia, with a streak gonad on one side and poorly formed testicular tissue on the other. In some instances the phenotype is more male, with a hypospadias and bifid scrotum. The majority of patients with either male or female pseudohermaphroditism have a gene-determined problem rather than a chromosome aberration, although chromosome studies are frequently needed to help in diagnosis, for example, XY karyotype in androgen insensitivity (testicular feminization) syndromes.

Sex Chromatin

The detection of a difference in the nuclei of somatic cells of males and females was described by Barr and Bertram well before chromosomes were understood as they are today. A small darkly staining chromatin mass at the edge of the nuclear membrane was found in 20 to 50 percent of the cells of a normal

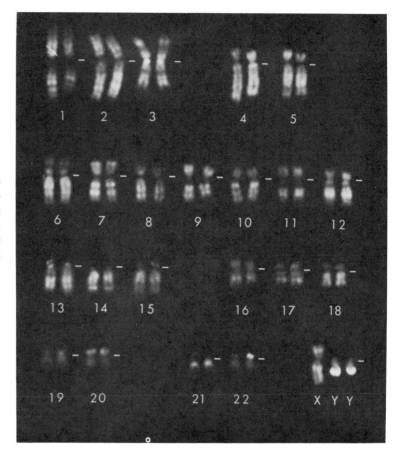

Fig. 8.8 Q-banded karyotype of a male with XYY sex-chromosome complement. Note the brightly fluorescent long arm of the Y chromosome (2,200×). (Courtesy of Lin CC, University of Calgary.)

female (chromatin positive), whereas males did not show such a mass. It was further found that patients with Turner syndrome (45,X) also lacked this chromatin mass and hence were called chromatin negative, as were normal males. It is now evident that the number of chromatin masses reflects one less than the total number of X chromosomes. Thus, a triple X female has two chromatin masses, and a Klinefelter male has one chromatin mass and is chromatin positive.

The most convenient place to obtain somatic cells is a scraping from the inside of the cheek, hence the term buccal smear. This is only a preliminary screening test in those individuals who present with symptoms suggestive of an X chromosome abnormality. In view of the large number of mosaic or isochromosome states, any female who is seriously suspected of having a Turner syndrome or variant should have a full chromosome analysis.

A similar screening test has been developed to detect the presence of the Y chromosome, which is shown by a special fluorescent staining, but this test does not replace a full chromosome analysis when a thorough assessment is called for (Fig. 8.9).

INDICATIONS FOR CHROMOSOME ANALYSIS

Clearly, if any of the well-described chromosome syndromes are suspected, such as Down syndrome, Turner syndrome, Klinefelter syndrome, or others, then chromosome analyses should be performed. In other instances the following indications for chromosome analysis may be of help to the physician: (1) A female whose stature falls below the third percentile for height in whom there is no other obvious diagnosis such as achondroplasia, hypopituitary dwarfism, or the like. (2) Primary amenorrhea. (3) A male with mild mental retardation in whom no other cause has been found. (4) A male with infertility involving azoospermia. (5) Intersex states or inappropriate changes at the time of puberty. (6) Patients with multiple congenital anomalies, particularly when mental retardation is involved.

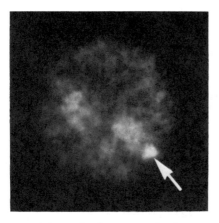

Fig. 8.9 Bright fluorescent Y-chromatin mass in nucleus of a normal male (1,900×). Courtesy of Lin CC, University of Calgary.)

MENDELIAN INHERITANCE

In the last 15 years the number of phenotypes due to single-factor inheritance has risen from 1,500 to nearly 3,000 (Table 8.3). The three major categories to be discussed are autosomal dominant, autosomal recessive, and X-linked inherited disorders.

If a pair of genes at the same locus on homologous chromosomes are identical they are termed *homozygous* with respect to that locus. If they are not identical they are termed *heterozygous*. Alternative forms of genes at the same locus are termed *alleles*. Many alleles exist for some loci. The terms *homozygous* and *heterozygous* do not infer normality or abnormality; this has to be specified separately. If the presence of a gene is manifest in a clinical way, that is, generally, as an abnormality in either single dose (heterozygous) or double dose (homozygous), then it is customary to refer to this as a *dominant* gene. When it is on one of the 44 autosomes, it is further categorized as an autosomal dominant gene or trait. If the ab-

normality shows up only when the gene is in double dose, that is, when it is homozygous, then the condition is known as *recessive*.

AUTOSOMAL DOMINANT

Since most dominant-gene disorders are rare, an affected individual usually has only one copy of the mutant gene, that is, the person is heterozygous. That person could be homozygous for a dominant gene, but this is far less common. Thus, at the time of reproduction, a person affected with a dominant gene disorder can transmit the trait to approximately half of his or her offspring as demonstrated in Figure 8.10. A typical autosomal dominant pedigree is shown in Figure 8.11. Note that the disorder can be transmitted by either sex to either sex, and that if data from large families are pooled the ratio of affected to unaffected is approximately equal, that is, 1:1. Persons in the pedigree who do not display the trait can be reassured that they will not develop it nor will their offspring. One exception to the above is the condition of *nonpenetrance* of the gene. If a person has an affected parent and an affected child and yet shows no physical signs despite detailed scrutiny, then we say this person has the gene but it is nonpenetrant. Closer inspection may reveal that the person does show some minor signs of the disorder that have escaped casual observation. In such a case the gene is fully penetrant, even if there are only minor signs, and is said to show *variable expressivity*.

These two concepts, namely nonpenetrance and variable expressivity, are frequently confused, and it is probably best that the clinician equate variable expressivity with clinical severity, keeping in mind that instances may arise when clinical severity is so minimal that present tests and examinations cannot detect the presence of the gene. On the other hand, close inspection by modern methods frequently shows that there are very few conditions in which

Table 8.3 **Mendelian Inheritance in Humans**

Phenotype	Verschuer 1958[b]	1966[c]	1978[c]	Aug 1979 (unpubl.)
Autosomal dominant	285	269(+568)[a]	736(+753)	841(+832)
Autosomal recessive	89	237(+294)	521(+596)	570(+662)
X-Linked	38	68(+52)	107(+98)	115(+180)
Total	412	574(+913)	1364(+1447)	1526(+1595)
Grand Total	412	1487	2811	3121

[a] Numbers in parenthesis refer to loci not yet fully identified or confirmed.
[b] Lehrbuch der Humangenetik. Munich, Urban and Schwartzenberg, 1958.
[c] Adapted with permission from McKusick VA: The anatomy of the human genome. Journal of Heredity 71:370–391, 1980.

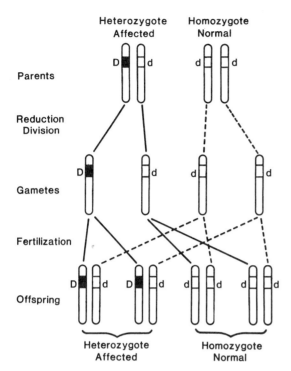

Parents

Heterozygote
Affected

Homozygote
Normal

Reduction
Division

Gametes

Fertilization

Offspring

Heterozygote
Affected

Homozygote
Normal

Fig. 8.10 Autosomal dominant segregation pattern. The recurrence risk is 50 percent. (Adapted with permission from Roberts JAF: An Introduction to Medical Genetics. 7th ed. London & New York, Oxford University Press, 1978.)

true nonpenetrance occurs. The term *forme fruste* is sometimes used to denote either variable expressivity or nonpenetrance, and implies no clinical consequence; but it is a term without precision and is probably best avoided. A dominant trait that is referred to as fully penetrant is one for which the literature records no example of the gene having skipped a generation. Other mechanisms of inheritance, such as X-linkage or multifactorial inheritance, should be excluded, since it is not uncommon to find skipped generations in those categories.

By convention the capital letter is used for a dominant gene and the lower-case letter for a recessive gene. Hence, a person with the dominant gene disorder achondroplasia would have the genotype written as Aa.

There are instances when a new dominant gene disorder appears within a pedigree and physical examination plus pedigree analysis disclose no other cases. This indicates that the condition has likely arisen because of a new mutation in one of the germ cells of the parents. It is likely that the mutation is confined to this germ cell alone, and thus further

children of those parents are not likely to be affected. The affected person will transmit the trait with the usual 50 percent frequency. Before a conclusion is reached ascribing the condition in question to a new mutation, the possibility of genetic heterogeneity should be considered. This will be discussed in a later section of this chapter.

Sometimes pedigrees are obtained for dominant disorders in which the severity and age of onset appear to change from one generation to another. In each succeeding generation the problem arises earlier and is more severe. Such a phenomenon is called *anticipation*, and is an artefact of ascertainment. Persons who are more mildly affected are more likely to reproduce, and their conditions are more likely to be recognized much later in life. In fact, the discovery of their conditions may come about because of their severely affected offspring. Severely affected persons are less likely to reproduce at all; hence, the reverse phenomenon is rarely seen, that is, the disease rarely becomes milder.

Co-dominance is said to occur when both alleles of a heterozygous pair can manifest themselves in the phenotype. A good example of this is the blood group AB.

The properties of autosomal dominant inheritance can be summarized as follows:

1. Usually the disorder appears in every generation (vertical transmission).

2. Affected persons will transmit the disorder (on the average) to half of their children.

3. If the gene is fully penetrant, then unaffected persons in the pedigree can be reassured that they will not develop the disorder nor will they transmit it.

4. Fresh mutations may account for the apparently sporadic case.

5. Since these genes are on the autosomes, it follows that either sex may be affected and can transmit it to either sex.

AUTOSOMAL RECESSIVE

Autosomal recessive disorders are those in which the mutant allele is recessive and hence does not show itself as disease unless the person has received a double dose, or, in other words, is homozygous. It follows, therefore, that both parents of an affected person must have the mutant allele in single dose, that is, they are heterozygotes, or carriers. The segregation ratio for such heterozygote parents shown in Figure 8.12 indicates that such parents have a 1 in 4

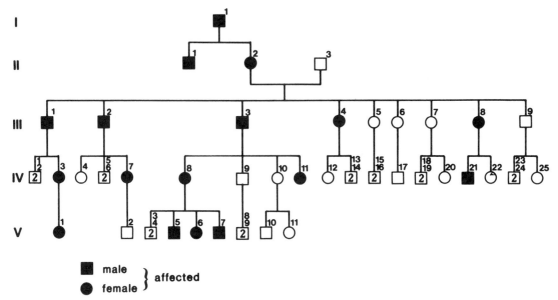

Fig. 8.11 Autosomal dominant pedigree from a family with congenital cataract. Note male-to-male transmission (I^1 to II^1). Some daughters of affected males are unaffected (IV^4 and IV^{10}). These two details make X-linked dominant inheritance improbable. Penetrance is full, thus unaffected persons can be reassured that the risks to their children are close to zero (the actual risk is the risk of a mutation).

or 25 percent risk of having an affected child with each pregnancy. It is important to realize that chance has no memory, and just because parents have one affected child does not mean that the next three will be normal. The risk is the same for each conception. A typical recessive pedigree is seen in Figure 8.13.

Individuals who are affected with a recessive gene disorder will be unlikely to have an affected child despite the fact that they must transmit at least one copy of the mutant gene. To have an affected child, an affected individual would have to mate with a carrier. For some recessive disorders it is possible to test normal individuals to see if they are carriers. In those recessive disorders in which carrier testing is not available, one has to rely on the statistical frequency of carriers in the population to get an idea of the actual risk. The frequency of carriers can be calculated by using a mathematical principle known as the Hardy-Weinberg formula. This consists of calculating the number of affected persons in the population, or incidence, and using the following abbreviated formula:

$$\text{carrier frequency} = 2\,(\text{incidence})^{1/2}$$

Parental consanguinity is more likely when the recessive trait in an affected patient is an extremely rare one. There are many genetic isolates who have high frequencies of certain recessive genes, for example, Ashkenazi Jews having the gene for Tay-Sachs dis-

ease, tyrosinemia in French Canadians from the Chicoutimi region of Quebec, and the Ellis-van Creveld syndrome among the Amish of Pennsylvania.

The term *recessive* is not entirely appropriate, since the presence of the abnormal gene in the heterozygous state can often be identified by special biochemical testing.

Compound Heterozygotes

There are some conditions in which there is more than one abnormal allele possible at a particular locus; when both of these mutant genes are present the person is said to be a compound heterozygote. An example of this is seen in hemoglobin SC disease. If one parent has the mutant gene for hemoglobin S and the other has the mutant gene for hemoglobin C, it is evident that both parents are heterozygotes, and so they function essentially as normal persons. Their offspring, however, could have hemoglobin SC disease, a disorder which is similar to sickle cell disease but somewhat milder (Fig. 8.14).

The properties of autosomal recessive inheritance can be summarized as follows:

1. The disorder is usually seen only in siblings, and so it is termed a disorder of horizontal inheritance. Parents and other relatives are usually normal.

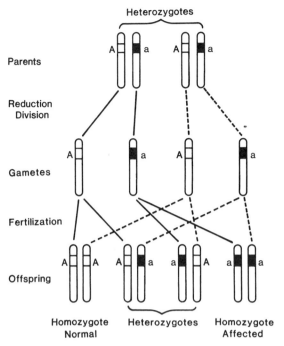

Heterozygotes

Parents

Reduction
Division

Gametes

Fertilization

Offspring

Homozygote
Normal

Heterozygotes

Homozygote
Affected

Fig. 8.12 Autosomal recessive segregation pattern. The risk of an affected child is 1 in 4 (25 percent). Note the risk of an unaffected child being a heterozygote (carrier) is 2 in 3, not 2 in 4, because the affected person can be identified whereas usually the heterozygote (Aa) cannot be distinguished from the homozygous normal (AA). (Adapted with permission from Roberts JAF: An Introduction to Medical Genetics. 7th ed. London & New York, Oxford University Press, 1978.)

2. Once parents have had one affected child, the risk in subsequent conceptions is 25 percent.

3. The more rare the condition, the greater the chance of consanguinity.

4. Since the genes are on autosomes, there is an equal sex distribution.

X-LINKED DISORDERS

Recessive

In many disorders the abnormal phenotype is almost totally confined to males, and a pattern of inheritance has been deduced that shows that females can be carriers of a recessive gene but they are seldom affected (Fig. 8.15). In other words, females having two X chromosomes can carry the mutant gene on one of them, and the normal or wild-type gene on the other, and thus can still function as normal persons. Males, in contrast have only one X chromosome; they are described as hemizygous. The genes on the X and Y chromosomes are not homologous, and hence any mutant gene on the X chromosome of a male will be fully expressed. Examples of such diseases include Duchenne type muscular dystrophy, hemophilia A (factor VIII deficiency), as well as less disabling conditions such as red and green color blindness. A carrier or heterozygous female will transmit the mutant gene on the average to half of her sons, who will be affected; her other sons will receive the normal allele and be normal. Half of her daughters will receive the gene and become carriers, and half will not.

Fig. 8.13 Autosomal recessive pedigree from a family with congenital glaucoma (buphthalmos). II[11] and II[12] are heterozygotes and have a 1 in 4 risk for each child. Their healthy children's risk is as follows: 2/3 chance of being a heterozygote × spouse's chance of being a heterozygote (that is, population risk, which is unknown but is likely to be less than 1/100) × 1/4 (segregation risk for two heterozygotes). 2/3 × 1/100 × 1/4 = 1/600. If the heterozygote frequency is 1/500 then their risk = 1/3,000.

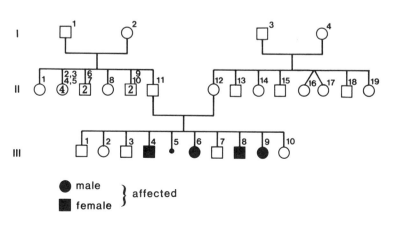

● male
■ female } affected

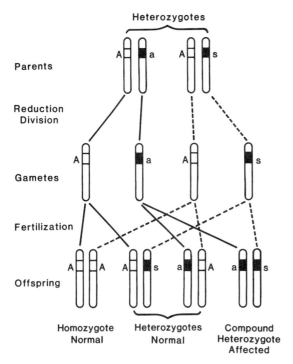

Fig. 8.14 Segregation pattern when each parent is heterozygous for a different allele. The usual 1 in 4 risk of an affected child applies. (Adapted with permission from Roberts JAF: An Introduction to Medical Genetics. 7th ed. London & New York, Oxford University Press, 1978).

If the condition is a lethal one, such as Duchenne type muscular dystrophy, where males have not reproduced, it follows that the condition appears by one of two mechanisms: either the mother is a carrier or the condition has arisen as a result of a mutation. It has been estimated in the past that approximately one third of the cases of Duchenne type muscular dystrophy in boys are the result of a new mutation. Carrier detection is obviously of the utmost importance in females, particularly when a sporadic case appears. There have been many attempts to delineate carriers, but despite a variety of methods only about 70 percent can be detected reliably, usually by serum creatine phosphokinase (CPK) estimation. Sometimes the success rate for identifying carriers can be improved by physical examination and electrodiagnostic testing of muscles by an experienced neurologist. Risk estimates can sometimes be refined by using a statistical technique known as Bayes theorem, which allows for the inclusion of data such as the number of unaffected males who have been born to a suspected carrier.

In instances of other X-linked recessive disorders that allow the affected male to survive and reproduce, as in hemophilia, all sons will be normal, since the affected male transmits a Y chromosome to his sons, whereas all of his daughters will be carriers, since the father has only one X chromosome and this contains the mutant gene.

Thus, in X-linked recessive disorders there may appear to be one or more skipped generations if only female infants are born into families in which the mutant gene is segregating. Clearly it would be desirable to have reliable carrier detection tests available on a routine screening basis and methods for detecting affected infants in utero.

It has been known for many years that there is a disproportionate number of males among the moderate and severely mentally retarded persons. Pedigrees supporting X-linked recessive inheritance can be found in the literature, and this is now an established entity. In fact, there are probably several different genes on the X chromosome that cause mental retardation. One of these is associated with enlarged testes (macro-orchidism). In some X-linked recessive forms of mental retardation there is a recognizable difference in the X chromosome, a secondary constriction near the long end, also known as a fragile X. In some families with X-linked mental retardation, there are females who have learning difficulties or who are slow learners. Occasionally they are also retarded. This does not contradict the method of inheritance but is likely to be due to selective inactivation of one X chromosome in the female, a phenomenon known as the *Lyon principle*.

The Lyon Principle

When a female infant is conceived, both the paternally derived X (X^p) and the maternally derived X (X^m) are fully active in all cells. About the 16th day after conception, one of the X chromosomes in each cell becomes inactivated and moves to the edge of the nuclear membrane to become the chromatin mass, also known as the Barr body. This is the mass that is studied in the buccal smear test. Inactivation of the X chromosome is a random event in each cell, but once the selection is made, all subsequent descendents of that cell will have the same inactive X chromosome. Hence, approximately half of a woman's X^p cells and half of her X^m cells are inactivated. With respect to genes on the X chromosome, a woman is a functional mosaic. If the X^p chromosome contains a mutant gene in a woman whose inactive X chromosomes by chance belong mostly to the X^m

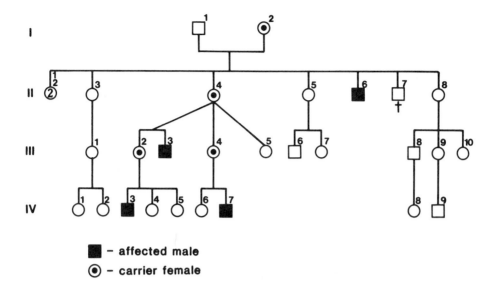

■ – affected male

◉ – carrier female

Fig. 8.15 X-linked recessive pedigree from a family with mental retardation. All affected persons are male. Note I^2 is an obligatory heterozygote because she has an affected son and at least one other affected male descendent via one of her daughters. II^4 has an affected son and two grandsons via her daughters, and the fact that the daughters have different fathers further substantiates the X-linked recessive nature of the disorder. Note the risk of IV^1 and IV^2 being carriers is 1/2(chance for II^3) × 1/2(chance for III^1) × 1/2(IV^1 and IV^2) = 1/8. The risk for IV^4, IV^5, and IV^6 is 1/2. The risk for II^5 is modified slightly because she has one unaffected son. Using Bayes theorem[6] the risk of her being a carrier is 1/3, which is derived as follows:

Risk for II^5		Carrier	Not a Carrier
A Prior probability		1/2	1/2
B Conditional probability (1 normal son)		1/2	1
Joint (A × B) probability		1/4	1/2
Posterior probability		$\dfrac{1/4}{1/4 + 1/2} = 1/3$	$\dfrac{1/2}{1/4 + 1/2} = 2/3$

The risk of III^7 being a carrier is half of her mother's risk, that is, 1/6. However III^9's risk is modified further because she has one unaffected son. Her risk is 1/11. The risk of IV^8 being a carrier is zero (actually the mutation rate) because she is the offspring of an unaffected male. (From Herbst DS, Pedigree P.: Am J Med Genet Nonspecific x-linked mental retardation: A review with information from 24 new families. 7:443, 1980, with permission. Copyright 1980, Alan R. Liss, Inc.)

class, then most of her functional X chromosomes will be X^P chromosomes, and hence she may express some of the abnormalities associated with the mutant gene. The Lyon principle is an important one because it helps explain the occasional case or partial manifestation of clinical findings in female hemophiliacs, females with slow learning in X-linked mental retardation, and an occasional woman with some pseudohypertrophy or muscular weakness in Duchenne type muscular dystrophy. It also explains why it is not possible to detect carriers of Duchenne type muscular dystrophy with a 100 percent certainty by current methods.

The properties of X-linked recessive inheritance may be summarized as follows:

1. The disorder is usually seen in males.

2. With the exception of new mutants, the gene is transmitted by carrier females.

3. The offspring of a carrier female face a 50 percent risk of being affected if they are male, and a 50 percent risk of being carriers if they are female.

4. In nonlethal conditions, the offspring of an affected male will all be normal and will not transmit the gene if they are male, and will all be carriers if they are female.

5. Because of the Lyon principle, an occasional carrier female may manifest some of the symptoms or signs.

X-Linked Dominant

The features of X-linked dominant inheritance are often hard to differentiate from autosomal dominant inheritance, since the pedigrees may often be very similar. In X-linked dominant disorders, either sex can express the mutant phenotype; an affected man cannot transmit the trait to any of his sons, but he will transmit the trait to all of his daughters because he has only one X chromosome. Therefore, the absence of male-to-male transmission is an important feature. The affected female, in contrast, can transmit the condition to either sex with the usual 50 percent frequency. In looking at large pedigrees with this pattern of inheritance, or in pooling the data from many pedigrees, there should be an excess number of affected females, compared with males, in a ratio approximating 2:1.

MULTIFACTORIAL INHERITANCE

The term *multifactorial inheritance* is used to imply an interaction between a gene and its environment. It is sometimes used synonymously with polygenic inheritance, although polygenic inheritance implies several genes with additive effects but virtually no environmental component. An example of polygenic inheritance is the dermatoglyphic pattern on fingertips, which is not known to be influenced by any environmental factors. Height is an example of a polygenic trait, although it might be more accurately described as multifactorial, since postnatal events can influence the ultimate outcome. Nevertheless, it is accepted that a trait such as height shows a continuous variation in the form of a Gaussian (or "normal") distribution within a population.

There are many diseases that appear to "run in families" for which examination does not support single gene inheritance, nor does a chromosome or an environmental factor appear to be operative. In such instances multifactorial inheritance should be suspected. One method of investigating this is to assess the frequency in monozygous twins compared with dizygous twins, and then do further family studies examining the frequency of the disorder in first-, second-, and third-degree relatives (first-degree relatives are parents and siblings, second-degree relatives are uncles, aunts, nephews, and nieces, and third-degree relatives are first cousins). For example, in autosomal dominant inheritance there is a regular decline in frequency from first- to second- to third-degree relatives, from 50 percent to 25 percent to 12.5 percent. In multifactorial inheritance, the risk falls off in an abrupt fashion from first- to second-degree relatives, and then drops much more slowly between second- and third-degree relatives, with the frequency in the latter group resembling that in the general population. Examples of these are seen in Table 8.4.

Two major problems with many multifactorial disorders are their lack of precise definition and the lack of methods for diagnosing them. Several models of a multifactorial system have been proposed, one of which is depicted in Figure 8.16. This proposes that in the general population there are risk factors composed of both genes and environment, which together constitute total liability. This total liability has a normal distribution, and those persons to the extreme right of the curve have a greater liability for the disorder in question, and hence express it. An arbitrary line, called the threshold, has been exceeded in these individuals. The model further proposes that first-degree relatives of affected persons do not have the liability curve of the normal population but one that is shifted to the right, with the mean standing approximately halfway between the mean for the normal population and the mean for affected persons. If the distribution curve for relatives is shifted to the right, it can be seen that more of them will be beyond the risk threshold and hence will show the disorder.

Congenital malformations are present in approximately 2 to 5 percent of newborns depending on the criteria used. Although the etiology is most often not known, some are due to chromosome and single-

Table 8.4 **Increased Frequency of Some Congenital Malformations in Relatives Compared with the Population Incidence**

	Cleft Lip and Cleft Palate	Talipes Equinovarus
General Population	0.001	0.001
First-Degree Relatives	×40	×25
Second-Degree Relatives	×7	×5
Third-Degree Relatives	×3	×2

(From Carter CO: Genetics of common disorders. Brit Med Bull 25:52–57, 1969, with permission.)

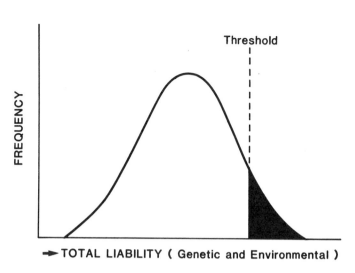

Fig. 8.16 Falconer model of multifactorial inheritance. Persons to the right of the arbitrary threshold are affected. First-degree relatives have a distribution curve that is shifted to the right, hence more are affected. (Adapted with permission from Carter CO: Genetics of common single malformations. Brit Med Bull 32:21, 1976.)

gene factors, and others are due to environmental factors such as rubella in pregnancy or teratogenic drugs. A large number are due to multifactorial inheritance. The multifactorial model has been worked out for many of the more common disorders such as cleft lip with or without cleft palate (CL ± CP), neural tube defects such as spina bifida and anencephaly, talipes equinovarus, and the more common forms of congenital heart defects. One of the features of many of these is a different incidence in males, compared with females, that is hard to explain on the basis of single-factor inheritance. The multifactorial model proposes a different distribution of liability for the two sexes, hence the threshold line will be at a different point on each of their curves. If the male is more frequently affected, as in CL ± CP, it can be appreciated that since females are less commonly affected, those who are affected will have more of the total liability factors. One would expect, therefore, that the risk to first-degree relatives of the less commonly affected sex, in this instance the female, would be higher than the risk to first-degree relatives of an affected male. Using similar reasoning, it can be appreciated that a person whose defect is more severe will likely have a greater number of the total liability factors; and again, using the example of CL ± CP, it is seen that persons with bilateral cleft lip and cleft palate are more likely to have affected first-degree relatives than are mildly affected persons who only have a unilateral cleft lip. Similarily, if two normal parents have two affected children, it can be expected that their liability factors are more to the right of the distribution curve than parents with only one affected child. Thus, their risk for a third affected child is higher than that of parents with one affected child.

Many of the common adult-onset disorders are also thought to be due to multifactorial inheritance, although they are less precisely defined when compared to congenital malformations. For example, there is no question whether someone has a cleft lip, whereas it may be difficult to say whether a person has schizophrenia, since there is no precise objective sign or laboratory test. Despite these problems, conditions such as schizophrenia show definite genetic tendencies and yet do not appear to conform to a single gene model. Twin studies have definitely shown that there is a considerable genetic component in schizophrenia, as do the studies of offspring of schizophrenic parents who are raised apart from their parents, that is, they are adopted. The risk for such children developing schizophrenia is approximately 10 percent, and is not too different from the risk for a child who is raised by his own schizophrenic parent.

Ischemic heart disease, essential hypertension, and diabetes mellitus are also thought to have genetic components, and some of them fall in the multifactorial category. However, there are very definitely single-gene categories within each of the examples. For instance, in ischemic heart disease some of the high-risk families will have one of the hyperlipidemias that may be inherited in a Mendelian manner. In diabetes mellitus, there are now more than 30 loci for genetically determined syndromes that have diabetes as a component. As with schizophrenia, it is often difficult to give a precise definition of what diabetes is, and for purposes of analysis diabetes is often divided into insulin-dependent and non–insulin-dependent groups. The former are commonly referred to as juvenile-onset diabetes (Type I), and the latter as maturity-onset diabetes (Type II). Every single gene model has been proposed for Type I, but in fact most studies clearly do not support such an etiology. There is tremendous heterogeneity not only within diabetes as a whole but also within Type I, with increasing evidence for a possible viral source acting on a genetic susceptibility in some cases. Studies of HLA antigens also demonstrate heterogeneity within Type I diabetics.

In some younger persons, diabetes is non-insulin dependent and thus appears to more closely resemble maturity-onset diabetes. This is one group of diabetics in whom single-factor inheritance may well be responsible, as pedigree analysis supports a theory of autosomal dominance.

A number of multifactorial genetic diseases have been found to be associated with one or more of the HLA loci. These are situated on the short arm of chromosome 6, and each locus has many different alleles. There are four major loci: HLA-A, HLA-B, HLA-C, and HLA-D. The best known example of a disease and association with an HLA antigen is that between ankylosing spondylitis and the B27 allele. The population frequency of B27 is about 7 percent, whereas it is present in about 90 percent of persons with ankylosing spondylitis. In certain Canadian Indians such as the Haidas, the frequency of the B27 allele is about 50 percent, and ankylosing spondylitis and sacral iliitis are extremely common in their adult males.

A number of other disease associations with one of the HLA loci are listed in Table 8.5. Some of the alleles are associated more frequently than one would expect, based on population frequencies. Such an increased association is termed linkage disequilibrium, and this mechanism may account for the disease associations.

Properties of multifactorial threshold traits may be summarized as follows:

1. Family risks are greater than population incidence but less than 50 percent or 25 percent.

2. With lower population incidence, the risks for relatives are relatively higher.

3. Family risks drop sharply with degree of relationship (from first to second to third degree).

4. Risks may vary from one family to another.

5. Risks vary with the severity of the index case.

6. When there is a sex difference in incidence, the risk to relatives depends on the sex of the index case.

GENETIC HETEROGENEITY

Closer inspection of one entity frequently reveals that it is composed of several different entities, all of which have some common sign or symptom. For example, the disorders that are now known as the mucopolysaccharidoses were originally lumped together as the Hurler-Hunter syndrome, as if they were one entity. About 25 years after the first description, an X-linked recessive pattern was described for one of these, while autosomal recessive proved responsible for the other. Many more years elapsed until it was demonstrated that mucopolysaccharides were excreted in the urine. Gradually the classification expanded as a result of improved clinical, genetic, and urinary excretion studies, until finally studies of cultured fibroblasts demonstrated the actual enzyme defects that were responsible for these widely varied disorders.

Thus it has become an established principle that when the patient facts do not seem to fit the existing knowledge, it is wise to consider the possibility of genetic heterogeneity and further subclassifications of an original syndrome. Prior to the discovery of homocystinuria, patients with this condition were grouped with Marfan syndrome patients, as were many other patients with arachnodactyly. Arachnodactyly is a very heterogeneous sign, and Marfan syndrome is one of a number of syndromes with this feature (Table 8.6). Another well-known genetic entity that has been shown to be heterogeneous is the Ehlers-Danlos syndrome (Table 8.7). All forms of short-limbed dwarfism were once labeled achondroplasia. There are now so many forms of short-limbed dwarfism that there are textbooks on this subject alone. It is especially important to remember genetic heterogeneity when dealing with any of the multifactorial diseases or malformations because within those categories there will be some that are determined by single genes, some by chromosomal im-

Table 8.5 Some Examples of HLA Locus and Disease Association

B27	Ankylosing spondylitis
A3	Hemochromatosis
B8 ⎫	
B15 ⎬	Juvenile Diabetes Mellitus
DW3 ⎭	
DW4	
B8 ⎫	Celiac Disease
DW3 ⎭	Graves Disease

Table 8.6 Syndromes with Arachnodactyly

Marfan
Homocystinuria
Congenital Contractural Arachnodactyly
Achard
Stickler
Frontometaphyseal Dysplasia

Table 8.7 **The Ehlers-Danlos Syndromes**

Type		Clinical Manifestations	Genetics[a]	Biochemical Defect
I	Gravis	Bruising, hyperelastic skin	AD	not known
II	Mitis	Milder than above	AD	not known
III	Benign Hypermobile	Mainly joints	AD	not known
IV	Ecchymotic or Arterial	Severe bruising, danger of ruptured arteries or bowel		
	Subtype A	Joint hypermobility	AD	not known
	B	Mainly restricted to hands	AR	not known
	C	Thin skin, some differences between subtypes	NK	Intracell accumulation of collagen
	D		NK	not known
V	X-Linked	Striking skin features, minimal joint hypermobility	XLR	? Deficiency of lysyl oxidase
VI	Ocular	Scoliosis, severe retinal detachments	AR	Deficiency of lysyl hydroxylase
VII	Arthrochalasis Multiplex Congenita	Short stature, congenital dislocations, joint laxity	AR	Deficiency of procollagen protease (or peptidase)
VIII	Periodontosis	Early loss of teeth, periodontosis, fragile skin	AD	not known

[a] AD = autosomal dominant; AR = autosomal recessive; XLR = X-linked recessive; NK = not known.
(Adapted with permission from McKusick VA: Mendelian Inheritance in Man. 5th ed., 1978. Baltimore, Johns Hopkins University Press, and Byers PH, et al: Clinical and ultrastructural heterogeneity of Type IV Ehlers-Danlos syndrome. Hum Genet 47:141–150, 1979.

balance, and some by environmental agents, leaving the vast majority within the multifactorial group. A well-established example is CL ± CP, of which there is an autosomal dominant form, a chromosomal form (trisomy 13), and a teratogenic form caused by diphenylhydantoin (Dilantin). The large remaining group is classified as multifactorial, but there is almost certainly further heterogeneity.

PHARMACOGENETICS

Many patients show undesirable responses when given drugs; however, the majority of these are probably sporadic, idiopathic events with no hereditary implications. A number, however, are the result of the patient having a mutant gene that causes a different or abnormal response to the drug. The study of such inherited drug reactions is termed *pharmacogenetics*. A number of them are listed in Table 8.8. Those that are of special importance are related to anesthetics, since an abnormal reaction may lead to death unless treatment is instituted promptly. In some of these heritable disorders the abnormality is due to an enzyme that is involved in the metabolism of the drug. The mutation presumably has been present for many generations or even centuries, and it is only the development of the particular drug that has uncovered the phenotype.

The best known of these disorders is *porphyria* variegata, also known as South African porphyria. This is an autosomal dominant trait showing skin photosensitivity, abdominal pain, neuritis, and psychosis. The attacks are intermittent, but those persons who have the gene can generally be diagnosed by measurement of porphyrin excretion in urine and stools. Drugs of the barbiturate series are likely to precipitate attacks, including pentothal and related short-term anesthetics. Unfortunately, these patients may unknowingly be given these drugs for symptomatic treatment. This may aggravate the disease, causing paralysis and death.

Malignant hyperthermia (MH) is usually precipitated by an anesthetic, particularly of the halothane, fluothane, or ether series. Sometimes muscle relaxants such as suxamethonium may induce the hyperthermia. The symptoms are those of a very rapid rise in body temperature and increasing muscular rigidity, which leads to metabolic acidosis, hyperkalemia, and hypocalcemia. Death due to cardiac arrest is not uncommon. Prompt recognition of the symptoms, followed by cooling measures and correction of the metabolic acidosis, is usually life-saving, and this can be augmented by use of the drug dantrolene.

Once such a patient has been identified, the family should be screened for the presence of this autosomal dominant disorder. Some persons who carry the gene can be identified by means of the serum creatine phosphokinase (CPK). The most reliable way of determining a person's genetic status with regard to MH is a test for contracture in response to caffeine, performed on a muscle biopsy. Occasionally, for unexplained reasons, persons with the gene can withstand anesthetics using the proscribed agents without

Table 8.8 Examples of Genetic Disorders Precipitated by Previous Drug Exposure

Disorder	Inheritance	Symptoms	Examples of Precipitating Drugs
Malignant Hyperthermia	AD	Hyperpyrexia, rigidity, metabolic acidosis	Anesthetics such as halothane, fluothane, ether
Porphyria Variegata	AD	Abdominal pain, paralysis, psychosis	Barbiturates
Pseudocholinesterase deficiency	AR	Apnea	Suxamethonium type of muscle relaxant
Slow Acetylator—Isoniazid	AR	Polyneuritis	Isoniazid, hydralazine, certain sulfa drugs
Glucose-6-phosphate Dehydrogenase Deficiency	XLR	Hemolysis	Antimalarial compounds, sulfonamides, some analgesics

suffering an attack. If the family history is positive for this disorder, a history of no reaction to certain anesthetics should not prevent further investigation by the two tests mentioned. Finally, it should be appreciated that there are safe anesthetics available for persons who carry the MH gene.

Other patients who may have problems with anesthetics are those with *pseudocholinesterase deficiency*. This is an autosomal recessive trait in which there are several different mutant alleles. No symptoms occur unless the person is subjected to the muscle relaxant suxamethonium, which is normally hydrolyzed by pseudocholinesterase. In the patient who is homozygous, prolonged respiratory paralysis may last for several hours. All siblings of an affected patient should be tested for pseudocholinesterase levels.

Metabolism of drugs frequently involves a process known as acetylation, controlled by the enzyme N-acetyltransferase. This is an important mechanism, as the kidney can excrete an acetylated drug more easily. Individuals can be classified into those who are rapid acetylators and those who are slow, and the rapid allele is dominant compared with the slow allele. Thus, persons who are slow acetylators are homozygous for the slow allele, indicating that this is an autosomal recessive disorder. (see Chapter 10, Adverse Drug Reactions.)

The best screening test for an abnormal genetic response to drugs is the family history. Once an individual at risk is found, then appropriate family members should be warned about the disorder and screened by whatever methods are available. Those persons who actually have the genetic disorder should wear a bracelet or necklace with this information, so that in the event of an accident the information is readily available. Undoubtedly, there are many more mutant genotypes awaiting recognition by some abnormal reaction to a drug, and when a patient has a very abnormal reaction, the physician should give consideration to the possibility of a gene effect.

PREVENTION

GENETIC COUNSELING

Genetic counseling is designed to inform the patient (or parents, in the case of a child) about the hereditary factors in the pertinent disorder to explain the biologic mechanisms, to help the patient cope with the problem, to reduce anxiety and guilt, to provide recurrence risk figures for offspring and other relatives, and to help with family planning decisions while encouraging patients to make their own decisions. Not only is the geneticist concerned about the hereditary aspects, but also with the psychologic impact the disorder may have on the patient or family. Counseling is less successful at the bedside or in hospital corridors, and ideally should take place in an unhurried atmosphere with adequate privacy. One of the goals of genetics is to make sure that all persons at risk are offered the option of genetic counseling. This ideal is not realized in most centers.

The importance of a correct diagnosis cannot be overemphasized, particularly remembering the possibility of genetic heterogeneity. The natural history of the disorder should be discussed if the patient is not totally familiar with it. There is little point in quoting recurrence risks unless the condition is understood. This seems self-evident but in fact is a recurring problem. For example, a female who has a distant male cousin with Duchenne type muscular dystrophy and has not grown up in close proximity to this boy, may not realize the seriousness of the condition, particularly if he is in the preschool age group. Another disorder that may pose a problem in this regard is Huntington's disease, since the physician is usually consulted by unaffected relatives of a patient. Frequently the counselor has the unpleasant task of informing these individuals, often the children of an affected person, of the 50 percent risk that they will develop the disorder. Despite these difficulties, it is best to inform families once a definitive

Table 8.9 Examples of Disorders for Which Prospective Genetic Counseling Could Be Given

Autosomal Dominant	Autosomal Recessive	X-Linked Recessive
Polyposis Coli	Tay–Sachs—Ashkenazi Jews	Some X-L mental retardation
Polycystic Kidneys	Sickle cell—blacks	Some Duchenne type muscular dystrophy
Neurofibromatosis	Thalassemia—Italians, Greeks, etc.	Some hemophilia

diagnosis has been made, and to discuss the genetic pattern of inheritance with all of those who are at risk.

Prospective Genetic Counseling

Conditions suitable for prospective genetic counseling are listed in Table 8.9. Ideally, the genotypes of a couple would be tested before reproduction to determine what mutant genes they may have, particularly with respect to autosomal recessive or X-linked recessive disorders. In fact, this is rarely possible, except for a few selected cases. For example, the Tay-Sachs gene is common in Ashkenazi Jews, and a blood test is available to determine heterozygosity. The frequency of carriers in most of the Ashkenazi population is approximately 1 in 28. Almost all other autosomal recessive disorders are so rare that it would not be feasible to screen for them even if biochemical tests were available.

For certain autosomal dominant disorders prospective counseling can be offered once an individual has been identified as having a condition, such as Marfan syndrome, adult polycystic kidney disease, or the like.

Retrospective Genetic Counseling

Retrospective counseling is the more usual event; couples identify themselves to be at risk because of an affected child.

When the disorder is due to Mendelian inheritance, recurrence risks are fairly straightforward, and these should be explained with the aid of tables that the patient can keep. For chromosome and multifactorial disorders, reliance is placed on empiric recurrence risks from the published literature (Table 8.10), and the family pedigree should be studied, since the risk may be based on this rather than the literature.

A sporadic case may be just as genetically determined as one for which there is a strong positive family history. A number of different mechanisms may be responsible, as listed in Table 8.11. The absence of previously affected members in the family may indicate a new dominant gene mutation. In families with small numbers of children most autosomal recessive disorders appear as sporadic events, as do the majority of cases due to multifactorial inheritance.

It should be emphasized that not all genetic counseling is gloom and doom. There are many positive aspects, particularly for the group of persons who are concerned about a genetic risk when in fact they do not have one. Even those who are at risk or who have a genetic problem frequently derive comfort from an understanding of the basic biology of the clinical disorder. For parents who have had a child with a genetic disorder, counseling often relieves guilt feelings. The approach of most medical geneticists is to try and help individuals and their families, and not to determine what is best for society. The latter emphasis has an overtone of eugenics, which is not the point of genetic counseling. In contrast to

Table 8.10 Some Empiric Recurrence Risks in Multifactorial Disorders

Disorder	Percentage Risk for Subsequent Children			
	Normal Parents 1 Affected Child	1 Affected Parent No Children	1 Affected Parent 1 Affected Child	2 Affected Parents No Children
Anencephaly Spina Bifida	2–5	2–4	11–14	30
Cleft Lip ± Cleft Palate	3–5	3	10	30–35
Cleft Palate	2	6	15	
Congenital Heart Defect All Types	1–4	1–3		
Congenital Pyloric Stenosis	3–4	3–5	10–15	27–30
Clubfoot	3	3	10	

(Adapted with permission from Bonaiti-Pellie C, Smith C: Risk tables for genetic counseling in some common congenital malformations. J Med Genet 11:374–377, 1974; Nora JJ, Nora AH: Evolution of specific genetic and environmental counseling in congenital heart disease. Circulation 57:205–213, 1978.)

Table 8.11 Possible Etiology in the Sporadic Case

1. Chromosomal	Mental retardation and congenital malformations suggest autosomal abnormality. Signs of Turner or Klinefelter—X chromosome.
2. Autosomal Dominant	New mutation. Check paternal age.
3. Autosomal Recessive	Check parental consanguinity and ethnic origins.
4. X-Linked Recessive	Unlikely if patient is female. If male, check maternal uncles and brothers.
5. Multifactorial	Use empiric risks and family history.
6. Environmental	Check history.

many other clinical situations, physicians should avoid giving direct advice as to whether to reproduce or not. If the disorder is serious and the recurrence risk 10 percent or greater, past experience has shown that few couples will take such a risk.

Although the physician is the most obvious person to provide genetic advice for his patients, it should be appreciated that the increasing complexity of genetic disorders, rapid expansion in knowledge, and the problem of genetic heterogeneity make it very difficult. In order to provide correct advice it is necessary to be up-to-date with the literature. Because of this, increasing reliance is placed on the services of the medical geneticist.

GENETIC SCREENING

The term *genetic screening* refers to the development of tests that can be applied to whole populations, and implies that the tests be relatively simple, inexpensive, and reliable. The greatest application is in the newborn. Most infants in developed countries are screened by means of a blood test for phenylketonuria (PKU) and many other inborn errors of metabolism. The success of the PKU program is enhanced by the fact that there is specific treatment available, namely dietary restriction, which will usually bring about normal mental development in the PKU child with deficiency of phenylalanine hydroxylase. In some of the inborn errors of metabolism there is no specific treatment available, but identification at an early stage permits genetic counseling so that parents understand the recurrence risk.

Screening for heterozygotes, that is, carriers of recessive disorders, is also carried out, but only on specific populations, for example, Ashkenazi Jews for Tay-Sachs disease, sickle cell anemia in blacks, thalassemia minor in Italians and Greeks. Although the aims of these programs are laudable, there can be undesirable repercussions. For example, in American Blacks who were screened for sickle cell trait, there were social consequences with respect to service in the armed forces, airplane travel, and insurance coverage. In addition, some heterozygous persons confuse this with homozygous and think that they, themselves, will become affected. In certain populations, screening may mean that a person is virtually ineligible for marriage should such heterozygosity be found. Before screening programs are initiated there needs to be widest possible discussion about the possible repercussions; provision for educational and counseling services are an essential part of screening. Unfortunately, screening often takes place without such preparation.

Despite these negative aspects, there are many advantages to having information about one's genotype, and it seems highly likely that in the future, ways will be available through molecular genetics to identify more recessive genes in humans. If specific treatment is not available, there may at least be the option of prenatal diagnosis.

PRENATAL DIAGNOSIS

Prenatal diagnosis refers mainly to the procedure of transabdominal amniocentesis, although other methods such as ultrasonography and fetoscopy may be used. The aim is to detect the disorder early in pregnancy to allow parents the option of having a therapeutic abortion if that is consistent with their ethical and philosophical attitudes. Amniocentesis also allows many couples to proceed with a pregnancy when they would not otherwise do so, particularly those who are at high risk for having another affected child. The indications for prenatal diagnosis are listed in Table 8.12.

Prior to the procedure, every couple should have adequate obstetric and genetic counseling so that they

Table 8.12 Indications for Prenatal Diagnosis

1. Maternal age 35 years or over
2. Previous child with trisomy
3. Either parent translocation carrier
4. Proven carriers of autosomal recessive disorder that can be diagnosed by a prenatal technique
5. Previous child with a neural tube defect
6. For fetal sexing—mother a carrier for x-linked recessive disorder

can make an informed decision about the issues. Ultrasonography is almost always performed prior to amniocentesis. Not only may it be diagnostic for anencephaly and some cases of spina bifida, it also may elicit important information such as the biparietal diameter (for calculating gestational age), the presence of twins, intrauterine death, and the position of the placenta. About 15 ml of amniotic fluid is removed, and after centrifuging, the cells are prepared for sex determination and cultured for chromosome analysis. The supernatant fluid is examined for α-fetoprotein, which is elevated in neural tube disorders, omphalocele, some cases of intestinal obstruction, and in congenital nephrosis. Biochemical testing for an inborn error of metabolism can only be applied to couples who are proven heterozygotes, that is, those who have had a previously affected child or, in the case of Tay-Sachs disease, couples who are proven heterozygotes by blood tests.

Fetoscopy is the visualization of parts of the fetus by means of a small telescope-like instrument. It will also permit the obstetrician to obtain a sample of fetal blood that can be used in the prenatal diagnosis of disorders such as the hemoglobinopathies. Direct visualization is useful in those genetic disorders in which there is invariably an external manifestation in association with a serious problem.

It seems likely that there will be further advances in prenatal diagnosis, particularly using noninvasive methods such as ultrasound. Serious disorders such as microcephaly and hydrocephaly have been detected in some centers by this method. Hopefully, methods will be found to actually correct or ameliorate the effects of the harmful gene, so that therapeutic termination of pregnancy will not remain the only option.

TREATMENT

The treatment of disorders that are totally or partially determined genetically, includes the use of glasses for refractive errors, hearing aids for deafness, and insulin for diabetes mellitus. An increasing number of genetic disorders are potentially treatable, examples of which are shown in Table 8.13. The classic prototype of dietary treatment is the low phenylalanine diet for the phenylalanine hydroxylase deficient form of phenylketonuria. This highly successful program is an interesting example of how an advance in one decade can lead to new problems two or more decades later. For example, it is impractical to keep phenylketonuria children on a low phenylalanine diet

Table 8.13 **Examples of Treatment for Genetic Disorders**

Replacement of Product	
Hemophilia A	Factor VIII
Congenital adrenal hyperplasia	Cortisol
Pituitary dwarfism	Growth hormone
Dietary Control	
Phenylketonuria	Low phenylalanine diet
Galactosemia	Lactose restriction
Lactase deficiency	Lactose restriction
Familial hypercholesterolemia	Low cholesterol and saturated fats
Hypertriglyceridemia	Low cholesterol and saturated fats
Vitamin therapy	
Homocystinuria (one form)	B_6 (pyridoxine)
Hypophosphatemia	D + phosphate
Surgery	
Familial polyposis coli	Colectomy
Fabry's disease	Kidney transplant
Polycystic kidney	Kidney transplant

throughout their lifetime; since brain maturation and myelinization have been largely completed in the childhood years, most authorities permit an unrestricted diet by the age of 7 years. There is no precise agreement as to the actual age of cessation of the diet; by teenage years, however, every PKU child is on an unrestricted diet. When PKU women have a high serum phenylalanine during pregnancy, fetal brain damage may develop. When the serum phenylalanine is greater than 20 mg percent, the chance that the offspring will be mentally retarded is nearly 100 percent. In these circumstances mental retardation is on an environmental basis, not a genetic one, that is, the child is likely to be heterozygous for the PKU gene (having received the mutant gene from the mother and probably the wild-type or normal gene from the father).

Therefore, adult females treated with the low phenylalanine diet should be aware of their PKU status, since they will need some form of dietary restriction from the time of conception in order to keep their serum phenylalanine at lower levels. The diet has to contain enough phenylalanine to permit normal growth of the fetus.

Galactosemia is another inborn error of metabolism in which effective dietary control can result in a normal person. It is important to exclude all forms of lactose, although this can be difficult, since many proprietary foods do not list their contents. Because of the danger of cataract development, it is recommended that affected persons eat a lactose-restricted diet for life.

Vitamin supplementation is important in disorders such as hypophosphatemia (vitamin D-resistant rickets). In these patients, large doses of vitamin D will overcome the basic metabolic defect. One of the several different forms of homocystinuria is responsive to vitamin B_6 (pyridoxine) therapy. This will induce some activity in the enzyme cystathionine synthetase, because vitamin B_6 is a cofactor. Frequently, a small increase in the level of enzyme activity will permit relatively normal metabolic balance. One form of methylmalonic acidemia can be treated in utero with vitamin B_{12}.

The gene product may be supplied in certain disorders such as hemophilia A (Factor VIII deficiency) and dwarfism due to growth hormone deficiency. Surgical reconstructive therapy is used for many congenital malformations that are commonly multifactorial in origin. Surgery may be useful for some single-gene disorders such as Fabry's disease, an X-linked recessive disorder causing rash, recurring fever, pain in the extremities, and kidney dysfunction. Kidney transplants in such patients may be a viable method of therapy, since the deficient enzyme is made in renal tissue. Kidney transplants are also used in adult polycystic kidney disease, an autosomal dominant disorder.

It is important to realize that all of the above methods have not changed the mutant gene. They have merely modified it, enhanced it, or replaced it. The possibility of actual gene therapy awaits further developments.

ETHICAL CONSIDERATIONS

Advances in genetics have brought many moral, legal, and ethical problems to the fore. Many issues are the result of the development of prenatal diagnosis. If a pregnant woman, aged 35 years or over, is not informed by her doctor about the diagnostic value of amniocentesis, could this be construed as negligence and is the physician liable? Suppose the patient is under 35 and is advised against amniocentesis, if she subsequently has a Down syndrome baby, is the physician or hospital liable? Does every woman have the right to demand an amniocentesis? Should it be done for selection of sex, that is, for couples wishing to plan the sexes of their children? For many physicians and geneticists these are serious problems that must include concern about inappropriate use of scarce resources.

Screening individuals for genetic disorders also has a number of problems. While screening should not be done unless informed consent has been obtained, such consent may be harmful even if it is easily obtained. Screening of newborn infants for disorders such as phenylketonuria or hypothyroidism is deemed to be desirable because treatment is available that will prevent a life-long handicap. What about newborn screening for Duchenne type muscular dystrophy for which no specific treatment is available? Early identification may seriously impair the parent-child bonding and result in rejection. Suppose the test was a false positive? Nonetheless, by alerting the parents to the problem, prevention of a second affected child could occur. Some of these issues appear during newborn chromosome screening with respect to the XYY karotype. It is not certain what proportion of such males will have any handicap, and consequently it is difficult to provide counsel to the parents. If the parents are not told, this complicates matters further.

Maternal serum α-fetoprotein screening is a current problem. Not all women will want to be screened; the time taken to explain it will be considerable; and if the test is sufficiently sensitive, it will generate a large number of unnecessary amniocenteses. This is not only expensive but likely to increase anxiety in women who undergo it.

Genetic counseling of the mildly mentally retarded raises particularly difficult ethical issues. Frequently there is a very small genetic risk for the offspring of such persons, but the social consequences may be great.

These issues and questions have no simple answers. It is most important that the level of genetic knowledge in the general public be increased to permit greater participation in decision-making by the patient. Awareness of this kind may also defuse the anxiety that surrounds genetic testing. Advances in technology should not be applied in the medical setting unless many of the issues have been thoroughly discussed and measures have been taken to minimize any harmful effects.

REFERENCES

1. Emery, A.E.H.: Elements of Medical Genetics. 4th ed. Edinburgh, Churchill Livingstone, 1975. (A good introductory text, available in paperback.)
2. Emery, A.E.H.: Methodology in Medical Genetics: An Introduction to Statistical Methods. Edinburgh, Churchill Livingstone, 1976. (The best available short text on this subject.)
3. McKusick, V.A.: Mendelian Inheritance in Man. Catalogs of Autosomal Dominant, Autosomal Recessive and X-Linked Phenotypes. 5th ed. Baltimore, Johns Hopkins University Press, 1978. (An essential reference text.)

4. Nora, J. J., Fraser. F. C.: Medical Genetics: Principles & Practice. 2nd ed. Philadelphia, Lea & Febiger, 1981. (A good introductory text).

5. Smith, D.W.: Recognizable Patterns of Human Malformation. 2nd ed. Philadelphia, W.B. Saunders, 1976. (An essential reference text.)

6. Thompson, J.S., Thompson, M.W.: Genetics in Medicine. 3rd ed. Philadelphia, W.B. Saunders, 1980. (A good introductory text.)

7. Vogel, F., Motulsky, A.G.: Human Genetics: Problems and Approaches. New York, Springer-Verlag, 1979. (The most comprehensive text available on this subject.)

9

Disorders of Fluid, Electrolytes, and Acid-Base Balance

Alan R. Hull, M.D.

The human body is equipped to maintain fluid volume in its various compartments and control the major electrolytes within an appropriate range, under a wide variety of circumstances. Abnormalities of fluid volume or electrolyte concentrations reflect dysfunction of the control mechanisms or undue physiological stress. Patients who present with abnormalities of fluids, electrolytes, or acid-base balance can be identified and treated appropriately, but the problem will recur unless the underlying mechanism is also recognized and corrected.

ABNORMALITIES OF FLUID VOLUME

The normal distribution of volume in the body compartments is outlined in Table 9.1. An excess of fluid may develop in any of the body compartments but, if present for a prolonged time, tends to be distributed to include each of the body compartments. For example, hyperinfusion of intravenous fluids will initially expand the plasma volume, but if diuresis does not remove that fluid, it will be transferred initially to the interstitial spaces and subsequently to the intracellular spaces. The mechanisms of such fluid accumulation in the body tissues are discussed in Chapters 11 and 16 in relation to mechanisms of edema formation.

Depletion of fluid volume may be a result of simple dehydration consisting of a loss of water without electrolytes, or hypovolemia due to combined losses of water and sodium. Simple dehydration will result in hypernatremia, as discussed below. The combined loss of water and sodium may occur with electrolyte concentrations well maintained. In many instances the mechanism of fluid loss is obvious.

Circulatory shock is said to be present when the blood pressure is markedly reduced while at the same time there are other manifestations of decreased peripheral circulation, such as oliguria or anuria. All of the definitions are arbitrary. Occasionally hypotension may occur in patients on vasodilating drugs or in patients widely vasodilated for other reasons, when shock is not present. Patients with septic shock frequently have warm and vasodilated extremities, whereas patients with pure hypovolemic shock generally have peripheral vasoconstriction. Altered sensorium due to poor cerebral perfusion and the development of metabolic acidosis are frequent accompaniments.

A mechanistic classification of the causes of shock can be outlined as follows:

1. Pump failure (cardiogenic shock): myocardial infarction or severe congestive failure.
2. Severe outflow obstruction: massive pulmonary embolism, aortic stenosis.
3. Reduced venous return: hypovolemia, septic shock with dilated vascular bed, overdose of drugs, neurogenic factors with peripheral vasodilation.

The therapeutic approaches must be based on a clear understanding of the cause. The most treatable form of shock is that due to hypovolemia, and patients having shock of this kind will respond to volume replacement. (Cardiogenic shock is discussed in Chapter 16.) For patients who are hypovolemic or

Table 9.1 Fluid Volume in the 70 kg Man

	Volume	Percentage Body Weight
Total Body Water	42 L	60
Intercellular Fluid	28 L	40
Extracellular Fluid	14 L	20
Interstitial Fluid	10.5 L	15
Plasma Volume	3.5 L	5

who are considered to be hypovolemic, a trial of fluid administration is important. Intravascular volume can be monitored by central venous pressure or pulmonary capillary wedge pressure. If the pressure is initially normal or low, 200 ml of fluid should be administered in 10 minutes, and the pressure should be reassessed. If the volume replacement does not cause the venous pressure to rise, the procedure should be repeated at regular intervals until the central venous pressure rises by 3 mm Hg or more, or until the blood pressure, cardiac output, and urinary output are restored. The management of shock requires rigorous monitoring and should be done by a physician with intensive clinical experience.

Gastrointestinal losses due to vomiting, diarrhea, or bowel fistulas are easily identified. Renal losses due to chronic renal failure, diuretic phase of acute tubular necrosis, adrenal insufficiency, osmotic diuresis, or use of diuretics may only be apparent after a careful history and examination of the urine flow. Skin losses due to excessive burns are readily apparent, but losses due to sweating may be difficult to assess. Finally, physicians must be particularly attentive to fluids lost by frequent thoracentesis or large volume paracentesis.

Hypovolemia may present clinically as orthostatic hypotension, weakness and fatigability, or with symptoms resulting from the associated electrolyte disturbances. Most frequently, hypovolemia accompanies other more prominent illnesses that are responsible for the fluid loss.

Volume depletion results in decreased skin turgor, particularly over the arms, the legs, and the face, a demonstrable postural drop in blood pressure, a dry tongue, decreased tension of the eyeballs, resting tachycardia, and often profound weakness. There is no simply available laboratory test to document hypovolemia. Measurements of blood volume and total body water require laboratory sophistication not commonly clinically available.

The urgency of volume replacement depends on the severity of the problem. When volume depletion results in circulatory collapse (shock) volume replacement is urgent and should consist of intravenous isotonic fluids, at least until the blood pressure is increased, or until the venous filling pressure of the heart is increased. Volume replacement must always be tailored to correct deficiencies in electrolytes or blood constituents.

THE MAJOR ELECTROLYTES

The concentrations of electrolytes are reported in different units by different laboratories. It is therefore essential to appreciate the different terminologies that are employed and to be able to relate one to another.

Perhaps most important is the relationship between weight and ionic strength.

One millimole of a substance equals its molecular weight expressed in milligrams: for example, 1 mmol Ca = 40 mg.

Since substances do not combine on a weight basis but rather do so in proportion to their ionic valence, it is useful to describe the amount of an ion that can combine with or replace 1 g of hydrogen. This amount is referred to as an equivalent (Eq). 1 millimole (mmol) of a substance multiplied by its valence equals the number of milliequivalents (mEq):

$$Na^+: \quad 1 \text{ millimole} = 1 \text{ milliequivalent}$$

$$Ca^{++}: 1 \text{ millimole} = 2 \text{ milliequivalent}$$

This allows us to convert from commonly used milligrams percent, (mg/100 ml or mg/dl) to milliequivalents per liter.

Examples:

1. Calcium: 10 mg% = (?) mEq/L.

$$\text{mEq/L of a substance} = \frac{\text{mg/dl}}{\text{atomic weight}} \times \text{valence}$$

$$\times \text{ conversion from 100 ml to 1,000 ml}$$

$$\text{mEq/L} = \frac{10}{40} \times 2 \times 10$$

$$\text{mEq/L} = \frac{200}{40}$$

$$\text{mEq/L} = 5$$

2. Sodium:

A 10 mEq sodium diet = (?) mg of Na^+

$$\text{mEq} = \frac{\text{mg}}{\text{atomic weight}}$$

$$\times \text{ valence}$$

$$10 = \frac{\text{mg}}{23} \times 1$$

$$10 \text{ mEq} = 230 \text{ mg}$$

Table 9.2 shows the primary location and approximate total body stores in mEq/kg of the major electrolytes of the body. In clinical medicine, Na, K, Cl, and HCO_3 are often viewed as a group, and in this way frequently give much more information than when viewed individually. We will consider their interactions in the way that they would be reported as laboratory results from a patient.

SODIUM (NORMAL 140–144 mEq/L)

The human body has a great ability to conserve sodium when kidney disease is not present. Normally, the kidney can limit Na losses to about 10

Table 9.2 Normal Body Electrolytes

Electrolytes	Serum Value Mg/dl	Serum Value mEq/L	Total Body Store	Major Location
Sodium (Na⁺)		140	(60 mEq/kg) 4,200 mEq	Extracellular
Chloride (Cl⁻)		100	(33 mEq/kg) 2,300 mEq	Extracellular
Potassium (K⁺)		4	(42 mEq/kg) 3,000 mEq	Intracellular
Bicarbonate (HCO₃⁻)		26	(20 mEq/kg) 1,400 mEq	Extracellular Intracellular
Calcium (Ca⁺⁺)	10	5	(800 mEq/kg) 56,000 mEq	Bone
Magnesium (Mg⁺⁺)		2	(15 mEq/kg) 1,000 mEq	Intracellular Bone

mEq/24 hours (about 250 mg of Na). If dietary sodium intake is restricted to 10 mEq/day, the body responds by losing sodium and body weight for a period of 3 to 5 days, at which point the kidney is able to balance loss and intake and a new stable state is attained. Blood pressure decreases slightly because of reduced extracellular volume, but the glomerular filtration rate (GFR) is ordinarily not decreased; this new steady state of a reduced Na intake can therefore continue indefinitely.

In contrast, the kidney has an almost unlimited ability to excrete large sodium loads. When given orally, up to 15 g of Na can be handled in normal subjects without any elevation of blood pressure or serum sodium levels and without the production of edema. The body's ability to perform such renal gymnastics indicates that the kidney is able to handle within reason whatever one's intake is. The fact that the body performs normally on very low sodium intake will be discussed later under blood pressure control.

Sodium is an extracellular cation. Serum sodium levels are only a measure of the extracellular concentration of the cation, and they give no information about either the total body sodium values or the amount of water in the body.

Hypernatremia

Hypernatremia is defined as a serum Na exceeding 145 mEq/L. Hypernatremia can result from either water loss in excess of Na loss, or an excess intake of Na into the body (Table 9.3). Water can be lost from three major sites: (1) The mucocutaneous structures, particularly skin and lungs. Sweating, fever, and hyperventilation due to any cause increase the losses. (2) The GI tract. Vomiting or diarrhea increase losses. (3) The kidneys. An osmotic diuresis, as in glycosuria, or diabetes insipidus may increase renal fluid losses.

Excess Na intake usually occurs through overzealous intravenous sodium administration.

The major clinical manifestations of hypernatremia are weakness and confusion. As the serum Na approaches 170 mEq/L, coma may supervene.

Replacement of "free" water is usually adequate therapy for hypernatremia. Correction of the underlying disturbance will then allow the body to return to its usual steady state of Na balance.

Hyponatremia

Hyponatremia is defined as a serum Na of less than 135 mEq/L. It may result from water retention in excess of salt or replacement of salt and water losses with solutions deficient in sodium.

The retention of water with salt, or of water alone, is commonly due to normal renal mechanisms trying to compensate for pathology in other organ systems. In congestive heart failure, cirrhosis, or nephrosis, the kidney retains salt and water in an attempt to expand the effective arterial blood volume and maintain blood pressure. Unfortunately, the fluid retained does not expand the appropriate body compartment and merely overloads the whole system. For example, the heart in congestive failure is unable to pump properly, and an increased vascular volume only increases the load on the heart and worsens the

Table 9.3 Hypernatremia
(Serum Na Greater Than 145 mEq/L)

Total Body Sodium	Mechanism	Example
High	Increased intake of sodium	NaHCO₃ given during cardiac arrest
Normal	Pure water loss	Diabetes insipidus
Low	Combined losses but water exceeds sodium loss	Sweating

situation. The kidneys response, however, would be appropriate if the cardiovascular system were normal; with a truly inadequate vascular volume, fluid should be retained to reduce the deficit.

Another example in which a physiologic renal response produces hyponatremia is the syndrome of inappropriate antidiuretic hormone secretion (SIADH). Under normal circumstances, ADH is secreted in response to a rise in serum osmolality, permitting the kidneys to retain fluid and thus expanding volume and reducing osmolality. ADH, however, can be secreted under a number of abnormal conditions, for example, central nervous system infection, tumor, or trauma. It can also be produced in states of disordered pulmonary function induced by a variety of drugs, and can be elaborated by ectopic tumors (typically oat cell carcinomas of the lung). In these situations, the kidney responds physiologically and retains water. The resultant volume expansion and dilution would normally stop the secretion of ADH, but in these abnormal conditions such feedback control is missing. Hyponatremia, therefore, progresses because the kidney continues to retain water due to the sustained ADH level, and the fluid retention causes volume expansion that triggers proximal tubular rejection of salt, and further dilution of serum sodium levels ensues. In SIADH, the total body sodium may be normal (since volume is increased) or low. The syndrome of inappropriate ADH secretion is one indication that volume sensors override osmolarity, and that maintenance of extracellular volume takes precedence over maintenance of serum osmolality.

Table 9.4 shows the relationship of total body sodium to the various mechanisms producing hyponatremia.

The clinical manifestations of hyponatremia are varied and relate to the underlying etiology and the effect of the sodium-to-water ratio. When both sodium and water are retained but water is retained in excess of sodium, edema results. When total body sodium is normal and only water is retained, there are few symptoms until the serum Na decreases below 120 mEq/L, particularly if the evolution of hyponatremia has been gradual. Below 120 mEq/L, however, confusion and seizures may result. Finally, when salt is lost and replaced by sodium deficient fluids, the primary manifestations are those of volume deficiency as described above.

Hyponatremia rarely requires therapy other than correction of the underlying condition. When necessary, water restriction or diuresis will usually return the total body sodium to normal. In congestive failure, for example, diuretics can be used to block renal salt and water retention, and digitalis is given to correct the pump failure. By contrast, where sodium has been lost, oral salt replacement usually permits the kidney to correct the abnormalities.

POTASSIUM (NORMAL 3.5 TO 5 mEq/L)

It is generally accepted that the nephron reabsorbs most if not all of the filtered potassium, and the potassium that appears in the urine does so by secretion and distal exchange. However, the human kidney is not able to handle potassium nearly as efficiently as it can sodium. This is particularly true in regard to conservation, and a gradual, continual loss may produce significant potassium depletion. Similarly, even in good health, but especially in renal disease, sudden, large loads of potassium may overwhelm the kidney and raise the serum potassium to dangerous levels. Such an event is perhaps better understood when one realizes that the normal daily intake of potassium may be 150 mEq, and that this exceeds the total amount of potassium in the extracellular fluid by a factor of 2.

Hyperkalemia

Hyperkalemia is defined as a serum potassium exceeding 6 mEq/L. The various etiologies of hyperkalemia are outlined in Table 9.5. When levels exceed 6 mEq/L, they should be followed with repeat studies, the cause should be determined, and emergency measures should be undertaken immediately.

The major clinical manifestations of hyperkalemia are muscle weakness, paralysis, and characteristic EKG changes. These include increased T wave voltage (peaked T waves), prolongation of the PR interval and decreased P wave voltage, widening of the QRS complex, and eventual appearance of a "sine wave" configuration as the widened QRS and peaked T wave merge.

Therapy is determined by the severity of hyper-

Table 9.4 **Hyponatremia (Serum Na Less Than 135 mEq/L)**

Total Body Sodium	Mechanism	Example
High	Both water and sodium added but water exceeds sodium	Congestive heart failure
Normal	Addition of water only	Syndrome of inappropriate ADH
Low	Loss of sodium and water and predominant replacement with water.	Diarrhea

Table 9.5 **Etiology of Hyperkalemia**

1. Pseudohyperkalemia
   A. Delayed analysis of blood
   B. Elevated platelets (greater than 1,000,000) or increased WBC (leukemia)
2. Increased Intake in the Presence of Renal Impairment
   A. Ingestion—food or drugs
   B. Blood transfusion
3. Shift from Cellular Space
   A. Acidosis[a]
   B. Tissue trauma—may become a problem if blood supply is restored to damaged area
4. Renal Causes
   A. Acute renal failure[a]—often associated with acidosis
   B. Potassium sparing diuretics—especially when linked with potassium supplements
   C. Hypoaldosteronism, Addisons' disease
   D. Chronic Renal Failure—especially with volume depletion

[a] The most common causes

kalemia. When the serum potassium exceeds 7 mEq/L, or when the EKG indicates severe hyperkalemia, rapid correction (seconds to minutes) should be accomplished with intravenous $NaHCO_3$ to correct acidemia; insulin and glucose to shift potassium back into the cells; and calcium gluconate to reverse the cardiotoxic effects of hyperkalemia. Alkali and calcium should never be given in the same intravenous solution, since calcium carbonate (limestone) may precipitate.

Intermediate therapy, effective over minutes to hours, can be accomplished by sodium-potassium exchange resins, given either orally or rectally.

Dialysis is the slowest means of correction, primarily because of the time required to establish adequate dialysis. Hemodialysis is carried out with a "zero" potassium bath, and is effective in virtually all cases of hyperkalemia except some cases resulting from massive tissue breakdown. Peritoneal dialysis can remove only 30 mEq/hour, but is very effective over 12 to 24 hours.

In emergency situations, one ampule (44 mEq) of $NaHCO_3$ given by intravenous push should produce an almost instantaneous lowering of the serum potassium (monitored by EKG), and the other parenteral drugs should permit stabilization until resins or dialysis become effective.

Hypokalemia

Hypokalemia is defined as a serum potassium less than 3.5 mEq/L. It is generally a more chronic problem than hyperkalemia. A basic rule of thumb is that for every 0.5 mEq/L decrease in serum potassium (if the pH is normal), the body is deficient by 100 mEq of K. This generalization only holds to a serum value of 2.0 to 2.5 mEq/L. Below this value, even severe total body losses may not be reflected by further reduction in serum level.

Potassium can be lost through the GI tract (diarrhea, intestinal or biliary tract fistulas, vomiting, nasogastric suction, and laxative abuse) or through the kidneys (diuretic abuse, renal tubular disorders, hypoaldosteronism, and ureterosigmoidostomy). Hypokalemia can also result from inadequate intake (rare), cellular shifts due to alkalosis, hypokalemic periodic paralysis, and profuse sweating (especially in poorly conditioned individuals). Laxative and diuretic abuse are the most common etiologies. Nasogastric suction causes hypokalemia not only through direct GI loss, but also by production of a metabolic alkalosis that increases urinary losses.

Clinical findings include muscle weakness, ileus, areflexic paralysis, and occasionally, hypertension. Characteristic EKG changes include flattening of the T wave and the appearance of a U wave. These manifestations of cardiac toxicity are rarely life-threatening. Sudden hypokalemia also predisposes to digitalis toxicity, and digitoxic arrhythmias may appear without an increase in serum digitalis levels.

Oral potassium replacement is usually satisfactory. Potassium chloride has an unpleasant taste but few side effects. On rare occasions, enteric tablets have been associated with small bowel perforation.

If intravenous replacement is desired, EKG monitoring should be established and potassium should be given at rates not exceeding 40 mEq/hour, especially in patients with impaired renal function.

Despite rapid normalization of serum potassium levels with both oral and intravenous replacement, obligate urinary losses result in delayed restoration of total body stores.

Hypokalemia and Hypertension

A small but significant group of patients with hypokalemia have elevated blood pressures (see chapter 3). In most cases this is thought to be associated with mineralocorticoid excess, either due to increased aldosterone production or to some substance that acts similarly. When hypokalemia and hypertension are observed and diuretic abuse has been ruled out, the physician should look for the following syndromes:

1. Primary aldosteronism
2. Cushing's syndrome
3. Tumors secreting ACTH-like substances (aldosterone levels may be normal)
4. Adrenogential syndrome
5. Renin producing tumors
6. Licorice abuse (aldosterone will be low or normal)

7. Accelerated hypertension

8. Renal artery stenosis (level of aldosterone, when measured, does not always correlate)

CHLORIDE (NORMAL 100 TO 104 mEq/L)

The physician should look at serum chloride levels for two pieces of information:

1. A low or high chloride value proportional to the serum sodium suggests that the cause is related to excess water intake or loss.

2. A chloride value that is disproportionately elevated or decreased compared with the sodium level, suggests an acid-base problem.

For example, with a sodium level of 128 mEq/L and chloride of 89 mEq/L, dilution is likely; with a sodium of 128 mEq/L and a serum chloride of 96 mEq/L, the chloride is disproportionately elevated compared with the sodium, and a metabolic acidosis is probably present. By contrast, the physician should suspect a metabolic alkalosis if the sodium were 140 mEq/L and the chloride 89 mEq/L.

When the chloride is abnormal but proportional to sodium, therapy is the same as described for hyponatremia and hypernatremia. If hyperchloremia or hypochloremia exists in disproportion to sodium, the underlying acid-base problem must be treated to correct the chloride.

BICARBONATE (NORMAL 24 TO 28 mEq/L)

The kidney filters over 4,000 mEq of bicarbonate every 24 hours, but maintains a normal serum bicarbonate level by two mechanisms:

1. In the more proximal area of the tubule, aided by the enzyme carbonic anhydrase, the kidney "reclaims" most of the filtered bicarbonate.

2. In the more distal areas of the tubule, when all the filtered bicarbonate has been reclaimed, the kidney begins to excrete hydrogen in exchange for sodium and to generate bicarbonate in the process. It is essential to realize that these two events, hydrogen excretion and bicarbonate generation, are synonomous.

THE ANION GAP

Having assessed four of the major electrolytes individually, we can now review them collectively for some additional "free" information (Fig. 9.1).

The sum of the ionic constituents of blood results in approximate electrical neutrality. Therefore all measureable cations should equal all measureable an-

140	4
SODIUM	POTASSIUM
CHLORIDE	BICARBONATE
100	26

Fig. 9.1 The Anion "Gap"

ions. Since sodium is by far the most measureable and quantitatively important cation, it can be considered to represent the cation pool. Chloride and bicarbonate are the most readily measured, quantitatively important anions and might be considered to represent the anion pool. The difference between the anions and cations measured has been termed the *anion gap*. A normal anion gap exists because of unmeasured anions such as phosphate, sulfate, and others. Clearly from the measured electrolytes outlined above a clinically useful estimate of the anion gap can be readily calculated.

$$Sodium - (Chloride + Bicarbonate) = Anion\,Gap$$
$$140\,mEq/L - (100 + 26)\,mEq/L = 14\,mEq/L$$

In general the range of 10 to 14 mEq/L is accepted as normal, but this value will vary from hospital to hospital. Anion gaps much outside this range must be considered abnormal, and should suggest one of the etiologies listed in Table 9.6.

ACID-BASE BALANCE

The body controls acid-base interaction by several systems with varying capacity that affect different components of acid production or elimination. The transition from one of these systems to another is

Table 9.6 **Abnormal Anion Gap**

High Anion Gap
  1. Metabolic acidosis
  2. Infusion of unmeasured anion (acetate)
  3. Dehydration (hemo concentration)[a]
  4. Alkalosis[a]
  5. Other sodium salt, for example, antibiotics[a]
Low Anion Gap
  1. Reduced concentration of unmeasured anions
      Dilutional
      Hypoalbuminemia
  2. Systematic *under*estimation of the serum sodium
      Hypernatramia (severe), hyperviscosity
  3. Systematic *over*estimation of serum chloride
      Bromism
  4. Increase nonsodium cations
      Paraproteins, for example, myeloma, calcium, magnesium, lithium

[a] These cause minor increases, less than 3 mEq/L.

smooth and overlapping, as they function to "defend" the normal hydrogen ion concentration.

The buffer system Intracellular and extracellular substances, for example, bicarbonate, phosphate, hemoglobin, and proteins, react together and in a series of pH ranges (usually relative to their pK) to stabilize minor fluctuations in hydrogen ion concentration. Since a change in any one buffer also results in a change in the others, we can monitor any one to follow acid-base changes. The buffer system that is generally employed is the bicarbonate-carbonic acid system with a pK of 6.1. It is an open-ended system in that one of the products, carbon dioxide, can be excreted by the lungs, and another, H_2CO_3, by the kidney.

The lungs The lungs act more slowly than the buffer systems but much more rapidly than the kidney. In normal man, the lungs remove carbon dioxide in proportion to the rate of production in the body. During periods of excess acid production (diabetic acidosis) the lungs may transiently be called on to eliminate much more carbon dioxide than that which is produced, thereby depleting body stores.

The kidneys The kidneys, although slower than the respiratory system, are more versatile in their ability to produce a stable acid-base environment (pH 7.4). When an alkalosis develops, the kidneys respond by excreting less acid, resulting in the loss of some filtered bicarbonate until the pH returns to normal. By contrast, the response to an acidosis is to reabsorb all the filtered bicarbonate and to generate new bicarbonate as the acid is excreted. To accomplish this, titratable acid and amonium production increases and can be measured in the urine.

The Henderson-Hasselbach equation relates pH to the buffer systems and reflects the contributions of the kidney and the lungs.

$$pH = pK + \log \frac{[HCO_3^-]}{[H_2CO_3]}$$

Since H_2CO_3 is directly proportional to PCO_2, by a conversion factor (f) the denominator can be converted to PCO_2. The pK is 6.1 (the pH at which the buffer operates most effectively; with 50 percent as acid form and 50 percent as base).

Therefore:

$$pH = 6.1 + \log \frac{HCO_3^-}{f \times PCO_2}$$

One can then think of the numerator (HCO_3^-) as the kidney control mechanism and the denominator (PCO_2) as the lung control mechanism. Conceptually, then, this becomes:

$$pH \text{ varies by } \frac{kidney\ mechanism\ (metabolic)}{lung\ mechanism\ (respiratory)}$$

SPECIFIC ACID-BASE DISTURBANCES

We can now look at acid-base regulation in regard to metabolic and respiratory causes of acidosis and alkalosis. In each section we will outline the initial event that triggers the primary results (labeled 1 and 2), followed by the compensatory event (labeled 3) that returns the pH toward normal (7.4). Note that the compensation is never complete. The situations with an increase in serum pH above 7.45 are called *alkalosis*, and the high pH (low H^+ concentration) is called *alkalemia*. Similarly the conditions with pH below 7.35 are called *acidosis* and the low serum pH (high H^+ concentration) is called *acidemia*. In general, the adverse effects of acid-base disturbances are determined by the severity of the acidemia or alkalemia, which depends on the effectiveness of compensatory mechanisms.

Alkalemia with a pH ranging from 7.45 to 7.50 is rarely symptomatic. Levels above 7.55 require urgent consideration, and levels over 7.60 may be associated with arrhythmias, tetany, and seizures. Acidemia ranging from pH 7.35 to 7.25 is generally well tolerated, but levels below 7.20 require urgent treatment. The hazard to the patient depends on the renal and respiratory compensatory results and associated problems such as coronary disease or underlying seizure disorders.

Metabolic Acidosis (Fig. 9.2)

Initial reaction:
  Addition of acid, for example, endogenous lactic acid production
  Loss of base, e.g., diarrhea
Primary result
  ① Decrease in the serum bicarbonate
  ② Fall in serum pH
Compensation
  ③ Increase in alveolar ventilation with decreased PCO_2 and pH returns *toward* normal

It is clinically useful to note that pure metabolic acidosis with respiratory compensation can be recognized because the PCO_2 generally equals the pH minus 7.0. For example, at pH 7.20, PCO_2 should be 20.

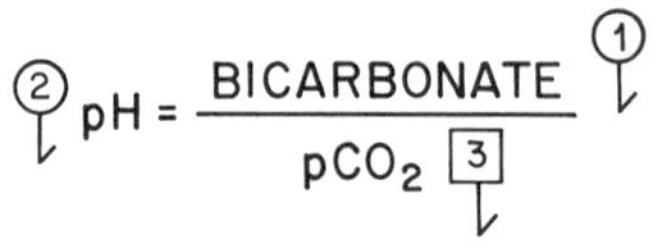

$$② \; pH = \frac{BICARBONATE \; ①}{pCO_2 \; ③}$$

Fig. 9.2 Metabolic Acidosis

Metabolic acidosis is most commonly associated with an increased anion gap, but may occur with a normal anion gap. Table 9.7 lists the causes of metabolic acidosis.

The symptoms of metabolic acidosis generally relate to the etiologic agent or disease process. In mild acidosis only the respiratory compensation with deeper (Kussmaul) and more rapid respirations may be evident. As the acidemia becomes more severe, cardiovascular impairment becomes apparent, with decreased ventricular contractility, peripheral vasodilatation, and central venous constriction. The central nervous system may be depressed, with headache, confusion, and, finally, coma.

Volume depletion may be associated with many of the above causes and, as with lactic acidosis or diarrhea, volume replacement alone may be all the therapy that is required. In other situations specific therapy, for example, insulin for diabetes mellitus or dialysis for renal failure, is required. If bicarbonate is needed to correct severe acidemia, it should be given cautiously (one-half the estimated deficit), and the patient should then be reevaluated. If we assume bicarbonate to be distributed in total body water, then an appropriate calculation of the deficit would be 60 percent of normal weight (kg) × bicarbonate deficit (mEq/L). In severe cases, 50 percent of the calculated deficit should be given in a set time period, and the patient should then be reevaluated by remeasuring the electrolytes and the blood gases.

In patients with chronic metabolic acidosis, oral bicarbonate or Shohl's solution (citric acid, sodium citrate mixture) may be all that is required to keep the patient stable.

Metabolic Alkalosis (Fig. 9.3)

Initial reaction:
  Loss of acid, for example, nasogastric suction
  Addition of base, for example, intravenous sodium bicarbonate
Primary result
  ① Increase in the serum bicarbonate
  ② Rise in the serum pH
Compensation
  ③ Decrease in alveolar ventilation resulting in increased PCO_2 with a return of the pH *toward* normal
  Compensation rarely increases the PCO_2 above 55 and never above 60 mmHg.

The clinical findings of metabolic alkalosis are usually related to the underlying cause. In many cases, symptoms due to associated hypokalemia may be the

Table 9.7 Causes of Metabolic Acidosis

Increased Anion Gap (greater than 15 mEq/L)
  1. Renal failure
  2. Ketoacidosis
      a. Starvation
      b. Alcoholic
      c. Diabetes mellitus
  3. Lactic acidosis
  4. Toxins
      a. Ethylene glycol
      b. Salicylates
      c. Acetate
Normal Anion Gap (less than 10 to 14 mEq/L)
  1. Renal tubular acidosis
      a. Distal (classic type 1)
      b. Proximal
      c. Mixed
  2. Diarrhea
  3. Posthypocapnic
  4. Ureteral diversions
  5. Additon of HCL or other acidifying agents

only finding. Rarely, with alkali administration, tetany is induced. A measurement of urine chloride should always be obtained, since it can give guidance to the etiology of the hydrogen ion loss (Table 9.8). The absence of chloride in the urine (less than 10 mEq/L) suggests a "chloride responsive" etiology. These patients are volume depleted with avid proximal tubular bicarbonate reabsorption. On the other hand a disproportionately high urine chloride (greater than 20 mEq/L) in the absence of diuretics usually means a "chloride resistant" cause. These patients are volume expanded with distal tubular bicarbonate reabsorption that is increased with potassium depletion. In chloride responsive patients, replacement of volume as sodium chloride solution is sufficient to allow the kidney to correct the alkalosis. In chloride resistant cases, replacement of potassium is often required to correct the alkalosis. Potassium may be required, because severe depletion can increase proximal tubule bicarbonate reabsorption to such an extent that volume expansion will only partially overcome this avid increase in reabsorption, and the alkalosis will persist, although at a less intense level. In some instances, specific therapy, for example, mineralocorticoid antagonists (spironolactone) may be required. In rare cases, when there is failure of several organ systems, acidifying agents such as ammonium chloride or arginine hydrochloride may be required.

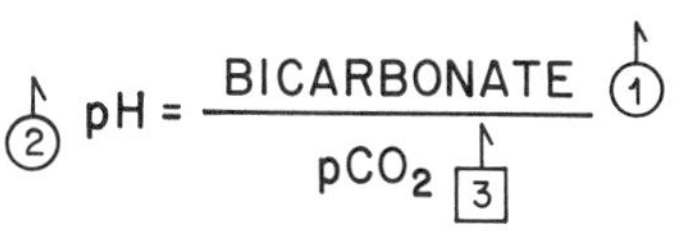

$$② \; pH = \frac{BICARBONATE \; ①}{pCO_2 \; ③}$$

Fig. 9.3 Metabolic Alkalosis

Table 9.8 **Mechanisms of Metabolic Alkalosis**

1. Increased Hydrogen Ion Loss
   A. Chloride responsive (urine chloride less than 10 mEq/L)
      a. Gastrointestinal Losses
         i. Vomiting[a]
         ii. Nasogastric suctioning[a]
         iii. Diarrhea with potassium and/or chloride loss
      b. Diuretic therapy[a]
   B. Chloride resistant (urine chloride more than 20 mEq/L)
      a. Mineralocorticoid excess
      b. Severe potassium loss
2. Excess Alkali Administration
   A. Intravenous bicarbonate—post-cardiac arrest
   B. Milk-alkali syndrome

[a] Most common and must always be considered

Respiratory Acidosis (Fig. 9.4)

Initial reaction:
  Decreased alveolar ventilation with retained PCO_2, for example, oversedation
Primary result
  ① Increased PCO_2
  ② Fall in serum pH
Compensation
  ③ Kidney produces bicarbonate and the pH returns *toward* normal
  In acute respiratory acidosis, for every 10 mmHg increase in PCO_2, the bicarbonate will increase 1 mEq/L due to effects on the buffer system. In chronic respiratory acidosis, for every 10 mmHg increase in PCO_2, bicarbonate will increase 4 mEq/L, reflecting the renal contribution to compensation.

Respiratory acidosis is discussed in chapter 15 in relation to respiratory failure. Lung disease, airway obstruction, central nervous system disease, drugs that depress ventilation, and disease of the respiratory muscles are all potential causes.

Acutely, the symptoms of respiratory acidosis are due to the acidemia; these include headache, blurred vision, delirium, and, finally, coma. Chronically, the patient may be asymptomatic until confusion develops; if untreated, coma may result (see Chapter 15, Table 15.1).

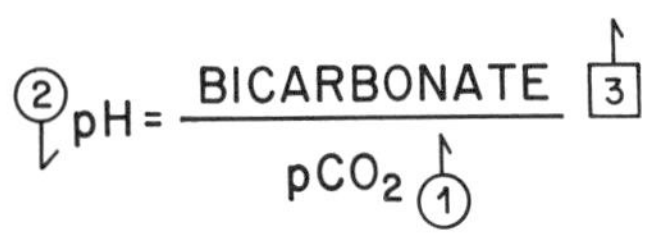

Treatment involves correction of the underlying problems, discussed in detail in Chapter 15.

Respiratory Alkalosis (Fig. 9.5)

Initial reaction:
  Increase in alveolar ventilation, for example, anxiety
Primary result
  ① Decrease in PCO_2
  ② Rise in serum pH
Compensation
  ③ Kidney excretes bicarbonate and the pH returns *toward* normal
  In respiratory alkalosis, for every 10 torr decrease in PCO_2, bicarbonate decreases 1 mEq/L. In chronic respiratory alkalosis, for every 10 torr decrease in PCO_2, bicarbonate decreases 5 mEq/L due to renal contribution to compensation.

The causes of hyperventilation and respiratory alkalosis include anxiety, fever, hepatic failure, central nervous system stimulants (for example, theophylline and salicylates), lung disease (asthma, pulmonary embolism, pulmonary edema), and hypoxemia due to any cause. This is a particularly common complication of artificial ventilation with mechanical respirators. Two clinical signs may raise suspicion of severe respiratory alkalosis: increased rate and depth of respiration, and symptoms of increased neuromuscular excitability (see Chapter 15, Table 15.2). Chronic hyperventilation may have no clinically recognizable features.

Mixed Acid-Base Disturbances

Patients frequently have more than one type of acid-base disturbance. These so-called mixed acid-base problems are most commonly seen in hospitalized patients. If the numbers do not correspond with the simple program outline above under initial reaction, primary results, and compensation, the physician should suspect a mixed disturbance. Offsetting disturbances, such as metabolic acidosis and respiratory alkalosis, will have a normal pH but abnormal PCO_2 and bicarbonate. In contrast, combined met-

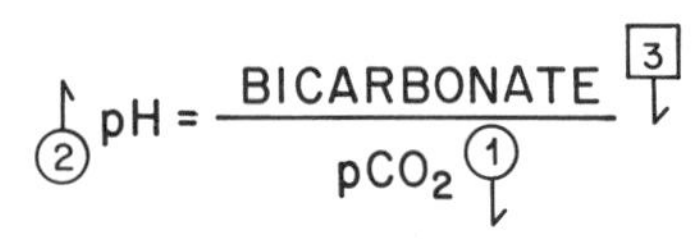

$$② \text{pH} = \frac{\text{BICARBONATE} \uparrow ③}{\text{pCO}_2 \uparrow ①}$$

Fig. 9.4 Respiratory Acidosis

$$② \text{pH} = \frac{\text{BICARBONATE} \downarrow ③}{\text{pCO}_2 ① \downarrow}$$

Fig. 9.5 Respiratory Alkalosis

abolic and respiratory acidosis or combined metabolic and respiratory alkalosis are marked by dramatic changes in pH, with only small changes in PCO_2 or bicarbonate.

Numerous nomograms have been developed to help unravel mixed disturbances, but none is foolproof. The severity and temporal relationship for each component of the acid-base disturbance must always be considered, and any simple nomogram will be inadequate to account for all possible variations.

OTHER ELECTROLYTES WITH COMMON CLINICAL DISORDERS

CALCIUM (NORMAL 9.5–10.5 mg/dl OR 4.7 TO 5.3 mEq/L)

The major discussion of calcium metabolism is presented in Chapter 13. Despite a very complicated control mechanism, serum calcium remains within a relatively narrow range. The most common cause of a low serum calcium level is a decreased serum albumin. Forty percent of the serum calcium is protein-bound, and a significant decrease in the serum albumin will lower the calcium level; for every 1 g/dl decrease of the albumin the serum calcium will decrease 1 mg/dl. The remaining 60 percent of the serum calcium is in complexed (10 percent) or ionized (50 percent) form and acts on nerves and muscle. This ionized portion is very pH sensitive. A rise in pH causes increased binding so that less calcium exists in the free or ionized form. Only the ionized calcium is both biologically active and filterable by the kidneys. The acceptable normal values for 24 hour calcium in the urine on a random diet is 250 mg/24 hours in females and 300 mg/24 hours in males.

The causes of hypercalcemia are listed in Table 13.13, in Chapter 13. Clinically, these patients have generalized nonspecific complaints and findings that are often hard to relate to hypercalcemia, for example, they may have, lethargy, nausea and vomiting, fatigue, constipation, decreased reflexes, and even psychiatric disturbances. With chronic hypercalcemia, disorders such as polyuria, kidney stones, and/or nephrocalcinosis may lead to renal failure. The causes of hypocalcemia (levels below 9 mg/dl) are discussed in Chapter 13. The signs and symptoms of hypocalcemia include muscle weakness, muscle cramps, and carpopedal spasm. Tetany should be tested for by Trousseau's sign; Chvostek's sign is too nonspecific to make the diagnosis. Sudden development of an alkalotic state can precipitate tetany in a normally asymptomatic person, due to increased protein binding of free calcium.

Therapy of hypocalcemia and hypercalcemia is discussed in Chapter 13 in relation to specific causes.

PHOSPHATE (NORMAL 3.5 TO 5.5 mg/dl)

Phosphate is an intracellular anion that interacts with a great many systems, including calcium for bone formation, urinary buffering of hydrogen ions, energy formation, and others. Hyperphosphatemia can be caused by renal impairment (a creatinine clearance of less than 25), increased intake associated with any degree of renal impairment, and shifts of phosphate out of cells. The latter rarely produces significant hyperphosphatemia unless there is massive cell lysis (for example, with chemotherapy for leukemia) or muscle breakdown, usually secondary to trauma.

The major problems of hyperphosphatemia are related to metastatic calcification, which, in the soft tissues, may cause itching, and in the heart may interupt the conducting system and cause arrhythmias. Therapy involves a low phosphate diet, which is usually difficult to maintain over the long term, and administration of phosphate-binding substances, most commonly antacids.

Hypophosphatemia usually only becomes a significant problem below 1 mg/dl. Clinical manifestations may then include rhabdomyolysis, hemolysis, weakness, and, chronically, bone pain. Causes include renal loss, dietary deficiencies, and cellular shifts, the last seen during parenteral hyperalimentation. Oral or intravenous phosphate replacement is the therapy of choice.

Calcium-Phosphorus Product

In clinical medicine, the calcium-phosphorus product serves as a rough guide to the tolerable limits of calcium and phosphate levels. Normally, the product is 40 when measured in mg/dl (calcium-10 × phosphorus-4). When the product is increased by 50 percent or more, metastatic calcification and soft-tissue deposition occur. Such levels must be avoided by lowering either the calcium or the phosphorus, or both. More controversial is the gray zone between a product of 40 and 60. Generally, clinicians attempt to keep the product as close to normal as possible, recognizing that chronically higher products appear to be associated with problems of soft-tissue deposition.

MAGNESIUM (NORMAL 1.5 TO 2.0 mEq/L)

Magnesium is mainly an intracellular cation, and is discussed in Chapter 13. A significant portion of an oral dose is absorbed by the gut until high serum levels (4 to 5 mEq/L) are reached. At this point, stool losses increase. Urinary loss also increases as the serum value rises. In normal humans, these two excretory pathways balance the usual dietary intake and maintain a normal serum level. Abnormal responses occur with changes in the renal handling of magnesium or with intramuscular administration.

Hypermagnesemia

Hypermagnesemia (levels exceeding 5 mEq/L) can occur in renal failure, probably secondary to the increased oral intake of magnesium-containing antacids. Because of the intestinal excretion mechanism above 4 mEq/L, symptomatic hypermagnesemia is rare. Intramuscular injections of magnesium used to treat pre-eclampsia can produce marked toxicity. Clinical manifestions include the loss of deep-tendon reflexes (above 6 mEq/L), paralysis (including respiratory paralysis), cardiac conduction abnormalities, confusion and coma.

Treatment of hypermagnesemia involves stopping all magnesium administration and giving calcium salts to block the effects of high magnesium on muscle cells, particularly cells of the myocardium. Dialysis can be used in extreme cases.

Hypomagnesemia

Hypomagnesemia (levels below 1 mEq/L) can result from decreased intake, malabsorption, extensive surgical bowel resection, and renal losses secondary to severe alcoholism or chronic renal failure. As is true of hypokalemia, serum magnesium levels may not disclose the true extent of the deficiency.

Clinical manifestations may include muscular weakness, progressing to carpopedal spasms and hyperreflexia, and, with extremely low levels, to enhancement of digitalis toxicity.

Treatment involves increasing oral intake and/or replacement with magnesium sulfate. In emergency situations, $MgSO_4$ can be administered intramuscularly.

REFERENCES

1. Arbus, G.S.: An *in vivo* acid-base nomogram for clinical use. Can. Med. Assoc. J. 109:291, 1973.
2. Davenport, H.W.: The ABC of Acid-Base Chemistry. (6th ed.). University of Chicago Press, Chicago, 1974.
3. Emmett, M., Narius, R.G.: Clinical use of the anion gap. Medicine 56: 38, 1977.
4. Jones, N.L.: Blood Gases and Acid Base Physiology. Brian C. Decker, New York, 1980.
5. Maxwell, M.H., Kleoman, C.R. (eds.): Clinical Disorders of Fluid and Electrolyte Metabolism. McGraw-Hill Book Company. New York, 1980.
6. Nevins, R.G.: Simple and mixed acid base disorders. A practical approach. Medicine 59:161, 1980.

10

Use and Assessment of Drugs

John K. Ruedy, M.D.

Successful drug treatment of a patient depends on precise diagnosis, an estimate of the anticipated course of the disorder (prognosis), and an understanding of the influence of the drug on the disease. In addition, the benefits and risks of alternative treatment must be considered, the dose requirements of the drug must be determined for the individual patient, and baseline and continuing observations essential to evaluation of the effects of treatment must be documented. Finally, response to treatment must be continually evaluated in an unbiased manner. Such seemingly complex prerequisites can appear overwhelming and impractical in the busy world of clinical practice. As with all skills, however, with practice the process of reaching decisions regarding drug therapy becomes rapid. Indeed, in many instances the process becomes virtually automatic, and the observer may misinterpret the efficiency of the experienced clinician as meaning that therapeutic decisions are reached intuitively and not determined by careful and critical analysis. Until skills have been developed to this level of proficiency, it is important that care be used to analyze the benefits and risks of therapy and to delineate therapeutic goals.

IDENTIFICATION OF TREATMENT GOALS

Similar deliberations are involved in reaching decisions regarding drug therapy, whether the goals of treatment are *preventive, curative, palliative,* or *symptomatic.* It is important to recognize, however, that there are characteristic constraints involved in achieving each of these particular goals. For example, the rewards of preventive treatment, although definite, are less tangible than the relief of suffering provided by symptomatic treatment. The side effects of the drug used for prophylaxis may well make the patient feel worse than he would feel without the treatment. Although the complications of stroke and cardiac failure can be partially prevented by treatment of arterial hypertension, the competence with which patients are provided such prophylactic treatment and the reliance with which they take their medication are poor. It has been estimated that only half of patients with diagnosed hypertension in the United States are being treated, and only half of these are receiving adequate treatment. The physician must realize the importance of prophylactic treatment, and the patient must understand that the treatment is not being provided to relieve symptoms, if treatment goals are to be achieved.

If curative treatment is available, particularly for disease that is likely to lead to permanent harm or death, much greater risks can be taken than when palliative treatment is the only resort. Acceptance of the severe suppression of normal hematopoietic function during curative drug treatment for acute lymphoblastic leukemia has resulted in permanent remission in over 90 percent of children and 70 percent of adults so treated. In chronic lymphocytic leukemia, however, such severe myelosuppression is unacceptable, since the goal of treatment is palliative—relief of mechanical and cosmetic effects of lymphadenopathy and splenomegaly, or modification of the severity of the anemia that attends the infiltration of lymph nodes, bone marrow, and spleen with leukemic cells. The amount of risk that is acceptable with treatment depends on the anticipated benefit.

Much treatment is symptomatic, the aim being to relieve symptoms without expecting to modify the course of the disease. In some situations, symptoms such as pain or fever are important markers of the nature and severity of the disorder, and the physician should withhold symptomatic treatment until the diagnosis is established or until the response to other therapeutic modalities has been assessed. Most fevers can be reduced with antipyretic drugs, but a failure of antibacterial drugs in bacterial endocarditis may be masked by such treatment. Relieving acute abdominal pain is humane, but can make accurate assessment of the underlying disorder impossible. These indiscriminate applications of symptomatic treatment are well recognized. What requires more emphasis, however, is that once the decision has been reached to provide symptomatic relief, the goal must be clearly understood and the drugs must be provided in an effective manner. Narcotic drugs are frequently needed to relieve moderate or severe pain due to a variety of conditions; however, the goal of symptomatic relief is frequently lost due to an interplay of attitudes and practices. Most physicians recognize that the average initial analgesic dose of meperidine in adults ranges between 75 and 100 mg, that the effect is short-lived and lasts between 3 and 4 hours, and that pain relief is achieved more easily if pain is continuously suppressed. A review of hospital practices, however, most often reveals that the dose prescribed for symptomatic relief of moderate and severe pain is smaller, is provided at longer intervals, and is repeated only after the pain recurs. Such patients generally receive about 150 mg of meperidine each day, and most will continue to suffer moderate or severe pain! Once the aim of treatment and the risks are identified by the physician and discussed with the patient and nursing staff, rational and effective analgesic treatment would be provided.

ESTABLISHMENT OF THE BENEFITS OF DRUG THERAPY

Therapeutics has outgrown the dominance of subjective impression and authoritarianism that characterized treatment until the middle of this century. Decisions regarding drug treatment are increasingly determined by disciplined evaluation of the benefits and risks of treatment, based on experience with the drug in large groups of patients and extrapolation to the individual patient. The major method of accumulating objective information on the efficacy of a drug is the clinical trial.

THE CLINICAL TRIAL

The objective of the clinical trial is to evaluate the effects of a single treatment (the maneuver), most often the use of a drug, on the course of a disease or disorder in a representative group of patients (the subjects). An unbiased assessment is only possible if all of the factors known to modify the result of treatment (the outcome) are identified and measured or equalized. This type of assessment has been referred to as a controlled clinical trial. Controlled clinical trials are ordinarily *prospective*; all factors likely to affect the outcome are identified before the study is begun, and the effects of treatment are followed over time. *Retrospective* studies involve initial identification of the outcome and a backward look to assess the contribution of treatment to the outcome. Such studies rarely permit adequate identification or measurement of variables other than the test treatment, which could affect the outcome. Another important characteristic of most controlled clinical trials is the inclusion of a comparison group to help to minimize observer bias. Such a group may receive no treatment, if this is ethically acceptable, or may receive standard treatment that does not include the test drug. Further, in many trials the test and comparison treatments are provided in a similar manner, making it impossible for the patient and the observer to identify whether the test or alternative treatment is being administered. The use of placebos is often necessary to accomplish such a blind trial. Thus, the standard method of evaluation (although clearly not applicable to all situations) is the double-blind, comparative, prospective, controlled clinical trial.

The function of the clinical trial is the validation of a therapeutic hypothesis that has been identified prior to the study. Unexpected outcomes of a trial may generate new hypotheses, which can only be evaluated by subsequent studies specifically designed for that purpose. Only under exceptional circumstances can a clinical trial provide unbiased support for a hypothesis that has been developed after the initiation of the study or during analysis of the data. It is also important that the emphasis on clinical trials not be permitted to diminish the detailed and critical clinical appraisal of the course of individual patients. New therapeutic approaches frequently are developed from intuitive deductions based on careful observations in a few patients. The basic feature of the controlled clinical trial is a comparison of the outcome of treatment in subjects receiving the treatment with an identical group of subjects receiving an alternative treatment.

In assessing the value of reported trials, the reader must consider each of the three fundamental features: the subjects, the maneuvers, and the outcome. Problems may arise in four categories: definitions, measurements, biases, and constraints. The quality of a clinical trial can be assessed by addressing the 12 questions outlined in Table 10.1.

The Subjects

Prior to the selection of subjects for a clinical trial, criteria for diagnosis of the disorder being treated must be specifically defined. For example, in clinical trials of treatment of angina pectoris, diagnosis could be based on the presence of characteristic chest pain alone, or in combination with specified electrocardiographic changes on exercise stress testing, or with angiographic evidence of narrowing of coronary arteries. The type of patient included will differ depending on the diagnostic criteria. With less detailed and rigid diagnostic criteria, nonaffected subjects will more likely be erroneously included, and heterogeneity of the subjects may mask differences between test and comparison drugs. With more restrictive diagnostic definitions, it will be more difficult to find subjects for study, and the population to which the results can be extrapolated will be more limited.

Careful examination must also be given to variables either associated or unassociated with the disease process that are likely to alter prognosis. It has become evident, for example, that symptomatic improvement of angina pectoris following coronary bypass surgery is most predicable if obstructive lesions are seen in at least two of the three major coronary arteries in the left anterior descending branch alone, if the obstructive lesion is severe and proximal, and if left ventricular function is normal or at most there is a single area of impaired myocardial contractility. Further, it is known that individuals having had one myocardial infarction are at greater risk for a second infarction than the general population. Smokers who continue smoking have a worse prognosis than those who discontinue smoking. Individuals in good physical condition appear to have a better chance of surviving a myocardial infarction than those who are less well conditioned. It may be necessary, therefore, in studies of coronary artery disease to define and measure a bewildering array of variables when identifying suitable subjects for study. In many studies, the relationship of the symptoms to the condition treated can affect the outcome. Patients with the same underlying disease may be identified because they present with symptoms primarily related to the disorder, or with complications of the disease, or fortuitously during investigation for an unrelated condition. The severity and duration of symptoms or of the disease and the presence of coexistent diseases and treatment, all require careful definition.

After diagnostic and prognostic criteria have been defined, it is important to consider the reliability of the measurements on which recognition of these features depends. In studies in which more than one individual is responsible for these measurements, interobserver variability is likely. This is particularly

---

Table 10.1 Twelve-Question Checklist to Assess Clinical Trials

Subjects

Susceptibility *bias*	1. Are *definitions* of diagnostic criteria and prognostic variables specific?
Entry *constraint*	2. Are *measurements* of diagnostic criteria and prognostic variables reliable?
Subject *diversion*	3. Are test and control groups of comparable susceptibility?
Exclusion *constraint*	4. Are there *constraints* on patient entry either through restrictions that limit the representivity of the study group or through exclusion of subjects for extraneous reasons, and have all subjects been included in the analysis?

Maneuvers (Treatments)

Cointerventions	1. Are test treatments and ancillary treatments specifically *defined?*
Compliance	2. Are *measurements* of delivery of the dose reliable, or is it possible that the control
Contamination	group inadvertently received treatment similar to that received by the test group?
Therapeutic *bias*	3. Are treatments applied with equal proficiency in test and control subjects?
Therapeutic *constraint*	4. Are inappropriate doses or dose intervals used, and does the treatment of controls meet presently accepted standards?

Outcome

Detection *bias*	1. Is a meaningful outcome specifically *defined?*
Type I and type II errors	2. Are *measurements* of outcome reliable and of appropriate sensitivity?
	3. Are all outcomes sought with equal assiduousness in test and control subjects?
	4. Is the difference between outcomes relevant or are there statistical *constraints* on conclusions?

so when entry is dependent on the evaluation of severity of symptoms. Instructions and rules must be specified for the ordinal scales frequently employed in such studies. In analgesic studies, for example, the distinction of severe from moderate pain may well vary from one patient to another, let alone one observer to another.

A major bias that commonly affects a clinical trial is that test and control subjects have different likelihoods of suffering undesirable outcomes. Protection against such bias is achieved by identification of prognostic variables, by randomization of assignment of treatment, and by stratification techniques. In a very large study designed to assess the effects of treatment of diabetes in cardiovascular disease (University Group Diabetes Project), such prognostic variables as smoking history, previous myocardial infarction, and intermittent claudication were inadequately identified, making it impossible to determine whether the greater incidence of complications of cardiovascular disease observed in the group receiving oral hypoglycemic drugs was affected by an inadvertent, unusual susceptibility. Randomizing the assignment of patients to test and control treatments minimizes bias that might otherwise enter into case assignment. Although randomization can do much to equalize the prognostic susceptibility of test and control groups, it cannot guarantee equality and does not obviate the need to identify and measure all of the known prognostic variables. An example of the many variables that must be identified is seen in a study on the effect of streptokinase in acute myocardial infarction in which 11 risk factors were identified (European Cooperative Study Group). When prognostic variables are few, stratification of case assignment can be used so that approximately equal numbers of subjects with each prognostic variable present will be assigned to each treatment. With multiple variables this may not be possible, and the influence of these factors can only be assessed by statistical analysis that attempts to compare results before and after the removal of the probable influence of prognostic variables, singly and in combination.

Various constraints limit the entry of subjects into clinical trials, and these must be identified. The necessity to avoid influences from a variety of prognostic variables, particularly those due to coexistent disease and treatment, may place such constraints on entry that the results in study subjects cannot be extrapolated to many individuals in the general population suffering from the same underlying disease. Two other avenues of loss of subjects can influence results. Extraneous factors may divert eligible patients from entering the study. In a prospective randomized study of coronary bypass surgery for stable angina, a steady decrease in the number of available patients occurred over a 5-year period probably due to changing attitudes among referring physicians toward coronary bypass surgery. The influence of such a diversional bias may result in the selection of individuals with a different prognosis for entry into the study, and may yield an unrepresentative sample. Loss of patients also occurs through selected exclusion of patients after entry. In a study comparing surgical and medical therapy for transient ischemic attacks (Joint Study of Extracranial Arterial Occlusion), some subjects in the surgical group were excluded from the analysis because of stroke or death occurring during or shortly after operation. The apparent better result with surgical treatment, compared with medical treatment, disappears if these patients are included. In a study comparing the nephrotoxic effects of gentamicin and tobramycin, many subjects were excluded because factors additional to the antibiotics were thought to have predisposed to renal failure. The apparent decrease in nephrotoxicity of tobramycin reported by the investigators disappears with the inclusion of all subjects. In general, there is no justification for the exclusion of subjects once they have been assigned treatment. A straightforward exception to this rule would be the situation in which treatment has been assigned but not administered. In a study of streptokinase in acute myocardial infarction (European Cooperative Study Group), a number of subjects assigned to the control heparin treatment were included, even though they died prior to receiving heparin. The results are quite different if these patients are excluded. It hardly seems justified to attribute deaths to a drug when the drug has not been given!

The Maneuvers (Treatments)

There must be similar care with definitions, measurements, and recognition of biases and constraints in regard to the maneuvers or treatments. Test treatments are usually specifically defined, although ancillary treatments are sometimes neglected. Such cointervention can modify results. In a second study of the effects of streptokinase on myocardial infarction (European Cooperative Study Group), a lower mortality rate is reported in the first 6 months following a myocardial infarction in the group who received streptokinase during the acute phase of treatment. The only information provided regarding other treatment is that all patients received standard ancillary treatment for a least 3 weeks after myocardial infarction. Other studies have provided evidence of beneficial effects of beta-adrenergic-receptor blocking drugs, sulfinpyrazone, prophylactic lidocaine, and anticoagulants in this clinical situation; therefore, it is important that their simultaneous use be identified. Further, measurements must be made to assess as accurately as possible the doses of test as well as cointervening drugs. Contamination of the study due to control subjects inadvertently receiving test treatment may further complicate studies. In long-term studies of the influence of acetylsalicylic acid or other drugs affecting platelet function on thromboembolic disease, it is very difficult to ensure that the control group does not receive drugs that affect platelets because of the widespread availability of salicylates and nonsteroidal anti-inflammatory drugs. The treatment group is also at risk of contamination by unplanned use of such drugs, so that the prescribed dose of antiplatelet drug may not be the dose consumed.

The double-blind technique protects against the unequal use of ancillary treatment by treated and control groups. In instances when the double-blind technique is not feasible, it is important that methods be included to ensure that test or control treatments as well as ancillary therapy are applied with equal proficiency to all subjects, in order to avoid a "therapeutic bias" favoring one or other group.

A now outmoded statistical idea was that all patients in a study group must receive the same dose of a drug if the results are to be combined and analyzed together. This has led to drug use in trials in a manner that is at variance with sensible and current clinical practice. In the study of the efficiency of hypoglycemic treatments in the prevention of vascular disease in maturity-onset diabetes mellitus (University Group Diabetes Project), two such distortions have been identified. A group of patients received insulin in a fixed dose as did all patients who received oral hypoglycemic drugs. No attempt was made to vary the dose according to the need of the patient. Clinical practice at the time this study was planned (1960) and still current is to titrate the dose of these drugs to the amount of sugar in the blood or urine. The trial, therefore, included treatments that did not meet the standards of ordinary clinical practice. Such a procedure raises ethical issues, but in addition places severe limitations on the therapeutic conclusions and generalizations that can be reached. Such constraints can be avoided if the control group receives treatment that is the current standard of practice.

The Outcome

It is important to define explicitly the outcome that will be assessed in a clinical trial and to validate the measurements that will be used to quantitate the results. Such prerequisites may seem obvious, but nothing is ever as straightforward as it appears. The relief of anginal pain is a desirable outcome that can be achieved by a variety of drug and surgical treatments. Such an outcome, however, may have a quite different meaning if the incidence of myocardial infarction is simultaneously decreased than if it is unchanged or increased. For example, nonfatal myocardial infarction can sometimes relieve an anginal syndrome. In these circumstances, the outcome of infarction during the trial becomes an important variable. Further, if relief of angina is associated with a reduced physical, mental, or emotional capability of returning to work (as has been observed in a number of patients who have had coronary bypass surgery), this must be balanced against the persistence of angina in other subjects who retain the capability of working. The outcome of a clinical trial should be defined so that results can be applied to treatment decisions in individual patients. Intellectual curiosity about related phenomena and methodological niceties should not divert efforts to specifically assess clinically applicable and practical outcomes.

The use of a double-blind technique that successfully prevents the patient and observer from recognizing whether test or control treatment is being used, reduces the possibility of bias in identifying benefits and risks of treatment. However, double-blinding does not provide protection against detection bias that may surreptitiously alter the assiduousness with which outcomes are detected. For example, the use of most nonsteroidal anti-inflammatory drugs is associated with anorexia, nausea, or vomiting in some individuals. If such symptoms lead to more rigorous investigation in these patients than in asymptomatic controls for the possibility of cholelithiasis or peptic ulcer disease, an erroneous conclusion may be reached. Both of these gastrointestinal disorders are common, and may be asymptomatic. Unless all study subjects undergo the same diagnostic tests to assess whether these disorders are present or absent, a detection bias may well lead to the conclusion that the drug with gastrointestinal side effects is associated with a higher incidence of cholelithiasis or peptic ulcer. The methods employed to assess all outcomes must be the same in all subjects if the outcomes are to be compared.

In the analysis of results of a clinical trial much

emphasis is placed on the statistical significance of differences in outcomes between test and control treatments. Unfamiliarity with arithmetic methods unfortunately may lead to neglect in the development of unbiased and reliable trial methodology, or to blind faith in poorly understood statistics. Further, statistical significance between differences provides no assurance that the differences are of practical importance or relevance. In a clinical trial with beta-adrenergic-blocking drug treatment of patients with hypertension, the percentage fall in blood pressure that was achieved with treatment was greater in those with high than in those with normal renin. However, in reviewing the data, it is evident that subjects with high renin activity had a higher initial blood pressure than did the comparison patients. Since drugs were used in increment doses until a predetermined blood pressure was achieved, the absolute blood pressure achieved by each group was not different (a relevant and predetermined desirable outcome); rather, those with high renin activity had a greater precentage fall because of their initial higher pressures.

Tests of statistical significance assess the likelihood that observed differences in outcome between treatment groups has occurred by chance. These tests are designed to test the hypothesis that there is no difference in outcome between treatments, that is the null hypothesis. By disproving this hypothesis, the alternative conclusion, that there is a difference, is accepted. In fact, tests are designed to assess the proportion of times a difference between treatments would be observed by chance if many groups of similar subjects were randomly selected from a large population in which no difference in outcome is expected. Most often, one accepts as a practical cutoff a 5 percent risk that the observed differences have occurred by chance. In almost all instances, one must assess the likelihood of a difference occurring in favor of either test or control treatment so that two-tailed or two-sided significance tests are employed. The erroneous acceptance of the conclusion that the observed difference is real and not due to chance is referred to as a false-positive result, or as a *type I error*.

If the null hypothesis cannot be rejected, there are two possible alternative conclusions: first, that there is no difference between treatments, and, second, that no conclusion can be made (the study was inconclusive). The distinction between these alternative conclusions is important and frequently missed. It is conservatively estimated that more than half of the clinical research papers currently published conclude there are no treatment differences, when it is more probable that no conclusion can be reached.

Further, in most instances the probability of this false-negative result, or *type II error*, could have been predicted before the studies were done. Suitable statistical tests exist to assess the probability of a type II error. The capacity of avoiding type II errors is sometimes referred to as the power of the experiment. A type II error is most likely if responses to treatment are variable and the number of subjects small.

ADVERSE DRUG REACTIONS

The selection of a drug in the treatment of a patient requires estimation of the benefits and the risks of therapy. Clinical trials, although fundamental to establishing the likely benefits of drug therapy, are less effective in determining the chance of adverse effects. In comparison with efficacy trials, the methodology for establishing the risk of drugs is less well developed.

For practical purposes, adverse reactions can be defined as any responses that are unintended and noxious. Such effects can occur in close temporal relationship to the administration of the drug, such as the acute bronchospasm that occurs when salicylate-allergic asthmatics take salicylates, or they can be delayed, sometimes occurring not in the subject herself but in her progeny, such as the occurence of adenocarcinoma of the cervix in the daughters of women who received diethylstilboesterol during pregnancy.

Adverse reactions to drugs have been classified in various ways. It is clinically useful to consider two broad types of reactions, those quantitatively abnormal effects that can be explained on the basis of the known actions of the drugs, and effects that are qualitatively abnormal and demonstrate some inherent anomaly in the response of the patient (Table 10.2).

Quantitatively Abnormal Adverse Effects

Pharmacokinetic Abnormalities

A variety of genetic, physiologic, pathologic, and extrinsic factors predispose patients to quantitatively unusual drug effects. Genetic factors have not been shown to be frequent determinants of differences among individuals in the processes of absorption, distribution, and renal excretion of drugs. The rate of drug metabolism, however, is commonly influ-

Table 10.2   Types of Adverse Reactions and Common Predisposing Factors

Types of Reactions	Predisposing Factors

1. Quantitatively Abnormal Effects
Adverse effects that can be explained by the known pharmacologic actions of the drug
  A. Pharmacokinetic
    Unusual absorption, distribution, metabolism, or excretion of drug or metabolite alters concentrations at site of action
  B. Pharmacodynamic
    Altered tissue responsivity alters effects of usual concentrations of drug or drug metabolite
	Genetic
	Physiologic
	Pathologic
	Exogenous
	Unknown

2. Qualitatively Abnormal Effects Adverse effects that differ in character from the known pharmacologic effects of the drug	Genetic Immunologic Pathologic Exogenous Unknown

enced by genetic variables (see Pharmacogenetics, Chapter 8). An example of such variability is seen in the metabolism of isoniazid. The rate at which isoniazid is acetylated under the influence of the enzyme acetyltransferase shows a bimodal distribution in the population, so that individuals can be characterized as "slow" or "fast" acetylators. Proportions in each category vary in different populations; over 80 percent of Inuit people (Eskimo), North American Indians, Japanese, and Chinese, 70 percent of Latin Americans, and 40 percent of white and negro North Americans are fast acetylators. Very slow acetylation characterizes 10 percent of the North American population. Wide differences in drug handling are observed between these two groups. In fast acetylators, 50 percent of the drug is excreted in about 1 hour, whereas in slow acetylators this proportion is 30 percent. The consequences of these pharmacokinetic differences are that slow acetylators are more liable to accumulate high concentrations of isoniazid and hence are more likely to develop pyridoxine-deficient peripheral neuropathy. Hydralazine, procainamide, and many sulphonamides are acetylated by the same enzyme system as isoniazid, and dose-related adverse effects are also more common in slow acetylators receiving these drugs.

Many drugs are metabolized by hepatic microsomal enzymes. The usual range of serum half-life of a variety of commonly used drugs is shown in Table 10.3. The wide variability in drug effects and adverse effects among individuals receiving these drugs is probably largely due to the wide differences in rates at which drugs are metabolized. Although the activity of these enzymes is influenced by a variety of extrinsic influences, most of the variability is determined by multifactorial genetic factors (see Chapter 8).

Variations in physiologic function accompanying aging and pregnancy, as well as changes in excretory organ function associated with renal or hepatic disease, frequently influence the concentration of a drug that reaches effector sites after a standard dose. Some of these changes result in decrease in the concentration of the drug: the apparent volume of distribution of ampicillin virtually doubles in late pregnancy, while that of theophylline increases markedly in acidemic states associated with chronic obstructive pulmonary disease. Most often, however, concentrations are increased: the patient in late pregnancy and the immature infant are virtually unable to metabolize caffeine and other xanthine drugs, including theophylline. Unless the intake of coffee and other caffeine-containing beverages is reduced, anxiety, restlessness, and insomnia are likely to be caused by these increased concentrations. Fortunately, either intuitively or in response to increases in the concentration of caffeine attained, most women drink less coffee in late pregnancy. In renal failure, the ability of the kidney to excrete gentamicin is impaired, and the interval between standard doses may have to be increased from the usual 8 hours to 48 hours or longer to avoid the dose-related adverse effects of tinnitus, vertigo, and hearing loss. The influence of physio-

Table 10.3   Difference Among Individuals in Rates of Metabolism of Some Commonly Used Drugs That Are Metabolized by Hepatic Microsomal Enzymes

Drug	Usual Range of Serum Half-Life (hours)
Carbamazepine	18–55
Dicumerol[a]	7–74
Diazepam	9–53
Phenytoin[a]	10–42
Phenylbutazone	24–175
Nortriptyline	15–90
Warfarin	15–70

[a] Rate varies with dose.

logic and pathologic factors on drug kinetics are discussed in more detail elsewhere in this chapter.

Exogenous factors, most commonly other drugs or foods, can increase the susceptibility of patients to adverse drug reactions. Drug interactions most often result in quantitatively abnormal adverse effects. Many are a result of additive effects on an organ system, such as the enhanced central nervous system depression often seen when alcohol is taken together with benzodiazepines. Others are a result of an influence of the second drug on the pharmacokinetics of the initial drug. Since the concentration of active drug reaching effector sites is a resultant of complex processes of absorption, distribution, and drug loss, other drugs influencing or competing with any of these processes can be expected to alter the amount of drug reaching the effector site and therefore the magnitude of drug effect. Examples of interactions are listed in Table 10.4. Among the most important factors of interaction between drugs is the process of drug loss, since the rate of loss determines the amount of drug that can accumulate during maintenance treatment. Since many drugs compete for common metabolizing enzymes, interactions at a hepatic site are of particular concern. Common drug interactions due to such mechanisms are summarized in Table 10.5.

Pharmacodynamic Abnormalities

Less is known about the factors that are responsible for the variability in sensitivity to drugs among individuals, which can lead to pharmacodynamically determined adverse effects. Many individuals have a genetically determined deficiency of red blood cell glucose-6-phosphate dehydrogenase, which renders their red cells less resistant to oxidant stresses. This renders the individual susceptible to hemolytic anemia after exposure to such drugs as primaquine, nitrofurantoin, and some sulphonamides. The inheritance of this characteristic is very variable, but the best known variant is inherited by sex-linked, incompletely dominant mechanism. The Mediterranean type of enzyme defect found in Greeks, Sephardic Jews, Sardinians, Asians, and North West Indian peoples is associated with the most severe and prolonged episodes of hemolysis. Angle closure glaucoma can be precipitated in some individuals due to an inherited increased susceptibility to the effects of atropine on raising intraocular pressure. Other less well-understood alterations in the magnitude of tissue response to standard drug doses that are not genetically determined are seen in the susceptibility of women to dysphoric states with narcotic drugs and of children and young adults to suffer dramatic dystonic reactions with phenothiazine drugs. The marked central nervous system depression seen after narcotic administration in patients with hepatic cirrhosis is probably due to an increase in sensitivity to the pharmacologic action of the drugs secondary to disease effects on central nervous system responsiveness. Perhaps the most familiar example of altered tissue susceptibility is seen with drugs or other factors that reduce the extracellular potassium concentration and hence increase the susceptibility of patients to the cardiac adverse effects of digitalis.

Quantitatively abnormal adverse effects are often predictable, and therefore preventable. Dose requirements vary among individuals, be they healthy or ill. An understanding of the known variables influencing the rate at which a drug is absorbed or lost from the body and of the variables affecting the sensitivity of the patient to the drug effects, combined with careful

Table 10.4   Examples of Adverse Pharmacokinetic Drug Interactions by Site of Interaction

Site of Interaction	Drugs	Interacting Drugs	Mechanism	Effect
Absorption (oral)	Thyroid hormones	Cholestyramine	Binding of hormone in intestine	Reduced thyroid effect
Binding (plasma)	Warfarin	Clofibrate Phenylbutazone Nalidixic acid	Displacement from binding sites	Increased anticoagulant effects
Renal excretion	Digoxin	Quinidine	Reduced renal clearance	Increased digoxin effects
	Diuretics	Lithium	Reduced renal clearance	Increased lithium effects
Hepatic metabolism				
Hepatic blood flow	Theophylline Lidocaine	Propranolol	Reduced hepatic flow	Enhanced drug effects
Hepatic enzymes		see Table 10.5		
Tissue distribution	Digoxin	Quinidine	Displacement from tissues	Increased digoxin serum concentrations

Table 10.5 **Examples of Adverse Pharmacokinetic Drug Interactions Due to Effects of Microsomal Enzymes and Other Mechanisms**

	Effects Increased by:		Effects Decreased by:	
	Inhibition of Microsomal Enzymes	Other Effects	Induction of Microsomal Enzymes	Other Effects
Anticoagulants (oral)	Allopurinol Chloramphenicol Cimetidine Disulfiram Metronidazole	Anabolic steroids Chloral hydrate Clofibrate Dextrothyroxine Nalidixic acid Phenylbutazone	Barbiturates Carbamazepine Glutethemide Griseofulvin Rifampin	Cholestyramine Contraceptives (oral)
Contraceptives (oral)			Ampicillin Barbiturates Carbamazepine Phenytoin Primadone	Rifampin Tetracylines
Corticosteroids			Barbiturates Phenytoin Rifampin	
Hypoglycemics (oral)	Chloramphenicol Dicumerol Methyldopa (c̄ tolbutamide) Phenylbutazone	Anabolic steroids Clofibrate Salicylates (c̄ chlorpropamide) Sulfonamides	Rifampin	Contraceptives (oral)
Phenytoin	Chloramphenicol Cimetidine Dicumerol Disulfiram Isoniazid Phenylbutazone	Imipramine		Diazoxide
Theophylline	Cimetidine	Erythromycin Influenza vaccine Propranolol Trioleandomycin		Smoking (tobacco or marijuana)

clinical observations, particularly during initial use of a drug in a patient, help to reduce the likelihood of such dose-related adverse effects.

Qualitatively Abnormal Adverse Effects

The second major type of adverse effects is less well understood, and the severity of adverse effect bears little or no relationship to the dose employed for pharmacologic effects. Hence, they are less predictable and less preventable. Fortunately they are less common than dose-related adverse effects.

Genetic Factors

A straightforward distinction is not always possible between qualitative and quantitative reactions, and this has somewhat frustrated practical classification of adverse effects. It might be argued, for example, that the hemolytic reaction of primaquine observed in patients with a deficiency of glucose-6-phosphate dehydrogenase represents a qualitatively abnormal response, although it can also be upheld that hemolysis could be produced in all individuals provided the dose of the oxidant drug was sufficiently large. Another example of a genetic variation in tissue responsiveness is seen in hepatic porphyria. A feature of this disorder, which is characterized by attacks of abdominal colic, constipation, vomiting, peripheral neuropathy, and anxiety or confusion, is a genetically determined overproduction of δ-aminolevulinic acid synthetase in the liver. The explanation of the particular symptoms that mark the disorder remains unclear. There can be little argument that the severe muscle contracture, hyperkalemia, acidemia, and hyperpyrexia that accompany halothane or succinylcholine administrations, so-called malignant hyperpyrexia, represents an adverse reaction that could not be produced in all subjects, even with very high drug doses. This disorder, which may be due to a deficiency of intracellular calcium binding, is inherited as a Mendelian autosomal dominant trait. Fortunately the trait is rare, occurring in about 1 in 20,000 individuals. A summary of the principal examples of genetically determined adverse effects is given in Table 10.6, and examples of genetic conditions that are only apparent after drug use are listed in Table 8.8, Chapter 8.

Immunologic Factors

The most frequent qualitatively abnormal drug effects are the immunologically determined or so-called allergic drug reactions. Most drugs are poor antigens because they are relatively small nonreactive molecules. In vivo, however, drugs can be metabolized to reactive byproducts and/or can bind covalently with protein, carbohydrates, and nucleic acid, and in such a form can cause antibody formation and can sensitize lymphocytes. A variety of pathogenetic processes underlie the many clinical manifestations of drug allergy (see Chapter 6).

Drugs comprise the most frequent cause of anaphylactic reactions. These reactions are due to antigen-antibody stimulated release of mediators from mast cells. These mediators induce bronchospasm, urticaria, and sometimes hypotension. Penicillin is the most frequently implicated drug. The allergen in penicillin anaphylaxis is probably a protein contaminant from the fermentation process used in the production of the drug, which interacts with penicillinic acid breakdown products of penicillin (the so-called minor determinants). Foreign antiserum, dextrans, iodine-containing radiologic contrast media, and intravenous anesthetics are among the more common drugs that cause anaphylactic reactions.

Drugs can also cause the serum sickness syndrome. This syndrome occurs due to damage from circulating immune complexes either with or without complement. Clinical manifestations are varied, with the following symptoms alone or together being the most common: fever, polyarthropathy lymphadenopathy, neutropenia, thrombocytopenia, and skin rashes. Almost all organ-systems may be affected, with the following consequences: meningoencephalitis, myelitis, neuritis, pericarditis, and glomerulonephritis. In addition, the features of anaphylactic reactions may be superimposed on the serum sickness syndrome, including bronchospasm, urticaria, and angioedema. Drugs known to be associated with immune-complex disorders include penicillin, sulphonamides, and the chemically related thiazides, sylphonylureas, and thiouracil.

Drugs can cause specific tissue damage due to antigen antibody reactions in a variety of ways. Drug may bind to tissues, and as a consequence of interaction with antibody, the cell may be destroyed. Such a reaction manifesting as a hemolytic anemia is seen with penicillin (particularly after high doses). Immune complexes may be absorbed passively to cells, which are then destroyed following activation of complement. Such an "innocent bystander" response has been described in the hemolytic anemia associated with sedormid. Still another mechanism is the modification of host cells by the drug, rendering a component antigenic and causing subsequent production of autoantibodies. Such a mechanism is responsible for the response to hydralazine and procainamide, which mimics lupus erythematosis. Apparently, some drugs can also induce the production of antibodies against unaltered tissues. Such a response is seen in the hemolytic anemia due to methyldopa.

Drugs can also induce cell-mediated allergic reactions. Drugs interacting with serum factors in skin components may interact with sensitized lymphocytes to cause a variety of forms of diffuse as well as localized (contact) dermatitis. Neomycin, and paraben derivatives used as preservatives in topical preparations, are commonly associated with contact dermatitis. Barbiturates and sulphonamides or their

Table 10.6 **Principal Examples of Adverse Drug Effects due to Genetically Determined Variations**

Type of Reaction	Drugs Causing Reactions
Quantitatively Unusual Effects	
Pharmacokinetic variations	
Acetyltransferase	Isoniazid, hydralazine, procainamide, sulphamethazine
Hepatic microsomal enzymes	Phenytoin, phenylbutazone, nortriptyline, warfarin
Pharmacodynamic variations	
Angle closure glaucoma	Atropine
Qualitatively Abnormal Effects	
Glucose-6-phosphate dehydrogenase	Primaquine, sulphonamides
Malignant hyperpyrexia	Anesthetics, neuromuscular blocking drugs
Hepatic porphyria	Barbiturates, benzodiazepines
	Oral contraceptives and others

chemically related derivatives, thiazides and sulphonylureas, are commonly associated with maculopapular allergic skin reactions.

Pathologic and Exogenous Predisposing Factors

Qualitatively abnormal drug reactions can result from host reactions due to disease or exogenous factors including other drugs or environmental variables. A classic drug reaction that only is evident in the presence of disease is the Jarisch-Herxheimer reaction. Within 2 hours of the initial treatment of syphilis, many patients (50 percent of primary, 90 percent of secondary, 25 percent of tertiary syphilis) suffer fever, chills, myalgias and other symptoms suggestive of a response to the release of toxin in tissues, and worsening of the local manifestations of syphilis may occur. Another example of a drug reaction dependent on an exogenous factor is the abnormal exaggerated sunburn, eczema, and urticaria occurring in patients sensitized by certain drugs who are exposed to sunlight. Some of these reactions can be elicited in almost all subjects with enough exposure, and are called phototoxic reactions. The photoallergic reactions, however, are due to a drug–induced immune response; skin proteins bind to drug in the presence of light and act as antigens (see Chapter 19).

Unusual drug reactions can be a result of an interaction between drugs. One of the most dramatic is the severe hypertension that can accompany the simultaneous use of drugs that inhibit the enzyme monoamine oxidase and drugs that release catecholamines (indirect-acting sympathomimetic drugs, pseudoephedrine, amphetamine), dopamine, or foods rich in tyramine (chianti wine, cheddar cheese). The most likely explanation of this reaction is that the indirect-acting sympathomimetic drugs release large amounts of noradrenaline that has accumulated in postganglionic sympathetic nerves due to inhibition of monoamine oxidase. A further mechanism in the case of tyramine-containing foods is that increased amounts of tyramine are absorbed because less is metabolized by monoamine oxidase in the gut and liver. Tyramine then acts to release noradrenaline from sympathetic nerve endings.

Establishment of the Risk of Drug Therapy

Methodology to predict adverse reactions to drugs and to provide an assessment of the risk is less developed than clinical trial methodology aimed at estimating the beneficial effects of drugs. Many chemicals, of course, are not used clinically because they have failed animal toxicology screening tests. There are no animal models, however, to assess a variety of adverse reactions that occur in humans, and it is impossible to recreate, in animal models, the many interacting variables that can be operative in the pathogenesis of adverse effects in humans. In human pharmacologic studies, the establishment of the risk of the drug prior to marketing is compromised by several factors inherent in clinical trial methodology. Because of the need for intensive observations on patients receiving a new drug, the number of individuals exposed to the drug prior to marketing is relatively limited. Therefore, rare though sometimes severe adverse effects may not be observed. In order to reduce extraneous influences, subjects for human pharmacologic studies include normal volunteer or carefully selected patients who have well-defined single diseases or disorders. They are chosen to avoid complications of the primary disease, other coexistent disease, constitutional factors known to alter drug responses, concomitant intake of other drugs, or the like. In a sense, subjects for initial clinical trials are selected on the basis of including only those who are *least* likely to suffer an adverse effect. Supervised observation during the early years of experience with the drug after it is available for widespread use (phase IV studies) is a logical methodologic development, which may yield a better assessment of the risk of drugs in the practical clinical world.

Some adverse effects are delayed, often occurring long after the drug has been stopped or even in the children of those who have received the drug. The establishment of causal relationships between these effects and a drug is often elusive. Whereas experimental trials of drug therapy to establish efficacy permit the use of a number of techniques to reduce bias and error, the architecture of studies to establish a relationship between a drug (or other environmental factor) and an adverse effect often does not permit similar safeguards.

An example of the difficulties in establishing such a relationship is seen with estrogen drugs and endometrial carcinoma. Although a prospective controlled trial could be established to test this hypothesis, the long period of time between exposure and outcome would mean many years of observation before conclusions could be reached. A further difficulty in such a study would be to assure that the outcome (that is endometrial carcinoma) was sought as rigorously in both control and treated subjects. Detection of the outcome is dependent in this example on histologic proof of carcinoma obtained from biopsy (or autopsy) material. Since vaginal bleeding is a complication not only of endometrial carcinoma but of estrogen treatment as well, women receiving estrogens would be more likely to undergo diagnostic dilatation and curettage than women not receiving the drug. In this way, asymptomatic endometrial carcinoma would more likely be detected in women receiving estrogens. Such a detection bias frequently mars studies of adverse effects of drugs or environmental substances when the time between exposure and outcome is long. Results of such trials are usually expressed in terms of the relative risk, which is the ratio between the proportion of individuals who were exposed to the drug and who suffer the outcome and the proportion of individuals who were not exposed and who suffer the outcome. This can be more easily understood by outlining the number of subjects in each of four categories as in Table 10.7.

More frequently, because of time constraints and logistic or ethical considerations, such prospective studies are impractical or unjustified and a retrospective case-control study is used. In this type of study the investigator begins by identifying subjects with the outcome (the cases), and thereafter assembles one or more groups of controls with as many characteristics identical to those of the cases as possible, except for the outcome itself. The prevalence of exposure to the putative drug is then compared in cases and controls. In this form of study not all subjects receiving the drug have been included nor has the study group been a representative sample, so that it is incorrect to express results in terms of relative risks. Results are expressed as an approximate relative risk, or odds ratio. The approximate relative risk is the ratio between the proportion of subjects exposed to the drug with and without the outcome and the proportion of subjects not exposed to the drug with and without the outcome. This is shown in tabular form in Table 10.7.

Table 10.7 Calculation of Risk and Odds Ratios

		Number of Subjects with Outcome (Adverse Effect)	
		Present	Absent
Number of subjects exposed	Yes	a	b
to the drug	No	c	d

$$\text{Relative risk or risk ratio} = \frac{a}{a + b} \div \frac{c}{c + d}$$

$$\text{Approximate relative risk on odds ratio} = \frac{a}{b} \div \frac{c}{d}$$

The potential for bias and error in such retrospective studies is, if anything, greater than in prospective studies, particularly in the estimation of exposure (and nonexposure) to the putative agent, although many of the constraints are raised by factors similar to those in controlled clinical trials.

Statistical analysis of the results of such studies permit an estimate to be made of the likelihood of differences in the risk or odds ratio being due to chance. As with clinical trials of drug efficacy, it is important that if the null hypothesis cannot be rejected, the likelihood of having missed an association should be tested statistically.

Even if an association is shown between exposure and outcome, this should not be accepted as proving that there is a causal relationship between the agent and the disease.

Many adverse effects that develop only after prolonged exposure or late after exposure are a result of more than one etiologic factor. For example, the increase in bronchogenic carcinoma observed in miners exposed to asbestos is only apparent in those exposed who also smoked cigarettes. The nonsmokers showed no increase in approximate relative risk; the approximate relative risk in those who smoked and were exposed, however, exceeded that of the nonexposed smoker. It is not uncommon for possible etiologic variables to be associated with one another, with any one having an additive effect or even enhancing the effect of another. Chronic exposure to methylmercury through the eating of contaminated fish in Northern Canada has been associated in native people with a neurological disorder consisting of incoordination, tremor, and sensory changes. Such a syndrome is difficult to differentiate clinically from the residual damage seen in a variety of nutritional deficiencies and some changes seen with aging. Separation of the outcome attributed to exposure of methylmercury from the influence of nutritional factors is difficult, since dependence on fish was greatest in individuals who could not afford alternative foods during periods of hunger, and estimation of nutrition available many decades ago is inaccurate.

Characteristics that support but do not prove that an outcome has been caused by the exposure include the following:

1. Dose-dependent relationship. Demonstration of an increasing effect with increasing exposure as well as a rational temporal relationship of the outcome to the exposure supports a causal relationship. Dose is frequently difficult to measure and cannot be controlled in retrospective studies. Further, the dose range may not be wide enough to result in different magnitudes of responses.

2. Consistency of association. The repeated demonstration of the same association in different settings by different strategies and by different investigators supports a causal association.

3. Uniqueness. The more frequent the outcome in the exposed group, and the more unusual or uncommon the outcome in the unexposed, the higher the risk or odds ratio. For example, the phocomelia following thalidomide exposure of pregnant mothers or the primary pulmonary hypertension that followed exposure of obese young women to the amphetamine-congener aminorex are unusual outcomes or very rare occurrences in the nonexposed population, and a causal relationship between outcome and exposure can be accepted with little doubt.

4. Rationality. A causal relationship is supported by a biologic explanation for the pathogenesis of the disorder. The liver damage associated with exposure to isoniazid will have more support regarding causality if it can be shown that the drug is metabolized to an active hydrazine metabolite. This would suggest that the disorder is due to an interaction of such a metabolite with components of hepatic cells.

When evaluating reports of adverse effects with drugs, guidelines previously outlined for the review of clinical trials can be used. In addition, the major criteria of causality, that is, dose-response relationship, consistency, uniqueness, and rationality, should be considered.

INDIVIDUALIZATION OF DRUG DOSES

The use of a drug in the treatment of an individual patient is determined by identification of the goals of treatment, knowledge of the results of clinical trials regarding efficacy of the selected drug, and understanding of the likelihood of adverse effects, and must include selection of the appropriate dose of the drug for the individual. Consequently, the physician needs an understanding of the time course of drug absorption, distribution, and loss (pharmacokinetics), as well as of the time course of drug effects.

The effects of most drugs are a result of an interaction between the drug and a component on or within a cell. Processes governing the delivery of drugs to their active sites differ among individuals and among drugs, and can be altered by functional and compositional changes in tissues and organs, which may be physiologic or pathologic. For practical therapeutic purposes, however, the principles underlying the pharmacokinetics of many drugs are easily understood and widely applicable.

DRUG LEVELS AFTER INTRAVENOUS ADMINISTRATION

After intravenous administration, a drug immediately mixes in the intravascular space and is distributed to a few richly vascular tissues (central compartment). This initial compartment is a functional rather than an anatomical space. Concentrations of drug in the serum can be used as an estimate of the drug content of the central compartment. Following mixing, concentrations in the serum progressively decrease, first quite rapidly and subsequently more slowly (Fig. 10.1). The initial rapid distribution phase, or α phase, of decline in serum concentrations, is largely explained by the distribution of drug from the central compartment into the tissues (the peripheral compartment). The overall rate of decline of serum concentrations can be estimated for the distribution phase, however it is a composite of many different rates of distribution into various tissues, influenced by the vascularity of the tissue as well as the avidity of the tissue for the drug.

An example of the complexity of the distribution phase for the drug thirpental is shown in Figure 10.2. The initial phase is dominated by the very rapid distribution of the drug into the viscera. After 2 minutes

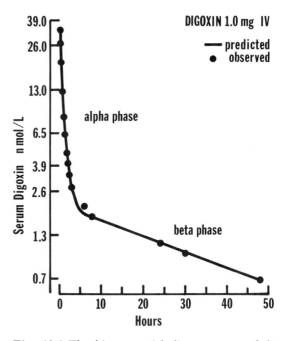

Fig. 10.1 The biexponential disappearance of digoxin after intravenous dosing in normal humans. This is a typical course of drug concentration in normal humans.

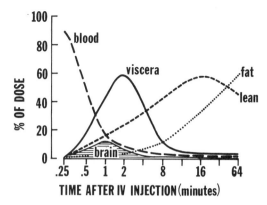

Fig. 10.2. The distribution of thiopental in blood and tissues after intravenous injection.

almost 60 percent of the dose is contained in the viscera while 25 percent has accumulated in skeletal muscle. Fortunately, concentrations of thiopental rise rapidly in the brain, reaching a maximum about 1 minute after injection. Other peripheral tissues therefore do not need to be "filled" prior to the time the drug reaches a maximum concentration in tissues in which the effect of the drug is required. Although the initial rapid phase of decline of serum concentrations of thiopental is explained by distribution of the drug out of the central compartment into tissues, it should be noted that during the subsequent slower phase of serum concentration decline, drug continues to accumulate in some peripheral tissues. Maximum distribution into skeletal muscle is reached at 16 minutes, and accumulation in adipose tissue continues for several hours. Although thiopental is lipid soluble, and adipose tissues have a high affinity for the drug, the limited vascular supply of adipose tissue delays distribution of thiopental to these tissues. The time course of effects of thiopental is further complicated because the drug is metabolized to an active metabolite, pentobarbital.

The second phase, or β phase, of decline of serum concentrations begins when the predominant drug movement is out of the peripheral compartment and back into the central compartment, that is, at equilibration between compartments. The curve depicting the β phase is a composite representing the sum of movement of drug; however, maximum concentration may only be reached in some tissues after overall equilibration has occurred. Thiopental, for example, continues to accumulate in muscle and fat even after net movement of drug from tissues to central compartment has begun. The β phase is predominantly determined by the loss of active drug from the body by metabolism and/or excretion.

These processes, of course, occur during the α phase, but contribute little to the rate of fall because the process of distribution of drug into peripheral tissue predominates during this early phase when there is a high concentration-gradient between the central and peripheral compartments.

The disappearance of most drugs from the serum can be described in a biexponential manner. It is important to realize that concentrations in the serum are not in equilibrium with concentrations in the peripheral compartment during the α phase of decline of drug concentrations, but that thereafter the ratio between the concentration in the peripheral compartment and that in the central compartment remains constant. In most patients the proportion of a drug in the body that distributes into tissue at and after equilibration is similar; thus measurements of drug in the serum after equilibration can serve as a useful guide to the amount of drug in the peripheral compartment.

DRUG LEVELS AFTER ORAL ADMINISTRATION

Most drugs are given by the oral route, which affects the time-serum concentration curve, due to the process of absorption. This process is relatively rapid in relation to the β phase of drug loss. Equilibration is reached more slowly after oral than intravenous dosing because of the delay in drug reaching the central compartment. Figure 10.3 shows the relationship between concentrations of digoxin in the central compartment and the peripheral compartment after

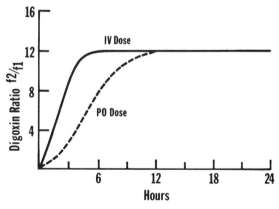

Fig. 10.3. The ratio of digoxin concentration in the peripheral compartment (f2) to that in the central compratment (f1) after intravenous and oral dosing.

oral and intravenous doses of digoxin. In normal humans, equilibration occurs approximately 6 hours after an intravenous dose of digoxin, but not until 12 hours after oral dosing. Disease processes, such as congestive failure, can decrease the rate of absorption of digoxin and further delay oral absorption and the time to equilibration.

Most drugs are absorbed from the portion of the gut supplied by the portal system; therefore, a drug must pass through the liver before it enters the systemic circulation. Some drugs are extensively extracted by the liver, including propoxyphene, pentazocine, lidocaine, propranolol, nortriptyline, and morphine. The extraction of drugs by tissues between the drug delivery site and the systemic circulation is referred to as the *first pass effect*. Oral doses of drugs with high hepatic extraction must be much larger than equipotent intravenous doses, and with some drugs oral dosing is impractical because of the very large amounts that do not reach the systemic circulation. A further consequence of the first pass effect is that dose requirements for drugs highly extracted by the liver are considerably reduced in the presence of liver disease, particularly cirrhosis. The rate at which the liver is able to metabolize drugs that are highly extracted is limited predominantly by the amount of drug delivered to the liver, and hence by blood flow to the liver. In diseases such as cirrhosis or hepatic schistosomiasis with shunting of blood from the portal to systemic circulation, the first pass effect is diminished and dose requirements are reduced.

APPARENT VOLUME OF DISTRIBUTION

The apparent volume of distribution of a drug (Vd) is a hypothetical volume calculated by assuming the body to be a single container in which the drug is distributed homogeneously at a concentration equal to that measured in serum:

$$Vd\,(L/kg) = \frac{\text{Amount of drug in body (mg/kg)}}{\text{Concentration of drug in serum (mg/L)}}$$

Vd is determined by tissue distribution and binding of the drug. Every drug has a characteristic Vd, ranging from 0.1 L/kg for drugs of restricted distribution such as phenylbutazone to 40 L/kg for drugs such as digitoxin. The Vd can often exceed the actual size of the individual, which emphasizes the conceptual (and unreal) nature of this concept.

THE SERUM HALF–LIFE

The β phase serum half-life (t½) of a drug is a useful characteristic of the many drugs that are metabolized or excreted at a rate proportional to their plasma concentration, that is, by *first order kinetics*. The β phase half-life is calculated by determining the time that it takes serum concentrations to diminish by one-half. Such estimates are made after equilibration has occurred, to avoid the early decrease in serum concentration that is predominantly due to drug distribution into tissues (α phase half-life). The serum half-life of a drug can be influenced not only by changes in the efficiency of drug-losing processes but by alterations in drug distribution. Thus, an increase in the half-life of a drug may be due to a decrease in the rate of drug metabolism by the liver or of excretion by the kidney, or to an increased amount of drug available in the tissues for diffusion back into the plasma as drug concentrations fall due to metabolism or excretion.

PLASMA CLEARANCE

Another useful pharmacokinetic concept is that of *plasma clearance* of a drug. The volume of plasma completely cleared of the drug per unit is usually calculated as follows:

$$\text{Clearance (L/kg/hour)} = \frac{Vd}{t\,½}\,(L/kg/hour)$$

$$Vd = \text{the apparent volume of distribution of the drug}$$

$$t½ = \text{the half-life}$$

Clearance is ordinarily determined using measurements of total drug in the plasma, but many drugs exist in the plasma space with an unbound portion and a portion bound to plasma proteins or lipids. Drug-loss processes are dependent only on the unbound portion of the drug; therefore, changes in binding of drugs can result in changes in plasma clearance. If the proportion of drug in the unbound form is increased, the calculated clearance will be increased, since less of the total drug is represented by the bound, less diffusible form. This could happen when drug is displaced from binding sites by other drugs sharing common sites.

It is important to understand the factors that modify clearance and t½ values. Clearance may be increased by (1) an increased rate of drug metabolism or excretion, or (2) decreased plasma binding of the drug. In comparison t½ may be decreased by (1) an increase in clearance, or (2) a decrease in Vd.

DRUG ACCUMULATION

Most drugs are not given in single oral doses but are given repeatedly. To avoid wide fluctuations in drug concentrations, doses are usually repeated prior to the complete disappearance of the preceding doses. Drug concentrations accrue progressively and result in an accumulation of drug in the body. Accumulation does not continue indefinitely, since most drugs are metabolized or excreted by first order kinetics. This means that the percentage of drug lost remains constant, and at higher blood levels increasing amounts of drug are lost. Accumulation ceases when the amount lost in the time between doses (dose interval) is equal to the amount absorbed from each dose. From this time on, if the dose and dose interval are constant and pharmacokinetic characteristics do not change, the amount of drug in the body will remain at a plateau or steady state. The characteristic drug time-course for maintenance doses of digoxin in an individual with normal renal function is shown in Figure 10.4. Fluctuations in body content and serum concentrations occur even at steady state, from a peak sometime after a dose to a minimum immediately prior to the subsequent dose.

Attainment of the steady state condition is determined by the amount of drug lost in each dosing interval. The greater the amount lost (that is, the greater the rate of loss) the less time it will take to accumulate enough drug so that the amount lost will equal the amount absorbed. The rate of loss, and therefore the time to plateau, can be expressed in terms of the t½ of the drug. In one t½, 50 percent, in two t½, 75 percent, and in five t½, 96.9 percent of plateau concentrations are attained. The time taken to reach plateau (steady state) will be approximately 5 times the t½ of the drug. Although only the rate of loss (t½) of the drug determines the *time* to plateau, the amount of drug that accumulates is also determined by the size of dose.

Average expected plateau concentrations can be estimated from drug concentrations achieved after the first dose of the drug from the following formula:

Average serum
concentration
at plateau

$$= 1.44 \times \frac{t½}{\text{dosing interval}} \times \begin{array}{l}\text{Serum concen-}\\\text{tration after}\\\text{first dose}\end{array}$$

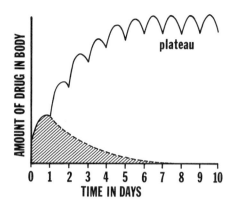

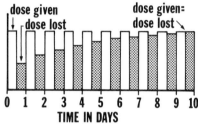

Fig. 10.4. The accumulation of digoxin in the body following administration of maintenance doses of digoxin. A steady state is achieved in 8 days.

For example, with digoxin (t½ approximately 36 hours) given in the same dose at intervals of 24 hours, plateau concentrations will be achieved in approximately 5 t½, or 7½ days (5 × 36 hours = 180 hours, or 7½ days) and plateau concentrations will be approximately twice the concentration achieved after the first dose (1.44 × $\frac{36}{24}$ = 2.16). If the patient receiving this dose of digoxin has impaired renal loss of digoxin and prolonged t½ to 72 hours, the time to plateau will be prolonged to 15 days (5 × 72 hours), and the concentration at plateau will be greater, approximately 4 times the concentration after the first dose (1.44 × $\frac{72}{24}$ = 4.32). Steady state concentrations in such a patient can be reduced by either reducing the size of the dose or prolonging the dosing interval.

Identical doses given repeatedly at the same dosing interval are referred to as maintenance doses. At times, the clinical situation may require more rapid attainment of concentrations equivalent to those expected at steady state. This can be achieved by giving a loading dose of the drug, and thereafter concentrations equal to those at steady state are sustained by continuing the maintenance dose. If concentrations equal to those anticipated at steady state are desired, the loading dose must be large enough so that the amount of drug absorbed is equivalent to the total body content of drug at plateau. This dose can be estimated from knowledge of the apparent volume of distribution of the drug and the desired steady state serum drug concentration:

Loading dose = Vd × steady state serum concentration

Since steady state serum concentrations are determined by the size of maintenance dose, the dosing interval, and t½, it should be clear that the loading dose can also be estimated from knowledge of the maintenance dose.

$$\text{Loading dose} = \frac{100}{\substack{\text{\% of drug eliminated} \\ \text{per dosing interval}}} \times \text{maintenance dose}$$

For example, if the average maintenance dose for digoxin in a patient with normal renal function is 0.25 mg every 24 hours (t½ approximately 36 hours, approximately 35 percent lost in each dose interval) the loading dose will be

$$\frac{100}{35} \times 0.25 = 0.71 \text{ mg.}$$

Some drugs may be excreted or metabolized by processes that can be saturated, in which case the kinetics are more complex and the above principles do not apply. Alcohol, phenytoin, and salicylates are examples.

THERAPEUTIC DRUG MONITORING

Many factors modify the proportion of administered drug that reaches the site of action, and therefore modify the relationship between the size of the dose given and the magnitude of effect. For some drugs, dosage can be titrated against a measurable therapeutic end point. The slowing of ventricular rate when digitalis is used to treat atrial fibrillation or the prolongation of prothrombin time when oral anticoagulants are used are examples of such drugs. For other drugs, the success or failure to reach therapeutic end points may be more difficult to assess.

When drugs are used to suppress symptoms, successful dosing can only be assessed by the absence of signs or symptoms of the disorder. Failure of therapy

may be life-threatening, making it unacceptable to risk reducing dosage until symptoms recur, as a means of establishing the minimum effect dose. Antiarrhythmic drugs for ventricular arrhythmias and anticonvulsant drugs for epilepsy require serum concentration measurements for the successful long-term management of patients. For many drugs serum concentrations have a closer relationship to the level of drug effect than does the dose of drug administered.

Increasing the dose of the drug until dose-related adverse effects appear is a well-established method for determining maximum dose, but is unacceptable if the adverse effects are severe. With such drugs as lithium, theophylline, and gentamicin, measurements of serum concentrations are essential when dose requirements approach those associated with toxicity.

BIOAVAILABILITY

Bioavailability of standard pharmaceutical preparations is reasonably predictable among individuals; however, absorption is more varied for products specially designed to delay or prolong absorption. Some of these products may be less completely absorbed than the standard formulation, and all are more likely to be affected by physiologic and pathologic variations in the absorptive process. For example, acetylsalicylic acid remains the drug of first choice in the treatment of rheumatoid arthritis, but many patients can only tolerate an enteric coated formulation. Such formulations are less predictably absorbed and failure of such products to control the symptoms of rheumatoid arthritis should not be considered drug failure without evidence that serum concentrations are in the therapeutic range.

The space into which a drug distributes and the rate at which it is lost from the body vary among healthy individuals, and are influenced by aging, pregnancy, and disease processes. The pharmacokinetic characteristics of drugs such as phenytoin, theophylline, lithium, and gentamicin are especially unpredictable, and drug measurements can provide assurance that optimal doses are being used.

SERUM–BINDING CHARACTERISTICS

Many drugs are loosely bound to plasma protein, predominantly albumin, but to lipoproteins and glycoproteins as well. Since it is the unbound drug that is in equilibrium with drug at cellular sites of action, and since most drug assays measure total drug (bound and unbound), it is important to be aware of situations in which drug binding is altered and total drug measurements can lead to erroneous conclusions. Phenytoin, for example, is approximately 90 percent bound to serum albumin. At a therapeutic concentration of 60 nmol/L, the free concentration would be about 6 nmol/L. In renal failure and hyperbilirubinemic states (serum bilirubin greater than 85 nmol/L) the albumin binding of phenytoin can be reduced to 50 percent. In such patients total serum phenytoin concentrations as low as 12 nmol/L may be asssociated with free concentrations that are therapeutically important and that approximate 6 nmol/L.

EFFECTS OF COMPLIANCE AND OTHER DRUGS

The dose prescribed is not always the dose taken by the patient, and drug measurements can assist in assessing patient compliance if treatment fails. Combinations of drugs are sometimes required to treat epilepsy, asthma or cardiac arrhythmias. Drug measurements can assist in determining which agents are being given in therapeutic doses. In addition, drug metabolism can be modified by a variety of environmental factors. For example, the common use of alcohol, known to enhance microsomal hepatic enzymes, can alter the rate of metabolism of phenytoin, and cigarette and marijuana smoking can increase the rate of metabolism of theophylline, thus contributing to the unpredictable pharmacokinetics of these drugs.

For a given drug, the serum concentrations that are associated with a measurable therapeutic effect and, at most, mild and acceptable side effects are frequently referred to as the therapeutic range of concentrations. It is important to realize that the magnitude of the therapeutic effect is related to the concentration within this therapeutic range but that the optimal cutoff points for minimum and maximum concentrations have large interpatient variability.

The predictive value of a serum drug concentration measurement in confirming that the drug is achieving therapeutic effects or causing dose-related toxic effects can be expressed quantitatively. This is dependent on the sensitivity and specificity of the cutoff concentration and the prevalence of the suspected state. This intuitive relationship has been expressed by Bayes theorem:

$$\text{Predictive value of test } (P(T/D)) = \frac{P(T/D) \times P(D)}{P(T/D) \times P(D) + P(T/\bar{D}) \times P(\bar{D})}$$

where $P(T/D)$ = proportion of individuals with disease and positive test

$P(D)$ = prevalence of disease

$P(T/\bar{D})$ = proportion of individuals without the disease and a positive test (false-positive ratio)

$P(\bar{D})$ = prevalence of nondisease

Sensitivity is defined as the proportion of individuals with the disease who have a positive test ($P(T/D)$) and *specificity* is defined as the proportion of individuals without the disease who have a negative test ($P(\bar{T}/\bar{D})$).

An example of the importance of considering these influences is seen in the use of digoxin measurements in confirming the diagnosis of digoxin toxicity. In several studies it has been found that approximately 80 percent of patients with digoxin toxicity have concentrations over 2.6 nmol/L, that is $P(T/D) = 0.8$, whereas 20 percent of patients without digoxin toxicity have concentrations more than 2.6 nmol/L. The predictive value of concentrations of more than 2.6 nmol in confirming toxicity can be calculated as follows:

$$\text{Predictive value of positive test in confirming toxicity} = \frac{0.8 \times P(D)}{0.8 \times P(D) + 0.2 \times P(\bar{D})}$$

In the patient being considered, the suspicion of digoxin toxicity is based on evaluating all information, except the serum drug measurement. If the index of suspicion is low, for example, 20 percent, then the predictive value of a concentration over 2.6 nmol/L can be calculated as follows:

Predictive value of concentration over 2.6 nmol/L in confirming toxicity

$$= \frac{0.8 \times 0.2}{0.8 \times 0.2 + 0.2 \times (1.0 - 0.2)} = 0.5$$

The predictive value of a serum concentration over 2.6 nmol/L in this case is no better than that which could be achieved by chance.

TIMING OF SERUM SAMPLES

The timing of serum sampling in relation to drug dosing is an important consideration in the use of drug measurements in modifying dose regimens.

The ratio between drug concentration in the plasma and that at the cellular site of action is only constant after equilibrium has been achieved between drug in the plasma and in the tissues. (see previous section Drug Accumulation). Variations in time to equilibrium are seen in particular disorders that influence tissue perfusion, such as low cardiac output states. Because of the variable time to equilibrium and the difficulty in estimating the time when peak concentrations are likely to be reached after a drug dose, trough concentrations, or concentrations immediately prior to the next dose, are most frequently used in estimating dose requirements. This timing provides the greatest assurance that equilibrium has been reached. If drug measurements are made before steady-state conditions have been achieved and mistakenly interpreted as steady-state conditions, an overestimate of chronic dose requirements is likely. When using drug measurements as a guide to chronic dose requirements, measurements are best made after the patient has received a constant dose of the drug over a period of at least 5 times the serum half-life to assure that steady-state conditions have been achieved.

The sensitivity of individuals to drugs is variable, as is the desired magnitude of drug effect, so that serum drug measurements cannot replace clinical evaluation of success or failure of drug treatment. Sensible use contributes to better treatment by avoiding both unnecessary toxicity and homeopathic dosing.

Therapeutic drug measurements are particularly useful with drugs having one or more of the following characteristics: unpredictable absorption, variable pharmacokinetics, therapeutic end-point difficult to quantitate, serious side effects, unreliable compliance, and combination drug therapy.

THERAPEUTIC DECISION-MAKING

The selection of optimal therapy for a patient with a proven disease is frequently based on balancing the anticipated benefits and risks of alternative treatments. The skillful physician extrapolates from published results of treatment in other patients, to predict the effect in the individual patient, and integrates this information with his experience in treating the particular disorder. This seems to be accomplished intuitively, and this is probably so. The stepwise deliberation in reaching therapeutic decisions, however, can be subject to analysis. Such decision analysis has not yet received whole-hearted support by clinicians or educators, probably because it readily lays bare the meager information on which decisions must be based. Nevertheless, it seems obvious that the more explicit the approach to decision-making, the more likely that the patient will be offered optimal treatment.

Problems that are to be subjected to decision analysis are usually expressed as a decision tree or matrix that exposes all of the possible actions and outcomes. A decision tree constructed to assist in reaching the optimal decision regarding the use of long-term anticoagulant treatment in preventing thromboembolic disease in a patient who has suffered a pulmonary embolus is shown in Figure 10.5.

The two possible actions, denoted by squares, are either to use or to withhold anticoagulants; and two possible "states of nature," denoted by circles, are either that the patient is susceptible to a recurrence of thromboembolic disease or that he is not. Four outcomes are identified: the individual susceptible to recurrence who receives anticoagulants will be anticipated to benefit from treatment, although the treatment carries a risk; the individual not susceptible to recurrence who receives anticoagulants gains no benefit but is subject to risk; the individual susceptible to recurrence who does not receive anticoagulants is exposed to the risk of thromboembolism; and the individual who is not susceptible and who does not receive treatment avoids needless risk of treatment.

The next step in decision analysis is the estimation of the probabilities of each state of nature. In this example, it is determined that the risk of a serious recurrent pulmonary embolus is 30 percent (probability 0.3); the probability of nonrecurrence is, therefore, 0.7. Subsequently, values must be placed on each outcome. In this example, it is determined that treatment provided a susceptible patient has a value of 1.0, and a similar value is given to avoiding treatment in the individual who is not susceptible. Treatment given without benefit to the nonsusceptible carries the risk of bleeding complications and is given as value of 0.9, while exposing a susceptible patient to thromboembolism is more serious and is assigned a value of 0.1. According to the theories of decision analysis, the utility of each outcome can then be determined by the product of the probability and the value of each outcome. The decision matrix showing the utility of each outcome summarizes the data in Table 10.8.

The utility of the decision to give anticoagulants in the example is 0.93, and the utility of not giving

ACTIONS   STATES OF NATURE   OUTCOMES

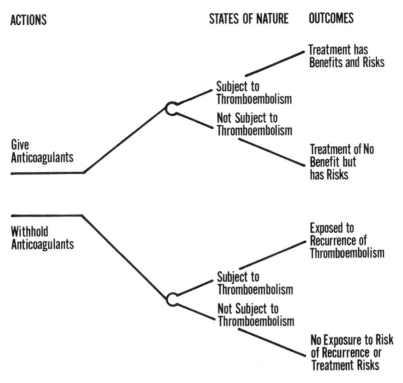

Fig. 10.5. Decision tree: the use of long-term anticoagulants in the prevention of thromboembolism.

anticoagulants is 0.73. Thus, giving anticoagulants would be the preferred course of action for this patient.

Each part of a decision analysis has inherent difficulties. An incorrect decision can be reached if some alternative course of action is omitted. The quantitation of each possible outcome can rarely be made from published information, since many variables in each situation modify the probabilities. The clinician must use clinical judgement as he does regularly in a less formal and less quantitative way. Outcome values frequently have different importance to different physicians, different patients, or different institutions. For example, a portocaval shunt to limit bleeding from esophageal varices in a patient with severe alcoholic cirrhosis may be considered of no value by

the physician since no prolongation of life can be anticipated, of some value to the patient since he may be spared the discomfort of alternative treatment for massive bleeding, and of some value to the community since the blood transfusions saved may be used for other purposes. Outcomes are often intangible as far as quantitation is concerned. In the use of anticoagulants, for example, the relative risk of the morbidity and mortality of a complication of retroperitoneal bleeding or acute blood loss from the gastrointestinal tract are difficult to balance against the discomfort of a nonlethal pulmonary embolism. Nevertheless, if one accepts that the information on which the analysis is based is imprecise, the use of a decision analysis approach is more rigorous than informed clinical judgement, and consideration of each

Table 10.8 **Decision Matrix: Long-term Anticoagulants in the Prevention of Thromboembolus**

	Utility		
Actions	Individuals Subject to Thromboembolus	Individuals Not Subject to Thromboembolus	Overall
Give Anticoagulants	$0.3 \times 1.0 = 0.3$	$0.7 \times 0.9 = 0.63$	0.93
Withhold Anticoagulants	$0.3 \times 0.1 = 0.03$	$0.7 \times 1.0 = 0.70$	0.73

component of the analysis should improve clinical decision-making. In particular, decision analysis includes consideration of the risk to the individual who receives unnecessary treatment, since he is not subject to the anticipated complication. Intuitive decisions seldom give sufficient weight to this possibility.

COMPLIANCE

Physicians not only overestimate the regularity with which patients act according to the advice they were given but are themselves unreliable in recognizing those patients most likely to be noncompliant. Compliance for short-term treatment with medications in symptomatic conditions averages about 75 percent, while the rate for short-term prophylaxis is 65 percent, and for long-term treatment is 50 percent in a variety of settings. These values are observed among patients of all socioeconomic backgrounds, of all ages, and with most disease states. Although a number of factors influencing compliance have been recognized, health professionals have been frustrated in their attempts to identify noncompliance. The intake of antacids by patients has been shown to be predicted as well by chance as by the prescribing physicians. Psychiatrists have been shown to be wrong 20 percent of the time in predicting which of their chronic patients will be noncompliant with their drug therapy. Frustrations over the inability to recognize noncompliance is coupled with disappointment in the results of attempts to improve compliance. Solutions to the problem of noncompliance will not be successful until an explanation for this form of behavior is clarified.

The most understandable model for explaining noncompliance is the "health belief" model. The basic postulate in this model is that compliance is determined by the patient's own perceptions of the seriousness or progression of the disorder and the patient's evaluation of the balance between the likelihood that treatment will reduce the threat and its cost, that is, expense, inconvenience, unpleasantness, and the like. The more conflict that exists between advantages and costs of treatment, the greater must be the perceived threat in order that the patient comply. The patient continuously reassesses the threat and benefit so that initial compliance may well differ from later behavior.

Several factors have been shown to modify compliance, including length of treatment and nature of the drug, side effects, complexity of regimen, and nature of the illness. The longer the treatment, the greater the likelihood of noncompliance. That this is not an independent variable, however, is shown by the generally high degree of compliance in patients taking digitalis, some of whom may even increase their medication without advice if symptoms worsen. Side effects, particularly those that are unexpected by the patient, diminish the likelihood that medications will be taken as directed. The more frequent the dose, the more medications involved, and the more inconvenient the dosage form, the more unlikely it is that the medication will be taken. Compliance is more likely to be low if drugs are being used prophylactically, if the disorder is asymptomatic or chronic. All of these factors can be explained on the basis of the health belief model, with the patient's perception of the balance of benefits and risks of treatment determining the likelihood of compliance.

Although patient characteristics would be expected to influence compliance, the results of studies are contradictory, and few investigations have identified all of the variables that can influence drug-taking behavior. Few studies have addressed the question of the patient's own perception of his disease and the advantage and risks of treatment.

The relationship between the patient and his physician (or other health professionals who are guiding treatment) is important. Compliance improves if the physician justifies the use of the medication to the patient and emphasizes (and reinforces) the need to continue to take the medication. If this is combined with the patient's view of the disease as serious, a concept that can be influenced by the physician, adherence to the regimen will improve. Community and family attitudes to treatment can significantly affect compliance.

It is important to recognize that compliance behavior varies during treatment as a result of new information gained by the patient. Reinforcement of an educated perception of the risks of the disease and rewards of the treatment are frequently necessary. Devices such as special pill containers, calenders, self-measurement of treatment response, and convenient treatment sites (for example, the workplace) have not been shown to be effective in isolation.

Physicians frequently fail to identify or recognize noncompliant behavior. Simple nonaccusatory questions asked of each patient regarding the dosage regimens for all regular medication taken during the preceding week, as well as the numbers of missed doses, is an important component of every medical history.

The patient may improve his own awareness of non-compliance if asked to record a daily, detailed medication diary.

REFERENCES

1. Albert, D.A.: Decision theory in medicine, a review and critique. Milbank Memorial Fund Quarterly, 56:362, 1978.
2. A study of the effects of hypoglycemic agents on vascular complications in patients with adult-onset diabetes. The University Group Diabetes Program, Diabetes, 19:(suppl. 2) 747, 1970.
3. Avery, G.S. (ed.): Drug Treatment, Principles and Practice of Clinical Pharmacology and Therapeutics. 2nd ed. Sydney, Adis Press, 1980.
4. De Wolff, F.A., Mattie, H., Brimer, D.D. (eds.): Therapeutic Relevance of Drug Assays. The Hague, Martinus Nijhoff Publishers, 1979.
5. European Cooperative Study Group for Streptokinase Treatment in Acute Myocardial Infarction: Streptokinase in acute myocardial infarction. N. Eng. J. Med., 301:797, 1979.
6. European Working Party: Streptokinase in recent myocardial infarction: a controlled multicentre trial. Br. Med. J., 3:325, 1971.
7. Kannel, W.B.: Some lesions in cardiovascular epidemiology from Framingham. Am. J. Cardiol., 37:269, 1976.
8. Kassirer, J.P.: The principles of clinical decision making: an introduction to decision analysis. Yale Journal of Biology and Medicine, 49:149, 1976.
9. Kloster, F.E., Kremkau, E.L., Ritzmann, L.W., et al: Coronary bypass for stable angina: a prospective randomized study. N. Engl. J. Med., 300:149, 1979.
10. Melmon, K.L., Morelli, H.F. (ed.): Clinical Pharmacology, Basic Principles of Therapeutics. 2nd ed. New York, Macmillan, 1978.
11. Murphy, E.A.: Probability in Medicine. Baltimore, Johns Hopkins University Press, 1979.
12. Sackett, D.L.: The diagnosis of causation. p. 106. In: Gent, M., Shigematsu, I. (eds.), Issues and Reported Drug-Induced Illnesses—S.M.O.M. and Other Examples. Hamilton, McMaster University Library Press, 1978.
13. Sackett, D.L., Haynes, R.B. (ed.): Compliance with Therapeutic Regimens. Baltimore, Johns Hopkins University Press, 1976.

11

The Genitourinary System

Alan R. Hull, M.D.

The kidneys, ureters, bladder, urethra, external genitalia, and, in the male, the prostate make up the genitourinary system. Since this system lies predominantly in the paravertebral retroperitoneal space and deep in the pelvis, it is not readily accessible to physical examination. The urinary meatus is readily visible in both male and female, but examination of the bladder and proximal urethra requires cystoscopy. The kidneys may become tender when infected, producing tenderness on deep abdominal palpation or on percussion of the costophrenic angle of the back. The prostate may be palpated informatively by digital rectal examination. Markedly enlarged kidneys can be palpated by abdominal examination. Auscultation of the upper abdomen and flanks may demonstrate vascular bruits in renal artery stenosis. Aside from these clues, however, the assessment of the genitourinary system depends largely on laboratory methods.

LABORATORY ASSESSMENT OF THE GENITOURINARY SYSTEM

URINE AND URINALYSIS

Urine is the end product of kidney function and should be looked at when the physician evaluates a patient generally or when there is a specific problem relating to the genitourinary tract. However, the physician should be aware that the kidney has a limited number of ways in which it can react to pathologic processes, and abnormal findings in the urine may be nonspecific. The urinalysis can be depended on to indicate if there is an abnormality in renal function but not to provide the specific diagnosis. In every case that a renal problem is suspected, the physician must personally examine a *fresh* urine sample and not depend totally on the laboratory report. Many hospital and clinic laboratories do an excellent job, but since urinalysis is a routine test, small but important findings can be missed when many dozens of specimens are examined in a day.

What To Look For In The Urine

A significant amount of information can be obtained by noting the urine even in a collecting bag or a specimen in the patient's bathroom. Always be sure it is fresh; the best clinical test for this is its temperature: *fresh urine is warm.*

Color

Normally fresh urine is a clear, pale yellow color.

1. Urine that is clear like water suggests the patient is diuresing or, rarely, that he or she cannot concentrate the urine.
2. An intense yellow color suggests that:
   A. The patient can concentrate the urine (confirmed by specific gravity test below).
   B. Some substance is coloring the urine:
      Intrinsic—bilirubin
      Extrinsic—vitamins or other drugs (such as rifampicin)
3. Cloudy urine suggests infection and/or that the specimen has stood for some time.
4. Pink, red or "smokey"—usually due to blood (see benzidine test below)
5. Other colors: A wide range of agents and diseases cause a variety of colors. Most standard nephrology textbooks list these.

Volume

The average 24 hour urine volume is said to be 1,500 ± 500 ml. It must be realized that a person can clear all the urinary waste products in as little as 300 ml urine/24 hours. By contrast, some water drinkers put out 6,000 ml daily without any known long-term ill effects. Such a wide range shows the kidneys concentrating and diluting ability, but alerts us to the fact that volume is an inadequate marker of renal function.

Concentration

This is measured in two ways, according to specific gravity and osmolality.

Specific gravity, by using a hydrometer or a refractometer, compares the mass or weight of urine against that of distilled water. This at present is the technique most clinical laboratories use to measure concentration. Abnormally high values are reported when glucose, protein, or radioopaque contrast material are present in the urine. A very rough correction for protein or glucose is to subtract .0035 for each 100 g/dl in the urine.

Osmolality records the freezing point of the urine. Since 1 mosm/mg of water depresses the freezing point by 1.83° C, we are able to measure the number of osmotically active particles present in the urine.

The osmolality is a more versatile measurement than the specific gravity, but either can be used to determine the kidneys' ability to concentrate or dilute the urine. The specific gravity of urine normally ranges from 1.002 to about 1.030, and this corresponds to urine osmolality of just under 50 to just over 1,000.

pH

Generally, nitrazine papers are used to assess the urine pH over a range of 4.0 to 9.0. Fresh urine pH is normally about 5, and depends somewhat on diet. An alkaline pH greater than 7 must be explained. The most common causes of an elevated urine pH include the following:

1. It is not a fresh sample.
2. Urea-splitting bacteria are present.
3. The diet is alkaline.
4. Drugs have been ingested.
5. Renal tubular defects are present.

A tubular defect should be suspected when blood analysis reveals systemic hyperchloremic metabolic acidosis. To test the kidney's ability to produce an acid urine, the specimen should be collected in a tube containing oil, and the pH should be measured anaerobically. (The oil will float on the urine sealing it off from air, thereby preventing the loss of carbon dioxide.)

Sugars

The urine is normally free of glucose. Paper test strips impregnated with glucose oxidase and a dye are useful to detect urine glucose when present in amounts greater than 100 mg/dl. This should be thought of only as a screening test for glucose, particularly useful in diagnosing diabetes mellitus. To detect the presence of other sugars one must use the Clinitest tablet or more sophisticated laboratory measures.

Foam

All urine foams when shaken, but two pieces of information can be suspected from this bedside test.

1. If it is white and the foam persists, look for proteinuria.
2. If it is yellow, check for bile.

The above tests are very general and must always be supported by actual measurements for the suspected substance.

Ketones

The kidney is very adept at clearing the serum of ketone bodies. It should be appreciated that adults who are starving and children overnight will often develop mild ketonuria. The test is useful during the treatment and control of diabetic ketoacidosis.

Benzidine Test for Blood

Generally a positive test indicates the presence of blood. Sometimes the "dip sticks" used to test for blood read positive but no RBCs are found in the urine to support this finding. Such a positive reading without RBCs can occur either when urine is clear or when it is red or pink. The following are possible explanations:

1. RBCs have hemolyzed; this can happen in very hypotonic urine. To be secure in this explanation,

the clinician should repeat the urinalysis with less dilute urine, and in addition should carefully examine the color of the plasma.

2. If the plasma is clear and the benzidine test is still positive with nondilute fresh urine, the reaction is probably measuring myoglobin, and rhabdomyolysis is present.

3. If the plasma is pink, free hemoglobin resulting from intravascular hemolysis is the most likely explanation.

Microscopy

Start with a *mid-stream clean catch specimen* and centrifuge it.

"Epithelial cells" mean the urine has swirled around the vagina and is therefore *not* a clean catch mid-stream urine. The specimen should be discarded and a new collection obtained if infection is the concern.

White blood cells (WBCs) up to 2 per high power field (HPF) in males and perhaps 4 per HPF in females can be considered normal on a centrifuged specimen. Greater numbers of WBCs, particularly if bacteria are present, usually indicate an infection, and a specimen for culture and sensitivity is indicated.

Red blood cells up to 1 per HPF is said to be normal, but if one sees RBCs in every high power field, it should be investigated. RBCs may be confused with fat, Phisohex, air, or yeast. The benzidine test commonly used to recognize RBCs in the urine is sensitive to about 5 RBC per HPF.

The presence of one or more *bacteria* per HPF on a noncentrifuged urine correlates in 95 percent of examinations with a positive culture (colony count greater than 10^5/ml). On a centrifuged specimen, 10 bacteria per HPF is suspicious, and 20 or more per HPF again has a 95 percent correlation with positive culture results.

Sloughed cells from the kidney tubules are usually excreted in the urine. In the presence of parenchymal damage or inflammation, increased numbers of cells may be sloughed. With decreased flow for any reason these cells often are trapped to form casts. *Casts* are cellular debris bound by mucoprotein. Under different conditions a variety of casts develop. *Hyaline casts* contain mucoprotein and carry little diagnostic significance, for example, they are present in parenchymal disease but also are produced by physical exercise. *Cellular casts* develop when cellular debris is sloughed and the cells are incorporated in the mucoprotein; this suggests a parenchymal process. *White blood cell and epithelial casts* may be seen alone or mixed, and they suggest the presence of an inflammatory or tubular degenerative process. If the progress through the tubules is slow, more degeneration of the cellular material takes place and a granular cast develops, which may be described as coarse or fine. *Red blood cell casts* are always regarded to be a marker of a glomerular inflammatory process. Acute glomerulonephritis results in pure RBC casts and not a mixture of RBCs, WBCs, and epithelial cells. Such mixtures of cells do not carry the same prognosis as casts made up only of RBCs. *Fatty casts* are *hyaline casts* which have incorporated epithelial cells that contain fatty material. These are seen where heavy proteinuria or the nephrotic syndrome is present. As chronic renal failure progresses the remaining nephrons and their tubules dilate. Often flow through such tubules is very slow. Therefore, casts under such conditions are broader and have undergone greater degeneration. In addition, proteinuria is often part of such renal failure. Hence, casts formed under these conditions are broader and appear waxy as they undergo prolonged degeneration; they are referred to as *waxy casts*, or *renal failure casts*.

Crystals are often seen in a concentrated overnight urine, and they vary with the pH of such urine. In acid urine, urates in their many forms may be seen, and they do not indicate gout or any other problem. In alkaline urine, the clincan often sees the prism-like phosphate crystals. While this may mean infection (urea-splitting organisms), they are present most commonly because the urine is stale and has become alkaline. The only abnormal crystal that may be present in a morning-concentrated specimen, and one that is easily recognized, is the six-sided cystine crystal. The presence of such crystals requires investigation to find their cause.

Hematuria

While hematuria can be benign, it should be looked at as a serious finding and one that requires a specific work-up. Gross hematuria requires immediate cystoscopy while the bleeding is present. Such an acute procedure, it is hoped, will localize the source. Information from cystoscopy permits the following conclusions:

1. A lesion may be present in the bladder.

2. If bladder urine is clear, the lesion is in the lower urinary tract below the bladder.

3. If blood is coming from one ureter and not the other, tumor must be ruled out as a cause, and therefore an angiogram or a renal scan is needed.

4. If the blood is coming from both ureters it indicates a generalized process affecting both kidneys.

Such findings almost always lead to a kidney biopsy for diagnosis.

When cystoscopy is not available, the three-bottle test may be useful. Have the patient void into one container at the start, into one in the middle, and into one near the finish of voiding. Gross hematuria in only the first bottle suggests that the bleeding is in the lower tract or urethra and is washed out with a large voiding. Blood in only the third bottle suggests that the lesion may be in the bladder, and bleeds with bladder contraction. Blood in all three bottles suggests the source is the upper tract including either or both kidneys.

Microscopic hematuria is often intermittent and its cause is more difficult to identify. Many nephrologists believe that this can be followed conservatively, provided that the GFR is normal, that there is no hypertension, and that proteinuria is normal or less than 1 gram. Such a conservative approach is not unreasonable if the patient is reliable and continues with medical follow-up. Preferably, however, a complete work-up is performed at the time persistant microscopic hematuria is found, and this commonly includes a kidney biopsy.

Proteinuria

See section entitled Nephrotic Syndrome and Edema, later in this chapter.

Summary

The urine should be looked at by a physician if abnormalities exist or are suspected. Careful examination of sequential urines in patients with renal impairment may at times give early indications of changes ocurring within the nephrons. However, major diagnostic revelations from the urine sediment are rare, and it should not be examined with that expectation in mind.

MEASUREMENT OF RENAL FUNCTION

The body's ability to remove toxins via the kidney is generally measured in two ways, (1) according to serum values of endogenous substances excreted by the kidney, for example, urea nitrogen (BUN) and/or creatinine, and (2) according to "clearance" of endogenous or exogenous substances, for example, creatinine, inulin, and Glofil.

Serum Measurement

Serum values of these substances provide a rough indication of kidney function or the glomerular filtration rate (GFR), and such measurements are affected by many other events in the body. The more common serum substances used to estimate renal function are discussed below, with the factors that cause variations in their measurement.

Blood Urea Nitrogen (BUN, normal less than 20 mg/dl) is measured relatively easily by most standard laboratories. Many factors besides changes in the glomerular filtration rate can cause major fluctuations in the BUN.

Factors influencing elevations of the BUN include the following:

1. High protein intake, especially protein of low biological value, such as beans
2. Blood in the GI tract, which may raise the BUN by as much as 4 times
3. Drugs, by blocking protein anabolism, for example tetracyclines and steroids
4. Decreased kidney perfusion, is referred to as "pre-renal" because the cause develops before flow reaches the kidney. (For any given decrease in GFR by this mechanism, BUN increases more than creatinine.)

Factors influencing reductions in the BUN include the following:

1. Starvation, leading to decreased urea production as a result of lowered food intake
2. High biological value protein diet. The body is able to utilize the essential amino acids from the diet along with nitrogen from urea to build protein.

When the BUN is used to estimate renal function, the clinician must realize that the serum value may reflect one or more of the above factors rather than a true change in renal function. Sometimes effects interact to give a false normal value, for example, a volume-depleted patient would normally have an increased BUN on the basis of a decrease in renal perfusion; if the patient is also starving, the BUN will be reduced toward normal and significant renal functional impairment may be overlooked.

In some areas of the world, conservative management of end-stage renal disease (ESRD) is extended by dietary manipulation. In such cases, a diet high in essential amino acids is given. The result of such dietary management is shown below. A patient with stable renal function (GFR 5 ml/min) is placed on a diet consisting of high–biological-value (HBV) protein in place of his or her normal diet for a 30-day period.

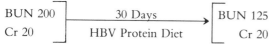

In such cases the body uses nitrogen from the urea and, with the essential amino acids, builds up protein. In the short term such dietary maneuvers result in the patients feeling better; however, in the long term, neuropathy and other problems produced by the "renal toxins" continue relentlessly. In the 1980s, dietary manipulation via a diet composed of less than 40 grams HBV protein should be restricted to a short period of time or to cases where no other therapy is available. It has been postulated that irreversible neuropathy can result from such therapy if it is continued for an extended period of time in the setting of impaired renal function.

Creatinine (Cr, normal less than 1.2 mg/dl in male, less than 1.0 mg/dl in female) can be measured accurately, and is included in most routine hospital automated chemical profiles. Creatinine is a normal breakdown product of striated muscle metabolism, and is influenced little by other extrarenal factors.

Factors influencing elevations of the serum creatinine include the following:

1. Decreased kidney perfusion, "prerenal" (see BUN, above)
2. Tissue breakdown. During rhabdomyolysis or crush injuries to muscle, marked elevation in the serum creatinine can occur.

Factors influencing reductions of the serum creatinine include the following:

1. Cachexia, loss of muscle mass
2. Loss of limbs

In most of the above factors influencing changes in the serum creatinine, the cause is readily apparent, for example, crush injury or loss of limbs. The clinician should be wary of the serum creatinine in obese individuals, especially females. Such patients often have a reduced muscle mass, and therefore renal function based on serum creatinine values is frequently overestimated.

Routinely, both the BUN and the serum creatinine values are ordered on patients, and often their comparison gives additional information. In the absence of renal disease, up to a 20:1 ratio of BUN to creatinine is acceptable. However, with impairment of renal function a ratio of 10:1 is more common, for example, BUN 50 mg/dl and creatinine 5 mg/dl. This ratio decrease probably relates to changes in

renal handling of these substances as well as to dietary protein variations.

In patients with impaired renal function, an elevated ratio of BUN to creatinine should suggest additional problems. For example, with BUN 120, creatinine 5, the ratio change could be the initial evidence of slow GI bleeding.

Clearance Technique

In contrast to measuring the level of some endogenous material in the serum as an estimate of renal function, the clearance technique actually determines what is removed or cleared from the body by the kidney. Therefore, over a prescribed time period, one measures the levels of a substance in both urine and blood and calculates the rate of removal, or clearance. This value is also known as the glomerular filtration rate (since it is assumed that tubular function plays no role).

$$\text{Clearance or GFR (ml/min)} = \frac{\text{Urine concentration (mg\%)} \times \text{urine flow rate (ml/min)}}{\text{Plasma concentration (mg\%)}}$$

Ideally, to accurately measure the GFR, the index substance should be unbound in the serum, filtered at the glomerulus, and neither secreted nor reabsorbed by the tubules. The closest we have come to this "ideal substance" is the inert sugar inulin, and this is the standard in research. However, for general use, it has two limitations: it is not easily measured, and to do so is expensive. In most hospitals and clinics, one of the following methods is used:

1. The 24-hour creatinine clearance. This determination is handled easily by most laboratories, and it requires no infusion since the substance is already present in the serum. There are, however, two difficulties with this procedure:

A. It is hard to get an accurate 24-hour urine collection in most hospitals. The best results are achieved by depending on the patient. In an attempt to determine the validity of *any* 24-hour collection of urine, one should always measure the amount of creatinine present. In males we demand at least 1 g of creatinine/24 hours and in females (because of less muscle mass) 900 mg/24 hours. Note that these are minimal values. Many wellmuscled people put out more than these amounts, but if we reach such minimal levels of creatinine we accept it as a complete 24-hour specimen.

B. Creatinine does not meet the ideal standards set out above to measure GFR, since it is secreted in varying amounts by the tubule. Fortunately, this error (approximately 20 percent) is balanced in the normal range of GFR by the presence of other chromogens in the plasma but not in the urine. As renal function decreases, measurements become less accurate.

2. Timed clearance. This is a more accurate method than 24-hour creatinine clearance because the patient and the conditions are under control. This technique can be improved further by using more ideal markers than creatinine, for example, Glofil (radioactive iodine tagged to the IVP dye iodothalamate). This exogenous substance is introduced into the blood stream intravenously (intramuscularly or subcutaneously are acceptable, but slower), and a steady plasma level is established. Urine is collected every 20 to 60 minutes (often under conditions of water diuresis) and blood samples are drawn around the mid-point of the timed collection period. Usually, the results of three time periods are taken and averaged. Glofil can be administered and "counted" rapidly and more easily than most other substances, and comes close to inulin in determining GFR at all levels of renal function.

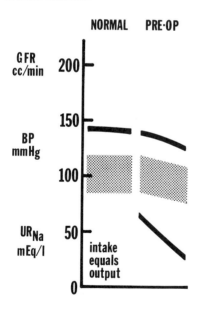

Fig. 11.1 Effects of upper G.I. Barium Enema I.V.P. "N.P.O." Cathartics. A schematic account of what generally occurs when patients are admitted to hospital. Studies and preoperative preparations can produce a volume-depleted patient.

Table 11.1 **Renal Function in 70 kg Man, 50 kg Woman**

	Normal		Impaired	
	Male	**Female**	**Male**	**Female**
Creatinine Clearance	120	100	14	10
Serum Creatinine	1.2	1.0	10	10
24-hour Cr Excretion	1 g	900 mg	1 g	900 mg

The serum creatinine is the best rapid screening method routinely available. However, the routine serum measurements cannot be utilized as proof of normal renal function. Such verification must be obtained by a clearance study. Figure 11.1 illustrates that there are patients with elevated serum creatinine (greater than 1.2 mg/dl) who have a normal GFR (greater than 120 ml/min). Unfortunately, there are also patients with normal serum creatinine values who have a reduced GFR.

The clearance concept holds regardless of the level of renal function. To demonstrate this, consider the usual 70 kg man or 50 kg woman without impairment of renal function compared with the same man or woman with decreased renal function. Let us assume there has been no loss of muscle mass, and no change in creatinine production or chromogen levels. Note that while the creatinine clearance value has decreased with renal failure and the serum values have risen, there has been no change in the amount of creatinine produced in the body and removed by the kidneys (Table 11.1). If the amount produced was not removed the serum level would merely rise further until the remaining kidney mass could clear the blood of the amount produced. Such a rise in the serum value would, of course, change the denominator in the equation and reduce the clearance value further. At some point with declining renal function, the remaining kidney tissue will fail to clear the blood of all the creatinine produced. In fact, as renal function decreases, other mechanisms affect creatinine production, such as caloric restrictions.

ACUTE RENAL FAILURE

EVALUATION

Acute renal failure (ARF) can be defined as a decrease in renal function manifested by (1) a rise in the serum levels of creatinine and/or BUN, or (2) a reduction in clearance values of these or other substances. ARF is usually, but not always, associated with a fall in urine output to less than 300 ml/24

Table 11.2   **Mechanisms of Acute Renal Failure**[a]

1. Blood Flow—To and from the Kidneys
   A. Pump Failure — Cardiac Problems
   - Congestive heart failure (severe)
   - Myocardial infarction (with cardiogenic shock)
   - Pericarditis with low cardiac output

   B. Flow to the Kidneys — Arterial Problems
   - Aorta (dissection)
   - Renal artery (stenosis or clot)
   - Renal vasculature (acute arteritis)

   C. Flow from the Kidneys — Venous Problems
   - Renal veins (Renal Vein Thrombosis)
   - Vena Cava (Clot or tumor in the vena cava)

   D. Inadequate Fluid in the System — Volume Depletion
   - Fluid loss decreasing vascular volume

2. Urine Flow—From the Kidney
   A. Upper Tract — Bilateral Ureteric Obstruction (rare)
   - Beware of patient with one kidney or previous undiagnosed kidney loss

   B. Lower Tract — Obstructions
   - Prostatic (males)
   - Neurogenic bladder (males & females)
   - Commonly seen with diabetes

3. Damage in the Renal Parenchyma — Acute Processes within the Kidney
   - Glomerulus (Rapidly Progressive Glomerular Nephritis)
   - Interstitium (Methicillin)
   - Vascular (Acute Vasculitis)
   - "Tubular" (ATN)

[a] Box = most common causes.

hours (oliguria); there is a subset of patients, however, in whom urine output does not fall although the clearance decreases. This is high-output, or non-oliguric, renal failure and these patients have a better prognosis for recovery of renal function without complications or dialysis. Table 11.2 lists the causes of oliguria and provides a simple mechanistic approach to acute renal failure. The major common causes should be dealt with immediately and ruled in or out. In addition, there are less likely causes that can be looked for with more complicated tests over time if the major etiologies are not the cause. Therefore, for most patients with decreased urine output, with or without an increase in the BUN or creatinine, the investigation and treatment is the same.

The treatment of decreased urine output is accomplished as follows:

1. Evaluate the volume status. If the lungs are clear and there is no evidence of elevated jugular venous pressure, it is reasonable to give fluids (saline is preferred). Such therapy becomes mandatory if the patient has vascular istability and orthostatic hypotension. The amount of fluid given depends on clinical judgement, but generally 1 to 2 L over 1 to 2 hours is adequate. Observation should continue during the period, and then the patient should be reevaluated by measurement of blood pressure and pulse while he or she is standing or supine.

2. Place a bladder catheter. To measure hourly urine output accurately and to rule out a lower urinary tract obstruction, a bladder catheter should be placed.

3. Send a sample of any urine for urinary electrolytes, osmolality, and creatinine values. This needs to be done before step 4; otherwise interpretation of such values becomes difficult, as outlined in Table 11.2.

4. Give intravenous furosemide and an osmotic diuretic such as mannitol. The urgency with which these are given depends on clinical judgement. Time may be an important factor; give these immediately if the patient does not have evidence of volume depletion. The usual doses are furosemide up to 100 mg IV and mannitol 12.5 g IV. Various indices have been devised to enable one to judge if such agents are necessary. However, in acutely "shut down" patients, one generally starts these agents early, often before urine electrolytes or other indices have returned from the laboratory.

5. Continue to monitor volume status frequently by physician examination; obtain a chest roentgenogram and electrocardiogram.

6. Evaluate blood tests as they become available.

A. The presence of anemia may suggest a chronic renal problem (provided that other causes of anemia are excluded).

B. A serum creatinine greater than 10 or 12 mg/dl without coma or seizures usually indicates underlying chronic renal insufficiency. A person with normal renal function cannot tolerate the acute rise to such levels over a few days without becoming very ill, whereas the same elevation attained over months or years often produces little or no symptoms.

7. Urinary Values. A great deal has been made of the urinary elecrolytes and osmolality. However, one must be careful how such electrolyte values are interpreted and always obtain more than one set of values if possible. Table 11.3 indicates how such values can be used to interpret the status of the renal function.

In summary, these steps allow one to estimate the patient's condition, initiate general treament, and form a base of comparison for future evaluation. In addition, such treatment, although somewhat non-specific, may stabilize the patient and perhaps even correct the basic problem if it is due to obstruction or volume loss. From Table 11.2 it is evident that there are three major causes of acute renal shutdown as seen in emergency rooms and other acute settings: (1) volume depletion, (2) obstruction, and (3) acute tubular necrosis. Volume depletion and obstruction can be ruled out clinically if we have addressed these causes in the seven steps during the initial evaluation. The third major cause is harder to prove immediately and at present we have no specific treatment other than time for acute renal failure of parenchymal origin, often referred to as *acute tubular necrosis.*

ACUTE TUBULAR NECROSIS

Acute tubular necrosis (ATN) is a very common term in the renal literature but it is really a misnomer; however, its use as a diagnostic category continues by default, since no other name seems to describe better this category of renal failure. Nevertheless, in using this descriptive phrase it should be realized that tubular changes or damages may not always be demonstrable when acute renal failure of parenchymal origin exists. Further, volume expansion can preserve renal function in the face of tubular lesions that we generally associate with renal shutdown. ATN consists of two general types:

1. Sudden onset. A rapid decrease in the urine output to less than 300 ml/24 hours. In this setting the serum creatinine rises rapidly at a rate of 1 to 2 or more mg/dl/day. These changes are associated with a markedly decreased or often zero renal clearance.

2. Gradual onset: a gradual rise in the serum creatinine, perhaps averaging 0.5 mg/dl/day. Urine output does not decrease until much later when serum creatinine approaches 10 mg/dl or greater. The most common form of this type of ATN in man is associated with aminoglycoside antibiotic toxicity.

A variety of etiologic agents produce the same end result; the pathway producing ATN is apparently common because the kidney only has a limited number of ways it can respond to a variety of insults.

Etiology of ATN

There are four major hypotheses regarding the etiology of ATN:

1. Tubular obstruction. Tubular obstruction may be either intrinsic from tubular debris or extrinsic due to interstitial edema.

2. Tubular "back leak." Damage to the tubular epithelium allows filtered substances to leak back into the interstitium of the kidney, leading to distal tubular collapse.

3. Vasoconstriction. Renin produced in the macula densa causes afferent arteriole vasoconstriction and a markedly diminished volume of tubular filtrate.

4. Glomerular membrane changes. This mechanism applies to experimental causes of decreased ultrafiltration; its role in human ATN is unknown at present.

The major difficulty with any theory new or old is that it must be compatible with the measured events in the various models of ATN. Two changes that all investigators agree on are the initial decrease in renal blood flow that occurs early during the development of ATN and the persistence of ATN after the reduced renal blood flow has returned to normal at approximately 24 hours. Unfortunately, no single hypothesis can explain the persistence of decreased urine output and/or GFR once the blood supply has

Table 11.3 **Urine Evaluation: Pre-Renal Azotemia vs. Acute Tubular Necrosis (ATN)**

	Pre-Renal	A.T.N.
Specific Gravity:	> 1.020	< 1.010
UNa$^+$	<10 mEq/L	>20 mEq/L
UCl$^-$*	<10 mEq/L	>20 mEq/L
U/P Creatinine	>14.	<10.
U/P Osmolality	> 1.5	< 1.0
U–Urine	P–Plasma	

* More specific test than Na.

stabilized. At present the summation hypothesis, that some or all of the above four etiologies may be involved but at different times with various models, is most campatible. For example, we know obstruction plays little if any role early during the initiation of ATN, but once ATN is established, obstruction probably becomes significant and could be a major factor after a few days in the maintenance of ATN.

In the kidneys, it is believed that prostaglandins regulate flow through the superficial or cortical nephrons. This regulation or shunting is particularly important as renal reserve is lost and renal insufficiency progresses.

The Non Steroidal Antigen-Inflammatory Agents (NSAIA) all appear to share the property of blocking prostaglandins. In the impaired kidney this interference produces renal failure, while in patients with normal renal function interstitial nephritis often develops with proteinuria and renal failure. The treatment is stopping the use of these drugs, and, in most cases, the damage appears to be reversible (the role of steroids in treatment is not clear). It should be a rule that such agents are not used in patients with renal impairment.

Clinical Manifestations

In order to understand this functional type of renal failure a little better, let us look at the development or progression of the most common acute type that we see, that is, postoperative ATN.

Development of ATN During Surgery

It has become evident that renal failure occurs postoperatively only when certain events are present before and/or during surgery. Figure 11.1 displays schematically what happens to patients as they are admitted to hospital and prepared for surgery. Patients who are admitted to the hospital are usually afraid and often decrease their fluid intake. In addition, we submit these patients to various radiographic contrast studies, such as intravenous pyelography, and gastrointestinal investigations that require interruption of fluid intake. The order "nothing per ora" (NPO) is common on the charts of these patients. Such fluid restriction is aggravated by additional fluid loss due to the osmotic effects of the radioopaque dyes. Finally, to complete our scenario, most frightened people don't eat, and in some hospitals patients find the food unpalatable when compared with their usual diet. The frequent result of this combination of dread, deprivation, and dislike is a volume-depleted patient. Such patients are avidly retaining sodium, and this retention appears to be the first one of the three necessary components to produce ATN. The second component is hypotension; however, we know from clinical experience that hypotension alone does not produce ATN. For example, patients suffering from gastrointestinal bleeding rarely, if ever, develop ATN, even if they come to the emergency room in shock. Finally, a third component, a circulatory toxin of some type, appears to be necessary to produce ATN. In the wars in Korea and Vietnam it was noted when soldiers were brought to the aid stations in shock that those with significant muscle trauma were more likely to develop ATN.

In summary, postoperative ATN occurs most often in patients who are volume depleted and who have a hypotensive episode during the surgery. These problems can be avoided by preoperative volume expansion and careful volume monitoring during the procedure.

Prevention of Postoperative ATN

1. Assume all patients are volume depleted, and after careful clinical evaluation, before major surgery, give 1 to 2 liters of normal saline intravenously, preferably the night before surgery. If you have questions concerning the patient's volume state, a spot urine sodium and chloride measurement may help. Values less than 20 mEq/L strongly suggest a salt-retaining state and volume depletion. Results above 40 mEq/L with normal renal function effectively rule out significant volume depletion (in the absence of diuretics).

2. Once volume is adequate, give 12.5 grams of manitol by IV push 1 hour before the patient goes to the operating room, and administer a further 12.5 grams of manitol with the IV fluids given during surgery (fluid administration in most operating rooms rests with the anesthesiologist). The use of furosemide 10 mg IV for any decrease in urine output below 0.5 ml/min should be considered. In hospitals where such a protocol is common practice for surgery in which the renal blood supply will be compromised, postoperative ATN is infrequent.

Clinical Course of ATN

Figure 11.2 shows a typical course of postperative ATN. Several significant points should be noted.

1. The serum creatinine rises at a rate of 1 to 2 mg/100 ml/day during the initial oliguric phase.

2. The serum creatinine continues to rise even after the urine output increases to the normal range (1,500 ml/day). Often urine output must go above

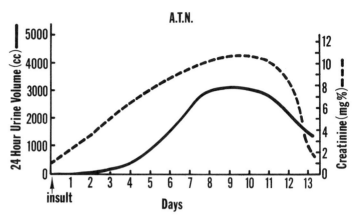

A.T.N.

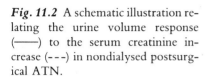

Fig. 11.2 A schematic illustration relating the urine volume response (——) to the serum creatinine increase (---) in nondialysed postsurgical ATN.

3,000 ml/day before the kidney can adequately clear creatinine. Such a high output is required due to the kidney's loss of concentrating ability; only a large volume of unconcentrated fluid can remove the creatinine and other toxic products produced in the body.

3. As a general rule, once oliguria is established (in the absence of dialysis or volume depletion) any urine output will approximately double for each succeeding day. This is of major importance in deciding when to dialyze. For example, let us consider two patients with a rising serum creatinine of 6 mg/dl on day 6. Patient A has an output of 100 ml in the previous 24 hours, and you can be almost certain that you will have to initiate dailysis, because the subsequent increases in urine volume will be too small and too late to reduce the creatinine safely. Contrast this with patient B, whose output is 1,900 ml on the previous day. While you know patients B's creatinine will continue to climb, you can also predict that you will probably not be required to dialyze such a patient.

4. Concentrating ability is the last parameter to return to normal following ATN.

Patients in the recovery phase of ATN are protected from developing further ATN because of a high osmotic load of phosphate, creatinine, and other substances, which in turn produce tubular volume expansion, as manitol does in the normal undamaged tubule. However, it is important to realize such patients can concentrate their urine to some degree when they become severely volume depleted, and such a situation may produce irreversible damage to the already impaired nephrons.

Return of Function after ATN

By definition, ATN patients always recover function. If they do not, most authors or clinicians would consider some other diagnosis. However, we have seen rare cases where function does not return, and yet the kidney biopsy is compatible with ATN. This phenomenon is seen in cadaver transplant patients and in patients with significant underlying chronic renal impairment who clinically develop ATN but who fail to recover necessary function. In this last example, the ATN is probably a final insult to already severely damaged nephrons.

CLINICAL MANIFESTATIONS OF ACUTE RENAL FAILURE

The patients often have no symptoms over the first 3 to 5 days of renal shutdown. There is, however, an immediate change in body chemistry. Since renal clearance is often zero, the BUN and serum creatinine begin to rise by whatever amount the body produces. By definition, these patients have *azotemia*, and by day 5 or 6 the creatinine is often approaching 10 mg/dl with a BUN of greater than 100 mg/dl. At this point, or even earlier, symptoms of uremia (nausea, vomiting, myoclonic muscle jerks, and drowsiness) begin to develop. While symptomatology is not caused by the BUN level and probably not even by the creatinine, it is thought that other "uremic toxins" accumulating at a similar rate cause these uremic symptoms. Other laboratory changes seen in conjunction with the decreased GFR are an immediate rise in the serum phosphate, either accompanied or closely followed by a significant decrease in the serum calcium. None of the above changes initially cause severe problems, although a rise in the serum potassium can trigger lethal arrhythmias (see Chapter 9). This rise in potassium depends on potassium intake, acid-base status, and/or cell breakdown. It is the one early clinical change that must be observed closely, because it can be controlled and is fatal if it is not regulated. If renal failure progresses unchecked from a previously normal state, most patients develop seizures and coma before the serum creatinine has reached 15 mg/dl. Again, this is thought to be due to the effect of the "uremic toxins," not of the creatinine itself. Years ago, more than 50 percent of such acute renal failure patients developed "uremic pericarditis" at this stage, which often played a role in the terminal event.

Generally, patients with ATN recover function, and this confirms the clinical diagnosis; biopsies are rarely done on these patients. The amount of function that patients recover seems to be related to two factors:

1. Age of subject. Younger patients recover almost complete return of function with those under 20 years of age having clearances in the normal range. This contrasts with patients over 40 years of age who appear to have only a partial return of their GFR. As a rule, the older the patient, the less return of function but it is usually enough to avoid chronic dialysis.

2. Underlying renal disease. Return of function in this group may not only be less but also follows a slower course and in some severe cases, recovery does not occur.

CHRONIC RENAL FAILURE

ETIOLOGY

Frequently the etiology of end-stage renal disease is not known because a diagnostic workup was never undertaken or, more commonly, the patient was unaware that he or she had serious kidney disease until symptoms developed. Such patients often are labeled with the diagnosis of chronic glomerulonephritis if they are caucasians, and nephrosclerosis if they are black, but one can never be sure at this stage in the absence of a diagnostic medical history. Such patients present the question of whether the initiating event was systemic hypertension eventually leading to renal failure and proteinuria, or whether glomerular lesions led to secondary hypertension. In the absence of a diagnostic history or previous tissue diagnosis, the following are the most common reasons for patients reaching end-stage renal disease:

1. Glomerular disease
2. Diabetes mellitus (25 percent of new patients reaching end-stage in the U.S.)
3. Hypertension (varies with the percentage of blacks in the population)
4. Interstitial nephritis (mostly due to analgesic abuse)
5. Hereditary renal disease (including polycystics)
6. Systemic lupus erythematosus
7. Myeloma and amyloid

8. Obstructive etiology
9. Other minor causes

THE ROLE OF RENAL BIOPSY IN RENAL FAILURE

Since only certain renal diseases can be diagnosed accurately by clinical means, the physician must then turn to other techniques to confirm clinical impressions. The most informative of these techniques, at present, is the renal biopsy. Since biopsy of the kidney is an invasive procedure with known complications, its use must be reserved for situations when an answer will influence therapy and therefore the risk is worthwhile. The renal biopsy can be performed either open (in a surgical suite under general anesthesia) or closed (percutaneously at the bedside or with the patient on a stretcher, utilizing flouroscopy or ultrasound). While the complications are greater with the open procedure, sometimes this technique must be used to obtain adequate tissue. Table 11.4 lists complications and contraindications for renal biopsy.

Proteinuria as an Indication for Renal Biopsy

If the patient has documented abnormal proteinuria by two adequate 24 hour collections, then biopsy is probably indicated. The following criteria can be

Table 11.4 **Complications and Contraindications—Renal Biopsy**

Complications
  1. Mortality—(less than 1 percent)
  2. Irreversible damage to the kidney (rare)
  3. Hematoma
      a. as demonstrated by IVP or ultrasound—common
      b. causing pain or a fall in hematocrit—5 percent
      c. requiring surgical intervention—rare (less than 1 percent)
  4. Gross hematuria 5 percent
  5. Transient microscopic hematuria and/or pain during the procedure—common (25 percent)
Contraindications
  Percutaneous
      1. Uncooperative patient
      2. Bleeding problems
      3. Hypertension (diastolic greater than 110 mm Hg)
      4. Infection
      5. One kidney
      6. Chronic advanced disease
  Open
      None

applied to urine protein as the sole indication for biopsy:

1. Less than 1 g/24 hours. The physician probably can follow the patient clinically, particularly if renal function is normal.

2. One to 3 g/24 hours. Such patients can be followed clinically, but biopsies frequently help regarding prognosis or therapy.

3. Greater than 3 g/24 hours. Biopsy is definitely indicated, except in children. The usual approach in children because of the high incidence of lipoid nephrosis is to try steroid therapy first and, if the response is inadequate, then biopsy.

CLINICAL COURSE OF CHRONIC RENAL FAILURE

Figure 11.3 is a schematic representation of how renal diseases progress. The purpose of the chart is to relate symptoms to the degree of renal failure and to understand the course of such signs and symptoms over time. It should be realized once again that the kidney has a limited number of ways it can respond to disease, and that almost regardless of the etiology the progression of the disease produces a predictable group of symptoms culminating in the uremic syndrome.

Generally, the progression to end-stage renal disease (ESRD) is slow, taking perhaps 10 to 20 years, and the symptomatology develops very gradually. While there are numerous exceptions to this prolonged course, they fortunately do not constitute a major segment of chronic renal failure patients. The importance of diagnosing this small subgroup of exceptions early is that some are reversible, such as vasculitis or interstitial disease secondary to drugs. Another smaller subgroup of these disorders can be improved with surgery, such as renal artery obstruction with collateral vessels. Therefore, when one is following progressive renal failure it is important to be aware of the markers of uncommon etiologies, on the rare chance of finding a reversible or correctable lesion.

The time course can be estimated roughly by using the reciprocal of the creatinine (1/Cr) against time. As shown in Figure 11.4 the progression of the renal failure can vary depending on the type of disease. Diabetes, once renal impairment is evident, is said to advance more rapidly than most glomerular diseases, whereas polycystic kidney failure has perhaps the slowest progression. These guidelines must be considered only as rules of thumb, but such an understanding can be helpful in dealing with patients and in helping them prepare for dialysis or transplantation. Most people seem to be able to handle ESRD better if they have been expecting it for some period of time and, as it were, had prepared themselves. Whereas, patients who are suddenly told they have rapidly progressive disease frequently do not handle their chronic renal failure state as well.

Early (Asymptomatic) Chronic Renal Failure

This initial period, which usually takes years, covers renal function loss from a normal clearance down to around 25 ml/min (Fig. 11.3). While this major

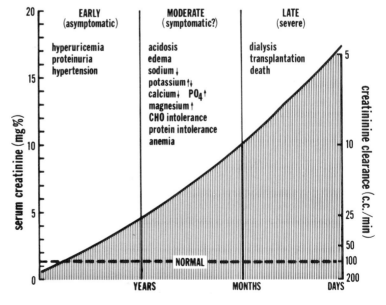

Fig. 11.3 The course of chronic renal failure is shown, emphasizing changes in serum creatinine and creatinine clearance associated with early, moderate, and severe renal failure.

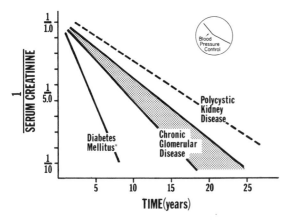

Fig. 11.4 Chronic renal failure progresses to end-stage renal disease at different rates. Patients with diabetes mellitus (———) progress much more quickly than patients with glomerular disease (shaded area), and these progress more quickly than patients with polycystic kidneys, (---). The rate of progression can commonly be predicted by plotting the creatinine ratio $\left(\dfrac{1}{\text{serum Cr}}\right)$ against time.

loss of reserve nephron function and mass is taking place, the body generally can compensate for the changes that occur. Serum phosphate does not rise, because the remaining kidney tubules excrete greater phosphate loads under the stimulus of an increased parathyroid hormone secretion. This occurs at the expense of progressive bone disease that does not become apparent until later. The development of symptoms is retarded during this period because in most organ systems, including the kidney, there is tremendous reserve capacity.

On examination, patients during this early period of nephron loss may only be identified by a decreased GFR. However, three other important findings are frequently present and require consideration with respect to treatment.

1. Hyperuricemia. The serum uric acid rises early as renal failure progresses. Despite the fact that some of these patients have gout, it should be noted that the uric acid, unlike creatinine, does not continue to rise but appears to reach a plateau. There is no solid evidence in the literature that an increased serum uric acid accelerates the decline of renal function. Therefore, unless patients develop stones or systemic symptoms of gout they should not be treated as renal failure progresses. Allopurinol and the uricosuric agents are expensive and have significant side effects.

2. Proteinuria. This is the common marker of glomerular disease, and at this early stage it should not be treated unless a specific diagnosis is made implicating a disease for which therapy is known to be effective, for example, membranous glomerular nephritis. At this early asymptomatic stage, protein loss can produce the nephrotic syndrome, or such spillage can also undergo spontaneous remission while the underlying glomerular disease progresses.

3. Hypertension. Approximately 75 percent of patients who reach ESRD have an elevated blood pressure. The range of such elevations varies from mild to severe. However, all hypertension should be considered harmful to kidney function, regardless of the etiology of the disease, and therapy should be utilized to lower blood pressure to normal. The evidence to support such strong statements is three-fold. The rate of progression of any type of renal failure can be modified by controlling elevated blood pressure. The serious complications of hypertension, for example, stroke, myocardial infarction, and renal failure can be reduced significantly if blood pressure is controlled (see Chapter 3). Control of accelerated or malignant hypertension, even after renal failure has developed, frequently allows a partial return of renal function. Such recovery is seen even when the serum creatinine is greater than 5 mg/dl.

It has recently been proposed by Brenner that as patients lose renal mass the normal high protein diet of North America may cause hyperfusion of the remaining nephrons. This increased flow is postulated to affect nephron survival and perhaps allow the development of hypertension and glomerulonephritis. At present this is being vigorously investigated. If supported, it may lead to marked modification of diet in patients with a creatinine clearance of less than 50 ml/minute.

Moderate (Sometimes Symptomatic) Renal Failure

When the serum creatinine increases to 4 or 5 mg/dl and the renal clearance approaches 25 ml/min, the patient enters a period in which many symptoms develop and progression to end-stage is often measured in months rather than years. It is during this time that the physician begins to recognize phenomena that have been slowly progressing but that have remained under cover of the body's reserves.

Bone Disease

As the first nephrons are lost, a fall in the GFR results. This decrease in the filtration rate, even if small, causes the serum phosphate to rise slightly and calcium to concomitantly decrease. These events trigger an increase in parathyroid hormone secretion, which allows the renal tubule to reabsorb less phosphate and which by at least three known mechanisms returns calcium to its previous level. Therefore, we are left with a stable but slightly decreased GFR, a normal calcium and phosphate, but a marginally elevated parathyroid hormone level. This "trade off" continues until the remaining renal tubules are rejecting 85 percent of the filtered phosphate, and parathyroid hormone cannot correct the serum calcium or phosphate values any longer. At this point (approximately a GFR of 25 ml/min) an elevation in serum phosphate begins to appear. During this same period, as the GFR decreases the skeleton becomes more resistant to parathyroid hormone, partly due to changes in vitamin D metabolism. The end result is that the metabolic system is no longer corrected but is producing progressive bone disease. In other words, a compensatory mechanism is now functioning beyond its ability to regulate the various components and is producing a new complication of renal failure, metabolic bone disease.

Treatment to avoid metabolic bone disease includes the following:

1. Oral antacids can be used to maintain the serum phosphate below 6 mg/dl.

2. Vitamin D can be used to increase the serum calcium level if the hyperphosphatemia is controlled below 6.0 mg/dl.

Anemia

As the GFR approaches 40 ml/min, a mild normochromic, normocytic anemia begins to develop. This anemia gradually progresses until end stage, when the GFR is 5 ml/min. The presenting hematocrit in such end-stage patients tends to range from 17 to 22 percent. This anemia may be due to reduced production of erythropoeitin as well as a decrease in marrow responsiveness to what erythropoeitin there is, a slight shortening in RBC life span in about one third of cases, and blood loss from skin excoriation and GI tract erosions.

Treatment of the anemia includes adequate iron and folate in the diet, but transfusions should be avoided unless the patient has an acute bleeding episode or becomes symptomatic due to the anemia.

Acidosis

As the GFR decreases, the body retains certain fixed acids, such as sulfate and phosphate. Despite the build up of these products the body compensates

with a pH that is almost always above 7.35. Usually, this retention of metabolic products does not cause problems, but it should be realized that there is less buffer capacity available if an acute stressful situation develops.

Treatment is tailored with Schohl's solution or sodium bicarbonate to maintain the serum bicarbonate above 20 mEq/L.

Edema

The kidneys' ability to handle large sodium loads decreases as renal failure progresses. If the serum albumin remains above 3 mg/dl and salt intake is reasonable, edema is not usually a problem. However, in the presence of a lowered serum albumin or when the GFR is less than 20 ml/min, patients who are unable to limit their sodium intake will develop edema.

The treatment consists of thiazide diuretics above a GFR of 20 ml/min. At a clearance below 20 ml/min or in the presence of anasarca, a loop diuretic such as furosemide may be required.

Late (Severe) Chronic Renal Failure

As ESRD progresses through its various stages the "trade-off" process described above for calcium and phosphate metabolism takes place in its various forms throughout the other body components.

Initially reserve is lost in the organ systems affected. As this occurs, the compensatory mechanisms begin to produce secondary side effects, frequently beyond the area of their compensation. Finally, as the metabolic by-products normally excreted by the kidney rise to toxic levels and compensatory elements are produced and retained, the body essentially becomes a new environment. This uremic environment affects all organ systems, probably starting at the cellular level.

These effects may be temporary and partially corrected with dialysis, with respect to the bone, or such abnormalities may become permanent if therapy is not initiated quickly, as occurs in the peripheral nerves. The actual mechanism of these uremic processes is unclear. A large variety of uremic toxins have been described, however, to date no specific substance has been universally recognized and accepted as the agent. Regardless of whether it is one or many substances, the renal toxin(s) does appear to at least initially be dialysable and the effects are completely reversible.

Symptoms and signs of late (severe) chronic renal failure include the following:

1. *Azotemia*: the elevation of the blood urea nitrogen above normal values for any reason. In the early stages and up to roughly a 5-fold increase (100 mg/dl) there are no associated symptoms. BUN is not the uremic toxin.

2. *Uremia*: the general state as renal failure progresses and toxins accumulate that affects all organ systems producing impaired function

3. *Uremic syndrome*: generally considered the end stage of the accumulation of uremic by-products normally excreted by the kidney. This is a complex of symptoms that usually include but are not limited to the following:

   A. Nausea and vomiting
   B. Myoclonic jerks
   C. General malaise
   D. Weight loss (even with edema)
   E. Itching
   F. Numbness and tingling

These symptoms may be due to long-standing renal disease or acute renal failure. The finding of any or all of these signs or symptoms means dialysis should be instituted.

TREATMENT OF END-STAGE CHRONIC RENAL FAILURE

When the serum creatinine rises to 10 mg/dl and/or the clearance falls to 10 ml/min, a point of decision-making has been reached. Either the patient is or is not a candidate for major support therapy.

Conservative Therapy

It must be recognized that there are patients who, because of age, other medical conditions, or family support, are not able to undergo regular chronic renal failure therapy. While such a decision is difficult and should be made only after discussion with the patient and family, it is often the correct decision because it prevents unnecessary suffering by the patient in a treatment modality he or she cannot master. It is important to realize that the heroic therapies that we now have available are for prolonging life and not for prolonging death. If long-term chronic therapy is not chosen then conservative therapy should include the following:

1. A 40-gram HBV protein diet
2. Intermittent peritoneal dialysis for as long as the patient is enjoying life

Table 11.5 **Results of Therapy in ESRD Patients**

	Dialysis	
	Survival 1 year	50 Percent Survival
All patients	89%	6 years
Diabetics	83%	3 years
Over age 55 years	87%	3.5 years
CAPD	(not enough long-term data)	
Self-care	95%	greater than 10 years
Transplantable group[a]	93%	10 years

[a] This represents a select group of patients who finally obtain or could obtain a kidney transplant. Such patients include those who are under 55 years of age, who do not have diabetes mellitus or cancer, and who have successfully dialyzed for 3 months. The 3-month limit eliminates patients who die suddenly or recover.

3. Admission for terminal care or, better yet, well-organized home care. In this often-neglected approach to the dying, medical and social support of the family and the patient is given at home until death occurs or until the home is no longer able to handle the situation.

Since the above supporting therapy requires time and intense interaction with the patient and the family, it is often "easier" to place the patient on dialysis and allow complications to terminate care. This "easy approach" should be avoided. We, as physicians, must recognize that death may be an acceptable choice for very debilitated patients.

Long-term Chronic Therapy

For most patients, the decision will be dialysis and/or renal transplant (see Table 11.5, 11.6). This decision should be made when the patient is still functional (Cr clearance greater than 5 ml/min), and the following course should be undertaken:

1. Establish vascular access.
   a. Arteriovenous fistula—always the first choice
   b. Foreign graft, either bovine artery or synthetic material

Table 11.6 **Renal Transplantation**

	Kidney Graft Survival		Patient Survival	
	1 year	5 years	1 year	5 years
Living related donor	80%	65%	95%	80%
Cadaveric kidney	55%	30%	90%	65%

c. Peritoneal catheter—if the patient chooses a form of outpatient peritoneal dialysis
2. Initiate dialysis to stabilize the patient.
3. Long-term care—dialysis and transplantation

Dialysis and Transplantation

As of this writing, most patients in the United States who reach end stage renal disease (ESRD) are considered for chronic therapy. An unrestricted acceptance policy such as this results in approximately 100 patients/million population/year entering therapy. This entrance rate is higher than elsewhere in the world for two reasons: age and other diseases such as diabetes are not an absolute contraindication, and hypertension is very common, particularly in our black population.

For patients under age 55 years, a kidney transplant from a living related donor is the best form of therapy. If no related donor is available, then cadaver transplant should be considered, based on two criteria:

1. Under age 30 years, most people have problems with the restrictions of dialysis, and cadaver transplant should be the preferred form of therapy.
2. For patients between age 30 and 55 years, dialysis should be tried and the patient should decide regarding cadaver transplantation, based on how they are able to function on dialysis. The closer one gets to 55 years the poorer the results with transplantation due to other age-related complications.

For patients over age 55 years, despite a few optomistic anecdotal reports, dialysis is the treatment of choice. If the patient is able, home dialysis or some form of "self-care" is the preferred form of therapy. For the 1980s, if abdominal infection can be controlled, continuous ambulatory peritoneal dialysis (CAPD) or some variation may become a major form of long-term dialysis care. At present, it comprises about 10 percent of the dialysis population at any one time in the United States, with up to one third of new patients utilizing CAPD in Canada.

There are continual improvements in the results of renal transplantation. At this time, donor-specific blood transfusions will probably increase related donor transplants and improve results significantly. In the current protocols, the recipients receive three transfusions of 200 ml each, 2 weeks apart, from the donor. If no cross-match reaction develops, the transplants are 95 percent successful.

Cadaveric transplants will probably continue, with the recent trend showing the following characteristics:

1. Random transfusions are given to all recipients (which probably select out the "high" and "low reactors").
2. Low reactors receive an unmatched graft (in the United States).
3. Failures and high reactors are given specific immunotherapy. Thus, both graft selection and management of immunologic rejection are undergoing continual refinement.

PROTEINURIA, NEPHROTIC SYNDROME, AND EDEMA

SIGNIFICANT PROTEINURIA

Normal subjects (males and females) deliver less than 150 mg of protein into the urine in a 24-hour period; greater than 300 mg on a consistent basis is definitely abnormal. Because of the kidneys' ability to concentrate, "spot urines" are an unreliable way to report and/or follow urine protein. Urinary excretion of protein should be based on one or more 24-hour collections, preferably out of hospital and in the absence of fever. The accuracy of every 24-hour specimen should be supported by calculating the amount of creatinine present in the specimen. See discussion of 24 hour creatinine excretion under Measurement of Renal Function above, and in Table 11.1. Incomplete 24 hour urine specimens underestimate the protein loss.

While spot urines are the common way we first recognize urine protein abnormalities, they are notoriously inaccurate in the very range we need to observe, that is, 200 to 1,000 mg/24 hour range. This inaccuracy results from two factors:

1. "Dip sticks" are frequently used, and they carry a 50 percent inaccuracy in the trace-to-1+ range. This problem is said to be greater in male observers because of red-green color blindness.
2. The kidneys ability to concentrate and dilute the urine is another factor. Table 11.7 demonstrates how a normal person may show significant proteinuria in the average concentrated-overnight specimen. Of more concern is the patient with significant proteinuria of, let us say, 1 g/24 hours who is also a water drinker and masks the amount of protein in a dilute urine when seen later in the day at a physician's office. To prevent such errors a 24-hour urine must be performed to evaluate urine protein losses. Spot urines can be somewhat more accurate if the specific gravity is checked as well as the protein. This permits

Table 11.7 Urine Volume, Concentration, and Proteinuria

| | | | Protein | | Dip Stick Reading |
Time	Vol.	Sp. Gr.	mg/dl	Total (mg)	
7 AM–3 PM	600	1.015	8	48	−
3 PM–11 PM	700	1.012	7	49	−
11 PM–7 AM	200	1.028	25	50	+
24 hours	1,500	1.014	10	147	−

an assessment of whether the urine is diluted or concentrated and permits a qualitative judgement about overestimation or underestimation.

False-Positive Tests

Although 3 percent sulfosalicylic acid is the easiest agent to use routinely in an office or a clinic, it does produce more false readings, especially false positives, compared with the dip sticks. While such false readings are rare, their causes should be noted. The most significant substances in this regard are radiographic contrast material, penicillins (including methicillin), and most non steroidal anti-inflammatory agents. Many of these same drugs can also produce false positives with the more sophisticated techniques (heat and acetic acid and the nitric acid ring test) used by the hospital or commercial laboratories.

How the Kidney Handles Protein

Small molecular weight proteins (less than 50,000 molecular weight) pass through the glomerular basement membrane normally yet do not appear in the final urine because they are reabsorbed in the tubules. When such small molecular weight protein (light

chains, microglobulins) appear in a urine sample, there are really only two possible mechanisms: an increased load has been produced by the body, for example, dysproteinemia, or there is tubular damage and the normally filtered small molecular weight protein cannot be reabsorbed (for example, β_1-microglobulins in ATN) By contrast, large molecular weight proteins (greater than 50,000 daltons) including albumin (69,000 daltons) appear in the urine only when there is a glomerular abnormality, since this size protein is not filtered by a normal basement membrane. Proteinuria consisting of low molecular weight proteins is said to be "selective" proteinuria; when large and small molecular weight proteins are represented it is termed "non-selective." These facts should direct studies to the proper area of the kidney to determine the etiology of the protein loss. Figure 11.5 presents the renal tubular handling of protein in normal subjects.

Causes of Proteinuria

Proteinuria without Primary Renal Disease

Orthostatic proteinuria Particularly in adolescents and young adults, protein may be found routinely in the urine of 10 percent of the population.

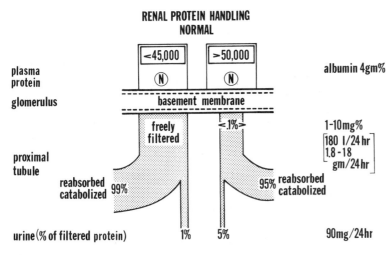

Fig. 11.5 The normal renal protein handling is illustrated. Small amounts of low molecular weight protein (<45,000 m.w.) in the serum permit total tubular reabsorption. The higher quantities of albumin (>50,000 m.w.) in the serum are largely retained because of very low permeability of the normal glomerular basement membrane.

This percentage increases to 75 percent when the same age group assume a lordotic position for 20 minutes. The etiology is thought to be increased venous pressure produced by lordosis; however, the evidence for this is minimal. Orthostatic proteinuria is found equally in both sexes, and in a 10-year follow-up in military recruits, it was transient in many but persistent in just under 50 percent. The most important finding was that in no case was such proteinuria an early marker of progressive renal disease. Such proteinuria generally causes spillage of less than 1 g protein/24 hours; however, in one extensive series, 35 percent of 350 cases excreted greater than 1.5 g/24 hours. Orthostatic proteinuria never produces the nephrotic syndrome, and other measures of renal function are always normal. Orthostatic factors as a cause of proteinuria must be ruled out before any invasive or harmful diagnostic techniques are performed. To do this the patient is asked to lie down, and 30 minutes later while still supine is asked to void. This specimen is discarded thereby removing any urine produced while in the upright position. Then for a timed period, the urine is collected while the patient remains continuously supine. The procedure can be performed overnight at home, or for shorter periods in an office or clinic. If one assumes that less than 150 mg of protein/24 hours is normal, then in 2 hours in an office there should be $\frac{1}{12}$ of 150 or less than 12.5 mg of protein in the specimen collected (for 8 hours supine at home, less than 50 mg). Since proteinuria is decreased in the supine position even in patients with glomerular disease, to diagnose proteinuria as orthostatic and not due to disease, the amount passed in the urine while supine must return to the normal range for that time period.

Other Probable Causes of Proteinuria

Below are listed a number of alleged causes of proteinuria. The mechanisms for this mixed group are not well studied.

1. Lordosis
2. Post prandial
3. Obesity
4. Effort (Exercise)
5. Circulatory: CHF, Constrictive Pericarditis
6. Cerebral Trauma
7. Infection with fever

Effort, constrictive pericarditis, cerebral trauma, and infection with fever are relatively common causes seen in patient care.

Renal Causes of Proteinuria

Tubular proteinuria   Any agent or disease process that causes damage to the renal tubule can be and usually is associated with small molecular weight proteinuria. Such protein loss is frequently but not always less than 1g/24 hours. This is presented schematicaly in Figure 11.6. In addition, production or "overflow" proteinuria can produce variable amounts of protein in the urine as in light chain disease in the presence of normal tubules. Therefore, the appropriate serum values must always be obtained when investigating tubular proteinuria. Table 11.8 lists a few of the many possible causes.

Glomerular proteinuria   will be discussed below in greater detail. It is because this group of glomerular diseases tends to progress to end-stage renal disease that proteinuria is such a significant marker. Proteinuria accompanied by hypertension carries a much worse prognosis in any of these diseases, compared with proteinuria alone.

THE NEPHROTIC SYNDROME

The nephrotic syndrome includes:

1. Twenty-four hour urine protein of 3.5 grams or greater
2. Hypoalbuminemia of less than 3.0 g%
3. Edema
4. Frequently hypercholesterolemia

The causes are many but can be grouped as follows:

1. Lipoid nephrosis—benign, particularly common in childhood
2. Systemic disease—for example, amyloidosis, drug-induced renal disease, connective tissue disease
3. Progressive renal disease—for example, membranous glomerulonephritis

The common etiology appears to be a change in the glomerular basement membrane that allows large molecular weight molecules (greater than 50,000 daltons) to be filtered. Such changes can be biochemical,

Table 11.8   **Causes of Renal Tubular Proteinuria**

Fanconi's syndrome	Potassium depletion
Cystinosis	"Acute tubular necrosis"
Cadmium poisoning— chronic	Myoglobinuria
Renal allograft rejection	Analgesic abuse
Wilson's disease	Balkan nephritis
Myeloma	Almost any condition with
Galactosemia	a renal tubular defect

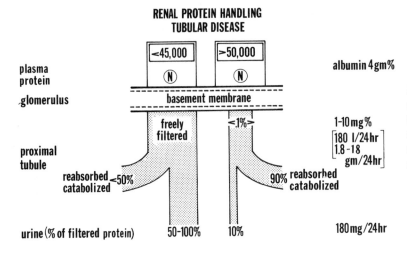

RENAL PROTEIN HANDLING TUBULAR DISEASE

Fig. 11.6 Renal protein handling in tubular disease. Note that reduced reabsorption results in high urine protein concentration. Compare with Figure 11.5.

as with lipoid nephrosis, or structural in other etiologies. Even the structural changes can sometimes be reversed with specific therapy, or such improvement may occur spontaneously.

Treatment of the Nephrotic Syndrome

Whenever possible, a specific diagnosis should be established and treated. The first line of treatment of idiopathic nephrotic syndrome is *restricted salt intake and diuretic therapy*. In many cases this will control the swelling until a treatable etiology is found or a spontaneous remission occurs. The second major treatment regimen is the use of steroids and/or immunosuppressive drugs. While such agents may be associated with a remission or perhaps partial improvement, they do have serious side effects and their use should be restricted to situations when the hypoalbuminemia secondary to protein spillage is causing serious systemic problems (see Glomerular Disease, following section).

GLOMERULAR DISEASE

CLASSIFICATION OF GLOMERULAR DISEASE BASED ON RENAL BIOPSY

Methods of renal biopsy, contraindications, and complications have been described under Chronic Renal Failure. An adequate renal biopsy samples enough tissue to allow three types of examination:

1. Light microscopy. Histology can be stained and looked at under a common microscope.
2. Electron microscopy. When specimens are fixed with special preservatives, much higher power resolution discloses structural changes that can be diagnostic, for example, amyloid deposition.
3. Immunofluorescent staining. Kidney slices are incubated with fluorescein labeled antisera to demonstrate the presence of immunoglobulins, complement, fibrin, or other material attached to tissue structures.

These methods of tissue examination together with the clinical manifestations generally permit a diagnosis of one of the following glomerular abnormalities:

1. Lipoid nephrosis
2. Focal glomerular sclerosis
3. Idiopathic membranous glomerulonephritis
4. Proliferative glomerulonephritis
    A. Acute post infectious
    B. Membranoproliferative (mesangiocapillary)
    C. Focal segmental glomerulonephritis
    D. Rapidly progressive glomerulonephritis (RPGN)
5. Other diseases presenting as the nephrotic syndrome

The following terms are often used in describing biopsy specimens:

1. Diffuse—all glomeruli are involved
2. Focal—some but not all glomeruli are involved in the process
3. Segmental—only a part of the glomerulus is affected
4. Global—a whole segment of the glomerulus involved
5. Proliferative—an increase in the number of cells in the glomeruli
6. Exudative—polymorphonuclear leukocytes have moved into the glomeruli

7. Membranous—increase in the glomerular capillary wall thickness

8. Sclerosis—fibrosis from previous glomerular damage

Role of Immune Complexes in Glomerular Disease

Glomerular disease leading to ESRD is composed of some well defined etiologies plus a large number of ill defined or undiagnosed causes. Glomerular disease is thought to be secondary to antigen-antibody deposition in the kidney with secondary responses that are variable and in some cases as yet unrecognized.

Normally if an antigen is released into the blood stream, the animal responds by producing an antibody to that antigen. The antigen and the antibody combine forming a soluble complex which is filtered out by the kidney and the reaction that occurs in the glomerulous produces transient kidney disease. The human example of this would be post streptococcal glomerular nephritis. Gradually the complexes are removed by macrophages and the kidney generally returns to normal and little if any scarring or damage results.

By contrast however if the antigen release becomes chronic, the kidney may not respond as well depending on the chronicity, size, and amount of antibody production as well as other factors.

Factors that may relate to the development of kidney disease:

1. Antibody production:
   a. When it approximates the amount of antigen, renal disease is more likely.
   b. Too much or too little antibody appears to allow sparing of the kidney. This probably is a size related phenomena and is influenced by 2 & 3 below.
2. Size of the antigen-antibody complexes. Large complexes are removed by the reticuloendothelial system.
3. Number of binding sites on the antigen can effect the ultimate size of the complexes.
4. Individual patients genetic make up.
5. Secondary response of the animal to the presence of antigen/antibody complexes:
   a. complement   b. leucocytes   c. platelets   d. non-specific antibodies
6. Glomerular Basement Membrane Antibodies:
   For unknown reasons the body may begin producing antibody that reacts against substances within the glomerular or tubular basement membrane. This phenomenon becomes evident when one utilizes the immunoflourescence technique on a biopsy specimen and demonstrates the presence of linear staining (e.g., Goodpastures' syndrome). It is theorized that this process may be related to tissue damage and/or viral infection exposing an antigenic site which the body reacts to by producing antibody.

Lipoid Nephrosis (LN) (Nil Change or Minimal Change Disease)

Etiology

Lipoid nephrosis represents a nonimmunologic process of unknown cause. Experiments suggest that a majority of findings in lipoid nephrosis can be explained on a biochemical basis. The loss of negatively charged sialoproteins from the region of the foot processes and the basement membrane allows large molecular weight protein ($> 50,000$ daltons), including albumin, to pass through into the urine. This change in charge along the basement membrane is not associated with structural changes that may be viewed by microscopy. This lesion has also been observed in patients with the nephrotic syndrome due to Hodgkin's disease.

Clinical Manifestations

Patients are usually discovered when peripheral edema appears and the patient is found to have proteinuria and a low serum albumin. This is the most common cause of the nephrotic syndrome in children. Because of this high incidence, particularly between the ages of 2 and 6 years, most pediatricians treat such patients first and investigate only those who do not respond. Lipoid nephrosis occurs in adolescents and in patients over age 20 years, but is less common.

Hypertension is reported in up to 10 percent of cases in children, but its presence should raise the question of another diagnosis. Impaired clearances and even renal failure may occur in children as a result of severe vascular volume depletion, but such hypoperfusion probably does not occur in adults.

True lipoid nephrosis should be considered a self-limiting disease that generally remains in remission once adulthood is achieved. Exacerbations in adults are less frequent and seem to be more easily controlled. In children exacerbations are the major concern.

One third of these patients have a permanent remission (> 1 year) with administration of oral steroids. Of the remaining two thirds that relapse, one third have infrequent exacerbations than can be controlled with higher doses, prolonged tapering, or chronic use of low-dose steroids. Two thirds of those that relapse have frequent exacerbations and are difficult to manage, often requiring cyclophosphamide along with the steroids to produce a prolonged remission. Infection, perhaps due to low IgG levels, is the major cause of death, particularly in the relapsing groups. Pneumococcal infection is the most common.

Laboratory Assessment

Twenty-four hour urine protein ranges from 2 to 3 grams up to greater than 20 grams and tends to be selective. Microscopic hematuria is seen in about 25 percent of cases if one looks diligently. The serum albumin is usually less than 3 g/dl and there is commonly hypercholesterolemia. The serum complement is normal.

The renal biopsy is most helpful in excluding other disease processes. Light microscopy reveals normal glomeruli or very mild segmental mesangeal hypercellularity in some glomeruli (focal). Electron microscopy demonstrates foot process fusion. This finding is probably related to protein spillage rather than to any specific disease process. Immunofluorescent stains are negative.

Treatment

1. If the edema can be controlled with salt restriction and diuretics, adult patients can be followed this way until a remission occurs.

2. Generally, oral steroids (for example, prednisone) are initiated on a daily basis (children 60 mg/M²/day, adults 1.5 mg/kg/day) until a remission occurs or until 4 weeks have passed. At that point many physicians switch to alternate-day therapy (children 40 mg/M², adults 1 mg/kg) and continue treatment for another 4 to 8 weeks. We generally taper the dose for a further 4 weeks in adults at ½ mg/kg every other day.

3. Exacerbations occurring while the dose is being tapered are treated with higher doses (1 mg/kg) on a daily basis for 6 weeks, followed by a slower taper.

4. Frequent exacerbations can be treated with cyclophosphamide recognizing its important side effects.

Since lipoid nephrosis is not a fatal disease and remissions almost always occur with increasing age, a patient, particularly a child, must be severely disabled by the edema and hypoalbuminemia before the physician utilizes toxic agents such as cyclophosphamide or chlorambucil. Patients whose conditions exacerbate while still on drugs or immediately after stopping therapy, appear to make up a special group. They should always be biopsied and followed closely for complications and the possibility of another diagnosis.

Focal Glomerular Sclerosis

Etiology

Focal glomerular sclerosis (FGS) is seen in 15 to 20 percent of the cases of adult idiopathic nephrotic syndrome. At present it is thought to be an immune complex disease; however, it is also observed in heroin addicts and post–renal-transplant patients. Two views have developed regarding the etiology of FGS: it may be a separate entity from lipoid nephrosis, perhaps of viral etiology or even secondary to continued protein spillage, or it may merely be a more severe form of minimal change disease that for some unrecognized reason has progressed. The only strong evidence to support the latter hypothesis is from the experimental puromycin model of renal disease, in which high doses of puromycin produce a persistent lesion like FGS, whereas low doses give a reversible lesion like lipoid nephrosis. Therefore, FGS is probably an immune complex disease but could be a form of lipoid nephrosis that for unknown reasons progresses to end-stage renal failure (see contrasting features Table 11.9.) As more cases are diagnosed and followed, subgroups with a better prognosis are being recognized.

Table 11.9 Clinical Comparison of Lipoid Nephrosis versus Focal Glomerular Sclerosis

	LN	FGS
Selective Proteinuria	Highly selective	Nonselective
Hematuria		
Microscopic	20%	50%
Gross	Rare	50%
Hypertension	Rare	50%
Renal function impaired	No	1/3 to 1/2
Response to:		
Steroids	95% Initially	10%
Immunosuppressives	Good	None
Prognosis	Excellent	Poor

Clinical Manifestations

Patients usually have significant proteinuria, with over 50 percent having the nephrotic syndrome. Approximately 50 percent of all cases have hematuria, hypertension, and impaired renal function at the time of diagnosis. It is now evident that certain findings appear to carry a better prognosis:

1. Children do not progress as rapidly as adults.
2. More children develop remissions than adults.
3. Remission with steroids is an excellent prognostic sign, and this subgroup is unlikely to ever develop renal failure.
4. A few "nonresponders" to steroids may later develop a spontaneous remission, and this appears to carry a better prognosis.
5. Patients who never develop the nephrotic syndrome do better.

Laboratory Assessment

Proteinuria is almost invariably present with FGS and tends to be nonselective. Microscopic hematuria is present in 50 percent of cases, and gross hematuria, while rare, can occur. Twenty-four–hour urine protein values vary from 1 gram to over 10 grams. Serum albumin is reduced in proportion to protein spillage. Serum complement is normal, and BUN and creatinine both rise as the disease progresses.

The renal biopsy has several distinctive features. On light microscopy, mesangial changes are seen early in segmental areas of some glomeruli, particularly those in the juxtamedullary area. Tubular changes and interstitial involvement may be present initially, and when present they support the diagnosis. As the disease progresses, more glomeruli become affected throughout the kidney, and the most involved ones become completely sclerosed. Electron microscopy reveals mesangial hyperplasia and foot process fusion if protein spillage is heavy. Electron-dense deposits appear in involved gomeruli. Immunofluorescent staining demonstrates IgM and complement in a granular pattern, particularly in the more affected gomeruli. IgA and IgG are observed less commonly. The presence of IgM with a minimal change lesion essentially makes the diagnosis of FGS.

Treatment

A relatively small proportion of patients with FGS respond to treatment. However, it is becoming evident that a subgroup with a better prognosis may be recognized depending on their response to treatment as outlined under clinical manifestations above. Most physicians try one course of steroids in the same dosage used for the lipoid nephrosis. If a remission does not occur in 2 to 4 weeks the steroid therapy should be stopped and salt restriction and diuretics continued. Treatment of renal failure and associated problems should be conducted as described in the section Chronic Renal Failure.

Membranous Nephropathy

Etiology

As of this writing, membranous nephropathy (MN) accounts for more than 50 percent of cases of the idiopathic nephrotic syndrome in adults. The pathogenesis of membranous nephropathy is still controversial. While it is probably immunologic, whether idiopathic MN is due to exogenous or endogenous antigens or immune-complex formation is not clear. What is clear is that there are a number of other causes that must be kept in mind when the diagnosis is made by renal biopsy. It should be recognized that the renal lesion may be recognized first in systemic diseases, such as lupus erythematosus, in chronic infections including hepatitis B and secondary syphillis, in certain neoplasms, and in a variety of other systemic diseases.

Clinical Manifestations

Approximately 75 percent of cases will present as the nephrotic syndrome, with the remainder being discovered on routine examination because of mild proteinuria and/or hypertension. Progression is variable and difficult to predict early in the course. In review of the literature and our own experience, we eventually can recognize three groups, each of which accounts for approximately one third of all cases of this disorder:

1. A rapidly progressive group that progresses to ESRD in 2 to 5 years
2. A group that slowly loses renal function over a much longer period, perhaps averaging 15 to 20 years
3. A group, perhaps less severely involved, that develops remissions and in some cases shows improvement on biopsy. These patients do not develop progressive renal disease.

Whether these three groups are all the same disease or whether they merely represent different processes linked by the kidneys' limited histologic response, is not known.

Laboratory Assessment

Proteinuria is almost always present with membranous nephropathy, and tends to be nonselective. Microscopic hematuria is present in more than 90 percent of cases, while gross hematuria is rare (< 5 percent). The 24-hour urine protein is greater than 3.5 grams in 75 percent of cases, with a range from trace proteinuria to over 20 g/day. Hypoalbuminemia is common, due to the urine protein loss. Serum complement levels are usually normal, and, if reduced, systemic lupus erythematosus should always be considered.

The renal biopsy reveals distinctive features. On light microscopy early in the disease, capillaries may be normal or may show evidence of what are probably immune deposits. Later the capillary walls thicken and deposits become more distinct. With silver stain at this stage, characteristic spike and dome projections are seen. In the final stage, marked thickening of the capillaries is present in all glomeruli, and gradual atrophy occurs. Electron microscopy in the early stages reveals small subepithelial deposits. These progress to distort the basement membrane, and projections reach out around the deposits, corresponding to the spikes seen on light microscopy. Finally, the deposits lose their denseness and are completely incorporated into the basement membrane. Immunoflourescent staining demonstrates IgG and C3 in the involved areas of the glomeruli. These phenomena advance as the disease progresses, but in the final stages distinct fluorescence is not clear.

Treatment

A large inter-hospital collaborative study in 1980 reported a controlled trial with alternate day steroids (prednisone) of up to 125 mg for 2 months, followed by a 1-month taper. Such treatment produced a significant response when compared with the control group. This form of treatment should be used on all patients with biopsy-proven membranous nephropathy with a creatinine clearance greater than 40 ml/min. For more advanced renal failure, sporadic reports suggest a similar response can be expected. The use of alternate-day steroids for 2 months every year, although in common use, has no basis in the collaborative study report. For patients with steroid failure or advanced cases of idiopathic membranous glomerulonephritis, cytotoxic agents have not been shown to be effective.

Proliferative Glomerulonephritis

Proliferative glomerulonephritis constitutes a category used to classify the various remaining glomerular lesions. Most of these disease states are currently being clarified through research. One exception to this statement is acute postinfectious glomerulonephritis most commonly due to streptococcal infections.

Post-streptococcal Glomerulonephritis (PSGN) (Post-infectious)

Etiology   Usually the patient has a pharyngeal infection, or a skin infection with type A beta-hemolytic streptococci 7 to 10 days before the onset of the kidney involvement, the so-called latent period. Post-streptococcal organisms are the major etiologic agents in producing this type of acute diffuse proliferative glomerulonephritis. There are two major groups that vary somewhat in course and perhaps even in prognosis. Pharyngitis due to types 1, 2, 3, 4, 12, 18, 25, 49, 55, 57, and 60 beta-hemolytic streptococci classically produce a 7- to 10-day latent period and are associated with increases in serum antistreptolysin (ASO) titer. Infected throats are the more common etiology in sporadic cases of post-streptococcal kidney disease. Skin infections due to types 2, 49, 55, 57, and 60 have a longer latent period of up to 20 days, and the ASO titer usually does not rise. Other serum antibodies such as antihyaluronidase, however, may rise. Impetigenous infections are the common cause of many epidemic outbreaks, particularly in undeveloped countries.

It is now recognized that many other infectious agents produce an almost identical pathologic picture, and these must be considered when determining the etiology of a diffuse proliferative glomerulonephritis. Other bacterial agents include pneumococcus, staphylococcus, and many others. Viral agents include common viruses as mumps, cytomegalovirus, and hepatitis B. Parasitic infections include the common agent of malaria. While there are an almost endless number of single-case associations, it is sometimes difficult to be certain of an absolute relationship. The physician must always rule out a low-grade streptococcal sore throat, and sometimes this is difficult since antibiotic therapy will decrease or eliminate the serological ASO response. Although it is thought that such infections trigger antigen-antibody reactions resulting in an immune complex disease, the exact nature of such an interaction is still unclear.

Clinical manifestations In classic post-streptococcal pharyngeal infection a latent period (7 to 10 days) is followed by the development of cloudy or "smokey" urine. A shorter latent period suggests previous infectious episodes. On microscopic examination, the smokey color of the urine is shown to be the presence of red blood cells. Such changes in the urine may be the only evidence of disease, and in fact many patients, especially in epidemics, may have completely subclinical courses (even negative urinalysis with classical changes on biopsy). The majority of cases, however, will develop further manifestations. Edema develops initially in the face and especially around the eyes, and is most evident on first rising in the morning. This may progress to generalized edema. Proteinuria is commonly in the range of 1 to 2 g/24-hours, but the nephrotic syndrome has also been reported. Oliguria is seen commonly and is not of major concern; however, anuria (less than 350 ml/24 hours is worrisome, and if it persists, crescentic glomerulonephritis should be considered. Hypertension develops commonly, and is volume related due to fluid retention. Digitalis and diuretics are rarely indicated, since diuresis occurs spontaneously in a few days. In children, this elevation of blood pressure seems to be more severe, but pulmonary edema is extremely rare if fluid restriction is instituted.

In almost all cases, these findings disappear in 2 to 3 weeks after the onset of the throat or skin infections, and the only findings that remain are in the urine. Persistence of clinical symptoms beyond 4 weeks raises the probability of another etiology.

There are two major schools of thought regarding the prognosis of post-streptococcal glomerulonephritis. One group holds that PSGN is an acute process and 98 percent of affected people recover completely with no long-term risk of renal failure. This view is supported by large epidemiologic studies in Red Lake, Minnesota, and in Trinidad, but the population of these studies tends to be younger than that of sporadic cases. The second view is that many patients following a bout of sporadic PSGN develop chronic glomerular nephritis over time (5 to 20 years). This is also supported by several large studies.

Some of the confusion regarding treatment and progression may arise because a patient may have well-recognized PSGN, and this can be considered the cause when future renal disease develops, even though undetected renal disease due to other cause is the true problem. Even if a biopsy is taken at the time of the PSGN, a mild chronic process may be missed because of the extreme proliferation. Until further proof is forthcoming, the clinician has to assume that either a few cases progress for some as yet undetermined reason or else such patients had previously undiagnosed renal disease.

Laboratory assessment Red blood cells are common in the urine of these patients and RBC casts are often present especially in the early morning specimen. Proteinuria is also common, but over 50 percent have less than 1 gram in a 24-hour collection. Only 20 percent have greater than 3 g/24 hours, and it is always nonselective. While the nephrotic syndrome is reported in up to 4 percent of cases, the physician should be cautious and always look for another etiology when the nephrotic syndrome is observed in post-streptococcal glomerulonephritis. The GFR, when measured, is found to be decreased in almost every case. The concomitant rise in serum creatinine is somewhat masked by the fluid retention.

The throat culture will usually be positive for group A beta-hemolytic streptococci. Serologic evidence of antistreptococcal antibodies may be most helpful. In classic untreated throat infections, 85 percent of patients will develop a significant rise in antistreptolysin O or antihyaluronidase antibodies. These values vary depending on the type of infection; ASO is not elevated with skin infection. If the pharyngitis is treated with antibiotics in the first few days, only 15 percent of patients will demonstrate an increase in these titers. The serum levels of these antibody responses bare no significance to the severity of the renal disease. They may continue to rise over the course of the disease and then slowly decline over weeks or months.

A much better marker of kidney involvement in post-streptococcal disease is the serum complement, which is reduced in 85 to 95 percent of cases. The degree of the complement decrease does not correlate with severity or duration of renal involvement. Normally, C3 is decreased by the end of the latent period and slowly returns to normal over the next 8 weeks. If the complement level remains depressed beyond this period, a different etiology should be looked for and a renal biopsy should be obtained.

The renal biopsy demonstrates diffuse proliferation in all glomeruli. It is very easy, with such diffuse changes, to miss some other mild underlying renal disease. By light microscopy the glomeruli appear uniformly enlarged and "full," due to the cellular proliferation of both mesangial and endothelial cells. There is variable infiltration with polymorphs, eosinophils, and mononuclear cells. Rarely a single crescent will be seen in a glomerulus, and this is considered insignificant if most of the glomeruli observed are non-crescentic. The diagnosis is confirmed by the presence of electron-dense "humps" sitting on the epithelial side of the basement membrane. These humps will gradually resolve over a period of 1 to 3 months. Immunofluorescence is not diagnostic and, in fact, is sometimes completely negative. If immunoglobulins are present, the clinician sees IgG and/or complement in a granular pattern more frequently than IgA or IgM.

Treatment   Only significant symptoms should be treated. Restrict salt and fluid intake to prevent fluid overload in oliguric patients. Steroids and other agents have no place in the therapy, and diuretics are not really effective while the GFR is depressed. Early treatment of the sore throat or skin infection probably does not decrease the incidence or severity of nephritis, in contrast with what is true for rheumatic fever, but this is still not absolutely certain. Until a vaccine is invented, nothing is available to prevent pharyngeal streptococcal infections. Cleanliness does appear to decrease the incidence of skin infections.

Membranoproliferative Glomerulonephritis (Mesangiocapillary GN)

Membranoproliferative glomerulonephritis, a type of renal pathology of unknown etiology, makes up 10 percent of the glomerular diseases, and has an overall poor prognosis, with a 10-year survival of approximately 50 percent. As in almost all glomerulonephritis, the presence of hypertension, persistent nephrotic syndrome, or a reduced GFR at the time of diagnosis are associated with a worse prognosis. At present, no form of treatment is recommended. Almost all cases have proteinuria (50 percent will have or develop the nephrotic syndrome) and hematuria. The most important diagnostic laboratory finding is a reduced serum complement (C3) found in over 75 percent of cases at the time of diagnosis or as the disease progresses.

The membranoproliferative group is composed of two major idiopathic types plus a number of diseases in which the pathologic biopsy findings of mesangial cell proliferation and "tram tracking," or splitting, of the basement membrane are present. Type I, with subendothelial deposits, affects an older age group (early 20s) and has a slightly better than 10-year survival. Type II, dense deposit disease, has dense deposits in the basement membrane and an average age of onset of about 15 years. Secondary causes of membranoproliferative changes are numerous and generally relate to infectious processes, for example, "arteriovenous-shunt" nephritis, and hepatitis B virus. A long list can be found in any standard nephrology text.

Focal and Segmental Glomerulonephritis

Focal and segmental glomerulonephritis is probably the least well defined of the glomerulopathies, and there is some question whether it is a distinct subgroup. Recurrent episodes of gross hematuria are often associated with upper respiratory or other infections, suggesting a link between these diseases. On biopsy, the clinician often finds mild focal segmental change, and in the most important types in this group, finds IgA on immunofluorescent staining.

1. Benign recurrent hematuria almost always presents with a normal GFR and does not progress to ESRD. Spontaneous remissions are characteristic.

2. IgA nephropathy (Berger's disease) is a geographically distributed disease (France and South East Asia have the greatest incidence) affecting predominantly males. IgA is present in kidney biopsies and, frequently, in skin biopsies. There is no treatment known, and progression to renal failure varies from 25 percent in France to somewhat less in other areas.

3. Henoch-Schönlein purpura is considered here not because of the biopsy or clinical findings but due to the presence of IgA in biopsies of kidney and skin. There is usually associated skin purpura with GI bleeding and joint pain not seen with pure IgA nephropathy (see Chapter 19.) In children the course tends to be benign and self-limited. Our experience in adults has been worse than that reported in the literature, with crescent formation and progression to ESRD being common.

It must be recognized that depending on the time of biopsy in relation to the onset of the disease, the clinician can see similar focal segmental lesions early in many systemic diseases, such as the vasculitis in Wegener's granulomatosis or Goodpasture's syndrome.

Rapidly Progressive Glomerulonephritis

Rapidly progressive glomerulonephritis (RPGN) is a descriptive clinical term used to describe the rapid progression over days or months to end-stage renal disease. *Crescentic GN* is the descriptive term used when a biopsy is obtained showing extensive marked proliferation of cells in Bowman's space of the glomerulus. A simple classification of crescentic GN shows two main groups with varying prognoses.

1. Primary or idiopathic crescentic GN. Immunoglobin deposits are demonstrated by fluorescent staining and can be either linear or granular.

2. Secondary crescentic GN

A. Infections. A variety of infectious processes have been related to crescentic GN, the more common being post-streptococcal processes, bacterial endocarditis, and hepatitis B virus. Post-streptococcal processes appear to carry the best prognosis, with up to 50 percent of cases getting some return of function.

B. Systemic diseases. While a large number of diseases have been implicated in sporadic case reports, some significant associations seem definite.

a. Goodpasture's syndrome—linear immunoglobulin deposition in the glomeruli with pulmonary hemorrhage

b. Systemic lupus erythematosus—less common

c. Henoch-Schönlein purpura—infrequent

d. Wegener's granulomatosis

For all types of crescentic GN, prognosis is improved if crescents involve less than 60 percent of the glomeruli, if urine output remains good (greater than 350 ml/24 hours) and if post-streptococcal infection is the etiology. Treatment of such a mixed group of diseases is not uniform and depends on the underlying cause. Plasmapheresis is considered the treatment of choice for Goodpasture's syndrome (based on early uncontrolled data). It appears reasonable to try plasmapheresis in systemic lupus erythematosus that is unresponsive to steroid therapy. Evidence for its use in other renal diseases is at present unproven.

Other Diseases That Can Present as the Nephrotic Syndrome

Systemic Lupus Erythematosus

Systemic lupus erythematosus (SLE) is a disease of unknown etiology with circulating immune complexes affecting most if not all organ systems. The presence of kidney disease is usually confirmed by abnormal renal function tests. If they are normal, then an abnormal urine sediment, a decrease in the serum complement level (C3), and/or a rise in the anti-native DNA level will confirm renal involvement. If all of the above tests are negative, in our experience renal biopsy will still probably display some involvement if other chemical tests for lupus are truly positive. Urinalysis generally shows red blood cells and protein varying from slightly abnormal to 25 g/24 hours. The World Health Organization report presented nine different subtypes; however, these can be condensed into three major

types, based on renal biopsy. These have features in common with the idiopathic glomerular abnormalities described above.

1. Mesangial and focal GN. There is little evidence that such abnormalities progress; however, a certain percentage (10 to 15 percent) will transform to a more serious lesion. At present, treatment is not recommended for this lesion, except if any extrarenal manifestations are present.

2. Membranous GN. Membranous GN is a lesion that is slowly progressive over years in some patients. Again, in controlled studies treatment appears to be unnecessary; however, many physicians use intermittent steroids for a 3-month period, as in idiopathic membranous GN described above.

3. Diffuse proliferative GN. This is a progressive lesion in SLE, and it requires treatment. Most authors now believe intermittent or daily steroids are the treatment of choice. Cytotoxic drugs have been studied but were shown to provide no added benefit and were associated with serious side effects. Only 50 percent of the patients treated with steroids will lose renal function within 5 years.

Patients with chemical evidence of SLE and urinary abnormalities generally require a kidney biopsy if renal function is impaired. Treatment is limited to those patients exhibiting extrarenal manifestations or a diffuse proliferative lesion on biopsy. The treatment of choice is steroids (prednisone) in a range of 60 to 100 mg per day. We add Azothiaprine after a few months and taper the steroids to avoid side effects, but this is not a widely established regimen. Plasmapheresis is utilized by many when deterioration occurs abruptly or when the disease process accelerates.

Goodpasture's Syndrome

Goodpasture's syndrome usually presents as mild to moderate renal disease accompanied by pulmonary hemorrhage. Lung bleeding may be slow and chronic, or can be of sudden onset and fatal in rare cases. While the pulmonary disease usually follows renal function abnormalities, it can be the presenting symptom and may even precede the presence of renal disease. Once established, the renal disease in most cases follows a relentless, rapidly progressive course.

Goodpasture's syndrome affects mostly males in early adulthood. Up to 50 percent report a previous respiratory infection, but the significance of such a common ailment is not clear. On biopsy, crescentic glomerulonephritis is found with linear fluorescent staining of IgG and complement.

The clinical course of such patients is generally to ESRD in a matter of weeks or months. No specific treatment produces uniform results. Transient and even permanent recoveries, which have been reported, usually are associated with large doses of steroids and cytoxic agents. However, there are many more failures than successes with similar treatment regimes. Nephrectomy is no longer considered acceptable therapy for the prevention of severe lung hemorrhage. At present, plasmapheresis along with high-dose steroids and immunosuppressive agents is the treatment of choice. Long-term controlled trials are not available to evaluate this approach.

Diabetes Mellitus

Type 1 diabetes is a slowly progressive disease that leads to renal failure in up to 50 percent of cases. (see Chapter 13). In the 1980s, over 25 percent of all patients entering ESRD have diabetes mellitus. Proteinuria generally does not appear until the disease has been present for at least 10 years. Once it occurs, it usually progresses, and by 15 years the nephrotic syndrome will develop followed by progressive renal failure. Conservative management with diuretics as well as fluid and salt restriction is the only recommended treatment until dialysis is required. The recent view that keeping the blood sugar under rigid control prevents or retards the microvascular complications of diabetes, may well be correct, but it has not been tested over time with controlled studies. These patients with end-stage renal disease accept transplanted kidneys as well as nondiabetics; however, patient survival is decreased markedly because of the continued progression of the other side effects of diabetes.

Type 2 diabetes, which occurs in older patients, has a much lower incidence of renal disease. In this form the major lesion appears to be associated with atheromatous disease.

Amyloidosis

Amyloidosis is a common cause of the nephrotic syndrome, particularly in older patients (older than 50 years). Most frequently it is associated with multiple myeloma, and the physician should be alerted by the triad of anemia, back pain, and proteinuria. Secondary amyloid associated with chronic, usually debilitating infections is a more obvious cause of amyloid.

The kidneys are usually large and may have a tendency to bleed more on biopsy. The diagnosis is confirmed by the classic fibrillar structure in the mesangium and basement membrane on electron microscopy sections.

Treatment, once amyloid is present in the kidney, is really limited to preventing volume depletion and renal shutdown due to cast formation. This is particularly important in multiple myeloma. Patients do not respond well to chronic dialysis, but instead usually die with infectious complications. Transplantation has been tried in a small number of patients with only limited success.

Renal Vein Thrombosis

The literature suggests that renal vein thrombosis may be present in up to one third of cases of idiopathic nephrotic syndrome. Many centers, including ours, have not been able to support this contention, and the reason for such a major descrepancy is not known. Clinically, patients present in two ways: sudden onset of renal impairment and often pain due to renal infarction, or slow onset where venous occlusion is partial (as is most frequently our experience), with hematuria and proteinuria as the major signs. The most common associated findings or causes include the following:

1. Obstruction due to extrinsic or intrinsic tumor
2. Nephrotic syndrome, particularly membranous glomerulonephritis
3. "Hypercoagulability state," Tumors and oral contraceptives may be in this category, but the condition is hard to verify by measurement.
4. Other causes. These include a long list of possible associated causes. The major one may be decreased blood flow, as occurs with severe dehydration.

Treatment is directed toward any known cause, for example, stopping oral contraceptive pills. Surgery is not indicated, but anticoagulants appear to stop progression. Whether anticoagulants can reverse the condition once renal function has already been lost, is not clear.

GENITOURINARY TRACT INFECTIONS

Robert Heptinstall realized the difficulty with kidney infection probably better than anyone when he said, "It is the failure to recognize that the kidney has a limited number of ways in which to respond to a large number of stimuli that has caused so much confusion over the diagnosis of chronic pyelonephritis." It must be acknowledged that many things other than infection may produce an interstitial inflammatory lesion in the kidney. The following definitions are helpful in clarifying our view of genitourinary tract infections.

DEFINITIONS

Urinary Tract Infection UTI: a symptom complex (dysuria, fever, flank or abdominal pain) associated with bacilluria and pyuria. This term deliberately attempts no localization between the upper and lower urinary tracts.

"Urethral Syndrome": a term usually applied when the symptoms compatible with pyelonephritis or cystitis are associated with a negative urine culture. It is believed by many authors to be a localized chronic infection of the urethral glands.

Pyelonephritis: Inflammation of the kidney parenchyma initiated by bacteria. Clinically it is portrayed by a variety of symptoms (none of which are in themselves essential for the diagnosis) associated with bacteria and/or white blood cells in the urine.

Cystitis: Generally refers to infection of the lower urinary tract. The symptoms are usually thought of as less severe and more localized than acute pyelonephritis. Studies show considerable overlap in clinical diagnosis.

Urine Collection: Males: A "clean-catch mid-stream" urine is a satisfactory method, provided that proper cleansing has been performed before collection. Females: "Clean-catch mid-stream" urines are always suspect if they are positive. If there is a real question regarding the presence of infection and treatment is to be based on the result, a careful "in and out" catheterization should be done.

Pyuria: more than 5 white blood cells per high power field on a centrifuged urine.

Bacilluria: the presence of greater than 100,000 ($>10^5$) bacteria/ml in the urine is said to denote infection. However, 10,000 to 100,000 (greater than 10^4) may indicate a significant infection, particularly in males.

Intrarenal Reflux: the refluxing of urine into the renal parenchyma from below on voiding. This phenomenon is demonstrated by placing dye in the bladder by a catheter and recording the subsequent voiding by taking roentgenograms of the kidneys.

THE GENITOURINARY TRACT

It should be recognized that the genitourinary tract is normally sterile and very resistant to infection. A review of the anatomy and its protective mechanisms is listed below.

Lower Urinary Tract

The Urethra

The proximal urethra is normally sterile and is claimed to have antimicrobial characteristics. The distal urethra normally contains organisms. This distal site is the major source of urinary tract contamination during instrumentation such as catheterization or cystoscopy.

The causes of bacilluria at the urethral level include the following:

1. Instrumentation—good correlation particularly in males.

2. Sexual—between ages 15 to 40 years, bacilluria is 8 times more common in females. The very short female urethra is said to offer less protection, particularly in relation to trauma such as during sexual intercourse. Prostatic fluid is believed by some workers to have an antimicrobial action in the male, although evidence for this view is weak. Perineal hygiene is an important factor; wiping after defecation should always be from front to back, especially in females.

The Bladder

The bladder is normally sterile, and if organisms are introduced experimentally into a normal bladder they will be eradicated in 3 or 4 days. This antimicrobial action depends on at least three mechanisms:

1. Bacteriostatic effect of normal urine. While urine will support bacterial growth both in vivo and in vitro, certain conditions may be present that inhibit growth. These include an osmolality greater than 600 milliosmols, and a pH less than 6.0. These conditions are found more commonly in male urine, and this probably explains the "magical powers" some authors have attributed to men's urine. One can readily see that if bacilluria and/or previous infection affect the kidney's concentrating ability, it could promote bacterial survival. This would be potentiated if the bacteria are urea splitters and raise the pH above 6.0.

2. Voiding with complete emptying. This probably only dilutes the number of organisms present. Normally a thin layer of urine containing organisms would be left on the bladder wall. However, if the residue is small, any organism remaining would be in contact with the mucosa, thus allowing mucosal factors to exert their effect.

3. Mucosal factor. A mucosal factor may exist that promotes neutrophil migration and subsequent phagocytosis of organisms. This appears to be abol-

ished by outflow obstruction and/or increased bladder pressure.

Therefore, normally most of the lower urinary tract is sterile and has mechanisms to eradicate or at least decrease bacterial multiplication. However, even if all the above mechanisms fail, a normal person can have a continuously infected bladder urine without developing upper-tract infection. The most important protection of the kidneys is at the uretero-vesical junction. During normal voiding, the bladder essentially contracts around the ureters and prevents urine from refluxing up to the kidney.

The known causes of bladder infection include the following:

1. Residual urine not only leaves more organisms to multiply, but bacteria that do remain will have less direct contact with the bladder mucosa surface.

2. Increased pressure in the bladder
   A. At high levels this may cause ureteral reflux.
   B. It may inhibit normal mucosal antimicrobial mechanisms.
   C. It chronically causes hypertrophy and changes the bladder wall surface.

3. Inadequate voiding probably causes a combination of 1 and 2 above.

4. Foreign body such as bladder stones

5. Previous inflammatory disease may reduce the mucosal defence mechanisms, and can allow reflux to develop.

The Upper Urinary Tract

Bacteria can move from the bladder or elsewhere to the kidney by three possible routes:

1. Lymphatic spread. At present, there is little evidence to support this as a major route from the bladder to the kidney.

2. Hematogenous spread. In clinical experience this probably is only significant for group A streptococci and coagulase-positive staphylococci. The hematogenous route may be more significant in patients with already damaged kidneys from any cause.

3. Ascending infection. This is the major route of kidney infection. The theory is that organisms from our own GI tract infect the urine and can then ascend to the kidney. This form of contamination is most common in females because of the closer anatomical relationship of the anus and urethra. As has been described above, various defense mechanisms in normal individuals prevent this. The major deterrent to the ascending route of infection is a competent vesicoureteral orifice. If this mechanism is intact, there is probably a negligible incidence of ascending infection. It must be remembered that cystitis itself can cause mild reflux and thus allow bacteria to reach the kidney. A few organisms may get up to the kidney even in a competent system; however, the kidney has significant defense mechanisms as well, and such a small inoculation of bacteria from time to time probably causes little problem in most people.

The kidney and urinary tract have many defense mechanisms, and except for anatomical abnormalities or obstructions, pyelonephritis should not occur. This is true in adults, but it must be realized that the major damage to the kidney by bacteria and/or reflux probably occurs before the age of 5 years.

Acute Pyelonephritis

Clinical and Laboratory Findings

Acute pyelonephritis is characterized by the sudden onset of chills and fever accompanied by flank or abdominal pain, usually associated with severe dysuria and frequency. Tenderness may be present on the affected side on deep abdominal palpation, or on percussion of the costovertebral angles.

The urine may be cloudy or even have mild to gross hematuria. On microscopic examination an uncentrifuged drop should show many bacteria. A centrifuged sample should have greater than 5 WBC per HPF. Peripheral blood leukocytosis with a left shift may be present. Urine concentrating ability is decreased. However, except in pregnancy, there is little if any decrease in GFR that cannot be accounted for on the basis of body fluid volumes.

Unfortunately, careful studies with urine cultures have shown that many times the above symptom complex cannot be linked to bacteria in the urine. In such patients the terms *cystitis* (infection of the bladder only) or *urethral syndrome* have become popular; many cases are due to localized chlamydia infections. Because of the difficulties in defining these terms clinically, we will hereafter use the term *urinary tract infection* (UTI) to refer to this symptom complex. If there is one finding or test that confirms a UTI it is bacterial growth in a fresh urine specimen. It is now well established that in a non-centrifuged urine sample, 1 or more bacteria per high power field on microscopy corresponds to a urine culture of greater than 100,000 bacteria/ml, with 95 percent reliability.

It should be recognized, however, that bacteria in the urine may occur without symptoms and probably in most cases without progression to ESRD.

Treatment

Appropriate antibiotics should be administered for 10 days. Since *E. coli* is the most common offending organism, ampicillin or a sulfa drug are generally effective (see Chapter 7). The urinalysis should be repeated one week after stopping drugs to make sure bacteria have been eradicated. Even without treatment, uncomplicated acute pyelonephritis is a self-limited disease. In the absence of obstruction it does not progress to chronic pyelonephritis.

Asymptomatic Bacilluria

Figure 11.7 shows the incidence of asymptomatic bacilluria at various ages in men and women. The finding of bacteria in male urine is unusual and requires investigation; usually a cause is found. The most common finding is previous kidney damage or past urinary tract instrumentation. In females in the child bearing years, somewhere between 4 and 7 percent are found to have asymptomatic bacilluria. Another 1 to 2 percent develop it during pregnancy. Most women with asymptomatic bacilluria have had one or more previous UTIs going back to childhood. As a group, they have slightly higher blood pressure

and somewhat less urine concentrating ability. They tend to have more abnormal pyelograms, compared with nonbacilluric control populations. Fifteen years of careful follow-up of such women by Kass has not shown any progression to renal failure. During pregnancy, one third of asymptomatic bacillurics will develop a UTI, usually in the second or third trimesters or at term. The major complication of asymptomatic bacilluria is in a small subgroup of patients that get recurrent infections and develop septicemia.

Treatment

During pregnancy, short-term antibiotic therapy will eradicate 90 percent of asymptomatic bacilluria and will reduce the incidence of clinically apparent UTI from greater than 25 percent to less than 2 percent. Patients with recurrent infections should be worked up to discover and correct any anatomical abnormalities. If no abnormalities are found, and recurrent UTI and/or septicemia continue, chronic suppressive antimicrobial therapy should be initiated. At present trimethoprim-sulfa is the agent of choice.

Chronic Pyelonephritis

Chronic pyelonephritis is an uncommon entity that has frequently been diagnosed incorrectly. Chronic pyelonephritis must be thought of as two separate and distinct types: (1) obstructive, and (2) nonobstructive. The diagnosis of either of these two enties is now made by radiographic procedures, since it has been shown repeatedly that the presence of organisms in the urine does not correlate well with chronic pyelonephritis.

I. *Chronic obstructive pyelonephritis* will show a dilated pelvis and calyceal system that generally affects the whole kidney equally. Usually a cause and/or location of the obstruction can be demonstrated in the renal pelvis, ureters, or lower urinary tract, and then can be surgically repaired. If undertaken early, this course will produce a good response. This form of chronic pyelonephritis progresses to end-stage renal disease if it is bilateral and remains untreated. Therefore, the obstructive form of chronic pyelonephritis is treatable if found early enough before pressure damage and/or infection cause tissue destruction or atrophy.

2. *Chronic nonobstructive pyelonephritis* will show no obstruction radiographically but a scar is usually present in the upper and/or lower polar regions, in

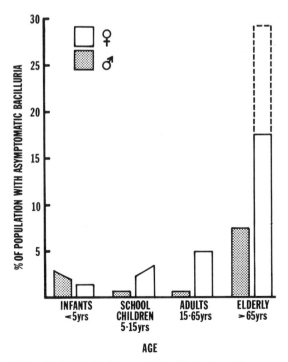

Fig. 11.7 The incidence of bacilluria in various age groups, by sex. The sloping bars indicate an approximate range.

one or both kidneys. The lesion does not appear to be progressive, at least in the older adult population. Just as acute pyelonephritis in the absence of obstruction does not progress to chronic pyelonephritis, so chronic pyelonephritis in the absence of obstruction does not progress to ESRD. There may or may not be infected urine. Hypertension appears to be increased in this population and the increased blood pressure in adults is probably the major concern.

Pyelonephritis should be considered merely as one type of interstitial nephritis, as outlined in Table 11.10.

Interstitial Nephritis

At present the most common cause of interstitial nephritis is analgesic abuse. It may account for as much as 5 percent of ESRD patients. Such patients tend to be middle-aged females with a dependent personality. Generally they have consumed greater than one kg of phenacetin over a period of years, often for headache or backache. Strangely, such patients usually deny use of these agents. They frequently present with anemia, hypertension, and peptic ulcer disease. If the physician can get them to stop taking the drugs, their renal disease will moderate and the

Table 11.10 Interstitial Nephritis

1. Pyelonephritis
   A. Bacilluria
   B. Reflux
      a. Vesicoureteral
      b. Intrarenal
   C. Obstruction
      a. With infection
      b. Without infection
   D. Immunologic
      a. Antigen-antibody complexes
      b. Anti-tubular basement membrane antibodies
2. Drugs
   A. Acute—for example, methicillin
   B. Chronic—for example, analgesics [a]
3. Toxins
   A. Heavy metals
   B. Balkan nephritis
4. Hereditary
   A. Alport's disease
   B. Medullary cystic disease
   C. Sickle cell disease
5. Metabolic
   A. Gout
   B. Nephrocalcinosis
   C. Hypokalemia
6. Iatrogenic
   A. Irradiation
   B. Transplant rejections

[a] This probably represents the most important subgroup, and should be checked for in every history.

hypertension will go away. However, keeping such patients away from the apparent "high" they get from these drugs is difficult, especially if other stress is present. As renal disease progresses, one often finds papillary necrosis either as an acute obstruction or chronically by the "ring sign" on intravenous pyelograms. There is no treatment other than stopping drug intake. Often because of the denial pattern, the diagnosis is confirmed by measurement of salicylate levels. Recent studies suggest that phenacetin or phenacetin and salicylates are necessary to develop the lesion. Acetaminophen, the breakdown product of phenacetin, does not appear to cause the same renal pathology when taken alone.

Primary Atrophic Pyelonephritis

The etiology of this form of pyelonephritis is probably due to intrarenal reflux of urine into the polar regions of one or both kidneys. It is still not clear if the damage occurs because of pressure reflux alone or if infected urine is essential. Depending on the severity of the reflux and the scarring produced, the physician may see four groups evolve:

1. Children who develop renal failure before age 10 years
2. Children who develop renal failure with the "growth spurt"
3. A group that survive the growth spurt but in their early 20s develop problems with hypertension or recurrent infection, usually associated with pregnancy
4. A group with polar scarring but normal or slightly impaired renal function.

In each of the last three groups there may be no evidence of reflux at the time of diagnosis. This does not mean that reflux was not present at an earlier time. Studies of young children who reflux show that 50 percent have recovered by age 6 years, and 70 percent by age 14 years. This is most likely due to maturation of the ureterovesical junctions (see below). Unfortunately the scarring often occurs early, before this maturation takes place. Treatment of chronic atrophic pyelonephritis is almost totally dependent on making the diagnosis before 5 years of age. Once it has been determined that severe reflux is present causing intrarenal damage, reimplantation of the ureters is indicated to stop the refluxing. Such treatment, if renal function is normal, may halt progression. In less severe reflux without scarring, close observation and eradication of infection may be sufficient until refluxing stops due to maturation of the system.

INVESTIGATION, THERAPY, AND LONG-TERM MANAGEMENT OF UTI

If complete investigation was carried out on all patients who have a UTI then the cost of medical care would rise significantly, since it is a common problem. Therefore, patient selection for investigation is important. The indications for performing a work-up of patients with UTI include the following:

1. Recurrent attacks in females
2. All children. Infants: Often the very young do not present with a fever or the usual signs of a UTI. All infants with "failure to thrive" or unexplained vomiting and/or diarrhea should have their urine cultured.
3. Males, after the 1st attack
4. Pregnancy, if pyelonephritis develops before or at term. (Forty percent of pregnant women with UTI will have an attack of acute pyelonephritis if the bacilluria is not eradicated.) Work-up is also indicated if treatment does not irradicate bacilluria even if no UTI results.
5. Fever associated with UTI. In older children and adults with UTI, fever greater than 101°F (38.5°C) has been shown to correlate with intrarenal reflux in several studies.

An Approach to Investigation of UTI or Bacilluria

1. Treat acute UTI when the patient presents with an infection.
2. Consider additional investigations when indicated (see list above).

A. Intravenous pyelography (IVP)—for kidney size and shape, for appearance of ureters, and for signs of obstruction and/or stones. Cystitis can cause transient ureteral reflux and it takes 6 weeks for dilated ureters to normalize following pregnancy.

B. Voiding cystoureterogram—if ureters are not well visualized, if there is any question regarding reflux, and in all children.

C. Retrograde pyelography can be performed during cystoscopy but should be reserved for specific problems, such as stones, nonvisualizing kidney, or unexplained abnormality in ureters on IVP. Sonography is replacing the retrograde study as the first-line approach for investigation of obstruction. It may not be quite as accurate, but it is much less invasive.

D. Aortography is reserved for nonvisualizing kidneys or when looking for a specific renal abnormality such as a tumor. Computerized axial tomography (CT scan) is less invasive, and many centers are using it and avoiding aortography except when absolutely necessary.

3. Perform a clearance study to determine baseline renal function.

4. Repeat cultures off antibiotic therapy and with any exacerbation of symptoms.

Principles of Treatment

1. Acute infections: Ampicillin or gantrisin are drugs of choice to eradicate organisms. In females, first UTI are not cultured because of the high incidence of *E. coli* infection.

2. Recurrent infections: The appropriate therapeutic agent is determined from culture and sensitivity data.

3. If investigation shows no correctable lesion and recurrent infections are either debilitating or, more importantly, producing septicemia, then suppressive agents should be considered. However, before initiating suppression, attempts to localize the infection by bladder washout and ureteric cultures should be undertaken, and a prolonged course (4 to 6 weeks) of appropriate antibiotics should be initiated. If this fails to eradicate the organism or prevent recurrence, then suppression therapy should be utilized. The choice of a selective agent probably does not matter, because these patients will have breakthrough infections on any agents. At present trimethoprim-sulfa in low doses seems to be the antimicrobial of choice, and the incidence of breakthrough infection is low.

4. Reflux: Mild reflux can probably be observed and not treated surgically, since 50 percent of children studied stopped refluxing by age 6 years and 70 percent by age 14 years. However, certain children are at risk even though observation is continued. Children with any of the following conditions will probably not resolve with age and will require surgical repair.

A. Severely dilated ureters
B. Shortened mucosal tunnel
C. Laterally placed ureteral orifices on cystoscopy
D. Any patients with intrarenal reflux
E. Recurrent infections in the presence of reflux

Surgical reimplantation of the ureters is 85 percent successful in stopping reflux in selected children. However, renal scarring may develop or progress, and renal failure may develop despite a successful repair.

In summary, pyelonephritis should be thought of as three entities:

1. Acute Pyelonephritis: Acute pyelonephritis is a hard-to-diagnose constellation of symptoms and findings that may be more correctly called urinary tract infection (UTI). In the absence of obstruction this is a self limited disease.

2. Chronic pyelonephritis: Without obstruction over the age of 20 years, this form of interstitial nephritis remains either stable or is very slowly progressive. If obstruction is present, it must be corrected or infection and progression to end-stage renal disease will result.

3. Primary atrophic pyelonephritis: This must be diagnosed early (probably before age 5 years). If intrarenal reflux is present, the treatment is surgery. Medical treatment alone in intrarenal reflux is not sufficient in patients younger than 5 years of age.

CONGENITAL KIDNEY DISEASE

The major causes of congenital or inherited renal disease are listed here.

POLYCYSTIC KIDNEY DISEASE

Clinical Manifestations

Adult-type polycystic kidney disease (PCKD) is transmitted as an autosomal dominant trait; however, this mutation occurs frequently, and about 5 to 10 percent of cases in our experience may have no reliable family history. The juvenile form is rare, and probably is recessively inherited. The diagnosis is usually made in the third or fourth decade of life because of the following occurrences:

1. Other older family members are diagnosed.
2. Signs and symptoms develop, for example, pain, bacilluria, or hematuria.
3. An abdominal mass is found.
4. Systemic hypertension is diagnosed.

Renal failure develops at different times in different families; however, within a given family, the age at which renal failure occurs tends to be similar. The progression of renal failure generally is slow, with rapid loss of function occurring only when obstruction and/or infections occur. Patients with PCKD tolerate volume restriction poorly and often appear to be "salt loosers." Stones occur in 15 to 20 percent of patients with PCKD.

Extrarenal manifestations may play an important role in this disease. Fifteen percent of patients with polycystic kidney disease have basilar artery berry aneurysms, but cerebral angiograms and surgery are reserved for those with an episode of bleeding. However, these aneurysms represent an important reason to control blood pressure. Cysts may also involve the liver and pancreas, but only rarely do they compromise liver function. Polycythemia occasionally develops due to increased erythropoietin production.

Treatment

1. Control blood pressure.
2. When infection occurs, antibiotics should be used early, and in most cases the infection will be controlled. When obstruction is present, on rare occasions it is necessary to operate and drain an infected cyst or perinephric abscess. Many of the cysts contain bacteria in an almost symbiotic relationship, without causing a significant inflammatory reaction.
3. Recurrent hematuria usually responds to decreased exertion and, in some cases, to bed rest for a few days.
4. Dialysis for end-stage disease usually works well, since these patients tend to have higher hemoglobin values (probably due to high erythropoietin levels from the remaining compressed renal mass) and continued urine output.
5. Following transplantation, the polycystic kidneys may be removed, but now more commonly such patients are observed and the kidneys appear to shrink and do not cause further problems.

MEDULLARY CYSTIC DISEASE

Clinical Manifestations

There are probably two major types of medullary cystic disease:

1. An autosomal dominant form, with renal disease developing between 20 and 30 years of age with very rapid progression to ESRD
2. An autosomal recessive form, with the disease occurring in the teen years and with slower progression

Multiple cysts develop in both kidneys, but the kidneys shrink as renal disease progresses. There are dual hallmarks of this form of disease:

1. Severe salt wasting
2. Anemia out of proportion to the degree of renal failure

Treatment

1. Prevention of volume depletion with adequate salt intake
2. Transfusion only when absolutely necessary (HCT below 15 percent or symptoms of severe anemia)
3. Dialysis and transplantation

MEDULLARY SPONGE KIDNEY

This condition is not hereditary and does not progress to ESRD in the absence of other complications. The diagnosis is usually made by chance with an IVP, in which contrast media fills dilated collecting ducts entering the calyces. Infection may be more common, but unless obstruction occurs, renal function remains normal throughout life.

ALPORT'S SYNDROME

The renal findings in Alport's syndrome include hematuria, proteinuria (usually nonnephrotic), and late mild hypertension. Males tend to develop renal failure between the third and fifth decade of life, whereas females often do not reach end stage. Inheritance is not clear, but an X-linked transmission seems most likely. Neurosensory deafness with initial high tone loss is common (35 to 50 percent), particularly in males, and a lesser number will have eye changes. On biopsy, tubular basement membrane splitting is apparent on electron microscopy; characteristic "foam cells" are helpful, but commonly are not seen. No treatment is known to arrest progression; however, such patients do well with a kidney transplant and the lesion does not recur.

THE FANCONI SYNDROME

The Fanconi syndrome is postulated to be due to a defect in proximal tubular reabsorption marked by amino-aciduria, phosphaturia and glycosuria. An increased urine loss of other substances normally reabsorbed mainly in the proximal tubule sometimes accompanies the syndrome, for example, uric acid. Simplistically, these substances are not reabsorbed in the proximal tubule and since the distal tubule has no recovery mechanism, these substances are lost in the urine.

The Fanconi syndrome can be either a congenital problem perhaps on an autosomal dominant basis or, more commonly, an acquired disorder. Causes of the acquired type are varied, such as multiple myeloma and heavy metal toxicity, and may be permanent or transient, depending on the agent.

Treatment involves removal of the offending agent, in the acquired form if possible, and dietary support.

DIABETES INSIPIDUS

Diabetes insipidus is a tubular defect in concentrating ability due to absence of endogenous vasopressin or to the inability of the renal tubule to respond to vasopressin.

1. "Central" diabetes insipidus is due to a failure of the pituitary gland to secrete vasopressin.
2. "Nephrogenic" diabetes insipidus is a failure of the renal tubule to respond to vasopressin. This form can be either inherited (X-linked recessive trait) or, more commonly, acquired. The acquired form can be permanent when associated with systemic diseases, such as amyloid. Fortunately, it is most often transient in association with renal toxins or drug therapy. For detailed discussion regarding diagnosis and treatment see Chapter 13.

TUMORS OF THE URINARY TRACT

Tumors of the urinary tract are common, particularly in the male.

CARCINOMA OF THE PROSTATE

Carcinoma of the prostate in men is common over the age of 60 years. More than 20 percent of males at autopsy have histological evidence of carcinomatous changes. Urinary tract obstruction may be the first symptom of this cancer. About half of the cases are diagnosed by identifying firm nodules on rectal examination, while half are incidentally diagnosed at the time of prostate resection for obstruction that has been clinically diagnosed as benign hypertrophy of the prostate. The tumor commonly metastasizes to regional lymph nodes, bone, and distant organs. Consequently, bone pain is a common presenting symptom. At this stage the serum acid phosphatase is elevated in about two thirds of patients, and metastatic spread may be identified by lymphangiograms or bone scans.

Treatment consists of surgical resection of the prostate, and this, with or without radiation therapy, is the only opportunity for cure. The tumor has a highly variable course and may be rapidly progressive and fatal, or indolent and slow growing over many years. Relief of pain can commonly be achieved by hormonal manipulation. The tumor is dependent on androgens, and consequently estrogen therapy and castration are sometimes helpful to relieve pain.

TUMORS OF URETHRA, BLADDER, URETERS, AND RENAL PELVIS

The most common tumor of the urinary tract is transitional cell carcinoma of the bladder. Bleeding causing hematuria and obstruction are the common presenting findings. Carcinoma of the bladder has been linked to numerous occupational carcinogens. Aniline dye precursors are the best documented. The only useful treatment is surgery, and complications resulting from local spread are most prominent.

RENAL TUMORS

In childhood the most frequent renal tumor is the Wilms' tumor. Generally this presents as a mass, and metastases are common at the time of diagnosis. Surgical resection and radiation may be curative, and chemotherapy now results in an improved prognosis.

Adenocarcinoma of the kidney (hypernephroma) is a common renal tumor that may be unilateral or bilateral. Hematuria is usually the earliest sign, but fever, a palpable mass, flank pain, or symptoms of distant metastases are common. Lung, liver, bone, and brain are frequently sites of metastatic involvement.

Nonmetastatic manifestations including fever, polycythemia, and hypercalcemia are particularly common systemic manifestations of this tumor.

Surgery is the only method of cure. Radiation therapy, chemotherapy, and immunotherapy remain under active investigation.

OBSTRUCTIVE DISEASES OF THE GENITOURINARY SYSTEM

Table 11.11 lists the major causes of obstruction to urine flow for each anatomic region. The causes of obstruction depend on the age group. Obstruction that is unrelieved may result in recurrent infection, structural changes such as dilatation or hypertrophy, or, eventually, reduced renal function.

Table 11.11   **Causes of Obstructive Uropathy**

Level of Obstruction	Common Causes
Urethral	Inflammatory strictures
	Prostatic Hypertrophy
Bladder	Carcinoma of the bladder
	Bleeding into urinary tract with clot obstruction
Ureteral	Ureteropelvic junction strictures or vessel bands
	Ureteral calculi
	Retroperitoneal fibrosis
Renal	Renal papillary necrosis
	Renal pelvis calculi, clot
	Renal tubular obstruction in dysproteinemia, hyperuricemia

In children, urethral obstruction may result from congenital anomalies or from stricture formation following manipulation of the urethra with foreign bodies. In adults urethral strictures more commonly result from venereal disease. The aging male develops high urethral or bladder neck obstruction due to benign prostatic hypertrophy or carcinoma of the prostate. All of these will result in a slowed urinary stream, commonly with dripping on cessation of voiding, and when obstruction is severe there may be a distended bladder with "overflow voiding." These patients are particularly prone to urinary tract infections, as outlined above. While acute obstruction may result in a large distended bladder, chronic obstruction causes hypertrophy and trabeculation of the bladder wall.

Obstruction within the bladder may result from carcinoma of the bladder, bladder calculi, or blood clots. The clots generally result from surgery involving the genitourinary tract, or from trauma.

Ureteral obstruction is most commonly unilateral. It may result from strictures or fibrous bands at the ureteropelvic junction or ureteral calculi. Rarely, severe interstitial nephritis results in necrosis of the renal papillae (renal papillary necrosis) and obstruction of the ureter with sloughed renal tissue. The rare condition of retroperitoneal fibrosis and, occasionally, tumors involving the retroperitoneal lymph nodes may result in extrinsic uretral obstruction. Such obstruction may cause pain that radiates to the groin and recurrent infection, and when prolonged may result in dilatation of the proximal urinary tract. Such dilation may involve the ureters, renal pelvis, and calyces, with eventual compression and destruction of renal tissue and hydronephrosis.

Occasionally obstruction will arise within the renal pelvis due to large calculi or blood clots.

Obstruction of the tubules within the kidney may develop in patients with dysproteinemia and hyperuricemia.

RENAL CALCULI

Renal calculi are concretions that include crystals and a matrix of organic material. The etiologic factors of the various types of calculi are not well established. Calculi are more common in patients with hypercalcemia due to any cause, hyperoxaluria, hyperuricemia, and several renal tubular defects. Normal urine contains all of the constituents for stones, but most individuals do not develop urinary calculi except when some factor results in increased tendency to crystal formation. Infection, increased alkalinity of the urine, and increased concentrations of crystalloids all play a role.

Patients with renal calculi may be asymptomatic, may present with infection, or with the severe pain of ureteral colic. Pain in the flank suggests an upper ureteral location, if the pain radiates to the scrotum the obstruction may be in the lower ureter. When the stone lodges at the uretero-vesical junction, symptoms often mimic cystitis or prostatitis, presenting as frequency or dysuria with urgency. Patients with small stones due to uric acid lithiasis frequently pass sand-like material in the urine.

The laboratory findings may be helpful. Urate crystals are common in patients with uric acid calculi, and the octahedral crystals of calcium oxalate may be present in patients with oxalate stones. Microscopic hematuria is frequent, and an alkaline pH may indicate urinary tract infection. Radioopaque stones generally indicate a high calcium content. These may be recognized on a plain film of the abdomen or on renal tomography. More often the stone is identified at the time of intravenous pyelography. Patients presenting with renal calculi should have thorough investigation for underlying metabolic disease causing hypercalcemia (see Chapter 13), evidence of obstruction of the genitourinary system, and evidence of urinary tract infection.

Therapy includes efforts to maintain a continuously dilute urine (3 to 4 liters fluid intake per day). Every effort should be made to relieve obstruction and irradicate infection promptly. When possible, the tendency for nephrolithiasis should be modified by diet and control of pH (Table 11.12.)

Table 11.12 **Characteristics and Treatment of Renal Calculi**

Type of Stone	Causes	Treatment
Calcium oxalate	Hypercalcuria	Thiazide diuretics
	Hyperoxaluria	Reduce hypercalcuria
	Hyperuricemia	Allopurinol
Calcium phosphate	Alkaline urine	Eradicate infection
	(Renal tubular acidosis, infection)	
Magnesium ammonium phosphate	Infection	Eradicate infection
Uric Acid	Urine hyperacidity	Reduce hyperuricemia
	Hyperuricemia	Urine alkalinization
Cystine	Cystinuria	Urine alkalinizaion

REFERENCES

1. Brenner, B.M., Rector, F.C., Jr.: The Kidney. 2nd ed. Philadelphia, W.B. Saunders Co., 1981.
2. Coe, F.L., Favus, M.J.: Treatment of renal calculi. Adv Int Med 26:373, 1981.
3. Culpepper, M., Andreoli, T.E.: The pathophysiology of the glomerulonephropathies. Adv Int Med 28:161, 1983.
4. Gutman, R.A., Stead, W.W., Robinson, R.R.: Physical activity and employment status of patients on maintenance dialysis. N Eng J Med 304:309, 1981.
5. Harrison, J.H., et al. (eds): Campbell's Urology. 4th ed. Philadelphia, W.B. Saunders Co., 1979.
6. Kim, Y., Michael, A.F.: Idiopathic membranoproliferative glomerulonephritis. Ann Rev Med 31:273, 1980.
7. Stamm, W.E., Turck, M.: Urinary tract infection. Adv Int Med 28:141, 1983.

12

The Gastrointestinal System

*Eldon A. Shaffer, M.D., Hugh J. Freeman, M.D.,
and Wilfred M. Weinstein, M.D.*

Part 1: The Hepatobiliary System and the Pancreas

LIVER STRUCTURE AND FUNCTION

STRUCTURE

The liver in an adult is the largest body organ, constituting approximately $\frac{1}{50}$ of the entire body weight (1500g). It is located beneath the ribs in the right upper quadrant of the abdomen.

Liver blood flow (1500 ml/min) comes from two sources: 25 percent from the hepatic artery, which is a branch of the coeliac axis, and 75 percent from the portal vein, a confluence of the superior mesenteric and splenic veins. The portal venous blood has a high oxygen content, averaging 80 percent saturation. These vessels enter the liver through a fissure, the porta hepatis, and divide into branches to the right and left hepatic lobes. The vascular beds of the hepatic artery and the portal vein interact hemodynamically, thus maintaining a constant total blood flow regardless of perturbations in the other system. The venous drainage from the liver is via the right and left hepatic veins which enter the inferior vena cava.

Biliary drainage is into the right and left hepatic bile ducts which join to form the common hepatic duct. The cystic duct connects the gallbladder to the common hepatic duct forming the common bile duct (choledochus) which then descends towards the duodenum. The common duct and the pancreatic ducts fuse in the duodenal wall to enter the second part of the duodenum through the ampulla of Vater. The sphincter of Oddi ensheathes the submucosal segment of the common duct. Tonic contraction causes the gallbladder to fill; relaxation permits bile to discharge into the duodenum.

A functional organization divides the liver into microcirculatory units: the hepatic acini. Hepatocytes in this unit receive their blood supply from an axis formed by a terminal hepatic arteriole and a terminal portal venule. Sinusoids radiating from this axis distribute blood throughout the cells of the acinus in a sequential manner. That is, the liver lobule may be divided into three zones: Zone 1, a portal zone located close to the supplying vessels; Zone 3, a hepatic region around the central vein far from the supplying vessels; and Zone 2, an intermediate area between the central and peripheral regions. Zones 1, 2 and 3 thus represent areas with blood containing an oxygen-nutrient content of first, second and third quality respectively. The peripheral portions of zone 3 of several adjacent acini are most vulnerable to toxic, anoxic or metabolic injury.

FUNCTION

Biliary Excretion

Bile is necessary for efficient intestinal digestion and absorption of lipids, and it provides the main excretory pathway for toxic metabolites, bilirubin, cholesterol and lipid waste products.

Bile formation begins in the canaliculus, independent of the vascular perfusion pressure. Rather it is related to energy-dependent transport processes. Bile salt secretion is the major factor causing the transfer of water and solutes from the liver cell into the canalicular lumen (Fig. 12.2). Distally in the biliary collection system, ductular secretion modifies canalicular bile by adding sodium bicarbonate and water and absorbing sodium chloride. Ductular flow is

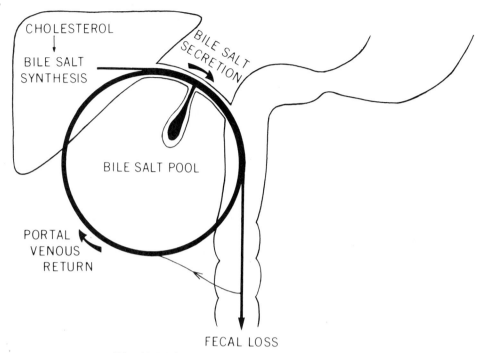

Fig. 12.1 The enterohepatic circulation of bile salts.

controlled by the hormone secretin. In man, bile flow amounts to almost 600 ml each day with over 400 ml being formed in the hepatic canaliculi and the remainder being added distally by ductular secretion. The limited storage capacity of the human gallbladder, about 33 ml, is compensated by active absorption across its mucosa. Its lining epithelium very rapidly transports electrolytes, primarily sodium and chloride, removing 90 percent of the water content. During the interdigestive period, over 50 percent of the hepatic bile enters the gallbladder to be stored. Gallbladder contraction occurs in response to food, particularly fatty acids and amino acids which release the intestinal hormone cholecystokinin. With gallbladder contraction the sphincter of Oddi relaxes reciprocally, and 75 percent of the gallbladder contents empty into the duodenum.

Bile salts, the most abundant organic solute in bile, are the driving force behind bile flow and the principal determinant of bile composition. They are synthesized in the liver from cholesterol. Degradation occurs solely in the intestine, the sole excretory route being fecal. Bile salts undergo an enterohepatic circulation (Fig. 12.1). Secreted by the liver, they are stored mainly in the gallbladder during the interdigestive period. Bile salts in the jejunum act as detergents to promote fat digestion and absorption. Later, in the terminal ileum, bile salts are actively and efficiently absorbed. Bile salts return via the portal vein to the liver, where they once more are ef-

fectively secreted into bile, completing the cycle. Bile salts recirculated from the intestine, then, are the major source of hepatic secretion; only a small portion is derived from *de novo* synthesis. Gallbladder storage and intestinal transit are the slow points in this circuit, whereas hepatic clearance and intestinal absorption are rapid and efficient. The total mass of bile salts within the enterohepatic circulation represents the bile-salt pool. The size of this pool multiplied by the rate at which it cycles gives the bile salt secretion rate. This efficient recycling system allows a small pool of bile salts to recirculate 5 to 15 times a day, while losing only 3 to 5 percent with each circuit. These small losses are accurately replaced by hepatic synthesis. Synthesis is regulated, in a negative feedback manner, by the rate at which bile salts return to the liver: low rate stimulates synthesis, a high rate inhibits it. The hepatic capacity for synthesis can only rise 5–10 fold, so that excessive losses in the feces cannot be adequately replaced. Synthesis of the primary bile acids, cholic acid and chenodeoxycholic acid, occurs exclusively in the liver, where a glycine or taurine moiety must also be added before the now conjugated bile salt is secreted into bile. Normal human bile has a molar ratio of glycine:taurine of about 3:1. Conjugated bile salts undergo bacterial degradation in the ileum and colon. Deconjugation breaks the peptide linkage yielding free bile acids, and bacterial dehydroxylation then removes hydroxyl groups from the primary bile acids forming second-

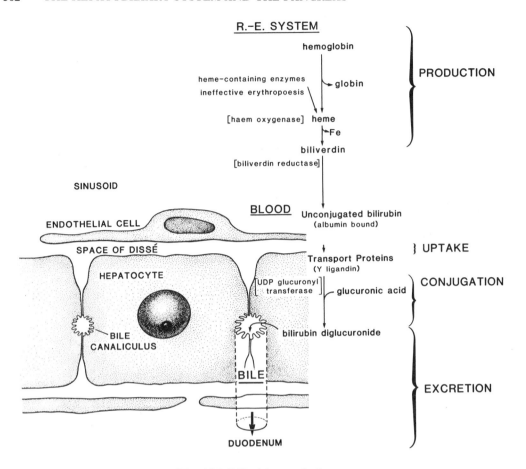

Fig. 12.2 Bilirubin metabolism, see text.

ary bile acids. Cholic acid is converted into deoxycholic acid. Chenodeoxycholic acid becomes lithocholic acid. Considerable dehydroxylation must occur, since human bile normally contains more than 25 percent of the total bile salts in the secondary form, chiefly as deoxycholic acid. Deoxycholic acid and any unconjugated (free) primary bile acids are passively absorbed from the colon, conjugated once again in the liver, and then resecreted into bile. Lithocholic acid with only one polar hydroxyl group is insoluble in water and so is trapped in the intestinal lumen and excreted in the feces.

Bile salts, as they cross the canaliculae, self-aggregate, forming small molecular packets called "simple micelles". The phospholipid lecithin can be dissolved by these bile salt aggregates creating "mixed micelles". This results in bilayer discs, resembling stout drums with a water-soluble coat and a water-insoluble core. Cholesterol can then be dissolved within the fat-loving core. In this manner the biological detergent bile salts can transport two water-insoluble lipids, lecithin and cholesterol, in bile which is 90

percent water. Because of this physical interaction, the flux of bile salts through the hepatocyte and into the bile canaliculus profoundly influences the secretion of lecithin and cholesterol. The liver is central in processing the heterogeneous sources of free cholesterol and in determining the portion of cholesterol converted into bile salts or excreted in bile.

Bilirubin, a linear tetrapyrole, is derived solely from haem catabolism (Fig. 12.2). Haem, a compound of iron and protoporphyin, is found mainly in hemoglobin and myoglobin. Small quantities are also present in cytochrome enzymes and haem compounds in the liver. The major source of bilirubin, about 80 percent, is the breakdown product of hemoglobin from senescent circulating red blood cells. Ineffective erythropoiesis within the bone marrow and spleen also contributes. In the reticuloendothelial cells of the spleen, liver, and bone marrow, haem is converted by haem oxygenase to biliverdin. Biliverdin reductase then changes biliverdin into free or unconjugated bilirubin. Unconjugated bilirubin is not water-soluble and must be carried in plasma tightly bound to albumin. As 1 mole of human albumin can bind at least 2 moles of pigment, the capacity to bind bilirubin in normal adults is never exceeded unless unconjugated bilirubin rises above 40 mg/dl (>680 mmol/L). Since albumin-bound bilirubin cannot diffuse across cell membranes, unconjugated bilirubin remains within the plasma compartment and is not excreted into urine. Unconjugated bilirubin is rapidly taken up by the liver via a carrier mechanism and then bound to a cytoplasmic acceptor protein, Y-protein or ligandin. Within the hepatocyte, bilirubin is conjugated with glucuronic acid making it more water soluble and allowing excretion into bile. The microsomal enzyme UDP glucuronyl transferase transfers glucuronic acid (UDPGA) onto one of the two proprionic acid groups forming an ester monoglucuronide which undergoes a second glucuronidation before exiting into bile as a diglucuronide. Biliary excretion is the rate-limiting factor in the transfer of bilirubin from plasma to bile. Conjugated bilirubin is not absorbed from the small intestine, but is hydrolyzed in the colon by bacterial beta-glucuronidases and then reduced to urobilinogen. Urobilinogen is well-absorbed from the ileum but not the colon. The small amount that is absorbed is re-excreted by both liver and kidney. Urobilinogen and its oxidation product, urobilin in the urine, are identical respectively with sterocobilinogen and its oxidation product, sterocobilin in the feces. Urobilinogens are colourless, whereas urobilin is pigmented.

Metabolism

Carbohydrate Metabolism

The liver plays a central role in intermediary metabolism. It maintains a stable blood glucose by taking up and storing glucose as glycogen (glycogenesis), breaking down this glycogen to glucose (glycogenolysis) when the need arises, and forming glucose from noncarbohydrate sources such as amino acids (gluconeogenesis). Since the storage capacity of the liver is limited and glucose consumption is continuous, hepatic glycogen stores are exhausted by one day of fasting. Hypoglycemia is an infrequent consequence of liver injury, usually arising only in severe, near-terminal liver disease where glycogen stores are depleted. It can also occur under other conditions: acute ethanol intoxication, where glyconeogenesis is inhibited; hepatocellular carcinoma with increased plasma insulin-like activity and increased glucose utilization; or hereditary deficiencies involving the enzymes responsible for glycogenolysis-like

glycogen storage diseases where excess glycogen accumulates in the liver. Hyperglycemia and an abnormal glucose tolerance test is common with chronic liver disease despite normal or elevated plasma insulin.

Protein Metabolism

The liver synthesizes the majority of proteins that circulate in the plasma. Serum albumin is the major protein produced in the liver, along with most of the globulins, other than gammaglobulins. Globulins include the coagulation factors: fibrinogen (factor I), prothrombin (factor II) and factors V, VII, IX, and X. Factors II, VII, IX and X are vitamin D-dependent. The prothrombin time may be prolonged with fat malabsorption as in marked biliary obstruction or cholestasis, but it should respond to parenteral vitamin K. In hepatocellular disease, deficiencies in these coagulation factors are not corrected by vitamin K. The liver is also the site for most amino acid interconversions, catabolism and degradation. Amino acids taken up from the portal vein are largely catabolized to urea by the liver. Ammonia, a product of nitrogen metabolism, is utilized and hence detoxicated in this process of urea synthesis.

Lipid Metabolism

Fatty acids taken up by the liver and esterified to triglyceride are derived from the following: *dietary triglyceride*, entering the circulation as chylomicrons and very low density lipoproteins from the thoracic duct (long chain fatty acids) or portal vein (medium chain fatty acids); *adipose tissue fat*, which is mobilized as free fatty acids during stress or starvation; and *hepatic synthesis* of fatty acids from acetate, a 2-carbon precursor. Most of the triglyceride produced in the liver combines with cholesterol, phospholipid, and an apoprotein moiety to form a lipoprotein moiety before being exported into the blood. Excess triglyceride can accumulate as fat droplets producing a fatty liver ("steatosis"). This occurs when the supply of fat exceeds the livers capacity for metabolism and lipoprotein secretion. *Increased influx* can result from an excessive load of fat, as in obesity, or enhanced mobilization of fatty acids from adipose tissue stores as occurs with stress, fasting, alcohol, drugs such as corticosteroids, or diabetic ketoacidosis. *Reduced efflux* occurs with either a block in fatty acid oxidation (e.g., from alcohol) or suppressed apoprotein synthesis for lipotrotein formation (e.g., chemicals like tetracycline), phosphorus or carbon tetrachloride.

Alcohol, the most common agent to produce steatosis, may act through several of the above mechanisms.

Most cholesterol synthesis takes place in the liver while a lesser site is the intestine. Cholesterol may also be derived from the diet, while HDL cholesterol is an important source of cholesterol in bile. In severe liver cell disease, total serum cholesterol is reduced, whereas in obstructive liver disease serum cholesterol can be elevated.

Many hormones, such as thyroxine and adrenalgonadal steroid hormones, are conjugated in the liver, partly excreted in bile, circulated enterohepatically, and eventually eliminated in the urine. The liver also synthesizes alpha globulins which bind hormones in the plasma. The fat soluble vitamins, A, D and K, along with vitamin B_{12} and folate are stored in the liver. Metabolic events include 25-hydroxylation of vitamin D.

Drug Metabolism

The liver plays a central role in drug metabolism by virtue of its rich enzyme systems and its position in the splanchnic circulation, defending the body from incoming noxious agents. Drugs and chemicals are either water soluble (hydrophilic) or lipid soluble (hydrophobic). Water-soluble or polar agents can be easily excreted unchanged in the urine or bile. Those that are lipid soluble are readily absorbed across the intestinal mucosa which functions as a lipid layer, but this lipid solubility prevents effective renal excretion. Lipid soluble materials must therefore be converted into more water-soluble compounds which can be excreted, or else metabolized to less active agents. Conversion of lipid-soluble substances to water-soluble compounds involves two major steps. First, microsomal enzymes located on the membrane surface of the smooth endoplasmic reticulum (SER) cause *oxidation, reduction or hydrolysis* of the parent compound. These reactions involve several enzyme systems of low specificity, including the mixed function oxidases containing cytochrome P-450. Such transformation may lead to activation (e.g., cortisone is activated to cortisol, prednisone to prednisolone), inactivation (e.g., insulin, barbiturates) or an altered effect (e.g., imipramine, a depressant, becomes desmethylimipramine, an antidepressant). The drug-metabolizing enzymes may also be increased ("enzyme induction") by treatment with certain lipid-soluble drugs such as phenobarbital or alcohol, or they may be inhibited by other drugs such as cimetidine. The hydroxyl or other radical so created makes the product more readily able to undergo

the next step, *conjugation*. Conjugation with glucuronic acid is a common pathway. As with bilirubin metabolism, UDP-glucuronyl transferase serves as a transfering enzyme. The conjugated product, besides being pharmacologically inactive, is more water soluble and can be excreted in urine and bile. The liver can also create its own poisons, toxifying drugs by converting them to chemically hepatotoxic metabolites. Severe liver disease and aging may decrease cytochrome P-450 and other oxidizing enzymes. Drug metabolism may then be reduced predisposing to drug overdosage unless the altered pharmacokinetics are recognized.

DIAGNOSIS OF LIVER DISEASE

CLINICAL FEATURES

History

The patient profile—age, sex, background—provides important clues. In youth, viral hepatitis and congenital hyperbilirubinemias are the most common causes of liver disease or jaundice, whereas cholelithiasis and malignancy predominate in the middle years. Women are more prone to develop chronic hepatitis and primary biliary cirrhosis, but not hemochromatosis. Any environmental exposure to potential hepatoxins or contact with animals or humans capable of transmitting a hepatitis agent should be noted. The onset of the illness may be characteristic. Sudden onset of malaise, anorexia and aversion to smoking followed by jaundice suggests acute viral hepatitis. The gradual appearance of pruritus and jaundice indicates cholestasis. Ankle swelling and increasing abdominal girth suggests chronic liver disease. Fever and chills point toward cholangitis from biliary tract obstruction. Abdominal pain, localized to the right upper quadrant, can result from hepatic inflammation or stretching of Glisson's capsule. Tense ascites can stretch the abdominal wall causing discomfort over the costal margin. The drug history should include all oral and parenteral agents plus a careful inquiry into alcohol consumption which often needs confirmation by family and friends.

Physical Examination

Patients with liver disease generally appear well-nourished. Cachexia is associated with malignancy, malnutrition from any cause, such as alcoholism, and advanced cirrhosis. Jaundice can be detected early in the light-protected membranes such as the sclerae under the eyelids or the palate of the mouth. Stigmata of chronic liver disease such as in cirrhosis from alcoholism include: spider angioma especially when found in men, parotid gland enlargement, Dupuytren's contracture, palmar erythema, gynecomastia and testicular atrophy. On abdominal examination one should examine the liver, estimate its size in the midclavicular line by palpating the lower and percussing the upper border, feel its edge to assess smoothness and regularity, and listen for bruits and rubs.

Splenomegaly suggests portal hypertension. Ascites may be detected by shifting dullness, a fluid wave, or periumbilical dullness on assuming a prone position leaning on the knees and outstretched hands (the "puddle" sign).

LABORATORY ASSESSMENT AND INVESTIGATIVE PROCEDURES

Biochemical Tests

Biochemical assessment seeks to detect and quantitate hepatic dysfunction and discern from the pattern of the abnormality the nature of the underlying disorder. Laboratory tests can be simply classified.

Indices of Cell Injury or Necrosis

Excessive leakage of intracellular enzymes, such as the transaminases, occurs in acute necrosis or injury. Aspartate aminotransferase, AST (previously known as glutamic oxaloacetic transaminase, GOT), is mitochondrial-bound and present in heart, skeletal muscle and kidney. Alanine aminotransferase, ALT (glutamic pyruvic transaminase, GPT), in the cytosol is present in the liver in greater amounts compared to the heart and skeletal muscle. ALT increase is more specific for liver damage than AST and rises higher unless extensive cell death releases the mitochondrial-bound AST. The transaminases increase briskly often above ten times normal in any form of acute liver injury such as viral hepatitis, drug-induced liver injury, ascending cholangitis, or hypoxic/ischemic events in the liver as with acute heart failure. Lesser elevations, below 5–10 times normal, are usually found in cholestasis, chronic necrosis and alcoholic hepatitis. In most instances of acute liver injury the AST/ALT ratio is less than 1, but with alcohol-induced liver injury the ratio may increase to 2 or more. The high ratio reflects two factors: (1) damage by alcohol to liver mitochondria (the site of AST), and (2) damage to non-hepatic tissues, such as muscles,

which contain AST but little ALT. Lactic dehydrogenase (LDH) is a rather insensitive index, but tends to be elevated with liver metastases.

Serum iron and serum B_{12} are also elevated in hepatocellular damage. Serum albumin, which is synthesized exclusively in the liver, is reduced in chronic liver disease. Because of its long half-life, about 20 days, serum albumin levels change slowly and may remain normal in acute parenchymal injury. The prothombin time (PT), although too insensitive to detect mild disease, reflects the severity of the liver injury. For routine purposes it reflects the severity of liver disease best, if parenteral administration of vitamin K has failed to correct the prolongued PT.

Indices of Reaction to Cell Injury or of an Inflammatory Process

Serum globulins reflect the nature of the disease process. The hyperglobulinemia in chronic liver disease is a reticuloendothelial reaction to intestinal antigens not cleared by the damaged liver. In chronic hepatitis it represents a nonspecific portion of the inflammatory process. IgG is elevated in chronic active hepatitis whereas IgM is high in primary biliary cirrhosis. Various tissue antibodies may be detected in chronic liver disease. Of these, the most useful is the anti-mitochondrial antibody which is necessary to diagnose primary biliary cirrhosis.

Indices of Cholestasis

Failure of bile secretion, either as extrahepatic obstruction or as intrahepatic cholestasis from diffuse or focal disease, causes increases in alkaline phosphatase, 5' nucleotidase, and gammaglutamyl transpeptidase. Any disorder in bile flow and bile salt secretion causes hepatic synthesis of alkaline phosphatase to increase. This enzyme is produced by other tissues, particularly bone, placenta and intestine, so that elevations occur in normal growing children, pregnancy and bone disorders associated with increased osteoblastic activity. Alkaline phosphatase is a relatively sensitive index of cholestasis and infiltrative diseases, characteristically showing marked elevation and often being the only abnormality on routine testing. Lesser elevations can occur with parenchymal liver damage, as in cirrhosis or hepatitis. 5' nucleotidase, another phosphatase, is more specific for the liver being normal in bone disease. Gammaglutamyl transpeptidase levels are increased in cholestasis, hepatocellular disease, and in response to alcohol abuse. Total bilirubin may also increase, but usually not with partial biliary obstruction (e.g., an obstructed hepatic duct) or focal cholestasis (e.g., metastases or granuloma in the liver). Although moderate cholestasis produces hyperbilirubinemia with dark, tea-coloured urine testing positive for bilirubin, serum bilirubin is a rather insensitive index for hepatic disease. Fractionation of serum bilirubin into indirect (unconjugated) or direct (conjugated) components helps differentiate unconjugated hyperbilirubinemia (see section on Jaundice, Table 12.1). Urine urobilinogen has limited usefulness. In complete cholestasis, when no bilirubin enters the gut, no urobilinogen appears in the urine. Here the urine is dark from bilirubin, but the stool colourless or acholic (no bile). Excessive urobilinogenuria, as detected by a dipstik (Urobilistix), occurs either with conditions of increased bilirubin production like hemolysis or with hepatocellular dysfunction like hepatitis or cirrhosis when hepatic clearance into bile is reduced and the excess spills into the urine.

Serum bile acid levels are the most sensitive and specific test to detect mild cholestasis or hepatocellular disease; however, this test is not routinely available. The Bromsulphalein (BSP) test measures the ability of the liver to take up this dye, partially conjugate it with glutathione, and excrete it into bile. Because of the risk of hypersensitivity reactions, the lack of specificity, and the fact that the test is invalid and unnecessary in jaundice, BSP excretion test has little use today except for the Dubin-Johnson syndrome.

Specific Tests

These laboratory tests provide specificity as to the nature of the disease process.

Viral markers Hepatitis B surface antigen (HBsAg) is located on capsular material of the hepatitis B virus. Its presence in the serum indicates that the individual is infected with hepatitis B virus. A positive test can occur with acute type B hepatitis, chronic hepatitis B, the carrier state or hepatocellular carcinoma. Other markers of this virus are discussed later (Table 12.5). Type A hepatitis is detected by IgM antibody (IgM anti HAV).

Metabolic markers These tests are rather specific in certain liver disorders: serum iron, iron binding capacity and ferritin which indicate iron overload in hemochromatosis; ceruloplasmin, a copper-containing serum alpha-globulin, which is very low in Wilson's disease; alpha-1-antitrypsin, a metabolic disorder which can result in liver disease.

Tumour marker Alpha-fetoprotein is useful in diagnosis and follow-up as discussed below under

Hepatic Tumors. The best known tumor-associated antigen, the carcinoembryonic antigen (CEA), represents a heterogeneous group of glycoproteins of fetal origin. CEA is associated with GI malignancies, but elevated values appear in many types of liver disease unassociated with neoplasia so that its value is quite limited.

The following simple tests are of established value in screening for liver damage.

Routine Laboratory Tests

1. Serum bilirubin
2. Serum alkaline phosphatase
3. AST (SGOT)
4. Serum albumin and globulin
5. Prothrombin time

Radiology

Abdominal plain films can detect splenic enlargement, ascites, and may reveal calcified densities in the gallbladder, liver (as a cyst or hemangioma), or pancreas. Upper gastrointestinal contrast series can demonstrate esophageal varices in over 70 percent of cases although endoscopy is more accurate. Contrast studies which depend on hepatic extraction and excretion of radiopaque iodine-containing dyes either by intestinal absorption (oral cholecystography) or by injection (intravenous cholangiography) may outline the biliary structures but provide limited information in the presence of hepatobiliary dysfunction (bilirubin 40 μmol/L). Better visualization of the biliary system comes from direct introduction of the contrast agent at surgery, via duodenoscopy or by needle injection. The vascular system may be assessed by the arterial or venous phase of selective arteriography, and this may be helpful to diagnose liver tumor masses. Portal pressure measurements can be performed indirectly by wedging a catheter in a branch of the hepatic vein (wedged hepatic venous pressure) or inserting a needle into the splenic pulp (splenic pulp pressure). Injection of contrast material during these procedures can also yield anatomical information about the hepatic vein and splenic-portal venous system, respectively.

Liver Scan

Radionucleotide imaging of the liver is usually performed with gamma-emitting agents like Technetium (^{99m}Tc) labelled sulphur colloid. The colloid is phagocytized by the reticuloendothelial cells of the liver and spleen and the radioactivity displayed on a gamma camera. The technique delineates liver size, shape and position. Neoplastic masses, abscesses or cysts over 2 cm in diameter can be detected as "cold", space-occupying mass lesions. False-negative scans occur with small infiltrates while false-positive filling defects occur in cirrhosis from distorted liver architecture. Diffuse liver disease, such as cirrhosis or hepatitis, causes decreased liver visualization with preferential uptake in the spleen and bone marrow. Gallium scans with ^{67}Ga show "hot" spots over neoplastic and inflammatory infiltrations. Gallbladder scans use radiopharmaceuticals which are taken up by liver cells and excreted into bile.

Ultrasonography

This safe, non-invasive procedure can detect 1 to 2 cm space-occupying lesions, differentiate cystic versus solid masses within the liver, and accurately diagnose cholelithiasis. It is particularly useful in patients with impaired liver function in detecting the presence of a dilated common duct during the investigation of cholestasis and evaluating the head of the pancreas as a cause of extrahepatic obstruction.

Computerized Axial Tomography (CT Scan)

The CT scan of the abdomen provides detailed anatomy in cross-sectional images. Its accuracy and sensitivity exceeds ultrasound in obese individuals and in the presence of excessive bowel gas. CT scanning diagnoses mass lesions in the liver, pancreas and retroperitoneal area. It distinguishes intrahepatic fluid collections such as cysts and abscesses by determining fluid density. In cholestatic jaundice, it can detect a dilated biliary tract and any pancreatic lesion, but its cost-effectiveness is less than ultrasonography.

Liver Biopsy

Percutaneous needle biopsy of the liver is a safe, simple bedside procedure that provides a tissue diagnosis. The major indications are: suspected diffuse parenchymal disease such as cirrhosis or hepatitis; unexplained cholestasis, hepatomegaly or splenomegaly; disseminated focal diseases such as tumors or granulomas; storage disease, and unexplained fever with suspected granulomatous hepatitis. Although the biopsy specimen represents only $\frac{1}{50,000}$ of the total liver weight, this minute sample picks up

about 95 percent of those diseases which diffusely involve the liver and 75 percent of hepatic neoplasms. Contraindications include an uncooperative patient, a coagulopathy (prothrombin time prolonged 2 sec or more, platelet count under 100,000), a vascular tumor, infection in the right upper quadrant or a right lower lobe pneumonic consolidation, tense ascites, suspected amyloidosis or hydatid disease (Echinococcus).

Peritoneoscopy and Laparotomy

Peritoneoscopy, which can be done under local anaesthetic, allows direct inspection of the abdominal organs and directed needle biopsy of any lesion. This procedure has less risk than an exploratory laparotomy in patients with marked hepatocellular necrosis. Generally, diagnostic laparotomy is reserved for those cases in which the clinical, laboratory and other investigative studies have failed to reveal the basis of the hepatobiliary disease.

JAUNDICE

The liver normally excretes about 200–250mg of bilirubin each day, but it is capable of handling more than three times this load. Hyperbilirubinemia is therefore a relatively insensitive index of hepatic function. Jaundice is a clinical term describing the yellow appearance of the skin and mucous membranes, usually becoming evident when serum levels of this orange material exceed 3 mg/dl (50µmol/L). As bilirubin is altered by ultraviolet light to colourless products, jaundice is most evident in light protected areas such as that portion of the sclerae covered by the eyelids or the soft palate. With prolonged cholestasis, the skin becomes greenish due to the formation of biliverdin, a green pigment.

A classification of jaundice comes from the fractionation of bilirubin into direct (conjugated) and total concentrations which yields two patterns: (1) *unconjugated hyperbilirubinemia* where less than 15 percent of the total bilirubin is direct, the urine is acholic (no bile) and the routine laboratory tests are commonly normal, and (2) *conjugated hyperbilirubinemia* in which more than half is direct. A mixed picture occurs between these two (Table 12.1).

UNCONJUGATED HYPERBILIRUBINEMIA

The plasma concentration of unconjugated bilirubin is determined by the balance between bilirubin synthesis versus hepatic clearance of bilirubin, uptake

Table 12.1 Laboratory Features of Jaundice

Bilirubin Disorder	Serum Bilirubin		Urine		Serum Bile Salts
	Unconjugated (indirect)	Conjugated (direct)	Bilirubin	Urobilinogen	
Overproduction	↑	normal	0	↑	normal
Hemolysis					
Ineffective erythropoesis					
Defective Uptake and conjugation	↑	normal	0	normal	normal
Gilbert's syndrome					
Crigler-Najjar syndrome					
Drugs					
Cholestasis	↑	↑ ↑	+	↓ to 0	↑ *
Intrahepatic					
Extrahepatic					
Hepatocellular Disease	↑	↑ ↑	+	↑	↑ *

* can be elevated even when bilirubin is normal

and conjugation. Indirect hyperbilirubinemia occurs when total bilirubin is elevated >1.5 mg/dl (25 μmol/L), with the ratio of direct/total bilirubin being less than 20 percent or a direct bilirubin less than 0.3 mg/dl (5 μmol/L). In the absence of other laboratory evidence of hepatocellular or biliary tract dysfunction, the usual cause is either overproduction (e.g., hemolysis) or decreased hepatic clearance and conjugation of bilirubin (e.g., Gilbert's syndrome).

Hemolysis

Overproduction of bilirubin results from either rapid red cell destruction or rarely ineffective erythropoiesis with increased red blood cell breakdown in the bone marrow. The clinical and diagnostic features of a compensated hemolytic anemia have been reviewed in Chapter 17. The presence of reticulocytosis, abnormal blood smear, reduced serum haptoglobin, increased LDH and shortened red cell survival all indicate hemolysis. Serum bilirubin rarely exceeds 5 mg/dl (85 μmol/L), unless severe anemia, sepsis or hypotension compromise the liver's ability to handle the pigment load. There generally are no clinical or laboratory features to suggest liver disease. Increased bilirubin formation can also arise from tissue infarction (e.g., pulmonary infarction) or from extravascular accumulation of blood (e.g., hematoma).

Gilbert's Syndrome

The most common cause of non-hemolytic hyperbilirubinemia, appearing in 2–5 percent of otherwise healthy individuals, Gilbert's syndrome is inherited as an autosomal dominant trait with low penetrance. It somehow occurs more frequently in

men. The cause of the mild unconjugated hyperbilirubinemia, in which serum total bilirubin rarely exceeds 3 mg/dl (50 μmol/L), is due to reduced hepatic clearance of bilirubin. Not only is the conjugating enzyme UDP glucuronyl transferase deficient but also there is a reduction in hepatic uptake of bilirubin. Some patients exhibit an additional problem: reduced red blood cell survival with the low grade hemolysis increasing the bilirubin load. Patients generally are asymptomatic, being discovered fortuitously on routine investigation. Others experience non-specific episodes of malaise, anorexia and upper abdominal discomfort. During periods of intercurrent illness, especially if associated with fasting, jaundice may become more pronounced. This feature of Gilbert's Syndrome is useful diagnostically. Following a subtotal fast of 400 cal per day for 36–48 hours, their serum bilirubin will double. Phenobarbital, by inducing microsomal enzymes, will do the opposite: restore serum bilirubin to normal. Some patients may be incidently detected following recovery from acute viral hepatitis (posthepatitic hyperbilirubinemia); others develop unconjugated hyperbilirubinemia associated with chronic persistent hepatitis. Here there is no family history.

Physical examination and other liver tests are normal, as is liver morphology. The diagnosis is therefore based on exclusion of overt hemolysis and significant hepatocellular disease, often with a family history. This benign disorder has an excellent prognosis. Treatment is not necessary.

Crigler-Najjar Syndrome

Severe unconjugated hyperbilirubinemia can rarely occur as a result of complete (Type I) or partial (Type II) deficiency of glucuronyl transferase. In

Type I newborns develop very high serum levels of bilirubin, over 25 mg/dl (>400 μmol/L) and usually die of bilirubin encephalopathy (kernicterus) within the first year. In these patients, bile lacks conjugated bilirubin and is colourless. Inheritance is autosomal recessive. The milder form, *Type II,* is autosomal dominant and has lower serum bilirubin values, 4–20 mg/dl (70–350 μmol/L). Jaundice is usually detected at birth, although occasionally not until adulthood. Bile is pigmented and contains conjugated bilirubin. As some conjugating enzyme is present, phenobarbital is capable of lowering serum bilirubin. Ultraviolet light in the form of sunlight or phototherapy also lowers serum values by photo-oxidation to water-soluble products which are then excreted in urine and bile. With such therapy, the disorder is easily controlled. Although neurological damage is not common, fasting and stress can raise bilirubin to dangerous levels.

Neonatal Jaundice

Transient unconjugated hyperbilirubinemia below 5 mg/dl (85 μmol/L) regularly occurs in newborn infants during the first few days of life. Such *physiological jaundice of the newborn* is primarily due to the immaturity of the hepatic conjugating enzymes, which attain adult activity levels 1–2 weeks after birth. In infants with superimposed hemolysis (e.g., erythroblastosis), the excessive bilirubin load can drive bilirubin to above 20 mg/dl (350 μmol/L) causing kernicterus. Therapy includes phototherapy and exchange transfusions to lower the bilirubin, and albumin infusion to increase bilirubin binding. In *breast milk jaundice,* unconjugated hyperbilirubinemia develops 1 to 2 weeks postpartum and then disappears either when breast feeding stops or after 1 to 2 months despite continued breast feeding. Milk from these mothers contains a steroid metabolite which inhibits glycuronyl transferase.

CONJUGATED HYPERBILIRUBINEMIA

Disorders of bilirubin excretion can either involve bilirubin selectively so that routine laboratory tests show only elevated conjugated bilirubin, or more commonly, the hyperbilirubinemia is just one feature of a generalized bile secretory failure from cholestasis. In cholestasis, there is reduced bile flow and decreased output of a variety of organic solutes, most notably bile salts and bilirubin.

Familial Causes

The *Dubin-Johnson Syndrome* is a rare, familial disorder, characterized by a specific failure to excrete certain organic anions into bile. Besides bilirubin, BSP and the contrast agents for oral cholecystography and intravenous cholangiography are poorly excreted. The standard BSP test is characteristic; the dye has an abnormal secondary rise after 45 minutes, being initially taken up by the liver but later released causing a higher serum level at 120 minutes. Other than a conjugated hyperbilirubinemia of 3 to 10 mg/dl (50–175 μmol/L) and bilirubinuria, conventional liver function tests are normal. The hepatocytes from these patients are filled with melanin-like pigment, producing a black liver on gross inspection. Chronic intermittent jaundice is the only feature of this benign disorder. *Rotor syndrome* is similar in many respects except there is no hepatic pigment, the BSP test does not show a secondary rise and the gallbladder opacifies on oral cholecystography.

In *cholestasis of pregnancy,* there is an increased sensitivity to the hepatic effects of estrogens which normally increase during pregnancy. The result is cholestasis. Pruritus followed by jaundice with dark urine usually develops in the third trimester of an otherwise normal pregnancy. In milder cases, generalized itching occurs without jaundice. The patient is otherwise clinically well, while the biochemical tests show only cholestasis with increased alkaline phosphatase and only a modest rise in transaminase. As alkaline phosphatase is also produced by the placenta, confirmation of its origin can be documented by an increased 5′ nucleotidase. Within a few days of delivery, the pruritus disappears, and the biochemical abnormalities return to normal by 1–2 weeks. Although there may be a risk of premature delivery and fetal wastage, the prognosis is excellent. Recurrences are common (about 60 percent) in subsequent pregnancies or if oral contraceptives are used. Cholestasis of pregnancy tends to run in families and is more frequent in Scandinavia and Chile. The diagnosis must be differentiated from more serious forms of liver disease such as acute fatty liver of pregnancy or tetracycline-induced fatty liver, in which fulminant hepatic failure supervenes in the last trimester. Both the Dubin-Johnson syndrome and primary biliary cirrhosis may appear for the first time during pregnancy. The most common cause of jaundice during pregnancy, however, is viral hepatitis.

Table 12.2 **Intrahepatic Cholestasis**

Cause	Diagnostic Features
Viral hepatitis (cholestatic phase)	General: Painless jaundice, pruritus Specific: Exposure, prodrome, HBsAg, (IgM anti-HAV) biopsy
Drug-induced	History of drug use. biopsy
Alcoholic hepatitis★	Alcohol abuse, fever, tender hepatomegaly wbc, biopsy
Postoperative jaundice	Jaundice 48 hrs. after surgery, drugs, hypotension, sepsis
Primary biliary cirrhosis★	Onset pruritus, female, antimitochondrial antibody, biopsy
Cholestasis of pregnancy	Third trimester, onset pruritus
Associated with other diseases	Carcinoma: primary or secondary Hodgkin's disease without hepatic involvement septicemia, pneumonia, abscess

★ may also have features of chronic liver disease (e.g., spider angioma, palmer erythema, ascitis, splenomegaly) or in primary biliary cirrhosis, chronic cholestasis (xanthomas, bone pain, bruising)

Mild pruritus responds to simple measures such as oatmeal baths. In more severe cases, cholestyramine ingestion will relieve itching.

Acquired Causes

Conjugated hyperbilirubinemia, which is due to acquired causes, is best considered in the general context of *cholestasis.*

CHOLESTASIS

Cholestasis can be defined in various ways. Physiologically, it means a reduction in canalicular bile flow commonly related to decreased secretion of bile salts. The defect in bile secretion can occur in the liver cell, the collecting system within the liver or the bile duct system outside the liver. Liver injury from viruses, drugs, alcohol or toxins commonly results in cholestasis being part of most *hepatocellular disease.* Cholestasis may also be caused by developmental, inflammatory or neoplastic processes affecting the duct system within the liver, termed *intrahepatic cholestasis.* Biliary obstruction can result from tumor, stones, inflammatory strictures or developmental failure of the large bile ducts outside the liver, called *extrahepatic cholestasis.*

Clinically, cholestasis describes the retention of substances normally excreted in bile such as bile salts and bilirubin. Pruritus is often prominent while jaundice and deepening pigmentation develops slowly. The urine becomes dark and if obstruction is complete, the stools turn pale, clay-coloured. Jaundice may be absent in localized or incomplete cholestasis. The onset of pure intrahepatic cholestasis is usually gradual with the patient feeling well, unlike the malaise and fatigue associated with hepatocellular disease or the fever and pain of extrahepatic obstruction. When chronic retention of lipids results in xanthomas. Intestinal bile salt deficiency eventually produces steatorrhea and malabsorption of the fat-soluble vitamins A, D and K.

Morphological evidence of acute cholestasis can be seen at three levels: (1) macroscopically, the liver is green and enlarged; (2) microscopically, stagnated or inspissated bile is present in the form of bile plugs or thrombi in canaliculi, and bile pigment in Kupffer and liver cells and (3) ultrastructurally, the bile canaliculi are dilated and the microvilli disappear. Chronic cholestasis can be associated with biliary cirrhosis. Biochemically cholestasis results in increased serum conjugated bilirubin, alkaline phosphatase and 5' nucleotidase, bile acids and cholesterol values. The urine contains bilirubin. The prothrombin time may be elevated but should respond to parenteral vitamin K, if significant hepatocellular disease does not exist.

The clinical presentation and especially the biochemical features do not always lead to a clear differentiation between liver cell disease versus small duct or large duct obstruction. The importance of this distinction is the need to select those cases amenable to surgical treatment. Not only is operating on patients with intrahepatic cholestasis unnecessary but also, in the case of viral hepatitis, dangerous. Some diagnostic features become evident when cholestasis is classified into intrahepatic and extrahepatic causes (Table 12.2, 12.3). More often, the diagnostic approach rests on demonstrating the presence or absence of dilated bile ducts (Fig. 12.3). Ultrasonography is the safest and simplist method to screen for biliary tract dilation, gallbladder disease, and any mass lesion in the pancreas. Computerized tomography (CT Scan) is also non-invasive, but is limited by expense and availability. These new techniques

Table 12.3 **Extrahepatic Cholestasis**

Cause	Diagnostic Features*	
	General:	pain, fever, pruritus, RUQ tenderness, enlarged liver
Extrahepatic Bile Duct Obstruction		
stone (choledocholithiasis)	Specific:	biliary colic, cholangitis
stricture		previous biliary surgery, cholangitis
cyst		young female, intermittent jaundice
Caroli's disease**		recurrent cholangitis, stones
suppurative cholangitis**		rigor, fever, RUQ pain
sclerosing cholangitis**		associated ulcerative colitis. Duct biopsy
carcinoma (cholangiocarcinoma)		progressive cholestasis, afebrile. Duct biopsy
Pancreas		
pancreatitis	Specific:	vomiting, abdominal pain, amylase ↑
pseudocysts		abdominal pain, tenderness, mass, persistent amylase ↑
carcinoma (pancreaticoduodenal)		weight loss, enlarged gallbladder

* Specialized radiographic and scanning techniques are often necessary for a diagnosis
** Caroli's disease (focal dilation of the intrahepatic bile ducts), suppurative and sclerosing cholangitis may also be categorized under intrahepatic cholestasis

are good but not infallible. Ducts, for example, are not always dilated in mechanical obstruction. If dilated ducts are seen, visualization of the biliary tree is essential to confirm a mechanical obstruction and delineate the lesion for the surgeon. The two most popular techniques are percutaneous transhepatic cholangiography (PTC) and endoscopic retrograde cholangiopancreatography (ERCP). In PTC, contrast agent is directly injected via a thin needle inserted under fluoroscopic control through the skin into bile ducts within the liver substance. Visualization of a dilated biliary tree is readily accomplished in over 90 percent of cases. With non-dilated ducts, the success of demonstrating the duct system drops to 60 percent. In experienced hands, the common duct will be visualized by ERCP in 70 to 85 percent of patients. Both procedures can result in cholangitis and sepsis; PTC can also cause bile peritonitis and hemorrhage, while ERCP can precipitate pancreatitis. With dilated ducts, PTC is the procedure of

choice. With undilated or narrowed ducts (as with sclerosing cholangitis), or when pancreatic or gallbladder disease is suspect, ERCP should be done. ERCP also views the stomach and ampulla and permits biopsies of any suspicious lesion. If there is no evidence of duct dilatation or biliary tract stones and blood coagulation is normal, then liver biopsy is a safe way to establish the diagnosis (Fig. 12.3). When doubt exists as to the appropriate invasive test, clinical observation with a repeat ultrasound study carries no hazard apart from the delay, which in itself may be revealing.

INFLAMMATORY DISEASES OF THE LIVER

Hepatitis means inflammation of the liver which is accompanied by hepatocyte injury. This may be diffuse, as in viral and toxic hepatitis, or focal, as in

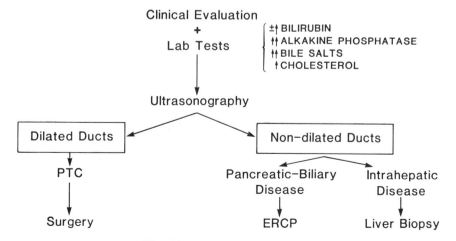

Fig. 12.3 Diagnosis of Cholestasis.

Table 12.4   **Features of Hepatitis A, B, and Non-A Non-B**

	A	B	Non-A Non-B
Virus	RNA	DNA	DNA
Transmission route	fecal-oral (contact associated)	parenteral, venereal, maternal-fetal	parenteral, other
Incubation period (weeks)	2–6	7–24	2–20 weeks
Age distribution	children	any age	any age
Onset	acute	insidious	insidious
Severity	mild	can be severe	mild
Clinical features:			
fever >38°C	common	less common	uncommon
anorexia	extreme	mild	mild
nausea, vomiting	common	less common	less common
rashes, arthralgia	infrequent	common	rare
Chronicity	no	yes (10%)	yes
Liver carcinoma	no	yes	?
Serology	anti HA	HBsAg	none available
Immunoglobulin prophylaxis	effective	hyperimmune serum globulin better with massive exposure	probably effective

granulomas. The extent of liver cell necrosis and inflammation determines the clinical manifestations which range in severity from mild dysfunction with a subclinical illness, to severe widespread damage with fulminant liver failure and coma.

ACUTE VIRAL HEPATITIS

Etiology and Pathogenesis

Acute viral hepatitis is a common infection in which acute necrosis and inflammation of the liver is caused by at least three different viral agents: type A, type B and type non-A non-B. Whereas these agents primarily affect the liver, other systemic viral infections, such as the Epstein-Barr virus which causes infectious mononucleosis, the cytomegalovirus, herpes simplex 1, coxsackie and yellow fever, can also cause hepatitis. This section will focus on the three viruses which predominantly affect the liver (Table 12.4).

Hepatitis A Virus (HAV), a 27nm RNA picornavirus, usually causes a mild hepatitis after a short incubation period and often appears in epidemics, especially among school-age children: hence, its previous terminology, "infectious hepatitis" or "short-incubation hepatitis." Transmission is by feces in which the associated antigen has been experimentally detected during the late incubation period and early clinical illness (see Fig. 12.4). It is not detectable in serum. Virus and antigen usually disappear by the time jaundice peaks. Hence infectivity is short-lived: from 2 weeks before to 1–2 weeks after jaundice begins. A carrier state has never been identified. Soon after the clinical illness begins, two an-

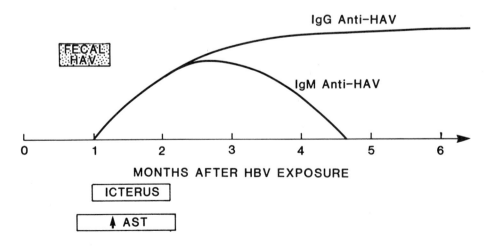

Fig. 12.4 Typical course of acute Type A hepatitis. HAV, hepatitis A Virus antigen; anti-HAV, antibody to hepatitis A virus; AST, aspartate aminotransferase.

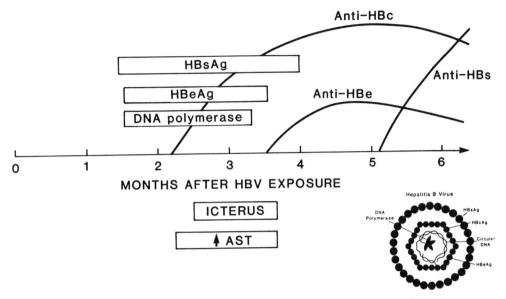

Fig. 12.5 Typical course of acute type B hepatitis. (See text for discussion). The important structures of the virus or Dane particle are drawn in the lower right: core antigen (HBcAg), e antigen (HBeAg), double-stranded DNA and DNA polymerase. The surface contains HBsAg.

tibodies to HAV (anti-HA) appear: first an IgM anti-HAV, then an IgG anti-HAV. The IgM antibody falls within 8 weeks, whereas IgG persists providing homologous immunity. The presence of IgM anti-HAV is diagnostic of a recent infection. The IgG antibody suggests a previous infection with immunity now being present. Since many adults (up to 97 percent) have IgG anti-HAV, this infection must commonly pass unrecognized in childhood. Indeed, the disease is frequently so mild that without jaundice (anicteric), it may be passed off as a "flu-like" illness or gastroenteritis. Mortality is low with no chronicity. Hepatitis B Virus (HBV) is a 44nm double stranded DNA virus which causes a more severe form of acute hepatitis and can lead to chronic disease. Symptoms appear after a longer incubation period and the usual route of transmission was previously considered to be blood products accounting for the term "serum hepatitis" or "long-incubation hepatitis." Transmission is parenteral, although intimate contact may be a factor in many situations, such as venereal spread which causes this disease to be quite prevalent among male homosexuals. Maternal transmission to the newborn may occur parenterally at the time of delivery or by close contact thereafter.

Hepatitis B virus (Fig. 12.5) consists of an outer coat containing hepatitis B surface antigen (HBsAg) and an inner core with two related antigens: core antigen (HBcAg) and "e" antigen (HBeAg). Inside the core is a small, circular, double-stranded molecule of

DNA which has a unique single-stranded region. Also inside is an enzyme, DNA polymerase. Once the virus has invaded the liver cell, DNA polymerase repairs the single-stranded gap during viral replication. The host cell manufactures the various viral components, producing core in the nucleus and coat in the cytoplasm. HBsAg is produced in excess. Its incorporation into the hepatocyte wall may cause an altered self which possibly leads to liver cell destruction by the host's immune system. The excess HBsAg in the serum allows easy detection. The presence of HBsAg in body fluids other than blood does not necessarily mean infectivity; the complete viral genome is necessary. HBcAg is released when core particles are disrupted, but free HBcAg does not circulate.

HBsAg is the most readily measured, and it is also the first detectable marker. It appears within 6 weeks of exposure, preceding biochemical change and symptoms by 2–4 weeks, and normally disappears within 6 months (Fig. 12.5). The presence of HBsAg indicates HBV infection: either as acute hepatitis even before the disease becomes evident or as a chronic viral infection when HBsAg persists beyond 6 months. Blood from sick patients is therefore infectious. HBeAg and DNA polymerase denote high viral levels and infectivity. They appear soon after HBsAg but are cleared early before HBsAg disappears. Their persistence suggests continued viral replication and the eventual development of chronic hepatitis. Normally, patients become HBeAg negative and anti-HBe appears indicating that infection and disease are beginning to resolve. Anti-HBc rises just as symptoms begin, unlike anti-HBs which develops months later. A short "window" is left between the disappearance of HBsAg and the appearance of anti-HBs. Some individuals never develop anti-HBs even though the disease resolves. If HBsAg is no longer present, anti-HBc can still serologically detect the infectious process.

Hepatitis B virus is not particularly cytopathic. The outcome of infection is probably determined most by the host's cell mediated response. A vigorous response produces acute hepatitis, the host recovers and the virus disappears within 12 weeks. A few may be overwhelmed by fulminant hepatitis. Sometimes the hepatitis virus persists without significant liver damage such as might occur in an immunosuppressed patient. Here the virus proliferates without any response from the host, producing excess surface antigen, HBsAg. There may be an intermediate response in which the cellular response produces liver damage but does not destroy the virus; this may lead to chronic active hepatitis. The *delta agent*, a small RNA protein, may be associated with HBV. It is reputed to be a major cause of progressive liver damage in chronic HBsAg carriers, such as drug addicts, or highly endemic areas.

Non-A non-B hepatitis became recognized when investigators found that a significant proportion of transfusion-associated hepatitis could not be serologically attributed to identifiable viruses: hepatitis B, hepatitis A, cytomegalovirus or Epstein-Barr (EB). There are currently no serological markers for non-A non-B hepatitis, and the responsible agents have not been identified. The diagnosis is made on clinical and biochemical evidence of viral hepatitis, with serological exclusion of recent hepatitis A, B, cytomegalovirus or EB virus infection. Non-A non-B hepatitis is the leading cause of post-transfusion hepatitis, now that hepatitis B virus-containing blood is being eliminated by screening for HBsAg. The disease is quite similar to type B hepatitis: transmission is largely parenteral, a carrier state exists, and chronic hepatitis can develop. The clinical illness, however, tends to be milder, two-thirds of reported cases having few or no apparent symptoms. Person-to-person spread may cause sporadic disease.

Pathology

The morphological features of hepatitis types A, B, and non-A non-B are identical. The basic lesion is an acute inflammation of the entire liver. Liver cell degeneration and necrosis predominantly involve the centres of the lobule ("centrilobular necrosis"). Mononuclear cells accumulate, but polymorphonuclear leukocytes and fatty changes are absent. The reticulin framework is usually well maintained, providing the scaffolding on which liver cells later regenerate. Occasionally, large areas of hepatocytes drop out, collapsing the reticulin framework and resulting in confluent or "bridging necrosis." Such *subacute hepatic necrosis* may have prognostic importance suggesting a more severe course or the development of cirrhosis. Certainly extensive necrosis involving many adjacent lobules carries a poor prognosis, while massive necrosis results in fulminant liver failure.

Clinical Features

Although certain distinctive features separate hepatitis type A, type B and type non-A, non-B it is impossible to differentiate these viral illnesses on clinical grounds alone. The typical course can be divided into incubation, prodromal, icteric and convalescent phases. The *incubation period* lasts from days to several months depending upon the viral type. A short incubation period suggests hepatitis A, although non-A non-B infection can follow exposure within as short a time as 2 weeks. The *prodromal period* begins a few days to 2 weeks before jaundice appears. Onset is abrupt in hepatitis A; more insidious in B and non-A non-B. Constitutional symptoms resemble any acute systemic infection, with anorexia, nausea, vomiting, malaise, arthralgia and weight loss. There may also be a peculiar aversion to smoking and altered taste sensation. A low grade fever may occur but usually without rigors. Fever, anorexia, nausea, and vomiting are more common in type A, whereas a "serum sickness-like" syndrome with arthralgia and rashes are more common in type B. The latter may be the result of circulating immune complexes involving HBsAg, anti-Hbs, and complement activation. As the inflamed liver enlarges stretching Glisson's capsule, the patient may experience a right upper quadrant ache. Soon the urine becomes dark and the stool lightens, heralding the development of jaundice within a few days. In the *icteric phase* jaundice develops, but the constitutional symptoms recede as the appetite improves. Jaundice deepens over the next week or two, sometimes accompanied by pruritus, and then disappears within 6 weeks. During the early icteric phase the liver can become enlarged and tender. The spleen is also palpable in some instances. Tender, enlarged cervical lymph nodes may be present. Spider angioma may become transiently

Table 12.5 **Clinical Forms of Viral Hepatitis**

I. Common
  A. Inapparent hepatitis–asymptomatic
  B. Anicteric hepatitis–asymptomatic
  C. Icteric hepatitis–symptomatic
II. Atypical
  A. Cholestatic viral hepatitis
  B. Fulminant viral hepatitis
  C. Benign sequelae
      prolonged hepatitis ⎫
      relapsing viral hepatitis ⎬ chronic lobular hepatitis★

      posthepatitis hyperbilirubinemia
      chronic persistent hepatitis★
      chronic carrier
  D. Serious sequelae
      chronic active hepatitis★
      cirrhosis
      hepatoma

★ Three forms of chronic hepatitis

evident without signifying chronic liver disease. The majority of patients show complete clinical and biochemical recovery within 6 months, even though lassitude and fatigue may persist.

Laboratory Assessment

The most striking laboratory abnormality is raised serum transaminases (AST and ALT), which increase during the late prodromal phase even before the rise in bilirubin. The absolute level reached, up to several thousand U/L, does not reflect the degree of liver damage. Transaminase values peak during the early icteric phase when serum bilirubin and alkaline phosphatase are also increased, and then fall to normal. Bilirubin appears in the urine in the prodromal period, just before the onset of clinical jaundice when serum bilirubin exceeds 3 mg/dl (50 umol/L). In anicteric hepatitis, there may only be a mildly elevated transaminase. Serum prothrombin time is usually normal except during prolonged cholestasis or with marked liver disease. Leukopenia is transient, being followed by a relative lymphocytosis often with atypical lymphocytes. Immunological findings are presented in Fig. 12.4 and 12.5).

Prognosis

The natural course of viral hepatitis is quite variable but most commonly appears in three forms (Table 12.5): *inapparent hepatitis*, in which the patient is totally asymptomatic but is later revealed to have markers indicating a previous infection with viral hepatitis; *anicteric hepatitis*, in which only the prodomal phase of an acute viral illness is manifest; and

lastly, *icteric hepatitis*, typical viral hepatitis with jaundice. Occasionally, the course may be atypical. There may be a prolonged cholestatic phase, *cholestatic viral hepatitis*, with jaundice and pruritus lasting for weeks to months. The patient otherwise feels well, whereas liver biochemistry reveals a bland cholestasis with high bilirubin and alkaline phosphatase values but near-normal transaminase. In such cases, extrahepatic causes of jaundice should be excluded. Clinical and biochemical features eventually subside without sequelae. The mortality of acute viral hepatitis is less than 1 percent, the rare case having a fulminant course with massive necrosis.

Fulminant viral hepatitis occurs when acute hepatic failure occurs abruptly during the course of otherwise typical viral hepatitis, sometimes even before jaundice becomes detectable. Fever, hyperventilation, and an altered sensorium may develop within a few days, only to be followed by somnolence, vomiting, a coagulopathy, coma and then death. Management should be undertaken in an intensive care unit (see later section on Hepatic Encephalopathy). If survival occurs, the liver usually returns to normal.

More benign sequelae can also occur, especially after type B hepatitis. In *prolonged viral hepatitis* clinical and laboratory abnormalities persist beyond 3–6 months. The lengthening represents a more protracted illness rather than a different disease. Prognosis is usually considered excellent. *Relapsing viral hepatitis* indicates that after an apparent complete recovery from typical acute viral hepatitis, the individual manifests a recrudescence of the original illness on at least one occasion. It is sometimes difficult differentiating relapsing viral hepatitis from more chronic forms of liver injury or from a second attack due to another agent. In fact, both prolonged and relapsing viral hepatitis may be morphologically characterized as *chronic lobular hepatitis.* (see Chronic Active Hepatitis below).

Chronic persistent hepatitis, the most common sequel, develops in about 10 percent of patients with acute type B hepatitis. From a different perspective, 75 percent of patients with chronic persistent hepatitis give an antecedent history of symptomatic hepatitis. It is best considered a slowly resolving, delayed healing phase of viral hepatitis which persists for at least 6 months after the initial episode of liver injury. In some, the disease may be associated with inflammatory bowel or collagen diseases. Episodic malaise and hepatic tenderness occur, but there are no stigmata of chronic liver injury and no hepatomegaly. Most patients are asymptomatic, being detected by routine blood tests which show mildly elevated transaminase levels (< five times normal) Serum globulin is normal. A mild unconjugated hyperbilirubinemia is sometimes present. Diagnosis can best be secured by a liver biopsy. Liver morphology shows a mononuclear cell infiltration in the portal tract without destruction of the surrounding outer plate of liver cells, the "limiting plate." There may be a few residual findings within the lobule suggesting acute viral hepatitis, but lobular architecture remains intact. Since the course is benign, treatment other than reassurance and periodic re-evaluation is not warranted.

A *chronic carrier state* develops in 5 percent of adults following recognized hepatitis B virus infection. Few carriers, however, give a history of acute viral hepatitis. These individuals are identified by the continuing presence of HBsAg in the serum, while infectivity is suggested by HBeAg. Prevalence of chronic carriers in the community ranges from 0.1 percent in western countries to almost 100 percent in South East Asia. Most HBsAg-positive individuals are healthy. Others develop chronic hepatitis, cirrhosis and/or hepatocellular carcinoma. Special problems arise when health care personnel, especially those involved in dialysis or oncology units, are HBsAg positive. The mode of transmission is usually from patient to staff, rather than from staff to patient. Isolation of such patients on dialysis units and use of special precautions by staff in handling infected patients or their blood products have reduced the incidence of outbreaks. A chronic carrier state may also follow non-A non-B hepatitis virus infection, whereas type A has never been implicated.

Management

The management of uncomplicated acute viral hepatitis is supportive as no specific therapy exists. Most patients can be readily handled at home rather than in the hospital, unless dehydration results from vomiting or any features suggest fulminant hepatitis. Whether at home or in hospital, common-sense enteric precautions are warranted for patients with suspected hepatitis A, whereas blood precautions should be used in patients who are HBsAg positive or have suspected type non-A non-B hepatitis. Bed rest is traditional but not essential, except for patient comfort when fatigue is overwhelming. Patients should be mobilized when they feel well enough for physical activity. No specific dietary regimes are warranted except to encourage an adequate caloric intake. Corticosteroid therapy has no role in uncomplicated acute hepatitis and may be detrimental. During the convalescent phase, liver tests should be followed until normal.

Prevention of viral hepatitis depends on: prevention of spread through standard public health measures such as good sanitation; proper disposal and cleansing of parenteral instruments; screening for HBsAg in blood donors; immunization of high risk groups with hepatitis B vaccine; and control of disease by use of passive immunoprophylaxis. Conventional gammaglobulin is effective in preventing or ameliorating type A viral hepatitis and should be administered to household contacts of patients with hepatitis A or travellers to endemic areas such as the tropics. Any individual with IgG anti-HAV presumably is already immune. The value of immune globulin against hepatitis B depends on its anti-HBs titer. Standard immune serum globulin with modest anti-HBs titers is considered adequate for pre-exposure prophylaxis in an endemic setting. Hepatitis B immune serum globulin with high anti-HBs is recommended as prophylaxis for persons who have sustained a definite exposure such as a needle stick containing HBsAg-positive material, sexual contacts of type B hepatitis patients and infants born to HBsAg positive mothers. Immune serum globulin should also be given to contacts of non-A non-B hepatitis.

CHRONIC ACTIVE HEPATITIS

Chronic parenchymal liver disease exists in two major forms: (1) *chronic hepatitis*, defined as continuous inflammation of the liver without improvement for at least 6 months which as chronic lobular hepatitis or chronic persistent hepatitis represents a harmless sequence to viral hepatitis but in the form of chronic active hepatitis predisposes to cirrhosis, and (2) *cirrhosis*, end-stage scarring of the liver with widespread fibrosis and an attempt at regenerative hyperplasia of the remaining liver cells forming nodules.

Chronic lobular hepatitis is an uncommon but benign

form of chronic hepatitis. The clinical onset and histology are similar to acute viral hepatitis except that it persists beyond 6 months. In some cases, there may be a succession of remissions and relapses with markedly increased serum transaminase. This differs from chronic active hepatitis in which spontaneous remissions are uncommon and relapses are associated with moderate increases in serum transaminase. There is no progression to cirrhosis.

Chronic persistent hepatitis, the most common form of chronic hepatitis, has mild clinical and laboratory features which usually are quite distinct from chronic active hepatitis (see Acute Hepatitis, Prognosis).

Chronic active hepatitis, is typified by: (1) chronicity of at least 10 to 12 weeks duration, although 6 months is the arbitrary minimum accepted by some, (2) biochemical activity featuring at least a ten-fold elevation of the serum transaminase or a five-fold elevation of this enzyme with a two-fold rise in gammaglobulins, and (3) evidence on liver biopsy of chronic active hepatitis characterized by "piecemeal necrosis": the destruction of liver cells which form the limiting plate around the portal triad. Mononuclear cells, fibroblasts and collagen extend from the portal tract into the necrotic areas, isolating the surviving hepatocytes in small islands. Extension of this process to connect adjacent portal areas or central veins results in "bridging necrosis". If this process leads to wide fibrous septa and a thwarted attempt at hepatic regeneration cirrhosis develops. Several factors can initiate chronic active hepatitis (Table 12.6).

Etiology of Chronic Active Hepatitis

An autoimmune process was originally suggested because some patients had a positive L.E. cell phenomenon: hence, the term "lupoid hepatitis". These individuals do not have S.L.E., a condition in which liver involvement is rare. Most cases probably have a viral etiology; serum HBsAg, for example, is present in about 25 percent. Many features are also found in metabolic disorders affecting the liver, such as Wilson's disease, alpha 1-antitrypsin deficiency, alcohol and drug-related liver injury.

Table 12.6 Etiology of Chronic Active Hepatitis

Viral hepatitis	Alcohol
Type B	Drugs
Type non-A, non-B	Methyldopa
Autoimmune or "lupoid"	Oxyphenistin
hepatitis	Nitrofurantoin
Wilson's Disease	Aspirin in rheumatic
α_1-antitrypsin deficiency	diseases

Two major forms of chronic active hepatitis should be distinguished because of their different response to corticosteroid therapy (Table 12.7). "Non-viral associated" hepatitis (i.e. HBsAg negative hepatitis) usually appears in young women. Onset is insidious in about two-thirds of patients leading to anorexia, slowly progressive jaundice, acne, amemorrhea, persistent fever, arthralgia, and asymptomatic hepatomegaly. In others, the onset is abrupt, like acute viral hepatitis. Multisystemic manifestations are common, ranging from a non-deforming arthritis, various skin manifestations, keratoconjunctivitis, to ulcerative colitis. Hypergammaglobulinemia and nonspecific tissue antibodies are frequently evident. HBsAg is negative. Patients are more symptomatic and serum transaminase levels higher. In such cases, corticosteroid therapy can be expected to produce a clinical, biochemical and morphological remission. Conversely, chronic active hepatitis which is HBsAg positive and presumably "viral associated" also presents a mild progressive disease, frequently without a prior history of acute hepatitis. Extrahepatic manifestations and immunological markers are absent, whereas HBsAg is positive. Disease activity is less and prognosis better, even though many go on silently to develop postnecrotic cirrhosis. Corticosteroids are of no value. There is, as yet, no way to identify those cases due to chronic virus infection with type non-A non-B hepatitis.

GRANULOMA OF THE LIVER (GRANULOMATOUS HEPATITIS)

The commonly used term "granulomatous hepatitis" is perhaps a misnomer because the lesion is not really a hepatitis and does not cause significant hepatic dysfunction. Hepatic granulomas are rather common, being found in up to 10 percent of liver biopsy specimens. Their importance is not the very mild liver dysfunction they produce, but rather the underlying disease with which they are associated. The commonest causes are sarcoidosis, histoplasmosis, tuberculosis, schistosomiasis and primary biliary cirrhosis, although one-quarter of cases are idiopathic. Fever may be a prominent feature. In such cases liver biopsy will reveal granuloma, although this is not necessarily the underlying cause.

LIVER ABSCESS

Pyogenic abscess of the liver, a collection of pus, most commonly results from obstruction and bacterial infection of the biliary tree (cholangitis). Less frequent

Table 12.7   **Two Forms of Chronic Active Hepatitis**

	Non-Viral Associated ("lupoid" or autoimmune hepatitis)	Viral Associated (HBV)
Age	young	young to middle aged
Sex	women	men
Clinical		
onset	insidious	insidious
systemic disease	common	common
Laboratory Tests		
serum globulins	↑ (polyclonal)	lower
antinuclear antibody	66%	rare
smooth muscle antibody	66%	rare
antimitochondrial antibody	25%	no
LE cell	15%	no
HBsAg	—	+
Prognosis	cirrhosis	better
Response to Coricosteroid	yes	no

causes are direct infection following blunt trauma, spread from an adjacent septic focus, or pyogenic contamination of an amebic abscess. Infection in the abdomen or pelvis may also cause portal pylephlebitis or septic emboli to the liver. Presentation is rather dramatic: severe continuous pain in the right upper quadrant associated with fever and general toxic manifestations. Jaundice may be present with multiple abscesses or acute suppurative cholangitis. The liver is enlarged and tender. Leukocytosis, anemia and cholestasis with elevated serum alkaline phosphatase are common. The abscess is best localized by radionucleotide imaging, ultrasonography, or CT scanning. There may be secondary evidence of an abscess with an elevated immobile right diaphragm and a pleural effusion. Plain films may reveal the presence of an air fluid level in the abscess cavity caused by gas-producing organisms. Needle aspiration of the abscess and multiple blood cultures are necessary to identify the causal organism(s), usually enteric gram negative bacteria. Management requires adequate drainage either by percutaneous needle aspiration under ultrasonographic guidance or at laparotomy. The choice of antibiotics should be based on the organisms isolated from the abscess or blood.

Amebic abscess of the liver is caused by *Entamoeba histolytica*. Amebae, ingested as cysts, pass to the colon where they change into trophozoites. This form invades the colonic mucosa causing intestinal amebiasis. In only a small portion of such patients are amebae carried via the portal venous system to the liver creating an abscess. The centre of these abscesses can contain liquified necrotic debris as a thick, reddish-brown pus appearing like anchovy paste. Secondary bacterial infection may supervene causing the material to become greenish and foul smelling.

The onset may be acute with fever, rigors, sweating, and right upper quadrant or right pleuritic chest pain. In others, the onset is more gradual with symptoms developing over a month or longer. Occasionally patients present with pleuritic pain with or without copious sputum production due to transdiaphragmatic rupture of the hepatic abscess into the pleural space or a bronchus. Amebic dysentery is present in only a very few cases, most having had asymptomatic intestinal amebiasis. *Entamoeba histolytica* is usually absent from the stools. The liver is enlarged and tender. A right sided pleural effusion may also be present. Leukocytosis, a mild anemia, and an elevated serum alkaline phosphatase are not very specific, but a positive hemagglutination inhibition test is extremely useful. Liver scan will show the filling defect, while ultrasound demonstrates the hollow cavity of the abscess. Needle aspiration yields chocolate-like or "anchovy paste" fluid. Trophozoites may not be present in the aspirate but can be identified if a needle biopsy is taken of the cyst wall.

Treatment with metronidazole for 10 days is usually quite effective for both amebic dysentery and liver abscesses. If secondary infection of the abscess cavity occurs, surgical drainage and appropriate antibiotics become indicated.

TOXIC AND DRUG-INDUCED LIVER INJURY

Just as the liver is the main organ responsible for the metabolism of drugs, particularly those absorbed from the gastrointestinal tract, so is it susceptible to injury from drugs and other chemicals taken into the body. The two principle mechanisms for liver injury associated with drugs and chemicals are listed in Table 12.8.

Table 12.8 **Mechanisms of Drug-Induced Liver Injury**

Classification	Examples	Effect
I. Intrinsic Hepatotoxin		
A. Direct	CCl₄, phosphorus	fatty liver, liver cell necrosis
B. Indirect		
1. Metabolite mediated	Acetaminophen	liver cell necrosis
2. Interference with cell metabolism	Tetracycline, antimetabolites	fatty liver, cirrhosis
3. Impaired bile secretion	C-17 alkylated steroids	cholestasis
II. Host Idiosyncracy		
A. Hypersensitivity	Halothane	liver cell necrosis
	Chlorpromazine★	cholestasis
B. Metabolic	Isoniazid★	liver cell necrosis

★ may also have intrinsic hepatotoxic potential

MECHANISMS OF DRUG-INDUCED LIVER INJURY

Intrinsic hepatotoxins predictably cause dose-dependent toxicity in all individuals after a brief latent period following exposure and can reproduce the liver damage in experimental animals. *Direct* hepatotoxins are agents which directly attack liver cells destroying both their structure and function. There are obviously no known direct hepatotoxins used as therapeutic agents. *Indirect* hepatoxins produce their effect either by (1) forming a toxic metabolite, (2) interfering with cell metabolism, or (3) depressing bile secretion. Toxicity may be mediated by the parent drug or by intermediate compounds formed in the process of hepatic metabolism. Even in the case of the few known "direct" hepatotoxins such as carbon tetrachloride (CCl₄), the liver injury may be mediated by a toxic metabolite. The first phase of drug metabolism not only makes the drug more polar in preparation for conjugation, but may also activate the drug to a toxic metabolite. Hence, any individual who genetically possesses a specific metabolic pathway or is concomitantly receiving other enzyme-inducing drugs which enhance hepatic transformation will be more likely to produce increased quantities of the toxic metabolite. Metabolic activation of chemically stable drugs may also produce potent alkylating or arylating agents which then covalently bind to tissue macromolecules. Binding of such reactive agents to hepatocytes can result in liver cell necrosis and death. Acetaminophen (paracetamol), which unfortunately has become a popular means of suicide, especially in the U.K., is a good example of a safe drug being metabolized to toxic products. In therapeutic doses, acetaminophen is normally conjugated with glucuronic acid and sulfate. Small amounts are oxidized via the enzyme system containing P-450 producing active metabolites. These are then detoxified in the liver by preferential conjugation with glutathione and safely excreted in the urine. When glutathione is depleted by large doses (above 10g) of acetaminophen and is no longer available for conjugation, the toxic metabolites then irreversibly react with macromolecules in the liver cell leading to hepatic necrosis. Concomitant ingestion of alcohol or barbiturates beforehand "induces" the hepatic microsomal mixed-function oxidase system, which augments the formation of toxic metabolites. Understanding this mechanism has led to a specific therapy for acetaminophen poisoning: enhanced conjugation. Exogenously administered glutathione is unable to penetrate hepatocytes. N-acetylcysteine (Mucomyst) a sulfhydryl compound, ameliorates severe liver damage when administered within twelve hours of acetaminophen ingestion. It is unknown whether acetylcysteine works by inhibiting the mixed-function oxidase system, increasing hepatic glutathione or trapping free radicals which might otherwise attack vulnerable sulfhydryl groups of essential proteins and enzymes. It probably acts like glutathione and prevents the toxic metabolites from binding to liver cell macromolecules. Drugs like cimetidine which inhibit the mixed function oxidase system, perhaps lessening the formation of toxic metabolites, may also have a role.

The second *indirect* mechanism involves drugs such as tetracycline or antimetabolites which impair cellular metabolism. Tetracycline interferes with protein synthesis leading to fat accumulation. Cytotoxic agents such as azathioprine and mercaptopurine can cause liver damage even though these drugs are sometimes given to treat chronic liver disease.

The third *indirect* effect is cholestasis, particularly that associated with C-17 alkylated anabolic and contraceptive steroids. The best recognized of these is estrogen, which inhibits bile formation within the bile canaliculi. Certain individuals are particularly sensitive to estrogens and develop cholestasis during pregnancy or when on oral contraceptives. Patients with diseases such as primary biliary cirrhosis and the Dubin-Johnson syndrome are also abnormally sensitive to estrogen. There is therefore an element of host idiosyncracy which brings out unknown pharmacological effects.

Host idiosyncracy accounts for hepatic injury which occurs in a small portion of exposed individuals given therapeutic doses of the offending drug. The basis may be a hypersensitivity reaction or a metabolic abnormality. The toxicity produced by the agent is not dose-dependent and the lesion can not be produced in experimental animals. There is no constant temporal relation to the institution of drug therapy, and extra-hepatic manifestations of hypersensitivity, such as fever, rash, arthralgia, and eosinophilia, may occur. An accelerated reaction on re-exposure to the drug with a recurrence of fever, rash, and eosinophilia is commonly associated with this type of allergic response. As with the intrinsic hepatotoxins, injury may also be mediated by an idiosyncratic reaction to a metabolite rather than the parent drug. This may be the mechanism of drug reaction with isoniazid, halothane and chlorpromazine.

The reaction from a metabolic aberration may take much longer to develop than a hypersensitivity response and does not show an accelerated response on re-exposure. The susceptible individual may have an underlying immunological defect or may have inherited an abnormality of hepatic enzymes responsible for metabolizing the drug. The distinction between a drug which is an intrinsic hepatoxin as opposed to liver injury produced in a susceptible host is well-illustrated by isoniazid. Although previously thought to cause hepatic injury on the basis of "hypersensitivity", this drug is now known to produce mild hepatic injury in as many as 20 percent of recipients. Even those who develop isoniazid hepatitis lack the usual hallmarks of allergy: rash, fever, and eosinophilia. The basis for the hepatic injury is metabolic; the host susceptibility lies in a unique metabolic pathway. Isoniazid is first acetylated, then hydrolyzed and eventually converted by P-450 oxidases to a chemically reactive acylating agent which is hepatotoxic. Hepatotoxicity is more common in persons who are genetically fast acetylators of isonidazid, such as orientals (see Chapter 8). The production of a toxic metabolite is hastened when another antituberculous drug, rifampicin, which is an enzyme inducer, is also administered.

TYPES OF LIVER INJURY

Acute hepatic injury produced by some drugs may be cytotoxic with overt damage to liver cells, whereas others are predominantly cholestatic with relatively little parenchymal injury. Some agents produce a mixed type with features of both.

Cytotoxic injury involves either liver cell necrosis or occasionally fatty infiltration (steatosis). Hepatic necrosis leads to hepatocellular jaundice in a syndrome resembling viral hepatitis. In fact, the clinical, biochemical (high transaminase, modest alkaline phosphatase elevations), and morphological picture are almost indistinguishable from viral hepatitis. The spectrum ranges from mild liver damage, distinguished only by elevated transaminase levels, to fulminant hepatic failure, with rapid deterioration occuring within days. Steatosis, as occurs with high dose parenteral tetracycline, can cause hepatocytes to become filled with small droplets of fat. There is little necrosis or inflammation. The resulting illness resembles acute fatty liver of pregnancy or Reye's Syndrome in children. Jaundice is slight, transaminase levels are only moderately elevated but prognosis is often grim with an acutely fatal outcome. Direct hepatotoxins can produce both a fatty liver and liver cell necrosis.

Cholestatic injury resembles obstructive jaundice with pruritus, jaundice and elevated alkaline phosphatase. The prognosis is excellent. A mixed picture occurs in some instances with features of both cholestasis and hepatocellular injury. Estrogenic agents can produce a bland cholestasis. Pruritus is followed by jaundice with dark urine weeks to months after initiating this medication. Withdrawal of the agent causes the cholestasis to disappear. Women who have experienced idiopathic jaundice of pregnancy are particularly susceptible to estrogenic agents. Like estrogen, chlorpromazine also causes cholestasis in some patients. Chlorpromazine, however, has both an intrinsic hepatotoxic effect, depressing bile secretion, and also exhibits some features of a drug allergy. The onset may simulate viral hepatitis with fever, rash, arthralgia and nausea. Pruritus, dark urine and jaundice soon follow. Eosinophilia may be present. Liver biopsy not only reveals cholestasis but also shows a portal inflammatory reaction. Cessation of therapy is followed by a slow but complete resolution of the cholestasis. Phenothiazines, oral hypoglycemics, and erythromycin produce a similar cholestatic reaction with associated portal triaditis in a non-dose related reaction.

Other drugs can specifically interfere with bilirubin metabolism without causing a general suppression of bile secretion. The effects range from altered serum binding of bilirubin caused by organic anions, such as salicylates or sulfonamides, hemolytic reactions which increase the bilirubin load resulting in an indirect hyperbilirubinemia, interference with bilirubin uptake, as occurs with cholecystographic contrast agents and rifampicin, to inhibition of bilirubin conjugation, as with novobiocin.

Chronic liver injury can occur in a number of forms. Some drugs such as oxyphenisatin, alphamethyl dopa, and nitrofurantoin can cause chronic active hepatitis leading to cirrhosis. Biliary cirrhosis has been reported to follow the use of chlorpromazine. Granulomatous hepatitis has been associated with allopurinol, indomethacin, and phenylbutazone. Prolonged administration of methotrexate can cause steatosis and fibrosis leading to cirrhosis. Oral contraceptives have been incriminated in hepatic vein thrombosis (Budd-Chiari Syndrome), peliosis hepatis with multiple blood cysts, and hepatic tumors in the form of adenomas, focal nodular hyperplasia, or hepatocellular carcinoma. Exposure to vinyl chloride has been associated with the development of angiosarcoma. These tumors are often asymptomatic with a right upper quadrant mass being found incidently. Hemorrhage into the tumor can lead to acute abdominal pain, while rupture is associated with intraperitoneal bleeding.

TREATMENT OF DRUG INDUCED LIVER INJURY

The management of drug-induced liver injury is largely supportive. Removal of the offending agent in most instances will lead to regression of liver dysfunction. Prevention is an obviously important concept, be it the avoidance of tetracycline during pregnancy or early institution of N-acetylcysteine in acetaminophen overdose.

In unpredictable drug reactions, there may be difficulty in proving a relationship to liver injury. Definitive proof of the drug etiology may depend on a rechallenge with the offending agent and demonstration that the abnormalities have returned. Such a test is only justifiable in the case of a cholestatic reaction where the risk is small. There is seldom any justification for a trial re-exposure to a drug which may have produced hepatic necrosis.

ALCOHOLIC LIVER DISEASE

Alcoholic liver disease includes all types of liver injury associated with heavy alcohol ingestion. What constitutes excess alcohol intake is a moot point. As little as 20g of ethanol (slightly more than one pint of beer) per day can cause liver damage in women; 60g per day suffices for men. Most alcoholics with cirrhosis have imbibed over 160g of alcohol daily (equivalent to 10 pints of beer, 13 ounces of spirits, or two bottles of wine) for at least 10 years. Not everyone who drinks excessively, however, develops liver damage: only 50 percent of those consuming 160g alcohol daily for 25 years will develop cirrhosis. Although the basis for variations in individual susceptibility to the hepatotoxic effects of alcohol are unknown, there is no question that the incidence of alcoholism and alcoholic liver disease is steadily increasing (see Chapter 1). The absence of a history of repeated drunkenness, alcohol withdrawl symptoms or blackouts does not eliminate alcohol abuse. The concept of the alcohol equivalent: 1 beer (12 oz) = 1 glass of wine (6 oz) = 1.5 oz of spirits, provides useful quantitation in establishing a detailed history of alcohol consumption.

Alcohol-induced liver disease appears in three forms: alcoholic fatty liver, alcoholic hepatitis, and Laennec's cirrhosis (Fig. 12. 6). Fatty liver probably is quite common among alcoholics, whereas alcoholic hepatitis and Laennec's cirrhosis occur less frequently but are more severe. The three histological entities can appear independently or may coexist within the same liver.

ALCOHOLIC FATTY LIVER

Alcoholic fatty liver. Ethanol has a direct toxic effect on the liver, the earliest and most common change being fat deposition. It may develop as soon as 8 days after the start of heavy drinking and is an almost invariable finding in the early stages of alcohol abuse. The lesion is benign and reversible and does not lead

Fig. 12.6 Relationships between the three types of liver injury in the alcoholic.

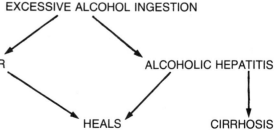

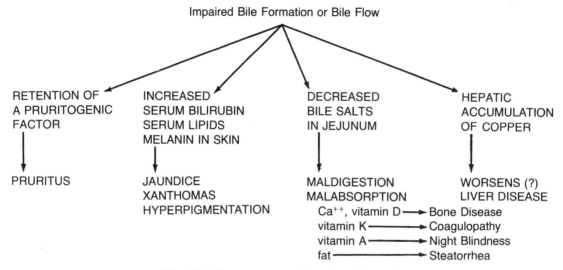

Fig. 12.7 Consequences of chronic cholestasis.

to chronic liver injury. Triglyceride is the fat which accumulates in the liver cells. The source of this fat could be either increased triglyceride synthesis from an influx of fatty acids, mobilized from adipose tissue or from the diet, or increased fatty acid synthesis in the liver, or decreased output from reduced incorporation of triglyceride into very low density lipoprotein. Although the fat laid down in the liver is mainly dietary in origin, a major factor may be accelerated triglyceride formation due to ethanol depressing mitochondrial function and hence decreasing fatty acid oxidation. Malnutrition can also cause a fatty liver and may contribute to the evolution of cirrhosis, even though a nutritious diet does not necessarily protect the liver from the ravages of alcohol abuse (see Metabolic Consequences of Alcohol, Chapter 1).

Morphologically, the liver exhibits diffuse infiltration with lipid droplets of various sizes. The fat is usually present in liver cells as macrovesicular (large-droplet) steatosis, in which the fat forms a single intracellular globule tending to displace the nucleus to the periphery of the cell. Less commonly, the fat may accumulate as microvesicular (small-droplet) steatosis.

There is often a striking lack of clinical symptoms, the most common clinical finding being hepatomegaly. Intrahepatic cholestasis can occur but the presence of encephalopathy, ascites, or other features of chronic liver disease suggests the existence of a more severe form of alcoholic liver disease. Usually liver function tests are only mildly abnormal with a modest elevation in transaminase, alkaline phosphatase and γ glutamyl transpeptidase.

The fatty liver will heal with abstinence from alcohol. The only treatment necessary is that directed at alcoholism.

ALCOHOLIC HEPATITIS

Alcoholic hepatitis is a more severe form of liver injury, which probably represents a transitional lesion leading to the development of cirrhosis. In the absence of cirrhosis, it is probably a reversible lesion (Fig. 12.7). There are no specific clinical or laboratory features of alcoholic hepatitis so that liver biopsy is usually necessary to confirm the diagnosis. The essential histological components of alcoholic hepatitis are liver cell damage, inflammation and fibrosis, which are most pronounced near the terminal hepatic venules (central veins). Liver cell damage appears as swelling of the liver cell and the appearance of characteristic Mallory bodies. Mallory bodies are clumps of eosinophilic, hyaline material in the cytoplasm, which represent degeneration of several cytoplasmic constituents. The inflammatory infiltrate is mainly polymorphonuclear leukocytes, which accumulate in the areas of liver cell damage. Fibrosis is also present and is an important factor in the transition to cirrhosis. Initially, fibrosis surrounds individual cells near the central veins. Later necrotic bridges and fibrous septa link central veins to portal tracts. The presence of inflammation and necrosis suggests that there may be an immunological mechanism for liver cell destruction and the development of cirrhosis. Fatty infiltration and cirrhosis may also be present, though neither are essential for the diagnosis.

The clinical features of alcoholic hepatitis vary from a relatively asymptomatic illness to severe liver disease. In symptomatic patients, anorexia, nausea and vomiting, malaise, upper abdominal pain, weight loss and fever are characteristic features. Morning nausea with dry retching represents a withdrawal phenomena. The most frequent physical findings are fever and tender hepatomegaly, sometimes associated with an arterial bruit. Two features of alcoholism may be present: Dupuytren's contracture of the palmar fascia and bilateral parotid gland enlargement from malnutrition. Other findings of more significant liver disease may be evident: splenomegaly, ascites, edema, spider angiomata, palmer erythema or jaundice. Cholestasis frequently worsens even while patients appear to be recovering clinically, but eventually improves. Hypoglycemic episodes can also occur. The more symptomatic cases are associated with a mortality ranging up to 30 percent. Death may result due to fulminant hepatic failure from progression. Most cases resolve over a period of weeks to months.

Laboratory tests show a polymorphonuclear leukocytosis and a modestly elevated serum transaminase, about 4–5 times normal. The rise in aspartate aminotransferase (AST, SGPT) is not accompanied by much of an increase in alanine aminotransferase (ALT, SGOT). Thus a AST/ALT ratio greater than 2 is more frequent in patients with alcoholic hepatitis than viral hepatitis. Elevated serum gammaglutamyl transpeptidase (γGT) is a good screening test for excessive drinking although not specific. Marked intrahepatic cholestasis takes place in 25 percent of patients, resulting in elevated alkaline phosphatase, bilirubin and cholesterol levels. The serum may be lipemic with high triglycerides.

Other causes of liver injury in patients with heavy alcohol consumption exist. Such liver disorders as cholangitis, acute hepatitis, or some form of chronic hepatitis can occur in alcoholic subjects. Liver biopsy is often necessary to confirm the alcoholic nature of the lesion, because the clinical and biochemical features frequently do not distinguish between alcoholic and nonalcoholic liver injury. In the presence of pain, fever, and cholestasis, alcoholic pancreatitis and choledocholithiasis must also be considered as possible causes.

Treatment is largely empirical. Patients should be hospitalized when jaundice, features of hepatic failure, or unexplained fever are present. An adequate diet, bedrest, and abstinence from alcohol are traditional. Because immunological mechanisms may play a role in the pathogenesis of alcoholic hepatitis, corticosteroids have been tried, but studies have so far given conflicting results. No specific therapy for this disease exists as yet.

ALCOHOLIC CIRRHOSIS

Of the estimated 9,000,000 alcohol abusers in North America, 10 percent will develop cirrhosis, making alcoholic cirrhosis the leading cause of chronic liver injury and a major cause of death. Cirrhosis results from widespread death of liver cells which results in its two morphological ingredients: fibrosis and nodular regeneration. Fibrosis implies an excess of collagenous tissue resulting from collapse of pre-existing fibres (passive) or by the formation of new fibres (active). Hepatic fibrosis can occur because of either augmented collagen synthesis or reduced connective tissue biodegradation. Although newly formed collagen fibres distort the liver architecture in many forms of chronic liver disease, fibrosis does not equal cirrhosis. The presence of regenerative nodules are necessary to define cirrhosis histologically. In cirrhosis, the normal lobular architecture is lost, being replaced by regenerating nodules separated from one another by connective tissue layers. Within the nodules, the hepatocytes form plates more than one cell thick. Cirrhosis has been morphologically classified into *micronodular* cirrhosis, which is characterized by nodules of fairly equal size, usually less than 1 cm in diameter and septa of almost equal width, and *macronodular* cirrhosis, with nodules of up to 5 cm in diameter and with broad septa. Micronodular or Laennec's cirrhosis appears to be the early lesion which can then progress to macronodular; many cases show features of both. Despite apparent waves of necrosis followed by regeneration with increased collagen formation, progressive liver cell loss results in a small, shrunken, hard, liver. The fibrosis and regenerating nodules cause vascular distortion, which increases pressure in the portal vein resulting in portal hypertension.

Alcoholic cirrhosis may be clinically silent but can present with features of alcoholic hepatitis, portal hypertension and/or hepatocellular failure. The patient with established cirrhosis often shows a round abdomen loaded with fluid, thin extremities reflecting muscle wasting, jaundice, spiderlike telangiectasia (spider angiomata) over the upper extremities, and features of malnutrition with multiple vitamin deficiencies.

Hepatic Effects

The following features may be evident, being directly related to cirrhosis and excessive alcohol intake.

1. *Altered sexual function*: in men, hypogonadism is characterized by impotence, infertility, testicular atrophy, decreased body hair and beard growth, and reduced size of the prostate. Feminization features gynecomastia, spider angioma, palmer erythema, and even a female body habitus and distribution of body hair. In women, there is a high incidence of secondary amenorrhea, infertility and reduced libido. These endocrine phenomena may be related to alcohol directly causing gonadal failure, hypothalamic-pituitary dysfunction and/or increased estrogen with reduced testosterone levels. The relative importance of alcohol versus hepatic dysfunction are not clear.

2. The *liver* may be enlarged early on as in fatty liver or alcoholic hepatitis, but it later becomes shrunken, firm, and irregular with regenerating nodules. The presence of a bruit in the absence of alcoholic hepatitis suggests the development of hepatocellular carcinoma.

3. *Jaundice*, if progressive, suggests either alcoholic hepatitis is superimposed or the cirrhosis is at an end-stage.

4. *Ascites* features fluid retention within the abdomen, along with peripheral edema.

5. *Portal hypertension* is evident by splenomegaly, abdominal wall collateral veins, hemorrhoids and upper gastrointestinal bleeding from varices.

6. *Hepatorenal syndrome* results in progressive renal failure.

7. *Extremities*: digital clubbing is usually seen in more chronic forms of cirrhosis such as primary biliary cirrhosis; leukonychia (white nails) has been related to protein catabolism and hypoalbuminema; periungual erythema and palmer erythema may result from the hyperestrogenemic state, while Dupuytren's contracture is alcohol-related.

8. *Hepatocellular carcinoma* may supervene in 5–15 percent of patients with alcoholic cirrhosis, usually as the macronodular form.

9. *Iron overload* can occur with iron deposits mainly in parenchymal liver cells but also in reticuloendothelial (Kupffer) cells (hemosiderosis). Hemosiderosis has no pathological significance, being possibly due to increased iron absorption, the iron content of alcohol beverages, hemolytic episodes, or portocaval shunting. Idiopathic (familial) hemochromatosis may occur in alcoholics with coexistent features of hemochromatosis and alcoholic liver disease.

10. *Gallstones* develop in up to 30 percent of patients with alcoholic cirrhosis, twice that found in a comparable non-cirrhotic population: usually as pigment stones.

Systemic Effects

Alcohol abuse, attendant malnutrion, and cirrhosis can also have systemic effects:

1. *Gastrointestinal*
   a. esophagitis, gastritis, duodenitis, and peptic ulcer disease have been associated with alcohol use.
   b. Mallory-Weiss syndrome, the tear at the gastroesophageal junction being due to vomiting.
   c. diarrhea, steatorrhea. A variety of substances are malabsorbed in chronic malnourished alcoholics: D-xylose, folic acid, vitamin A., thiamine, glucose, sodium and water, fat, nitrogen, and vitamin B_{12}. Mild steatorrhea, usually less than 10 g per day, occurs in 50 percent of patients with cirrhosis. In 10 percent, however, steatorrhea can be more severe, exceeding 30 gms a day. The possible causes include pancreatic insufficiency, reduced intraluminal bile salts below the critical micellar concentration, altered small intestinal absorptive function and the use of drugs such as antacids, neomycin or cholestyramine.
   d. chronic relapsing pancreatitis.

2. *Hematological*
   a. Anemia is commonly due to folate deficiency, hemolysis, or iron deficiency as a result of gastrointestinal bleeding.
   b. Pancytopenia may result from a direct suppressive effect of alcohol on the bone marrow or from hypersplenism. Thrombocytopenia is common.
   c. Coagulation disorders may occur secondary to inadequate vitamin K absorption or metabolism. Disseminated intravascular coagulopathy can accompany acute hepatic necrosis.

3. *Cardiac effects* may be present as a cardiomyopathy due to alcohol depressing ventricular function, or secondary to thiamine deficency (beriberi heart disease).

4. *Respiratory complications* occur in the form of aspiration pneumonia, trauma, and a heightened risk of infections especially with tuberculosis and Klebsiella pneumonia.

5. *Metabolic effects* include hypoglycemia, hyperuricemia, or hypertriglyceridemia.

6. *Alcoholic myopathy* can present acutely during heavy drinking, with pain, tenderness, weight loss,

or progressive proximal weakness. Hypokalemia or hypophosphatemia contribute to muscle weakness.

7. *Nervous system.* The wide range of acute and chronic disorders of the central nervous system are detailed in Chapter 1. Peripheral neuropathies are common. Hepatic encephalopathy is discussed below and in Chapter 14.

Alcoholic cirrhosis should be suspected in a patient with a history of alcohol abuse who develops features of liver disease. Laboratory tests may reveal hepatic dysfunction, with the prothrombin time and serum albumin particularly reflecting the severity of liver disease. Liver scan may show decreased and irregular hepatic uptake, an enlarged spleen, and increased uptake by the spleen and bone marrow. The definitive diagnosis of cirrhosis, however, requires morphological evidence of the disease. If no contraindication exists, most cases warrant a percutaneous liver biopsy to confirm the diagnosis and stage the disease process.

The prognosis for patients with alcoholic cirrhosis definitely improves when they stop drinking. The 5 year survival in one series rose from 40 percent in those who continued to drink to over 60 percent in patients who abstained. Whether or not total abstinence is necessary for such improvement is unknown. Survival is less in individuals from lower socioeconomic groups and in those with severe liver disease causing variceal bleeding or ascites. Survival rates are only 10–30 percent 5 years after the onset of ascites and 5–10 percent after the occurrence of hemorrhage from esophageal varices. *Sudden deterioration in a patient with stable cirrhosis should raise the possibility of a complicating condition* such as a gastrointestinal bleed, infection (such as pneumonia or spontaneous bacterial peritonitis), hepatocellular carcinoma, or portal vein thrombosis. The cause of death in most cirrhotic individuals is related to bleeding esophageal varices or hepatic failure. The predictive features implying a poor prognosis include: abnormal liver function tests with prolonged prothrombin time and low serum albumin; jaundice, ascites, esophageal varices, hepatic encephalopathy, or hepatorenal failure.

Therapy is largely directed at eliminating the cause, alcohol, and treating the complications. Hospitalization is often necessary for an initial evaluation or for a complication. Adequate dietary intake with vitamin supplements is often necessary. Sedatives such as the benzodiazepines may be necessary to control alcohol withdrawal symptoms. Alcohol induces the liver enzymes used in its own catabolism so that the alcoholic may be able to metabolize drugs more rapidly until such time as the liver is significantly damaged. In addition, a tolerance to the sedative

properties of many drugs develops. Once significant liver disease supervenes, the pharmacokinetics of those drugs in which liver metabolism is involved becomes disturbed so that drug therapy may have to be individually tailored.

OTHER CAUSES OF CIRRHOSIS

Cirrhosis is best defined morphologically as a diffuse process characterized by fibrosis and the conversion of normal liver architecture into structurally abnormal nodules (1975 WHO definition). The morphological features of cirrhosis, nodular regeneration of the parenchyma and formation of new connective tissue, does not necessarily reveal the original cause. By the time cirrhosis becomes established, the pathogenetic events in terms of inflammation, necrosis or fibrosis may no longer be evident. Although the clinical, functional and morphological aspects of cirrhosis frequently overlap, some entities have distinctive features.

CRYPTOGENIC CIRRHOSIS

Termed "postnecrotic cirrhosis," it is a catchall category for cirrhosis of unknown etiology. As the name implies, the etiological factors have not been established. In North America, it is second only to alcohol as the most common cause of cirrhosis, and may be even more frequent in the United Kingdom. This entity probably represents the aftermath of viral hepatitis which has progressed to chronic active hepatitis, either as hepatitis B or hepatitis non-A, non-B. Some patients with cryptogenic cirrhosis may have been exposed to toxins or drugs associated with chronic active hepatitis. Others may be covert alcoholics or have α1-antitrypsin deficiency.

The morphological picture is not distinctive. Most times it resembles macronodular cirrhosis with large regenerative nodules surrounded by broad bands of fibrous tissue irregularily distributed throughout the liver.

There are no characteristic clinical features. The disease is often latent, being unrecognized during life or presenting late in the form of portal hypertension with splenomegaly and esophageal varices. Liver biopsy is necessary for a diagnosis. Unless its cause can be found there is no specific therapy.

PRIMARY BILIARY CIRRHOSIS

This is an immunological disease affecting the small bile ducts leading to features of chronic cholestasis. The synonym, "chronic nonsuppurative destructive cholangitis", is perhaps more appropriate from a pathogenic viewpoint as cirrhosis only appears at a late stage. It may also be considered a "dry gland" syndrome with damage primarily involving ductular epithelium in many organs, causing biliary and pancreatic hyposecretion, xerostomia and keratoconjunctivitis (the sicca complex). The chronic cholestasis causes retention of copper, which is normally excreted in the bile. Whether or not increased concentrations of hepatic copper contribute to the continuing liver damage is unknown, but chelation therapy does not appear to prolong life. The copper levels in primary biliary cirrhosis often reach those found in untreated Wilson's disease, sufficient to be deposited as Kayser-Fleischer rings in the cornea.

The basic histological lesion is bile duct destruction by granulomatous inflammation (non-suppurative destructive cholangitis). Later, bile duct proliferation appears and portal inflammation extends beyond the limiting plate in a pattern like chronic active hepatitis. As the inflammation subsides, fibrosis links adjacent portal areas. Ultimately cirrhosis supervenes; the liver is entirely converted to nodules by fibrous septa. Few bile ducts remain.

Predominantly a disease of middle aged women, primary biliary cirrhosis typically begins insidiously and progresses very slowly, ultimately leading to death from hepatic failure after many years. The earliest symptom is generalized pruritus, followed within 2 years by jaundice. Hyperpigmentation from melanin deposition may appear even earlier than the jaundice. Some may be totally asymptomatic, being detected by finding unsuspected hepatomegaly or an elevated alkaline phosphatase on a routine evaluation. Some 20 percent present with fairly advanced liver disease: jaundice, bleeding esophageal varices or ascites.

Patients appear healthy and surprisingly well-nourished throughout most of the course of their disease. Hepatomegaly is a rather constant finding, while splenomegaly appears a few years later reflecting the development of portal hypertension. Features of chronic cholestasis soon become apparent (Fig. 12.7) in the form of dark urine, pale stool, deepening jaundice (often to a greenish color), and the development of steatorrhea and xanthomatous lipid deposits. Disordered bone and calcium metabolism is particularly distressing. Osteodystrophy including both osteomalacia and osteoporosis primarily reflects the reduced vitamin D and calcium absorption in the gut. Finger clubbing occurs in one-quarter of patients, often accompanied by periostitis which causes tenderness over the bones of the lower legs (hypertrophic osteoarthropathy). Gallstones, present in nearly 40 percent, are usually asymptomatic. Primary biliary cirrhosis has been associated with several collagen disorders including scleroderma.

Liver function tests reveal a cholestatic pattern, the earliest abnormality being an increased alkaline phosphatase and 5' nucleotidase. Serum transaminases are usually only increased 3 to 4 times. IgM is frequently elevated. The mitochondrial antibody is very sensitive being positive in more than 99 percent of cases, but not specific, also being present in 30 percent of cases with chronic active hepatitis and in collagen diseases.

The diagnosis of primary biliary cirrhosis rests upon a characteristic setting of a middle aged woman with cholestasis who has a positive mitochondrial antibody. A liver biopsy should be performed as the findings may be diagnostic. Extrahepatic bile duct obstruction must be excluded by an ultrasound examination or, if anicteric, an oral cholecystogram. In doubtful cases, transhepatic or endoscopic cholangiography should be performed.

The prognosis for the early stages of primary biliary cirrhosis is extremely good. Treatment should be directed at symptoms which are largely due to chronic cholestasis. Early on, pruritus can often be controlled with topical therapy in the form of oatmeal baths or a trial of a choleretic agent such as phenobarbital to improve bile output. Cholestyramine binds bile salts and/or the pruritogenic agent within the intestine, interrupting the enterohaptic circulation. It will relieve the itching so long as some bile enters the intestine, as evidenced by colored stools. Methyl testosterone, a C-17 alkyl substituted androgen, can also relieve itching. Because of its adverse effects like masculinization and worsening cholestasis, the drug should be reserved for intractable cases. Phototherapy in the form of a simple sunlamp may help improve the jaundice. Steatorrhea can be managed by restricting the dietary fat to less than 40 gm per day and adding pancreatic enzyme replacement and vitamin-calcium supplementation. There is as yet no proven therapy for the disease itself. D-penicillamine is currently undergoing trials because of its copper-chelating and immunological effects.

SECONDARY BILIARY CIRRHOSIS

This is produced by prolonged mechanical obstruction of the large intrahepatic or extrahepatic bile ducts. The most common cause of this type of biliary cirrhosis in adults is chronic bile duct obstruction from post-operative stricture or by choledocholithiasis often with infectious cholangitis superimposed. In infants, congenital atresia of the intra-or-extrahepatic bile duct system can rapidly lead to cirrhosis.

Pain, fever, and a previous history of biliary surgery are the characteristic historical events, which suggest the diagnosis of secondary biliary cirrhosis. The mitochondrial antibody is negative, while ultrasonography may show dilated bile ducts in the liver and indicate cholelithiasis. A definitive diagnosis may require cholangiography. Treatment is by surgical relief of mechanical obstruction.

Table 12.9   Causes of Hemochromatosis

I. Idiopathic Hemochromatosis
II. Secondary Hemochromatosis
   due to:
   A. Anemia and Ineffective Erythropoiesis (Erythropoietic hemochromatosis) thalassemia major, sideroblastic anemia
   B. Liver Disease
      alcoholic cirrhosis, after portocaval anastamosis
   C. High Oral Iron Intake
      medicinal iron, in alcoholic beverages ("Bantus siderosis")

HEMOCHROMATOSIS

Hemochromatosis refers to a generalized increase in body iron storage with resultant tissue damage, in contrast to *hemosiderosis* where there is either a focal or general increase in iron storage without evidence of tissue damage. The original description of hemochromatosis described a triad of diabetes mellitus, skin pigmentation, and hepatomegaly with eventual cirrhosis ("bronze diabetes"). The term has now been broadened to include a group of disorders characterized by a progressive increase in total body iron with deposition of iron in parenchymal cells (Table 12.9).

This is an iron storage disease in which the excess iron causes parenchymal damage. Total body iron in normal humans is approximately 5 gm, of which less than $1/3$ is in a storage form. One-third of the stored iron is found in the liver, principally wrapped up as a colloid inside a protein shell termed ferritin. This internal reservoir not only supplies iron when needed, but also being stored as ferritin, protects against iron toxicity. When excessive iron is introduced into the body, both hepatocytes and Kupffer cells accumulate large amounts of ferritin. Kupffer cells tend to store relatively more of the excess non haem iron in forms other than ferritin, such as hemosiderin. The reticuloendothelial system normally has only a limited role in iron storage unless iron is administered intravenously, when it becomes the preferred site for deposition.

Idiopathic Hemochromatosis

This is an uncommon entity, occuring in less than 1 in 10,000 births. It is characterized by failure to control intestinal iron absorption. The result is a progressive accumulation of iron so that total body iron rises to 20–50 gm. Iron is deposited in the liver, primarily in the parenchymal cells, and also in other organs including the pancreas, heart, pituitary, adrenals, spleen and gastric mucosa. The basic metabolic defect for increased intestinal absorption is unknown but appears to be inherited. For example, 25 to 50 percent of first-degree relatives show abnormalities of iron metabolism. There is also an association with two HLA types, A3 and B14. The exact genetics are unknown, although the pattern appears to be autosomal recessive. The entity occurs ten times more frequently in males, women presumably being protected by iron loss from menstruation, pregnancy and lactation.

Secondary Hemochromatosis

This condition can be associated with anemia and ineffective erythropoiesis. Anemias, such as thalassemia major and sideroblastic anemia, have a defect in red cell production associated with normal or increased iron absorption. Increased iron absorption is a major component to iron accumulation and probably is stimulated by the increased erythropoietic activity. Since the iron is not properly utilized, it is preferentially stored in the liver and reticuloendothial system. In addition, these patients may also receive multiple blood transfusions, which only enhance iron accumulation. More than 100 units of blood must be transfused before excess iron accumulates, usually in the reticuloendothelial system and only later in the parenchymal cell. Simple parenteral administration of iron in the form of transfusions or as iron preparations results in reticuloendothelial cell overload, hemosiderosis. The patients with abnormalities in erythropoiesis are different in that iron is also deposited in parenchymal tissues.

Iron overload may occur in alcoholics. The cause of increased iron accumulation is multifactoral: alcohol beverages especially red wine often contain large quantities of iron; alcohol itself may enhance iron absorption; hemolysis or ineffective erythropoiesis with folate deficiency may be an added factor, and increased iron deposition occurs after portacaval anastamosis. The Bantu natives of South Africa brew their beer in iron vessels and so develop hemochromatosis by consuming excessive iron in an alcoholic beverage. Whether or not prolonged ingestion of oral iron in a normal subject can produce hemochromatosis is unknown.

The major histological feature is increased iron deposition in many organs particularly the liver and pancreas, but also in endocrine glands and the heart. Increased melanin in the epidermis causes the bronze pigmentation, whereas the iron tends to impart a slate-grey colour. In the early stages of liver involvement, hemosiderin is deposited first in parenchymal cells and later in Kupffer cells. As fibrous septa develop the picture progresses to the pattern of fibrosis, and eventually with parenchymal regeneration, an irregular multilobular cirrhosis. The pancreas also exhibits fibrosis and parenchymal degeneration with iron deposition. Many endocrine glands are involved, but testicular atrophy is secondary to the pituitary involvement.

The classical picture is a lethargic middle aged male exhibiting hepatomegaly, diabetes mellitus and excessive skin pigmentation either bronzing or as a metallic grey. Many of the features of chronic liver disease are present; splenomegaly and portal hypertension eventually develop. Testicular atrophy and loss of libido are common. Arthropathy, starting in the small joints of the hand, may progress to a polyarthritis involving larger joints in about half of all patients. Acute synovitis may occur in the knees with deposition of calcium pyrophosphate (pseudogout or chondrocalcinosis). Hepatocellular carcinoma develops in about 15 percent, twice as frequently as with other types of cirrhosis.

Laboratory investigation should include standard liver tests and blood examinations for evidence of anemia and abnormal erythropoiesis. Certain tests best screen for excessive parenchymal iron stores, including: (1) serum iron concentration, (2) percent transferrin saturation and (3) serum ferritin. These tests are not infallible. Elevated ferritin concentrations unrelated to increased iron storage may be found in such diseases as acute and chronic liver damage, infection, and neoplastic disorders. Bone marrow iron may give an index of iron overload, but liver biopsy is necessary to diagnose hemochromatosis. It not only assesses the extent of tissue damage, but permits histochemical estimation of tissue iron. One way to quantitate iron storage involves the chelating agent, desferrioxamine. In hemochromatosis, parenterally administered desferrioxamine greatly increases urinary iron excretion to above 10 mg iron per 24 hours.

The definitive test and treatment of iron overload is repeated phlebotomies. A 500 ml unit of blood contains slightly more than 200 mg iron. In the presence of excess iron stores, blood regeneration is rapid with hemoglobin production rising 6 to 8 fold. If a few phlebotomies at weekly intervals precipitate an anemia then iron stores were probably normal. Conversely, with iron stores above 20 gm, 2 to 3 years of weekly phlebotomies would be required to deplete such large stores. Relatives of patients with idiopathic hemochromatosis should be screened with serum iron, percent transferrin saturation, and serum ferritin levels. Although phlebotomy therapy prolongs life in established hemochromatosis, it may not prevent the development of hepatocellular carcinoma and may not improve the hypogonadism, arthropathy or portal hypertension.

WILSON'S DISEASE

Also called hepatolenticular degeneration, this is a rare disorder of copper metabolism which is inherited as an autosomal recessive trait. The metabolic defect is characterized by a decreased synthesis of ceruloplasmin (the copper-carrying protein in serum), an abnormal copper binding protein in the liver, and decreased biliary excretion of copper. This results in the accumulation of copper in the liver and the subsequent release of free copper into the circulation allowing it to accumulate in other organs such as the basal ganglia of the brain, the cornea and the renal tubules. Clinical manifestations of copper excess usually appear in adolescence or early adulthood, rarely before the age of 6 years.

Hepatic manifestations often precede the neurological signs especially in the child or adolescent. Liver involvement can manifest as acute hepatitis similar to viral hepatitis, fulminant hepatic failure, chronic active hepatitis or cirrhosis identical to that of postnecrotic (macronodular) cirrhosis. Liver biopsy may not be distinctive even with special copper stains.

Neurological features tend to predominate in adults and may not necessarily be accompanied by liver disease. Disorders of movement predominate with tremor, incoordination, rigidity and dystonia. Awkward gait, drooling, slurred speech, dysphagia, and mental deterioration may develop.

Proximal renal tubular damage results in the Fanconi syndrome. The most dramatic expression of copper accumulation is the appearance of Kayser-

Fleischer rings, a golden-brown or greenish-yellow discoloration in the limbic region of the cornea due to deposition of copper in Descemet's membrane. If not detected with the unaided eye, a slitlamp examination can establish their presence. These are not always present or specific for the diagnosis of Wilson's disease: they appear in primary biliary cirrhosis as well.

Diagnosis of Wilson's disease is made by finding reduced serum ceruloplasmin (less than 20 mg/dl), elevated urinary copper excretion and increased liver copper concentration obtained at the time of biopsy. None of these tests are infallible. There are various loading tests with radiocopper which measure incorporation into ceruloplasmin; these sometimes can discriminate the more difficult cases.

Therapy uses D-penicillamine to remove the excess copper quickly while monitoring the response with urinary copper excretion. Therapy can be life saving, but must be life long. A definitive diagnosis of Wilson's disease also mandates the screening of siblings and other relatives for possible asymptomatic Wilson's Disease.

α_1-ANTIPROTEASE DEFICIENCY

This deficiency is due to failure of abnormal α_1-globulin (α, antitrypsin) to be excreted by the liver. A point mutation causes a single amino acid alteration, affecting the molecule's ability to attach sialic acid during glycosylation. In the most severe deficiency, the PiZZ molecule is retained in the liver causing the characteristic appearance of eosinophilic globules which are readily detected by a positive periodic acid-Shiff (PAS) stain. The liver damage may result not from an excessive accumulation of an abnormal glycoprotein but rather uncontrolled proteolytic digestion by cellular (lysosomal) enzymes.

About 10 percent of children with the homozygous deficiency (PiZZ) will develop significant liver disease making alpha 1-antiprotease deficiency a common factor in cirrhosis of infancy and childhood. Emphysema is uncommon in these younger patients, however, pronounced alpha 1 antiprotease deficiency can be associated with severe panlobular emphysema in adults (See Chapter 5).

COMPLICATIONS OF CIRRHOSIS

The key effect is reduced liver cell mass and altered hepatic hemodynamics in which blood flow is diverted past the liver parenchyma.

PORTAL HYPERTENSION

Portal hypertension is a sustained elevation of pressure in the portal vein above the normal level of 5–10 mm Hg. Portal pressure can be directly measured by transhepatic or umbilical vein catheterization, both technically difficult procedures, or indirectly by determining intrasplenic or wedged hepatic vein pressure. Intrasplenic pressure estimates portal pressure from a needle inserted into the pulp of the spleen. Wedged hepatic vein pressure is recorded via a catheter introduced from an arm vein through the vena cava into a hepatic venous radical unit; it is tightly wedged against the liver. Values above 20 mmHg are indicative of portal hypertension.

Portal hypertension can occur from increased blood flow or increased vascular resistance anywhere along the course of portal blood flow from the portal vein to the heart. Table 12.10 is a classification of portal hypertension based on the level at which the abnormality occurs.

In *presinusoidal* portal hypertension the wedged hepatic vein pressure is normal. Since portal pressure is elevated, a significant pressure gradient exists between the portal and hepatic venous systems (>5 mm Hg).

In *sinusoidal* portal hypertension both the wedged hepatic vein and portal pressures are elevated resulting in only a small pressure gradient (<5 mm Hg). Hepatic blood flow is diminished because sinusoidal flow is hindered at different levels of the sinusoidal bed.

Hepatocellular function is usually not impaired in presinusoidal portal hypertension. Otherwise, the underlying liver disease tends to dominate the clinical picture, even though certain features can be specifically attributed to portal hypertension *per se*:

1. *Portal-Systemic Venous Collaterals.* The resultant collateral flow between the portal and systemic beds produces dilated veins around the gastroesophageal junction (esophageal and gastric varices), the rectum (hemorrhoids) and the falciform ligament of the liver (periumbilical or abdominal wall collaterals). Anterior abdominal wall collaterals especially around the umbilicus ("caput medusae") are a helpful sign of portal hypertension. Their radiation is centrifugal, away from the umbilicus, in contrast to the dilated abdominal wall vessels from inferior vena cava obstruction in which drainage flows upward above the umbilicus to reach the superior vena cava. The presence of a loud venous murmur at the umbilicus in association with dilated abdominal wall veins is termed the "Cruveilhier-Baumgarten syndrome".

Table 12.10　**Classification of Portal Hypertension**

Types	Causes	Portal Pressure Measurement* Wedged Hepatic Venous Pressure	Intrasplenic Pressure
I. Presinusoidal			
A. Extrahepatic (Prehepatic)	—Portal or splenic vein thrombosis	normal	↑
	—Increased splenic flow with massive splenomegaly or A-V fistula in splanchnic bed		
B. Intrahepatic	—Schistosomiasis	normal to ↑	↑
	—Portal infiltration sarcoidosis, lymphomas, granulomas		
	—Toxins arsenicals, vinyl chloride		
II. Sinusoidal			
A. Intrahepatic	—Cirrhosis	↑	↑
	—Alcoholic hepatitis		
	—Fatty liver		
	—Veno-occlusive disease		
B. Extrahepatic (Posthepatic)	—Hepatic vein occlusion (Budd-Chiari Syndrome)	↑	↑
	—Congestive heart failure		
	—Constrictive pericarditis		

★ When the liver is normal, the wedged hepatic venous pressure measures sinusoidal pressure. In cirrhosis, wedged hepatic venous pressure reflects portal pressure. Intrasplenic pressure measures portal venous pressure.

The murmur is due to flow through a congenitally patent umbilical vein.

2. *Splenomegaly.* An enlarged spleen is an important diagnostic sign of portal hypertension, being detected either by palpation, most sensitively performed with the patient in the right decubitus position or on radionucleotide scan. The spleen enlarges from passive congestion and may cause secondary hypersplenism with anemia, leukopenia and thrombocytopenia ("Banti's syndrome").

3. *Ascites.* Peritoneal fluid accumulation can only develop when portal hypertension is associated with some element of intrinsic liver disease. Ascites is therefore not commonly a feature of presinusoidal portal hypertension.

The diagnosis of portal hypertension is usually indirect, based on the findings listed above. Esophageal varices are best detected by fibroptic endoscopy but can also be seen on barium swallow. Liver scan may be of some help in identifying diffuse liver disease and portal hypertension. Portal pressure measurements will document that portal hypertension exists and generally locate the obstruction to either a pre-sinusoidal or sinusoidal (intrahepatic) site. Anatomic definition of the site of obstruction and the collateral circulation comes from splenic or portal venography. The venous phase of a mesenteric angiogram will often demonstrate the enlarged portal vein, as can ultrasonography. Liver biopsy will detect any intra-hepatic cause of obstruction.

Bleeding from esophageal and/or gastric varices, the major complication of portal hypertension, may vary in severity from slow and chronic to massive exsanguination with hematemesis and melena. In most instances the bleeding will spontaneously cease but the prognosis depends on the underlying liver disease. In the presence of jaundice, ascites, and encephalopathy the mortality easily reaches 80 percent. In fact, almost half of all deaths in patients with cirrhosis result from bleeding gastroesophageal varices.

In managing acutely bleeding varices, the primary effort must be directed at adequate blood replacement and correction of any bleeding diathesis. An accurate endoscopic diagnosis is necessary, especially in alcoholic cirrhosis, because the bleeding site is frequently another lesion: acute erosive gastritis, peptic ulcer disease or the Mallory-Weiss syndrome. If bleeding does not stop spontaneously, two immediate but temporary forms of therapy are available. Vasopressin intravenously constricts the splanchnic resistance vessels, lowering portal venous pressure. Use of vasopressin reduces the amount of blood replacement necessary but does not change the eventual outcome. Unfortunately, tachyphylaxis soon develops after repeated systemic injections and vasopressin administration can precipitate coronary artery spasm. An alternative form of therapy is local compression of varices with the double-balloon, Sengstaken-Blakemore tube. The principle is to produce gastroesophageal tamponade by applying traction to the tube and pressing the inflated gastric balloon against the cardia. The esophageal balloon may also be inflated to a pressure of 20 to 30 mmHg to compress the esophageal varices. Nasopharyngeal secretions are aspirated through a lumen opening above the esophageal balloon. Such compression is often quite successful in controlling bleeding from esophageal varices, but carries many complications including airway obstruction, aspiration pneumonia or ulceration-rupture of the esophagus. Such tubes require meticulous care, and this procedure should only be undertaken in intensive care units. Thus, vasopressin with its short-acting effect is probably the preferred initial mode of therapy, even though there is some question of its efficacy. The aim of emergency management of patients with bleeding varices is to first maintain an adequate circulating blood volume and stop the hemorrhage by a non-operative approach since any emergency surgery has a high mortality.

Prevention of variceal bleeding has largely involved surgical decompression of the portal system, diverting portal blood into the systemic circulation through a portal systemic anastamosis. Prophylactic shunts in patients with varices, who have not yet bled, is unwarranted; life is not prolonged and not all patients with varices will bleed. Elective surgery should be reserved for patients with a documented variceal bleed. In these people, there is a 66 percent chance that bleeding will recur and each bleed carries a mortality of about 50 percent. Visualization of the portal vein and its two tributaries, the superior mesenteric and splenic veins, is essential preoperatively; a thrombosed portal vein dramatically changes the surgical approach. Various modifications of portacaval anastamoses have been tried. The standard procedure is a portacaval shunt in which the portal vein is joined to the inferior vena cava. Operative mortality is low in good-risk patients. Such surgery is extremely effective in preventing recurrent variceal hemorrhage so long as the shunt remains patent. Loss of portal blood flow to the liver and progression of the chronic liver disease lead to further deterioration in liver function. Portal systemic encephalopathy develops in one-third to one-half of patients after a standard portacaval shunt, presumably because toxic products from the intestine are shunted past the liver to affect the brain. An even higher percentage can be shown to have subclinical encephalopathy. Long-term survival is, in fact, no better in shunted patients who die from liver failure, compared to non-shunted patients who die from variceal bleeding. With bilirubin <2 mg/dl (35 umol/L), albumin >35 gm/L, no ascites, no encephalopathy and normal nutrition, the operative risk is low; with bilirubin >3 gm/dl (50 umol/L), albumin < 30 g/L, poorly controlled ascites, advanced encephalopathy and poor nutrition, the operative risk is high. The recent use of a splenorenal shunt has reduced the frequency of postoperative encephalopathy to 10 percent. The operation itself is technically difficult, and a full evaluation of the long-term results are still pending. Portal caval shunt surgery is warranted in patients with presinusoidal hypertension where liver involvement is minimal and in patients with non-alcoholic liver disease, such as primary biliary cirrhosis, especially if their clinical status is good.

Newer less aggressive approaches to prevent recurrent variceal bleeding are currently under investigation. Foremost among these is injection scleroptherapy in which sclerosing solutions are injected into or near the esophageal varices under direct vision through an endoscope. There may also be a place for chronic lowering of the portal pressure using β adrenergic blocking agents like propranolol.

ASCITES

Ascites is the accumulation of free fluid in the peritoneal cavity. The ascitic fluid can be characterized as either a transudate which is clear and amber, or an exudate likely to be turbid or bloody, or chylous which is creamy and contains triglycerides (Table 12.11). Ascites is a cardinal manifestation of decompensated cirrhosis, although it may be associated with congestive heart failure, the nephrotic syndrome, disseminated carcinomatosis, or pancreatitis. Ascites usually appears in a setting of portal hypertension combined with hepatic insufficiency. The complex mechanism of free peritoneal fluid formation consists of general factors which cause salt and water retention, plus the presence of portal hypertension and hepatic lymph overproduction which localize the edema to the peritoneal cavity. Portal hypertension increases capillary hydrostatic pressure while hypoalbuminemia reduces plasma oncotic pressure. This imbalance of Starling forces drives fluid out of the liver capsule and splanchnic bed into the peritoneal cavity. The site of portal venous obstruction is an important factor in ascites formation. In presinusoidal hypertension, such as portal vein thrombosis, ascites rarely occurs in the absence of liver disease. Conversely, hepatic vein occlusion commonly percipitates ascites. In posthepatic sinusoidal hypertension, hepatic lymph production is increased and leaks into the peritoneal cavity producing free fluid with a high protein concentration. In cirrhosis, despite the element of sinusoidal obstruction, the ascitic fluid protein levels are low, suggesting that

Table 12.11 **Differential Diagnosis of Ascites**

Type	Characteristics
I. Transudate	
A. Sinusoidal intrahepatic portal hypertension: cirrhosis	Clear appearance, Protein <25g/L, s.g. < 1.015 wbc <300/mm^3 (<25% polys)
B. Sinusoidal extrahepatic portal hypertension: (posthepatic) Hepatic vein obstruction Constrictive pericarditis Congestive heart failure	Variable protein content
C. Other: Nephrotic syndrome Meig's syndrome (benign ovarian tumor)	May be chylous
II. Exudate	Clear-cloudy, protein >25g/L, s.g. > 1.015
A. Neoplasia: peritoneal carcinomatosis	Bloody, ↑LDH, positive cytology, peritoneal biopsy
B. Lymphatic obstruction: trauma, tumor, tuberculosis	Chylous (Sudan-stain for fat)
C. Pancreatitis	Increased amylase
D. Spontaneous bacterial peritonitis	Wbc > 300/mm^3 (>75% polys), culture positive
E. Tuberculosis	Positive peritoneal biopsy, culture
F. Other: myxedema	

fluid loss from the mesenteric capillaries is probably more important than leakage of hepatic lymph.

In ascites, urinary sodium excretion is usually less than 5mEq per day which tends to produce a positive salt and water balance. The traditional concept proposes that fluid accumulation in the peritoneal space from portal hypertension and hypoalbuminemia reduces the "effective" circulating volume. This then decreases renal blood flow and glomerular filtration rate; renin and aldosterone levels increase, producing salt and water retention. Alternatively, the "overflow" theory suggests that the primary event is an inappropriate retention of excessive sodium by the kidneys with resultant expansion of plasma volume. This theory suggests that the initial disorder is renal dysfunction; the portal hypertension then localizes the excess plasma in the peritoneal space. No matter what the origin, secondary hyperaldosteronism initiated by the renin angiotensin system is further promoted by impaired metabolism of aldosterone. There may also be a loss of the "third factor" effect which normally blocks tubular reabsorption of sodium in response to expansion of extracellular volume. Reduced free water clearance occurs; perhaps it is related to excessive antidiuretic hormone activity. Intrarenal blood flow is redistributed, decreasing superficial renal cortical flow while increasing flow to the sodium-retaining juxtamedullary nephrons.

The presence of small amounts of free peritoneal fluid may be difficult to detect, especially in obese patients. Ascites can usually be clinically demonstrated when about 500 ml of fluid are present. On examination, there is dullness to percussion in one or both flanks which shifts when the patient is turned on one side. A fluid thrill may be present. A ballotable, enlarged firm liver and/or spleen may also be palpated. A pleural effusion appears in up to 10 per-

cent of cases. For small amounts of ascites, dullness can be demonstrated in the periumbilical region ("puddle sign") when the patient assumes the knee-chest position. The most sensitive way to confirm the diagnosis is by ultrasonography in which the liver is separated from the abdominal wall by fluid. Abdominal paracentesis not only confirms the diagnosis, but the 50 to 100 ml of fluid obtained can be characterized leading to a more precise diagnosis (Table 12.11). The fluid should be examined for specific gravity, protein content, WBC and RBC count, LDH (lactic dehydrogenase), amylase, gram stain, culture and cytology.

The development of ascites in patients with cirrhosis is an ominous sign, being associated with a five year survival of only 10 to 30 percent. Increased salt intake, a fresh bout of alcoholic hepatitis, an unsuspected complication such as portal vein thrombosis or development of a hepatoma could precipitate or worsen ascites. Its appearance in chronic active hepatitis also carries a poor prognosis.

Effective management of ascites should be directed at its two principle causes, hepatocellular disease and portal hypertension. Because few specific therapies exist for the liver disease, and surgery for portal hypertension does not appear to prolong life in alcoholic cirrhosis, physicians tend to zealously treat ascites with potent diuretics, seeking rapid weight loss and clearing of edema as signs of a dramatic response to therapy. Too rapid a diuresis may precipitate electrolyte imbalance, the hepatorenal syndrome and liver failure. There are only two circumstances in which therapeutic paracentesis with the removal of 1–2 litres of fluid may be warranted: massive ascites causing abdominal pain and respiratory embarassment, and an umbilical rupture, a complication with a very high mortality rate. Therapeutic paracentesis is otherwise of little value and may be hazardous causing protein loss, hypokalemia, and shock. The best guide to a therapeutic response is a weight loss of 0.5 kg per day, as only 700 to 900 ml of ascites can be maximally mobilized in 24 hours. In the presence of peripheral edema, a 1 kg loss per day is quite acceptable.

Initial therapy should be bed rest and dietary sodium restriction. In moderate ascites, dietary sodium should be reduced to 50 mEq/day. If this fails to initiate fluid loss within 4–7 days, a diuretic acting on the distal renal tubule such as the aldosterone antagonist, spironolactone (100 mg/day) is a reasonable first choice, because its potassium-sparing effect offsets any hypokalemia from the secondary hyperaldosteronism. The dose should not be increased until maximum therapeutic action is achieved, about 4 days. Spironolactone can be eventually increased to 600 mg daily. If the ascites is still refractory, a diuretic acting on the proximal tubule ("loop" diuretic) such as furosemide (40 to 80 mg/day) may be added. If hyponatremia becomes a problem, fluid intake should be restricted to 1500 ml per day or less. If hypokalemia or azotemia develop stop all diuretics. Occasionally a patient will be totally resistant to diuretic therapy, with a continually low sodium excretion (10mEq/day). Large abdominal paracentesis with filtration and reinfusion of the ascitic fluid to conserve protein has been attempted, but is cumbersome. Infusion of salt-free albumin may also initiate a transient diuresis. Subcutaneously implanted peritoneal venous shunts, such as the LeVeen shunt, allow one-way flow through a special valve from the peritoneal cavity to an intrathoracic vein. Such reinfusion of ascitic fluid is contraindicated in sepsis and tends to precipitate a chronic, occasionally lethal, disseminated intravascular coagulopathy. The overall safety and efficacy of such procedures are uncertain especially as the shunts tend to become blocked once the ascitic fluid is drained.

Spontaneous bacterial peritonitis is a recently recognized, often fatal complication which develops in cirrhotic patients with ascites. The setting is appropriate for bacterial infection to occur. Not only is ascitic fluid an ideal bacterial culture medium, but portal-systemic collaterals which bypass the filtering action of the liver permit intermittent bacteremias to seed the peritoneal fluid. The responsible organisms are usually Gram negative bacilli or *Streptococcus pneumonia*. Although spontaneous bacterial peritonitis is typified by rapidly accumulating ascites, general deterioration, fever and abdominal pain, the disorder may appear with little or no fever and none of the usual signs of peritonitis. Sometimes the only manifestation is fever. The ascitic fluid is characteristi-

cally cloudy with an increased white blood cell count above 1000 per cu mm (normal <300) predominantly polymorphonuclear cells. Since the fluid can be clear with overlap in the normal range of number of leucocytes the diagnosis of spontaneous bacterial peritonitis may only be possible from bacterial culture. Appropriate broad spectrum antibiotics should be used in all suspected cases with counts over 500. A more specific antibiotic can be selected once the results of culture and sensitivity become availabe.

HEPATORENAL SYNDROME

Hepatorenal syndrome is progressive functional renal failure occuring in patients with severe liver disease. It is characterized by oliguria, with urinary output under 400 ml/day, azotemia and often hyponatremia. The renal impairment is considered "functional" because there is no morphological evidence of kidney damage. The mechanism of renal failure in the presence of advanced liver disease may be related to a redistribution of renal blood flow from the outer cortex to juxtamedullary and medullary nephrons. The substance(s) responsible for this inappropriate renal vasoconstriction are unknown.

The usual setting is severe liver disease with ascites, jaundice and encephalopathy. Precipitating causes of the hepatorenal syndrome commonly involve a decrease in circulating blood volume from a gastrointestinal bleed, vigorous diuresis, or sepsis such as spontaneous bacterial peritonitis. As the renal blood flow and glomerular filtration rate fall, urine volume falls (<500 ml/day) and serum creatinine rises. The urine is concentrated (being hyperosmolar with urine:plasma osmolality ratio up to 3.5). There is no abnormal sediment. Urinary sodium concentration is low. The high urinary osmolality with low sodium concentration is biochemically similar to prerenal failure. Acute tubular necrosis (ATN) may be present initially or may follow a period of functional renal failure (see Chapter 11). Hyponatremia is usually present in the hepatorenal syndrome, and a measurement below 125 mEq/l is associated with an ominous prognosis. The usual problem is telling whether the hepatorenal syndrome from azotemia is due to volume depletion, urinary obstruction, acute tubular necrosis, drug-induced interstitial nephritis, or pyelonephritis.

Management should begin with correction of the precipitating causes of renal failure, particularly hypovolemia. A trial of volume expansion is often warranted. Conservative measures should include stopping diuretics, treating any infection, and carefully monitoring fluid and electrolyte balance. There is no

Table 12.12   **Factors Precipitating Portal-Systemic Encephalopathy**

Cause	Mechanism
Gastrointestinal bleed	Blood protein provides nitrogenous substrate
	Hypoxia impairs cerebral and hepatic function
Azotemia	↑ Urea nitrogen in gut converted to ammonia
Diuretics, diarrhea	Alkalosis favors transfer of ammonia across the blood-brain barriers
	Hypokalemic, alkalosis ↑ renal ammonia production
	Hypokalemia
Sedatives, hypnotics, narcotics, anaesthetics	Direct depression of brain
	↓ Liver metabolism alters drug pharmacokinetics
Other Factors:	
Excess dietary protein	Substrate for ammonia
Constipation	More time for production and absorption of ammonia
Infection	Tissue catabolism provides endogenous nitrogen
Renal tubular acidosis (distal)	Kaliuresis causes hypokalemia
Hypoglycemia, hypoxia, hypomagnesemia, hypophosphatemia	Deterioration in intracellular metabolism

specific treatment. Acute dialysis allows time for assessment of an individual patient, but chronic intermittent dialysis does not affect the high mortality rate.

HEPATIC ENCEPHALOPATHY

Etiology and Pathogenesis

Hepatic encephalopathy is an organic brain syndrome associated with acute or chronic liver disease which has a wide spectrum of neuropsychiatric features. *Portal-systemic encephalopathy* is a neuropsychiatric syndrome which may develop during the course of chronic liver disease associated with portal systemic shunting. The mechanism is presumably a metabolic disorder as there are no important morphological lesions and the encephalopathy is reversible. Because the usual setting is severe liver dysfunction with shunting of portal blood into the systemic circulation, the pathogenesis of this syndrome has been largely attributed to a cerebral toxin which is absorbed from the intestine but not detoxified by the liver. Altered ammonia metabolism is the archetype for this toxic hypothesis. Ammonia levels may rise due to decreased urea synthesis, excessive nitrogenous material in the intestine from blood or dietary protein, renal failure with elevated blood urea nitrogen, or hypokalemic alkalosis with reduced urinary ammonium loss. Children with congenital abnormalities of the urea cycle can also exhibit encephalopathy. Further, hepatic coma can be precipitated in decompensated cirrhotic patients when they ingest excess dietary protein or increase their endogenous production of ammonia from the gastrointestinal tract or kidney. Other putative toxins include mercaptans, fatty acids, and various amino acids. One or more of these agents could depress brain metabolism. Alternatively, the liver could normally produce a protective factor, the absence of which might further increase the risk of encephalopathy. The second hypothesis concerning hepatic coma involves the amino acid precursors of those chemicals which make the central nervous system work, the neurotransmitters. The true pathogenesis of this reversible syndrome is likely multifactorial.

Clinical Features

Portal-systemic encephalopathy may arise spontaneously during the course of acute or chronic liver disease, or it may have a clearly identifiable precipitating factor. As the extraneous factors frequently respond to therapy, these should be carefully identified (Table 12.12). The diagnosis of hepatic encephalopathy is based on presence of significant liver disease in conjunction with three findings: alterations in behaviour, asterixis, and an abnormal electroencephalogram. It may begin abruptly, rapidly leading to coma especially in fulminant hepatic failure, or insidiously, with a subtle deterioration in mental function progressing to coma. The early stages of the syndrome ("hepatic precoma") are characterized by slight alterations in judgement, personality and affect: euphoria, depression or agitated confusion. Disturbed consciousness begins with hypersomnia leading to an inversion of the sleep pattern. As the disease progresses, the patient becomes more confused, is difficult to arouse and finally passes into coma. The most specific clinical feature is *fetor hepaticus*, a musty, fishy, sweetish odour to the breath probably produced by mercaptans. *Asterixis*, an irregular tremor, is the most characteristic neurological sign, best demonstrated as a flapping tremor with the patient's arms outstretched, wrists hyperextended and fingers separated. It can be elicited in the closed eyelids, protruded tongue, pursed lips and in the toes. The flap is bilateral but asymmetrical, occurring in bursts about once every 1–2 seconds. It is absent at rest. The flapping tremor reflects an inability to maintain sustained posture. This results from impaired inflow of joint position and other afferent information to the reticular formation in the brain stem. Asterixis is not specific for encephalopathy, being also present in uremia, hypocalcemia, congestive heart failure, hypercarbia, sedative overdose, hypoglycemia, and hypokalemia. Intellectual deterioration in the form of constructional apraxia may be elicited.

The hepatic encephalopathy associated with acute fulminant hepatic failure may produce asterixis, fetor hepaticus, and delirium which may quickly progress to deep coma, convulsions, and even decerebrate rigidity. Cerebral edema occurs in up to 50 percent of these patients.

Laboratory Assessment

The electroencephalogram (EEG) shows slowing of cerebral activity in the delta range below 4 cycles/sec. The CSF pressure and protein levels are usually normal. Laboratory tests frequently reveal an elevated blood ammonia but this does not necessarily correlate with the degree of coma. Respiratory alkalosis may occur secondary to hyperventilation. Standard liver and coagulation tests reflect the underlying liver disease. Hypoglycemia, electrolyte and acid-base disturbances are common.

Management

Management is aimed at decreasing ammonia production in the colon while eliminating or treating any precipitating factors (see Table 12.12). Diuretics and sedatives should be stopped, and any hypokalemia corrected. At the same time, other conditions which can mimic hepatic coma (especially in an alcoholic), such as altered consciousness from a subdural hematoma, hypoglycemia, or confusion and tremor as in alcoholic withdrawal and Wernicke's encephalopathy, should be ruled out.

Gut cleansing with laxatives and enemas removes the nitrogen load from a dietary or a blood source. Protein intake should be restricted until the encephalopathy is controlled but not to the extent that caloric intake and nutrition become jeopardized. Only 0.7 g of protein per kg ideal body weight is necessary to prevent endogenous protein catabolism under normal circumstances. Protein derived from milk and vegetables appears to be tolerated better than that from animal sources. With recovery, protein intake can be gradually increased from 20 to 60g or more per day. Supportive measures should include careful monitoring of fluid and electrolyte balance and good nursing care for comatose patients. Treatment of the underlying liver disease should be attempted whenever possible.

Specific drug therapy has also been directed at reducing the ammonia production and absorption from the gut. Neomycin, a relatively non-absorbable antibiotic, is effective in hepatic encephalopathy, whether administered orally or rectally. The presumed mechanism is through its antibacterial activity although the drug can also adsorb substances within the lumen of the intestine. A small but significant absorption of neomycin does occur, potentially leading to ototoxic, neurotoxic, and nephrotoxic side effects particularly in the presence of renal failure. An alternative form of therapy to reduce ammonia formation and absorption came from the introduction of lactulose which was intended to qualitatively alter the enteric flora. Its efficacy is more likely related to metabolism of this synthetic disaccharide by the enteric flora. When administered orally, lactulose passes unchanged into the colon where lactulase-containing intestinal bacteria hydrolyze the disaccharide into lactic and acetic acid. This sugar fermentation acidifies the stool, favoring the conversion of ammonia (NH_3) to ammonium ($NH4+$), trapping the polar form in the bowel. The excretion of nitrogenous compounds is also enhanced by the fermentation, which produces osmotic diarrhea. Carbohydrate may inhibit bacterial metabolism of amino acids. In ambulatory patients with chronic hepatic encephalopathy, lactulose along with a restricted protein intake is effective and safe. Other therapeutic approaches have been tried following the hypothesis that plasma amino acid abnormalities can cause the accumulation of false neurochemical transmitters leading to impaired cerebral neurotransmission. Two approaches have had trials with some limited success: L-DOPA, a precursor of the neurotransmitters, norepinephrine and dopamine; and bromocriptine, a dopamine receptor agonist. Their clinical efficacy has not been proven.

Management of fulminant (acute) hepatic failure generally involves attention to details of good sup-

Table 12.13.   **Primary Tumors of the Liver: Etiologic Associations**

Tumor Type	Factor
I. Malignant Tumors	
A. Hepatocellular carcinoma	cirrhosis and chronic inflammation
	chronic hepatitis B infection
	mycotoxins (aflatoxin)
	drugs and chemicals: sex hormones, arsenic
B. Cholangiocarcinoma	parasites: liver flukes
C. Angiosarcoma	chemicals: vinyl chloride, arsenic
	radioactive agents: Thorotrast
II. Benign Tumors	
A. Hepatic adenoma	sex hormones

portive care and treatment of complications. These cases are complicated by coagulopathy requiring fresh frozen plasma, hypoglycemia, and gastrointestinal hemorrhage from stress ulceration. Sepsis is often silent, requiring constant surveillance but no prophylactic antbiotics. The "adult respiratory distress syndrome" can also occur in fulminant hepatic failure. Cerebral edema, a potential major cause of coma and death, is becoming increasingly recognized in this acute encephalopathy. It is not necessarily manifest by papilledema, but rather a sudden deterioration in the level of consciousness.

Attempts to support the liver have led to heroic measures, including exchange transfusions, plasmapheresis, cross-circulation (either with a primate or human volunteer), and extracorporeal liver perfusion. None have been consistently successful. More recently "artificial livers" have been developed using absorbents or special dialysis membranes in an attempt to remove cerebral toxins. These hemoperfusion techniques and the possibility of liver transplantation are still in experimental stages. The aim of therapy overall is to support a failing liver and allow time for it to regenerate.

HEPATIC TUMORS

Hepatocellular carcinoma (primary liver cell carcinoma), originating from hepatocytes, is the most common (>75 percent) primary tumor of the liver usually appearing in the setting of cirrhosis. *Cholangiocarcinoma* (cholangiocellular carcinoma, a less common (5–10 percent) intrahepatic malignant tumor, is derived from bile duct epithelium. The frequency of primary liver cell cancer varies from a rare condition in the West, being found in less than 1 percent of autopsies, to an extremely high prevalence in Africa and Asia. Worldwide it is a leading cause of death from cancer. The incidence is higher in men and peaks in the latter decades of life, although it appears earlier in areas with a high prevalence.

A number of etiological factors have been implicated in causing primary liver cell tumors (Table 12.13). Most patients (75 percent) with hepatocellular carcinoma have an underlying cirrhosis indicating chronic liver injury. The more prolonged the duration of chronic injury, the greater the frequency of liver carcinoma. Postnecrotic cirrhosis is the most common, but alcoholic cirrhosis, hemochromatosis and congenital liver disease (α_1-antitrypsin deficiency, hereditary tyrosinosis) are also associated. Even chronic parasitic infestation of the biliary system leads to a neoplasm: cholangiocarcinoma. Perhaps carcinoma would develop in all forms of chronic liver damage if patients were to live long enough. Evidence is mounting that hepatitis B virus is oncogenic. The mycotoxin, aflatoxin, is the best known liver carcinogen. These toxic metabolites of fungi are found in a variety of foods and may act synergistically with chronic viral infection to increase the risk of malignant transformation.

About one-third of patients present with clinical features of malignancy: weakness, weight loss, and anorexia. Others will present as an unexplained deterioration in a known cirrhotic. Hepatomegaly with vague pain and tenderness is common. The liver may contain a tender mass, sometimes with a friction rub or bruit. Ascites, if present, is frequently blood-stained with an increased protein and LDH content. Fever, splenomegaly and jaundice may also occur. Less common features include a Budd-Chiari syndrome, portal vein thrombosis with esophageal varices, hypoglycemia, polycythemia, acquired porphyria, hypercalcemia, or another of the paraneoplastic syndromes. Hypercholesterolemia occurs in about 30 percent of cases.

The most diagnostic laboratory test is the detection of serum alpha fetoprotein. In utero, this component of fetal serum alpha globulin is derived mainly from embryonal liver cells, but disappears a few weeks after birth. Alpha feto protein reappears in over 80 percent of patients with hepatocellular carcinoma, usually exceeding 500 ng/ml. Values over 2,000 ng/

ml are virtually diagnostic. Alpha fetoprotein levels can be elevated up to 500 ng/ml in other conditions: neonatal hepatitis, acute or chronic viral hepatitis, embryonic tumors (testis, ovary, and hepatoblastoma), gastrointestinal tumors with hepatic metastases, and pregnancy especially with fetal malformations.

A variety of radiological techniques help localize the tumor: chest films revealing abnormalities of the right hemidiaphragm, angiography showing a hypervascular mass with distorted vessels, and ultrasound, CT scan or liver scan demonstrating a mass lesion. A gallium scan will reveal increased uptake. Definitive diagnosis, however, comes from needle biopsy which gives a positive result in 75 percent of cases. This yield may be increased with peritoneoscopic or ultrasound guidance.

Prognosis is grim in hepatocellular carcinoma with death commonly occuring within 6 months of diagnosis. Extensive replacement of liver tissue by neoplastic cells leads to death from hepatic failure, massive gastrointestinal bleeding from esophageal varices, or from progressive cachexia. The only hope of therapy is an aggressive surgical approach: partial hepatectomy which is usually only attempted in young patients, without obvious metastases and without cirrhosis. Chemotherapy has been rather disappointing. In the future, prevention should come in the form of worldwide control of hepatitis B infection with a vaccine.

No treatment is necessary for benign tumors. Adenomas associated with oral contraceptive therapy often regress after discontinuing the pill.

DISEASE OF THE GALLBLADDER AND THE BILIARY TRACT

CHOLELITHIASIS

Etiology and Pathogenesis

Gallstone disease is the most common disorder of the biliary tract and a major health problem in North America, cholecystectomy being one of the most frequently performed abdominal operations. The reported frequency of gallstones in different countries varies widely, from being quite rare in the Masai tribe of East Africa and in Canadian Eskimos, to being very common (more than 30 percent) in Northern Europeans. The rate in North American whites ranges from 10 to 30 percent.

Human gallstones are usually composed of either cholesterol or pigment material.

Cholesterol gallstones: the majority of stones (over 80 percent) in the West are composed of free cholesterol. Their formation involves abnormalities in cholesterol and bile salt metabolism. In fact, cholesterol originally meant bile solid. Bile is over 90 percent water. Of the solids present, three organic components predominate: bile salts, lecithin and free cholesterol. The latter two lipids are insoluble in water. Bile from healthy persons is a homogenous liquid, in which bile salts combine with lecithin in the form of "mixed micelles" to keep cholesterol in solution. The solubility of cholesterol in bile is limited, being dependent upon sufficient bile salts and lecithin to maintain cholesterol in micellar solution. When the relative concentrations of bile salts and lecithin are insufficient to solubilize the cholesterol in bile, the excess cholesterol either remains as an abnormal supersaturated solution or else precipitates as solid crystals.

Cholesterol gallstone formation begins with the liver producing chemically abnormal or "lithogenic" bile. The liver can produce such bile either by decreased secretion of the solubilizing agents, bile salts or lecithin, or by an increased secretion of cholesterol, or both. In fact, the hepatic defect involves several mechanisms, perhaps representing several diseases. Non-obese patients have a decreased amount of bile salts and reduced secretion of bile salts and lecithin. In contrast, morbidly obese people produce and secrete excessive cholesterol. Most overweight patients with cholesterol gallstones probably have a combined defect: reduced bile salt plus increased cholesterol secretion. Abnormal bile production may begin as early as the teens: in females this may be associated with some degree of obesity combined with the increased estrogen output of puberty. There are other risk factors predisposing to lithogenic bile formation (Table 12.14). Next comes a physical change in this abnormal bile in which microscopic crystals precipitate from solution. This process is hastened and more likely to occur in the presence of a nucleating agent, such as desquamated epithelial cells, calcium salts, precipitated bile acids or a foreign body. Ultimately, the microcrystals aggregate and grow producing a macroscopic stone. Gallstones develop either as a simple stone or by adherence of several simple stones to form complex mulberry stones. Gallstones finally produce symptoms by blocking the cystic or common duct, or by irritating the gallbladder. The tendency to cause symptoms is unrelated to the size, number or type of stones present.

Pigment stones are composed of bile pigment, calcium and a matrix of organic material. They contain only trace amounts (less than 20 percent) of cholesterol. These small, dark, amorphous stones result

Table 12.14 **Risk Factors for Cholelithiasis**

Risk factor	Mechanism
I. Cholesterol Gallstones	
A. Demographic: American Indian, probably familial	increased cholesterol secretion
B. Obesity	increased cholesterol synthesis
C. Diet factors: high-calorie, polyunsaturated fats, high cholesterol, high carbohydrate, low fibre	
D. Female sex hormones (estrogens)	increased cholesterol secretion
E. GI diseases: cystic fibrosis, ileal disease	bile salt malabsorption
II. Pigment Gallstones	
A. Demographic: oriental	infections of the biliary tract
B. Chronic hemolysis	increased bilirubin load
C. Cirrhosis	? abnormal bile pigment

from abnormal metabolism of bile pigment. In the gallbladder they form tarry concretions, whereas stones in the common duct resemble reddish brown mud. Over half of pigment stones have sufficient calcium to be radiopaque, and therefore are visible on plain films of the abdomen.

Most pigment stones are associated with infection and can be found anywhere in the biliary system including the intrahepatic tree. This may account for their high incidence in the Far East where parasitic infections such as *Ascaris lumbricoides* or *Clonorchis sinensis* are not uncommon. The associated stasis with coliform infection can elaborate hydrolytic enzymes which deconjugate bilirubin, transforming a soluble bilirubin diglucuronide into insoluble free bilirubin. The latter then combines with calcium in bile forming calcium bilirubinate which polymerizes forming a pigment stone. It can also act as a nidus for cholesterol precipitation. Pigment stones are also associated with chronic hemolysis and alcoholic cirrhosis.

Clinical Features

About 50 percent of gallstones are clinically silent. The remainder are discovered because of specific biliary tract manifestations: biliary colic, cholecystitis, cholangitis, or obstructive jaundice. Nonspecific dyspepsia, flatulence or fatty food intolerance often prompt cholecystography or ultrasonography which results in a fortuitous discovery of cholelithiasis. The symptoms are likely coincidental and should not be attributed to the stones. This is the most common cause of the *postcholecystectomy syndrome* in which the preoperative complaints persist despite cholecystectomy. In such cases, the symptoms are usually due to another cause such as reflux esophagitis or an irritable bowel syndrome.

Gallstones can impact in the cystic duct or common duct causing *biliary colic* without acute cholecystitis. The pain of biliary colic onsets abruptly, peaks very quickly and maintains a maximum, steady intensity for up to 4 hours before easing. The steadiness of the pain is characteristic. If the pain waxes and wanes like a true colic, a different diagnosis such as small bowel obstruction should be entertained. If the pain persists beyond 5–6 hours another complication such as cholecystitis or pancreatitis probably has developed. Biliary tract pain is commonly located in the right upper quadrant or epigastrium, but can present anywhere from the right shoulder to either iliac crest, or even the back. Radiation occurs through to the interscapular area, the angle of the right scapula, the right shoulder, arm or neck. Nausea is frequent but vomiting uncommon, except with a stone in the common duct or with pancreatitis. There is no evidence that fatty food ingestion specifically precipitates biliary colic.

Acute cholecystitis in over 90 percent of cases results from stones in the cystic duct or Hartman's pouch. Cholecystitis is unusual in the absence of gallstones, although acalculous cholecystitis can occur in association with congenital anomalies of the biliary system, infections in children and diabetics, after trauma or burns with bacteremia, or with vasculitis. The pain of acute cholecystitis lasts longer than that of simple biliary colic, subsiding in most by 72 hours but progressing in the rest to perforation or gangrene. The pain is more generalized and has a peritoneal component being worse with deep breathing or movement. Jaundice occurs in one-quarter of cases from passage of stones into the common duct with brief obstruction at the sphincter of Oddi. Pancreatitis, which can complicate cholelithiasis, is also a cause of cholestasis. After a single episode of acute cholecystitis, chronic cholecystitis supervenes. Right upper quadrant tenderness and guarding are frequent. Other findings include local cutaneous hyperesthesia, a palpable gallbladder, Murphy's sign with point tenderness in the right upper quadrant on deep inspiration causing inspiratory arrest, or Boas's sign with hyperesthesia between the ninth and eleventh ribs posteriorly on the right side. Fever, dehydration and paralytic ileus may also occur. The gallbladder is generally enlarged, but palpation can be difficult because of guarding.

Elderly patients may look and feel well without fever or leukocytosis even when the gallbladder is gangrenous and perforates. Local abscess formation may occur or a biliary fistula develop to the duodenum. Indeed, gallstone ileus with the stone passing through a choledochoduedenal fistula, impacting at the ileocaecal valve is a not uncommon cause of small bowel obstruction in the aged.

Chronic cholecystitis almost invariably is accompanied by cholelithiasis even in asymptomatic patients. Chronic inflammation of the gallbladder may follow an episode of acute cholecystitis or biliary colic, but frequently has rather non-specific complaints, such as flatulence and vague abdominal discomfort. The presence of right upper quadrant tenderness is a helpful, though not consistent sign.

Choledocholithiasis occurs in 15 percent of patients with stones in the gallbladder and leads to biliary colic and/or cholangitis in three-quarters of these people. Nonsuppurative cholangitis produces Charcot's triad (pain, fever and jaundice) which spontaneously subsides after 1 to 3 days or in response to antibacterial therapy. The episodic nature of cholangitis, even with a gram-negative bacteremia, is related to intermittent impaction and dislocation of stones within the common duct. Recurrent or prolonged obstruction can lead to secondary biliary cirrhosis with chronic cholestasis. Common duct obstruction can occasionally produce acute suppurative cholangitis, a severe illness with pus accumulating under pressure in the biliary tract, and leading to liver abscess and endotoxic shock. Jaundice or cholangitis can also result from a stricture of the common duct, which may develop months after the original duct injury from biliary tract surgery.

Laboratory Assessment

During the acute attack, the leukocyte count is raised with increased band forms, and cholestasis may be manifest by an elevated alkaline phosphatase. Serum aminotransferase may also be mildly increased. The serum amylase levels may be significantly elevated even in the absence of pancreatitis.

The standard oral cholecystogram is the principle method of establishing gallbladder pathology. Ingestion of an iodinated dye (iopanoic acid) is followed by its absorption in the intestine, excretion into bile, and concentration by the gallbladder. A problem in any one of these steps results in failure of the gallbladder to opacify. X-ray films can be obtained 12 hours later. A better result comes from ingesting the dye on two consecutive evenings. Radiolucent gallstones, usually of cholesterol type, appear as filling defects. Demonstrating gallstones is diagnostic, while even a non-visualized gallbladder after two doses conveys a greater than 85 percent accuracy for biliary tract disease. Reliability of ultrasonography to detect abnormal echoes from within gallbladders harbouring gallstones may exceed 95 percent, but only in the best hands. A plain film may demonstrate radiopaque stones, limy bile or air in the right upper quadrant. Limy bile results from precipitation of calcium salts in the lumen of the gallbladder whose cystic duct is completely obstructed. Air in the biliary tree is produced by a fistulous communication with the intestine or after sphincterotomy. Intravenous cholangiography, in which the dye is given intravenously, has too many risks from adverse reactions for common usage, and it is best replaced by transhepatic cholangiography or endoscopic retrograde cholangiopancreatography in the more difficult cases with jaundice. Cholescintigraphy, a radionuclear scan of the gallbladder, is valuable in acute cholecystitis: a non-visualized gallbladder is virtually diagnostic of acute cholecystitis with cystic duct obstruction. Here, the radionucleotide is excreted by the liver but does not enter the gallbladder. The test is obviously less valuable with cholestasis.

Management

Surgery continues to be the mainstay of management of biliary tract disease. Cholecystectomy is clearly indicated for patients with acute cholecystitis, gallstone associated pancreatitis, cholangitis or recurrent biliary colic, unless the patient's general medical condition precludes an operation. Supportive measures in acute cholecystitis include nasogastric suction, IV fluid replacement, analgesia, and close monitoring. The role of proplylactic antibiotics is not completely resolved. If pain, fever, tenderness, and leukocytosis progress, as occurs in some 25 percent of cases, urgent surgery is warranted. If the patient responds to nonsurgical therapy, then a definitive diagnosis by oral cholecystogram and/or ultrasound is indicated before elective surgery 6 weeks later. This way the operative mortality is low ($<.5\%$), and the diagnosis of cholelithiasis secure. Some surgeons champion immediate cholecystectomy once the clinical diagnosis is made. This certainly reduces the length of disability and duration of hospital stay. Surgery for asymptomatic cases, the "silent stone", is debatable as most never develop symptoms or serious complications.

Medical dissolution of cholesterol gallstones became a reality with the hypothesis that the excessive cholesterol saturation of bile resulted from a small bile salt pool. Two bile acids promote gallstone dissolution: chenodeoxycholic acid at 12 to 15 mg/kg daily and ursodeoxycholic acid at 8 to 10 mg/kg. Bedtime administration of chenodeoxycholic acid and perhaps a diet low in cholesterol may enhance the desaturating effect and presumably accelerate dissolution. These two bile acids appear to act by suppressing cholesterol synthesis in the liver and secretion into bile. Bile acid therapy is effective in many cases. Small stones, especially if they float on oral cholecystography, are more amenable to dissolution. A nonvisualized gallbladder or radiopaque stones are absolute contraindications. The efficacy and absolute safety of medical therapy remain to be proven. The most obvious indication would be relatively asymptomatic patients, especially in the older age group or those with a high operative risk.

OTHER DISORDERS OF THE BILIARY TRACT

Cholangitis is characterized by inflammation of the bile duct system. Acute cholangitis occurs when large duct obstruction leads to bacterial infection of the biliary tree, often termed "ascending cholangitis". Partial abrupt obstruction as with a stone or duct stricture leads to cholangitis more frequently than complete or gradual bile duct obstruction from malignancy. The clinical features are dominated by pain, jaundice, and fever. Management centers on determination of the presence and cause of the obstructing process, adequate supportive care with antibiotic coverage and prompt surgical relief of the obstruction whenever possible.

Sclerosing cholangitis is an uncommon disorder manifest by episodic cholestasis often with acute cholangitis, resulting from inflammation and progressive fibrosis which obliterate the biliary tree. Most cases are associated with ulcerative colitis. The usual clinical features are jaundice, fever, pruritus and abdominal pain. The biochemical picture is cholestasis with an elevated serum alkaline phosphatase. Diagnosis comes from endoscopic retrograde cholangiography, which shows diffuse irregular narrowing of the extrahepatic bile duct system with beading and stricture of the intrahepatic duct. Prognosis is variable but eventually progressive secondary biliary cirrhosis complicated by portal hypertension and liver failure develops. Management is usually palliative. The only surgical approach available is dilatation and stenting of the bile ducts by passing prosthetic tubes through the narrowed areas.

Pericholangitis, an inflammatory process involving small bile ducts in the portal tracts, is usually associated with ulcerative colitis or Crohn's disease. It may merely represent a non-specific reaction secondary to inflammatory bowel disease or else a minor variant of sclerosing cholangitis. The usual manifestation is merely an asymptomatic elevation of the serum alkaline phosphatase. Prognosis is considered excellent, depending on the natural course of the colitis.

Cholangiocarcinoma and other tumors can affect the gallbladder and extrahepatic biliary tract. Malignant tumors of the gallbladder are frequently associated with gallstones, although there is no evidence that chronic gallstone disease predisposes to the development of neoplasia. Extrahepatic bile duct carcinoma is associated with liver flukes and with ulcerative colitis. The clinical picture depends upon the site of origin of the tumor. Tumors of the gallbladder present with an upper abdominal mass with persistent pain, jaundice, and weight loss. Tumors of one hepatic duct produce a minimally elevated bilirubin and high alkaline phosphatase. Tumors of the common duct or head of the pancreas cause progressive unrelenting jaundice and an enlarged gallbladder. Epigastric pain, anorexia and weight loss are common. Although slow growing, prognosis is quite hopeless as most are inoperable.

PANCREATIC STRUCTURE AND FUNCTION

The pancreas, an elongated gland located retroperitoneally in the upper abdomen, is capable of both exocrine and endocrine functions. The exocrine cells, arranged in an acinar pattern, produce polypeptide enzymes for digestion. The duct system, a tree-like structure, not only drains pancreatic acini but also elaborates bicarbonate for the neutralizing of hydrochloric acid passing from the stomach. The pancreas also contains numerous endocrine cells located in groups: the islets of Langerhans. The islets do not connect with the lumen of the pancreatic ducts but are separated from the surrounding acinar tissue by fine reticular fibres.

The exocrine pancreas is under both hormonal and neural control. Regulation of pancreatic secretion is primarily through two gut hormones: secretin and cholecystokinin (CCK). Secretin, released from the duodenal mucosa in response to acid emptied from the stomach, stimulates the pancreatic and biliary ductal systems to secrete large volumes of fluid, rich in bicarbonate. CCK is released by intestinal mucosa in response to fatty acids and amino acids. This gut hormone causes the gallbladder to empty and also stimulates the pancreas to produce juice with a high enzyme content. As for neural control, eating and gastric distention stimulate the vagus nerve resulting in a high pancreatic output with fluid rich in enzymes.

The endocrine secretions are hormones: glucagon, produced by the alpha cells, and insulin, elaborated by the beta cells of the islets.

DIAGNOSIS OF PANCREATIC DISEASE

CLINICAL FEATURES

This deep seated organ often presents with vague symptoms in the early stages of disease. The *pain* is usually severe, persistent and located in the midepigastrium. It may also occur in the left upper quadrant when the tail of the pancreas is affected or bore directly through to the back. Characteristically, the pain is worsened when the patient lies flat, stretching the posterior peritoneum over an inflamed pancreas, but is relieved when curled up or leaning forward. Recurrent *vomiting* frequently accompanies the pain but does not relieve it, unlike the pain caused by most gastroduodenal disorders. *Anorexia and weight loss* are quite characteristic of pancreatic carcinoma. Pancreatic disorders involving the head frequently obstruct the distal common duct causing *jaundice*. A *mass* may also be present. The pancreas has a large function reserve. Greater than 90 percent of the pancreas must be damaged before *maldigestion* of fat and protein becomes evident. The islets appear even more resistant to common pathologic insults. *Diabetes* develops late in most pancreatic diseases.

LABORATORY ASSESSMENT

Tests of Pancreatic Inflammation

The hallmark of pancreatic inflammation is an increased *serum amylase*, the result of spillage when the gland is damaged. Values exceeding five times the upper limit of normal are quite characteristic of acute pancreatitis. Unfortunately, hyperamylasemia appears in other disorders, some of which can be confused with acute pancreatitis (Table 12.15). Furthermore, hyperlipemic serum can mask this diagnostic test of acute pancreatitis. Despite its relative lack of sensitivity and specificity, elevated serum amylase is the most widely used and readily available test to identify acute pancreatitis as the cause of an acute abdomen. It is not helpful in diagnosing chronic pancreatitis or pancreatic carcinoma, and its absolute value does not correlate with the amount of gland destruction, being occasionally normal even in fulminant pancreatitis.

Urinary amylase excretion is also increased in acute pancreatitis. Because of intermittent elevations from hour to hour, a single specimen is inadequate. A 2 or 6 hour collection is quite accurate and more practical than the usual 24 hour measurement. Amylase clearance by the kidneys can be increased in conditions other than pancreatic inflammation. Macroamylasemia, which occurs in 1 to 2 percent of the population, is characterized by a low or normal urinary amylase but increased serum amylase. This condition results from an amylase-globulin complex too large to be cleared by renal excretion, and it is usually discovered during the investigation of abdominal pain. *Ascitic* and *pleural fluid amylase* values are increased in fluid collections associated with pancreatitis.

Serum lipase also rises in parallel with the amylase and tends to persist longer (up to 14 days) after an attack of acute pancreatitis. Lipase elevation suggests the source of hyperamylasemia is from the pancreas and not the salivary glands.

Table 12.15 Causes of Hyperamylasemia and/or Hyperamylasuria

I. Pancreatic disease
  A. Acute pancreatitis
  B. Chronic pancreatitis
  C. Complications of pancreatitis
    phlegmon, abscess
    pseudocyst
    ascites
  D. Pancreatic carcinoma
II. Other abdominal diseases
  A. Biliary tract disease: cholecystitis, choledocholithiasis
  B. Peritonitis: any source
  C. Peptic ulcer: penetrating or perforated
  D. Intestinal obstruction or infarction
  E. Ruptured ectopic pregnancy
III. Non-pancreatic disease
  A. Renal failure
  B. Salivary gland disease: mumps, calculus
  C. Macroamylasemia
  D. Burns
  E. Diabetic ketoacidosis
  F. Cerebral trauma

Tests of Exocrine Pancreatic Function

In these tests, duodenal intubation collects the exocrine secretions either in response to exogenous stimulus, such as injection of secretin (*secretin test*) or secretin plus cholecystokinin, or endogenous stimulation, such as a standard meal (*Lundh test*). The volume of aspirated juice and its enzyme content, usually amylase or trypsin, are measured. To quantitate sodium bicarbonate during the secretin test, the stomach is aspirated separately to prevent gastric acid from neutralizing the pancreatic sodium bicarbonate. In severe pancreatic insufficiency, there is a reduced volume with low concentrations of bicarbonate and enzymes. When carcinoma involves the head of the pancreas, total flow is greatly diminished, while bicarbonate concentration is normal. Cytological examination of the fluid may help separate carcinoma from chronic pancreatitis. The low specificity of these tests limits clinical usefulness, except to diagnose pancreatic insufficiency as a cause of malabsorption.

Pancreatic exocrine failure results in *maldigestion*. Microscopic examination of the stool may reveal undigested meat fibres and, when properly stained, fat droplets. Steatorrhea is best detected by a significantly elevated 72 hour fecal fat determination. Tests of mucosal absorptive function, such as the D-xylose test, are generally normal. Damage to the endocrine islets is assessed by tests for carbohydrate intolerance; chemical diabetes mellitus only appears after extensive destruction.

Anatomic Studies

Definition of pancreatic disease is best made through anatomic studies. Conventional plain roentgenograms of the abdomen may reveal localized ileus suggesting acute pancreatitis or pancreatic calcification signifying chronic disease. On barium contrast studies, enlargement of the head of the pancreas can cause anterior and superior displacement of the stomach, widening of the duodenal C-loop, or downward displacement of the colon. Ultrasound is the simplest and least invasive test to detect pancreatic disease. In acute pancreatitis, an enlarged, inflamed pancreas is seen in 90 percent of cases. Ultrasound will also detect the majority of mass lesions, be they inflammatory, cystic, or neoplastic. It can also detect pancreatic calcification. Excessive intestinal gas and obesity interfere with ultrasound studies. In equivocal cases, computerized tomography (CT scan) is useful, especially in obese subjects, to detect mass lesions of the body and tail of the pancreas. As the x-ray absorption values of normal, inflamed and cancerous tissues are quite similar, CT scan cannot always distinguish between these conditions. Endoscopic retrograde cholangiopancreatography (ERCP) can define the pancreatic and biliary duct systems. Cholelithiasis, a frequent cause of pancreatitis, can often be detected simply with an oral cholecystogram. Abdominal angiography will identify pancreatic neoplasms by the presence of arterial irregularities or tumor vessels. Lastly, percutaneous fine-needle aspiration biopsy can be performed under ultrasound or fluorscopic guidance to detect pancreatic malignancy.

In general, suspected pancreatic disease can be screened with a few simple blood tests, such as amylase and glucose, and by a non-invasive anatomic visualization with ultrasonography. In more difficult instances, CT scan and ERCP may be quite revealing and a laparotomy definitive.

PANCREATITIS

Acute inflammatory disease of the pancreas contains a wide spectrum of pathology ranging from interstitial edema and minimal necrosis, termed *edematous pancreatitis*, to more severe hemorrhage or suppuration, designated as *necrotizing pancreatitis*. These two forms of acute pancreatitis are frequently difficult to distinguish on a clinical basis, particularly at the onset. In chronic pancreatitis, proteinaceous material precipitates in the duct system, becomes calcified and obstructs the lumen.

The best classification of pancreatitis was developed at the Marseille Symposium (Fig. 12.8). In this definition, acute pancreatitis is always reversible even in the relapsing form. Pain may appear, enzymes may rise, and dysfunction occur but these always return to normal. By contrast, the chronic form invariably leaves some residual deterioration in pancreatic exocrine and endocrine function even after the first attack.

ACUTE PANCREATITIS

Etiology and Pathogenesis

An attack of acute pancreatitis is commonly associated with either the presence of cholelithiasis or alcohol abuse. The causal factor is otherwise unknown or infrequent (Table 12.16). The initial event is presumably some form of acinar cell injury. This is followed by activation of pancreatic proteolytic enzymes, particularly trypsinogen to trypsin. This triggers an enzyme cascade which culminates in autodigestion and pancreatic necrosis. Trypsin activates

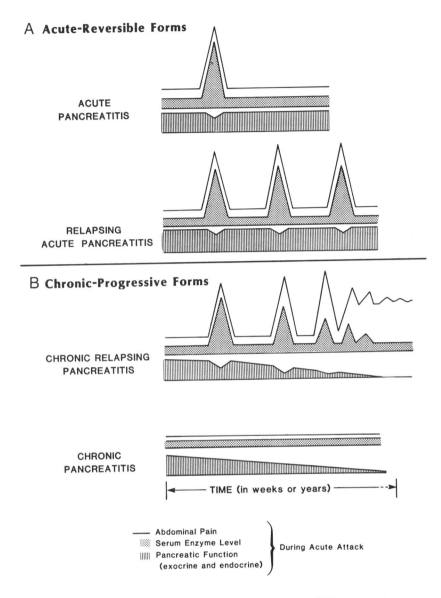

A **Acute-Reversible Forms**

ACUTE
PANCREATITIS

RELAPSING
ACUTE PANCREATITIS

B **Chronic-Progressive Forms**

CHRONIC RELAPSING
PANCREATITIS

CHRONIC
PANCREATITIS

|←————— TIME (in weeks or years) ————--→|

—— Abdominal Pain
▦ Serum Enzyme Level
‖ Pancreatic Function   } During Acute Attack
   (exocrine and endocrine)

Fig. 12.8 Classification of pancreatitis with clinical and laboratory features.

other digestive enzymes resulting in proteolysis, fat necrosis, and destruction of the elastic fibre in walls of blood vessels. The sequence, if limited, causes only edema. With enzyme activation, cell injury and death liberate more activated enzymes setting up a vicious cycle which causes the pancreas to self-destruct by autodigestion. Vasoactive peptides are also released compounding the inflammatory process. How the various etiological factors initiate pancreatitis is largely unknown. Migrating gallstones may transiently lodge in the ampulla of Vater while spasm or fibrosis of the sphincter of Oddi could either obstruct the pancreatic duct or allow bile to reflux into the pancreas thus activating proenzymes. Drugs, vi-

ruses, ischemia and trauma could also activate trypsinogen to trypsin, setting off the autolytic chain of events. Alcohol, a metabolic toxin to the liver and many other tissues, may directly damage the acini and secondarily obstruct small and large ducts.

Clinical Features

Severe, steady abdominal pain penetrating through to the mid-back is the most characteristic symptom. There may also be nausea, vomiting and a low-grade fever. The patient appears quite ill and uncomfortable, preferring a bent-over position with

Table 12.16   **Causes of Acute Pancreatitis**

I. Alcohol }most common	
II. Gallstones	
III. Idiopathic	
IV. Trauma: postoperative, after motor vehicle accident, after duodenal endoscopy.	
V. Duodenal ulcer—penetrating	
VI. Drugs: azathioprine, thiazides, estrogens, sulfonamides, tetracycline	
VII. Metabolic: hypercalcemia, hyperlipidemias, cystic fibrosis, uremia	
VIII. Infectious: viral (mumps, viral hepatitis), parasitic infestations (ascaris)	
IX. Carcinoma of pancreas	

the knees flexed. The abdominal findings are moderate compared with the severity of the pain. Tenderness with some guarding in the upper abdomen is usual, but rebound or rigidity is not. Bowel sounds are reduced or absent. Fever, if present, is usually only 1 to 2°C above normal. A high fever indicates another process such as pancreatic abscess, ascending cholangitis, pneumonia or other complicating infection. A palpable epigastric mass becomes evident with the development of a pseudocyst or marked peripancreatic fat necrosis. Cholestatic jaundice appears in about 20 percent of patients; it is caused by pancreatic inflammation compressing the common bile duct. A similar number of cases have pulmonary complications, such as atelectasis or a pleural effusion, usually on the left. The peritoneal exudate is small, but occasionally pancreatic ascites possessing high amylase activity becomes evident. In severe cases, tachycardia, hypotension and shock result from hypovolemia due to massive retroperitoneal exudation and from release of vasoactive peptides like the kinins. The inflammatory process can extend to adjacent structures causing thrombosis of the splenic or portal vein. Seldom does sufficient blood accumulate in the fascial planes to discolor the skin around the umbilicus (Cullen's sign) or the flanks (Grey Turner's sign). Metastatic fat necrosis can produce reddish nodules on the leg and bone pain from medullary infarcts.

Laboratory Assessment

Laboratory diagnosis of acute pancreatitis is primarily based on an elevated serum amylase concentration, which is abnormal in most cases. The rise occurs within the first 24 hours of onset but then falls towards normal within a few days, unless inflammation continues or a pseudocyst forms. Urinary amylase excretion rises higher than serum amylase and persists longer. Unfortunately, false-positive amylase elevations in serum and urine occur in many situations other than pancreatitis (Table 12.15), while false-negative values turn up particularly in chronic

relapsing pancreatitis. Elevated serum lipase helps corroborate the pancreatic origin. Hypocalcemia is common in acute pancreatitis. A serum calcium value below 7 mg/dl (< 1.75 mmol/L) is associated with severe pancreatitis and an ominous prognosis. The hypocalcemia results from several events: insoluble calcium soaps being deposited in areas of fat necrosis, impaired parathormone response to decreased ionized calcium, elevated glucagon causing calcitonin release which deposits calcium in bone, and/or a parathormone-resistant state associated with the hypomagnesemia of alcoholic patients. The presence of a high normal serum calcium in patients with pancreatitis should arouse the suspicion that the acute episode has masked an underlying hypercalcemia. Hyperglycemia may result from low insulin and high glucagon levels. Hypertriglyceridemia can transiently produce a cloudy serum, especially in alcohol-induced pancreatitis. In addition, the hyperlipidemias associated with chylomicronemia (types I and V) can produce recurrent pancreatitis. Serum lipids should be monitered once the acute phase has resolved. Transitory cholestasis results in hyperbilirubinemia and slightly elevated alkaline phosphatase.

Radiological signs are generally nonspecific but help eliminate other diagnoses such as a perforated viscus with free intraperitoneal air. Plain films of the abdomen frequently reveal abnormalities, often in the form of a localized ileus related to adjacent inflammation: a "sentinal loop" formed by a dilated segment of upper small intestine, or a "colon cut-off sign" from dilation of the ascending colon and hepatic flexure proximal to a spastic segment of transverse colon. Paralytic ileus may be generalized with air-fluid levels. Ultrasonography commonly will show pancreatic edema or occasionally a complication like a pseudocyst formation which warrants further monitoring. Ultrasound may also uncover the origin of the attack, such as cholelithiasis. Oral cholecystography should be performed in the early recovery period just before discharge, as the gallbladder will visualize in more than 90 percent of nonjaundiced patients without biliary tract disease. Nonvisualization can occur but suggests a follow-up evaluation to rule out cholelithiasis.

Complications

Complications may affect many organ systems. Most often an inflammatory mass develops locally, up to 2 weeks after the acute episode either as a phlegmon, pseudocyst or abscess. Phlegmon, a solid mass composed of the swollen, inflamed pancreas, appears within a few days, and usually subsides spontaneously after 1 to 2 weeks. The phlegmon will present as a solid mass on ultrasound. If the adjacent blood vessels thrombose, it may become necessary to surgically debride the chronic inflammatory tissue and resect infarcted colon. A *pancreatic abscess* may arise from secondary infection due to invasion of the necrotic pancreas by Gram positive or enteric flora. Fever, toxicity and a palpable mass develop 1 to 4 weeks after apparent recovery from the initial episode of acute pancreatitis. Abdominal roentgenograms occasionally reveal gas in the abscess as a "soap bubble" sign. Although pancreatic abscess is an infrequent complication of acute pancreatitis (less than 10 percent of cases), it carries with it an extremely high mortality. Prophylactic antibiotics have not been shown to prevent their occurence. Once the diagnosis of a pancreatic abscess is made, antibiotic coverage and surgical drainage become necessary. Following acute pancreatitis, the exudate from the surface of the gland and any collection of pancreatic fluid may be walled off by the adjacent serosal, mesenteric and peritoneal surfaces. The inflamed membranes become thickened and form a fibrotic wall, termed a *pseudocyst* because unlike a true cyst, it lacks an epithelial lining. Ultrasonography has demonstrated that pseudocysts develop in one-half of all episodes of acute pancreatitis. During the early phases of development when they lack a mature fibrous capsule, pseudocysts can resorb spontaneously. One-third do so when monitored by ultrasound. The capsule once formed is permanent. In chronic pancreatis, pseudocysts arise from obstruction of the pancreatic duct, behind which functioning acinar tissue produces digestive juices. Pseudocysts can present as abdominal pain, a mass or merely an abnormality detected by ultrasound. Non-specific symptoms like abdominal pain, nausea and vomiting, and weight loss are often present, but an abdominal mass, ascites (with high amylase content) and/or jaundice are more obvious features. Serum amylase is persistently elevated. Catastrophic complications such as free perforation into the peritoneal cavity, secondary infection, intestinal obstruction or rupture into a viscus with gastrointestinal hemorrhage can also occur. Management can be expectant in those cysts without symptoms, which frequently resolve spontaneously. Otherwise laparotomy with permanent internal drainage into the stomach (cystogastrostomy) or into an adjacent loop of small intestine becomes necessary.

Management

Initial management of acute pancreatitis includes restoration of effective plasma volume with parenteral electrolyte solutions or plasma, and pain relief using potent analgesics such as meperidine hydrochloride (Demerol). Total fluid replacement should be assessed by monitoring pulse rate, blood pressure, urinary output and, in severe cases, central venous pressure or occasionally pulmonary capillary wedge pressure. Calcium replacement may become necessary with symptomatic hypocalcemia below 7 mg/dl (<1.75 mmol/L). It seems reasonable to "put the pancreas at rest" by interrupting all stimuli to exocrine secretions, eliminating oral intake and perhaps emptying the stomach with nasogastric suction. The use of nasogastric aspiration, is best reserved for more severe cases as clinical trials have not shown any advantage in mild to moderate cases. It may be valuable in patients with severe nausea and vomiting due to ileus. Anticholinergic drugs and prophylactic antibiotics have no clear-cut value, while their side effects and risks outweigh any possible benefits. Specific therapeutic agents such as the antikallikrein (Trasylol) and glucagon have not proven effective. Surgery is indicated in three instances:

1. diagnostic laparotomy when the illness is critical and the diagnosis insecure;
2. development of certain complications, such as a pancreatic abscess or a pseudocyst which fails to resolve; and
3. elective surgery after full recovery for biliary tract disease.

Peritoneal lavage via a percutaneous dialysis catheter has been attempted in more severe cases; its value has not been established.

The course of acute pancreatitis is unpredictable but in most instances the disease is benign with evidence of recovery occurring within a few days. In necrotizing pancreatitis the mortality approaches 50 percent especially if some of the following features are present early: severe hemoconcentration and hypovolemia with the need for massive fluid-colloid replacement, pronounced hypocalcemia, and hypoxia with respiratory failure.

CHRONIC PANCREATITIS

Etiology and Pathogenesis

Chronic pancreatitis implies irreversible damage from the fibrosis and acinar atrophy due to duct obstruction. Inflammation is not necessarily present. Recurrent attacks cause progressive destruction, fibrosis, calcification and loss of exocrine and endocrine functions. Chronic pancreatitis then contains two ingredients: permanent morphological damage sometimes appearing on abdominal roentgenograms as calcium deposits (termed *chronic calcific pancreatitis* or as irregular ducts on cholangiography, plus impaired function perhaps leading to steatorrhea or diabetes.

The most common cause in the western world is alcoholism characterized by a chronic alcohol intake averaging 150 g per day (about 13 ounces of spirits or two bottles of wine). Ethanol has been postulated to be toxic to the pancreas by causing it to produce a very concentrated pancreatic juice in which enzymes precipitate, become calcified and plug the duct system. Less frequent causes include hyperparathyroidism, hyperlipidemia and uremia. Cystic fibrosis is the most common basis for pancreatic insufficiency in childhood, while protein-calorie malnutrition is a quite prevalent cause in third world countries. Unlike acute pancreatitis, gallstone disease does not cause chronic pancreatitis.

Clinical Features

More than 90 percent of patients experience repeated painful attacks with nausea and vomiting, each lasting days to weeks and not always necessitating hospitalization. The intervals between attacks may progressively shorten until pain becomes almost continuous. In alcoholic men, chronic calcific pancreatitis begins in the late thirties, an average of 8 years after the initial acute attack. Very occasionally, following a single attack of pain, chronic pancreatitis develops painlessly and years later leads to steatorrhea and diarrhea. Physical examination may be quite unremarkable in mild attacks or show the typical features of acute pancreatitis with abdominal tenderness and a low grade fever. Any palpable mass likely represents a pseudocyst rather than a carcinoma.

At first, there may be episodes of mild jaundice with dark urine, temporary steatorrhea or transient symptomatic diabetes mellitus. Later, when more than 90 percent of the pancreas is destroyed, steatorrhea and diabetes become permanent. Malabsorption supervenes causing weight loss, oily stools, and other clinical features of malnutrition. Surprisingly there are few problems related to malabsorption of the fat soluble vitamins. The diabetes is usually mild, requiring little more than dietary therapy.

Other complications include pseudocyst formation which may be a common cause of persistent pain in chronic pancreatitis. Massive ascites may also occur, usually associated with a pseudocyst. Pleural effusions, also with elevated amylase values, may present with dyspnea, chest pain or cough. Drainage by thoracentesis or a chest tube should similarly be tried before managing the internal pancreatic fistula surgically.

Laboratory Assessment

Investigation may show only a modestly elevated serum amylase, hyperglycemia and transient cholestasis with increased bilirubin and alkaline phosphatase values. The 72 hour fecal fat may be elevated. The most prominent radiological finding is the presence of pancreatic calcification on plain film. When present, the classical triad of pancreatic calcification, diabetes mellitus and steatorrhea establishes the diagnosis of chronic pancreatitis. Pancreatic function tests will demonstrate a low volume and low bicarbonate and enzyme concentration only when a major portion of the gland has been destroyed. Better definition comes from anatomical studies: with ultrasound, the pancreas looks irregular, sometimes with a dilated pancreatic duct; ERCP can define the pancreatic duct system better, and demonstrate the changes of chronic pancreatitis.

Management

Management is directed at prevention, pain control and pancreatic replacement therapy. As alcohol is presumably toxic to the pancreas, total abstinence is advisable in alcohol-related pancreatitis. In the early stages this should reduce exacerbations. Unfortunately it is difficult to demonstrate conclusively that abstinence slows disease progression, especially when the process is advanced.

Pain is a major problem in chronic pancreatitis. During milder relapses, analgesics, bed rest and a reduced oral intake are effective. In more severe cases with persistent pain, hospitalization becomes necessary, particularly in order to monitor narcotic use and search for another cause such as a pseudocyst. Pain relief may require narcotics, with a judicious choice between relief and abuse. Painful attacks have been attributed by some to duct obstruction, best identified by pancreatography (ERCP). This may necessitate aggressive surgical drainage procedures or resection of major (>85%) portions of the pancreas in selected patients. These procedures have limited success and considerable risk. Fortunately the pain tends to lessen as the disease progresses with fibrosis and atrophy.

The nutritional consequences of pancreatic insufficiency can usually be controlled with a low fat diet and oral pancreatic enzyme replacement therapy. Within limits, the more enzyme ingested with meals, the greater is the effect. Pancreatic replacement therapy is not necessary in mild cases where nutrition is adequate, at least in adults. Diabetes mellitus occasionally will require insulin replacement.

CYSTIC FIBROSIS

Cystic fibrosis is the commonest lethal genetic disease of whites occurring in 1 in 2,000 live births. Inherited as an autosomal recessive trait with the heterozygote parents displaying no clinical symptoms, it exhibits a wide variation in severity suggesting the presence of modifier genes or a closely linked multigenic locus. It affects primarily the exocrine glands which produce a thick sticky mucus. The mucus secretions precipitate and obstruct organ passages leading to chronic pulmonary disease, pancreatic insufficiency, hepatic cirrhosis, intestinal obstruction, and obstruction of the male genital tract. The eccrine sweat glands exhibit defective tubular reabsorption of electrolyte and/or water resulting in a striking increase in the levels of sodium and chloride in sweat. The cornerstone of diagnosis is based on the quantitative pilocarpine iontophoresis sweat chloride test which should be performed on at least two separate occasions. Sweat chlorides which exceed 60mEq/L are virtually diagnostic, although there is no clear agreement about the upper limits of the normal range in adults. With better long-term care and improved screening, cystic fibrosis is no longer confined to childhood and adolescence. Ten percent of patients are over 25 years of age.

There is a heterogenous assortment of presentations with variable degrees of organ dysfunction. Chronic obstructive pulmonary disease is eventually present in all cases accounting for much of the morbidity and most of the mortality associated with cystic fibrosis beyond the neonatal period. Gastrointestinal symptoms are only slightly less consistent; pancreatic insufficiency occurs in 85 percent of patients with cystic fibrosis, making it the most common cause of pancreatic insufficiency in the pediatric age in the western world. In children, pancreatic insufficiency results in weight loss, muscle deterioration, and growth retardation. Nutritional deficiencies are common. In adulthood presenting features may be diarrhea and steatorrhea. Recurrent episodes of pancreatitis may occur. The endocrine pancreatic dysfunction manifests as glucose intolerance in 30 percent of patients although only a few develop symptomatic diabetes mellitus. The intestinal tract is also commonly involved. Meconium ileus is the initial symptom in 15 percent of infants with cystic fibrosis, appearing within 48 hours of birth as intestinal obstruction. Beyond the neonatal period tenacious bowel contents and fecal impaction can produce distal intestinal obstruction with abdominal pain and a palpable caecal mass. This "meconium ileus equivalent", once a surgical problem, usually responds to the administration of a mucolytic agent like N-acetylcysteine via a nasoduodenal tube. Hepatic complications are common but symptoms are rare. Reversible cholestasis can occur in neonates and young children. When prolonged, perhaps from excessive biliary mucus, cholestasis is termed the "inspissated bile syndrome", and may be associated with meconium ileus. In children focal biliary fibrosis develops later on as a morphological lesion. These focal lesions coalesce in a few individuals progressing to biliary cirrhosis and portal hypertension. Biliary tract abnormalities occur in approximately one-third of patients. Gallbladders may be small ("microgallbladders") or nonfunctioning on oral cholecystography due to cystic duct obstruction. Bile salt malabsorption in cystic fibrosis leads to cholesterol gallstone formation.

Management is directed at preventing the progression of pulmonary involvement. Pancreatic enzyme replacement using enteric-coated microspheres is the mainstay of gastrointestinal therapy. If bicarbonate secretion from the pancreas is deficient, maximal enzyme function may not be achieved without the addition of sodium bicarbonate. Even with this, malabsorption of fat is never completely corrected in cystic fibrosis. Oral supplementation of essential fatty acids with linoleic acid monoglyceride and the fat soluble vitamins A, D, K and E is sometimes necessary.

PANCREATIC TUMORS

CARCINOMA OF THE PANCREAS

The incidence of carcinoma of the pancreas is rising steadily in all western countries, trebling in North America since 1930 and doubling in the UK over the same period. Pancreatic cancer is now the second most prevalent gastrointestinal malignancy and the fourth most frequent cause of all deaths from cancer. Despite this rapid increase, treatment is as unsuccessful as ever. The 5-year survival rate is one of the worst of all cancers (1 percent). The dismal prognosis, where most patients die within 6 months of diagnosis, presumably results from its late presentation with metastases. Early symptoms are vague, while evaluation of this deep-seated organ is difficult. The major risk factors are smoking, diabetes mellitus and perhaps coffee consumption. Diabetes mellitus and chronic pancreatitis have been associated with pancreatic carcinoma, yet pancreatic carcinoma itself can induce both conditions. The causal relationship is therefore not clear.

Carcinoma of the pancreas commonly involves the head in three-quarters of patients, and the body and tail in the remainder. Carcinoma can also arise in periampullary tissues other than the pancreas (i.e., the lower 2 cm of the common bile duct, the ampulla of Vater, and the duodenum adjacent to the papilla of Vater). These tumors present clinically in the same way as carcinoma of the head of the pancreas but have a slightly more favorable prognosis.

The major symptoms are pain, jaundice, and weight loss. Some patients may present insidiously with depression followed by progressive painless jaundice. Over half, however, present with pain and almost 90 percent have pain at some time in the course of the disease. The *pain* is typically a boring, epigastric ache which is progressive and worse at night. The pain may be aggravated by eating or reclining; relief may come from sitting forward. Pain is usually referred to the back. *Jaundice* may be the first symptom of carcinoma of the head of the pancreas or periampullary tumors, but pain soon follows. The cholestasis is progressive although spontaneous fluctuations sometimes occur. Pruritus can be particularly troublesome. *Weight loss* is perhaps the commonest symptom and is also rapid and progressive. It likely results from anorexia rather than malabsorption because steatorrhea occurs in only about 10 percent of patients. Other symptoms include epigastric bloating and flatulence, malaise, altered bowel habits and vomiting. In carcinoma of the head of the pancreas, jaundice and an enlarged smooth liver are common. The gallbladder is enlarged and painless (Courvoisier's Law) in up to one-third of cases. In carcinoma of the body and tail of the pancreas, an abdominal mass is found in 50 percent. Thrombophlebitis occurs in less than 10 percent of cases.

Laboratory investigations may show an elevated serum amylase and lipase, fasting hyperglycemia or glycosuria, or an anemia. The stools can be positive for occult blood in periampullary carcinoma. The tumor mass is best identified by duodenoscopy and ERCP. Duodenoscopy with a side viewing endoscope allows visualization and biopsy of the ampulla of Vater. Cannulation of the pancreatic duct allows injection of contrast media, to outline the biliary and pancreatic duct system, and collection of pancreatic juice for cytological analysis. Ultrasonography and CT scanning are valuable non-invasive tools to detect mass lesions in the pancreas. Pancreatic function tests and radionucleotide pancreatic scan are either nonspecific or insensitive. Percutaneous aspiration biopsy of the pancreas under ultrasonic guidance can be diagnositic. Commonly, laparotomy is required for both a tissue diagnosis and assessment of tumor resectability.

The results of surgical treatment of carcinoma of the body of the pancreas have been uniformly discouraging. Most surgeons now opt for a palliative bypass procedure to relieve any cholestatic jaundice or duodenal obstruction. In early cases of periampullary carcinoma, surgical excision carries a slightly more favorable result. Medical management is directed at reducing pain, improving nutrition and general support.

PANCREATIC ENDOCRINE TUMORS

Pancreatic endocrine tumors arise from islet cells. As discussed elsewhere, these include either tumors that exert no perceptable hormonal effect, or the following hormone-secreting tumors:

1. insulinoma: beta-cell islet tumor producing insulin;
2. Zollinger-Ellison syndrome: non-beta cell islet tumor producing gastrin;
3. glucagonoma: alpha-cell islet tumor producing glucagon;
4. pancreatic cholera: delta cell islet tumor producing vasoactive intestinal peptide (VIP);
5. somatostatinoma: delta-cell islet tumor producing somatostatin
6. carcinoid syndrome: non-beta-cell islet tumor producing serotonin and prostaglandins.

Part 2: The Gastrointestinal Tract

ACUTE ABDOMINAL PAIN

History

In patients who are markedly distressed by severe abdominal pain the history must focus quickly on certain key questions to determine potential cause. Table 12.17 provides a general outline of the causes of abdominal pain.

Pain location is best defined by having the patient point to the region. The character of the pain is more typical (e.g., burning in peptic ulcer) when symptoms are milder. When pain is severe the patient will often not provide a hoped-for classical description. The question of duration must include rate of onset and periodicity. The abrupt onset of excruciating pain is characteristic of perforation of a hollow viscus or aneurysm. Pain that regularly waxes and wanes over minutes is colic and indicates an obstructed viscus or severe spasm. Pain related to mealtimes is more representative of peptic ulcer, cholelithiasis and pancreatic diseases. Specific aggravating and relieving factors to question are position, relationship to eating and to bowel movements. Associated features often help narrow the differential diagnosis. For example, the coexistence of fever indicates an inflammatory process in the abdomen. Hematemesis and melena suggest peptic ulcer. Concomitant diarrhea suggests inflammatory bowel disease. Urinary frequency may indicate an inflammatory process adjacent to the bladder as in appendicitis, diverticular disease and peptic inflammatory disease.

Physical Examination

Certain physical signs have diagnostic implications. The physical examination begins with auscultation of the abdomen to determine whether there is an ileus. Prior palpation may create pseudo-bowel sounds. Absence of bowel sounds indicates ileus and if accompanied by board-like rigidity of the abdomen the condition is termed an acute abdomen. This commonly results from widespread peritoneal inflammation (generalized peritonitis). High-pitched intermittent bowel sounds are characteristic of bowel obstruction. A venous hum may accompany portal hypertension and a systolic arterial murmur over the liver may be found in hepatoma. A bruit near the mid-line accompanied by a pulsating abdominal mass is characteristic of an abdominal aortic aneurysm. A gastric succussion splash present four or more hours after a meal suggests gastric outlet obstruction.

Generalized abdominal distention may be due to a partial bowel obstruction or ascites. If abdominal distention is suspected but the patient is corpulent, ask the patient directly whether the shape of the abdomen is different than usual.

An enlarged gallbladder may often be more apparent by visual inspection from a tangential plane than by palpation. This is caused most frequently by carcinoma of the head of the pancreas or at the ampulla of Vater. Edema of the flank may indicate a perinephric abscess.

Table 12.17 **Causes of Abdominal Pain**

I. Intra-abdominal Structures
  1. Generalized peritonitis (acute abdomen)
    a. Perforated viscus
    b. Primary bacterial peritonitis
    c. Ruptured ovarian cyst
  2. Localized pain
    a. Above umbilicus e.g. peptic ulcer, cholecystitis, biliary colic, pancreatic disease, hepatitis
    b. Periumbilical—e.g. small bowel obstruction, Crohn's disease
    c. Below umbilicus—e.g. appendicitis, diverticular disease, inflammatory bowel disease, pelvic inflammatory disease
    d. Back and abdominal—e.g. retroperitoneal neoplasms, renal and ureteral obstruction
II. Extra-abdominal Causes
  1. Muscle wall—e.g. hematoma
  2. Neurogenic—e.g. radiculitis from spinal osteoarthritis, *Herpes zoster*
  3. Thoracic—e.g. myocardial infarction, pneumonia
  4. Metabolic—e.g. diabetes, lead poisoning, uremia, porphyria, adrenal insufficiency

---

Laboratory Investigation

The initial selection of laboratory tests is based on information derived from the history and physical examination. Certain studies will be discussed briefly because they deserve special emphasis in the context of evaluating the patient with abdominal pain.

Plain x-ray films of the abdomen are often obtained very early because a wealth of information may be obtained. Some of the diagnostic findings in plain films of the abdomen are outlined in Table 12.18. *Ultrasound* is especially useful for abscesses, cysts, aneurysms, and gallstones. An *abdominal tap* and analysis of peritoneal fluid may provide a quick answer in some acute abdominal conditions and should be performed when free peritoneal fluid is suspected on the basis of the physical examination. A white blood cell count greater than 250/mm^3 in peritoneal fluid is usually associated with intra-abdominal trauma, acute pancreatitis, ruptured aneurysm, ruptured spleen and some neoplasms. Exudative ascites is found in the presence of bacterial peritonitis, pancreatitis, and peritoneal malignancy. An elevated ascitic fluid amylase is characteristic of pancreatitis. *Contrast radiographs* with water soluble media are done for suspected perforation or to localize the site of an intestinal obstruction. In chronic abdominal pain conventional barium studies will provide much more specific information.

Initial Management

In acute abdominal conditions supportive care must often begin prior to institution of any investigations. It may be necessary to resuscitate the patient quickly with fluid, electrolytes and blood. Opiate analgesics should only be given in moderate doses until the precise nature of the abdominal pain has been established. When an ileus is present or when intestinal obstruction is suspected, nasogastric suction should be instituted promptly. In patients with an acute abdomen, electrocardiograms and chest radiographs should be performed early for two reasons: (1) surgery may be required on an emergent basis; (2) there may be accompanying pneumonitis in older patients who have been confined to bed for a long time, or myocardial ischemia may have resulted from hypotension.

SEVERE GASTROINTESTINAL BLEEDING

Bleeding from the gastrointestinal tract may be severe, with visible blood in vomitus or stools; the overall mortality is 10 percent. The major complications of massive gastrointestinal bleeding, especially in the elderly, are myocardial ischemia, stroke and renal failure.

The patient may present with hematemesis, melena, hematochezia (red bloody stools) or shock. The basic steps in management are to resuscitate the patient, institute initial nonspecific therapy, localize the bleeding site and institute specific therapy.

Resuscitation and Initial Assessment

The first step is to determine the patients volume status. A markedly reduced circulating blood volume is reflected by symptoms of faintness and thirst, and by signs of postural hypotension and tachycardia.

Resuscitation entails frequent monitoring of vital signs, fluid intake and output. Intravenous fluids (normal saline or lactated Ringer's solution) are given until blood is available for transfusion. In most instances, packed red blood cells can be used. Platelets must be supplemented with every five units of blood transfused and fresh frozen plasma should be added after every 4 to 6 units of packed red blood cells. Serial hematocrit determinations are required because the initial values may reflect hemoconcentration. The hematocrit level usually falls after plasma volume is expanded. Nasal oxygen may be required and an electrocardiogram must be obtained promptly in all patients with hypotension.

The next step is to determine whether the patient has upper versus lower gastrointestinal tract bleeding. Brisk bleeding from sites proximal to the duodenojejunal junction (ligament of Treitz) results in hematemesis and/or black (melena) stools. Black stools may also be produced by the ingestion of iron,

Table 12.18 **Diagnostic Findings on Abdominal Plain Films**

Findings	Example
Calcifications	
Right upper quadrant	Gallstones
Midline linear	Aortic aneurysm
Midline mottled	Chronic pancreatitis
Lateral to spine	Renal, ureteric calculi
Dilatation of hollow organs	Obstruction, ileus
Gas collections	
Free air under diaphragm	Perforated viscus
Circumscribed and mottled	Abscess
Sentinal loop in small intestine	Acute pancreatitis
Masses	Tumors, abscesses
Loss of colonic haustra	Ulcerative colitis
Thumbprinting of bowel	Ischemia, Crohn's Disease

charcoal, large amounts of spinach or bismuth. Stool is usually maroon-colored when bleeding is from distal small bowel or right side of the colon and is reddish when lesions of tranverse and distal colon bleed massively. Since stool color is affected by transit time, massive bleeding from the stomach or proximal duodenum with rapid transit may result in maroon or red-colored loose stools, not melena.

With repeated hematemeses the patient usually vomits bright red blood. However, if blood has been in the stomach for an hour or more and digestion has begun, then the blood will appear as "coffee grounds". In the patient with melena but no vomiting, a nasogastric tube is passed to determine whether "coffee grounds" are present in gastric contents. If they are, then upper gastrointestinal bleeding is confirmed.

The history may help identify a cause of bleeding. Has the patient bled before and was a diagnosis established? Does the patient take aspirin, anticoagulants or excessive alcohol? Is there a prior history of any of the common causes of gastrointestinal bleeding and the associated clues shown in Table 12.19? If no clues are evident then more exotic causes must be considered. These include primary bleeding disorders (coagulopathies) and vascular disorders such as hereditary hemorrhagic telangiectasia (Osler-Weber-Rendu syndrome).

Nonspecific Therapy

Gastric lavage with iced saline is usually performed if there is blood in the stomach. It is not known whether it helps stop bleeding but it provides the additional potential benefit of clearing the region for endoscopic examination. Indwelling nasogastric tubes are not required to monitor bleeding rate or detect rebleeding. They are necessary only if there is repeated vomiting. Careful monitoring of vital signs and bowel sounds is essential. Hyperactive bowel sounds suggest active bleeding whereas ileus in association with bleeding suggests an intraabdominal catastrophe.

Most patients stop bleeding soon after admission to hospital. Five to 10 percent continue to bleed. If esophageal varices are suspected, intravenous vasopressin can be tried, at a rate of 0.2–0.4 units/min. This is contraindicated if there is evidence of current or recent myocardial, cerebral, or renal ischemia. After upper gastrointestinal tract bleeding ceases and before a specific diagnosis is established, cimetidine 300 mg every 6 hours and liquid antacids 30 cc/h can be started. There is no evidence however that this therapy alters the natural history of the bleeding.

Table 12.19 **Common Causes of Overt Gastrointestinal Bleeding**

Causes	Clues
Upper gastrointestinal bleeding	
Peptic ulcer	Epigastric pain
Erosive gastritis/ duodenitis	Aspirin ingestion, stress "ICU" setting, alcoholism
Esophagitis	Heartburn
Esophageal varices	Alcoholism; signs of chronic liver disease
Gastric carcinoma	Weight loss
Esophageal (Mallory-Weiss) tear	Repeated "dryheaves"
Lower gastrointestinal bleeding	
Carcinoma of colon	Change in stool habit and calibre
Diverticular disease	Longstanding symptoms; previous radiographs
Angiodysplasia	Elderly; aortic stenosis murmur
Ischemic bowel disease	Ileus; abdominal pain
Inflammatory bowel disease	Diarrhea; previous symptoms
Hemorrhoids	Bright red rectal bleeding; physical examination
Polyps	History of previous finding; family history

Tests to Make a Specific Diagnosis

Endoscopy is the most accurate first test for upper gastrointestinal bleeding. It is best deferred until bleeding stops, in order to optimize visualization in a clear field. If surgery appears imminent because active bleeding continues or is life-threatening, then endoscopy should be done because even suboptimal visualization may aid the surgeon's operative approach.

For patients with hematochezia anoscopy and sigmoidoscopy may reveal hemorrhoids, inflammatory bowel disease, carcinoma, or polyp. A barium enema may reveal diverticular disease, colonic tumor or inflammatory bowel disease.

Angiography is only of limited value but is sometimes used when bleeding is massive. It requires special skills not generally available and the bleeding must be brisk at the time of the test to localize the site.

Colonoscopy for lower intestinal bleeding is currently being evaluated.

Specific Therapy

This will be detailed in the sections that deal with specific disorders.

Certain therapeutic measures are employed to help

"buy time", so that a patient can be stabilized prior to surgery and in high-risk surgical candidates where the hope is that bleeding ceases and surgery can be avoided. Esophageal balloon tamponade for esophageal varices is risky and requires skilled personnel. Intra-arterial vasopressin infusion, delivered after angiography sometimes reduces the rate of bleeding. A number of novel techniques are being evaluated to determine whether they affect outcome and prevent the need for surgery. These include endoscopic hemostasis with laser or electrocautery for ulcers and for vascular lesions such as angiodysplasia of the right colon. Endoscopic sclerosis of esophageal varices is being evaluated to determine whether it helps control re-bleeding.

Surgery is reserved for patients who fail to stop bleeding or who rebleed in hospital. The decision when to operate is based on the underlying cause and the patient's general condition. It should be deferred as long as possible in patients with diffuse erosive gastritis associated with aspirin ingestion. On the other hand, an elderly patient in good general health might have surgery earlier (e.g., after a 6 unit bleed from a duodenal ulcer). This is because the risks of rebleeding and mortality are greatest in the elderly.

THE ESOPHAGUS

Structure and Function

The esophagus is a 20–25 cm long tube that is bound at each end by muscular sphincters. The primary function is to transport material from the mouth to stomach. The mucosa is lined by stratified squamous epithelium. The muscle layer consists of an inner circular and an outer longitudinal component. The inner bundle obliterates the lumen when it contracts and the outer bundle shortens the esophagus during contraction. The upper esophageal sphincter (cricopharyngeus) consists of striated (skeletal) muscle. Distal to this is a transition zone that extends for one-quarter of the esophagus. It consists of variable amounts of striated and smooth muscle. The lower half to two-thirds of the esophagus and the lower esophageal sphincter contain a smooth muscle wall.

The esophagus can be divided into thirds when considering venous and lymphatic drainage. This breakdown helps to understand the development of esophageal varices and the lymphatic spread of cancer. Blood drains through the superior vena cava, azygous, and gastric (coronary) veins. The latter are part of the portal venous system. Lymphatic drainage is to cervical nodes from the upper esophagus, to mediastinal nodes from the mid-third and to the celiac nodes from the lower third.

The voluntary act of swallowing is initiated by relaxation of the upper esophageal sphincter and the initiation of peristalsis. This is controlled by the swallowing center in the brain stem and cranial nerves V, VII, IX-XII.

Innervation of the esophageal body and lower esophageal sphincter is via 3 systems: parasympathetic cholinergic, sympathetic adrenergic, and neurons neither cholinergic nor adrenergic. Peristalsis refers to a series of sequential stripping waves from proximal to distal esophagus usually culminating with relaxation of the lower esophageal sphincter. The intrinsic control of peristalsis and lower esophageal sphincter function is from intramural neurons whose specific neurotransmitter has not been identified. Although vagal stimulation can stimulate peristalsis, vagotomy does not abolish it. Cholinergic drugs stimulate peristalsis and lower resting esophageal sphincter pressure. Anticholinergics have the opposite effect.

The lower esophageal sphincter is located at the level of the diaphragmatic hiatus, occupies a zone of 2–4 cm and is approximately 38–42 cm from the incisors. There are no grossly thickened or specialized collections of muscle as is seen in other sphincters. This sphincter has two major functions: to maintain a high pressure zone and to relax after swallowing (in order to permit material to pass from esophagus into stomach). The resting tone of the lower esophageal sphincter is controlled by direct myogenic action. β adrenergic drugs, nitrates and calcium channel blockers inhibit peristalsis and reduce esophageal sphincter tone.

Major Symptoms of Dysfunction

Chest Pain

The cardinal symptom of gastroesophageal reflux is heartburn, characteristically a retrosternal burning. In some patients the pain is localized only to the epigastrium and thus mimics peptic ulcer pain.

Patients with motor disorders of the esophagus (esophageal spasm) may describe a gripping type of retrosternal pain that mimics pain of myocardial ischemia. Odynophagia refers to painful swallowing. This may be associated with dysphagia. It is commonly reported by patients with severe erosive esophagitis or strictures due to gastroesophageal reflux, or by those with esophageal infections such as candida and herpes.

Dysphagia

This means difficulty in swallowing. These patients must be investigated thoroughly because of the risk of pulmonary aspiration and malnutrition resulting from fear of eating or inability to swallow. There are two broad categories. One is produced by an abnormality in the neuromuscular function of the striated muscle portion of the esophagus including the upper esophageal sphincter. This results in a transfer problem characterized by difficulty in initiating a swallow and moving material from the mouth to esophagus. Often there is associated nasopharyngeal aspiration and choking coughs. Clinical examples are seen in some patients with strokes, myasthenia gravis and those with local lesions such as carcinoma.

Esophageal dysphagia is produced by a transport problem. The patient describes the food as sticking behind the sternum and surprisingly can often pinpoint the actual site of the lesion. Table 12.20 outlines the esophageal causes of dysphagia. The clinical challenge is to determine whether the dysphagia is due to mechanical obstruction, chiefly benign strictures and carcinoma, or a motor (neuromuscular) disorder such as achalasia or diffuse esophageal spasm.

If the dysphagia has progressed from an initial difficulty only with solids through to problems with liquids, then a benign stricture or carcinoma is most likely. If heartburn has been a prominent accompaniment then benign stricture is more likely.

If the dysphagia has been intermittent at the outset for *both* solids and liquids and progression has been slow then the diagnosis favors a primary neuromuscular disorder such as achalasia.

Finally, if the dysphagia has been intermittent, longstanding and only for solids then an esophageal web or ring is the favored diagnosis.

Table 12.20 **Esophageal Causes of Dysphagia**

I. Mechanical obstruction
  1. Intraesophageal lesions
     Benign strictures
     Tumors
     Lower esophageal (Schatzki) rings
     Webs
  2. Extraesophageal compression
     Mediastinal tumors
     Vascular lesions (aneurysm, aberrant right subclavian artery)
II. Neuromuscular Disorders
  1. Primary
     Achalasia
     Diffuse esophageal spasm
  2. Secondary
     Scleroderma

Gastroesophageal Reflux (Reflux Esophagitis)

This is the most common esophageal disorder. Symptoms of gastroesophageal reflux are among the most common gastrointestinal complaints.

Pathogenesis

Reflux of gastric contents is a normal event and most people have experienced its major symptom, heartburn. In healthy, asymptomatic persons brief (several minute) episodes of asymptomatic reflux may occur several times a day. These brief episodes of physiologic reflux occur most commonly within 2 hours after meals, and at night when sleeping.

The patient with symptomatic gastroesophageal reflux has a condition that represents an intensification of physiologic reflux. A number of factors contribute to its development but no single factor can be implicated as primary. Lower esophageal sphincter pressures in patients with symptomatic reflux are lower than in healthy controls but there is a great deal of overlap. One-third of patients may have normal sphincter pressures. Acid clearance from the esophagus is often delayed after a reflux episode and this permits prolonged contact of the esophageal mucosa with acid and pepsin. In patients who develop esophageal reflux symptoms after gastric surgery, refluxed duodenal contents may be the primary injurious agents to the esophageal mucosa. When intraabdominal pressure increases, as in pregnancy or with weight gain in general, reflux symptoms may first appear. Other factors that have been implicated in some patients are asymptomatic delayed gastric emptying and the sliding hiatal hernia. The presence of a hiatal hernia is no longer considered a prerequisite for the development of symptomatic reflux but it may represent a risk factor. An important factor that is poorly understood is that of mucosal sensitivity. Some patients have severe symptoms with little evidence of mucosal damage. Other patients have minimal symptoms, yet they may develop severe complications of reflux such as ulceration and esophageal stricture.

Clinical Features

Heartburn is the cardinal symptom of gastroesophageal reflux. If may be provoked by eating, lying down or bending forward. Temporary relief is achieved by drinking fluids to clear the esophagus or by taking antacids. Certain foods may provoke

Table 12.21   **Tests Used in Gastrointestinal Reflux Disease**

	Comment
I. Tests that indicate possible reflux	
Barium radiograph	Poor predictor; main value is to exclude other conditions and document complications of reflux
Esophageal motility study	Manometric recording of lower esophageal sphincter pressure and esophageal peristalsis; *very low*, lower esophageal sphincter pressure is suggestive of gastroesophageal reflux
II. Tests that show effects of reflux	
Endoscopy and biopsy	Pathognomonic if ulcers, exudates or strictures found; many patients have normal appearing mucosa
Acid Perfusion (Bernstein test)	0.1N HCl dripped into the esophagus to try to mimic patients' symptoms; sometimes yields positive but unrelated symptoms
III. Tests that show actual reflux	
Acid reflux (Tuttle) test	pH probe in distal esophagus and pH recorded before and after intragastric instillation of 0.1N HCl
24 hour pH test	pH probe in lower esophagus records number and duration of reflux episodes; clinical utility requires more evaluation
Gastroesophageal scintiscan	Monitor reflux and quantity of radioactive technetium instilled into the stomach

heartburn, typically citrus juices and coffee. Some patients have the accompanying symptom of regurgitation of bitter-tasting fluid into the throat. If this occurs at night the patient may wake up coughing or may have liquid gastric contents staining the pillow. Some patients present with the complications of chronic gastroesophageal reflux. They may have overt or occult (anemia) gastrointestinal bleeding from esophageal ulceration, or dysphagia from a stricture. Occasionally their pain is more akin to that of angina pectoris. This is believed due to esophageal spasm induced by the reflux. Some patients have pain only localized to the area of the xiphisternum. In these individuals peptic ulcer is the major consideration in differential diagnosis.

Laboratory Investigation

The syndrome of symptomatic gastroesophageal reflux requires a clinical diagnosis, based on the history and response to therapy.

When tests are deemed necessary they are usually barium radiographs and endoscopy. Table 12.21 outlines the tests that may be used in gastroesophageal reflux disease. The first test that is usually done is a barium radiograph, preferably with cine esophagram so that esophageal motility can be assessed simultaneously. The same examination helps exclude peptic ulcer, carcinoma and esophageal stricture. Demonstration of barium reflux into the esophagus is not a discriminating point because a normal person may reflux barium and conversely a patient with chronic reflux symptoms may not reflux at the time of the examination. The finding of a hiatal hernia is unimportant in diagnosis because this finding is so common in the general population.

The other most commonly used test, when tests are deemed necessary, is endoscopy and biopsy. This helps exclude other conditions but in addition can confirm the presence of mucosal injury if ulcers, exudates or strictures are found. However, three-quarters of unselected patients with symptomatic reflux may have a normal mucosal appearance at endoscopy. Even on biopsy only one-fifth of patients have inflammatory change with polymorphonuclear leukocytes. Others may have the histologic findings of elongated dermal papillae and basal cell hyperplasia in the stratified squamous epithelium. These changes however may be patchily distributed and are also found in normal persons within 2 cm of the lower esophageal sphincter.

None of the tests listed in Table 12.21 is ideal in terms of sensitivity or specificity. They should be reserved for patients with atypical symptoms who are suspected to have gastroesophageal reflux, patients who have a suboptimal response to therapy, and those in whom surgery is contemplated.

Treatment

The two goals of therapy are to control symptoms and to help prevent recurrences. The latter is difficult and pertains largely to weight loss for the overweight and cessation of smoking. Smoking decreases lower esophageal sphincter pressure.

Liquid antacids taken as 15–30 cc, 1 and 3 hours

after meals and at bedtime control symptoms in most patients. Full-dose H$_2$-receptor antagonist therapy should be reserved for those with severe symptoms, or with complications. However, a single dose of cimetidine at night may be useful for the patient who continues to be wakened despite daytime therapy with antacids. Patients should be encouraged to continue antacid therapy for at least one week after all symptoms have cleared.

A number of foods have been shown to reduce lower esophageal sphincter pressure. However the most important dietary advice is to have the overweight patient lose weight. Often a very modest weight reduction will dramatically reduce symptoms, presumably because it results in a reduction of intraabdominal pressure. Coffee is a potent stimulant of gastric secretion and should only be taken in moderation and then only in conjunction with food. Alcohol intake should be reduced or eliminated during the active treatment period. The only other dietary advice is to have the patient avoid specific foods that provoke symptoms and to avoid food binges.

Nocturnal reflux is reduced by having patients elevate the head of their bed on 6 inch blocks and by avoiding food and fluids for two hours before bedtime.

Patients who do not respond within a week or two to this initial approach require four times a day H$_2$-receptor antagonist therapy. This can be given in addition to antacids. For the intractable patient, either urecholine or metoclopramide can be used as adjunctive therapy. Both increase lower esophageal sphincter pressure and accelerate gastric emptying. The urecholine dose is 25 mg and the metoclopramide dose is 10 mg; given one-half hour before meals and at bedtime. The major side effects of urecholine are increased salivation, urinary frequency, tachycardia and bronchoconstriction. The major side effects of metoclopramide are drowsiness, anxiety and rigidity or tremors.

How long should therapy be continued? Several weeks suffices if symptoms come under control quickly and especially if the patient is motivated to lose weight and curtail smoking. For patients with more intractable symptoms or with complications such as bleeding from esophageal erosions or ulcers, therapy should continue for several months, including one of the adjunctive drugs. Specific recommendations for therapy duration are hampered by a lack of a specific end point. The patient with frequent recurrences should continue elevation of the bed head, avoidance of evening food and fluids and may require a night-time dose of an H$_2$-receptor antagonist for many months after completion of the initial intensive course of therapy.

Most patients will respond to therapy. Thereafter they may have periodic brief flares and will control their symptoms with antacids on a p.r.n. basis. A smaller group of patients has frequent major flareups or develops complications of reflux.

The small number of patients who have frequent major recurrences and/or complications that cannot be controlled with medical therapy require surgery. The fundoplication operation is the most common antireflux operation performed. The principle is to wrap the gastric fundus around the distal esophagus. Its major side effect is a gas-bloat syndrome.

Complications

Aspiration   Aspiration pneumonia or frequent bronchitis episodes may complicate chronic gastroesophageal reflux. Sometimes the accompanying heartburn is only mild relative to the severity of the regurgitation.

Stricture   These patients present with dysphagia that has progressed slowly from solids to liquids or with a sudden food impaction. They are generally older and have had reflux symptoms for a long time. They have a history of aspiration pneumonia or frequent bronchitis. Barium radiographs and endoscopy with biopsy will define the extent and severity of the stricture and exclude carcinoma. Surgery can be avoided in many of these patients with intermittent peroral mercury bougie dilatation combined with medical therapy for reflux.

Ulcers and erosions   These are detected at endoscopy in patients with very severe symptoms or in patients with gastrointestinal bleeding. Esophageal carcinoma must be excluded. Therapy must be prolonged and titrated to ensure endoscopic evidence of healing.

Barrett's esophagus   This is an unpredictable mucosal response to chronic reflux in which variable lengths of the lower esophageal squamous lining epithelium are replaced by a columnar lining. Its prevalence in chronic reflux may be as common as 10 percent. Barrett's esophagus is recognized increasingly because of the greater utilization of endoscopy. These patients have a greater risk of developing adenocarcinoma of the esophagus, a tumor that is otherwise rare in this organ. They also are at greater risk from developing peptic strictures and ulcers.

There is controversy concerning the efficacy of medical or surgical therapy in causing regression of the Barrett's epithelium and also in relation to how often surveillance for adenocarcinoma should be done.

Uncommon Forms of Esophagitis

Dysphagia and odynophagia are the major symptoms in these patients. Endoscopy, with cultures, smears or biopsies, is required to establish a specific diagnosis.

Candida-associated esophagitis is seen increasingly in immunosuppressed patients on chemotherapy or antibiotics, and in patients with the acquired immunodeficiency syndrome. Oral nystatin is the initial drug used. Herpes simplex esophagitis may occur in previously healthy as well as immunosuppressed individuals. Oral lesions are not always evident. Symptoms usually subside within several weeks.

Radiation esophagitis is a major side effect of intrathoracic irradiation. Symptoms subside after the course of irradiation.

Corrosive esophagitis may develop from lye ingestion; an uncommon poison or suicidal agent. Esophageal dilatation may be required to prevent strictures.

Pill-induced esophagitis is an increasing problem, perhaps due to taking pills hurriedly without liquids. Tetracyclines, potassium chloride and ascorbic acid are among the drugs incriminated.

Esophageal Motility Disorders

Symptoms due to these disorders may result from primary neuromuscular involvement of the esophagus or be secondary to a systemic disease.

Primary Motility Disorders

Achalasia   This uncommon (1/100,000 per year) disorder may present at any age. Its cause is unknown. Achalasia is characterized by a loss of peristalsis and a lower esophageal sphincter that has a high resting pressure and an impairment of relaxation. Early on, patients have intermittent dysphagia for both solids and liquids and later they have progressive dysphagia for all foods. The esophagus becomes dilated and they develop overflow symptoms of coughing and aspiration.

Barium radiographs show a dilated food or fluid-filled esophagus with a short smooth narrowed distal segment. The dilated food-filled esophagus is often detectable on chest roentgenograms. These patients require endoscopy to rule out malignancy. Tumors of the proximal stomach may create a secondary type of achalasia, presumably by neuromuscular invasion.

Achalasia can be effectively treated by peroral pneumatic bag dilatation-rupture of the gastroeso-phageal junction or by surgical lower esophageal sphincterotomy, the Heller procedure.

Diffuse esophageal spasm   This is a puzzling disease or group of diseases. The clinical features, chest pain, dysphagia or both, overlap with other esophageal diseases and with coronary artery disease. The chest pain is squeezing and lasts minutes. If dysphagia is present for solids, liquids, or both, then an esophageal cause for the pain is more obvious. During pain and dysphagia episodes, even water may be regurgitated.

A barium swallow during symptomatic periods may reveal simultaneous contractions and a corkscrew appearance. Manometry may reveal large amplitude simultaneous contractions in the body of the esophagus, elevated resting pressures and impaired relaxation of the lower sphincter. If the patient is asymptomatic at the time of testing, x-ray studies and manometry may be normal.

Patients with squeezing chest pain, dysphagia or both may not have the typical manometric features of either achalasia or diffuse esophageal spasm. Some have isolated manometric features that overlap with both syndromes.

Therapy for presumed diffuse esophageal spasm includes antireflux therapy in the event that reflux triggers the spasm. Nitrites and anticholinergics are used with variable and unpredictable effectiveness. Calcium channel blocking agents are being assessed.

Secondary Motility Disorders

Scleroderma   Esophageal involvement in scleroderma is common and results from smooth muscle atrophy and fibrosis. These changes are manifested by weak or absent contractions of the smooth muscle portion of esophagus and a diminished lower esophageal sphincter pressure. This results in gastroesophageal reflux and markedly delayed acid clearance. Once the esophageal hypomotility is established then erosive esophagitis is common. These patients are at greater risk for developing strictures and aspiration pneumonia. They require a chronic maintenance antireflux program with the hope of avoiding stricture formation (see Chapter 17).

Other Secondary Motility Disorders   The elderly, diabetics, and patients with intestinal pseudoobstruction may have esophageal motility disturbances, but they are rarely symptomatic. Chagas disease due to infection with *Trypanosoma cruzi* is an important cause of abnormal gastrointestinal motility in certain parts of the world. Esophageal motility abnormalities with this infection are identical to those of achalasia!

Esophageal Cancer

Squamous cell carcinoma is the most common tumor of the esophagus. It is increasing in incidence in North America. Smoking and alcoholism are factors that increase risk. Progressive dysphagia is the most common presenting manifestation. Occasionally the presenting manifestation is anemia from occult bleeding. Accompanying weight loss is usually commensurate with the amount of dysphagia and reduced food intake that has occurred.

Every patient with dysphagia must be carefully evaluated for evidence of an organic lesion (Table 12.20). Even if a barium radiograph is negative, endoscopy must be done in patients with dysphagia. Endoscopic biopsy establishes the diagnosis in intramural obstructing lesions or excludes cancer in benign strictures. If an adenocarcinoma rather than a squamous cancer is found, the most likely site is the gastric cardia or alternatively an underlying Barrett's epithelium. Other tumors of the esophagus, such as leiomyomata, are rare.

Only 20 percent of the patients with squamous carcinoma of the esophagus have potentially resectable lesions, and five-year survival after operation is only 10 percent. Similarly dismal results are obtained with radiotherapy. There is no chemotherapy that significantly alters outcome.

The most important advance in patients with obstructing untreatable tumors has been the development of tubes that can be positioned through the obstructed lumen under direct-vision at endoscopy. This permits the patient to swallow and to eat. Formerly, many of these patients literally drowned in their secretions or had to have major palliative surgery when their condition was otherwise hopeless.

Other Esophageal Disorders

Esophageal Tears

The Mallory-Weiss syndrome is a tear at the gastroesophageal junction that causes upper gastrointestinal tract bleeding. It is not rare and occurs more often in alcoholics who experience prior vomiting and/or retching. The diagnosis is made at endoscopy. Most patients stop bleeding spontaneously once vomiting is controlled.

Diverticula

Zenker's diverticulum arises in the region of the upper pharyngeal sphincter. It may be asymptomatic, but when the diverticulum fills and enlarges, dysphagia and a mass in the neck may result. Barium radiographs make the diagnosis and surgery cures the condition.

Other esophageal diverticula are usually asymptomatic and are discovered incidentally. Sometimes they arise proximal to an obstructing lesion of the esophagus.

Rings and Webs

The Schatzki ring is a 1–3 mm thick firm narrowing at the squamocolumnar junction. It consists of fibrous tissue under the squamous epithelium. If it produces symptoms of dysphagia or food bolus impaction it can often be ruptured with a mercury-filled bougie or an endoscope.

Congenital muscular rings and webs secondary to iron deficiency are rare.

THE STOMACH

Structure

The wall of the stomach and the gastrointestinal tract distal to it have the same general arrangement—an inner mucosal lining, submucosa, circular and longitudinal muscle layers and a serosa.

The anatomic divisions of the stomach are shown in Figure 12.9. These landmarks are used to describe the location of lesions on barium radiographs and at endoscopy. The *cardia* is the region of the gastroe-

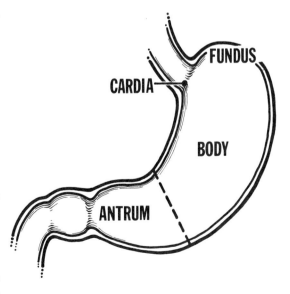

Fig. 12.9 Anatomic divisions of the stomach.

sophageal junction. The *fundus* is the dome of the stomach. The *body* occupies most of the stomach and ends at the region demarcated by a line drawn from the angularis (incisura) on the lesser curvature. The gastric *antrum* ends at the pyloric sphincter. This sphincter separates gastric antrum from the duodenal bulb, the small conical shaped area of the proximal duodenum.

From a mucosal histologic point of view the stomach has three different zones. Each zone is classified according to the histology of the mucosal glands beneath the columnar surface epithelium. The *cardiac gland* mucosa corresponds to anatomic cardia and contains clear staining mucus glands. The *fundic (oxyntic) gland* mucosa occupies both the anatomic body and fundus of the stomach. These glands contain the parietal cells which secrete acid and intrinsic factor, and the chief cells which secrete pepsinogens. The *antrum (pyloric) gland* mucosa corresponds to the anatomic antrum. The glands are of the clear-staining mucus type and contain gastrin-producing cells. The antal gastrin cells and other endocrine cells of the stomach such as those which contain somatostatin, serotonin, and glucagon-like activity require special immunocytochemical techniques for identification.

The extrinsic innervation is sympathetic from the celiac plexus and parasympathetic from the vagus. Blood supply is from the celiac trunk and venous drainage is conveyed to the liver by the portal vein.

Function

Motor Activity

The major function of the stomach is to act as a reservoir for solids and liquids and to control delivery into the duodenum. Most of the mixing of food occurs in the antrum. The antrum, pylorus and proximal duodenum must function in synchrony to permit controlled delivery of gastric contents into the small intestine. More than 50 percent of a mixed solid-liquid meal empties within 90 minutes.

Acid and Pepsinogen Secretion

Acid secretion is stimulated by sights, smells and chewing of food (cephalic phase), by the presence of food within the stomach and distension (gastric phase), and by food within the intestine (intestinal phase). Vagal stimulation, local cholinergic reflexes and gastrin play an important role in the stimulation of acid secretion. The primary chemical transmitters that regulate parietal cell function are acetylcholine, gastrin and histamine. They are delivered via neurocrine, endocrine and paracrine pathways respectively. The combination of histamine with H_2 receptors on the parietal cells is blocked by H_2 antagonists but not by H_1 antagonists.

Pepsinogens are the major secretory proteins of the gastric mucosa and are converted to the pepsin enzymes by hydrochloric acid. There are two major immunochemically distinct types of pepsinogen in man: pepsinogen I, located primarily in chief cells and pepsinogen II produced by chief cells and antral glands.

Gastric juice initiates the process of dispersion and digestion of a meal but achlorhydric man suffers no adverse nutritional consequences, except for possible vitamin B_{12} malabsorption. On the other hand, major changes in the reservoir or motor functions of the stomach, as after gastric surgery, may result in impaired absorption.

PEPTIC ULCER

Peptic ulcer affects the mucosal lining of the digestive tract that is exposed to gastric juice containing acid and pepsin; including lower esophagus, stomach, proximal duodenum, small intestine adjacent to a surgically produced connection with the stomach, and Meckel's diverticula that contain functioning gastric glands. Gastric and duodenal ulcers will be considered here. An ulcer is a mucosal break that extends the full thickness of the mucosa through the muscularis mucosa. Erosions are more superficial and do not penetrate the muscularis. They will be considered in the section on gastritis.

Risk Factors

Smoking increases the risk for duodenal and gastric ulcers. Aspirin clearly increases gastric ulcer and possibly duodenal ulcer risk. Close relatives of gastric or duodenal ulcer patients have three times the expected number of ulcers. Certain diseases pose an increased risk, especially for duodenal ulcer; chronic obstructive pulmonary disease, alcoholic cirrhosis, renal transplantation and possibly chronic renal failure. The incidence of gastric ulcer is increased in rheumatoid arthritis; antiarthritic drugs may contribute to the risk. The association of hyperparathyroidism and duodenal ulcer may be largely due to patients with Type I multiple endocrine adenomatosis who have both hyperparathryoidism and gastrinoma.

Pathogenesis and Pathophysiology

Peptic ulcer is a final common pathway of injury and represents a group of disorders in which different mechanisms are operative in a given patient. Ulcers occur when there is an imbalance between acid–pepsin and mucosal resistance. Increased acid–pepsin secretion, decreased mucosal resistance or the two acting together are ulcerogenic. The factors that contribute to mucosal resistance are poorly understood. They include mucosal blood flow, mucus and bicarbonate secretion, rate of cell renewal and the capacity of epithelial cells to resist autodigestion.

One-third of patients with duodenal ulcer secrete more acid in the basal state and in reponse to stimuli, however, there is great overlap with normal persons and those with gastric ulcer. Other defects that may be operative in duodenal ulcer in some patients are increased vagal drive, increased parietal cell sensitivity to stimuli and reduced acid inhibitory mechanisms. High levels of serum pepsinogen I are found in some duodenal ulcer patients and their relatives. Accelerated gastric emptying is also observed in some patients.

An important underlying defect in gastric ulcer appears to be impaired mucosal defense. Many gastric ulcers occur at the junction of gastric antrum and body on the lesser curvature and are associated with a diffuse nonerosive antral gland gastritis. It has been postulated that this diffuse antral gastritis reflects injury from increased reflux of duodenal contents into the stomach. Prepyloric gastric ulcers refer to those located within two cm of the pylorus. Physiologically, they behave more like duodenal ulcers.

There are certain ingrained beliefs that ulcers may be caused by stress, type of occupation, diet and alcohol. None have been proven.

Clinical Features

Duodenal ulcers occur more commonly than gastric ulcers and both are more common in men than in women. Duodenal ulcers affect approximately 10 percent of men and 4 percent of women during their lifetimes.

Upper epigastric pain is the main mode of presentation. It is usually located in the midline or just to the right. Sometimes it extends along the costal margin to the right edge of the rectus sheath. Some patients describe a burning quality but many others will use terms like boring, gnawing or hunger pains. In duodenal ulcer, pain relief will often occur within 30 minutes after eating or taking antacids. Eating sometimes worsens the pain, especially when ulcers are located near, or in the pyloric canal. Pain may be provoked or worsened by ingestion of aspirin, coffee or alcohol, and heavy smoking.

Some patients present *de novo* with few previous symptoms and with the complications of ulcer, such as bleeding or perforation. Some ulcers are detected incidentally and serve to remind us of the common discrepancy between the amount of pain experienced and the size and location of peptic ulcers.

The physical examination is often normal. The most important abnormal finding is localized tenderness to palpation in the upper or midepigastrium.

Peptic ulcer may mimic gastroesophageal reflux, symptomatic cholelithiasis or recurrent pancreatitis. The latter is not usually an important diagnostic consideration unless the patient is an alcoholic or has had recurrent bouts of pancreatitis in the past. Severe peptic ulcer disease with multiple ulcers, or failure to heal may occur in patients with the Zollinger-Ellison syndrome.

Laboratory Investigation

Patients with typical symptoms who are having a first or second attack of apparently uncomplicated peptic ulcer can be treated on the basis of a clinical diagnosis. Stools should be tested for occult blood and the plasma hemoglobin level assessed.

When a test is chosen, the first is usually a barium radiograph of the esophagus, stomach and duodenum (upper GI series). X-ray examination has a combined false-positive and false-negative rate of at least 20 percent. It is being replaced as the first test in many centres by endoscopy.

Endocrine causes of ulcer may need further investigation. (See Zollinger-Ellison Syndrome.)

Management

The objective of therapy is to control symptoms and to help accelerate healing. The average course of therapy is 6 weeks. Patients must be forewarned that their symptoms will generally vanish within a few days or weeks but that therapy must be continued.

Drugs

In duodenal ulcer an effective drug is one that is associated with an 80 percent or greater healing rate after 6 weeks of therapy. Healing rates are generally slower for gastric ulcer. The choices (Table 12.22) are basically between locally-acting drugs (antacids,

Table 12.22 **Classes of Drugs For Treatment of Peptic Ulcer**

Drug Class	Examples	Mechanism of Action
Reduce Acid		
1. Antacids	Many magnesium and aluminum-containing compounds	Neutralize gastric acid
2. Histamine H_2-receptor antagonists	Cimetidine; ranitidine	Block action of histamine on H_2 receptors
3. Anticholinergics	Atropine cogeners; Pirenzepine†	Block muscarinic action of acetycholine
Enhance Mucosal Defense		
1. Sulfated disaccharides	Sucralfate	Coats ulcer crater; may bind pepsin and bile acids.
2. Colloidal bismuth*	Tripotassium dicitrate bismuthate	Coats ulcer crater; may simulate mucus

† Structurally related to tricyclic antidepressants; undergoing trials.
* Undergoing trials.

sucralfate) and H_2-receptor antagonists (cimetidine, ranitidine). Anticholinergics are used little because of unpleasant side effects.

For uncomplicated peptic ulcer, local therapy is preferable as the first choice because of fewer side effects than with systemically absorbed drugs. All drugs used for peptic ulcer should be considered capable of interfering with the absorption of other drugs. Therefore, it is judicious practice to have patients on life-sustaining drugs such as digitalis or antiarrhythmics take these drugs at separate times from the drugs used to treat ulcers.

Antacids The potent antacids are those in liquid form that contain magnesium and aluminum hydroxides. An average dose is 30 cc, and the regimen is given 1 and 3 hours after meals and at bedtime. This postprandial timing prolongs the buffering capacity. The magnesium promotes diarrhea and the aluminum may result in constipation. The sodium content of some antacids is sufficient to warrant caution in patients with heart failure. Calcium-containing antacids are potent but are in disrepute because they may cause greater acid rebound than non-calcium containing antacids.

Sucralfate This disaccharide-aluminum hydroxide complex has only a minimal buffering effect and absorption. It binds to the ulcer base. Sucralfate provides an option for local therapy, without the compliance problems of frequent-dose antacid therapy; one gram is given 1 hour before meals and at bedtime.

H_2-receptor antagonists Cimetidine is the most widely used drug in this class. Ranitidine has been tested less but appears to be comparably effective and may have fewer side effects. The standard dose of cimetidine is 300 mg 4 times a day. The dose should be reduced in renal failure to 300 mg 3 times a day for a serum creatinine of 2–4mg/dl, and to 300mg every 12 hours for a serum creatinine greater than 4mg/dl.

Side effects of cimetidine are rare. They include confusion in the elderly, gynecomastia, and granulocytopenia. There may be important drug interactions with sedatives, propranolol and anticoagulants. When these drugs are prescribed concomitantly with cimetidine it may be necessary to reduce their dose.

Other drugs Colloidal bismuth is another promising locally-active drug undergoing trials. Certain prostaglandins remain experimental in ulcer therapy. They illustrate an important mechanism because some cogeners promote ulcer healing by a mechanism other than reduced gastric acid, presumably by shoring up mucosal defense.

General Approach to Treatment

During the course of therapy patients should avoid foods that predictably precipitate or aggravate attacks of pain. Coffee, even the decaffeinated form should be taken only in moderation because it is a potent stimulus of acid secretion. Aspirin-containing compounds and alcohol should be avoided. Patients should be strongly encouraged to stop smoking or at least drastically reduce the number of cigarettes they smoke. Patients will often ask about the relationship between stress and ulcer disease. They should be reassured that they have not brought the condition upon themselves, however, inordinate stress may provoke symptoms of ulcer disease just as it may provoke symptoms of most other conditions.

Duodenal ulcer therapy can be discontinued after 6 weeks and no further tests are required. The approach to gastric ulcers is different since a small number are malignant at the outset and may heal partially on medical therapy. Therefore documentation of healing is required either with a repeat X-ray examination or preferably with endoscopy. Endoscopy at the time of initial workup of a patient with gastric ulcer affords the opportunity to obtain biopsies and help rule out malignancy. In addition, if initial endoscopy was performed, the treatment course for gastric ulcers can be extended to about 2 months before a healing test is done, since they tend to heal more slowly than duodenal ulcers.

After the initial course of treatment is complete it is essential to explain the natural history to patients. The pain may return but this does not necessarily reflect a full-blown return of the ulcer itself. They may take p.r.n. antacids for occasional pain, and antacids several times a day as outlined previously for pain clusters. Patients should reconsult the physician if the pain occurs frequently. At that point another formal course of therapy may be required.

H_2-receptor antagonists may be considered for maintenance therapy. The main indication for chronic maintenance therapy with reduced dosages of cimetidine or with ranitidine is patients who have frequent symptom flares but who are high-risk surgical candidates because of associated diseases. The long term side effects of maintenance therapy are unknown, and it is also not known whether prolonged maintenance therapy actually reduces the complications of peptic ulcer. The patient with a rheumatic disorder who requires aspirin or other nonsteroidal anti-inflammatory drugs and has recurrent ulcers may require maintenance therapy with H_2-receptor antagonists.

Approximately 75 percent of duodenal and gastric ulcers will heal during this 6-week course of therapy. Symptoms will usually disappear much earlier. Endoscopic studies in duodenal ulcer have shown that more than half of patients have a return of the ulcer crater within a year after cessation of therapy. Thus pain may return in the absence of an ulcer crater or the crater may return and frequently be asymptomatic. This waxing and waning nature of the disease probably accounts for the considerable number of patients who have healed on placebo therapy in controlled trials.

Complications

With the exception of perforation, endoscopy is very helpful to accurately define the nature of the complication and exclude other causes.

Intractability

The most common form of intractability is characterized by such frequent relapses that repeated formal courses of therapy seriously interfere with a patient's life. Rarely do patients fail to achieve symptom-control or fail the healing test for gastric ulcer with a single-drug approach. The combination of local drugs and H_2-receptor antagonist therapy may help in this setting.

Bleeding

Approximately 20 percent of all patients with duodenal or gastric ulcer will bleed at some time in their lives. Bleeding is a more common complication than obstruction or perforation. The bleeding may be massive or may be occult and present as anemia. The management of the patient with overt bleeding has been discussed earlier. When bleeding is brisk, the decision concerning timing of surgery is based on the patient's condition and age. In younger patients surgery is usually deferred until the patient bleeds a second time.

Obstruction

This occurs because of progressive scarring in the region of the pyloric canal. Sometimes it is associated with swelling from an active ulcer. Vomiting is the principal symptom but more subtle complaints include early satiety and even the first development of heartburn. The latter is presumably due to the increased amount of gastric contents available for reflux into the esophagus. For complete obstruction with repeated vomiting, fluid and electrolyte replacement and nasogastric suction are instituted. Endoscopy is done to differentiate benign causes of outlet disease from cancer. Medical therapy for incomplete obstruction can be monitored with a saline load test or radioisotope (technetium-99 meal) emptying test. The saline load test is done by instilling 750 ml of normal saline into the stomach. A residual volume greater than 400 ml, 30 minutes later suggests persistent obstruction.

Perforation

If a duodenal ulcer on the anterior wall perforates, the patient will present with symptoms of generalized peritonitis. A duodenal ulcer on the posterior wall may present with *penetration*, characterized by symptoms of boring pain radiating to the back. This reflects penetration into the lesser sac and pancreatic bed. Perforations of gastric ulcers usually present with generalized peritonitis. A gastric ulcer rarely penetrates into the colon causing a gastrocolic fistula.

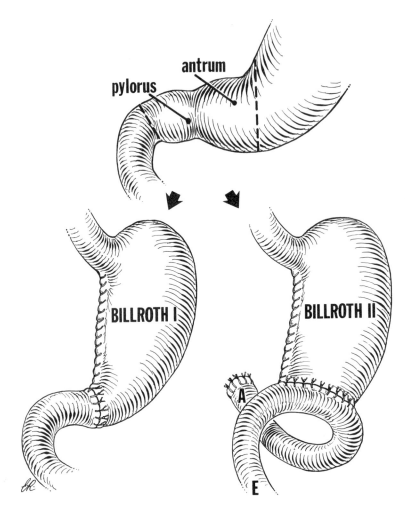

Fig. 12.10 Anastomoses after antrectomy. The Billroth I is a direct end-to-end hookup of the gastric remnant to the duodenum. The Billroth II entails oversewing the proximal duodenum and performing a gastrojejunosotomy. The afferent and efferent limbs are labeled A and E, respectively.

Surgery for Peptic Ulcer

Surgery is reserved for the complications of peptic ulcer. The objective in duodenal ulcer is to reduce acid secretion. Truncal vagotomy and pyloroplasty, or truncal vagotomy and antrectomy are the most commonly used procedures for duodenal ulcer. Antrectomy further reduces acid secretory capacity by removing the gastrin-secreting mucosa. With antrectomy the gastric remnant is joined directly to the first part of the duodenum (Billroth I). If there is excessive duodenal scarring, a Billroth II (gastrojejunostomy) is performed (Fig. 12.10). Parietal cell (highly selective) vagotomy is gaining acceptance for duodenal ulcer. This technically demanding operation involves transection only of the vagal branches to the acid-secreting portion of the stomach, leaving the nerves to the antrum intact. A drainage procedure (pyloroplasty) is not required because normal gastric emptying is preserved. Recurrent ulcer rate is greater with parietal cell vagotomy than with other operations, but post-surgical side effects are fewer.

For gastric ulcer, antrectomy alone or antrectomy with vagotomy is chosen.

Emergency surgery for perforation with generalized peritonitis often consists of simply oversewing the perforation.

Side Effects of Surgery

Only 5–10 percent of post-surgical patients develop troublesome symptoms. Those related to eating are most common and they can usually be improved with simple dietary maneuvers. (Table 12.23).

The early postprandial symptoms are abdominal fullness during or shortly after a meal, with variable accompanying nausea, crampy abdominal pain, feelings of weakness and sweating. Late postprandial symptoms are similar to those of hypoglycemia and can be relieved by eating sweets. Multiple factors contribute, including "dumping" of food and fluid into the small bowel, disturbances in gastric motor function associated with rapid gastric emptying, and functional hypoglycemia. Such patients should take frequent small meals, reduce the carbohydrate intake and take liquids between meals rather than with meals. When early satiety and vomiting predominate, metoclopramide taken before meals may improve symptoms.

Symptoms of prominent pain or vomiting require endoscopy to rule out recurrent ulcer and mechanical obstruction. Barium radiographs for recurrent ulcer may be inaccurate because of the surgical deformity. Recurrent ulcers usually occur at the site of the anastomosis in patients with a previous antrectomy. They often respond to H_2-receptor antagonist therapy. Antacids are ineffective because they empty too rapidly. Healing should be documented with follow-up endoscopy. If the ulcers recur promptly then another operation may be necessary. However, many of these patients can now be managed with intermittent courses of H_2-receptor antagonists. For the elderly and infirm, maintenance H_2-receptor antagonist therapy may be the most useful option.

A small group of patients has persistent postoperative pain and vomiting with no defined cause. The term symptomatic *alkaline reflux* has been applied to some of these patients. It is presumed that they are sensitive to the increased reflux of duodenal contents into the stomach after surgery. Empiric trials with antacids, bile salt binding agents, metoclopramide and reoperation (Roux-en-Y diversion) are only variably and unpredictably successful.

Iron deficiency anemia is the most common type of anemia after gastric surgery and the most common reason for it is failure to replenish iron stores after

Table 12.23   **Side Effects of Surgery for Peptic Ulcer.**

I. Multiple postprandial symptoms
    Early ("dumping")
    Late ("dumping")
II. Predominant pain and/or vomiting
    Defined Causes
        Recurrent ulcer
        Mechanical obstruction
        Bezoar (retained food concretions)
        Afferent loop syndrome
    Ill-defined Syndromes
        Nonobstructive delayed emptying
        Reflux "gastritis"
III. Other problems
    Anemia
    Diarrhea/Malabsorption
    Gastric cancer

operation. This is further compounded by the fact that iron absorption is reduced after surgery for peptic ulcer in many patients. These patients should be investigated as any other patient with iron deficiency anemia. Only if no cause is found should the anemia be attributed to the prior ulcer surgery. Vitamin B_{12} malabsorption is much less common after gastric surgery and is usually due to bacterial overgrowth (see Malabsorption section).

Many patients have more frequent and less-formed stools after surgery for peptic ulcer. Sometimes severe diarrhea occurs and persists. It has been termed *postvagotomy diarrhea*. If it is unaccompanied by symptoms of malabsorption and weight loss, dairy products can be removed from the diet because relative lactase deficiency may have been unmasked by surgery because of more rapid transit. If this fails, an empiric trial of a broad spectrum antibiotic such as tetracycline can be employed as a diagnostic-therapeutic test for bacterial overgrowth. If symptoms of malabsorption are dominant then other causes of malabsorption should be excluded.

A slight but definite risk of gastric cancer in the gastric remnant becomes apparent 15 years after antrectomy. Opinion is divided concerning how intense the surveillance should be.

NON-ULCER DYSPEPSIA

Non-ulcer dyspepsia represents a poorly understood group of disorders, even more common than peptic ulcer. These patients have epigastric discomfort similar to that of peptic ulcer but no ulcer is present. Sometimes there is endoscopic evidence of *duodenitis*, mainly duodenal bulb inflammation with swelling or tiny erosions. Often there are no abnormal findings at endoscopy. A clear-cut response to ulcer therapy is observed in some of these patients. When ulcer-type pain remains unexplained it is tempting to label such patients as "functional" or "psychosomatic". However, the absence of a crater in someone with ulcer-like symptoms is not sufficient evidence for the label of a psychological disorder.

ZOLLINGER-ELLISON SYNDROME

This rare disease is caused by a slow-growing non-beta cell gastrin secreting tumor of the pancreas. The syndrome is characterized by severe peptic ulcer disease and, sometimes, by diarrhea. The latter is due to large volumes of gastric acid that produce small bowel mucosal injury and malabsorption resulting from inactivation of bile acids and pancreatic juice. A gastrinoma should be suspected in patients with intractable ulcer disease, multiple ulcers or frequent recurrences in a given patient with diarrhea. Suspicion should be heightened when there is a strong family history of ulcer disease or when other family members have had pancreatic or parathyroid endocrinopathy (multiple endocrine adenomatosis-type I syndrome). The best tests to screen for this syndrome are a fasting serum gastrin and a one-hour basal gastric acid secretion test. A basal gastric acid output greater than 15 mmol/h and an elevated fasting serum gastrin strongly suggest this syndrome. Gastric acid secretory tests are used rarely and reserved primarily for patients suspected to have the Zollinger-Ellison syndrome.

Treatment is laparotomy with the hope of finding a resectable tumor (minority), and total gastrectomy to remove the target tissue and source of massive acid hypersecretion. An alternative is parietal cell vagotomy and maintenance H_2-receptor antagonist therapy.

GASTRITIS

Erosive Gastritis

Erosive gastritis is also known as acute or hemorrhagic gastritis. This important cause of upper gastrointestinal tract bleeding is usually associated with little or no abdominal pain. Barium radiographs are usually negative and the diagnosis is established with endoscopy. Underlying conditions include severe illness ("stress ulcers") such as burns, trauma, multiple organ system failure, aspirin and possibly other nonsteroidal antiinflammatory drug ingestion, and alcoholism. Rarely, erosive gastritis occurs without any obvious association and in this instance may represent a variant of peptic ulcer disease.

In seriously ill patients the pathogenesis is poorly understood and may relate to mucosal ischemia. The risk of bleeding in the seriously ill (ICU patient) has decreased dramatically in recent years. This is probably due to better cardiorespiratory and nutritional support. Use of prophylactic antacids or H_2-receptor antagonists for seriously ill patients may be a further contributor to the reduced frequency of bleeding in this category of patients.

Aspirin may contribute to both chronic low-grade gastrointestinal blood loss and more overt bleeding by inhibition of prostaglandin synthesis because prostaglandins play a role in mucosal defense. In addition, the low pK_a of aspirin facilitates gastric mucosal absorption in an acid environment and this may promote back diffusion of acid and pepsin. Aspirin taken on a full stomach or in the enteric-coated form is associated with a lower incidence of gastric erosions. In alcoholism a number of factors may be operative, including the effect of alcohol itself, malnutrition and heavy smoking.

The role of corticosteroids in this condition and in ulcer disease in general is unclear.

Most of these patients cease bleeding spontaneously and surgery for continued bleeding is only rarely required. When bleeding stops the patient should be treated as for ordinary peptic ulcer disease.

Nonerosive (chronic) Gastritis

This is a histologic diagnosis and is not a clinically recognizable entity. There is no proof that histologic nonerosive gastritis can cause symptoms. The inflammatory change is usually more prominent in the antral gland mucosa than fundic gland mucosa, but both histologic zones are often involved. The incidence increases with age so that some degree of nonerosive gastritis is virtually inevitable after the age of 50. Antral gland gastritis is a frequent accompaniment of gastric ulcers and gastric cancers of the body of the stomach. After antrectomy the gastric remnant develops an accelerated nonerosive gastritis which in part may contribute to the decreased acid secretion following surgery.

Severe fundic gland inflammation with atrophy is not uncommon in older persons and is associated with hypochlorhydria or achlorhydria. Achlorhydria refers to total absence of acid in the gastric juice aspirated after injection of a stimulant such as pentagastrin. It is important to recognize that most elderly patients who have severe atrophic fundic gland gastritis and achlorhydria do not have pernicious anemia. They have residual tiny nests of parietal cells and are still capable of secreting enough intrinsic factor to absorb vitamin B_{12} normally. In classical pernicious anemia there is total achlorhydria, fasting serum gastrin levels are elevated if the antrum is spared, and two-thirds or more of patients have serum parietal cell antibodies.

Specific Types of Gastritis

Several *specific* varieties of gastritis are rare and occur as part of a defined clinical syndrome restricted to the stomach or as part of a systemic disease. Radiation may produce antral or prepyloric ulcers or scarring. Menetrier's disease is characterized by thick, inflamed mucosal folds, hypochlorhydria and chronic hypoalbuminemia. Mucosal infection may occur in immunosuppressed patients (e.g., Candida or herpes) or as part of generalized infection in tuberculosis or syphilis. Crohn's disease and sarcoidosis may result in mucosal disease.

TUMORS OF THE STOMACH

Adenocarcinoma of the Stomach

Adenocarcinoma is the most common tumor of the stomach. In North America there has been a dramatic decline in incidence in the past 4 decades. This cancer is still very common in Japan, parts of Central and South America, and in parts of Eastern Europe.

Risk Factors

Patients with severe inflammation and atrophy of gastric glands (atrophic gastritis) have a slightly increased risk. In patients with pernicious anemia risk is estimated to be three times that of the general population. Adenomatous benign gastric polyps, larger than 2cm, may contain a carcinoma or may be associated with carcinoma elsewhere in the stomach. Fifteen years or more after surgical antrectomy, the risk is increased, especially in patients with a Billroth II anastomosis.

Clinical Features

Most patients have incurable lesions when they first present to physicians. The most common symptoms are indigestion, upper abdominal pain and weight loss. Anorexia and vomiting occur in at least half of the patients. Hematemesis is unusual but occult bleeding and anemia are common. The nature of the symptoms also relates to the location of the tumor and its growth pattern. Most of the tumors grow either as ulcers, as intraluminal masses or both. Rarely they grow along the gastric wall layers and result in reduced distensibility. The ulcerating type might present just as a benign gastric ulcer; mass lesions at the cardia or pylorus may be characterized by dysphagia and symptoms of gastric outlet obstruction respectively.

The physical examination may reveal epigastric tenderness. Signs of metastatic spread may include hepatomegaly or jaundice indicating hepatic metastases, an epigastric diffuse mass indicating local extension, or supraclavicular adenopathy.

Laboratory Investigation

The diagnosis is established with barium radiographs, endoscopy and biopsy. The main differential diagnosis is from benign gastric ulcer and other gastric tumors, especially lymphoma.

Iron deficiency anemia and stool positive for occult blood are common. Liver test abnormalities suggest metastatic deposits in the liver.

Treatment and Outcome

Surgical removal offers the only hope for cure. Unfortunately only half of the patients have a resectable lesion and many of them already have regional lymph node involvement. Operative mortality may be as high as 10 percent, in part because many patients are malnourished. The overall five-year survival is 10 percent. The tumors that have a more favorable prognosis are those confined to mucosa and submucosa without lymph node involvement.

There is no chemotherapy for metastatic disease that significantly increases overall survival. Very occasionally there are individuals who have worthwhile responses to chemotherapy or adjunctive therapy.

Other Tumors

Primary gastric lymphomas account for 5 percent of gastric malignancies. Most are the histiocytic or lymphocytic type. Secondary gastric involvement in disseminated lymphoma is more common than the primary form. The modes of presentation and investigation are similar to those of gastric adenocarcinoma. Treatment consists of surgery for excision and staging, and chemotherapy or radiation therapy. Thirty to 50 percent of patients survive 5 years or more.

Leiomyomas are often small and are detected incidentally. When they are large or when there is *leiomyosarcoma* central ulceration may develop in the overlying mucosa. In this setting anemia and overt bleeding is common.

Benign polyps are less common than in the colon and are often detected incidentally. They are most commonly hyperplastic or cystic in type. Adenomatous polyps are a less common form. Some of the larger ones can be removed by endoscopic polypectomy. Other tumors are endocrine cell (carcinoid) tumors, secondary metastases to stomach and rare tumors of the other elements of the gastric wall (i.e., vessels, nerves, etc.).

Abnormal Gastric Emptying

Acute Gastric Dilatation

This may occur after trauma, the use of body casts and in association with diabetic ketoacidosis and other causes of ileus. Vomiting and abdominal distension are the principal symptoms. Plain films of the abdomen reveal a dilated stomach filled with gas and fluid. Therapy is nasogastric suction.

Nonmechanical Delayed Emptying

This may occur after truncal vagotomy or as a complication of systemic disease, especially severe diabetes and severe scleroderma. Characteristically patients with gastric motility disorders have large stomachs that contain food seen on plain films or barium radiographs. Endoscopy is done to rule out mechanical obstruction due to benign ulcer or malignancy. Metoclopramide is beneficial in some patients.

Bezoars may be found in some of these patients. These mass-like concretions most commonly consist of retained food. Therapy to break them up consists of vigorous gastric lavage, fragmentation at endoscopy and trials of enzymes such as cellulase. Surgery is required if these measures fail.

Foreign Bodies

Foreign bodies may be swallowed inadvertently or intentionally. Small smooth objects pass through the intestines and can be spotted with the naked eye in stool or be detected in radiographs of stool if they are radioopaque. Sharp objects such as pins and needles should be removed endoscopically if possible. Some pass without incident. Others require surgical removal if they cause ulceration or perforation.

SMALL AND LARGE INTESTINE

Structure

General Features

The adult small intestine is approximately 8 m long and is divided into the duodenum, jejunum and ileum. The ligament of Treitz is the anatomic and radiologic landmark that corresponds to the region of the duodenojejunal junction. The large intestine measures approximately 1.2 m in length. The cecum is at the proximal end and the appendix arises from it. The ascending colon extends from the cecum to the hepatic flexure. The transverse colon is bounded by the hepatic and splenic flexures. The descending colon extends from the splenic flexure to the sigmoid colon. The sigmoid colon terminates distally in the rectum. The region of the mid-transverse colon is an arbitrary point used to separate the colon semantically into right and left portions.

The superior mesenteric artery supplies most of the small intestine and the colon up to the region of the splenic flexure. Distal to that zone, blood supply is mainly from the inferior mesenteric artery. Venous drainage follows a similar pattern.

The walls of the intestines have the same general arrangement as the rest of the gastrointestinal tract. The mucosa consists of a columnar surface epithelium, a lamina propria and a thin strip of muscularis mucosa. The longitudinal muscle of the colon is gathered into three bundles called teniae coli leaving the remainder of the colon wall with only circular muscle fibers.

In the small bowel, surface amplification is achieved by mucosal folds (valvulae conniventes), by finger-like villi which project into the lumen and also by microvilli (brush border) at the apical surfaces of epithelial absorptive cells. A glycocalyx ("fuzzy coat") sits on the surface and overlying it is an unstirred water layer.

In the colon there are no villi. The epithelial invaginations called rectal glands or crypts are packed with mucus-secreting goblet cells.

Cellular and Regional Specialization

Columnar absorptive cells are the most numerous cell-type in the small bowel epithelium. The next most common are the mucus-secreting goblet cells. In the colon, goblet cells are more numerous and the microvilli are less well developed. Microvilli contain carrier proteins to facilitate absorption, hydrolytic enzymes, hormone receptors, and specific receptors for nutrient absorption such as vitamin B_{12}. Specialized function of the lining epithelium is acquired during the process of cell differentiation. In the small intestine the crypts, located at the bases of villi, are the proliferative zones. Newly-born cells migrate out of the crypt compartment onto the villus and are shed from the villus tip after 5 or 6 days. Cell differentiation and maturation occur during the migration upward from the crypt towards the villus tip.

Endocrine cells in the small intestine secrete cholecystokinin and secretin, essential for triggering gallbladder contraction and pancreatic secretion. In addition, nerves in the lamina propria, submucosa and muscle layers contain various neuropeptides.

Specialized cells in the epithelium may be localized only to certain segments of the gut. In the ileum there are epithelial "membrane-like" (M) cells located over Peyer's patches. They appear to be important in immunological recognition. In addition to cellular specialization of the surface epithelium there is regional specialization, especially within the small intestine. Certain substances such as iron are absorbed primarily in the proximal small bowel whereas others such as vitamin B_{12} and bile salts are absorbed primarily in the distal small bowel.

The lamina propria contains plasma cells, lymphocytes and macrophages The predominant immunoglobulin in lamina propria plasma cells is IgA but smaller amounts of IgG and IgM are also present. These cells are important as immune modulators and have a protective role. The blood vessels and lymphatics within the lamina propria serve to transport absorbed materials from the intestine.

Movements

Throughout the intestine, the inherent rhythmicity of smooth muscle is the major determinant of intestinal movement. This myogenic control is tuned by neural and hormonal factors.

The most important movement of the small intestine is segmentation because it prolongs contact for absorption. Small peristaltic contractions move a few centimeters at a time. Between meals, an interdigestive migratory motor activity sweeps the small intestine in cycles that average 90 minutes.

The ileocecal valve permits controlled delivery of residual small bowel contents into the cecum. They are churned in the cecum and ascending colon and passed slowly to the rectum by haustral contractions and mass movements. Eating stimulates colonic motility.

Defecation is controlled by anal sphincters and pressure sensors. The internal smooth muscle sphincter relaxes in response to rectal distention. When stool enters the anal canal mucosal receptors are stimulated. The outer anal sphincter (striated muscle) then controls defecation. If the time and place to have a bowel movement are inappropriate the outer sphincter remains "tight", rectal pressure falls and the internal sphincter closes by a return of high resting tone.

Digestion and Absorption

The sites of assimilation of major nutrients are shown in Figure 12.11. The main function of the small intestine is to transport nutrients that have been digested, and to complete digestion and absorption. Absorption of carbohydrate, protein and fat involves luminal, intestinal (mucosal), and transport (delivery) phases. The luminal phase occurs mainly within proximal duodenum and jejunum due to the actions of secreted bile salts and pancreatic enzymes while the intestinal phase occurs on the surface or within the mucosal cell. The main function of the colon is to reabsorb most of the residual fluid and electrolytes, and to store the residual contents until it is convenient to evacuate them.

Carbohydrate Absorption

Much of our dietary carbohydrate is hydrolyzed to simpler forms prior to absorption. The major dietary sources are starch (60 percent), sucrose (30 percent) and lactose (10 percent). For starch the final end products are glucose; for sucrose, glucose and fructose; and, for lactose, glucose and galactose. Amylase secreted by the exocrine pancreas is the major source of hydrolytic activity for ingested starch. Amylase action produces oligosaccharides which in turn undergo further hydrolysis by enzymes in the brush border (microvilli) of the intestinal absorptive cells. Brush border disaccharidases also hydrolyze dietary sucrose and lactose. Glucose and galactose are coupled to active sodium transport. The sugars are ultimately transmitted into portal venous blood.

Protein Absorption

The average adult requires about 45 g of dietary protein daily. Endogenous protein is provided in the gut from secretions, desquamated cells and leakage of small amounts of plasma protein. The luminal phase is initiated in the stomach but contributes little to the overall process. However the products of gastric digestion may be potent releasers of hormones from endocrine cells, such as cholecystokinin and secretin, in the small bowel mucosa. These stimulate pancreatic enzyme release and gallbladder contraction. The pancreatic peptidases such as trypsin and chymotrypsin, and peptidases liberated from the intestinal brush border complete the luminal phase of protein digestion and produce small peptides and single amino acid residues. Next is the mucosal stage.

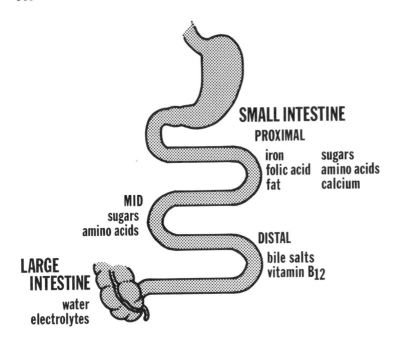

SMALL INTESTINE
PROXIMAL
iron   sugars
folic acid amino acids
fat   calcium

MID
sugars
amino acids

DISTAL
bile salts
vitamin B₁₂

LARGE
INTESTINE
water
electrolytes

Fig. 12.11 Sites of absorption in the small and large intestines.

Intestinal absorptive cells contain many enzymes for peptide hydrolysis and the final products are mainly free amino acids in portal venous blood. For amino acids, absorption rates are greater in the jejunum than in the ileum. Some dipeptides and tripeptides are not hydrolyzed at the brush border, but are absorbed intact to undergo hydrolysis within the mucosal cells.

Fat Absorption

North American adults eat 60–100 g of fat per day, mostly in the form of triglyceride. In the lumen, triglyceride must be converted to more water-soluble components before significant absorption can occur. Pancreatic lipase with the aid of colipase splits the triglyceride into two fatty acids and a β-monoglyceride. Bile acids cluster as micelles to incorporate fatty acids, β-monoglycerides and other lipids to render them soluble in the aqueous environment of the intestinal lumen. The mixed micelle serves as a shuttle to transport fats across the unstirred water layer to the absorptive cells.

In the intestinal cell, the fats are reesterified to triglyceride and are packaged with protein, cholesterol, cholesterol esters and phospholipid to form chylomicrons. These chylomicrons or lipoprotein complexes are delivered into the lymphatics (see Chapter 2, Hyperlipidemia).

Bile acid diffusion is slow and most bile salt reabsorption actually occurs in the distal ileum where an active transport mechanism exists. More than 90 percent of secreted bile salts are recycled via the liver. This enterohepatic circulation is essential because of the limited capacity of the liver to synthesize bile salts.

Shorter chain triglycerides (medium-chain triglycerides), composed of 6 to 10 fatty acids, have a different fate from long-chain triglycerides. These may be absorbed intact, or hydrolysed completely by pancreatic lipase. These are more soluble in water, form micelles more readily with bile salts, do not undergo intracellular esterification, and may traverse the intestinal cell directly to the portal venous system.

Water and Electrolyte Absorption

Unlike most other substances, water and electrolyte absorption involves both the small and large bowel. Besides ingested water, large volumes are added to gastrointestinal content through endogenous secretions. Although the total volume of fluid handled each day ranges from 5 to 10 liters, only 100-200 ml is finally excreted in stool. The small bowel is the principal absorptive site. Luminal content becomes isotonic in the duodenum and remains isotonic through the remainder of the small bowel.

The mucosa of the small bowel is permeable to sodium. In addition, sodium is actively reabsorbed. Flux from lumen to blood depends on active epithelial cell sodium transport; blood to lumen depends on luminal sodium concentration. Glucose and amino acids are also carried into cells with sodium.

During active sodium absorption, hydrogen is secreted into the lumen, reacts with bicarbonate and forms carbon dioxide which diffuses into blood. This effectively results in bicarbonate absorption.

The jejunal mucosa is exposed to osmotic changes created by ingested food. Thus absorption of water and electrolytes in the jejunum may occur secondary to absorption of organic solutes, a process called solvent drag.

Luminal bile acids and oleic acid from fat digestion inhibit sodium and water absorption, therefore the distal small intestinal content remains fluid. In jejunum and ileum, chloride absorption is coupled to bicarbonate secretion resulting in more alkaline content near the distal ileum. Potassium is absorbed by passive diffusion throughout the small bowel.

An average of 1500 ml of fluid is delivered to the colon each day. The colon normally absorbs sodium and water, but secretes potassium.

Iron Absorption

Dietary iron totals 10 to 20 mg each day but only 0.5 to 1.0 mg is absorbed in healthy adult men and slightly more in menstruating women. Normal iron balance depends on iron absorption in the duodenum and proximal jejunum. Gastric acid is not essential for iron absorption but prevents formation of insoluble iron complexes. The mechanism and control of iron absorption remain unclear. Initial uptake of iron into the mucosal cell probably depends on a specific iron receptor and active transport (see Chapter 13).

Absorption of Other Minerals and Vitamins

Calcium transport by the small bowel is an active energy-requiring process. The capacity for calcium absorption is greatest in duodenum. Absorption requires *vitamin D* (calciferol) and the accumulation of 1, 25-dehydroxy-vitamin D_3 in the small bowel parallels its regional capacity for calcium transport. In small bowel malabsorption, osteodystrophies may result, in part, related to impaired absorption of vitamin D.

Besides vitamin D, other fat soluble vitamins, *vitamin A* (retinol), *vitamin E*, (α tocopherol), and *vitamin K* are absorbed in the small bowel through mechanisms similar to other fats, namely micellar solubilization followed by passive diffusion. Vitamin K may also be derived from vitamin synthesis by microflora.

Folic acid occurs naturally conjugated to glutamic acid residues and undergoes hydrolysis to monoglutamyl folate prior to active absorption, especially in the proximal small bowel.

Cyanocobalamin or *vitamin B_{12}* combines with salivary and gastric binding proteins (R proteins). These are digested by pancreatic proteases to enable intrinsic factor, the glycoprotein synthesized in the parietal cells, to form a B_{12}-intrinsic factor complex. This complex binds to specific receptors in the terminal ileum and the vitamin B_{12} is absorbed (see Pernicious Anemia, Chapter 13).

Of the water soluble vitamins, thiamine or vitamin B_1 and vitamin C are actively transported. Most of the others diffuse passively into the mucosa.

DISORDERS OF THE SMALL INTESTINE

Malabsorption

Most disorders that produce malabsorption alter fat absorption and produce steatorrhea (i.e., excessive fat in the stools). Carbohydrate malabsorption may coexist with disorders that produce steatorrhea. Sometimes, as in lactase deficiency, carbohydrate malabsorption occurs without accompanying steatorrhea. Protein malabsorption and its consequences rarely dominate the clinical picture in patients with malabsorption.

The patient with malabsorption commonly but not invariably has diarrhea. The pathogenesis of the diarrhea depends on the underlying cause of the malabsorption. Diarrhea may be produced by the osmotic effects of unabsorbed materials that are dumped into the colon. In addition some of these unabsorbed substances such as bile acids, carbohydrates and hydroxylated fatty acids may also inhibit water and electrolyte absorption in the colon or actually promote secretion. Other mechanisms of diarrhea are dealt with in the section on the pathophysiology of diarrhea.

Causes and Mechanisms of Malabsorption

The classification of malabsorption and selected examples are shown in Table 12.24.

Insufficient pancreatic enzymes Pancreatic exocrine reserve is so great that output must be reduced by 80 percent or more before steatorrhea results. When it does, the steatorrhea is usually very severe and is associated with striking weight loss. However the absorption of fat soluble vitamins is less dependent on the action of pancreatic juice so deficiency of these vitamins is uncommon, even with severe pancreatic insufficiency.

Table 12.24   Classification and Selected Examples of Malabsorption Disorders

Insufficient Pancreatic Enzymes
   Chronic pancreatitis
   Cystic fibrosis
   Pancreatic cancer
Insufficient Bile Acids
   Cholestasis
   Ileal resection
Small Bowel Mucosal Diseases
   See Table 12.25
Impaired Lymphatic Drainage
   Lymphangiectasia
Multiple Defects
   Postgastrectomy
   Bacterial overgrowth (stasis syndromes)
   Zollinger-Ellison syndrome
   Crohn's disease
Uncertain cause
   Diabetes
   Hypogammaglobulinemia (common variable immunodeficiency)
   Hyperthyroidism

The most common cause of pancreatic malabsorption in adults is chronic pancreatitis due to alcoholism. In children it is due to cystic fibrosis. Pancreatic tumors that obstruct major pancreatic ducts may produce steatorrhea. Commercial pancreatic enzyme supplements given with meals reduce the steatorrhea. Sometimes the steatorrhea is further decreased by addition of antacids or H_2-receptor antagonists. The rationale is that buffering or reducing acid helps prevent inactivation of the pancreatic enzymes, especially lipase.

Insufficient bile acids   Mild steatorrhea is common when there is cholestasis associated with jaundice. In primary biliary cirrhosis, steatorrhea can occur without jaundice. As in other forms of liver disease, steatorrhea is mild but malabsorption of fat soluble vitamins is more prominent. Even when there is total bile acid diversion as in patients with T-tube drains after biliary tract surgery, only 20 percent of ingested fat is malabsorbed. This is somewhat puzzling considering the critical importance of the bile acid micelle in normal fat absorption.

Insufficient luminal bile acids may also result from chronic loss of bile acids into the colon after massive ileal resection (usually greater than 100 cm) or in the presence of extensive ileal disease as in Crohn's disease. Watery diarrhea is produced by the action of bile acids on the colon and may be treated with anion exchange resins such as cholestryamine. The diarrhea is thus controlled by binding the bile acids and minimizing their effects on the colon; however the associated steatorrhea may increase.

Small bowel mucosal diseases   The clinical features and laboratory abnormalities are dependent on the region of the small bowel affected (Fig. 12.11) and on the extent of small bowel involvement. The diagnosis is usually established with biopsy in mucosal diseases such as celiac sprue or with barium radiographs to determine residual small bowel length after massive resection. Celiac sprue, giardiasis, lactase deficiency and the short bowel syndrome are discussed separately below.

Impaired lymphatic drainage   When there is extensive obstruction from lymphatics in abdominal lymphoma and in association with certain small bowel diseases, such as the rare condition Whipple's disease, steatorrhea may develop. This is usually also accompanied by a striking loss of protein from the gut, a protein-losing enteropathy. The steatorrhea results from impaired transport of fat from absorptive cells to lymphatics and also from leakage of chylomicron fat from ruptured lymphatics into the bowel lumen.

Multiple defects   As indicated in the section on Peptic Ulcer, malabsorption may occur after gastric surgery. Steatorrhea is usually mild. The factors contributing to the malabsorption include poor gastric mixing and digestion, rapid emptying and enhanced intestinal transit. This may result in inadequate contact with pancreatic enzymes and bile acids. Certain susceptible individuals may have secondary lactase deficiency unmasked because of the reduced contact time. The diarrhea may decrease when dairy products are withdrawn from the diet. After certain types of operations especially antrectomy and Billroth II anastomosis, bacteria may flourish in the afferent limb, resulting in a bacterial overgrowth syndrome and steatorrhea.

Bacterial overgrowth syndromes may be associated with severe diarrhea and steatorrhea. There is almost invariably an underlying condition that promotes intestinal stasis, such as a blind loop of bowel (afferent limb of Billroth II), intestinal strictures from irradiation or Crohn's disease, atonic small bowel produced by scleroderma or severe diabetes, and rarely, multiple small bowel diverticula. Bacterial contamination results in deconjugation of bile salts rendering them less effective in fat absorption. Mucosal injury may also be associated, and may account for part of the total clinical picture. Bacteria also appear to compete directly for vitamin B_{12}, so that vitamin B_{12} malabsorption is almost invariably present in bacterial overgrowth syndromes. Intermittent short courses of broad spectrum antibiotics such as tetracycline result in marked improvement in these patients and are often used as both a diagnostic and therapeutic test.

Crohn's disease is a transmural inflammation that may affect the small bowel, especially the ileum. Malabsorption may occur although other features such as pain and systemic symptoms are usually more common. When malabsorption is present it may be due to direct involvement of the small bowel mucosa, loss of bile salts, fistula formation, altered bowel flora and lymphatic obstruction. The approach to treatment in these disorders, is to try to control the inflammatory process (see discussion of Crohn's disease), replace deficiencies and use nonspecific measures such as antidiarrheal drugs for diarrhea.

Uncertain cause   Patients with severe diabetes may have diarrhea and steatorrhea. The approach to these patients is to rule out other causes of malabsorption. When none are found, bacterial overgrowth is considered as a possibility and a trial of antibiotics is justified. The mechanisms however remain unclear in some patients even after specific causes of malabsorption have been ruled out and suspected bacterial overgrowth has been treated.

Patients with common variable immunodeficiency (adult-onset panhypogammaglobulinemia) may have malabsorption. *Giardia lamblia* infestation is the most common cause and bacterial overgrowth is the second most common. Some of these patients continue to have malabsorption even when giardiasis and bacterial overgrowth have been excluded.

In hyperthyroidism, accelerated intestinal transit is one of the postulated mechanisms to account for the diarrhea and mild steatorrhea that is sometimes observed.

Investigation of Malabsorption

History and physical examination   Malabsorption is obvious when patients have weight loss in the face of a normal or increased food intake (hyperphagia), and have bulky, pale stools. Stools may float, contain fat globules, and be more rancid than usual. However most patients with malabsorption do not have these textbook symptoms. Their diarrhea is often intermittent, or they may have no bowel symptoms at all. Instead, they may present with unexplained nutritional problems, such as anemia or less commonly with osteopenic bone disease or bleeding due to hypoprothrombinemia. Hyperphagia may be subtle presenting as increased food required to maintain the usual weight.

When diarrhea is the leading complaint it must be differentiated from idiopathic inflammatory disorders of the colon such as Crohn's Disease, ulcerative colitis, and infectious diarrheas. (See the section on Diarrhea below.) Severe lower abdominal pain is uncommon, but mild diffuse cramps, distension and excessive flatulence are common. These symptoms are caused by the effects of unabsorbed fats and carbohydrates on the colon.

The symptoms accompanying the underlying cause (Table 12.24) may be so prominent that the diagnosis is fairly obvious. When an underlying cause is not obvious, the major challenge is to determine whether the malabsorption is due to small bowel mucosal versus pancreatic diseases. In adults, pancreatic disease can usually be eliminated as a cause of malabsorption if there is no prior history of alcoholism or previous attacks of pancreatitis. It is rare for patients to present with painless steatorrhea as the first manifestation of a pancreatic carcinoma.

A history of previous abdominal surgery (e.g., gastrectomy or small bowel resection) should be obtained. Foreign travel, contact with overseas travellers or camping near mountain lakes should prompt a careful search for *Giardia lamblia*. A prior history of unexplained iron deficiency anemia is a common feature of celiac sprue. The sudden appearance of diarrhea, cramps and flatulence with ingestion of dairy products points to an underlying small bowel mucosal disease.

Abnormal physical signs may be related to the underlying cause but more commonly reflect the consequences of the malabsorption. Thus there may be obvious dehydration, weight loss, pallor, edema due to hypoalbuminemia, and more rarely signs of hypocalcemia.

Laboratory Assessment   The stool must be examined to see if the characteristic features of steatorrhea are present. Microscopic examination with a Sudan stain reveals large numbers of fat globules when steatorrhea is obvious. Unfortunately, the test often fails when the abnormality of fat excretion is only mild or moderate. Microscopic examination for parasites, especially *Giardia lamblia* is essential.

A very low fasting serum carotene suggests malabsorption especially of small bowel origin. The body stores of carotene are limited and are derived from ingestion of vegetables and fruits, eggs, and liver. The plasma concentration is therefore largely dependent on dietary intake and intestinal absorption. The D-xylose screening test is used to differentiate between small bowel and pancreatic disease. Xylose is a water soluble pentose that is absorbed mainly from the duodenum and upper jejunum and excreted by the kidneys. It is given by mouth, blood levels are measured and the urine is collected for 5 hours. Reduced excretion may indicate small bowel mucosal disease; however, delayed gastric emptying, bacterial overgrowth and renal failure may also cause low values.

A blood smear may demonstrate macrocytic or

hypochromic anemia. Tests to screen for nutritional deficiency states include serum albumin, calcium, magnesium, prothrombin time (vitamin K), iron, folic acid and vitamin B_{12}. When there is malabsorption of vitamin B_{12}; the serum levels may remain normal for 2–5 years until body stores are depleted.

Radiologic studies begin with a plain film of the abdomen. It may reveal calcification of the pancreas and the bone density may suggest osteopenic bone disease. The small bowel barium radiograph is often mistakenly used as a screening test for malabsorption. The typical "malabsorption pattern" consists of thickened mucosal folds, dilatation of the bowel lumen and flocculation of barium. This typical pattern is often absent even in the face of moderate steatorrhea. The main value of the small bowel barium radiograph is to define the anatomy when previous gastric or intestinal surgery was performed and to reveal specific disorders such as Crohn's disease.

Special diagnostic tests   A *small bowel biopsy* is performed when malabsorption is present but the cause is not obvious from the history and the tests referred to above. The most common diseases that are diagnosed with small bowel biopsy are celiac sprue and giardiasis. These conditions will be considered separately later in this section. Table 12.25 gives the classification of diseases that may be characterized by abnormalities on small bowel biopsy. The conditions listed are those encountered in a clinical setting when biopsy might be performed. Other conditions such as radiation enteritis can affect the small bowel mucosa, but biopsy is usually not performed. Biopsies are performed using peroral suction biopsy tubes positioned fluoroscopically at the ligament of Treitz. When suction biopsy capability is no available then endoscopic biopsies from the descending duodenum are obtained. They are generally less satisfactory because they are smaller.

A *fecal fat* determination is the most reliable method to detect steatorrhea. It is very laborious and is usually not required because the specific cause of malabsorption can be found without it. The patient must be on a fixed diet containing 80–100 g fat for 5 days and stools are collected for the last 3 days. The normal excretion is less than 6 g/day. The main value of this test is in two settings. One is to confirm steatorrhea when a patient is suspected to have malabsorption but screening tests and perhaps a small bowel biopsy fail to reveal a cause. The second circumstance is in the patient with a complicated type of malabsorption, due to two or three causes, in which various treatments need to be assessed objectively.

The Schilling's test for vitamin B_{12} absorption is very useful when ileal disease or bacterial overgrowth secondary to small intestinal stasis are suspected. If concomitant pernicious anemia is not suspected then the second stage with intrinsic factor is done initially. Normal subjects excrete more than 10 percent of the radioactive vitamin B_{12} in the 24 hours after ingestion of the isotope. In bacterial overgrowth the test should correct after a course of a broad spectrum antibiotic such as a tetracycline. The test may be abnormal in pancreatic insufficiency because of deficient proteases to split R proteins from vitamin B_{12}. In this circumstance the test should return to normal if the radiolabelled vitamin B_{12} is given with pancreatic enzymes.

Pancreatic function tests such as the Lundh or secretin tests are used to measure exocrine pancreatic secretory capacity. Duodenal luminal contents are aspirated for trypsin assays, after pancreatic stimulation with intravenous secretin or an oral Lundh test meal. For the secretin test, aspirates need to be collected continuously and are analyzed for volume, bicarbonate and enzymes. Maximal volume should reach 2 ml/min and bicarbonate concentration should reach 90mEq/1 within 90 min of secretin injection. The patient with obvious chronic alcoholic pancreatitis, steatorrhea and recent onset diabetes requires no further tests assuming there is a clear-cut response to oral pancreatic enzyme therapy.

A lactose tolerance test may be helpful to diagnose lactose intolerance; more often a clinical response to withdrawal of dairy products is sufficient. In normal nondiabetic adults, blood glucose levels increase by 20 mg/dl or more after ingestion of 50 g of lactose. Patients with lactose deficiency have a flat curve that does not peak to 20 mg/dl. A more important clinically relevant criterion for a positive test is that the 50 g of lactose should reproduce the patient's symptoms within 24 h of ingestion.

A variety of *breath tests* have emerged to provide non-invasive methods to assess malabsorption. They require measurement of specific bacterial metabolites in expired air. Their clinical value remains to be determined.

Malabsorbed carbohydrate is fermented in the colon, and the excessive gas produced is reflected in increased expired hydrogen. The ^{14}C-labelled glycocholic acid breath test is used for bacterial overgrowth; bacteria in the small bowel deconjugate the labelled bile acid so that $^{14}CO_2$ is expired.

Stool output tests are occasionally used for the clinical evaluation of patients. Total bile acids in stool can be analyzed. In protein-losing enteropathy the loss can be quantitated after the administration of intravenous ^{51}Chromium labelled protein.

Table 22.25 Diagnostic Usefulness of Small Bowel Biopsy in Adults

Disease	Histologic Features	Comment
USUALLY DIAGNOSTIC (diffuse involvement)		
Celiac Sprue	"Flat" avillous mucosa with elongated crypts and increased lamina propria round cells	Diagnosis requires confirmation by response to a gluten-free diet; in adults from certain countries similar lesions may be seen in tropical sprue but lesions more patchy and tropical sprue responds to folic acid and antibiotics
Giardiasis	Variably abnormal villi but organisms adherent to surface epithelium and adherent mucus	One third of cases have negative stool examinations for ova and parasites
Hypogammaglobulinemia (common variable immunodeficiency)	Lesion variable in severity but plasma cells reduced or absent; *Giardia lamblia* common; nodular lymphoid hyperplasia may be present	In these disorders IgA very low but IgG and IgM also reduced; suspected because of other features e.g. recurrent pulmonary infections
Whipple's disease	Lamina propria infiltration by macrophages that contain the Whipple's bacillus	Rare but treatable; usually elderly males with arthritis; treatment is successful with a variety of antibiotics
MAY BE DIAGNOSTIC (patchy involvement)		
Other parasites	Coccidioidosis (isospora belli), strongyloides, cryptosporidium in tissue sections; variable mucosal abnormalities	Suspect in immunosuppressed host; Southeastern U.S. is endemic area for strongyloides.
Intestinal lymphoma	Mucosal infiltrates of malignant lymphoid cells	May complicate celiac sprue; diffuse form in Middle East often associated with alpha chain disease
Eosinophilic gastroenteritis	Masses of eosinophils in mucosa	Rare syndrome, unknown etiology; recurrent severe abdominal pain and eosinophilia
Systemic infiltrates	Amyloid or macroglobulin deposits	Rarely present as a small bowel disease
Lymphangiectasia	Dilated mucosal lymphatics	Rare primary form in childhood; secondary form due to malignant obstruction of lymphatics; medium chain triglycerides are used as caloric support when steatorrhea is severe
SELDOM DIAGNOSTIC (histology nonspecific and lesions patchy)		
Crohn's disease	Noncaseating granulomata	Small bowel biopsy usually done in Crohn's only when a second or concomitant small bowel disorder suspected
Bacterial overgrowth	Patchy mild or moderate inflammation	Recovery follows treatment with antibiotics; biopsy not required for diagnosis but is done to exclude other diseases e.g. celiac sprue
Infectious gastroenteritis	Same as in bacterial overgrowth	After acute "viral gastroenteritis" some adults have prolonged but self-limited intermittent diarrhea

Selected Malabsorption Disorders

Celiac Sprue (syn. Celiac Disease, Gluten-sensitive Enteropathy)

Pathophysiology   The mucosal disease is always most severe in the duodenum and jejunum and generally decreases in severity towards the ileum. The mucosal surface appears flat and exhibits absent villi, increased crypts, an expanded lamina propria, and an abnormal cuboidal surface epithelium. The degree of malabsorption is dependent upon the length of intestine involved.

The mucosal injury is due to gluten, a group of proteins found in wheat, barley, rye, and oats. The etiology of the disease and the mechanism of the gluten injury are unknown.

The disorder is presumed to begin in childhood and either becomes clinically overt then or remains subclinical until adulthood. In adults it may present at any age, but usually after the second decade.

Ten to 20 percent of first degree relatives of patients with celiac sprue have the disease, often in a clinically occult form. There is a preponderance of HLA-B8 and HLA-Dw3. The prevalence of the disease in North America is not known. In certain parts of Ireland the incidence is as great as 1 in 300.

Clinical features   Two-thirds of the patients present with clinically overt symptoms, signs and laboratory features of malabsorption. Because of the striking changes in the proximal small bowel, iron and folic acid deficiency anemia are prominent features and often provide early clues. Clinically occult celiac sprue occurs in one-third of patients. These individuals may simply present with an unexplained iron deficiency anemia, intermittent abdominal distention or very mild alteration in bowel habit, possibly due to secondary lactase deficiency. They may be detected in the course of an evaluation for unexplained metabolic bone disease, hypocalcemia or the skin disease, dermatitis herpetiformis. Three-quarters of patients with this skin disease have the typical flat mucosa of celiac sprue. Most of them are asymptomatic with no clinical or laboratory features of malabsorption because the lesion is confined only to the duodenum and a short segment of upper jejunum.

Diagnosis and treatment   There are two diagnostic criteria for celiac sprue: typical mucosal changes on small bowel biopsy, and a response to a gluten-free diet. In patients with obvious clinical and laboratory malabsorption rebiopsy is not required. However, those who present with the clinically occult form of the disease must have rebiopsy to confirm that the gluten-free diet has resulted in an improvement of the severe mucosal lesion.

Ninety percent or more of patients with the characteristic flat mucosa of celiac sprue have a clear-cut sustained response to a gluten-free diet and must remain on the diet for life. In those who fail to respond to a gluten-free diet or who have a relapse, the most common reason is conscious or inadvertent ingestion of gluten. When this has been excluded, other conditions to consider are those that represent rare but definite complications of celiac sprue. They include small intestinal multifocal lymphoma, intestinal ulceration or stricture, and a rare condition called collagenous sprue.

A small percentage of patients have the typical mucosal appearance of celiac sprue, but do not respond to a gluten-free diet. This group is termed unclassified or refractory sprue, and they probably represent a heterogeneous group of disorders.

Giardiasis

Infestation with the parasite *Giardia lamblia* is common. This parasite resides in the small bowel but the mechanism whereby it produces symptoms is not clear; the degree of mucosal injury is sufficient to account for the symptoms. The major sources of infestation are food and water. Increased numbers of cases are seen in homosexual men presumably because of oral-fecal contamination. Children in daycare centers may also be at greater risk. The organism is endemic but is particularly common in some mountain lakes.

Severe steatorrhea is not a feature of giardiasis unless the patient also has common variable immunodeficiency. The symptoms range from acute, crampy diarrhea to low-grade intermittent diarrhea and abdominal cramps, and may mimic those of the dysfunctional bowel syndrome (see Large Intestine). Secondary lactase deficiency is common. Therefore, individuals who have a clinical response to dairy product withdrawal should have giardiasis considered as a possibility, in addition to celiac sprue.

In approximately two-thirds of cases the diagnosis can be established by examination of two or more stools. However, in one-third, stool examinations are negative, presumably because of intermittent excretion of the tryphozoites. The diagnosis in this group can be established by examining duodenal aspirates or by small bowel biopsy. The organisms will be evident either in the duodenal smears or in the tissue sections where they reside on the luminal surface epithelium at villous tips or between villi.

Therapy consists of either atabrine or metronidazole (Flagyl). Symptoms may resolve slowly in patients who continue ingestion of dairy products because of the associated secondary lactase deficiency. This lactase deficiency may persist for weeks after successful eradication of the parasite.

Lactase Deficiency

The clinical manifestations of carbohydrate malabsorption in adults are similar, irrespective of the underlying defect. The unabsorbed carbohydrate attracts water to the lumen of the small intestine, reaches the colon and is fermented by colonic bacteria. A variety of osmotically active short–chain fatty acids, carbon dioxide, and hydrogen gases are produced by the bacterial fermentation. The fatty acids create osmotic retention of the fluid in the colon and inhibit sodium and water absorption. The net effect is diarrhea, cramps and flatulence. Patients with carbohydrate malabsorption have intermittent symptoms which correspond to the amount and type of carbohydrate ingested.

In adults, lactase deficiency is by far the most common type of carbohydrate malabsorption. Congenital lactase deficiency is rare and occurs in the neonatal period. Most lactase deficiency is the primary acquired type that develops during childhood. More than 50 percent of Orientals, Blacks, Jews and many other races have lactase deficiency to a variable degree. This usually becomes apparent after the age-equivalent of "weaning" (i.e., between 5 and 10 years). Primary lactase deficiency in adults is common; however, in North America only 5-7 percent of non-Mediterranean Caucasians have lactase deficiency in adulthood.

Secondary lactase deficiency occurs when there has been injury to the small intestinal mucosa as in celiac sprue. It may be transient after treatment for giardiasis or resolve spontaneously after infectious gastroenteritis.

Dairy product withdrawal for several days may establish the presence of lactase deficiency if the patient notes an improvement in symptoms. In patients with lactase deficiency and watery diarrhea, the stool pH is often low because of the presence of the short-chain acids. Occasionally the lactose tolerance test is used to confirm a diagnosis. A flat lactose tolerance test by itself is not clinically relevant unless the ingested lactose reproduces the patient's symptoms. Other methods to establish the diagnosis are to actually measure the mucosal lactase or utilize the breath hydrogen test.

Most patients who have primary lactase deficiency on a genetic or racial basis recognize their food in-tolerance and have voluntarily restricted dairy products. In secondary lactase deficiency, correction of the underlying mucosal defect is associated with restoration of the ability to tolerate dairy products.

Isolated congenital sucrase deficiency or transport defects for glucose and galactose are extremely rare.

Short Bowel Syndrome

The short bowel syndrome reflects the inability of the remaining small bowel to cope with the daily load of nutrients and the endogenously produced secretions. Metabolic consequences depend on the site and extent of resection. The symptoms also depend upon the effects of unabsorbed material in the colon. Nutrient deficiencies may need to be replaced parenterally.

When the terminal ileum is resected, bile acid malabsorption may occur and can be treated with cholestyramine. When the resection is very extensive, hepatic synthesis is able to compensate for the loss of bile acids. Therefore, in addition to diarrhea produced by loss of bile acids in the colon, there is also fat malabsorption. Vitamin B_{12} deficiency may develop.

With time, the intestine undergoes a phenomenon called adaptation but this may take a year or longer. Adaptation is often incomplete in the sense that symptoms are fewer, but some remain. When steatorrhea is severe, medium chain triglyceride supplements can be given. In the presence of severe steatorrhea, the diarrhea component can often be improved with the use of a low fat diet. A reduced fat load is delivered to the colon so there is less of a cathartic effect. This is an important therapeutic maneuver in all types of untreatable steatorrhea.

Several complications of the short bowel syndrome may occur with time (see surgical treatment for obesity, Chapter 1). Cholesterol gallstones occur more commonly because of a reduced bile acid pool if the distal small bowel has been resected. Another important complication is hyperoxaluria and oxalate renal stones. Normally, ingested oxalate is bound by calcium and is eliminated in stool. In the presence of fat malabsorption the calcium is bound by free fatty acids leaving oxalate in a water soluble form in the colon. Oxalate is then absorbed. When oxalate renal stones have developed, a low oxalate diet is given together with citrate and magnesium supplements because these are related inversely to the urinary excretion of oxalate. Gastric acid hypersecretion occurs in some patients after major resection of the small bowel. The pathogenesis is unclear. Patients may require maintenance H_2-receptor antagonist therapy if they develop intractable peptic ulcers.

Small Intestinal Obstruction

This occurs when there is a failure of progression of intestinal contents due to abnormalities in intestinal muscular activity or mechanical causes. *Nonmechanical causes* are due to ileus associated with peritonitis, and reflex causes such as after abdominal surgery and spinal fractures. *Mechanical causes* result from structural blockage of the intestine from intrinsic or extrinsic bowel lesions.

The clinical features of mechanical obstruction are colicky abdominal pain, vomiting, abdominal distension and tenderness. Bowel sounds may be high pitched. Patients may have no passage of rectal gas or they may have an "overflow diarrhea".

Plain x-ray films of the abdomen reveal dilated loops of small bowel with air-fluid levels.

The principles of therapy are to provide nasogastric suction, correct fluid and electrolyte imbalances from vomiting and to correct the underlying cause.

Congenital Disorders of The Small Intestine

Cogenital Anomalies

These are usually diagnosed before the age of two. They include atresia, duplications and malrotations. The latter may be asymptomatic and detected in adulthood in the course of a barium radiograph obtained for other reasons.

Meckel's Diverticulum

Incomplete obliteration of the intestinal end of the vitelline duct (Meckel's diverticulum) is the most common congenital abnormality. Its prevalence is 2 percent. It measures approximately 2 inches in length and occurs about 2 feet from the ileocecal valve. Half the cases contain ileal mucosa. The remainder contain gastric, pancreatic or colonic mucosa. Among symptomatic patients, 40 percent are older children and adults. Complications are due to mechanical causes or due to ulcers in the gastric tissue. They include recurrent abdominal pain which may mimic appendicitis, rectal bleeding, intussusception, obstruction, inflammation and perforation with peritonitis. The diagnosis may be difficult to make preoperatively.

Tumors of The Small Intestine

Primary tumors of the small intestine are uncommon (fewer than 5 percent of gastrointestinal neoplasms). Adenomas, and lipomas are the most common benign tumors; adenocarcinoma, lymphoma, and carcinoid tumors are the most common malignant lesions of the small bowel. The benign lesions are usually asymptomatic. The characteristic symptoms of small bowel tumors result from obstruction or bleeding. The diagnosis of malignant tumors is made with barium radiographs and sometimes by angiography. These diagnostic procedures can be complemented by abdominal computerized axial tomography (CAT scan) to evaluate the extent of metastasis.

The objective in therapy is surgical resection when possible. For lymphomas, chemotherapy and radiotherapy may be beneficial.

Carcinoid Syndrome

Carcinoid tumors are endocrine cell tumors that arise from the intestinal crypts. The appendix is the most common site of origin but they may develop anywhere in the gastrointestinal tract. These tumors are similar in appearance to other endocrine cell neoplasms of the gastrointestinal tract and pancreas (e.g., gastrinoma).

Carcinoid tumors grow slowly and most patients survive for 5 to 10 years after the diagnosis is made. After metastasis to the liver, some patients may develop the *carcinoid syndrome* with diarrhea, bronchospasm, cyanosis, flushing, pellagra-like skin lesions and right-sided valvular heart lesions. These signs and symptoms are due to the increased production of a variety of active substances: 5-hydroxyindoleacetic acid (5-HIAA); 5-hydroxytryptamine (serotonin); catecholamines; and prostaglandins. The diagnosis is established by demonstrating increased urinary excretion of 5-HIAA and high blood levels of serotonin.

Surgical resection of isolated slow-growing hepatic metastases in selected cases may abort the symptoms of the carcinoid syndrome.

DISORDERS OF THE LARGE INTESTINE

Diarrhea

The objective definition of diarrhea is a stool weight that exceeds 300 g per day or a stool water content greater than 250 ml per day. Patients may describe it as any combination of increased stool frequency, increased volume or decreased consistency.

Table 12.26 Mechanisms of Diarrhea

Mechanism	Examples
Osmotic	
Poorly absorbed solutes	Magnesium-containing laxatives, antacids
Maldigestion and malabsorption	Celiac sprue, pancreatic insufficiency, lactase deficiency
Secretory	
Exudative (mucosal injury)	*Salmonella typhimurium*, Crohn's disease, ulcerative colitis
Active ion secretion	
Bacterial enterotoxins	*Vibrio cholera*, toxigenic *E. coli*
Hormonal secretagogues	Calcitonin (medullary thyroid carcinoma), gastrinoma
Other	Viruses, bile and fatty acids, certain laxatives, intestinal obstruction

Mechanisms of Diarrhea

Diarrhea results from excessive fluid and electrolyte loss in the gastrointestinal tract leading to fecal excretion of more than 250 ml daily. Active electrolyte secretion, decreased electrolyte absorption, increased luminal osmolality due to other solutes, and disordered motility are proposed mechanisms although in most disorders more than one is operational. The osmotic and secretory mechanisms are the most important. (Table 12.26).

If osmotically active solutes are poorly absorbed or not absorbed in the small bowel, they carry water with them into the colon. Magnesium and sulphate ions (i.e., Epsom salts) are only slowly absorbed, leading to watery diarrhea.

Toxins of *Vibrio cholerae* or *Escherichia coli* bind to specific microvillus membrane receptors, enter the cell, and activate adenyl cyclase leading to stimulation of fluid secretion and a volume too large to undergo colonic reabsorption. Infectious diarrheas are discussed in the large Intestine Section.

Combined osmotic and secretory mechanisms are common and the diarrhea may be generated both in the small bowel and colon. For example, in celiac sprue unabsorbed lactose may create an osmotic effect in small bowel and colon, while colonic bacterial fermentation of the lactose to short chain fatty acids creates a secretory diarrhea as well.

A classification of the causes is given in Table 12.27.

Approach to Investigation

History First one should determine whether the patient actually has diarrhea. Increased stool frequency, without increased stool weight is more common in the idiopathic variety (i.e., the dysfunctional syndrome or "irritable bowel"). Increased frequency

without actual diarrhea also results from a persistent sensation of the need to defecate (tenesmus). This may be due to anal fissures, large painful hemorrhoids, or a localized ulcerative proctitis.

The best indicators of severity are the daytime frequency and nocturnal bowel movements. If the patient is wakened at night to have a bowel movement, a cause of the diarrhea is likely to be found.

If blood is mixed in with watery diarrhea it points more to an infectious cause or to ulcerative colitis. On the other hand, pale large-volume stools point

Table 12.27 Causes of Diarrhea

Dietary
  Excess caffeine
  Alcohol
Drug
  Laxatives
  Antacids
  Antibiotics
  Lactulose
  Unpredictable reaction to many drugs
Infection
  Viral: Norwalk-like agents; rotaviruses
  Bacterial: Food poisoning agents (Table 12.28); *Shigella*; *Campylobacter*; *C. difficile*; *Yersinia enterocolitica*; enterotoxigenic *E. coli*
  Parasitic: *Giardia*, ameba
Idiopathic Inflammatory Bowel Disease
  Ulcerative colitis
  Crohn's disease
Idiopathic
  Dysfunctional bowel syndrome ("irritable bowel")
Malabsorption Disorders
  See Table 12.24
Mechanical
  Diverticular disease
  Colon carcinoma
  Obstruction from stricture, fecal impaction
Secretory Tumor Effects (rare)
  Carcinoid syndrome
  Villous adenoma
  Pancreatic cholera (VIP-producing tumors)
  Medullary carcinoma of thyroid (calcitonin)

more to a malabsorption disorder. The timing of onset helps in differential diagnosis. A chronically progressive diarrheal syndrome is not characteristic of the infectious causes, with the possible exception of giardiasis. When the onset is abrupt and infectious causes are suspected, it is important to determine whether other family members or contacts were similarly affected, whether there was recent foreign travel or contact with overseas travelers, and whether the timing of onset followed a specific meal.

In chronic diarrhea a careful dietary and drug history should be obtained, specifically in relation to dairy products, caffeine and alcohol. Dairy product intake should be evaluated in relation to symptoms. Patients may suddenly develop diarrhea despite a fixed intake of coffee and alcohol and may improve when these are withdrawn or reduced in amount. Artificial sweeteners (sorbitol) in chewing gums may provoke diarrhea if taken in large amounts. The most common drugs which produce diarrhea are laxatives, antacids, and antibiotics. Surreptitious laxative abuse is an increasingly recognized manifestation of serious underlying psychological disturbances. Patients may develop diarrhea on an idiosyncratic (unpredictable) basis with many drugs. It is important to determine whether the onset of diarrhea coincided with the institution of a new drug. Unless the drug is life sustaining, it should be withdrawn to see if the diarrhea subsides.

Symptoms that accompany or precede the diarrhea may provide a clue. In ulcerative colitis and Crohn's disease, the local manifestations, such as anal fissures, or systemic manifestations such as erythema nodosum, iritis or uveitis, and arthralgis may have preceded or accompanied the first presentation with diarrhea. A longstanding prior history of intractable constipation might indicate a mechanical obstruction or a fecal impaction, with so-called "overflow diarrhea".

When there is no obvious underlying cause of diarrhea the history must be used to determine whether investigations begin for malabsorption disorders or the colonic inflammatory bowel disorders. The issue is whether to begin the workup from "above" or "below". In the malabsorption group, stool volumes tend to be larger and there is a modest increase in their number. There is usually little or no associated urgency, tenesmus, or blood in the stool. In the colonic inflammatory disorders the reservoir capacity of the colon is decreased. Therefore, there are small amounts of stool with increased frequency, urgency, and tenesmus. Blood may be mixed in with the stool. A longstanding history of large-volume watery diarrhea associated with weakness and previously documented electrolyte disturbances points toward rare, pure secretory disease.

Diagnostic tests　　The most common form of diarrhea is a short-lived episode without associated systemic toxicity. These forms of infectious gastroenteritis require no further workup. If the diarrhea has persisted for more than 10 days or if it is very severe with signs of systemic toxicity, then investigations need to be performed. If the history and preliminary screening tests suggest malabsorption then the workup proceeds as outlined above.

Initial blood tests should assess the consequences of the diarrhea: electrolytes, blood urea nitrogen and serum creatinine for dehydration; hemoglobin concentration to screen for anemia or hemoconcentration; white blood cell count as an index of the severity of the inflammatory response. If persistent diarrhea is believed due to an infectious cause or inflammatory bowel disease, the specific workup begins with two or three stool cultures for the infectious causes, and stool examinations for ova and parasites. A stool examination for the presence of leukocytes is sometimes helpful. Large numbers of leukocytes may be seen in certain infectious diarrheas such as due to *Campylobacter* and *Shigella*, and in active acute ulcerative colitis. Variable numbers are seen in other bacterial infections but leukocytes in the stool are generally absent in diarrhea caused by viruses, Crohn's disease, and giardiasis.

Sigmoidoscopy should be carried out without prior cleansing laxatives or enemas. This provides an opportunity to obtain additional stool specimens for testing and prevents artifactual mucosal abnormalities caused by enemas. Mucosal biopsies are often helpful; inflammatory change may be present in inflammatory bowel disease, especially Crohn's disease, despite a normal mucosal appearance. Even when specific biopsy abnormalities are not found, the finding of mucosal inflammation at least points to the colon as the source of the diarrhea. Certain sigmoidoscopy appearances are fairly typical. A diffuse "skinned knee" appearance suggests diffuse ulcerative colitis. Solitary aphthous lesions suggest Crohn's disease. Adherent white plaques suggest antibiotic associated colitis. Inflammatory change limited to the distal 5 or 6 cm of rectum indicates a proctitis rather than a generalized colitis.

Barium radiographs are deferred during the acute phase of a patient's illness, and performed after symptoms improve with general supportive measures.

Under certain circumstances special tests may be performed for specific conditions. *Clostridium difficile* toxin assay may confirm the presence of an antibiotic-associated colitis. In suspected surreptitious laxative abuse the stool can be alkalinized to see if it turns pink as a result of the phenolphthalein contained in many laxatives. A search of patients' belongings may be required for non-phenolphthalein containing laxatives and diuretics. In high volume diarrhea associated with hypokalemia it may be necessary on rare occasions to determine whether the diarrhea is of the pure secretory type associated with tumors. Patients are fasted completely for 24 hours. In a secretory diarrhea stool volume usually remains greater than 500 ml per 24 h, the stool osmolality is in the range of 290 (stool Na + K concentrations × 2 approximates the recorded stool osmolality).

Therapy in the absence of a specific diagnosis   When a self-limited gastroenteritis is thought to be present, the principles of therapy are generally the same regardless of cause. Patients treated at home are advised to take abundant clear liquids with added sugar and salt. They should report back if they get dehydrated (thirst, decreased urine output), develop bloody stools or high fevers. Antidiarrheal agents should only be prescribed for patient comfort if bloody diarrhea and signs of toxicity are absent. The most potent antidiarrheal agents are codeine, loperamide, and diphenoxylate with atropine (Lomotil).

If hospitalization is required because of severe symptoms, intravenous fluids are given, oral intake is withheld to place the bowel at rest and investigations are undertaken. Upon refeeding, dairy products are introduced with caution in the event that the cause of the diarrhea was one that affected the small bowel to produce secondary lactase deficiency.

Infectious Diarrheas

These are characterized by an abrupt onset and are usually self-limited. Many patients simply "ride out" their symptoms. When symptoms are severe or prolonged, investigation should include stool cultures, examination for parasites and serology. If these are negative and the patient recovers, the diagnosis of "viral" or "nonbacterial" gastroenteritis is made. It is now recognized that some of these infections are due to newly recognized bacterial causes such as *Campylobacter* or *Yersinia*.

Viral Gastroenteritis

The rotaviruses and Norwalk-like viruses are the most commonly recognized types. *Norwalk-like viruses* cause epidemic gastroenteritis and generally in-

fect older children and adults. There are different antigenic strains. Approximately one-third of epidemics of gastroenteritis are produced by the Norwalk viruses or closely related types. The illness usually lasts 1 to 3 days with diarrhea and vomiting as the major symptoms. Accompanying symptoms may be low-grade fever, abdominal cramps and myalgias. Mild small intestinal lesions are produced and may be associated with a secondary lactase deficiency. It is not known whether the rectal mucosa is involved.

Rotavirus infection is a major cause of morbidity, especially in young children but infection may occur in any age group. In temperate climates there is a marked predominance of infection in the fall and winter months and a low incidence in the summer periods. Disease is also usually self-limited and symptoms are similar to those seen in infection with the Norwalk-like viruses. Respiratory symptoms are common accompaniments, especially in children. In adults, rotavirus infection may be an important cause of traveler's diarrhea. This virus directly infects intestinal epithelial cells on the villi and produces nonspecific patchy light microscopic findings.

Bacterial Infections

Food poisoning is a self-limited illness characterized by diarrhea, with or without vomiting, that occurs in a suspected temporal relationship to a meal. The most common causes in North America are due to *Salmonella*, *Staphylococcus aureus* and *Clostridium perfringens*. Illness is produced either by direct infection or by the effects of preformed toxins. With the latter, the incubation period is shorter. Table 12.28 lists the more common agents and potential food sources. For public health reasons it is important to determine whether a given patient represents part of a common source outbreak (e.g., a restaurant or catering firm).

Other bacterial causes of infectious diarrhea are listed in Table 12.29. All may be self-limited and subside within a week, without antibiotics. If they become severe or prolonged, with bloody diarrhea, then the clinical picture and the sigmoidoscopic findings may mimic acute-onset ulcerative colitis or, less likely, Crohn's disease.

Salmonella and *Shigella* enterocolitis both cause illness by direct infection (invasion) and toxin production. *Salmonella* acute gastroenteritis usually does not require antibiotic therapy. *Salmonella* syndromes such as typhoid (enteric) fever and localized infections do require antibiotic therapy. Both *Salmonella* and *Shigella* infections may be contagious in terms of person-to-person spread. Therefore negative stool

Table 12.28   **Food Poisoning**

Agent	Mechanism	Type of Food	Incubation Period	Duration
Salmonella	Infection; possibly preformed toxin	Poultry	12–24 hours	If uncomplicated, 1–7 days
Staphylococcus aureus	Preformed toxins	Creamy foods; puddings	2–6 hours	6–24 hours
Clostridium perfringens	Sporulation in intestine results in toxins	Meats; gravies	8–24 hours	1–2 days
Bacillus cereus	Preformed toxin	Rice; Chinese food	1–20 hours	12–24 hours
Vibrio parahemolyticus	Infection and toxin	Seafood (common in Japan; uncommon in North America)	12–18 hours	2–5 days

cultures should be documented after acute attacks, especially in individuals who are food handlers.

Campylobacter and *Yersinia* enterocolitis are more newly-recognized causes of bacterial gastroenteritis. They require selective culture techniques. Infection with *C. fetus subsp. jejuni* is now the most frequently recognized bacterial infection of the gastrointestinal tract in adults. It has been isolated in 5-15 percent of symptomatic patients with acute onset "infectious diarrhea".

Travelers' diarrhea and enterotoxigenic E. Coli   With increased worldwide travel, the problem of diarrhea in a strange land has become more important. The major pathogens in travelers' diarrhea are the enterotoxigenic *E. Coli*, which are isolated in 40 to 70 percent of travelers with diarrhea. Further down the list is *Shigella* with a frequency of 5 to 20 percent. Other organisms include *Campylobacter* and certain viruses. Often, more than one pathogen is involved, and in up to 30 percent of cases, no specific pathogen is identified.

Enterotoxigenic *E.Coli* are different than the enteropathogenic *E.Coli* which produce gastroenteritis in infants and children. Typically the traveler is well for the first 2 or 3 days after arrival and then the illness lasts 1-3 days. Only occasionally does the diarrhea persist for weeks. Because the major damage occurs in the small bowel, bloody diarrhea is not a feature. Investigations are not usually indicated because of the self-limited nature of the disease.

The major questions that travelers ask their physicians are whether prophylaxis helps, and what treatment to use once an attack begins. The risk of an attack and its severity can be reduced by certain antibiotics (doxycycline or trimethoprim-sulfamethoxazole). Another more laborious approach is to take bismuth subsalicylate in large doses. An alternative to prophylaxis is to see whether an attack develops and then treat it with a regimen shown to be effective, at least in Mexico, namely, trimethoprim-sulfamethoxazole. For mild cases opiates may also be taken. When the diarrhea is prolonged it is important to determine whether the patient has another condition, especially a parasitic infestation.

Table 12.29   **Infectious Diarrhea—Bacterial Causes**

Agent	Clinical Features	Comment
Food Poisoning Agents	See Table 12.28	See Table 12.28
Salmonellosis	Watery or bloody stools	Usually self-limited; antibiotics may prolong organism excretion
Shigellosis (Bacillary dysentery)	Similar to salmonellosis	Antidiarrheal drugs may prolong excretion of the organism; if severe illness use ampicillin or trimethoprim-sulfamethaxozole until sensitivities established
Campylobacter enterocolitis	Febrile illness precedes half the cases; sigmoidoscopic findings may mimic ulcerative colitis or Crohn's disease	Most frequently recognized bacterial cause of gastroenteritis (5–15 percent); if prolonged, use erythromycin or tetracyclines
Yersinia enterocolitis	Most are self-limited; some cases last months and may mimic Crohn's disease	Some types associated with mesenteric adenitis syndrome in children; serology may be helpful in prolonged cases; use tetracycline as first drug in prolonged cases until sensitivities established
Enterotoxigenic *E. coli* in travelers' diarrhea	See text	See text
Antibiotic-associated Colitis	See text	See text

Antibiotic-associated colitis   Diarrhea is a common, usually benign side effect of therapy with many antibiotics. When the diarrhea becomes severe, antibiotic-associated colitis must be considered. Most cases are related to treatment with clindamycin, ampicillin or cephalosporins, although almost every antibiotic has been implicated. Super-infection with *Clostridium difficile* has been established as the most important cause of the colitis. *Staphylococcus aureus* overgrowth is now rare in this setting. *C. difficile* is harbored in 3 percent of healthy adults and in 20 percent of patients who receive antibiotics but have no diarrhea. In patients with antibiotic-associated colitis it can be cultured in 80 to 100 percent. However, the culture, is of less value than is the demonstration of *C. difficile* toxin in stool; the toxin is found in only a small percentage of patients who have diarrhea without evidence of antibiotic-associated colitis.

The clinical manifestations of antibiotic-associated colitis consist of a profuse watery diarrhea, sometimes accompanied by fever and abdominal tenderness. In severe prolonged cases, toxic megacolon, hypoalbuminemia and edema may occur.

The diagnosis is established by visualizing the characteristic *pseudomembranes* at sigmoidoscopy. The pseudomembranes are 2–10 mm yellow-white adherent plaques with intervening normal mucosa. Rectal biopsy reveals a pathognomonic lesion with a focal cap of fibrin, mucin and inflammatory cells. Rarely the sigmoidoscopy and biopsy appearances resemble those of diffuse ulcerative colitis. No further diagnostic tests are required if the sigmoidoscopy and biopsy appearances are typical in the appropriate clinical setting. In atypical or prolonged cases, cultures for *C. difficile* and stool assays for the toxin may be useful. If a barium enema is done, the findings may be similar to those seen in Crohn's disease.

Most patients respond simply to withdrawing the antibiotics. Patients who are moderately ill and fail to respond to antibiotic withdrawal can be treated briefly with cholestyramine which is believed to bind the toxin and may accelerate recovery. Patients who are very ill or who fail to respond to cholestyramine require a course of vancomycin. Metronidazole may be an alternative therapy.

Some patients develop pseudomembranous colitis without prior ingestion of antibiotics. In some, ischemic bowel disease is implicated, *shigellosis* is detected in a few, and in others no incriminating cause of pseudomembranous colitis can be found. It has been suggested that *C. difficile* overgrowth and toxin production may be responsible for some flareups in patients with inflammatory bowel disease. This remains to be proven.

Parasitic Infestations

Giardiasis   See disorders of the small intestine above.

Amebiasis   This is an important parasitic infestation, endemic in the native population in northern Canada, in certain parts of the United States and is a risk for travelers to endemic areas.

Entameba histolytica exists in a trophozoite and cyst form. Trophozoites live and divide in the proximal colon and have time to encyst if they pass out into the feces of the asymptomatic patient. Amebic dysentery results from mucosal invasion. The symptoms are recurrent diarrhea, usually bloody, associated with lower abdominal crampy pain. Symptoms may persist for long periods and thus mimic ulcerative colitis. Sigmoidoscopy shows focal ulcerations with overlying exudate. Usually the mucosa between ulcers appears normal.

The diagnosis is established by examining stools for ova and parasites. Trophozoites are also easily demonstrated in wet preparations from scrapings of ulcers at sigmoidoscopy. Barium enema radiographs may be indistinguishable from ulcerative colitis. Sometimes a localized mass and stricture occur in the right colon (*ameboma*) and this may be confused with carcinoma or Crohn's disease. Serologic tests are helpful in diagnosis. The indirect hemagglutination (IHA) test is positive in 90 percent of cases of invasive colon disease and in 50 percent of patients with asymptomatic intestinal infections. It is positive in about 98 percent of extraintestinal amebic disease. A positive test does not necessarily indicate an active infection since elevated titers may persist for months or years.

Extra-intestinal amebiasis is most commonly found in the liver. Only half of these patients have a prior history of diarrhea and the stools may be negative for the parasites. (See section on amebic liver abscess above.)

Therapy for asymptomatic carriers is diiodohydroxyquin. For amebic colitis the therapy is metronidazole often followed by a course of diiodohydroxyquin.

Idiopathic Inflammatory Bowel Disease

Idiopathic inflammatory bowel disease refers to *ulcerative colitis, Crohn's disease*, and to an uncommon condition that shares features of both, called *indeterminate colitis*.

The etiology is unknown and the pathogenesis of both the local inflammatory change and the extraintestinal manifestations are poorly understood.

The incidence of Crohn's disease appears to be increasing. It predominantly affects young people in the second or third decades but can occur at any age. Ulcerative colitis usually appears after the third decade but childhood forms exist.

There may be familial aggregation of inflammatory bowel disease as well as the extraintestinal manifestations such as ankylosing spondylitis. Jews are more commonly affected and blacks have a decreased incidence. The psyche and underlying personality type are no longer held responsible for causing ulcerative colitis and Crohn's disease.

Pathophysiology

Ulcerative colitis   This is a mucosal disease confined to the colon. The rectum is always involved and the mucosal inflammation is generally more severe in the left colon than in the right. Histologically, the mucosa is diffusely inflamed with increased inflammatory cells, depleted goblet cell mucus, and crypt abscesses. With time, the colon shortens and becomes featureless due to loss of haustra. Pseudopolyps may develop. These are polypoid masses of inflammatory tissue that protrude into the lumen.

Crohn's disease   This is a transmural disease that may affect any part of the gastrointestinal tract. The most common patterns of localization are the ileum and right colon (ileocolitis), colon alone (Crohn's colitis) and the small bowel alone (regional enteritis). Involvement of esophagus, stomach and proximal small bowel is uncommon.

Transmural inflammation with accompanying granulomata are the characteristic features of Crohn's disease. Granulomata are not invariably present. The involvement is segmental and produces "skip lesions". The overlying mucosa may develop aphthoid or deep linear ulcers. Fistula formation is common and may persist as intramural tracks, result in localized abscesses, or extend into adjacent structures such as other parts of the bowel, bladder, vagina, or skin. Luminal narrowing is a regular feature, due to active transmural inflammation. In later stages it is due to strictures.

Clinical Features

In ulcerative colitis, because of the diffuse mucosal involvement, the main symptoms are diarrhea mixed with blood. The severity of bleeding is variable but it is rarely exsanguinating. Accompanying abdominal cramps are relieved by bowel movements. In moderate or severe disease there may be systemic signs of fever, volume depletion and anemia. Rarely, patients present with the syndrome of toxic megacolon and perforation. Extraintestinal manifestations may be present at the outset or may have preceded the development of the colitis.

In both ulcerative colitis and Crohn's disease intermittent low-grade diarrhea may have gone unnoticed over the preceding months or years.

In Crohn's disease the symptoms reflect the site involved and the fact that the disease is transmural and segmental. Although diarrhea may be present, rectal bleeding is not as common as in the diffuse mucosal disease of ulcerative colitis. Instead, symptoms of subacute obstruction are more prominent with colicky periumbilical and lower abdominal crampy pain that may be provoked by eating and is often not relieved by bowel movements. Weight loss and anemia may result from reduced food intake because of fear of eating, anorexia, and from malabsorption if a significant length of distal small bowel is involved. Concomitant anal fissures or fistulas may be present at the time of presentation or may be the presenting complaint.

The physical examination is often not helpful in pinpointing the specific kind of inflammatory bowel disease. There may be generalized abdominal tenderness in severe forms of ulcerative colitis. In Crohn's disease there may be an abdominal mass, especially in the right lower quadrant, because of the frequent involvement in the right colon and ileum. Extraabdominal signs of toxicity (fever, tachycardia, and dehydration) depend on the severity of the attack.

Laboratory Assessment

An essential principle in the investigation of inflammatory bowel disease is to exclude infectious causes with stool cultures, examinations for ova and parasites, and serology, when appropriate.

The diagnosis of ulcerative colitis is primarily made by sigmoidoscopy and a biopsy which reveals histological features compatible with this diagnosis. Sigmoidoscopy reveals a friable, oozing mucosa covered with thin patchy exudates. Discrete deep ulcers are not features of ulcerative colitis. The rectal biopsy is not "diagnostic of" but rather is "compatible with", and helps exclude amebiasis and the presence of granulomata. The plain X-ray film of the abdomen may suggest the colonic involvement. A barium enema radiograph should not be done when diarrhea is severe and signs of toxicity are present, because toxic megacolon may be precipitated. Positive signs on barium enema include tiny ulcerations, loss of haustra, shortening of the colon, and pseudopolyps, but radiographs may be normal in milder cases.

The diagnosis of Crohn's disease is made primarily by barium radiographs. A sigmoidoscopy is done to determine whether there is obvious involvement of the rectosigmoid area. Aphthous-like tiny mucosal ulcers suggest Crohn's disease. Anal fissures or fistulas may be present even when the rectum is spared. Sometimes granulomata are found in rectal biopsies from normal appearing areas. The barium enema in Crohn's disease may reveal signs of bowel wall thickening and mucosal irregularity, especially in the right colon. Other areas of the colon may also be narrowed in a segmental fashion with "skip" lesions. If barium refluxes into the terminal ileum there may be evidence of adjacent ileal involvement. When luminal compromise is marked, the classic ileal "string sign" is produced. Intramural fissures, fistula tracks and localized abscesses may be demonstrated. The small bowel barium radiographs help to define the extent of ileal involvement and to determine whether more proximal areas are affected. More precise visualization is achieved with small bowel intubation and a rapid infusion of barium, the enteroclysis examination.

Some patients, perhaps 5 percent, have a colitis without specific features of either ulcerative colitis or Crohn's disease. Their *indeterminate colitis* is treated according to the same principles.

Blood tests are designed to screen for fluid and electrolyte imbalance, anemia (bone marrow suppression and blood loss) and nutritional deficiency states.

Complications

Local complications (Table 12.30) result from direct involvement of the affected bowel or adjacent structures. Perianal complications and fistual formation are more common in Crohn's disease than in ulcerative colitis.

Rectal bleeding is more common in ulcerative colitis than in Crohn's disease. Massive exsanguinating hemorrhage is uncommon in both disorders.

Toxic megacolon is a dreaded complication that is more common in ulcerative colitis. There is progressive dilatation of the colon, especially on the right side, and it may result in perforation. Patients with toxic megacolon require close clinical followup by physicians and surgeons. Serial plain films of the abdomen are done and the patient is prepared for colectomy surgery in the event that the condition deteriorates.

Carcinoma of the colon represents a distinct risk after 7–10 years of ulcerative colitis, with risk rates in the range of 3 percent per annum. After 20 years

Table 12.30   Local Complications of Idiopathic Inflammatory Bowel Disease

Perianal Disease (more common in Crohn's disease)
  Anal fissure
  Anal fistula
  Perirectal abscess
Fistula (almost exclusively Crohn's disease)
  Vagina
  Bladder
  Entero-enteric
Hemorrhage
  Mild with anemia (more common in ulverative colitis)
  Massive
Toxic Megacolon (more common in ulcerative colitis)
Perforation
  Localized, with abscess (more common in Crohn's disease)
  Free perforation in toxic megacolon (more common in ulcerative colitis)
Carcinoma (more common in ulcerative colitis)
Stricture (more common in Crohn's disease)
Renal
  Hydronephrosis (Crohn's disease)

the risk is even greater. Colon cancer risk in Crohn's disease may be increased, but much less than in ulcerative colitis.

When Crohn's disease affects the right colon and terminal ileum (ileocolitis), it may involve the ureter and result in asymptomatic right-sided hydronephrosis. Renal calculi may develop as there is prolonged stasis in the renal pelvis.

Extraintestinal manifestations (Table 12.31) may precede the first overt symptoms, may accompany the initial bowel manifestations or may develop subsequently.

Table 12.31   Extraintestinal Manifestations of Inflammatory Bowel Disease

Joint
  Nondeforming arthritis
  Ankylosing spondylitis
Skin
  Erythema nodosum
  Pyoderma gangrenosum
Eye
  Conjunctivitis
  Iritis
  Uveitis
Anemia and Nutritional Deficiencies
  Reduced food intake
  Losses from inflamed bowel
  Malabsorption
Liver disease
  Fatty change
  Pericholangitis
  Sclerosing cholangitis
  Bile duct carcinoma
Other
  Amyloidosis
  "Hypercoagulable state"
  Clubbing of digits

A nondeforming fleeting arthritis may occur, especially in ulcerative colitis and in Crohn's disease of the colon. It often flares in association with the bowel disease. There is also an increased incidence of ankylosing spondylitis in both ulcerative colitis and Crohn's disease (see Chapter 18).

A variety of nutritional disturbances may result from reduced food intake, malabsorption, and from nutrient losses from the inflamed bowel. When anemia occurs it may be due to blood loss, bone marrow suppression from chronic inflammation and least commonly to vitamin B_{12} malabsorption in ileal Crohn's disease.

In the liver, mild fatty change is common. Uncommon liver complications are pericholangitis, sclerosing cholangitis, and bile duct carcinoma.

Therapy

The goals of therapy are to correct any electrolyte and nutrient deficiencies, control symptoms, and to help prevent relapses. It is important to recognize that no medical therapy alters the basic natural history in terms of preventing the need for surgery in either ulcerative colitis or Crohn's disease.

In mild cases of ulcerative colitis or Crohn's disease, sulfasalazine in a dose of 2–4 g/d is the initial drug used. Its value in controlling symptoms has not been established in controlled trials. If symptoms are more severe, with fever and multiple (8–10) stools each day, corticosteroids may be required. Very ill patients may also benefit from total parenteral nutrition in order to put the bowel at rest. When symptoms are controlled, the corticosteroids are slowly tapered to the lowest possible dose or are withdrawn completely.

Maintenance therapy consists of sulfasalazine. It has been shown to reduce the number of flare-ups in ulcerative colitis but its role in helping reduce subsequent flare-ups in Crohn's disease is not established. Other therapies that have been tried but remain unproven include metronidazole, azathioprine, and antibiotics.

Total colectomy for ulcerative colitis results in a permanent cure. The obvious disadvantage however is that the patient is left with a permanent ileostomy. If a patient has required maintenance corticosteroids for 1-2 years because of continuous symptoms then total colectomy is usually recommended. The decision to do colectomy in ulcerative colitis is more difficult in patients who have frequent long remissions.

In view of the increased cancer risk, some patients opt for colectomy after 10 years. Those without colectomy must have annual or semi-annual colonoscopy examinations with multiple biopsies to look for evidence of dysplasia or "precancer".

Surgery for Crohn's disease is reserved for complications, namely intractable fissures or fistulas, localized abscesses, and bowel obstruction. There is a tendency for Crohn's disease to recur after surgical resection. Therefore, operations are deferred until absolutely necessary.

Outcome

A small number of patients with ulcerative colitis have only one attack and the disease never recurs. It is possible that these patients actually have had an unrecognized infectious cause of colitis that mimics ulcerative colitis. In 10-15 percent, ulcerative colitis is continuous and may become fulminant. The remainder of patients have a course characterized by intermittent remissions and exacerbations. In Crohn's disease the clinical behavior of an individual patient is highly variable. In general, most patients will require at least one operative resection for a complication within the firts 5-10 years of disease. The prognosis in terms of avoiding the need for surgery seems to be most favorable in those with Crohn's disease confined to the colon.

Proctitis

This refers to inflammation usually confined to the distal 5 or 10 cm of the rectum. The major symptoms are rectal bleeding with normally formed stools, rectal urgency, and discomfort during passage of stools. Diarrhea is absent because most of the colon is intact.

Idiopathic ulcerative proctitis is a condition whose gross and microscopic appearances are identical to those of ulcerative colitis except that the lesion rarely extends to involve the rest of the colon. Therapy to control rectal bleeding consists of 7-10 day courses of rectal corticosteroid enemas and the use of stool softeners. In severe cases, sulfasalazine may be used for maintenance but there is no clear evidence that it helps to reduce flare-ups as it does in ulcerative colitis. The condition tends to wax and wane unpredictably and is often characterized by long symptom-free periods.

The diagnosis rests with demonstration that the typical sigmoidoscopic and biopsy features are confined to the distal rectum. A number of indistinguishable *infectious proctitis syndromes* are increasingly recognized as sexually transmitted disorders, especially in male homosexuals. The major cases are *gonorrhea*, *herpes simplex*, *syphilis*, and *Chlamydia* proctitis. Anorectal swab cultures and dark field examinations for syphilis exclude the infectious proctitides. Serology may be of value in *Chlamydia* proctitis.

In addition to proctitis syndromes, infectious diarrheas in general are recognized increasingly in male homosexuals.

Diverticular Disease

The term diverticular disease encompasses diverticulosis (the presence of diverticula) and diverticulitis (diverticula associated with signs of inflammation). Diverticular disease is present in about 30 percent of people over the age of 60.

Most diverticula occur in the sigmoid colon from herniations of mucosa and submucosa between bundles of circular muscle along the perforating branches of blood vessels. The hypothesis is that diverticula arise when intraluminal pressure rises abnormally, perhaps because of increased segmentation activity and the application of high pressure to the bowel wall. Epidemiologic studies have suggested that diverticular disease is rare in groups who eat high roughage diets.

Diverticular disease is usually asymptomatic. When symptoms occur in uncomplicated diverticular disease they are usually characterized by intermittent left lower quadrant abdominal pain that is relieved by passage of gas or a bowel movement. There may also be an alteration in bowel habit characterized by constipation alternating with diarrhea. The diagnosis is established with a barium enema study and other disorders must be excluded, particularly adenocarcinoma. Therapy in the uncomplicated case consists of encouragement to eat a normal diet with adequate fiber.

Complications of Diverticular Disease

The major complications of diverticular disease are *diverticulitis*, a severe localized inflammation, and *bleeding*.

Diverticulitis   Diverticulitis is characterized by intense left lower quadrant pain with altered bowel habits and fever. Physical examination reveals a palpable and intensely tender left colon with systemic features of inflammation such as leukocytosis. The goals of therapy are to place the bowel at rest with a liquid diet or nothing by mouth, use broad spectrum antibiotics and consider elective surgery when the attack subsides. Elective surgery is sometimes deferred until a second attack. This decision depends upon the patient's age and associated conditions.

The other manifestations of diverticulitis result from penetration or perforation and they present as pericolic abscess, fistula, free perforation and liver abscess.

A pericolic abscess may present as a painful mass, confirmed on an abdominal plain film or ultrasound test. In this situation barium contrast studies are avoided until symptoms subside. Patients are treated with intravenous fluids, antibiotics, and surgery. A fistula may communicate with the bladder (pneumaturia), vagina, or skin. Th diagnosis is established with contrast studies that demonstrate the fistula. Free perforation presents with clinical features of peritonitis. Liver abscess may be another reflection of perforation or penetration. For all complications of perforation, two-stage operations may be required. The first stage is to perform a diverting colostomy. When the inflammatory process has subsided then definitive resection and reanastomosis are performed.

Bleeding   Bleeding complicates diverticular disease in about 5 percent of patients and is rarely massive. The bleeding is either bright red in character or maroon-colored, depending on the rate of bleeding and the transit time. The principles of resuscitation were outlined in the earlier section Gastrointestinal Bleeding. Sigmoidoscopy, colonoscopy and air contrast barium studies help to eliminate other causes of bleeding. Only when other causes of lower gastrointestinal tract bleeding have been eliminated, should one attribute the bleeding to the presence of diverticular disease.

Constipation

Constipation refers to a reduced frequency of bowel movements and the passage of hard stools. At times constipation is almost physiological when associated with a reaction to unfamiliar toilets during travel, and to periodic stresses. A major concern in patients with no obvious underlying cause is the possibility of an organic colonic obstruction. Other causes include certain drugs, endocrine disorders such as hypothyroidism, metabolic disturbances such as hypercalcemia and neurogenic disorders associated with spinal cord damage.

If the condition is longstanding and the patient is a habitual user of laxatives and enemas, a vicious-cycle may have been created in which there is a dependence on these maneuvers.

The principles of investigation and the nonspecific approaches to therapy are similar to those outlined in the next section on the dysfunctional bowel syndrome.

Dysfunctional Bowel Syndrome ("Irritable Bowel Syndrome")

The dysfunctional bowel syndrome (DBS) is the most common symptom complex in the gastrointestinal system. It is characterized by any combination of abdominal pain (usually lower), constipation and diarrhea. Abdominal bloating is a common accompaniment.

The pathogenesis is poorly understood. Perhaps the most useful way to think of DBS is as a heterogeneous group of disorders which we are currently unable to sort out. Conditions that were formerly lumped into DBS prior to their elucidation are lactase deficiency, giardiasis, and early Crohn's disease. Abnormal bowel motility and underlying psychological disorders can be documented in some of these patients but there is clearly no single "lesion".

The decision to pursue laboratory investigation must be made on an individual basis, based on the duration and severity of symptoms. Ultimately, the diagnosis is one of exclusion. The investigation is focused on the predominant symptoms. For example, a patient with predominant constipation must have obstructing lesions of the colon, especially carcinoma excluded. In younger patients with alternating constipation, diarrhea, and abdominal pain, Crohn's disease would be a major consideration. If symptoms coincide with a psychological disorder such as an anxiety state or depression, these features may warrant further assessment. Patients should not be considered to have a psychological disorder simply because all the tests are negative.

The essentials of therapy include reassurance; no serious cause has been found and empiric therapy usually helps. The patient must understand that there may be periodic exacerbations. The best initial therapy is to add bulk to the diet in the form of 1 or 2 tablespoons a day of raw unprocessed bran and psyllium (Metamucil or related compounds). This regimen may worsen symptoms for the first 2–4 weeks. A trial of a high residue regimen should not be abandoned prior to 3 months. With this approach, bowel habit is usually regulated and the associated abdominal pain is often reduced in intensity. Patients will then often volunteer that they can live with their residual symptoms. If the patient also has a psychological disorder, it needs to be treated in parallel. Sedative drugs should not be prescribed simply because a patient has DBS.

Patients with chronic belching may have to be taught that they often do this as a result of air swallowing.

In patients with prominent complaints of bloating and excessive flatulence, certain therapeutic maneuvers may be helpful. Carbon dioxide is produced in the upper bowel from the neutralization of acid by bicarbonate. However, most of the carbon dioxide as well as hydrogen and methane in flatus is derived from colonic bacterial fermentation. Foods high in nonabsorbable carbohydrate content such as beans and cabbage should be eliminated. Since some normal individuals may not absorb all their ingested starches and lactose, it may be useful to reduce both the lactose and overall carbohydrate intake to reduce bacterial fermentation and gas production in the colon.

Vascular Disorders of The Small and Large Intestine

Angiodysplasia

Angiodysplasia lesions are ectatic veins and capillaries found most commonly in the cecum and ascending colon, but they may also be present in other parts of the gastrointestinal tract. Their cause is unknown but they appear to be related to advancing age and the prevalence may also be increased in patients with aortic stenosis.

Some of these lesions cause gastrointestinal tract bleeding without associated abdominal pain. It may be overt brisk bleeding or it may be detected because of anemia or stools positive for occult blood. The diagnosis is most often established with colonoscopy and is complemented by selective angiography. Because the lesions may be common in elderly patients, they should only be blamed as the cause of the gastrointestinal tract bleeding when they are seen to bleed or when no other cause is found. Because many of the patients are elderly, the decision concerning whether and when to operate depends on the magnitude of the bleeding.

Ischemic Bowel Disease

Ischemic bowel disease may be nonocclusive, as a result of hypoperfusion, or occlusive in nature. Vascular occlusion may result from mesenteric venous thrombosis and arterial embolism or thrombosis. The ischemic bowel syndromes usually occur when there is an underlying cause. These include associated myocardial or valvular heart disease, hypercoagulable states or vasculitis.

There are two categories of presentation. One is a catastrophic acute abdomen with actual perforation or with signs of impending perforation. There may be associated gastrointestinal tract bleeding. In the colon major target sites of ischemia are the flexures because these are the areas of marginal anastomotic blood supply between the superior and inferior mesenteric systems. The rectosigmoid is rarely involved except after previous reconstructive aortic bypass surgery. Plain films of the abdomen may show a gas filled bowel indented by a "thumb printing" pattern. This is due to localized hemorrhage and transmural swelling. When the presentation is acute, immediate surgical exploration and appropriate bowel resection are essential.

The second less dramatic syndrome is one in which delayed stricture formation appears. The symptoms are those of intestinal obstruction. When the small intestine is affected there may be postprandial abdominal cramps and abdominal distension. When the colon is affected symptoms usually begin with alternating bowel habits. Barium enema may reveal localized stricture, "thumb-printing" or a nondescript narrowing that might mimic Crohn's disease. Strictures in the small bowel are much less common. A more chronic syndrome of small bowel ischemia called "intestinal angina" is rare in its classic form. It consists of postprandial pain to the point of producing a fear of eating, and associated weight loss. The diagnosis is often difficult to make with these low grade presentations of ischemic bowel disease. The usual concern is to exclude other conditions that may produce segmental changes, especially in the colon, namely carcinoma and Crohn's disease. In these more chronic syndromes, surgery is reserved for evidence of clear-cut progression with evolving symptoms of peritonitis, or outright obstruction as a result of chronic stricture formation.

Appendicitis

The appendix is the remnant of the apex of the cecum. Appendicitis is an inflammation that involves all layers and the most frequent cause is occlusion of the lumen from food residues. The obstruction proceeds to ulceration and may terminate with necrosis and perforation.

The initial symptom of acute appendicitis is usually a periumbilical pain and variable accompaniments of nausea, vomiting and diarrhea. Within a few hours the pain shifts to the right lower quadrant because the inflammatory process involves the peritoneal surface of neighboring loops of bowel and the anterior parietal peritoneum. At that point the physical examination may reveal involuntary guarding and rebound tenderness, the signs of a localized peritonitis. There may be low grade fever and moderate leukocytosis. If perforation occurs then the signs are those of an acute abdomen. Some perforations are walled off and present as periappendiceal abscesses.

Generally the diagnosis is established on clinical grounds alone and is confirmed at surgery. Early diagnosis prevents the life threatening complications of perforation. If symptoms are atypical, a barium enema is sometimes performed. The rationale is that if the appendix is visualized on barium enema it is not obstructed and thus excludes appendicitis.

Radiation Injury of The Small and Large Intestine

Radiotherapy to treat malignancy may create side effects in any part of the gastrointestinal system. The most commonly affected regions are the small and large intestine because abdominal and pelvic irradiation are commonly used.

An early syndrome occurs during or shortly after the course of radiotherapy. The rapidly dividing cells of the small bowel and colon are susceptible. Diarrhea is a common side effect. Small bowel changes consist of villous blunting and reduced numbers of mitotic figures. In the colon a proctitis or colitis may be produced depending on the field of irradiation. Bloody diarrhea may ensue and the features may resemble those of ulcerative colitis.

A late syndrome may develop months or years after the radiation therapy. The manifestations are due to progressive scarring and stricture formation, in part due to small vessel fibrosis. Therefore, in the small bowel the presentation is that of subacute obstruction with stricture formation. The stasis may result in a bacterial overgrowth syndrome with steatorrhea. In the colon, the features may be those of stricture formation, or rectal bleeding due to a more chronic form of colitis. The exact reason for the colitis is not clear but it may relate to mucosal ischemia. The typical sigmoidoscopy findings in these patients are telangiectasia very similar in appearance to those observed on the skin of patients who have received radiation therapy for breast carcinoma.

There is no specific therapy for radiation injury. Surgery is performed for intractable or progressive strictures.

Tumors of The Large Intestine

Benign Polyps

Epithelial polyps are common and may be present in 10 percent of patients over the age of 40. The most common *hyperplastic* type is a simple proliferation of the epithelium in normal mucosal glands. These are usually less than 5 mm in diameter, do not cause clinical symptoms and have no potential for malignancy. *Adenomatous* (tubular), *mixed villo-adenomatous* and *villous adenoma*-polyps carry a greater risk of malignancy when they exceed 1 cm in diameter. These polyps may be either sessile or pedunculated with a stalk. Adenomatous (tubular) polyps are generally larger than hyperplastic polyps. Mixed villo-adenomatous polyps are less common than adenomatous polyps. Villous adenomas are the least common type of colonic polyp, may be larger than the others and are sometimes associated with a severe watery diarrhea syndrome with hypokalemia.

Benign nonepithelial polyps are rare in adults. Juvenile polyps associated with gastrointestinal bleeding usually present in childhood. These are lobulated and pedunculated lesions which contain disordered cysts and fibrous tissue. Hamartomatous polyps are seen in association with a rare syndrome, the Peutz-Jeghers syndrome which is characterized by mucocutaneous pigmentation and is inherited as an autosomal dominant trait. This syndrome does not carry a high risk of malignancy. Other types of polyps such as carcinoids, leiomyomas and lipomas are rare.

Clinical features   Polyps are usually found in asymptomatic individuals who have screening sigmoidoscopy or barium enema X-ray examinations for other reasons, or in individuals who are being evaluated for occult gastrointestinal bleeding. Very large polyps may cause symptoms of abdominal pain due to localized obstruction.

Investigation and management   These lesions require visualization with both barium enema (preferably with air contrast) and endoscopy. Approximately three-quarters of all polyps are within the distal 50 cm of the colon and are thus detectable by flexible sigmoidoscopy. When the polyps are detected, colonoscopy is useful to exclude companion lesions in the more proximal colon. Endoscopy provides the opportunity to biopsy polyps and to do endoscopic polypectomy for those polyps with a stalk. Sessile lesions greater than 1.5–2 cm in diameter should be removed surgically, and surgery should also be performed when endoscopic polypectomy specimens from pedunculated polyps reveal malignant invasion of the stalk.

After adenomatous polyps are detected, followup examinations should be performed after 1 year and if negative, every 2 or 3 years. The usual followup test is air contrast barium enema but colonoscopy is probably more sensitive. These patients should also be screened regularly for the presence of occult blood in the stool.

When the colon has many adenomatous polyps the risk of adenocarcinoma is great. Several inherited disorders should be considered. *Familial polyposis coli* and *Gardner's syndrome* are autosomal dominant conditions characterized by a predominance of adenomatous polyps in the colon. Gardner's syndrome is also associated with benign and malignant tumors and cysts of soft tissues and bone. Some patients have disseminated gastrointestinal polyps unassociated with a familial syndrome. All patients with multiple adenomatous polyps require colectomy because of the increased cancer risk. In a patient with multiple adenomatous polyps of the colon it is important to obtain a careful family history and to screen suspect relatives with a barium enema and sigmoidoscopy.

Adenocarcinoma

Adenocarcinoma of the large bowel is increasing in frequency in North America and is now the most common malignancy after skin cancer. It is important, because, of all gastrointestinal tumors it is the most amenable to early diagnosis and definitive cure. The majority of these tumors occur in the distal large bowel, but increasing numbers occur in the proximal colon. Multifocal tumors may occur.

Clinical features   The risk factors include stool positive for occult blood in a patient older than 40, recurrent adenomatous or villous polyps, long-standing ulcerative colitis, previous cholecystectomy, family history of colon carcinoma and the presence of an inherited polyposis syndrome.

The most common symptoms of carcinoma of the colon are altered bowel habit and occult or overt lower gastrointestinal bleeding. Tumors in the right colon, especially the cecum, grow larger before local symptoms develop so that blood loss anemia is often the first mode of presentation. In tumors of the descending colon, sigmoid colon, and rectum, symptoms of obstruction develop earlier. These are characterized by altered bowel habits (constipation, or alternating constipation and diarrhea) and abdominal cramps. In these left-sided lesions there may be accompanying bright red rectal bleeding, sometimes wrongly attributed to hemorrhoids. Serious bowel obstruction or localized perforation are uncommon features. The most common local physical findings are an abdominal mass or a palpable lesion on rectal examination. The stool guaiac test for occult blood is often positive if bright red bleeding is not obvious.

Some patients present with obvious metastases, especially to liver, and the primary lesion is only detected afterwards.

Laboratory Investigation The finding of anemia or occult blood in a patient over 40 mandates a complete evaluation with sigmoidoscopy and air contrast barium enema. If these are negative, a colonoscopy and biopsy of observed lesions should be done. Patients with diverticular disease may have a gross deformity in the region of the sigmoid colon and this requires direct visualization with endoscopy to rule out a carcinoma. In ulcerative colitis, benign strictures need to be differentiated from accompanying cancer. Other inflammatory lesions such as Crohn's disease may enter into the differential diagnosis.

Treatment Surgery for cure requires resection and reanastomosis. Tumors of the rectum usually require an abdominoperineal resection and a permanent colostomy. With advanced disease, colostomy proximal to the lesion may be required for the palliation of obstruction or severe bleeding.

An important aspect of therapy is *preventative screening*. It is recommended that patients over the age of 40 have annual stool guaiac tests and an annual digital rectal examination. After the age of 50, sigmoidoscopic examinations should be added every 2 years. Stool guaiac tests have been simplified with home kits. False positive results may occur in patients who consume meat. Therefore, initially positive tests need to be repeated on a meat-free diet. False-negative results may occur when samples age for 4 or 5 days. If two consecutive stools are positive for occult blood and continue to be positive on a meat-free diet then investigation for colon carcinoma should be instituted. Approximately 10 percent of these patients will have either a large polyp or an adenocarcinoma of the colon. Patients who have risk factors referred to earlier should have colonoscopy performed every few years.

Outcome Five-year survival depends on the site of the cancer, whether regional lymph nodes are positive and how far into the bowel wall the tumor has penetrated. There is an 80 percent 5 year survival for lesions confined to the mucosa alone and a 25 percent survival when there is lymph node involvement. If distant metastases are present, the 5-year outlook is 5 percent or less. Chemotherapy for colorectal cancer is not very effective but isolated dramatic responses may occur.

When surgery for cure has been performed, annual evaluations should include chest radiographs, hemoglobin determination, and stool guaiacs. Barium enema radiographs, and endoscopy may be performed every 1–2 years. Many use the carcinoembryonic antigen test (CEA) for followup evaluation after colorectal surgery for cure. A rise in the circulating CEA indicates the presence of recurrent disease.

Other Malignancies of the Large Intestine

These comprise less than 5 percent of all malignancies of the colon and rectum. The primary tumors include carcinoids and lymphomas. Secondary tumors may arise from an adjacent primary such as prostate or from remote primary sites.

Anal and Perirectal Disorders

Hemorrhoids

When vascular anal cushions are prolapsed through the anal canal as a result of straining, the condition of hemorrhoids may develop. In advanced stages permanent prolapse occurs. External hemorrhoids usually represent a thrombosis of the external hemorrhoidal plexus. Frequently these resorb leaving external anal tags.

The primary symptoms are bloody streaks coating the stool or a bloody discharge. There may be associated severe perianal pain.

The diagnosis is based on inspection of the perirectal region while the patient is straining and anoscopy. The main differential diagnosis is to exclude other causes of rectal bleeding, particularly anal fissures, ulcerative proctitis, and carcinoma.

Therapy is directed towards providing a high residue regimen as outlined earlier for the dysfunctional bowel syndrome and to add stool softeners such as dioctyl sodium sulfosuccinate. Hot baths may relieve the perianal pain.

The natural history is that of mild low grade intermittent symptoms. When bleeding is severe and recurrent or when there is intractable painful prolapse with thrombosis, other techniques are required. They include sclerosis with rubber band ligation at the base of the hemorrhoids to produce sloughing, and cryosurgery. Surgical hemorrhoidectomy is deferred until other measures fail because a small number of patients may develop the late complications of anal stenosis or mild anal sphincter dysfunction.

Pruritus Ani

This is a common complaint. Characteristically the pruritis is worse at night when the distracting stimuli of the day are absent. Sometimes patients scratch the perianal region during the night without being aware of it. Pruritis ani may be a manifestation of local disease such as fistula, fissure, and neoplasm. There may be a generalized dermatologic disorder with secondary involvement of the anus. Infections should be sought. These include candidiasis, pinworms, scabies, and condyloma acuminata. Candidiasis may develop in patients with gross obesity, in diabetics or in patients who are generally immunosuppressed. Pinworm ova can be found by touching the perianal area with a piece of transparent tape and examining it under the microscope.

Often no specific cause is found. General measures consist of adding bulk to the diet to provide larger softer stools. Patients should be advised not to wipe the perianal area vigorously nor to use strong soaps and detergents. The perianal region should be washed with water after bowel movements and patted dry. When there is severe associated dermatitis, topical ointments such as zinc oxide may be required. In more intractable cases a topical corticosteroid cream may be necessary.

Anal Fissures

These are tears in the anal canal and the most common cause is related to passage of hard stool. They usually heal promptly. The primary symptoms are bleeding and pain. The bleeding may only be appreciated as blood on the toilet tissue. The pain may become so excruciating that patients become fearful of having a bowel movement and constipation results. This creates a vicious cycle because subsequent passage of hard stool aggravates the fissure. The differential diagnosis is as for hemorrhoids. In patients with chronic fissures it is important to determine whether this represents the first manifestation of Crohn's disease. Treatment is with high residue diets and stool softeners. Warm baths help relieve the pain.

REFERENCES

Hepatobiliary

1. Alter, H.J. : Hepatitis B. Serminars in Liver Disease, Volume 1, Number 1, 1981.
2. Boyer, J.L.: Chronic hepatitis—a perspective on classification and determinants of prognosis. Gastroenterology, 70: 1161–1171, 1976.
3. Hanna, S.S., Warren, W.D., Galambos, J.T., et al: Bleeding varices. Can Med Ass J 124:29–47, 1981.
4. Isselbacher, K.J.: Metabolic and hepatic effects of alcohol. N Engl J Med 196:612–616, 1977.
5. Schmid, R.: Bilirubin metabolism: state of the art. Gastroenterology, 74:1307–1312, 1978.
6. Shaffer, E.A.: Gallstones: Current concepts of pathogenesis and medical dissolution. Can J Surg 23:517–532, 1980.
7. Sherlock, S. (ed.) Diseases of the Liver and Biliary System. 6th ed. Blackwell Scientific Publications, The C.V. Mosby Company, St. Louis, 1981.
8. Weber, F.L.: Therapy of portal-systemic encephalopathy: the practical and the promising. Gastroenterology 81:174–181, 1981.
9. Zimmerman, H.J.: Intrahepatic cholestasis. Arch Intern Med, 139:1038–1045, 1979.

Pancreas

1. Di Magno, E.P.: Pancreatic cancer: a continuing dilemma. Ann Int Med, 90:847–848, 1979.
2. Morgan, R.G.H., Wormsley, K.G.: Cancer of the pancreas Gut, 18:580–596, 1977.
3. Park, R., Grand, R.J.: Gastrointestinal manifestations of cystic fibrosis: a review. Gastroenterology, 81:1143–1161, 1981.
4. Salt WB, Schenker S: Amylase—its clinical significance: a review of the literature. Medicine 55:269–281, 1976.
5. Diagnosis of chronic pancreatitis. Lancet 1:719–720, 1982.

The Gastrointestinal Tract

1. Bengoa, J.M., Irwin, H. Rosenberg, M.D.: Parenteral nutrition therapy in gastrointestinal disease. Adv. Int. Med. 28:363, 1983.
2. Guth, P.M.: Pathogenesis of gastric mucosal injury. Ann. Rev. Med. 33:183, 1982.
3. Janowitz, H.D., Sachar D.B. Inflammatory bowel disease. Adv. Int. Med. 27:205 1982.
4. Jensen, R.T.: Zollinger-Ellison Syndrome: Current concepts and management. Ann. Int. Med. 98:59, 1983.
5. Kestenbaum, D., Behar, J.: Pathogenesis, diagnosis and management of reflux esophagitis. Ann. Rev. Med. 32:443, 1981.
6. Silva J. Jr., Fekety, R.: Clostridia and antimicrobial enterocolitis. Ann. Rev. Med. 32:327, 1981.
7. Tucker, H. Schuster, M.M.: Irritable bowel syndrome: new pathophysiologic concepts. Adv. Int. Med. 27:183, 1982.

13

The Endocrine System

Bernard Corenblum, M.D. and Robert Volpé, M.D.

PRINCIPLES OF ENDOCRINOLOGY

The word *hormone* is derived from the Greek word *hormaein*, meaning "to set in motion." A hormone is a chemical messenger that regulates preexisting cell function, but does not produce a new function in the cell. Certain principles that apply to all components of the endocrine system are related to synthesis, transport, degradation, and, most importantly, regulation of hormone release and action at the cellular level.

PRINCIPLES OF ENDOCRINE PHYSIOLOGY

Chemical Classes of Hormones

Three major chemical classes are present:

1. Polypeptide derived hormones may range from simple, such as TRH (a tripeptide), to complex molecules consisting of several hundred amino acids with more than one peptide chain, and these may also include carbohydrate components.
2. Steroid derived hormones are biochemically based on the typical steroid molecule, with variations in structure giving rise to glucocorticoid and mineralocorticoid activity, sex steroids (progesterone, androgens, and estrogens) and vitamin D.
3. Monoamines such as norepinephrine may function as hormones, and as neurotransmitters.

Biosynthesis of Hormones

There are two general mechanisms involved in the biosynthesis of hormones:

1. Ribosomal translation. Ribosomal translation gives rise to polypeptide hormones. Polypeptide synthesis is under genetic control, whereby transcription in the nucleus and translation on cytoplasmic ribosomes results in a polypeptide product called a *prehormone*. Subsequently, translocation across the rough endoplasmic reticulum and a number of further modifications of the hormone may occur.
2. Enzymatic transformation of precursors. A precursor undergoes enzymatic modification through specific biosynthetic pathways resulting in a final product—a steroid hormone or a thyroid hormone. The genetic control for this type of hormone is much more complex, since each enzyme required in the biosynthetic pathway itself has to be synthesized. For this reason, inborn errors of metabolism are much more common for steroid hormones, and quite uncommon for polypeptide hormones. In contrast, ectopic hormone production by malignant tissue usually results in the production of a polypeptide hormone.

Hormonal Storage, Secretion, Plasma Transport, and Peripheral Degradation

Polypeptide hormones are usually stored in cytoplasmic granules, in amounts sufficient for short-term requirements. Steroid hormones are not significantly stored, and for this reason features of steroid insufficiency (such as glucocorticoid insufficiency) can develop quite rapidly. Vitamin D is an exception, since it may be stored by incorporation into body lipid pools. Thyroid hormones are stored for longer periods of time within the thyroid follicles, bound to a large follicular protein, thyroglobulin.

Hormones are usually secreted at low or basal rates. Factors that enhance secretion usually result in release of any prestored hormone, as well as an increase in the biosynthesis of that hormone. Secretion may occur in pulsatile rhythms, episodic bursts, or in relation to certain biologic rhythms (such as ACTH and cortisol interaction).

Soluble hormones, such as polypeptides, are carried free in the blood. Hormones that are less soluble (steroid and thyroid) have carrier proteins. Usually the active form of the hormone circulates, but there also may be hormone precursors or even metabolic products of the same hormone in the circulation (such as with parathyroid hormone), and these may contribute to the assay recognition of plasma hormonal levels. Protein-bound hormones are not biologically active, but coexist in an equilibrium state with nonprotein bound ("free") hormone levels. It is the free hormone concentration that determines physiologic feedback and regulation. Changes in the levels of plasma binding globulins do not have any influence on endocrine function, nor do they enter the feedback control, but they may alter the diagnostic application of laboratory procedures.

The actual plasma level of a hormone is determined by the amount of binding by plasma factors, directly by the secretion rate, and indirectly by the metabolic clearance rate of the hormone. Degradation of each hormone may occur at the target cell, usually within the liver, and occasionally by the kidney. The inactive metabolic products are then excreted in the bile and in the urine. Some is excreted unchanged in the urine (such as urinary free cortisol, which may be assayed). The peripheral tissues may not only degrade hormones, but may alter the hormone to a form with different effects (such as conversion of testosterone to estradiol) or more potent effects (such as conversion of testosterone to dihydrotestosterone, T4 to T3, or cholecalciferol to 1,25 DHD$_3$). Because there also be may peripheral generation of a hormone, the production rate consists of the sum of the amounts of hormone secreted plus the amount produced by peripheral generation. If normal feedback regulatory mechanisms are intact, then abnormalities of degradation (such as liver or kidney dysfunction) will not produce endocrine abnormalities, since the site of hormonal regulation is at the level of biosynthesis and release.

Mechanisms of Hormone Action

Each hormone binds to a receptor that functions as the means for recognition and activation of the hormonal signal.

Cell Surface Receptors

Cell Surface receptors are protein macromolecules within the plasma membrane that selectively bind a hormone. The receptors may be species specific (such as growth hormone) or may not be species specific (such as insulin). The biologic response to a hormone depends on the concentration of receptors, the avidity of receptors for hormone, and the concentration of hormone. Variation in the percentage of receptor occupancy accounts for variation in tissue response; the tissue sensitivity (receptor occupancy) required for insulin to inhibit lipolysis is less than the receptor occupancy required for insulin to inhibit the release of amino acids from muscle. A hormone usually regulates the number of its receptors by altering the synthesis or degradation of receptors. A hormone may increase the number of receptors ("up" regulation, such as with prolactin) or decrease the number of its receptors ("down" regulation, such as with insulin). There also may be intracellular receptor sites for polypeptide hormones such as insulin, prolactin, and parathyroid hormone, which may enter the cells. End-organ resistance may result from absence of receptors, from postreceptor events (as in nephrogenic diabetes insipidus), or from antibodies directed against the receptor (such as diabetes mellitus associated with acanthosis nigricans).

The surface receptors may mediate postreceptor events by generation of another substance called a *second messenger*. Cyclic AMP is a second messenger that may mediate some responses of most peptide hormones. The peptide hormone activates plasma membrane adenylate cyclase, which then generates cyclic AMP from ATP. A coupling protein, N protein, is involved with the hormone-receptor activation of adenylate cyclase. This may have clinical implications, since, for example, some patients with pseudohypoparathyroidism type I have low levels of protein N and are unresponsive to parathyroid hormone. Cyclic AMP action is mediated by stimulation of protein kinases which result in the expression of several biologic effects of hormones. Cyclic AMP may:

1. Activate nuclear protein kinases, which results in phosphorylation of nuclear chromatin, with the production of messenger RNA, which then results in protein synthesis.

2. Activate a protein kinase in the cytoplasm, which may then phosphorylate an inactive enzyme, with resultant production of an active enzyme.

3. Activate a protein kinase that phosphorylates microtubule protein, with resultant release of secretory granules.

As an example, hypoglycemia is a release of epinephrine and glucagon, which circulate and then bind to a receptor in the liver to activate adenylate cyclase; this in turn increases the intracellular cyclic AMP concentration, with resultant activation of a protein kinase. This may activate phosphorylase B, which is then converted to phosphorylase A by a protein kinase; this then may produce glycogenolysis, with resultant release of hepatic glucose as a direct response to the initial plasma hypoglycemia. This complicated cascade system produces an amplification effect, so that the interaction of a few molecules will result in a larger biologic response; in this example, much glucose is generated and delivered to the circulation.

Cyclic GMP also may affect cellular processes, usually opposite to the action of cyclic AMP. These two mediators may relate to different hormonal systems. For example, the beta-adrenergic system may stimulate cyclic AMP, while the alpha-adrenergic system may stimulate cyclic GMP.

Some peptide hormones, such as insulin and growth hormone, have no intracellular effect on the generation of cyclic AMP. Rather, the hormone may act directly at the level of the plasma membrane to change transport of substances (such as insulin, thereby affecting the transport of glucose) or may use other second messengers, such as calcium. Further, some cells that respond to hormonal stimulation with the generation of cyclic AMP may also use calcium as a possible third messenger distal to cyclic AMP generation. Calcium exerts its biologic effect by binding to an intracellular protein, calmodulin, which produces the biologic action by activating enzymes such as phosphodiesterase.

Prostaglandins are complex lipids synthesized in cell membranes from fatty acids (such as arachadonic acid). Receptors for prostaglandins are present on cells, so prostaglandins may function either as local hormones or as intracellular messengers.

Peptide hormones may also be internalized to act directly on intracellular receptors, and then may be finally degraded by intracellular lysozymes.

Steroid Hormones

Steroid hormones enter the cell by diffusion or by facilitated transport, where they bind to cytosol receptors, and the complex is then translocated to the nucleus. The potency of the steroid is directly proportional to the avidity with which it binds to the receptor. Each class of steroid hormone binds to a relatively specific receptor. The net effect is the interaction of the hormone-receptor complex with nuclear chromatin, which results in a change in DNA transcription, with resultant new messenger RNA and new protein production by that cell.

Thyroid Hormones

Thyroid hormones cross cell and nuclear membranes to bind to specific nuclear receptors. This results in new messenger RNA with new protein production by that cell. Further, thyroid hormones may bind to mitochondrial receptors, which then may increase oxidative phosphorylation.

Regulation of the Endocrine System

The biologic activity of any given hormone is usually controlled within certain physiological ranges, with ability to develop increased or decreased biologic activity as necessary. Most endocrine disease processes are merely extensions in either direction beyond the normal range of biologic activity.

1. The negative feedback system. The negative feedback system is the most fundamental factor controlling hormone level. The level of the hormone itself, or some product of the hormone's action, modulates the secretion of that same hormone. For example, hypocalcemia results in increased parathyroid hormone secretion. The resultant rise of serum calcium then feeds back to inhibit parathyroid hormone secretion.

2. Regulation of receptor binding. A hormone may alter the concentration of its own cellular receptor by the process of up or down regulation, or by altering the affinity of its own receptor (negative or positive cooperativity).

3. Post receptor regulation. There may be intracellular interaction of one or more hormonal systems with a net effect of summative or inhibitory changes on the level of nuclear messenger RNA generation.

ENDOCRINE PATHOLOGIC STATES

Types of Endocrine Disorders

Disordered endocrine function may result from a net oversecretion of one or more hormones, a net undersecretion of one or more hormones, or the effects of a tissue mass within the gland. Endocrine hypofunction may also be due to tissue (end-organ) resistance to a hormone.

A mass within a gland may be producing hormonal hypersecretion, may impair the gland to induce hormonal hyposecretion, or it may be important due to the increased space it occupies. As an example, with pituitary tumors the position alone of an expanding space-occupying lesion may have clinical implications. Any growth may be benign or malignant, and a malignant mass has further implications regarding local and distant spread.

Clinical Approach to Endocrine Disease

The most difficult aspect of the approach to patients with endocrine disorders is to identify patients with nonspecific presenting features and to distinguish them from a general population. This may be especially difficult in the early phases of the natural history of the disease process. The clinical approach will vary depending on the status of the patient.

In urgent situations, such as with a comatose patient, it may be necessary to look quickly and specifically for certain disorders such as hypoglycemia and to treat on the basis of suspicion. In the more usual situation, clinical data may be obtained in a more systematic fashion. The patient himself acts as a bioassay for the end-organ effects of hormonal secretion. Hypersecretion or hyposecretion of one or more hormones should cause variations in the total somatic effects of that given hormone. Thus, the clinical challenge is to differentiate abnormal features from mere variations of normal. This approach must take into consideration elements of racial variation, such as variations in pigmentation or hair distribution. Taking a careful history is important in order to document the presenting aspects of the clinical problem and to isolate the features suggestive of endocrine dysfunction. Features such as birth weight, growth rate, family history (since many endocrine disorders are familial), and drug history (since drugs may simulate the disease, hide the disease, or alter diagnostic tests), all are of importance.

The physical examination should be performed with the clinician regarding the patient as a bioassay manifesting the biologic effects of an endocrine dis-order. For example, the finding of an obese patient with hypertension may suggest the possible presence of Cushing's syndrome, but if proximal muscle weakness is demonstrated, such a diagnosis is even more likely (as opposed to the more common problem of simple obesity with essential hypertension). Endocrine effects may be clinically assessed by examining the body proportions and stature, the fat distribution, the skin (texture, temperature, thickness, pigmentation, acne, fungal infection), the hair (texture, general and sexual distribution), the eyes, the blood pressure lying and standing, and the breasts, and by directly examining the only two palpable endocrine glands—the gonads and the thyroid.

The clinical assessment may be used to confirm hormonal integrity. For example, features suggesting the presence of a normal ovulatory menstrual cycle demonstrate the integrity of the brain-hypothalamic-pituitary-ovarian axis.

The initial clinical approach, even with laboratory aid, may fail to establish a definite diagnosis, because of the difficulty of separating endocrine dysfunction from variations of normal. Following the natural clinical course for several months or years may be necessary, for example, following a short child for 1 or 2 years to make a diagnosis of constitutional growth delay.

Laboratory Diagnosis of Endocrine Dysfunction

The laboratory is usually capable of providing a definite diagnosis that confirms or invalidates the clinical suspicion. As with all aspects of laboratory medicine, the diagnosis depends on the specificity and sensitivity of any given test, the care in collecting materials presented to the laboratory, and judicious interpretation based on general principles of endocrine physiology.

Principles of Hormonal Assays

1. Radioisotope hormone binding assays require a radiolabeled molecule that specifically binds to the hormone in question. This may be an antibody, endogenous binding protein, or a hormone receptor, which respectively are used for the radioimmunoassay, competitive protein binding assay, or the radioreceptor assay. A highly purified hormone is used as the assay standard, and a method is developed to separate bound from free hormone. Antibodies used are produced by conventional methods, which result in a heterogenous mixture of immunoglobulins with

different affinities and specificities for binding. This may result in variation from one laboratory to another. It may soon be possible to generate a single specific monoclonal immunoglobulin from the cells of antibody-producing tumors, known as hybridomas for use in various specific radioimmunoassays. This would provide more standardized results from different laboratories.

The radioimmunoassay measures the immunologic reactivity of the hormone, which may not be related to its biologic activity. Further, it may measure immunologically similar precursors and metabolic products of that hormone. The radioreceptor assay reveals the biologic activity of the hormone measured, since biologic potency and receptor binding are mechanistically related.

2. Bioassay is used to compare a test substance to that of a reference standard, in terms of a measureable biologic response. It is generally used prior to availability of pure hormone and radioimmunoassay techniques. With some exceptions, it is usually not adequately sensitive to measure hormone levels in most body fluids. Bioassays are still used in the standardization of hormone preparations.

3. Biochemical assay may be used to directly measure hormonal content of body fluids. Usually hormones are extracted and chemically converted to compounds suitable for colorimetric or fluorometric assays. These are used for some steroid measurements.

Principles of Testing

Hormones may be measured in different body fluids, taken as a single sample or collected over a period of time:

1. Blood levels. Basal measurements are adequate when the hormone levels are relatively constant over short periods of time, as is true of thyroid hormone. Single blood levels are not as useful for hormones whose blood levels are quite variable or episodic, for which the integration of several samples is more meaningful. If the hormone in question has rhythmic or diurnal variation, if it varies with the phase of the menstrual cycle, or if it may be altered by changes in plasma binding proteins, then even greater understanding of endocrine physiology must be utilized to interpret the values.

2. Urine hormone measurements. Urine hormone measurements usually provide integrated levels of a hormone over a long period of time, commonly 24 hours. The accuracy of the urine collection should be monitored by measurement of urine creatinine.

Changes in renal function or pharmacologic interference may alter urine hormone measurements. Most hormones excreted in the urine have been metabolically altered to produce a more soluble product for excretion. Some free hormone is filtered and excreted, and may reflect the secretion rate (such as urinary free cortisol).

3. Dynamic testing. The feedback control of hormone function allows more specific diagnosis by dynamic testing of hormonal hyposecretion or hypersecretion respectively, by stimulation and suppression tests. The failure of a gland to increase its secretion of a hormone despite direct and specific stimulation indicates decreased secretory reserve and reflects at least the early phases of hormonal hyposecretion. Generally this is used as definitive proof of glandular failure. Hypersecretion of a hormone usually is associated with abnormalities in suppression, either quantitatively or qualitatively. The failure of a gland to decrease its secretion despite the presence of a normal physiologic signal for suppression, is used to diagnose autonomous hypersecretion. This testing must be taken in clinical context, since, for example, growth hormone secretion is not suppressed in response to glucose administration in acromegaly, but may show a similar failure to be suppressed in patients with anorexia nervosa.

4. Anatomic localization. Anatomic localization of the source of endocrine hypersecretion may be necessary. Sampling of hormone levels from veins in different anatomic sites under radiologic guidance may be necessary to isolate the source of parathyroid, adrenal, ectopic, or metastatic hormone secretion. Various roentgenographic techniques, including contrast procedures and computerized tomography, may be required to suggest or definitively demonstrate a mass within or spreading from an endocrine gland.

THE HYPOTHALAMUS AND PITUITARY GLAND

ANATOMY AND CONTROLLING MECHANISMS

The main part of the hypothalamus forms the floor of the third ventricle and the anterior part of the lateral wall of the third ventricle below and in front of the thalamus. The hypothalamus lies between the optic chiasma anteriorly, and the mamillary bodies posteriorly. Demarcation of its boundaries is impossible, but it measures roughly 1.5×1.3 cm. It contains a number of nerve cell groups referred to as nuclei, and numerous and extensive neural pathways connect these with the rest of the brain.

The hypothalamus is involved in nonendocrine regulatory homeostatic mechanisms in body function, which include hunger, satiety, thirst, sleep, and temperature. The endocrine functions of the hypothalamus are subserved by two systems of neuroendocrine cells:

1. The neurohypophyseal system arises from the supraoptic and paraventricular nuclei and synthesizes antidiuretic hormone and oxytocin along with their carrier proteins (neurophysins). The secretory granules migrate along axons and are stored in the posterior lobe of the pituitary.

2. The tuberohypophyseal system arises from nuclei mainly in the medial basal hypothalamus; these neuroendocrine cells synthesize and release hypothalamic regulatory hormones that control the anterior pituitary. The tuberohypophyseal system is controlled by neural impulses (from the limbic system and other areas of the cerebral cortex and the brain stem, all mediated by neurotransmitters), by hormonal influences (from the anterior pituitary target glands), and by some metabolic fuels (such as glucose, amino acids, and fatty acids).

The pituitary gland weighs about 0.5 grams, but weighs more in pregnancy. It lies within the sella turcica of the sphenoid bone. The upper limits of its dimensions are 16 mm anteroposterior, 12 mm vertical, and 14 mm coronal. It consists of two lobes formed by the fusion of two separate embryologic processes, an evagination of the oral pharynx, which forms the adenohypophysis (anterior lobe), and an outpouching of the floor of the third ventricle, which forms the neurohypophysis (posterior lobe). The superior hypophyseal artery, a branch of the internal carotid artery, services the anterior lobe, while the inferior hypophyseal arteries, branches from the internal carotid artery, serve the posterior lobe. Venous blood from the median eminence region perfuses the pituitary through the hypothalamic-hypophyseal portal system. Blood from both lobes drains into the venous cavernous sinus.

The structures related to the pituitary gland include: anterosuperiorly, the optic chiasm; superiorly, the hypothalamus; inferiorly, the sphenoid sinus, and laterally, the cavernous venous sinuses containing cranial nerves III, IV, VI, and the first branch of V. The adenohypophysis contains several distinct cell types classified according to various staining characteristics.

The hypothalamus is controlled mainly by higher brain centers, in response to endogenous and exogenous stimuli. These then modulate the functions of the hypothalamus through neurosynapses. The hypothalamus is a neurotransducer, whereby neuroimpulses (electrical stimuli) are converted to chemical messages via hormonal secretion. Dopamine, norepinephrine, and serotonin are the main neurotransmitters modulating hypothalamic activity. Many other neurotransmitters have had some support indicating their modulation of hypothalamic function, but these are not as yet clearly delineated. Only dopamine has been shown to act directly on the pituitary to inhibit the release of prolactin. Otherwise, the biogenic amines appear to act at the hypothalamic level.

There appears to be a specific releasing hormone present in the hypothalamus for most pituitary tropic hormones. Both releasing hormones and inhibiting hormones appear to be present to regulate the secretion of prolactin and growth hormone, which do not have a target endocrine gland to act upon and therefore are not subject to the usual target hormone feedback system. Afferent neurons from various parts of the brain modulate neurosecretory neurones within the hypothalamus. These latter neurones contain neurosecretory granules, which are the releasing and inhibiting hormones; these are than discharged into the hypothalamic-pituitary portal circulation and transported to the anterior pituitary to act on specific separate pituitary cells. Gonadatropin releasing hormone (GnRH) stimulates the release of leutinizing hormone (LH) and follicle-stimulating hormone (FSH); thyroid-releasing hormone (TRH) stimulates the release of thyroid-stimulating hormone (TSH), but pharmacologic doses may also stimulate the release of prolactin. Somatostatin inhibits growth hormone release, but in pharmacologic doses has effects on other pituitary and nonpituitary hormonal secretion (Table 13.1).

The level of hypothalamic-pituitary function is subject to normal homeostatic physiologic controlling mechanisms, but this itself may be further influenced by endogenous and exogenous stimuli acting through the brain. This will result in diurnal variations in hormone secretion, biologic rhythms, and even certain influences overcoming the usual control system, such as the effect of stress on adrenocorticotropic hormone (ACTH) and cortisol secretion.

The *opioid peptides* also have a role in hypothalamic-pituitary function. It appears that enkephalins and endorphins are derived from a pituitary hormone, β-lipotropin. The opioid peptides may produce a release of prolactin, growth hormone, ACTH, and antidiuretic hormone (ADH), and decrease of LH, FSH, and TSH. They do not appear to have any direct effect on the pituitary, but rather

Table 13.1 Known Anterior Pituitary Hormones and Their Hypothalamic Regulations

Anterior Pituitary Cell	Anterior Pituitary Hormone	Hypothalamic Regulatory Hormone[a]
Somatotroph	Growth hormone (GH)	Growth hormone release-inhibiting hormone (GHRIH, somatostatin)
		Growth hormone releasing factor (GHRF)
Lactotroph	Prolactin (PRL)	Prolactin-releasing factor (PRF)
		Prolactin-inhibiting factor (PIF)[b]
Gonadotroph	Follicle-stimulating hormone (FSH)	Gonadotropin-releasing hormone (GnRH)
	Luteinizing hormone (LH)	
Corticotroph	Corticotropin (ACTH) β-lipotropin (β-LPH)	Corticotropin-releasing hormone (CRH)
Thyrotroph	Thyrotropin (TSH)	Thyrotropin-releasing hormone (TRH)

[a] "Hormone" nomenclature refers to a substance isolated and definitely identified. "Factor" nomenclature refers to a substance whose presence is strongly suspected but is not identified.
[b] PIF is likely dopamine

may alter hypothalamic-dopamine and serotonin concentrations with subsequent modulation of pituitary hormone secretion.

INDIVIDUAL HORMONES

Adrenocorticotropic Hormone

Adrenocorticotropic hormone (ACTH) is produced as a common preprohormone molecule that contains ACTH, MSH, and β-lipoprotein. It appears that MSH secretion parallels ACTH secretion and may be a major factor in the hyperpigmentation resulting from hypersecretion of ACTH. Corticotropin releasing hormone (CRH) appears to stimulate ACTH release. This then stimulates synthesis of adrenocortical hormones, mainly cortisol, by activating steroidogenesis. The resulting increasing plasma cortisol levels then feedback to inhibit CRH secretion and also directly inhibit the pituitary corticotroph cell from further secretion of ACTH. Adrenal androgens are secreted along with cortisol, but do not have any feedback control mechanism on CRH or the corticotroph cell. Aldosterone secretion will only be transiently increased, even though an intact pituitary is necessary for normal aldosterone secretion. The CRH-ACTH-cortisol pathway has a recognised diurnal rhythm, with peak levels occurring early in the morning just before awakening, and the system may be overridden by "stress" to produce increased ACTH and cortisol secretion.

Thyroid Stimulating Hormone

Thyroid stimulating hormone (TSH) stimulates the thyroid follicular cells to take up iodine and synthesize thyroid hormones, and then to release thyroid hormone. The subsequent increasing levels of serum thyroid hormones then inhibit TSH release by feedback inhibition, mainly at the level of the pituitary. TRH has been identified and synthesized, and is available for provocative testing of TSH reserve. Basal TSH levels are clearly elevated in primary hypothyroidism, and are reduced in hypothyroidism due to central causes.

Luetinizing Hormone

Luetinizing hormone (LH) and follicle-stimulating hormone (FSH) may come from the same cell or possibly also from separate cells within the pituitary. They both appear to be stimulated by hypothalamic gonadotropin-releasing hormone (GnRH) and, to date, a separate FSH releasing factor has yet to be identified. The release of LH and FSH in response to GnRH is modulated by peripheral steroid levels, as well as by proteins (inhibin) released by ovarian follicles, very immature spermatids, or Sertoli cells of the seminiferous tubules. LH acts on the testicular Leydig cell or the ovarian theca cell to produce androgens. FSH acts on Sertoli cells of the testicle with several effects; a major effect is the production of testosterone-binding protein, which results in the increased intratesticular testosterone concentration, which in turn stimulates spermatogenesis. In the ovary, FSH primarily stimulates follicle maturation, but also appears to act on the granulosa cells to aromatize locally produced androgen, thus converting it to estrogen. In the ovarian cycle, midcycle surges of LH stimulate ovarian synthesis of an ovulation-induction protein, with resultant ovulation; LH also causes luteinization of the theca cells with production of the corpus luteum, which primarily secretes progesterone and increasing amounts of estrogen. GnRH has a major function in initiating the pubertal state, by increasing gonadal steroid secretion, and is necessary for the maintenance of normal adult gonadal function. Its artificial production allows it to be used clinically as a stimulation test in order to demonstrate the integrity of the gonadotrophs of the pituitary, but the acute test does not differentiate pituitary from hypothalamic hypoganadotrophic states.

TSH, LH, FSH, and human chorionic gonadotropin (HCG) are all glycoproteins containing alpha and beta subunits. The alpha subunits are all identical, while the beta subunits differ and account for specificity of biologic activity.

Growth Hormone

Growth hormone (GH) secretion and synthesis is controlled by a not yet identified, but probable, growth hormone releasing factor, and is inhibited by somatostatin. Growth hormone levels fluctuate widely throughout the day and night, increasing in response to exercise, hypoglycemia, protein ingestion, stress, and early deep sleep. An increase of plasma glucose will suppress growth hormone levels. Since growth hormone is the most plentiful of the hormones in the anterior pituitary, a reduced growth hormone response to provocative stimuli is an important pituitary reserve test to demonstrate early pituitary hyposecretion. Thyroid hormone is essential for growth hormone synthesis, so growth hormone measurements cannot be interpreted in the presence of hypothyroidism. In prepubertal patients growth hormone responses to provocative testing may be subnormal, and these improve after estrogen treatment.

Growth hormone is not biologically active in vitro in physiologic concentrations. Growth hormone actions occur through the induction of other biologically active substances, the somatomedins. The primary biologic effects of growth hormone include stimulation of protein anabolism, which then results in an increased number and size of cells in most tissues such as cartilage, membranous bone, connective tissue, specific organ tissues, and exocrine gland tissue. These effects are associated with retention of nitrogen, water, chloride, magnesium, and phosphate. Growth hormone antagonizes glucose utilization through an anti-insulin effect at the cell receptor site. Growth hormone indirectly results in stimulation of lipolysis by the activation of hormone sensitive lipases. This results in peripheral fat mobilization and an increase in the level of plasma free fatty acids.

Prolactin

Prolactin (PRL) secretion by pituitary lactotrophs is normally inhibited by the continuous secretion of prolactin inhibiting factor, which likely is dopamine. Prolactin stimulates milk production by mammary glands if they have been suitably prepared for lactation by estrogen and progesterone. Very high levels of estrogens inhibit the action of prolactin levels, as occurs during pregnancy. TRH may be utilized to directly stimulate pituitary prolactin secretion; drugs with antidopaminergic action may be utilized to indirectly stimulate prolactin secretion. These two tests may be used to separate hypopituitarism resulting from primary pituitary disease from that due to suprasellar disease.

Serum levels of prolactin are high in the fetus, and relatively large quantities of prolactin are found in amniotic fluid. The role of prolactin in fetal growth and development is not clear. Maternal serum prolactin levels gradually rise throughout pregnancy, likely due to the increased estrogen stimulation. Suckling or breast manipulation, hypoglycemia, and "stress" will all increase prolactin levels, and there is also a sleep-related increase of prolactin secretion. Estrogens sensitize lactotrophs to produce increased prolactin synthesis, secretion, and lactotroph hyperplasia.

Melanocyte Stimulating Hormone

Melanocyte stimulating hormone (MSH) stimulates tyrosinase enzyme activity, which results in increased melanin production. In humans, melanocytes produce and store melanin as granules in melanosomes. MSH levels in plasma seem to fluctuate in parallel with ACTH levels. The primary control of MSH secretion is not well established.

Antidiuretic Hormone

Antidiuretic hormone (ADH) and oxytocin are produced by the hypothalamic supraoptic and paraventricular nuclei. Both are synthesized in association with another protein, referred to as a neurophysin. These hormones are then transported along with their neurophysin as secretory granules down the neurohypophyseal tract from the hypothalamus to the posterior pituitary. ADH increases the permeability of the collecting renal tubules to water, resulting in increased reabsorption of water. Oxytocin stimulates uterine muscle contraction and breast milk ejection in the female during late pregnancy, or during lactation in response to the suckling stimulus. There is no known function for oxytocin in the male, but the contraction of sperm ducts has been suggested.

The cell bodies of the hypothalamus that secrete ADH form synapses with afferent fibers from other brain areas, and these synapses are predominately cholinergic. The hypothalamic thirst centers are located in adjacent and overlapping areas in relation to the supraoptic and paraventricular nuclei. The thirst center nuclei have nerve fibers extending to the various parts of the brain, primarily to the cerebral cortex to affect behavior in response to thirst. ADH is probably continuously secreted at low basal levels.

The primary stimuli for ADH secretion are an increase of plasma osmolarity in the blood perfusing the hypothalamus (simulating osmoreceptors) and a decrease in extracellular fluid volume, which is a more potent stimulus than the osmotic stimulus. A decrease in blood volume will stimulate ADH release via baroreceptor afferents from the carotid sinus via the ninth cranial nerve, and via the tenth nerve from volume sensors in the left atrium and pulmonary vein. Other less significant stimuli to ADH release include pain, emotional stimuli, nicotine, and drugs such as barbiturates and narcotics. The same stimuli for the release of ADH will also increase the sensation of thirst, which represents a dual homeostatic mechanism to correct hyperosmolarity or volume depletion by decreasing water loss in the urine and by increasing water intake.

HYPOPITUITARISM

Hypopituitarism may involve a variable degree of deficiency of one or more, and occasionally all, pituitary hormones. Isolated deficiency of one hormone may only be one stage of progressive disease, with further deficiencies of other pituitary hormones developing at a later time. Hypopituitarism may result either from decreased hypothalamic control due to an anatomical disorder of the hypothalamus or interference with hypothalamic neurotransmission, or else from primary pituitary disease. The underlying cause may be congenital, such as isolated loss of growth hormone, GnRH, or several hypothalamic releasing hormone deficiencies, or may be acquired at any stage of life.

Clinical Manifestations.

The clinical signs and symptoms of pituitary hormone deficiency are those of deficient function of the target gland or tissue. Occasionally pituitary hormone deficiency may not be clinically recognizable, and may have to be elicited by evaluating pituitary hormone reserve after stimulation testing. The causes of hypopituitarism are shown in Table 13.2.

The clinical manifestations depend on the age of the patient when the disease first occurs, as well as on the extent of the hormonal deficiencies. Most commonly, growth hormone deficiency is first to occur, but this is only clinically evident in the prepubertal child. Such a patient will have short stature, hypoglycemia (which may also occur in adults), and delayed puberty. Loss of TSH with resultant hypothyroidism may contribute to the growth failure, as well as producing its own symptoms. Associated ACTH deficiency may be relatively clinically silent, since in the hypothyroid condition there is less need for cortisol, and the decreased ACTH secretory capacity may thus be relatively asymptomatic. It

Table 13.2 **Causes of Hypopituitarism**

Congenital pituitary aplasia
Idiopathic hypopituitarism (functional loss of hypothalamic releasing factors)
Pituitary or hypothalamic acquired disease
1. Trauma, surgery
2. Vascular—hemorrhage, infarction, sickle cell disease
3. Infection
4. Granulomatous disease, histiocytosis X
5. Autoimmune disease—glandular atrophy, vasculitis
6. Tumors and cysts

should be noted that aldosterone deficiency usually is not clinically evident in states of hypopituitarism. In patients with TSH and/or ACTH deficiency (thyroid or cortisol insufficiency), the clinical picture of associated diabetes insipidus resulting from ADH deficiency may not be clinically evident, but may only occur once thyroid and/or cortisol supplementation is given. Adults with hypopituitarism usually show regression of sexual function, with amenorrhea, decreased libido and sexual activity, and, after some time, regression of the already acquired secondary sexual characteristics. The elderly patient may not demonstrate any of these features and more commonly presents with symptoms related to the underlying cause of the hypopituitarism. Similarly, males show more subtle regression of sexual function and characteristics than females, and are more likely to present with the signs and symptoms due directly to the underlying cause of the hypopituitarism. The more dramatic presentation in adult females is especially evident in the situation of postpartum hemorrhage (Sheehan's syndrome); this disorder may rarely present in the antepartum period, and is not always a result of a severe hypotensive episode. The hyperplastic pituitary gland that results from pregnancy appears to be particularly susceptible to pituitary necrosis, and may result in a dramatic form of hypopituitarism, or may be present in an insidious form only to be discovered several years later.

Most patients with *chronic hypopituitarism* have nonspecific symptoms, such as fatigue, subtle mental changes, or even psychiatric symptoms. The patient usually appears somewhat ill and pale (due to anemia and loss of ACTH-MSH pigmentation). There may be fine wrinkling over the face (usually from growth hormone deficiency) as well as around the mouth and eyes (from loss of the sex steroids), and the classic findings of hypothyroidism may be observed. Relative hypotension with a postural fall in the blood pressure is a frequent finding. The patient may have symptoms resulting from fasting hypoglycemia due to decreased capacity for gluconeogenesis, and is susceptible to hyponatremia. With loss of ACTH, the patient shows regression of hair that is normally stimulated by adrenal androgen, failure of axillary hair to regrow, thinning of the pubic hair, and some decrease in beard growth. The male will have soft testes smaller than the lower limits of normal (less than 4 cm in length) as well as a small prostate. Prolactin insufficiency will only manifest itself by inability to initiate lactation.

The most common *isolated* hormonal deficiency is growth hormone deficiency, which likely is secondary to a congenital disorder in the hypothalamic releasing factor for growth hormone secretion. A child with this condition would have a normal birth weight but a progressive growth retardation, with the stature below the third percentile (Table 13.3). The body proportions would be close to normal, and the patient may have a delayed puberty. There may be greater retardation of appendicular growth compared to axial growth, often delayed dental maturity, small mandible, and increased subcutaneous fat. Assessment of bone age would reveal marked retardation, and radiologic comparison of the diameter of the cranial vault with the mandibular intercondylar diameter would reveal an increase in this ratio. Besides isolated growth hormone deficiency, patients with similar clinical manifestations may have apparently normal growth hormone secretory capacity, but inability to generate the peripheral somatomedin (Laron dwarf) in response to the growth hormone, while other similar persons (for example, pygmies) appear to have normal growth hormone and somatomedin secretion and likely have some not yet defined peripheral resistance to these hormones.

Occasionally patients may present with life-threatening problems. Patients with hypopituitarism of short or long duration may enter a decompensated stage as a result of stresses such as infection, cold exposure, trauma, surgery, or the administration of drugs. They usually manifest disturbed consciousness, weakness, hypotension with a postural fall of the blood pressure, bradycardia, hypoglycemia, and hypothermia, all of which may require urgent therapy and support. The underlying hypopituitarism may be diagnosed if the longstanding historical features are obtained, but otherwise signs of one or more target gland deficiency may have to be detected by bedside examination. Thus, the finding of males with small testes, signs of hypothyroidism without a palpable thyroid gland, and scanty sexual hair, may suffice to alert the physician to this situation. Electrolyte disturbances should be sought for and corrected.

Diabetes insipidus results from partial or complete deficiency of ADH secretion (Table 13.4). To produce symptomatic disease there must be a disorder involving the suprasellar area, since pituitary disease by itself usually is not extensive enough to produce total ADH insufficiency. The polyuria and polydipsia typically seen in ADH deficiency may also be seen in nephrogenic diabetes insipidus (deficiency in the renal response to normal levels of ADH), as well as in psychogenic diabetes insipidus (primary polydipsia with appropriate secondary polyuria). In the patient who is conscious with access to water, the serum osmolarity is usually normal (although it may be below the normal range in primary polydipsia), while the large volume urine shows a low osmolarity. This differentiates it from an osmotic diuresis. Only when the patient has decreased cerebral function or no longer has any access to water does the resultant loss of body water produce dehydration and eventually circulating volume depletion.

Table 13.3   Mechanisms of Short Stature

1. Decreased end-organ response (epiphyseal cartilage)
   A. Cartilage and bone disorders (for example, achondroplasia, osteogenesis imperfecta)
   B. Constitutional growth delay (most common of short stature)
   C. Acquired end-organ resistance (for example, chronic infection, renal failure, cortisol excess)
2. Decreased substrate supply
   A. Hypoxia (cardiopulmonary disease, chronic anemia)
   B. Malnutrition (for example, malabsorption)
   C. Emotional deprivation
3. Decreased hormonal stimulation
   A. Hypothyroidism
   B. Growth hormone deficiency
      Somatomedin deficiency (Laron dwarf)
      Resistance to somatomedin (Pygmy)
4. Excessive sex steroid stimulation—premature closure of epiphyses (for example, congenital adrenal hyperplasia)
5. Familial (short parents)

Table 13.4   Causes of Diabetes Insipidus

1. Physiologic diabetes insipidus (synonym: primary polydipsia)
   A. Psychiatric (synonyms: compulsive water drinking, psychogenic polydipsia)
   B. Nonpsychiatric (for example, tumors or postinflammatory lesions causing chronic stimulation of the thirst center)
2. Hypothalamic diabetes insipidus (synonym: true diabetes insipidus)
   A. Hereditary (probably autosomal dominant)
   B. Acquired
      a. Suprasellar tumors
         i. Primary, for example, carniopharngioma
         ii. Secondary, for example, carcinoma of the breast
      b. Traumatic, for example, car accident
      c. Neurosurgical procedures
      d. Granulomas, for example, sarcoidosis, syphilis, tuberculosis
      e. Infiltrative, for example, histiocytosis X
      f. Infection, for example, basal meningitis
      g. Vascular
3. Nephrogenic diabetes insipidus
   A. Hereditary (may be X-linked recessive)
   B. Acquired
      a. Involvement of renal medulla (for example, hypokalemia, hypercalcemia, sickle cell anemia, medullary cystic disease, amyloidosis, obstructive nephropathy, chronic renal disease, multiple myeloma, Sjögren's syndrome, posttransplantation
      b. Drugs (for example, methoxyflurane, lithium, demeclocycline)

Laboratory Diagnosis

The principle of diagnosis in hypopituitarism is to document end-organ hyposecretion (such as hypothyroidism) without the appropriate rise of the particular pituitary tropic hormone (such as TSH). This contrasts with primary target gland failure, in which the specific pituitary tropic hormone would be elevated. Minimal deficiency of pituitary hormones may not be clinically recognizable, and may have to be elicited by evaluating pituitary tropic reserves. Appropriate stimulation tests are utilized to determine whether or not the pituitary tropic hormone in question can respond to this stimulus; the failure to respond is ascribed to decreased reserve, which leads to the diagnosis of hyposecretion. Pituitary stimulation may be performed by agents that act directly at the level of the pituitary gland, via the systemic circulation, as well by agents that indirectly affect higher centers, with subsequent stimulation of the pituitary to increase hormonal secretion. Some pituitary stimulation tests may be combined and carried out simultaneously, such as TRH stimulation, GnRH administration, and the insulin hypoglycemia test. This will result in an entire evaluation of anterior pituitary function, and also will test the integrity of the hypothalamic pituitary axis. Table 13.5 indicates the more common tests presently used. The combination of these tests may be helpful in the delineation of primary hypothalamic from primary pituitary causes of hypopituitarism. Roentgenologic visualization of the area and other measures may be necessary to identify the underlying cause of the hypopituitarism.

Table 13.5   Common Pituitary Stimulation Tests

Stimuli acting directly at the pituitary gland via systemic vascular supply:
1. Thyrotropin-releasing hormone (TRH)—release TSH and prolactin
2. Gonadotropin Hormone Releasing Hormone (GnRH)—release LH and FSH

Stimuli acting at a functional level above the pituitary gland, requiring intact hypothalamic—pituitary control:
1. Insulin-induced hypoglycemia—release GH, ACTH, PRL
2. L-dopa-release GH
3. Glucagon—release GH
4. Arginine—release GH
5. Dopaminergic antagonists (for example, chlorpromazine, meclopropamide—release PRL)
6. Metyrapone—reduce feedback inhibitory release of ACTH
7. Clomiphene (estrogen-receptor antagonist)—release LH and FSH
8. Water deprivation—induce volume and osmolar release of ADH

Treatment

The treatment of hypopituitarism generally involves administration of target-gland hormones rather than pituitary hormones; unfortunately, pituitary hormones would need to be parenterally administered, since they would be digested if administered orally. However, pituitary hormones without target endocrine glands, such as growth hormone or ADH, must be administered specifically when required. In isolated GnRH deficiency, GnRH may be administered parenterally or intranasally. Treatment of the underlying cause should be specific to the particular entity encountered.

HYPERSECRETION OF PITUITARY HORMONES

The most usual underlying cause of hypersecretion of a pituitary hormone is a functioning pituitary adenoma, which usually produces one, but occasionally more than one, hormone. Less commonly, there may not be an obvious adenoma present; instead, diffuse hyperplasia of a single cell type may be manifest, with resultant hypersecretion of its hormone. It is yet to be established whether pituitary hypersecretory states arise primarily from pituitary disease or secondarily from hypothalamic dysfunction. Both forms of etiologies may occur. Relatively rarely, pituitary hormones or releasing factors such as GnRH may be secreted by nonpituitary endocrine and nonendocrine neoplastic disease (ectopic hormone secretion). Secreting pituitary adenomas usually present with symptoms of hormonal hypersecretion rather than symptoms due to the mass lesion itself, although these also may be present.

Hyperprolactinemia

Clinical Manifestations

The most common pituitary hypersecretory state is hyperprolactinemia, which may have an underlying prolactin secreting adenoma in approximately 90 percent of cases. Because prolactin cell hyperplasia and increased secretion occur directly in response to estrogen stimulation, it has been suggested that pregnancy and birth control pill administration may stimulate such adenomas to become clinically overt, and may possibly act as the cause of such adenomas, but this latter notion is much less accepted. The clinical manifestations of prolactin hypersecretion reflect the central, breast, and gonadal effects of this hormone.

Women may have inappropriate nonpuerperal galactorrhea, and menstrual abnormalities (usually amenorrhea). Their degree of estrogenization may vary, but most commonly they show the clinical signs of hypoestrogenization and usually do not have withdrawal bleeding after administration of a progestational agent. The menstrual abnormalities may result from suppression of the midcycle surge of gonadotropins; at a later stage the disorder appears to produce a picture similar to that noted before puberty, with low amplitude LH secretion and relatively low basal plasma LH levels. The male may manifest decreased libido and possibly decreased potency. Galactorrhoea may occur in the male, but occurs only with very high prolactin levels and relatively large tumors. This may occur without obvious gynecomastia. Oligospermia has been intermittently reported in males with hyperprolactinemia. The decreased libido is not due solely to decreased testosterone secretion, since replacement of testosterone does not restore libido; only when the prolactin is suppressed to normal is libido restored. This suggests the decreased libido is due to a central effect of the hyperprolactinemic state. Osteopenia, especially at an early age, may occur with hyperprolactinemia and the resultant decrease in sex steroids. Decreased bone mass has been documented in such patients.

Laboratory Diagnosis

Increased circulating prolactin levels can be readily demonstrated. Unless tumor mass tissue is visualized by procedures such as CT scanning, there is no diagnostic suppression or stimulation test that completely separates hyperprolactinemia due to pituitary adenomas from hyperprolactinemia due to nonadenomatous causes. The diagnosis then remains presumptive, but is usually correct in patients with documented hyperprolactinemia, the associated clinical and biochemical features, and with suggestive radiologic changes.

Treatment

Since the long-term effects of hyperprolactinemia are benign and the tumors often do not produce local symtoms due to the mass effects, the treatment should be equally innocuous. The two major forms of therapy currently are prolactin suppression with dopaminergic agonists (the most common being bromocriptine) or transsphenoidal microsurgery with resection of the prolactin secreting pituitary adenoma. If the serum prolactin is normalized and the patient does not have any hypopituitarism prior to or after surgery, usually the entire symptom complex reverts to normal. Besides having an effect on normalizing the serum prolactin, dopaminergic agonists have been shown to have an antitumor effect, with observed reduction in adenoma size, especially evident with macroadenomas.

Growth Hormone Excess

Clinical Manifestations

Acromegaly in adults and gigantism in prepubertal children result from hypersecretion of growth hormone, usually due to a hormone secreting pituitary adenoma. About one third of these tumors also secrete excess prolactin (mammosomatotrophic tumor), and appear to be mixed pituitary adenomas. The features of acromegaly are insidious, and often are not recognized by those in frequent contact with the patient. The changes are those of normal growth hormone action, present in an excessive amount. The most frequent symptom due directly to the tumor mass is headache. Both long-term cosmetic and metabolic abnormalities occur, and the latter may decrease longevity. There may be enlargement of certain parts of the skeleton, as well as of soft tissue in the parenchyma of organs. Because all growth-hormone–sensitive areas increase their responsiveness, some obvious physical findings appear. The skin becomes thickened due to the anabolic effect of growth hormone when compared with a normal person of similar age and sex. Other effects of growth hormone on the skin appendages result in oiliness, hypertrichosis, and increased sweating and body odor. The skull shows thickening of bony ridges; the mandible grows and changes the bite, with undercutting and spreading of the lower teeth. Laryngeal cartilages enlarge and the vocal cords thicken, with resultant deepening of the voice. Other soft-tissue enlargement may result in carpal tunnel symptoms resulting from median nerve compression. Arthralgia and osteoarthritis may occur from changes in joint bearing, as well as from synovial thickening and articular cartilage hypertrophy. These skeletal abnormalities are not reversible. There may be enlargement of the organs, most obviously of the salivary and thyroid glands, and of the liver. Cardiomegaly may occur, and the resultant hypertrophy and fragmentation of muscle fibers may result in a cardiomyopathy, eventually leading to cardiac decompensation. This may be aggravated by associated hypertension. There may be enhanced atherogenesis due to this hypertension, and possibly due to the increased lipolysis resulting from changes in lipid metabolism. Other metabolic changes include diabetes mellitus due to antagonism of insulin receptors by the growth hormone hypersecretion. Hypercalciuria may result in renal calculi. The hypercalciuria may be due to the increased glomerular filtration rate. The cosmetic changes, mostly irreversible, add another element of long-term morbidity.

Laboratory Diagnosis

Although the diagnosis is based on biochemical criteria, there may be radiologic features, such as increased skin thickness and increased heel pad thickness observed by soft-tissue techniques. Measurement of hand volume (usually by measuring the water displaced by hand immersion) is also useful to document and follow the course of the acromegaly. Visual-field changes due to the underlying pituitary adenoma may be present and the pituitary mass may be suspected from plain films of the skull or CT imaging.

The biochemical diagnosis depends on demonstration of abnormal growth hormone secretion. Because growth hormone is released in pulsatile bursts, as well in response to "stress," measurement of a single basal level is of little value. The principle applied is to demonstrate the failure of normal suppression. Normal subjects given oral glucose show appropriate suppression of the plasma growth hormone levels. In patients with gigantism or acromegaly, there is a failure to suppress their growth hormone to similar levels, and there may even be a paradoxical elevation of growth hormone levels in response to oral glucose administration.

Treatment

Treatment is directed toward ablative or medical suppression of the hypersecreting growth hormone cells. Ablative forms of therapy are surgery and/or various forms of irradiation. Because the natural history of acromegaly is associated with substantial morbidity and mortality, such ablative therapy is indicated usually as the primary form of therapy. Transphenoidal removal of the pituitary adenoma is often attended by a biochemical cure or significant improvement, and is considered the treatment of choice. Some acromegalics demonstrate a paradoxical suppression of growth hormone secretion in response to dopaminergic agents, which appear to act directly at the abnormal growth hormone pituitary cells. Such patients may show a biochemical and clinical improvement in response to continuous administration of such drugs, but their role in the overall management of acromegaly is not yet determined.

Excess ACTH Production

Clinical Manifestations

Cushing's disease due to ACTH secreting pituitary adenoma is the third most common pituitary hypersecretory state. As with the previously discussed tumors, the underlying cause is usually a corticotroph cell adenoma, but the majority do not display radiologic abnormalities. These patients present with the signs and symptoms of Cushing's disease, as well as hyperpigmentation in the Addisonian distribution within the skin and mucous membranes. These features will be described in the section dealing with the adrenal glands. The major features of Cushing's disease include reversible cosmetic changes, and increased morbidity and mortality due to metabolic and cardiovascular disease. Although these pituitary adenomas are usually quite small, occasionally they can become large and locally invasive and rarely have distant spread. Growth of these adenomas after bilateral adrenalectomy (Nelson's syndrome) is associated with marked pigmentation and may possibly be retarded by prior pituitary irradiation.

Laboratory Diagnosis

The principle of diagnosis is again to demonstrate the failure of normal suppression of ACTH and cortisol secretion. Screening tests are useful; an elevated 24-hour urinary excretion of cortisol (or its metabolites) failure to suppress with an overnight dexamethasone suppression test, indicate the possible presence of Cushing's disease. The failure to suppress serum and urine cortisol or metabolite secretion after 2 mg/24 hours of dexamethasone administered for 48 hours, with normal suppression in response to 8 mg/24 hours of dexamethasone indicates the likely presence of Cushing's disease. This test requires intact hepatic and renal function, the absence of drugs that change dexamethasone metabolism (such as dilantin), and the presence of normal dexamethasone pharmacokinetics.

Treatment

The treatment of a corticotrophic cell adenoma may be ablative therapy (surgery or irradiation) directed toward the pituitary, or surgical therapy directed toward the adrenals (adrenalectomy). The high incidence of an underlying corticotroph cell adenoma indicates that pituitary microsurgery is the preferred form of ablative therapy, in patients fit for this procedure. Medical therapy may be directed toward the adrenal glands by either adrenolytic drugs (o,p-DDD), or reversible antagonists against enzymes of steroidogenesis (aminoglutethimide or metyrapone); these may be used in patients not fit for ablative therapy or in patients who have had irradiation, but who still require medical therapy to alleviate the biochemical and clinical features of Cushing's disease while waiting for the beneficial effects of irradiation to occur. Recent application of neurophysiologic principles has been utilized with the drug cyproheptadine, which has both antiserotonic and anticholinergic actions, since both of these neurotransmitters have been implicated in the normal hypothalamic control of ACTH release. Although the role of cyproheptadine is still not clear, it appears that a third of patients with Cushing's disease show a clinical and biochemical normalization in response to cyproheptadine administration. Because the drug effects are not permanent, its role may be that of an adjunct to ablative therapy or a primary therapy in patients unfit for ablative therapy.

Excess Production of Other Pituitary Hormones

Very rarely pituitary tumors may be hypersecreting glycoproteins such as TSH, LH, or FSH. These may occur in situations of long standing target gland hypofunction, with secondary tropic cell hyperplasia, finally resulting in adenoma formation. These adenomas also may arise de novo and produce actual hyperfunction in the target glands. Approximately 30 patients with hyperthyroidism secondary to pituitary TSH excess have now been reported. About 10 percent of pituitary tumors are undifferentiated cell adenomas with apparent hormone secretion and granule formation, but no obvious clinical effects. Recently, some of these adenomas have been found to secrete alpha subunits, the protein chain common to the pituitary glycoprotein hormones. No clinical signs are produced, but this alpha subunit may function as a tumor marker.

Pituitary adenomas may be associated with adenoma or hyperplasia in other endocrine glands, as part of the familial multiple endocrine neoplasia (MEN) syndrome. Most frequently associated problems are hyperparathyroidism and insulinoma, or occasionally syndromes associated with hypersecretion of gastrin.

MASS: LOCAL EFFECTS OF PITUITARY ADENOMAS

Pituitary tumors rarely metastasize, but are potentially fatal by nature of their position, since the confined space may give rise to compression of surrounding structures. In addition to the possibility that they may be hypersecreting one or more hormones, such tumors may also impair normal pituitary function and produce partial or more widespread hypopituitarism. The local consequences are due to interference with the function of adjacent structures. Headache may arise from compression of sensitive structures such as the dura. Visual-field defects may occur, secondary to optic chiasm compression. Table 13.6 indicates the local effects, as well as the diagnostic approach. Changes on routine skull roentgenograms or even tomography may not be entirely diagnostic, since similar changes may occur on the basis of normal variations, or secondary to the empty sella syndrome, with changes in the pituitary fossa resulting from increased transmitted pressure. Only if the actual mass is demonstrated by methods such

Table 13.6 **Clinical Features of Pituitary Tumors**

Clinical Presentation
   Mass
      Headache
      Superior: visual field cuts, central scotoma, hypothalamic symptoms, increased intracranial pressure
      Inferior: CSF rhinorrhea, spenoid sinus mass
      Lateral: Cranial nerves III, IV, VI, V_I, dysfunction
   Hypersecretion
      Acromegaly, Cushing's, galactorrhea-amenorrhea/decreased libido
      Associated endocrine gland hyperfunction (MEN)
   Hyposecretion
      One or more deficiencies in end organ function (thyroid, adrenal, gonadal), short stature, diabetes insipidus
Diagnostic Approach
   Mass
      Skull x-rays/sellar tomograms
      Visual field examination
      CT scan, contrast studies
   Hypersecretion
      Glucose suppression for acromegaly
      Dexamethasone suppression for Cushing's disease
      Basal serum prolactin
      Screen for MEN (serum calcium, fasting serum glucose)
   Hyposecretion
      Basal pituitary hormonal levels along with basal target gland hormone levels
      Direct stimulation with GnRH, TRH
      Indirect stimulation with hypoglycemia, arginine, L-dopa, Clomiphene, metyrapone

as CT scanning or contrast studies, is the diagnosis of a pituitary mass lesion definitive.

Secreting pituitary tumors usually present with symptoms due to the hypersecretory state. The non-secreting pituitary adenomas present with an incidental finding on routine skull roentgenograms or else by their mass effects. Females tend to present earlier due to the onset of amenorrhea, while males and elderly patients tend to present later in the natural history of these adenomas (that is, with growth), usually with local neurological changes such as visual-field abnormalities.

Other tumors such as craniopharyngiomas or even carotid aneurysms may produce similar mass effects. Craniopharyngiomas develop from remnants of Rathke's pouch, and present with local mass symptoms such as visual-field changes and diabetes insipidus, usually in children. They are slow growing and frequently calcified. They may be cystic or solid.

Patients may be asymptomatic but have a roentgenologic abnormality in the sella turcica; the examination may have been requested because the patient had nonspecific headaches. The abnormal sellar shape may not be due to an intrasellar growth, but rather to the *empty sella syndrome*. This is especially common in obese hypertensive women. It appears to be due to a defect in the diaphragma sella (the dura above the sella), which allows herniation of the subarachnoid space, and the local increased pressure is transmitted to the sella with resultant alteration in the bony shape. Definitive diagnosis may require pneumoencephalography, which demonstrates air entering the sella, but more recent advances in CT scanning, especially with coronal cuts, allow this diagnosis to be made more readily. Usually the patients have normal pituitary function if stimulatory testing is performed.

The natural history of adenomas is usually one of slow growth, and unless there are already local effects, hypersecretion, or hyposecretion, they may be followed clinically without intervention. One potential dramatic complication, although quite rare, is acute massive hemorrhage or infarction within the pituitary tumor (*pituitary apoplexy*). Such patients complain of a sudden, severe headache in the retroorbital area, which is followed by alteration in consciousness and symptoms of visual field defects or cranial nerve palsy. Previous irradiation may make patients more susceptible to this rare acute complication. It may resolve with conservative management or may produce hypopituitarism, but may also require acute surgical decompression. Such patients must be given glucocorticoids throughout the acute episode, because of the hypopituitarism and the stress of the situation. Pituitary adenomas may be treated with ablative therapy by means of surgery or radiation, or may be followed without intervention, and treatment decisions may be deferred. Treatment must be suited to the individual patient. The decrease in tumor size seen in many prolactin adenomas and some acromegalics with bromocriptine now permits medical treatment for the mass problem of some pituitary adenomas.

DISEASES OF THE THYROID GLAND

PHYSIOLOGY, BIOCHEMISTRY, AND CLINICAL BIOCHEMISTRY

The thyroid gland begins embryologically as a midline descending evagination of the pharyngeal endoderm. The path of descent begins at an area that later becomes the junction of the posterior third and anterior two thirds of the tongue. Remnants of the thyroid, or thyroglossal duct primordia, along the path of descent, may form ectopic thyroid tissue or cysts. The thyroid lobes are connected by an isthmus that wraps around the front of the trachea below the cricoid cartilage. Two pairs of parathyroid glands and the recurrent laryngeal nerves lie behind and medial to the lateral lobes of the thyroid. The gland is easily palpable, and is proportionately larger in women than in men. The fascia enclosing the thyroid gland (the pretracheal fascia) is attached above to the thyroid cartilage, with the result that the thyroid moves upon swallowing. The primary functional unit of the thyroid gland is the follicle, which is lined by epithelial cells that accumulate iodine from the circulation. After iodide is concentrated it is oxidized and incorporated into tyrosyl residues to form monoiodotyrosine and diiodotyrosine, which are coupled to form thyroxine (T4) and triiodothyronine (T3). These active hormones are stored in peptide linkage to thyroglobulin. Thyroid stimulating hormone (TSH) promotes each of these steps in thyroid hormone synthesis and the activation of lysosome activity required to release the stored thyroxine into the circulation. Each of these biosynthetic steps may be inhibited by pharmacologic agents. The trapping of iodine (uptake) is inhibited by perchlorate and thiocyanate; the organification of iodine and the coupling steps are inhibited by thionamide drugs (propylthiouracil and methimazole); and the release of stored thyroid hormone into the circulation may be inhibited by large doses of stable iodide and by lithium (Fig. 13.1).

Thyroid hormones produce their biologic effect by changing metabolic activity and protein synthesis in target tissues. Some of these effects may be related to the direct binding of T3 and T4 to nuclear receptors within the cells. The rate of aerobic metabolism in mitochondria is enhanced. Further, protein synthesis may be induced by increasing the activity of the nuclear, DNA-dependent, RNA-polymerase. There appears to be an enhanced sensitivity to the peripheral action of catecholamines, possibly by thyroid hormone either altering the number of cellular receptors or the intracellular response to catecholamine-receptor interaction. The effects on metabolic processes are varied. Thyroid hormones may directly stimulate protein synthesis and may synergistically enhance the action of growth hormone as well; thyroid hormones may stimulate an increase in lipid and cholesterol turnover, and thereby affect all aspects of carbohydrate metabolism (modified by catecholamines and insulin action).

Thyroid hormones are transported in the circulation mainly bound to plasma proteins, the most important of which is thyroxine binding globulin (TBG). Less than 0.05 percent of the total circulating thyroxine (T4) is non-protein bound ("free") and 0.5 percent of triiodothyronine (T3) is free. The bound fraction is biologically inert and acts as a reservoir to help regulate and maintain normal plasma levels of free thyroid hormone. The free fraction is biologically active and binds to cell receptor binding proteins to initiate thyroid-induced metabolic activity. Circulating T4 has a half-life of about 7 days, and T3 has a half-life of 1.5 to 2 days. T3 has greater biologic activity than T4, and it now appears that T4 is deiodinated in the peripheral tissues to T3 to produce most of its biologic effects. The hypothalamic-pituitary-thyroid axis constitutes a homeostatic regulator of thyroid hormone secretion which tends to maintain a constant level of free thyroid hormone through the mechanism of feedback control. The feedback control of thyroid hormone is thought to be exerted primarily at the level of the pituitary gland. TSH then controls the rates of all steps of activity within the thyroid gland.

The serum concentrations of T4, and to a lesser extent T3, may be altered by changes in the serum concentration of TBG. An example would be the increase in TBG seen with estrogens, such as during a pregnancy or during birth control pill administration. This would then increase the total serum T4 concentration, but the free fraction of T4 would be maintained within homeostatic ranges. In some illnesses there may be an alteration in the affinity of TBG-T4 interaction, and in some pathologic states, such as those associated with starvation, there may be a change in the peripheral metabolism whereby there is an inhibition of the peripheral conversion of

T4 to T3, or an enhancement of the alternative pathway so that T4 is converted to reverse T3, a biologically inactive form.

The thyroid function tests may assess glandular function directly or indirectly, but due to inherent problems, they require one or more associated tests for appropriate interpretation. The usual measurement of plasma hormones (plasma T4 or T3) requires concomitant assessment of the plasma binding of these hormones. Thus, measurement of total serum thyroxine is usually accompanied by the T3 resin uptake, an indirect estimate of the plasma TBG. A combination of these two tests, the free thyroxine index, attempts to compensate for any changes in TBG affecting the total thyroxine level. Nevertheless, even the free thyroxine index must be interpreted cautiously in some patients with severe nonthyroidal illness. Another test of basal thyroid function is the radioiodine uptake, whereby a radioactive iodide tracer is administered and the percentage uptake is measured and compared with that in normal patients. This test reflects the uptake and, therefore, presumably the hormonogenesis within the thyroid gland, but is altered in an individual patient by that patient's total body iodine pool.

The integrity of the feedback control of the thyroid gland may also be tested. In primary hypothyroidism, the plasma TSH is elevated due to pituitary TSH secretion. This is the most sensitive indicator of the primary hypothyroid state. However, the plasma TSH concentration cannot be used to identify a hyperthyroid patient since some normal persons have low or undetectable levels of plasma TSH.

One provocative test entails measuring the TSH response to an injection of TRH. In hypothyroid patients without an elevation of TSH, their response to TRH may be useful in determining whether there is underlying pituitary disease (with no release of TSH) or possibly hypothalamic disease. This latter may be a result of severe nonthyroidal illness, and must be interpreted in the proper clinical context. The most useful application of the TRH test is in the diagnosis of borderline hyperthyroidism or even "euthyroid-Graves' disease." With autonomous thyroid function within the normal or barely elevated ranges, there is still feedback inhibition of TSH secretion, which is continued despite an injection of TRH. Thus, the failure to observe a release of TSH in response to TRH may indicate autonomous thyroid function. The TRH test is not useful in elderly patients, in whom normally there is a somewhat blunted TSH response to TRH stimulation.

The thyroid suppression test (using daily doses of T3 for 10 days) also may be used to help delineate borderline hyperthyroid function, although this is now being largely replaced by the TRH test. Failure to decrease the radioiodine uptake after administration of thyroxine, or to see a decrease in serum T4 values after administration of triiodothyronine, all support autonomous disease of the thyroid gland.

Immunologic tests in routine laboratories are usually restricted to the measurement of antibodies to thyroidal antigens (thyroglobulin and microsomes). The measurement of these antibodies is used to reflect the presence of autoimmune thyroiditis (Hashimoto's thyroiditis). Although still a research tool, measurement of thyroid-stimulating immunoglobulins may be used to give a definitive diagnosis of Graves' disease.

A variety of scintiscan techniques delineate the anatomy of the thyroid and differentiate functional from nonfunctional tissue. Ultrasound imaging is utilized to differentiate cystic from solid thyroid enlargements. On the basis of these procedures fine needle biopsy may be used to obtain diagnostic cells in solid masses, and a larger needle aspiration may be utilized to treat cysts.

HYPERTHYROIDISM (THYROTOXICOSIS)

Increased thyroid hormone may result from several different pathologic processes. The clinical features of hyperthyroidism reflect the two basic effects of thyroid hormone on peripheral tissues:

1. The increased thyroid-induced metabolic activity
2. Enhanced sensitivity of peripheral tissues to the actions of catecholamines.

Circulatory demands may increase due to the hypermetabolism and the need to dissipate the excessive heat produced. This is achieved by dilatation of peripheral vascular beds, and increased cardiac output with increases in both stroke volume and heart rate. Thyroid hormone further may affect the heart by direct action as well as by potentiating catecholamine sensitivity. This may produce sinus tachycardia (and may deteriorate into atrial fibrillation), systolic flow murmurs, and a prominent and forceful apex impulse. Both coronary blood flow and myocardial oxygen consumption increase, but efficiency of the myocardium may decrease. The patient may be aware of rapid or forceful heart beating, and angina pectoris may be aggravated. The cardiovascular symptoms may include arrhythmias and congestive heart failure in older persons or in patients with preexisting cardiac disease.

The skin is warm and moist due to cutaneous vasodilatation and sweating. The patient will feel uncomfortably warm at normal room temperatures, and may also experience increased thirst due to water loss from sweating. Skeletal muscle weakness and atrophy may occur due to impaired ability of the thyrotoxic muscle to phosphorylate creatine, as well as to the catabolic metabolism of body protein with negative nitrogen balance. The patient will notice muscle weakness, most notably in the proximal distribution. Ventilation may increase out of proportion to the increase in oxygen demands. Generalized weakness of respiratory muscles has been described. The patient may notice shortness of breath on exertion. Food intake is increased due to increased caloric requirements, but weight loss is common. The patient may notice hunger, although anorexia may predominate in severe forms of thyrotoxicosis. There may be an increased number of bowel movements due to smooth muscle catecholamine effects as well as increased food intake. Hyperkinesia (quick and jerky movements) and fine tremor of the hand may be present as a reflection of the increased sensitivity to catecholamines. Central nervous system effects may appear as emotional lability or even overt psychic disturbances. Chronic caloric insufficiency results in a net catabolism of body protein, which may result in muscular weakness and contribute to osteoporosis. This latter feature may also be exaggerated by the increased calcium excretion in the urine. There may be a change in the overall secretion and metabolism of steroids, with an increased ratio of serum estrogen to testosterone, which may be responsible for the findings of gynecomastia in some males.

Other clinical features may be more related to the actual etiology of the hyperthyroidism. In patients with autoimmune disease (Graves' disease), there may be associated vitiligo, and concomitant organ-specific autoimmune endocrine disorders or other autoimmune diseases such as myasthenia gravis. Associated ophthalmopathy and infiltrative dermopathy may coexist.

To some degree, the thyroid gland may reflect the underlying cause. Generalized enlargement, even asymmetrical, with a rubbery nature and associated bruit is typically seen with Graves' disease. A multinodular goiter is easily identifiable, and an autonomous single adenoma is palpable while the remaining thyroid tissue is very difficult to palpate. Subacute thyroiditis is usually associated with a painful, tender thyroid enlargement, but this is not always the case. In patients ingesting thyroid hormones (thyrotoxicosis factitia), the entire thyroid gland should be barely palpable, if at all. Diffuse thyroid enlargement is found in the rare forms of hyperthyroidism due to excess pituitary TSH or due to large amounts of HCG (choriocarcinoma or hydatidiform mole).

The thyroid eye signs may be nonspecific, merely reflecting the increased thyroid hormone or specific to the autoimmune process associated with Graves' disease. Hyperthyroidism, by potentiation of the sympathetic tone, will produce lid retraction with increased sclera visible above the iris, which results in the nonspecific stare. The same process results in the finding of "lid lag." The ophthalmopathy associated with Graves' disease is associated with retroorbital inflammation with resultant forward protrusion of the globe (proptosis), and inflammation within the extraocular muscles. This may be assymetrical or even unilateral. The extrocular muscle weakness may cause diplopia, and is evident by direct examination of the extraocular movements. Other signs associated with retroorbital inflammation are increased tearing, chemosis, and conjunctivitis. When such ocular symptoms are present with obvious hyperthyroidism, then the underlying cause of this oculopathy is evident. If evidence of associated thyroid disease is not present, then this cause of oculopathy can be inferred by detecting the presence of autonomous thyroid dysfunction (abnormal TRH release of TSH, abnormal thyroid suppression test), or by utilizing radiologic procedures such as CT scanning or sonography to visualize the presence of the enlarged extraocular muscles. The latter feature is very suggestive of Graves' ophthalmopathy, but not entirely diagnostic, since pseudotumor may show similar changes.

Elderly patients with thyrotoxicosis may not show typical clinical features. The ocular signs may not be present, or only the signs of lid retraction may be evident. These patients may have associated anorexia, and may present with unexplained weight loss or weakness. They frequently present with subtle features, with evidence of cardiac decompensation, arrhythmias, or with gradual inanition suggestive of the presence of an occult neoplasm.

The infiltrative dermopathy that is associated with Graves' disease is an uncommon feature. It usually occurs over the anterior lower legs and is referred to as pretibial myxedema. The skin is thickened and shiny and difficult to squeeze or raise. There may be some local discomfort.

Causes of Hyperthyroidism

The various causes of hyperthyroidism are noted in Table 13.7.

Graves' Disease

Graves' disease appears to be related to a primary abnormality within the immune system; the presence of a thyroid-stimulating antibody is detectable in most cases, which interacts with the TSH receptor on the thyroid follicular cell to then stimulate uncontrolled glandular hyperactivity. There is a genetic predisposition which is in linkage disequilibrium with HLA antigen DW3. This genetic abnormality is expressed as a specific disorder in immunoregulation; this in turn allows self-reactive lymphocytes (arising by random mutation during life) to survive, instead of being normally suppressed. This activates the immune response directed toward the thyroid antigen and results in production of a variety of immunoglobulins, some of which interact with the TSH receptor, causing thyroid overactivity. The associated ophthalmopathy appears to represent a very closely related, but separate autoimmune disease. Patients with Graves' ophthalmopathy appear to have a circulating factor which produces exophthalmos, by inducing deposition of retroorbital mucopolysaccharides. There also may be a more specific immune response directed toward extraocular muscle antigens. The course of the ophthalmopathy may not reflect the thyroid disease. The immunologic cause of the associated dermopathy is not clear.

The diagnosis of Graves' disease depends on the typical clinical features and the rubbery firm goiter. When the associated oculopathy is present, the diagnosis is certain. The serum T4 and T3 are elevated, and the radioiodine uptake is usually above the normal range. If the confirmatory biochemical tests are borderline, the TRH test or the thyroid suppression test may be necessary.

Table 13.7 **Causes of Hyperthyroidism (in Order of Frequency)**[a]

1. Graves' Disease
2. Nodular Goiter
   A. Multinodular
   B. Autonomous adenoma
3. Thyroiditis
   A. Chronic lymphocytic (Hashimoto's)
   B. Subacute thyroiditis
      Painful
      Painless
   C. Miscellaneous—radiation, suppurative and others
4. Hyperthyroidism due to choriocarcinoma or hydaditiform mole (excessive HCG)
5. Excessive thyroid hormone ingestion
6. Administration of exogenous iodide (Jod-Basedow)
7. Pituitary TSH secreting tumor
8. Thyroid carcinoma
9. Struma ovarii

[a] Only 1–3 are common.

Remissions in Graves' disease may occur spontaneously, but, if untreated, the disease process generally deteriorates. It is therefore necessary to treat the hyperfunctioning gland with either antithyroid drugs or with ablation of thyroid tissue with either a therapeutic dose of radioiodine or with surgery (Fig. 13.1).

The treatment of Graves' disease during pregnancy involves special principles designed to avoid fetal injury or wastage. Radioiodine is contraindicated, and surgery carries a risk of premature labor. Despite the fact that antithyroid drugs cross the placenta, the treatment of choice is to use relatively small dosages of antithyroid drugs to bring the hyperthyroid state into control (particularly in the last trimester), thus minimizing the amount of drug passed to the fetus. Goiter due to the thionamides thus can be avoided. Because the thyroid-stimulating immunoglobulins cross the placenta the newborn may be born with hyperthyroidism, but this spontaneously reverts to normal after several weeks. Treatment of the Graves' ophthalmopathy may require simple symptomatic measures (elevation of the head of the bed during sleep, methylcellulose drops), or, rarely, glucocorticoid therapy to decrease inflammation and to treat diplopia if detected early. Severe exophthalmos may require surgical orbital decompression.

Multinodular Toxic Goiter

Multinodular toxic goiter is usually an end result of a longstanding nontoxic goiter. Preexisting nodular goiters, initially TSH dependent, will ultimately undergo metaplasia, become autonomous, and finally develop hyperthyroid manifestations. If the multinodularity is not evident by palpation of the thyroid gland, it may be more evident on the thyroid scintiscan. Because these patients are usually older, and because the disorder is slow and subtle in development, cardiovascular symptoms may predominate. The treatment is the same as for the diffuse toxic goiter of Graves' disease.

Toxic Adenoma

Toxic adenomas consist of a single hyperfunctioning benign autonomous nodule. This appropriately suppresses the TSH and remaining otherwise normal thyroid tissue; the presence of a palpable nodule, with the remaining gland being impalpable, represents the typical clinical presentation in these hyperthyroid patients. A scintiscan confirms that the palpable nodule is hyperfunctioning and that the remaining gland is virtually nonfunctioning. If, however, the patient is injected with TSH, repeat scintiscanning demonstrates return of function in the previously suppressed part of the gland. The three choices of therapy that may be utilized for this clinical situation are the same as those noted above for Graves' disease.

Thyroiditis

Thyroiditis is the descriptive term for a number of inflammatory processes within the thyroid gland, resulting from various causes. Thyroiditis may arise from an autoimmune disorder (Hashimoto's thyroiditis), a viral infection, a bacterial infection (acute suppurative), or may result from chronic inflammation (sarcoidosis, amyloidosis). The most important form, subacute thyroiditis which has a hyperthyroid phase, may be clinically difficult to differentiate from Graves' disease. Subacute thyroiditis may present with pain in the thyroid area, often radiating up to the angle of the jaws towards the ears; the thyroid gland on palpation is usually quite tender. Another variation is silent thyroiditis, in which there is no localized pain and the gland is not tender. Both forms of this disorder are self-limited, with return to normal glandular function over a few months. The patient may have nonspecific systemic symptoms such as fever (especially in the acute cases), fatigue, and malaise. The erythrocyte sedimentation rate is usually elevated in the painful cases, but is normal or just above normal in the painless group. Because the inflammatory state results in release of thyroid hormone, the hyperthyroid state leads to feedback inhibition of the pituitary and suppression of uptake of iodine by the gland. Moreover, the follicular cells are disrupted, another reason for the low uptake. Thus, in hyperthyroid patients with an enlarged thyroid gland and an extremely low radioiodine uptake, the diagnosis is likely subacute thyroiditis. (The test results are similar in factitious hyperthyroidism and Jod-Basedow disease secondary to excess iodine administration.) Because the disease is self-limited, only symptomatic therapy is necessary. Beta-adrenergic blockers may alleviate symptoms of hyperthyroidism, and aspirin may help limit the pain in milder forms of thyroiditis. In several cases, glucocorticoid therapy (approximately 40 mg. of prednisone per day) will be required. In the recovery phase the patient may pass through a temporary hypothyroid stage before returning to normal. A certain percentage of these patients may show a relapse after months or years.

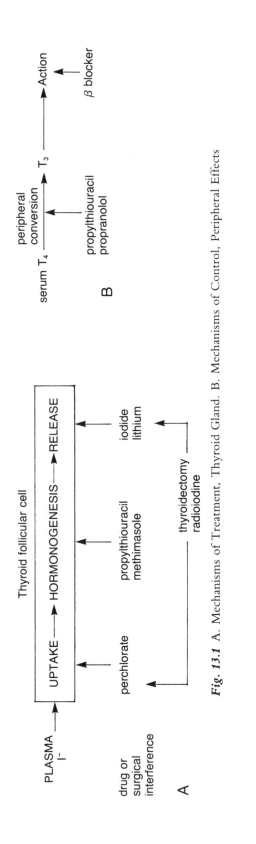

Fig. 13.1 A. Mechanisms of Treatment, Thyroid Gland. B. Mechanisms of Control, Peripheral Effects

Variant Expressions of Hyperthyroidism

Some patients in whom hyperthyroidism is clinically suspected may not demonstrate an elevated serum T4, and therefore an isolated elevation of T3 (T3 toxicosis) should be sought. In this situation T3 may be the predominant thyroid hormone secreted.

Thyroid storm is a rare clinical situation in which very severe hyperthyroidism is manifested as a life-threatening emergency, usually with organ failure. It generally occurs when there has been superimposed medical or surgical stress on previously unrecognized hyperthyroidism. The hyperthyroid state is more pronounced, and there are additional features; these include fever (to the point of extreme hyperpyrexia), possibly cardiac decompensation with hypotension, and a deterioration in cerebration usually presenting with delirium and coma. Therapy is directed toward treating the hyperpyrexia with a cooling blanket, returning the cardiovascular status toward normal, correcting circulating fluid volume deficiency, and treating the hyperthyroidism with high doses of antithyroid drugs (usually propylthiouracil and stable iodide). To alleviate the cardiovascular decompensation, propranolol and, occasionally, digitalis may be necessary. High doses of glucocorticoids have traditionally been given initially to meet the possibility of concomitant adrenal hypofunction. Whether or not this is necessary, glucocorticoids, propranolol, and propylthiouracil have all been demonstrated to have peripheral actions in decreasing the conversion of T4 to T3, which may help alleviate the severe hyperthyroid state.

DECREASED THYROID FUNCTION (HYPOTHYROIDISM)

Hypothyroidism results from decreased thyroid hormones, while myxedema refers to the more severe situation in which there is also obvious deposition of mucopolysaccharides in the skin and other tissues. Although the severity of the hypothyroid state is more marked as age progresses, the effects of hypothyroidism on various organs may be detected at any age. The basal cardiac output is decreased due to reduction in the heart rate and stroke volume. The decrease in cutaneous circulation is responsible for the coolness and pallor of the skin, and the increased sensitivity to cold that the patient may notice. In more severe myxedematous states the heart may be enlarged due to mucopolysaccharide deposition in the cardiac tissue and there may be pericardial effusion. The skin has an increased amount of mucoprotein, likely due to decreased catabolism of these substances. This produces a thick and puffy appearance of the skin, and the facial features may be coarsened due to thickening of the eyelids and lips. The associated hypercarotenemia produces a yellow-orange color to the skin. Secretions of sebaceous and sweat glands are reduced, producing dry, coarse skin and hair, while the nails are dry and brittle. Mucinous deposits in the median nerve in the carpal tunnel may produce an entrapment neuropathy with resultant paresthesiae. Other neurologic involvement may result in cerebellar, spinal cord, and auditory nerve dysfunction. Central nervous maturation (myelination and neuronal development) is dependent on adequate thyroid hormone and thus neonatal hypothyroidism may produce irreversible brain damage unless corrected at a very early stage. The adult patient may merely show general slowing of intellectual functions, with memory defects, lethargy, and somnolence. In some instances dementia or depressive reactions are present.

The patient may complain of stiffness, muscle cramps, and aching of the muscles. The decreased rate of muscle contraction and relaxation gives rise to a very useful clinical diagnostic sign of delayed relaxation phase of the deep tendon reflexes. Ventilation usually decreases, possibly reflecting the decreased oxygen comsumption. Appetite and food intake are both reduced, and weight gain is usually related to retention of fluids. Constipation may result both from decreased peristaltic activity and decreased food intake. Myxedematous infiltration of the larynx and tongue may give rise to hoarseness and slurred speech.

The metabolic effects of hypothyroidism are widespread. The decrease in protein anabolism is reflected by the retardation of skeletal growth. This also may result from a decrease in secretion and effect of growth hormone in hypothyroidism. Further, epiphyseal dysgenesis may occur in hypothyroid prepubertal children. These features produce severe impairment of linear bone growth, leading to dwarfism in which the limbs are disproportionately short in relation to the trunk. Bone age is usually retarded in relation to chronologic age.

Severe hypothyroidism beginning in infancy is termed *cretinism*, and early recognition is crucial if intellectual attainment and growth are to be normal. Early postnatal symptoms, within the first few months of life, may include the persistence of physiologic jaundice, feeding problems, constipation, somnolence, and a hoarse cry. Later, there is delayed eruption of deciduous teeth. The preadolescent child will manifest delay of growth and sexual development.

Myxedema coma is now a rare complication of long-standing hypothyroidism. It is usually precipitated by superimposed stress such as an infection, drug administration (such as major tranquillizers), cold exposure, or may merely occur as the end stage of severe longstanding hypothyroidism. Clinical manifestations include hypothermia and hypoventilation; this results in severe respiratory acidosis. Treatment consists of artificial ventilation, correction of fluid and electrolyte disturbances, and gradual reversal of the hypothermia. Parenteral thyroid hormone must be administered at once.

Congenital causes of hypothyroidism include congenital defects in embryogenesis, as well as inborn defects in thyroid hormone synthesis. The acquired causes comprise primary thyroid diseases or those secondary to pituitary or hypothalamic dysfunction. Primary thyroid diseases may be associated with thyroid enlargement due to increased pituitary TSH secretion, or may occur as a result of reduced thyroid parenchyma. Chronic lymphocytic thyroiditis (Hashimoto's thyroiditis) may be associated with goiter, or with an atrophic thyroid gland (idiopathic atrophy). Other goitrous forms of hypothyroidism include iodine deficiency, ingestion of goitrogens, and various cellular and noncellular infiltrations. Iatrogenic hypothyroidism, secondary to surgery or radioiodine ablation, are common causes of nongoitrous hypothyroidism.

Hashimoto's thyroiditis, the most common cause of spontaneous hypothyroidism, appears to be a response to an autoimmune process, very similar to that seen with Graves' disease. The thyroid function at any stage of this process may be euthyroid, hypothyroid, or occasionally hyperthyroid. The patient may thus be well, or may present with hypothyroid symptoms. There is usually no pain in the thyroid region. Systemic symptoms are absent, unless thyroid function is abnormal. The gland is found to be moderately enlarged, firm, and nontender by palpation, although this is variable. There is frequently a family history of autoimmune thyroid disease, and there is a higher incidence of concomitant autoimmune disease in other endocrine glands, or in other organ systems. Circulating serum antibodies directed toward thyroid antigens are usually detected, often in high titers. The course of Hashimoto's disease is variable, with about half of the patients progressing to hypothyroidism with end-stage fibrosis, while the remainder may remain stationary.

The most important clinical situation to differentiate biochemically from hypothyroidism is the "euthyroid sick syndrome." These patients are usually quite ill, and frequently are elderly. Measurement of the serum T4 and T4 index may be low, well into the hypothyroid range. If the free T4 (bi-ologically active fraction) is measured, this may be normal, but unfortunately this test is not readily available. The TSH is normal, a feature militating against primary hypothyroidism. If the TRH test is performed, the result is usually normal, a point against pituitary hypothyroidism. In this clinical state, especially if accompanied by decreased caloric intake, the serum T3 is decreased; in contrast the reverse T3 is increased, indicating an alteration in the peripheral conversion pathways of T4 and T3 in response to the clinical state. With recovery, the serum T4 and T3 return to normal. Recognizing this situation and differentiating it from true hypothyroidism requires careful interpretation of the laboratory results within the total clinical context.

Treatment

The treatment of hypothyroidism is to replace the thyroid deficiency by synthetic thyroxine, although other preparations and even T3 are available. The T4 dosage may be monitored by the normalization of the clinical state, the serum TSH, and the total serum T3, which is preferable to the serum T4 for this purpose. If there is preexisting heart disease, it may be rational to initiate treatment with very low daily doses and gradual incremental doses thereafter. In most situations, in younger patients, this is not necessary, and full daily replacement therapy may be administered.

MASS: ENLARGEMENT OF PART OR ALL OF THE THYROID GLAND

Goiter

A goiter is an enlargement of the thyroid gland, regardless of the overall functional capacity of the gland. If the gland is uniformly and symmetrically enlarged it is referred to as a diffuse goiter, and if composed of several nodules it is referred to as a multinodular goiter. A single localized area of enlargement is referred to as a thyroid nodule.

A goiter represents a compensatory response to a variety of etiologic factors (goitrogenic or genetic) that impair normal synthesis of thyroid hormone. Impairment of normal thyroid hormone synthesis results in hypersecretion of TSH, leading to increased thyroid hormone biosynthesis (compensation), leaving a euthyroid patient but with a goiter. If the degree of compensation is not adequate, the patient may have concomitant hypothyroidism. If there is a deficiency in normal thyroxine secretion, such as with iodine deficiency, the decreased ability to form T4 may be counterbalanced by preferential secretion of T3. The glandular enlargement associated with Graves' disease is not, of course, compensatory, and is not due to excessive TSH, but rather due to TSH-like thyroid-stimulating immunoglobulins. Multinodular goiters most likely arise from a longstanding preexisting diffuse goiter.

The actual enlargement may produce a mass effect, resulting in obstruction of the trachea or esophagus, which may result in stridor or dysphagia. Hoarseness may arise due to involvement of the recurrent laryngeal nerve, but this is quite unusual in benign goiters and more often suggests a malignant process. Marked thyroidal enlargement may impair venous return from the head and neck, especially when the arms are raised above the head. Occasionally the bulk of the goiter is retrosternal and may only be apparent on tracheal tomograms.

The diagnosis is usually obvious on physical examination, but scintiscanning may be necessary to differentiate diffuse from nodular goiters. Thyroid antibodies should be obtained to rule out Hashimoto's thyroiditis as the underlying cause, even if the patient is euthyroid. Some goitrogenic drugs may be implicated in causing thyroid enlargement, such as lithium, iodides, sulfonylureas, and the thiocarbamides.

The treatment depends on the clinical situation. If the patient is hyperthyroid, then drug or ablative forms of therapy are indicated. If the patient is hypothyroid, regardless of the underlying etiology of the goiter, thyroid hormone replacement is indicated, and usually the goiter will decrease in size due to suppression of TSH. The euthyroid goiter may be merely followed, or a decrease in size may be pursued by thyroxine administration. If there are significant obstructive symptoms, then surgical removal may be indicated, either prior to or after an attempt has been made to shrink the goiter with thyroxine therapy.

Thyroid Neoplasms

A thyroid nodule is a common finding on routine physical examination. Virtually any pathologic process involving the thyroid gland can manifest itself as a distinct nodule, and careful examination of the remainder of the gland is necessary to ensure that the single obvious nodule is not merely part of a multinodular process. Of all the processes that may produce a single nodule, the most important to consider and differentiate are benign adenomas (with or without cystic elements) from thyroid carcinomas. A simple cyst can often be readily differentiated from the above lesions.

The benign adenomas consist of different cellular types. In general they are hypofunctioning, however, follicular adenomas may show normal function on scintiscanning. The adenomas that are hypofunctioning on scintiscanning must be differentiated from carcinomas. Malignant neoplasms (carcinomas) may have different natural histories depending on whether the underlying type is papillary, follicular, medullary (arising from the parafollicular or C cells of the thyroid), or anaplastic. The vast majority are of the papillary or follicular histopathologic type. Only uncommonly are these latter tumors aggressive, but they may show local, lymphatic (usually with the papillary variety), or hematogenous (usually with the follicular type) spread. Nevertheless, it is quite uncommon for these carcinomas to result in death. Anaplastic carcinoma is locally invasive and very aggressive; death usually occurs within 6 to 12 months, with little regard to any form of surgical, radiation, or chemotherapeutic intervention. Medullary carcinoma may be familial in origin, and may coexist with pheochromocytoma or other hyperfunctioning endocrine states in other tissues (multiple endocrine neoplasia type 2). Because they arise from the C cells, plasma calcitonin is elevated and is useful as a tumor marker. It is important to screen all members of families in which a medullary carcinoma appears, by measurement of serum calcitonin.

One recognized thyroid carcinogen is low-dose irradiation. Prior exposure to external irradiation produces a greatly higher incidence of both benign and malignant thyroid nodules, which may even be multifocal.

The clinical presentation of a thyroid nodule, benign or malignant, is usually an asymptomatic finding on routine physical examination. However, if the nodule is large it may cause symptoms of local compression. Malignancy is more likely with the finding of unusual hardness and fixation (nonmobility) of the nodule, and especially if there is associated lymphadenopathy. In the euthyroid patient the next investigative step is thyroid scintiscanning, since the hyperfunctioning nodule is almost always benign, while the hypofunctioning nodule (relative to the remaining tissue) may be either benign or malignant. Even if the nodule is hypofunctioning, over 80 percent of these lesions are benign. Ultrasound examination should be performed next to differentiate a cystic from a solid lesion; cystic lesions are amenable to large needle aspiration, which may eliminate the nodule, and the fluid can be sent for cytologic examination. In hypofunctioning solid nodules, assuming the presence of an expert cytopathologist, fine needle aspiration biopsy is utilized to again differentiate malignant lesions. If, after this entire process, the nodule is still not clearly diagnosed as benign or malignant, it may be either arbitrarily surgically removed, or clinically followed with or without thyroid suppression with exogenously administered thyroxine.

If there is continued growth of the nodule, especially during thyroid hormone suppression, then the nodule should again be considered for surgical resection. Because the percentage of single nodules proving to be malignant is higher in children, males, postmenopausal females, or patients with a previous radiation exposure, earlier surgical removal should be considered in these groups.

In patients with thyroid carcinoma, the treatment of choice is a thyroidectomy, followed by ablation of any remaining thyroid tissue with radioactive iodine. Following this, a total body radioiodine scan should be performed to see whether there are functional metastases, and if this is the case, they also should undergo radioablative therapy. For patients with continued symptomatic clinical deterioration, chemotherapy has been utilized with moderate success.

Plasma thyroglobulin is elevated in some patients with well differentiated thyroid carcinoma. While this is not specific for malignancy, it may be utilized as a tumor marker in the long-term follow-up and management of patients who have undergone a total thyroidectomy, since a new elevation of thyroglobulin usually indicates tumor recurrence or metastases.

THE ADRENAL GLAND

THE ADRENAL CORTEX

The adrenal glands cover the superior pole of each kidney at the level of the first lumbar vertebra. They are supplied with arterial blood derived from branches from the aorta. The adrenal glands consist of two components, the mesodermal portion, which develops into the cortex of the gland, and the ectodermal portion, which forms the medulla. The cortex produces steroids while the medulla produces catecholamines. The fact that the two parts of the gland have different sites of origin yet become anatomically interrelated suggests an associated functional interrelationship. It is now recognized that the final step of catecholamine biosynthesis, the conversion of norepinephrine to epinephrine, requires a higher concentration of cortisol than is found in peripheral blood, and this requirement is present throughout the entire adrenal gland due to local production.

The adrenal cortex is divided into three zones, the product of each being a different family of steroids. The outer glomerulosa layer produces mainly mineralocorticoids, the middle fasciculata layer produces mainly glucocorticoids, and the inner reticularis produces mainly sex steroids.

The regulation of adrenocortical secretions varies among the three zones of the adrenal cortex. The regulation of cortisol secretion is the most complex; the first step is at the hypothalamus, which releases corticotropin-releasing hormone, (CRH), which travels to and acts upon the pituitary to release ACTH. ACTH then binds to receptors in the cells of the adrenal cortex to form intracellular cyclic AMP and cyclic GMP, which then stimulate steroidogenesis and adrenal cortical growth. In the absence of this endogenous ACTH stimulation, the adrenal cortex becomes atrophic. The secreted cortisol circulates bound to cortisol-binding globulin, in equilibrium with a certain amount of free cortisol that enters the cell to exert its physiologic effects. The mechanism of action of steroid hormones is described in the section Endocrine Physiology. One of the peripheral actions of cortisol is to perform as a feedback messenger at the level of the pituitary to inhibit further ACTH secretion, the negative feedback control mechanism. Overriding this simple control mechanism is an endogenous rhythm (diurnal variation) whereby ACTH and cortisol levels are highest on awakening in the morning and lowest on retiring, with a gradual fall throughout the day. Episodic secretion of ACTH and cortisol occurs, but the mean levels during 24 hours show the typical diurnal variation, and indicate the integrity of the hypothalamic input. Higher brain centers may override this system with input at the level of the hypothalamus so that under conditions of stress (such as surgery, hypoglycemia, fever, or the like) the entire system is stimulated, and more ACTH and more cortisol is produced to meet the now increased metabolic demands. The same ACTH also results in adrenal sex steroid output.

Aldosterone secretion is controlled by the renin-angiotensin system, serum potassium and to a minor degree by ACTH. Reduced blood volume and serum sodium are sensed at the level of the juxtaglomerular cells of the afferent arterioles of the kidney; renin is released from the storage grenules. Renin then acts enzymatically to convert angiotensinogen to angiotensin I, which is converted to angiotensin II by vascular endothelium. Angiotensin II directly stimulates the secretion of aldosterone. Aldosterone increases sodium reabsorption with concomitant potassium and hydrogen ion excretion in the distal nephron, salivary glands, sweat glands, and gastrointestinal mucosa.

The biosynthesis of adrenal cortical hormones is indicated in Figure 13.2. This is clearly a complex system, since it involves many steps and several different enzymes. This complexity may result in congenital deficiencies in the biosynthesis and lends itself to pharmacologic manipulation of the biosynthetic pathway.

Hyposecretion of Adrenal Cortical Hormones

Hyposecretion may involve all three layers of the adrenal cortex, either as a consequence of primary adrenal disorders or secondary to pituitary disease, or else may involve only one of the end products (such as isolated aldosterone deficiency due to hyporeninism or isolated inability to make cortisol following long-term iatrogenic suppression with pharmacologic doses of glucocorticoids).

Secondary adrenal cortical insufficiency results from any pituitary-hypothalamic disease process that inhibits CRH and ACTH secretion. Through the renin system, the aldosterone secretion remains close to normal. The major clinical effects are due to reductions in cortisol and androgen secretion, and the inability to demonstrate ACTH-induced pigmentation. Primary adrenal cortical insufficiency is most commonly due to idiopathic atrophy (Addison's disease), now considered due to immunologic destruction. This may coexist with other autoimmune diseases causing destruction or stimulation in other endocrine glands, or in association with immunologic diseases in other organ systems.

Clinical Manifestations

The manifestations of adrenal deficiency vary from an acute presentation that is potentially a fatal medical emergency, to a more insidious chronic presentation that requires considerable clinical acumen to be detected. Although both forms of adrenal insufficiency are quite uncommon, they must be considered in any of the common presentations of other disorders that may simulate adrenal insufficiency. In the form of disease that is slower in onset, the characteristic hyperpigmentation due to MSH-ACTH overproduction occurs as a diffuse tan over the body, greater in the exposed parts, and particularly prominent over pressure points such as knees, elbows, creases of skin, areolae, and newly acquired scars. In the patient with autoimmune adrenal disease, there may be areas of vitiligo (contrasting with the increased pigmentation) indicating associated autoimmune involvement of the melanocytes of the skin. Loss of adrenal androgens results in inability to maintain axillary and pubic hair in the female, but not in the male who has continued testicular testosterone secretion. Mineralocorticoid insufficiency results in salt wastage, with salt craving, muscular cramps, and postural lightheadedness. The clinical findings include hypotension with postural drop, and a small heart. Loss of glucocorticoid results in fatigability, changes in

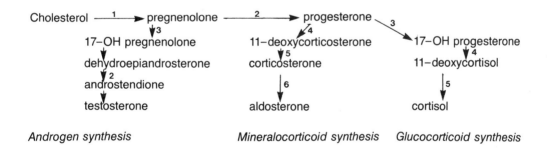

Fig. 13.2 Major Steps in Biosynthesis of Adrenal Cortical Hormones

mentation, nonspecific nausea and anorexia, and a tendency toward hypoglycemia in the fasting state.

The severely ill patient with acute adrenal insufficiency presents with a constellation of symptoms including fever, hypotension, nausea and vomiting, hypoglycemia, muscular weakness, diarrhea, hyponatremia, and hypercalcemia, which may culminate in hypothermia, shock, and death. Unless another obvious etiology for the presenting symptoms is evident, a presumptive diagnosis of acute adrenal insufficiency should be made and the patient given immediate parenteral glucocorticoids; these should be maintained until a definitive diagnosis of adrenal insufficiency can be either established or ruled out. While the patient is maintained on a synthetic glucocorticoid such as dexamethasone (which is not measured by the plasma cortisol assay), the patient should have an ACTH stimulation test. The presence of normal adrenal function should not be inferred by finding a "normal" basal plasma cortisol level prior to therapy, since under this stressful state, basal cortisol levels should be significantly elevated above the "normal" range.

In the patient with idiopathic Addison's disease, there should be clinical suspicion for concomitant autoimmune disorders, such as Hashimoto's thyroiditis, Graves' disease, pernicious anemia, diabetes mellitus, gonadal failure, and hypoparathyroidism. Most of these disorders can be ruled out clinically and by simple biochemical assays. The patient remains at risk for future development of such disorders, especially younger patients.

Patients with hypopituitarism are pale rather than pigmented, and do not have the hyperkalemia associated with mineralocorticoid deficiency. Hyponatremia may still coexist on a dilutional basis, reflecting the cortisol insufficiency with inability to excrete an ingested water load. Further, there may be evidence of other pituitary tropic hormone deficiency, such as concomitant hypothyroidism or hypogonadism. This may therefore simulate multiple autoimmune end-organ glandular failure. In endorgan failure, the pituitary tropic hormone is elevated, which readily distinguishes this condition from hypopituitarism.

Laboratory Diagnosis

Laboratory features reflect a decreased serum sodium and an elevated serum potassium with associated metabolic acidosis. The decreased blood volume may result in an elevated BUN and hematocrit, or cortisol deficiency may result in mild anemia, lymphocytosis, and eosinophilia. Basal measurements of cortisol in the plasma, in the 24-hour urine, or of cortisol metabolites (17-ketogenic or 17-hydroxycorticoids) in the urine may be low or low normal, but the definitive diagnosis depends on failure of basal levels of cortisol or metabolites to increase after appropriate stimulation with ACTH. In patients with adrenal disease due to hypothalamic-pituitary insufficiency, there is a normal or blunted response to ACTH, but an abnormally low response to stimuli such as hypoglycemia or metyrapone.

Hypoaldosteronism

Isolated hypoaldosteronism may result from congenital enzyme deficiencies, and from certain types of renal disease in the elderly population. Some forms of interstitial renal disease may impair renin secretion, and patients with autonomic neuropathy may have inhibition of release of renin, which may secondarily impair aldosterone release. The most common underlying cause is diabetes mellitus, which may result in renal disease and autonomic insufficiency; the insulin deficient state may also impair the control of aldosterone secretion by inhibiting the shift of potassium into the glomerulosa cells. Such patients with *hyporeninemic hypoaldosteronism* present with volume depletion, and hyperkalemia that occasionally is life-threatening. The management of such patients may involve mineralocorticoid replacement therapy.

Congenital Adrenal Hyperplasia—A disorder of Both Hyposecretion and Hypersecretion

Congenital adrenal hyperplasia actually represents not a single error but a group of genetically transmitted inborn errors of metabolism resulting from decreased function of an enzyme involved in the steroid biosynthetic pathway. The defect appears to be autosomal recessive in transmission, and occurs in 1 in 5000 to 1 in 50,000 births. With the net effect of decreased cortisol synthesis, there is enhanced pituitary ACTH secretion with resultant hyperplasia of the adrenal glands and overproduction of precursors prior to the enzymatic block. The clinical manifestations depend on the site of the block, and the symptoms reflect both the deficiency of the biologic activity of cortisol and the excess of the biologic activity of the precursors. Because the earliest branches of the steroid synthetic pathway lead to androgen synthesis, androgen excess forms an integral part of all of these syndromes, except when the enzyme deficiencies specifically inhibit androgen biosynthesis. Oversecretion of androgens may present in the newborn with virilization of females and ambiguous genitalia, but mild defects may result in precocious puberty of males or pubertal virilism in the female. The appearance of these genital abnormalities gives rise to the term *adrenogenital syndrome*. Other effects of the enhanced androgen secretion promote bone growth and early epiphyseal closure, resulting in short stature.

Six enzymatic defects are identified in Figure 13.2 and the specific syndromes are described below.

1. 20-Hydroxylase deficiency. The first step in corticosteroid synthesis is inhibited, so that cholesterol cannot be converted into pregnenolone. This results in the patient's inability to produce any form of adrenal steroid, presenting with severe salt wasting and cortisol insufficiency, as well as absence of any virilization in the newborn.

2. 3-β-Dehydrogenase deficiency. Pregnenolone cannot be converted to progesterone, and this prevents the formation of four major corticosteroids: aldosterone, cortisol, testosterone, and estradiol. Male infants will have ambiguous genitalia and both sexes will have severe salt losing.

3. 17-α-Hydroxylase deficiency. This will inhibit the production and secretion of cortisol, estradiol, and testosterone, but not of aldosterone, which leads to increased mineralocorticoid activity. Males will have ambiguous genitalia and hypogonadism, and both sexes will have hypertension with associated hypokalemia.

4. 21-Hydroxylase deficiency. This, the most common disorder, results in impairment of cortisol and aldosterone synthesis but not of androgen and estrogen synthesis, resulting in sex steroid overproduction. This will result in salt wasting in both sexes, ambiguous genitalia in females, and precocious puberty in males. The degree of sodium wasting and volume depletion reflects the severity of the aldosterone deficiency, which in turn relates to the degree of block in the biosynthetic pathway. The more severe the impairment, the more severe and earlier the presentation of the salt wasting. In some patients there may be no evidence of aldosterone insufficiency, resulting in no clinical signs of salt wasting.

5. 11-β-Hydroxylase. This impairs the last step in aldosterone and cortisol synthesis, but not androgen production. Another precursor that accumulates is 11-deoxycorticosterone, which produces hypertension and hypokalemia; virilism in females, and pre-

cocious puberty in males result from the increased androgens.

6. 18-Hydroxysteroid dehydrogenase deficiency. This impairs the last step in aldosterone synthesis, resulting in isolated salt wasting with hyperkalemia. Because there is no block in cortisol synthesis, there is no compensatory increase in ACTH.

Treatment

Treatment entails providing the missing steroids, mainly cortisol. Excessive cortisol therapy is to be avoided so as not to inhibit growth in children and young adolescents. Mineralocorticoid replacement may also be necessary.

Hypersecretion of Adrenal Cortical Hormones

The clinical manifestations of adrenal cortical hormonal excess relate to the particular type of steroid that is hypersecreted, and to the particular combination of hormones involved. Excessive cortisol secretion affects fat, protein, carbohydrate, and electrolyte metabolism. Increased androgen secretion will result in virilization of females, producing hirsutism, baldness, deepening of the voice, acne, alteration in the menstrual periods, clitoral enlargement, and an enlarged musculature. Pure estrogen secreting tumors of the adrenal gland are extremely rare, but would result in feminization of a male. Excessive mineralocorticoid biologic activity, usually due to aldosterone or desoxycorticosterone secretion, produces hypertension and hypokalemia (with suppression of the renin angiotensin system resulting in a low plasma renin activity).

Hypersecretion of Aldosterone

Primary aldosteronism occurs when the adrenal gland produces an excessive and inappropriate amount of aldosterone. This must be differentiated from secondary aldosteronism, in which adrenal gland hypersecretion of aldosterone occurs in response to an appropriate physiologic stimulus. Activation of the renin angiotensin system due to decreased effective circulating fluid volume or hyponatremia (as with ascites, congestive heart failure, and hypovolemia) or due to a primary hypersecretion of renin (as with renal artery stenosis, renal infarct, and estrogen-containing medications), all result in increased aldosterone secretion that will contribute to hypertension and may produce hypokalemia. Primary aldosteronism will secondarily suppress the renin angiotensin system, and therefore has associated low plasma renin activity along with the hypertension and hypokalemia (see Chapter 3). The hypokalemia affects neuromuscular excitability, producing fatigue, weakness, or frank paralysis. Reduced response to antidiuretic hormone, at a level beyond the binding of ADH to its receptor, results in polyuria, polydipsia, and nocturia. In susceptible patients the hypokalemia may impair insulin release and peripheral insulin action, and thereby bring about clinical diabetes mellitus. There is usually an associated metabolic alkalosis, likely secondary to the hypokalemia. Physical examination usually reveals hypertension and its end-organ changes, but with severe hypokalemia and alkalosis, there may be absence of deep tendon reflexes, and positive Chvostek's and Trousseau's signs.

The suppressed plasma renin activity must be determined under stimulatory conditions: if it remains suppressed despite an adequate stimulus, then the hyposecretion of renin is compatible with primary aldosterone hypersecretion. Because the major stimulus for renin secretion is that of plasma volume, various forms of volume depleting protocols are utilized for test purposes, for example, administration of a potent diuretic, such as furosemide, or a hypotensive agent, such as diazoxide. The most potent stimulus used for renin secretion is a 10 mEq sodium diet for 5 days. If, despite the low volume stimulus, the measurable plasma renin activity still remains low, then the renin is suppressed. This finding is observed in about 20 percent of the population having essential hypertension, and thus it is not specific for primary hyperaldosteronism. The next step is to measure the plasma or urinary aldosterone secretion. This again is usually performed on a protocol of fixed activity and sodium and potassium intake, so that the measured values can be compared with those of normal people on a similar regimen. Some protocols use suppressive tests, either with several days of sodium loading, saline infusion, or administration of a mineralocorticoid pharmacologic agent (Florinef); since patients with primary aldosteronism usually show nonsuppressible aldosterone secretion.

The differentiation of primary aldosteronism due to unilateral adenoma versus bilateral hyperplasia is the next step, and is discussed in Chapter 3. In normal people or in patients with essential hypertension, on arising from a supine state and walking around for 4 hours, there is an increase in renin and aldosterone secretion. Patients with bilateral adrenal hyperplasia, despite a suppressed plasma renin activity, generally retain the postural release of aldosterone; therefore, there is an increase in serum aldosterone levels after 4 hours of erect posture. The majority of patients with unilateral adrenal adenomas no longer have any postural response. This test is useful, but is susceptible to the "stress" response releasing ACTH and resulting in a surge of aldosterone, which may be inappropriately interpreted as a normal response to the upright posture. Therefore, concomitant measures of cortisol are necessary.

The treatment of a unilateral adenoma is surgical excision, while the treatment of bilateral adrenal hyperplasia is medical. A small percentage of patients with bilateral adrenal hyperplasia appear to respond to dexamethasone administration, for unknown reasons, but possibly due to suppression of ACTH. It may be rational to administer dexamethasone for 10 days and to then determine whether or not there is normalization of the serum potassium and blood pressure. If this is not the case, then treatment with spironolactone is indicated.

Hypersecretion of Cortisol-Cushing's Syndrome

The signs and symptoms of excessive cortisol secretion represent an exaggeration of the hormone's physiologic actions. Common manifestations include obesity, hypertension, hirsutism, and diabetes. Associated thinness of the skin and proximal muscle weakness reflecting the protein catabolism, may indicate which of the patients with the above common disorders should be further investigated for the possibility of cortisol excess. In some situations when there is a rapid fulminant onset of excessive cortisol secretion, as in ectopic ACTH secretion due to malignancy, the typical features of Cushing's syndrome are often not seen; the patient may merely have severe muscle wasting, psychosis, and electrolyte disturbances. In the usual cases of Cushing's syndrome, the manifestations of excessive cortisol secretion include changes in fat metabolism (truncal obesity, hyperlipidemia, and accelerated atherosclerosis), protein metabolism (muscle wasting with proximal muscle weakness, thin skin with striae and ecchymoses), and carbohydrate metabolism (clinical diabetes mellitus). Sodium retention and potassium excretion may produce hypertension, hypokalemia, and alkalosis. Additional effects of cortisol may include osteopenia (antagonism of vitamin D metabolism, and protein catabolism), growth hormone antagonism resulting in growth failure of children, increased MSH-ACTH resulting in hyperpigmentation, and androgen excess producing hirsutism and virilization in the female. Neurologic effects include emotional, neurotic, or psychiatric manifestations. Variations in the degree of these manifestations depends to some extent on the basic cause of the disorder.

The causes of Cushing's syndrome are indicated in Table 13.8. Increased pituitary production of ACTH is known as Cushing's disease. The ectopic ACTH syndrome may occur with malignant or benign tumors. The benign tumors usually result in all manifestations of Cushing's syndrome, but the malignant tumors usually are of rapid onset and are associated with a negative caloric balance, so that the patients do not manifest all the signs of Cushing's syndrome. Usually weakness, psychosis, pigmentation, and hypokalemic alkalosis are the obvious features. Although ACTH secretion has been found in virtually every tumor type, the most common is oat cell carcinoma of the lung. The most common benign tumors are bronchial carcinoids and thymus.

The diagnosis of Cushing's syndrome is based on the principle that autonomous hyperfunction is qualitatively or quantitatively nonsuppressible.

The presence of Cushing's syndrome may be suggested by one or more of the following screening tests:

1. The normal diurnal rhythm of cortisol excretion is altered, therefore comparison of an early morning and late evening (ideally 0800 and 2300 hours) basal plasma cortisol concentration is useful. However, stress may eliminate the diurnal rhythm.

2. A 24-hour urine collection for cortisol (urinary free cortisol) or its metabolites is useful to show an enhanced secretion. Patients under nonspecific "stress" can also have elevated levels, such as occur sometimes in a depressed patient. Since many of the hypersecretory states have episodic secretion, occasionally a patient with true Cushing's syndrome will have a normal 24-hour urine excretion.

Table 13.8   Causes of Cushing's Syndrome

ACTH Elevated
1. Pituitary-hypothalamic
   A. Pituitary tumor[a]
   B. No demonstrable pituitary tumor (? corticotroph hyperplasia)
2. Ectopic ACTH secretion

ACTH Suppressed
1. Adrenal adenoma
   A. Adrenal gland
   B. Adrenal rest tissue
2. Adrenal carcinoma
3. Nodular bilateral adrenal hyperplasia
4. Iatrogenic (use of glucocorticoids)

[a] Most common cause in adults (excludes iatrogenic)

3. The overnight dexamethasone suppression test is a more dynamic test to assess whether the hypothalamic-pituitary-adrenal axis is autonomous. One milligram of dexamethasone is taken at midnight, and a plasma cortisol is assayed at 0800 hours the next morning to see whether it is appropriately suppressed. Patients taking estrogen will have elevated cortisol binding globulins, and it may be difficult to use an absolute number as an indication of suppression. In this situation it is useful to measure the plasma cortisol at midnight and at 0800 hours; failure of the cortisol level to increase indicates that the dexamethasone did suppress the overnight surge of ACTH.

4. The response to insulin-induced hypoglycemia may be helpful. In patients who are depressed, obese, and under "stress," all three previous tests may give false-positive results, but such patients usually still demonstrate a normal cortisol response to hypoglycemia, in contrast to patients with true Cushing's syndrome who fail to increase plasma cortisol.

Once the screening test has demonstrated the likely presence of Cushing's syndrome, more definitive tests for the diagnosis and localization of the exact cause are necessary.

Plasma ACTH levels help differentiate primary adrenal tumors from pituitary or ectopic ACTH secretion. Ectopic ACTH secretion has a greater elevation of ACTH levels than pituitary ACTH hypersecretion, and with adrenal tumors ACTH levels are low.

The dexamethasone suppression test is also useful. Dexamethasone given in low dose (0.5 mg every 6 hours for 48 hours), which is only slightly hyperphysiologic, will be capable of suppressing adrenocortical function in normal persons but not in patients with Cushing's syndrome. This is followed by a high dose (2 mg every 6 hours for 48 hours). Plasma and urine cortisol measurements are taken again, and, at this dose, suppression generally indicates pituitary-dependent Cushing's syndrome, referred to as Cushing's disease. (Patients taking drugs such as Dilantin, and some severely depressed patients show this response.) Failure to suppress basal levels at this dose is more in keeping with ectopic ACTH syndrome, adrenal adenoma, and adrenal carcinoma.

At this stage more anatomic localization can be attempted, using skull roentgenograms, intravenous pyelograms with tomography, adrenal venography with bilateral adrenal venous sampling, iodocholesterol scans, ultrasonography, and CT scanning.

Metyrapone administration is useful as a test procedure; patients with pituitary-dependent Cushing's syndrome have an exaggerated response, while patients with ectopic ACTH syndrome usually fail to show any response, as do patients with adrenal tumors.

The urinary 17-ketosteroid measurement may suggest the site of the excessive cortisol excretion. Compared with the degree of elevation of the 24-hour urine cortisol, the 17-ketosteroids are relatively high in ACTH-dependent Cushing's, disproportionately higher in adrenal carcinoma, and relatively low in adrenal adenoma.

Treatment is adapted to the underlying cause. In Cushing's disease there have been high success rates with transphenoidal exploration and resection of the pituitary adenoma. This now appears to be the treatment of choice in patients fit for surgery, and has supplanted bilateral adrenalectomy as the surgical treatment for Cushing's disease. Because there is some evidence for the roles of both serotonin and cholinergic neurotransmission in the control of ACTH release, recent use of the drug cyproheptadine has met with success in one third of patients with pituitary-dependent Cushing's disease. However, when the drug is discontinued, Cushing's disease recurs. When the disorder is due to ectopic ACTH syndrome, ablative therapy is directed toward the primary tumor. In untreatable cases, adrenal cortisol synthesis may be impaired by the use of the adrenolytic drug o, p-DDD, or with the enzyme antagonists aminoglutethamide or metyrapone. The same drugs may be utilized with pituitary-dependent Cushing's syndrome either as a primary form of therapy in patients unfit for more invasive forms of therapy, to bring patients to a normal metabolic state prior to ablative therapy, or to allow the time required for procedures such as pituitary irradiation. The treatment of adrenal tumors is surgical removal, and in unresectable or metastatic adrenal carcinoma the adrenolytic drug o, p-DDD has been useful and has produced some prolonged remissions. The unusual patient with bilateral nodular hyperplasia is still treated by total adrenalectomy.

Adrenal Masses

Adrenal carcinomas are rare, and present either with the manifestations of hypersecretion, usually Cushing's syndrome, or with a palpable abdominal mass, which is present in the majority of cases. Because adrenal carcinoma tissue is not as efficient as normal tissue, the steroid molecules that are generated early in the biosynthetic pathway tend to accumulate. There is often inappropriate elevation of the urinary 17-ketosteroids when compared with the elevation of urinary cortisol. Similarly, accumulation of more immature mineralocorticoid steroids produces hypokalemia more commonly than seen in usual states of Cushing's syndrome. There is a special tendency toward hypoglycemia in some of these patients, possibly due to increased secretion of nonsuppressible insulinlike activity (NSILA), which simulates the peripheral action of insulin. Peripheral metastases tend to appear in lungs, liver, and bones.

The treatment of choice is surgical removal, with or without local irradiation. In nonresectable cases, treatment with o, p-DDD is sometimes effective in eliminating the symptoms of hypersecretion and has been shown to produce objective regression of tumor mass and metastases in some cases.

THE ADRENAL MEDULLA

The adrenal medulla is embryologically derived from the neuroectoderm, Because it is an extension of the sympathetic nervous system, its secretory products are catecholamines: the adrenal medulla has a unique ability to synthesize epinephrine from norepinephrine, due to the local high cortisol concentration (from the adrenal cortex), which is sufficient to induce the enzyme N-methyl transferase that produces this conversion to epinephrine. This enzyme is present only in the adrenal medulla and the organ of Zuckerkandl. The released epinephrine then acts on specific alpha and beta adrenergic receptors in the various target tissues throughout the body. Free catecholamines are measurable in the blood, and in the urine due to some excretion of the unchanged native hormone. The liver and kidney change much of the secreted hormone to inactive methylated compounds, metanephrine and normetanephrine, which are excreted in the urine, and which may be measured as an index of secretion. Some of these metabolites are further changed by oxidative deamination to produce vanillylmandelic acid, which also may be assayed in the urine as an index of adrenal medullary secretion.

The peripheral actions of epinephrine are hemodynamic: increase in heart rate and cardiac contractility and vasodilation in skeletal muscle vasculature. Epinephrine also increases glucose output from the liver via glycogenolysis, and inhibits insulin release. It promotes release of free fatty acids from adipose tissue. Norepinephrine acts on alpha receptors generally to produce vasoconstriction.

Hyposecretion of the adrenal medulla may result from destructive lesions of the adrenal gland (such as tuberculosis or intraadrenal hemorrhage) or due to an autonomic neuropathy syndrome, such as in patients with "idiopathic" postural hypotension.

Hypersecretion of the adrenal medulla results from the tumor, pheochromocytoma. Since the major clinical feature is hypertension, this condition is discussed in chapter 3 under Hypertension Secondary to Endocrine Causes. Pheochromocytoma may be associated with multiple endocrine neoplasia syndrome type 2 (medullary cell carcinoma of the thyroid and parathyroid hyperplasia). It is also associated with other neuroectodermal syndromes, such as neurofibromatosis, Lindau's disease, tuberous sclerosis, and Sturge-Weber syndrome.

Increased catecholamine secretion may also result in myocarditis and present with a cardiomyopathy. The psychiatric manifestations may dominate the picture, with suicide as a complication of this disorder.

After clinical suspicion is aroused, the diagnosis is made by assay of catecholamines in the plasma, or catecholamines and/or metabolites in a 24-hour urine collection. Therefore, an elevation of a urine catecholamine or metabolite should be followed by a repeat collection measuring an additional compound, to confirm the elevation. Patients who have clearly episodic symptoms may be normotensive and have normal urinary assay results between the episodes, so it may be worthwhile beginning a urine collection at the time of the onset of episodic symptoms.

Further investigation requires localization of the tumor; the vast majority will prove to be single benign tumors of the adrenal gland, with twice as many on the right side as on the left. Because the tumors may be bilateral or malignant, preoperative localization is useful. This may be carried out by arteriography, or by CT scanning. Adrenal vein catheterization is difficult and potentially dangerous. All stressful procedures should be performed after the patient has been given alpha-adrenergic blocking agents, so that the stressful state does not result in a sudden release of catecholamines producing a hypertensive crisis. A simple chest roentgenogram usually rules out a tumor of the sympathetic chain within the chest.

The treatment of these tumors is surgical removal, but due to functional inhibition of the sympathetic nervous system it is best to treat patients with alpha-adrenergic blockade one week prior to surgery to allow recovery of the sympathetic reflexes, and to eliminate postoperative hypotensive problems. Further, because the effective circulating fluid volume is lower in these patients, they usually require volume expansion postoperatively to maintain normal blood pressure. In patients who are secreting a significant amount of concomitant epinephrine, beta-adrenergic blockade may also be necessary. For inoperable tumors or metastatic carcinoma, constant alpha blockade with phenoxybenzamine has been useful. If there is associated medullary carcinoma of the thyroid or parathyroid hyperplasia (presenting with hypercalcemia), the treatment is surgical, and the entire family and future offspring should be examined at frequent intervals for the possible development of one or more of these hypersecretory states.

THE FEMALE REPRODUCTIVE SYSTEM

NORMAL FUNCTION

Disorders of the female reproductive system vary depending on the stage of sexual maturation. Abnormalities commencing in utero present with abnormal sexual differentiation or ambiguous genitalia. Anormalities occurring prior to puberty present as precocious or delayed puberty, and postpubertal disorders present as menstrual abnormalities, infertility, or hirsutism.

The infantile pituitary gland and ovaries are capable of full function if appropriately stimulated. However, the hypothalamus is extremely sensitive to the inhibitory effects of estrogen, which keeps the pituitary-ovarian axis almost completely suppressed throughout childhood. At puberty the excessive sensitivity to the feedback inhibition of estrogen apparently becomes diminished, resulting in enhanced episodic production of GnRH that approaches adult amplitude and frequency. This is apparently all that is necessary to produce adult levels of the pituitary secretion of gonadotropin, the ovarian secretion of estrogen, and follicular development. At this early stage of puberty there is not adequate development to allow the midcycle surge of LH required to produce ovulation (the "positive feedback" mechanism), which requires several months or even years to become operative. For this reason the initial menstrual periods after the menarche are anovulatory and only later become ovulatory. Thus, the key factor required for the change from a prepubertal to an adult reproductive axis is an increase in the amplitude and frequency of GnRH secretion, which appears to be a necessary but passive element in maintaining the normal menstrual cycle (see also preceding section on the Hypothalamus and Pituitary Gland and Table 13.1).

The normal function of the adult menstrual cycle

with resultant ovulation is an integrated action between the hypothalamus-pituitary-ovarian axis. The important effects of the higher areas of the central nervous system and psychic factors are poorly understood. Serious stresses can interfere with the menstrual cycle, so that a loss of body weight (usually to a weight less than what was present at the menarche), severe emotional upsets, or environmental changes may all override the episodic hypothalamic GnRH secretion and convert this to a prepubertal level, with resultant amenorrhea and hypoestrogenization. The hypothalamus is the source of the gonadotropin releasing hormone (GnRH), which is transmitted to the anterior pituitary gland to enhance the release of LH and FSH. The secretion of LH and FSH in response to GnRH appears to be modulated by ovarian steroids. The secreted LH and FSH act on the ovarian cells to produce new proteins, but in addition they increase the conversion of cholesterol to pregnenolone, which is converted to its steroidal products, that is, estrogens, progesterones, and androgens. Initially, FSH produces proliferation of granulosa cells and causes these cells to convert locally produced androgens to estradiol, which then acts synergistically with FSH to stimulate development of the follicle. LH acts on the theca cells to induce synthesis of androgens, which diffuse locally into the follicular fluid, and which are aromatized to estrogens by the FSH-stimulated granulosa cells. Both the sex steroid hormones and the ova are products of a follicular apparatus interacting with surrounding stromal elements under the stimulus of hormones secreted by the pituitary. The type and relative quantities of steroids secreted by the ovary will depend on the phase of the menstrual cycle. The follicle secretes mainly estradiol, the corpora lutea secrete mainly progesterone, and the stroma secretes mainly androgens. The secreted sex steroids develop the genital organs and secondary sex characteristics during childhood and puberty, and then prepare the genital tract for pregnancy during each cycle; they prepare for a single ovulation by participation in the interaction with the hypothalamus and pituitary. There are several metabolic effects of estrogen:

1. Estrogen increases the size of the internal sexual organs and external genitalia, changes the vaginal epithelium to a stratified form that is more resistant to trauma and infection, and produces proliferative changes in the endometrium.

2. Estrogen affects the breasts by producing fat deposition, development of stromal tissues, and growth of an extensive ductile system.

At the beginning of each cycle there is an elevation of FSH and LH because of the negative feedback mechanism. At midcycle, estrogen production from a fully developed follicle results in a surge of LH with resultant stimulation of ovulation (the so called positive feedback effect of estrogen in modulating LH secretion). It appears that estrogens alter the sensitivity of the anterior pituitary to GnRH secretion, and this accounts for the variation in response to GnRH, with the resultant variation in release of LH and FSH throughout the menstrual cycle. Further, estrogens have an effect directly at the level of the ovarian follicle to increase the responsiveness of the follicle to gonadotropins. This may be the mechanism whereby the dominant follicle continues to increase its own growth (due to its local, excessive secretion of estrogens) while the pituitary gonadotropin secretion is actually falling.

The Menstrual Cycle

Dynamic relationships between the hypothalamus-pituitary hormones and gonadal hormones allow for the cyclic nature of normal reproductive processes.

Early Follicular Phase

This actually begins in the later luteal phase of the preceding cycle, and is characterized by the growth of a new set of ovarian follicles. A decrease in the levels of circulating estrogens due to the decay of the corpus luteum results in a rise in the serum FSH by the negative feedback mechanism. The ovarian responses to this rise in FSH are cellular proliferation, formation of antral fluid, appearance of estradiol receptors, appearance of aromatase enzymes, and the formation of LH receptor molecules. At this stage LH acts on interstitial and thecal cells to produce testosterone, some of which is aromatized to estradiol, under the influence of FSH, in follicular granulosa cells.

Midfollicular Phase

The estrogen secretion increases due to follicular growth and increased numbers of granulosa cells. Concomitant with this rise in estrogen is a decrease in serum FSH due to the negative feedback response, yet the major follicle continues to mature because the number of FSH receptors increases, which is probably induced by estradiol.

Late Follicular Phase

The FSH continues to fall, but the dominant follicle is selected since it is protected from a fall in FSH by its increased local secretion of estrogen, which potentiates the action of FSH, while the other follicles that make less estrogen become atretic. At this time there are different effects of the gonadal steroids in modulating pituitary gonadotropin secretion, negative feedback continuing to suppress FSH but stimulating rise in LH. In response to the rise in LH there appears to be a rise of androgens, which may enhance atresia of the remaining nondominant follicles, and furthermore may stimulate libido.

Ovulatory Phase

A surging rise of serum LH leads to the final maturation of the follicle, follicle rupture, and ovulation. This may be accompanied by a surge in the GnRH, or might not be accompanied by a surge as long as the continuous pulsatile GnRH secretion is maintained. It appears that the ovarian message for the LH surge is the positive feedback mechanism that occurs with the peak in estrogens, 12 to 36 hours prior to the LH surge; thus, the ovary signals that a mature follicle is ready for ovulation. The rupture of the follicle occurs within 24 hours of the onset of the LH surge.

Luteal Phase

Development of the corpus luteum is initiated by the LH surge, and is maintained for 10 to 14 days if there is a small continuous LH secretion. The hormonal changes are reflected by an increase in plasma progesterone as well as estradiol, with conversion of the endometrium from a proliferative to a secretory phase.

In the normal menstrual cycle there appears to be little role for prolactin, but in patients with enhanced secretion of prolactin there are changes at various levels (see section on Hyperprolactinemia).

FEMALE HYPOGONADISM

If hypogonadism occurs at the time of adolescence, it presents as delayed puberty; but if this condition occurs in the otherwise sexually mature female, it will present as menstrual disorders (usually amenorrhea) or infertility. If the ovaries are not function-ing prior to the menarche, then female eunuchoidism occurs. Accompanying this will be failure to develop the usual secondary sexual characteristics, and sexual organs remain infantile.

Amenorrhea usually reflects cessation of cyclic hormone production. This by itself does not present any danger to general health, but prolonged estrogen deficiency at an early age may result in premature osteopenia. Further, patients with longstanding amenorrhea associated with continued estrogen production and, as a result, constantly proliferative endometrium, may have a higher incidence of endometrial carcinoma. The amenorrhea may be a symptom of an underlying disorder, and because of its inseparable connection with fertility it represents an important social and psychologic problem for the patient. Except for local diseases of the genital tract, amenorrhea is the result of primary lesions or malfunction of the hypothalamic-pituitary-ovarian system. Each morphologic and endocrine event in the ovary is initiated via FSH and/or LH after the ovary has signaled its readiness. If this signal is insufficient or absent due to ovarian causes, disturbed by metabolic aberrations, or misread by the hypothalamus or the pituitary, then normal cyclical ovarian function ceases, resulting in anovulation with oligomenorrhea or amenorrhea.

Primary Amenorrhea

Primary amenorrhea is present when there is no menstruation by age 14 years, with associated absence of development of secondary sexual characteristics, or by age 16 years, despite the appearance of secondary sexual characteristics. Primary amenorrhea presents the same diagnostic principles present in secondary amenorrheas but requires consideration of Müllerian abnormalities (imperforate hymen) or Müllerian agenesis, testicular feminization, and gonadal causes in over half of the cases.

Turner's syndrome, a major cause of primary amenorrhea, consists of a 45X chromosome single cell line, but mosaicism and partial deletions of one X chromosome may occur (see chapter 8). The clinical characteristics will vary from the typical short stature, hypoestrinism, webbed neck, shield chest, and cubitus valgus, to near normal features. There may be associated aortic coarctation, renal collecting system abnormalities, and Hashimoto's thyroiditis. Elevated serum gonadotrophins indicate ovarian disease. Replacement cyclical estrogen plus progesterone therapy is required at the time of late adolescence.

Secondary Amenorrhea

Secondary amenorrhea is a common symptom and should be approached in an organized fashion. The history may point directly to the etiologic factor, when amenorrhea is associated with severe weight loss (nutritional amenorrhea), severe emotional disorders (psychologic hypothalamic amenorrhea), severe postpartum hemorrhage (Sheehan's syndrome), oligoamenorrhea extending back to the menarche (suggestive of the polycystic ovary syndrome), a surgical procedure such as a uterine curettage (traumatic loss of endometrium), and other obvious associations. Physical examination may reveal evidence of a pituitary tumor, the presence of galactorrhea, or the presence of extensive hirsutism.

Etiology

Three common causes of amenorrhea are weight loss, hyperestrogenized amenorrhea (polycystic ovary [PCO] syndrome), and hyperprolactinemia.

1. The patient with weight loss is identified by history. Usually there is rapid and dramatic weight loss, to a level close to or even below what the weight was at the time of the menarche. Possibly on a nutritional basis there is resultant amenorrhea, and the physiology is very similar to the prepubertal state. The FSH and LH levels fall, with low LH to FSH ratio. The patient is hypoestrogenized and does not show a withdrawal response to progestational agents. The same abnormality appears to occur in other hypothalamic causes of amenorrhea, such as severe emotional stress. In anorexia nervosa the amenorrhea may precede the weight loss.

2. The hyperestrogenized amenorrhea associated with a high LH to FSH ratio and withdrawal bleeding after progesterone administration, indicates that the entire reproductive axis is functioning but no longer in a cyclic manner. This may reflect enhanced secretion of estrogens with an increase in LH without an increase in FSH, with resultant continued and enhanced stimulation of ovarian androgen and estrogen secretion. A vicious cycle is established with loss of the cyclical pattern, presenting with oligomenorrhea. This may occur in the PCO syndrome or severe obesity.

3. Hyperprolactinemic amenorrhea may be due to a primary hypersecretory prolactin state (pituitary adenoma or hyperplasia); prolactin may be secondarily elevated due to another cause (medications, hypothyroidism). The pattern usually simulates that of number 1 above, but with hyperprolactinemia (see previous section, Hyperprolactinemia).

In most instances, no specific underlying cause is identifiable, so that a logical sequential investigation is indicated as depicted in Figure 13.3. Women who do not have occasional spontaneous menstrual bleeding but who show withdrawal bleeding after the administration of a progestational agent, clearly have a uterus with an endometrium capable of responding to ovarian steroids, with evidence of some endogenous estrogen activity. In these patients there is evidence of at least some ovarian activity, and the presence of some normal hypothalamic GnRH activity sufficient for pituitary stimulation. Conversely, if after the administration of a progestational agent withdrawal bleeding does not occur, then combined treatment with both estrogen and progesterone is utilized to determine whether uterine bleeding can be induced. If bleeding occurs it indicates the presence

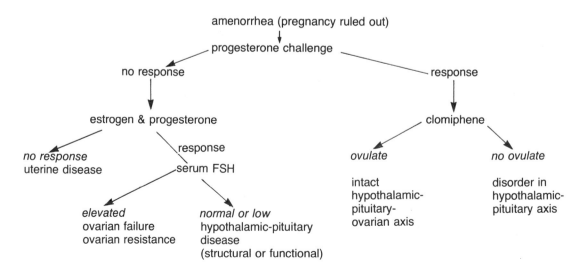

Fig. 13.3 Mechanisms and Assessment of Amenorrhea.

of a uterus capable of response and ovaries that do not provide the required estrogen. Failure of uterine bleeding indicates a local gynecologic cause.

Decreased ovarian secretion may be differentiated from central causes by the serum FSH, which is elevated in the former and inappropriately normal or even low in the latter. The group with elevated serum FSH levels may have ovarian failure (premature menopause), or the resistant ovary syndrome, which may only be identified by biopsy of the ovaries. The patients with inappropriately normal or low serum FSH levels have abnormalities of the pituitary or hypothalamus.

EVALUATION OF THE MENSTRUAL CYCLE

Investigation of Gonadotropin Secretion

1. LH and FSH levels may be measured in the serum at any time during the menstrual cycle. The absolute concentrations vary from day to day throughout the cycle, and, due to episodic secretion, they can vary from hour to hour. It is more important to estimate the LH to FSH ratio than the individual levels. Early in the menstrual cycle when the estrogen levels are the lowest, the serum FSH is relatively higher, and the LH to FSH ratio is relatively low. In the preovulatory phase, when the estrogen levels are the highest, the serum LH is relatively higher than the FSH, and the LH to FSH ratio is high.

2. The clomiphene test is used to evaluate the integrity of the hypothalamic-pituitary axis (see also Fig. 13.3, Table 13.5). This agent acts by stimulating the negative feedback response, since it is an estrogen antagonist. If there is a normal response of FSH and LH to clomiphene, then the hypothalamic-pituitary axis is intact (this requires pubertal maturation, since the prepubertal child or an adult whose "set point" has regressed to the prepubertal level will not respond). If ovulation and menstruation occurs in response to clomiphene, then the entire hypothalamic-pituitary-ovarian axis is normal, including the midcycle estrogen modulation to produce the LH surge.

3. Estrogen administration may be used to determine whether there is an LH surge 12 to 36 hours following the administration. This directly tests the estrogen-induced modulation of LH secretion.

4. The GnRH test involves the administration of synthetic GnRH, to determine whether there is release of LH and FSH. Since the gonadotrophic cells may lose their acute responsiveness to GnRH, a negative response may not distinguish a pituitary from a hypothalamic hypogonadotropic state.

Investigation of Ovarian Function

Estrogen secretion may be directly assessed by performing a maturation index on cells in the vaginal smear, studying the cervical mucus, endometrial biopsy, or by determining whether there is withdrawal bleeding in response to progesterone administration. This last test has a high correlation with the presence of normal adult serum estradiol levels. Direct methods measure estrogens either in the urine or plasma under basal conditions. Primary ovarian disease may be inferred by identifying decreased estrogen secretion despite an elevated serum FSH concentration.

Investigation of the luteal phase involves progesterone measurement in the serum or urine, daily measurement of basal body temperature as an indirect assessment of luteal function, or endometrial biopsy demonstrating secretory endometrium.

HIRSUTISM

Hair is regarded as excessive when it grows coarser, longer, or more profusely than is normal for the age, sex, and race of the individual. Hair follicles occur all over the body, except on the palms and the soles. The distribution is the same in both sexes, with only the degree of hormone-dependent hair growth distinguishing the male from the female pattern. In women, hirsutism generally means the excessive growth of sexual or hormone-dependent hair, and implies enhanced androgenic biologic activity. The degree of hirsutism that is considered unacceptable to the female is to some extent determined by the norm of the culture. Two basic types of hair occur in the human body, vellus hair, which is soft, nonpigmented, and rarely more than 2 cm long, and terminal hair, which is coarser and pigmented, and continues to grow. Hair follicles are merely dormant, and in certain circumstances may be stimulated to grow hair by the action of dihydroxytestosterone. *Virilization* refers to changes in androgen-sensitive structures (such as the external genitalia) in response to excessive levels of biologically active androgen, and invariably reflects a pathologic state with implications beyond simple hirsutism (see Chapter 19).

Etiology

The causes of hirsutism in the adult female include the following:

1. Idiopathic hirsutism is a heterogenous group. The diagnosis is usually one of exclusion. Menstrual abnormalities are usually not present, and fertility is

not impaired. Acne may be present, but is mild. There may be a positive family history of similar problems or a racial component. The present data suggests that mild ovarian hypersecretion of androgens underlies this cause, which may merely be a mild form of the spectrum of the polycystic ovary syndrome.

2. Adrenal causes. Typical patients with congenital adrenal hyperplasia usually present with prepubertal hirsutism, but milder forms, referred to as adult-onset adrenal virilism, may occur postpubertally; these are very difficult to differentiate from ovarian causes of hirsutism. Under normal circumstances, the adrenal cortex secretes a variety of androgens, most of which have little androgenic effect; but some of these are peripherally converted to testosterone. Measurement of plasma dehydroepiandrosteronesulfate (DHEA-S) may reflect any adrenal contribution to the androgen levels, since 95 percent of this steroid is derived from adrenal secretion. Primary hypersecretion of androgens may arise from adrenal carcinoma, or from Cushing's syndrome.

3. Ovarian causes. The polycystic ovary syndrome includes a group of physiologic and pathologic abnormalities consisting of menstrual irregularities, infertility, and microscopic ovarian changes. Mean blood levels of total testosterone (reflecting the bound and the "free" levels) may be normal, but the free testosterone levels and ovarian production rate are usually higher than in normal women. Peripheral conversion of these androgens to estrogens may occur. This extraglandular estrogen production may interfere with normal hypothalamic-pituitary-ovarian cyclical activity and result in oligoamenorrhea. Because of the hyperestrogenized state with resultant changes in gonadotropin secretion, the basal FSH is usually normal while the basal LH is usually elevated, producing a high LH to FSH ratio.

Other ovarian lesions producing hirsutism are rare, for example, ovarian tumors. The more dramatic onset and rapid progression of hirsutism, with associated features of virilization, indicate the ominous underlying nature of an ovarian tumor.

4. Medication-induced hirsutism occurs with two types of drugs:

    A. Drugs in which hirsutism is an unexpected complication, such as Dilantin, diazoxide, and minoxidil. These agents produce growth of hair primarily over the face, the trunk, and the extremities, and is usually reversible with drug withdrawal. The mechanism is unknown.

    B. Drugs in which hirsutism is an undesirable but predictable effect. These include anabolic agents, progestational agents, androgens, glucocorticoids, and ACTH.

5. Certain miscellaneous disorders have hair growth as an accompanying element, such as porphyria, juvenile hypothyroidism, acromegaly, and anorexia nervosa. The abnormal hair growth is not selectively concentrated over the areas of sexual (androgen) distribution.

Clinical Approach to Diagnosis

The investigation begins with a full history and physical examination to detect the presence of associated disorders and medication ingestion, as well as to assess the extent of severity of the hirsutism. Laboratory tests may be used to assess the biochemical abnormalities and possibly to localize the site of androgen excess. A high LH to FSH ratio suggests, but is not specific for, underlying polycystic ovary syndrome. The urinary 17-ketosteroids may be utilized to determine the possible presence of excess adrenal secretion of androgens, but ovarian androstanedione secretion may also produce this elevation. If Cushing's syndrome is suspected, then the urinary free cortisol may also be measured. Plasma testosterone may be measured, but does not adequately reflect the "free" testosterone. Measurement of the "free" testosterone, or even using saliva (an ultrafiltrate of plasma), to measure testosterone may serve as a better measurement of biologic activity. Generally, suppression and stimulation tests have not proven to be highly sensitive for localizing the exact site of the excessive androgen secretion, and have fallen out of favor.

Treatment

The treatment is generally frustrating, since once the hair follicle has been stimulated to change from vellus to terminal hair, it often requires many months after the stimulus is removed before any appreciable change in growth rate occurs. It takes 3 months for a hair to fall out and for a new one to form. Because 10 percent of hairs are in a resting stage at any one time, it may take 30 months to turn over all androgen-sensitive hair. Depending upon the underlying cause, the personal preferences of the patient, and the total clinical situation, the treatment may be in the form of adrenal suppression with glucocorticoids (usually administered at bedtime in physiologic amounts), ovarian suppression with either estrogen or progestational agents, or the utilization of androgen receptor antagonists. The most potent androgen receptor antagonist, cyproterone acetate, is not readily available; spironolactone and cimetidine have both been used in this regard with some success. Progesterone also has properties of androgen receptor antagonism, and may be useful, but it has the side effect of concomitant amenorrhea. When adequate therapy is being instituted, new hair growth may be suppressed and the growth rate of the hair already present may decrease. In order to obtain good cosmetic results with the existing hair, local depilation may still be necessary.

THE MALE REPRODUCTIVE SYSTEM

NORMAL FUNCTION

Normal reproductive and sexual function in males requires the integrated activities of a number of organ systems that make up the reproductive axis. Abnormalities of any one of these components may result in clinically apparent reproductive dysfunction. This dysfunction may become manifest at different times in the patient's life:

1. During embryogenesis, resulting in abnormal sexual differentiation of the genitalia
2. Before sexual maturation at puberty, resulting in failure to attain adult secondary sexual characteristics and reproductive capacity
3. After puberty, resulting in a decline in normal sexual and reproductive function

Embryologic Development

Chromosomal factors direct the differentiation of the indifferent gonad into either an ovary or a testis. The H-Y antigen on the Y chromosome appears to represent the testis-determining factor. The fetal testis, acting via hormones, is then responsible for differentiation of the internal ducts and external genitalia. Testosterone is responsible for virilization of the Wolffian duct system to form the epididymis, vas deferens, and the seminal vesicle. A second factor, Müllerian-inhibiting substance, is responsible for regression of the Müllerian ducts. These two testicular secretions act ipsilaterally. In the absence of a fetal testis, as in the normal female, neither of these substances is secreted, and consequently the Müllerian derivatives form and the Wolffian ducts regress. Testosterone appears to be the intracellular mediator necessary for differentiation of the Wolffian system, whereas dihydrotestosterone is the intracellular hormone responsible for virilization of the urogenital sinus and the external genitalia. The male external genitalia will develop when testosterone is converted to dihydrotestosterone at the target tissue. In the last trimester, testicular descent occurs as the testes move from the internal ring into the scrotum. Endocrine factors play an important part in this migration, and fetal gonadotropin and androgen are necessary.

At early puberty, the tubules enlarge, Leydig cells mature, and active spermatogenesis occurs. At this time the serum FSH concentrations have entered the adult range, and the serum LH concentration begins to slowly increase. There is a concomitant increase in serum testosterone. At midpuberty there is an increase in LH secretion at night, associated with sleep. The early sign of puberty is enlargement of the testicles, and when the testis reaches 2.5 cm in diameter, then growth of the external genitalia is imminent.

The adult testis normally measures 4.5 × 2.5 cm. Isolated damage of the seminiferous tubules produces a soft and small testis. Blood within the internal spermatic arteries cools as it approaches the testes, losing heat to the adjacent venous system by countercurrent heat exchange. This results in scrotal temperature being 2°C less than abdominal temperature, which promotes spermatogenesis. The Sertoli cells line the basement membrane about the seminiferous tubules, and appear to perform local functions necessary for spermatogenesis. One substance secreted by the Sertoli cell is a high-affinity binding protein for testosterone and dihydrotestosterone, called androgen-binding protein. This generates a diffusion potential that results in accumulation of androgen in the immediate environment of the germ cells. The secretion of this androgen-binding protein appears to be regulated by testosterone and FSH. The germinal epithelium consists of spermatogenic cells arranged in an orderly manner, and through a series of mitotic divisions the spermatogonia differentiate eventually into spermatids, each of which then matures into a spermatozoon. The time necessary to produce the spermatozoon is 74 days. The Leydig cells are the principle source of testosterone production. The local production of testosterone is important for spermatogenesis; testosterone levels about 20 times higher than plasma are necessary to induce and complete spermatogenesis.

The first sign of puberty is an increase in testicular size. Pubic hair appears early, initially stimulated by adrenal androgens and then by testicular androgens. The penis gradually increases in size, the scrotum becomes elongated, then rugose and pigmented, and the prostate and seminal vesicles enlarge. Testicular enlargement is primarily gonadotropin-induced, whereas the other changes are the result of increasing testosterone secretion. A linear skeletal growth spurt, axial greater than appendicular, occurs after the appearance of pubic hair and testis enlargement. Increasing androgen secretion also results in increasing musculature, deepening of the voice (due to an enlarged larynx), increase in body hair, increase in libido, and a change in behavior. Temporary gynecomastia may appear, may be asymmetrical, and may persist from one to two years.

THE REPRODUCTIVE HORMONAL AXIS

Areas of the central nervous system such as the amygdala have receptors for gonadal steroids, and may modify hypothalamic pituitary function. An example would be depressed serum testosterone levels in mentally stressed men. The hypothalamus translates neural messages from the CNS and humoral messages from the testes to modulate GnRH secretion and, thereby, gonadotropin secretion. The anterior pituitary secretes FSH and LH episodically throughout the day. The magnitude of these pulses is dependent upon factors such as age, sex, and steroid hormone levels. FSH primarily controls spermatogenesis. LH stimulates testosterone synthesis by the Leydig cells of the testes and thereby maintains spermatogenesis. There is a synergism between FSH and LH, as FSH stimulates the production of LH receptors. It is possible that in the adult male, nocturnal elevation of serum prolactin may act synergistically with circulating LH to produce the normal nocturnal rise in circulating testosterone. Otherwise prolactin in physiologic amounts does not appear to affect the reproductive axis.

Feedback control involves two substances. There is a negative feedback role for testosterone on LH; the role of steroids on FSH regulation is minimal. Present evidence suggests that the Sertoli cells secrete a substance called inhibin that specifically regulates FSH secretion. In situations of extensive testicular tubular damage (due to radiation, cancer chemotherapy, or the like) there is isolated elevation of serum FSH levels, but no changes in serum LH levels as long as the Leydig cells continue to secrete normal amounts of testosterone.

Testosterone circulates in the blood bound to sex-hormone–binding globulin. Only a small fraction circulates in the unbound form, but it is this "free" concentration that is responsible for the biologic activity. The urinary 17-ketosteroid secretion is not a reliable guide to the secretion of testosterone. A better measurement of testosterone production is the plasma testosterone levels, and the free component can be estimated by direct measurement, or by measurement in saliva, which is an ultrafiltrate of plasma. Androgens pass through the plasma membrane of the target cell, as do other steroids, to bind to a specific receptor protein in the cytosol; this complex is then transferred to the nucleus. Testosterone appears to be a prohormone and must first be reduced to dihydrotestosterone to exert its androgenic (but not anabolic) effects. This conversion occurs in most androgen-dependent tissue, with the exception of muscle anabolic action.

MALE HYPOGONADISM

Clinical Manifestations

If testicular failure occurs before puberty, then pubertal changes will not develop. In addition to sexual infantilism there is delayed epiphyseal closure, which allows continued long-bone growth resulting in the typical eunuchoid habitus. In this situation the armspan (fingertip to fingertip) is more than 5 cm greater than the height, and the measurement from the pubis to floor is 5 cm greater than the measurement from the pubis to the top of the head. Roentgenograms will demonstrate the delay in closure of the epiphyses. There will be a concomitant lack of adult male hair distribution, and failure of scalp hair to recede. A high pitched voice persists and the genitalia are prepubertal.

Hypogonadism in the adult male may be suspected by noting a beard distribution that is abnormally reduced or an abnormal distribution of body hair. Facial change occurs in the adult male, similar to the changes seen in an estrogen-deprived female. Typically, this consists of fine linear creases extending outward from the corners of the mouth and the eyes. Testicular size is decreased; any testis less than 4 cm in length is abnormal. In such a testis, tubular function would be expected to be abnormal, since 90 percent of the testicular volume is composed of spermatic tubules. Age of the adult does not influence the testicular size. There may be symptoms of impotence, decreased libido, and a decreased amount of fluid in the ejaculate that may indicate concomitant Leydig cell failure. Gynecomastia may also indicate decreased androgen secretion.

The causes of hypogonadism are set out in Table 13.9.

Abnormalities in Hypothalamic-Pituitary Function

Abnormal hypothalamic-pituitary function is implicated by the presence of clinically recognizable hypogonadism with concomitant low blood concentrations of LH and/or FSH. This may be part of a

Table 13.9 Male Hypogonadism

Site	Cause	Syndrome
Hypothalamus	GnRH deficiency	Kallman's
		Prader-Willi
	Hypothalamic disease	sarcoidosis, and others
Pituitary	LH/FSH deficiency	hypopituitarism
	LH deficiency	Fertile eunuch
	Prolactin excess	decreased libido, oligospermia
Testes	Leydig cell dysfunction	Klinefelter's, anorchia
		acquired destructive disease
	Enzyme deficiency	decreased testosterone synthesis
	Germinal cell failure	oligospermia—idiopathic,
		mumps, and others
Target Organs	Decreased receptors	complete or incomplete testicular
		feminization
	5-α-reductase deficiency	Imperato-McGinley

global anterior pituitary disturbance (panhypopituitarism) or due to isolated LH or FSH deficiency. Any patient with hypogonadism of this nature should be adequately studied for the ability of the pituitary to secrete its other tropic hormones. Isolated GnRH secretion may coexist with hyposmia or anosmia (Kallman's syndrome), which may be familial. Decreased hypothalamic GnRH secretion may also result from functional hypothalamic disorders (emotional changes, weight changes) or structural disease. Further, hyperprolactinemia will result in decreased hypothalamic GnRH secretion with resultant decreased stimulation of pituitary gonadotropin secretion. Isolated LH deficiency (the "fertile eununch" syndrome) may result in the absence of Leydig cell activity but the presence of some spermatogenesis on testicular biopsy; testosterone secretion improves after treatment with HCG (which has LH-like activity).

Primary Gonadal Abnormalities

Errors in Testicular Development

1. Klinefelter's syndrome is a common cause of male hypogonadism occurring in 1 of 500 newborn males. The syndrome is a spectrum ranging from men who seem almost indistinguishable from normal to men who are blatantly hypogonadal. All of these men have at least two X and one Y chromosomes in some of their cells. Classical karyotype for Klinefelter's syndrome is XXY. These patients may appear as phenotypic males with a body build varying from feminine to eunuchoid to normal male, depending on the time of onset and degree of decreased testosterone secretion. An increasing number of X chromosomes appears to correlate with a tendency to increased stature as well as to psychosocial behavioral problems. The main clinical features involve small

firm testes, gynecomastia, and some evidence of decreased androgen secretion. The patients usually present with infertility and delayed puberty, or failure to masculinize in a normal manner.

2. Testicular agenesis (vanishing testis) results in a phenotypic male who is eunuchoid, has no testes palpable, and no testosterone production after HCG stimulation. Postpubertally, the serum FSH and LH levels become elevated. The testes must have been present during embryogenesis to permit regression of the Müllerian ducts and stimulation of the Wolffian ducts, but have regressed after this stage of embryogenesis.

3. Noonan's syndrome (Male Turner's syndrome) results in a phenotypic male with short stature, mental retardation, right-sided cardiac lesions, webbed neck, low set ears, and other anomalies. Usually it is associated with hypogonadism, and undescended testicles.

Defective Testosterone Synthesis Six enzymatic defects have been described that result in impaired androgen synthesis, each of which is transmitted as an autosomal recessive trait. The degree of abnormality of the external genitalia depends on the completeness of the enzyme deficiency, and the clinical expression of such patients may range from nearly normal males with mild hypospadias to individuals having the appearance nearly of normal females.

Seminiferous Tubule Failure Adult seminiferous tubular failure may occur due to drugs, radiation, trauma, inflammation (such as mumps), cryptorchidism, or with developmental defects such as varicocele. Most often it is referred to as idiopathic oligospermia, since no underlying cause is identified. There usually is normal androgenization with normal adult levels of testosterone and LH. Due to isolated oligospermia the testes may be normal in size or small and soft; the serum FSH levels may be normal or elevated, depending on the severity of the defect of spermatogenesis. In the "Sertoli cell only" syndrome, there is total absence of sperm production. In adult seminiferous tubular failure the patient appears normal but presents with infertility.

Defects in Androgen Action   Defects in the tissue action of normally secreted androgens results in men who are not fully androgenized. The clinical spectrum will depend on the tissues affected and the severity of the end-organ defect. The defect is due to absent cytosol receptors for the androgen, to a defect in the transport and binding of the androgen-receptor complex to the nuclear chromatin, or to decreased cellular conversion of testosterone to dihydrotestosterone.

1. Testicular feminization syndrome is a recessive trait, the complete form of which results in the complete biochemical resistance to androgen action, so that XY males show no response to androgens during embryogenesis or throughout life. The patient will therefore present as a phenotypically normal female, will be psychologically female, but amenorrheic and infertile. They undergo feminization at puberty due to both testicular estrogen secretion and peripheral conversion of androgens to estrogens, which results in end-organ response to these estrogens. Axillary and pubic hair do not develop. On examination no cervix is found, due to a blind, short vaginal pouch, and there is no Müllerian duct system (hence no uterus). Often the patient has bilateral inguinal hernias with palpable testes in the inguinal canal. On investigation the patient will show an XY karyotype, normal or elevated serum testosterone, somewhat elevated serum estradiol (for a male), and elevated serum LH. Because of the high incidence of malignancy in these testes, removal of these gonads is recommended, once the patient has been feminized.

2. Male pseudohermaphroditism type I manifests a spectrum ranging from almost complete absence of virilization to moderately hypogonadal males. These patients have an XY karyotype and only incomplete end-organ resistance to androgen action.

3. Male pseudohermaphroditism type II is due to failure of conversion of testosterone to dihydrotestosterone, resulting in failure of external genitalia to differentiate along male lines. Because the genitalia appear female the patients are raised as females, but have male internal genitalia due to the stimulatory effect of testosterone, which is still intact. As these patients reach puberty they develop partial virilization resulting from the increased testosterone secretion. They also become quite muscular, reflecting the anabolic action of testosterone, which does not require conversion to dihydrotestosterone. At this time, absence of female internal genitalia is found, and failure of breast development is noted. Investigations find normal adult male blood levels of LH, FSH, and testosterone. Interestingly, many of these patients convert to a male psyche and go through life as males, despite being raised as females.

4. Some men with severe oligospermia have partial end-organ resistance to androgen.

Clinical Approach to Diagnosis

Investigations of men with hypogonadism begin with the clinical examination. The physical features of decreased testosterone secretion have been described. There may be evidence of somatic features associated with chromosomal abnormalities, signs of pituitary disease, decreased olfactory acuity, or changes in body habitus.

Spermatogenesis may be evaluated by a sperm count. A semen sample is analyzed for volume, number of sperm, motility and morphology, and is a good biologic index of the intact reproductive axis. If chromosomal abnormalities are suspected, then a chromosomal analysis is necessary, since the Barr body assay is too inaccurate, especially in view of the frequent mosaicism (see Chapter 8). Leydig cell function may be assessed by measurement of the plasma testosterone. If decreased plasma testosterone or sperm counts are found, then serum LH or FSH levels should be measured. These are subnormal in pituitary-hypothalamic disorders and elevated with primary testicular disorders. If all is normal and the patient has azoospermia, then a testicular biopsy is useful to see whether this is due to a disorder of spermatogenesis or an obstruction of the outflow tract of the sperm, which may be surgically correctable.

A stimulation test of the reproductive axis may be utilized, with clomiphene to stimulate the hypothalamic GnRH, GnRH injection to stimulate pituitary release of LH and FSH, and human chorionic gonadotropin (HCG) injection to see whether the Leydig cells respond with increased testosterone secretion.

Hyperprolactinemia may present with hypogonadism, and so measurement of the serum prolactin is indicated. If hyperprolactinemia occurs at the time of puberty, it may delay the onset and progression of puberty.

CRYPTORCHIDISM

This is the most common disorder of male sexual differentiation, and may be present in 1 in 200 births. It must be differentiated from present but retractile testes, which has no long-term problems. Patients with true cryptorchidism, either unilateral or bilateral, may have this as a presenting feature of underlying hypogonadism. Further, there is an increased incidence of infertility due to oligospermia as well as an increased incidence (20 times) of malignant testicular tumors. In the cryptorchid testis, Leydig cell function is usually normal, unless there is underlying testicular disease producing the cryptorchidism. Usually inguinal hernias coexist. If these testes remain cryptorchid into adulthood, then they only rarely develop normal seminiferous tubule function, but even if brought down in childhood they are associated with a higher incidence of adult onset oligospermia. To ensure the greatest potential for future fertility as well as to have the testis in a location where it is accessible to be examined for the possibility of tumor development, placement of the testis into the scrotum is usually performed before 6 years of age. Prior to a surgical procedure, it is worthwhile to initially give a trial of HCG injection, since up to 50 percent of testes respond to the increased local testosterone levels and subsequently enter the scrotum. If the testis has become ectopically placed in some subcutaneous pouch, then a surgical approach should be the initial form of therapy.

GYNECOMASTIA

Gynecomastia is a benign glandular enlargement of the male breast, unilateral or bilateral. It occurs in the majority of males at some time during their life span, but is only occasionally clinically significant. Unilateral changes must be differentiated from other causes of breast enlargement, especially local benign and malignant tumors. Tumors will be firm, infiltrating, and nontender. Furthermore, gynecomastia should be differentiated by palpation from a mere local increase of adipose tissue, which is diffuse, bilateral, and not localized just to the region of the areola. Gynecomastia varies in degree from a slight enlargement of tissue under the areola to a manifestation indistinguishable from the adult female breast. Any situation in the adult that results in an enhanced estrogen or decreased androgen secretion (with an increased estrogen to androgen ratio) may result in gynecomastia. This may result from excessive estrogen secretion, excessive peripheral conversion of androgens to estrogens, or decreased estrogen degradation. Excessive estrogen or androgen secretion usually results in an increase in ductal elements accompanied by lobule formation, but if the gynecomastia results from proliferation of the stroma, then usually the underlying sex steroid levels are normal. The causes of gynecomastia are listed in Table 13.10.

Table 13.10   Causes of Gynecomastia

1. Puberty
2. Refeeding—malnourished men with improved nutrition
3. Androgen deficiency—testicular failure, androgen resistance
4. Estrogen excess—iatrogenic, cirrhosis, adrenal tumor, hyperthyroidism
5. Testicular tumors—secrete HCG or estrogen
6. Nonendocrine tumor—secrete HCG
7. Drugs—antiandrogens, estrogens, steroids, phenothiazines
8. Klinefelter's syndrome
9. Idiopathic

When gynecomastia occurs at puberty it may result from rapid changes in hormonal levels, possibly due to a high estrogen to androgen ratio from the new secreting testicle. In situations when the reproductive axis has regressed toward the prepubertal state (such as with starvation or malnutrition), upon correction of this disorder the reproductive axis recovery again stimulates the events of puberty; these patients may develop "refeeding" gynecomastia, which is likely very similar to the pubertal state. Carcinoma of the breast in males with gynecomastia approaches the incidence in normal females, and therefore self-examinations should be taught to these patients.

Treatment

Treatment depends on the underlying cause. If self-limited, then only reassurance is necessary. Often for psychologic reasons, however, cosmetic surgery may be necessary. Antiestrogen agents may be used as an alternative to surgery.

SCROTAL MASSES

Testicular cancer, although uncommon, is the most common solid tumor in men between the ages of 20 and 35 years, and the incidence appears to be increasing. For this reason routine examination as well as home self-examination programs should be directed toward this problem. A scrotal mass should be identified with regard to whether it is a mass within the spermatic cord, a hydrocele, a mass within the epididymis, or a mass within the testicle itself. The most common cause of scrotal swelling is the hydrocele, and it is identified by transillumination. A varicocele produces a worm-like mass in the scrotum that disappears in a recumbent position. The benign varicoceles are invariably on the left side. If one is present on the right side, or if there is sudden development of a varicocele, an underlying obstruction of the inferior vena cava should be considered.

The malignant testicular tumors are usually found as palpable mass or unusual firmness of the testicle. If a suspicious mass is detected, then surgical exploration should be undertaken. There may be associated HCG secretion, resulting in gynecomastia, and this is useful as a tumor marker. If the mass is within an undescended testicle, the risk of malignancy is enhanced (see also Chapter 5).

DISORDERED CARBOHYDRATE METABOLISM: DIABETES MELLITUS AND HYPOGLYCEMIA

DIABETES MELLITUS

The metabolic consequences of decreased amounts of effective insulin action are recognized clinically as diabetes mellitus. *Type I* diabetes (ketosis prone) is usually associated with absolute deficiency of insulin due to degeneration of the pancreatic beta cells. *Type II* diabetes (nonketotic) is most often associated with a relative deficiency of insulin due to decreased insulin action.

Various factors may result in diabetes mellitus:

1. Loss of pancreatic beta cells due to surgery, trauma, inflammation, hemochromatosis, or the like. Type I or juvenile diabetes has an unknown etiology, but it is now thought that various immunologic, viral, or toxic factors may give rise to beta-cell degeneration in genetically predisposed people. Islet cell antibodies may be detected, and it is now clear that there is an autoimmune basis in many cases resulting in beta-cell degeneration. The risk of developing juvenile onset diabetes is highly associated with certain genetically determined histocompatibility antigens (HLA-Dw3 and Dw4).

2. Inadequate stimulus to insulin synthesis and release, such as with certain gut hormone deficiencies, or inhibition of insulin secretion by catecholamines, Dilantin, diazoxide, or other agents.

3. Factors that may decrease the effectiveness of insulin:

   A. Decreased numbers of insulin receptors, as seen in obesity, acromegaly, myotonic dystrophy, and other disorders.

   B. Insulin-receptor antibodies, as in acanthosis nigricans.

   C. Decreased insulin action after binding to the receptor, as in hypokalemia, uremia, and other disorders.

4. Increased insulin requirements, as seen in hyperthyroidism.

5. Increased insulin degradation, as occurs in the placenta during a normal pregnancy.

6. Factors that increase blood glucose levels as a result of gluconeogenesis and glycogenolysis, such as cortisol, glucagon, or epinephrine.

It is now recognized that diabetes mellitus is a heterogeneous disorder with respect to its clinical presentation, natural history, etiology, and genetics.

Carbohydrate metabolism involves hormone mechanisms in the intestine, stomach, and pancreas. This knowledge led to a concept of the gastro-entero-pancreatic endocrine system.

Insulin is produced in the endoplasmic reticulum of the beta cell and is stored in the granules as proinsulin; it is then split into the native insulin and C-peptide fragments, which are released into the portal vein and then passed to the liver (about 50 percent is removed) and to the general circulation. Insulin secretion is stimulated by nutrients (glucose, amino acids), or hormones (glucagon, beta andrenergic activity, gastric inhibitory polypeptide). Gastric inhibitory polypeptide has a role in enhancing the secretory response to ingested food. Insulin secretion is inhibited by the lack of nutrients (fasting, hypoglycemia) and by other hormones (somatostatin and alpha adrenergic activity). Glucose is the most potent stimulus for insulin secretion, but the response is biphasic, with an initial rapid secretory burst resulting from the release of preformed insulin within the storage granules, and then a later, more steady release from newly synthesized insulin. The peripheral action of insulin depends on the availability of receptor sites. As insulin binds to its receptor, it activates a transport system for glucose, amino acids, and ions. Further insulin effects appear to be mediated by internalization of the insulin-receptor complex, which then appears to act as a second messenger to affect intracellular enzyme function. Insulin sensitivity, therefore, depends on the number of receptors on the cells and the affinity of these receptors for insulin. Obesity, for example, results in a decreased number of receptors, and thus brings about a hyperinsulinemic state. But hyperglycemia still occurs in patients genetically predisposed to diabetes mellitus.

As an overall metabolic concept, insulin results in nutrient storage as it promotes synthesis of glycogen, protein, and fat, while preventing their mobilization. Thus, insulin action will result in decreased plasma glucose, fatty acids, amino acids, potassium, and inorganic phosphate.

In response to eating, there will be an elevation in blood metabolites and gut hormone release, which will result in the initial and later release of insulin. In response to this, the liver takes up glucose and synthesized glycogen, inhibits the processes of gluconeogenesis and ketogenesis, and changes over to lipogenesis. By this mechanism any excess calories are converted into triglycerides by the liver and then stored in adipose tissue. In the fed state with the rise of insulin, there is glucose uptake in the muscle and glycogen synthesis, as well as protein synthesis from the now available amino acids. The adipose tissue responds to the rise in insulin by increasing glucose uptake, lipid synthesis and storage, and by inhibition of lipid mobilization.

Glucagon is secreted from the alpha cells of the islets. It promotes hepatic glucose production both by glycogenolysis and gluconeogenesis. It also activates adipose tissue lipase, which results in lipolysis with subsequent release of fatty acids and glycerol. The primary stimulus for glucagon secretion is a decrease in plasma glucose, and it is suppressed by a rise of plasma glucose. Other influences such as amino acids, especially arginine and alanine, stimulate glucagon release. Thus, glucagon and insulin are the major modulators of plasma glucose levels. Glucagon secretion appears to be enhanced in diabetes, and it is not suppressed by glucose. Whether this represents a primary abnormality of diabetes, or whether it is just secondary to the uncontrolled carbohydrate metabolism, is not clear. The fact that glucagon levels and the suppressibility of glucagon normalize after vigorous control of the diabetes suggest that its hypersecretion is likely secondary to the altered metabolic state.

Recent studies have demonstrated that mechanical insulin delivery systems which reproduce normal patterns of insulin release, can normalize the disordered metabolism of glucose, fat, and protein. The abnormal basal and stimulated levels of glucagon, catecholamines, and growth hormone also were normalized. This indicates that decreased effective insulin action is the main underlying factor in the disordered metabolic state of diabetes.

In the fasting state, insulin levels fall appropriately, the adipose tissue releases free fatty acids, and the muscle releases amino acids. The liver responds with appropriate glycogenolysis and gluconeogenesis, to maintain normal concentrations of blood sugar for use by tissues such as the brain. The rise in circulating fatty acids allows them to be used as a fuel by muscle.

Clinical Manifestations

With the onset of decreased insulin action (diabetes mellitus), these normal control mechanisms deteriorate, first after feeding and eventually even in the fasting stage. Increased fatty acid and amino acid release from the adipose tissue and muscle, and gluconeogenesis by the liver, results in hyperglycemia, and then glycosuria. The loss of glucose in the urine is associated with loss of water, electrolytes, and, of course, calories. The patient suffers weight loss, polyuria, polydipsia, and nonspecific fatiguability. With a further decrease in effective insulin action, lipolysis and ketogenesis occurs with ultimate ketoacidosis. By this stage the patient becomes susceptible to infections, usually due to *Staphylococcus aureus*, as well as fungal infections such as moniliasis. Thus, the patient may present with recurrent furuncles or with moniliasis. The osmotic changes secondary to hyperglycemia may alter the shape of the lens, and the patient may present with blurring of vision.

With further deterioration in the effectiveness of insulin, more and more ketone bodies are produced. As these accumulate, the patient becomes ketotic; the symptom of polyphagia may change to nausea and anorexia. Because the ketone bodies are acidic, the patient becomes acidotic, and this stage is referred to as *ketoacidosis*. The patient is hyperglycemic, dehydrated due to the osmotic diuresis (which also removes sodium and potassium), and in a state of protein catabolism whereby the amino acids are utilized as gluconeogenic precursors. Uncontrolled lipolysis occurs, with glycerol used as a gluconeogenetic precursor, and the free fatty acids result in ketone production.

The clinical signs in patients with ketoacidosis are hypothermia (conversely, hyperthermia indicates an underlying infection as a possible precipitating factor), increased respiratory rate with an increased depth of respiration (Kussmaul breathing), acetone odor on the breath, and decreased effective circulating fluid volume (with tachycardia, postural hypotension, and collapsed neck veins in the supine position. This may progress to stupor, focal or generalized neurologic signs, and coma. Thus, electrolyte and water disturbances observed in this condition include volume depletion, acidosis, potassium abnormalities (typically hyperkalemia with total body potassium depletion), and hyperglycemia with its hyperosmolar state. With adequate treatment the prognosis is generally good, and is related more to the underlying precipitating cause than to the ketoacidosis itself.

Laboratory Diagnosis

In the presence of overt diabetic symptoms associated with glycosuria, an unequivocal elevation of the serum glucose is adequate to make the diagnosis of diabetes mellitus. In the absence of overt symptoms, a fasting serum glucose greater than 150 mg/dl is virtually diagnostic. If fasting hyperglycemia is not high enough to be diagnostic, then a random 2-hour postprandial serum glucose greater than 180 mg/dl is suggestive. An oral glucose tolerance test (OGTT) may be necessary to diagnose the presence of glucose intolerance. Thus, the indication for the OGTT includes those patients in whom there are borderline screening serum glucose levels, or, as a more provocative test, in patients at risk of becoming diabetic (such as obese patients, patients with strong family history of diabetes), or in patients who present with complications that may be secondary to diabetes (such as neuropathy, women with large babies, or other complications). Criteria for the interpretation of the glucose tolerance test should be obtained from the local laboratories. The patient should have adequate dietary preparation, since carbohydrate restriction may temporarily impair hepatic glucose uptake, and thus produce a somewhat abnormal OGTT. Certain drugs may impair glucose tolerance, such as thiazide diuretics (or their derivatives), diphenylhydantoin, and the glucocorticoids. Further, hypokalemia may produce the picture of glucose intolerance by impairing the beta cell response to the glucose load. An excessive amount of counterregulatory hormones may decrease the effective insulin action and impair glucose tolerance, as occurs with acromegaly, Cushing's syndrome, aldosteronism, glucagonoma, pheochromocytoma, and thyrotoxicosis. Because many factors other than diabetes may cause abnormal fasting serum glucose, or an abnormal glucose tolerance test, unless there is overt symptomatic diabetes mellitus, the abnormality should be demonstrated more than once to ensure the correct diagnosis.

Gestational diabetes refers to the onset of glucose intolerance during pregnancy, when the intolerance has not been present prior to pregnancy. In most cases, the glucose tolerance returns to normal after delivery. Such patients are at an increased risk of perinatal mortality and morbidity; clinical recognition of the gestational diabetes mellitus and appropriate therapy improves these risks. Further, these women are at a high risk for developing diabetes several years after delivery, and should be followed clinically with that in mind. Glycosuria is common in normal pregnancy due to changes in renal handling of glucose. Therefore, in patients suspected of having gestational diabetes, the fasting serum glucose concentrations as well as the OGTT are required. The criteria are somewhat altered during pregnancy. The fasting glucose concentration is generally lower than in the nonpregnant woman because the fetus utilizes maternal glucose, and the glucose clearance after OGTT is delayed.

Complications of Diabetes Mellitus

Acute complications include infection, ketoacidosis, or nonketotic hyperosmolar coma. The more chronic complications of diabetes mellitus are related to large- and small-vessel disease. Atherosclerotic changes seen in the large vessels of diabetics are qualitatively not different but quantitatively more extensive than in nondiabetics. The small vessel disease (microangiopathy) is relatively unique to diabetes. This involves accumulation of PAS-stainable material within the vessel walls, endothelial proliferation, and basement-membrane thickening. The actual mechanism for these microvascular changes is controversial; it has been suggested that they are related to the primary genetic nature of diabetes mellitus; but the generally held view is that they are secondary to the metabolic changes. High serum glucose with conversion to sorbitol and fructose within the lens of the eye, with the resultant osmotic changes within the cells, contributes to the cataracts that form with increased frequency in diabetics. Whether or not this mechanism is responsible for microvascular changes, or whether glucosylation of proteins has a role is yet to be determined. The microangiopathic changes may conspicuously involve the vasculature of the kidneys, the retina, and the nerves (resulting in nephropathy, retinopathy, and neuropathy).

Cardiovascular System

Coronary artery disease is present in a higher incidence in the diabetic population, and is a manifestation of the large vessel atherosclerosis. Females do not appear to have any singular resistance to coronary artery disease, unlike that observed in the nondiabetic population. Diabetic cardiomyopathy may contribute to heart failure in diabetes. More extensive atherosclerosis in the diabetic population produces cerebral and peripheral vascular disease.

Kidneys

The diabetic kidney has increased risk of infection (pyelonephritis), renal artery atherosclerosis with resultant hypertension, and diabetic glomerulosclerosis. This last complication is related to the duration of the disease, but may show rapid deterioration after clinical evidence of the nephropathy appears. Patients with progressive deterioration may initially develop proteinuria, and then hypertension, nephrotic syndrome, and finally renal failure. Such patients may either be treated with chronic dialysis or renal transplantation, while transplantation is the treatment of choice. It appears that patients on chronic hemodialysis have, if anything, an acceleration of their atherosclerotic state, worsening of the retinopathy, and generally a worse prognosis than the transplanted patients.

Eyes

Diabetic retinopathy appears to be a compensatory mechanism for retinal ischemia. It may occur as the initial presentation of diabetes, but usually has its clinical onset after several years of overt diabetes. Microaneurysms seen on ophthalmologic examination may be associated with neovascularization, and hemorrhages from rupture of new small blood vessels. Decreased visual acuity results from accumulation of edema at the posterior pole of the eye, and responds to photocoagulation therapy; photocoagulation is also useful for control of retinitis proliferans. Exudates result from plasma leakage and lipid accumulation due to ischemia of the vessel wall. Ingrowth of connective tissue may occur after hemorrhage into the vitreous fluid. Contraction of the fibrous tissue may give rise to retinal detachment. Cataracts may occur due to changes in lens metabolism.

Peripheral Nerves

Neuropathies usually involve the sensory nerves, resulting in impaired sensation or parasthesia. Such involvement of the peripheral nerves is usually symmetrical. There may also be a more segmental neuropathy arising from involvement of nerve roots, or a single cranial or spinal nerve. If motor endplates are involved, with a loss of muscle, amyotrophy may occur. The mononeuropathies are of a fairly sudden onset, are usually self-limited, and frequently involve the extraocular muscles, resulting in diplopia. The underlying cause may be a microinfarct. There may be diffuse involvement of the autonomic nervous system. Autonomic neuropathy may result in impotence, nocturnal diarrhea, gastroparesis postural hypotension, and less sweating. A severe deep unrelenting pain may result from neuropathies. This responds poorly to analgesics, but may respond to carbamazepine or tricyclic antidepressants.

Foot Complications

The *diabetic foot* may reflect a combination of several of these mechanisms. Neuropathy may alter the position of weight-bearing and blunt the sensation that would otherwise detect the early lesion. The change in weight bearing and painless injury may result in ulceration, with secondary infection and gangrene, which is potentiated by the vascular insufficiency. Ultimately amputation may become necessary.

Complications in Pregnancy

The pregnant diabetic woman is prone to more complications than the pregnant nondiabetic woman. It appears that the glucose intolerance in early stages of pregnancy predisposes to an increased incidence of congenital malformations; good diabetic control in the first two months of pregnancy (during organogenesis) decrease the incidence of congenital abnormalities. As pregnancy progresses, the diabetic woman is more at risk for preeclampsia and hydramnios. Poor control results in large babies, which tend to be somewhat immature at delivery and are more at risk for respiratory distress of the newborn. Proper obstetrical care of the diabetic patient requires close collaboration by various members of the health team; the timing of delivery is crucial, and needs to be monitored by modern assessments of amniotic fluid and by ultrasound. The delivery should be timed in relation to the severity of the woman's diabetes and diabetic complications.

Infectious Complications

Infection in the diabetic may have marked effects on the metabolic state, occasionally producing ketoacidosis. Therefore, any infection should be rapidly treated. Some studies have suggested that the poorly controlled diabetic has impairment in host defenses. The legs and feet are prone to infection, and ulcers due to local vascular and neurologic impairments are common. If not contained, the cutaneous infection may lead to osteomyelitis and even to amputation. Vigorous antibiotic therapy (usually a penicillinase-resistant penicillin and an aminoglycoside) and surgical debridement are needed. The skin is generally prone to staphylococcal furuncles, and mucous membranes often develop infections due to candida albicans.

Upper and lower urinary tract infections may occur, especially in the presence of a neurogenic bladder. Catheterization of diabetics should therefore be avoided if at all possible.

Whether the control of diabetes will prevent the chronic complications is not established. Because these complications may not have the same pathogenic basis, and since genetic factors as well as other unknown factors may have an important role in the pathogenesis of some of these complications, it is possible that treating the hyperglycemia itself may not prevent the long-term sequelae of diabetes mellitus. Even though there is no proof that hyperglycemia itself is responsible for these complications, there is enough suggestive evidence that most diabetologists recommend that control of the glucose intolerance be as rigid as possible (without producing an increased number of hypoglycemia reactions) in an attempt to decrease the development of chronic complications.

Treatment

The objectives for management of diabetes mellitus should be the following:

1. To relieve symptoms of hyperglycemia and uncontrolled diabetes mellitus
2. To avoid undesirable effects of therapy, mainly hypoglycemia
3. To maintain a mean serum glucose as close as possible to normal, with the hope of preventing or delaying the chronic complications of diabetes mellitus

The bases of therapy are diet and exercise, and if these are inadequate to normalize the blood glucose, then a hypoglycemic agent needs to be added, either an oral agent or insulin.

Since almost 90 percent of diabetics are obese, noninsulin dependent, and ketosis resistant (type II), weight reduction is the main aspect of management, and may be the only form of therapy that is required. Exercise is an adjunct to dietary therapy. The obesity decreases the effectiveness of insulin. Weight loss and decreasing size of the adipose tissue cells begins to reverse this abnormality, even with a small weight loss. The diet should comprise a balanced physiologic diet (low in simple carbohydrate, high in fiber), which may correct previously abnormal eating habits and decrease the caloric intake so that weight reduction may occur (if necessary) toward ideal body weight. The diabetic youth must have sufficient calories to allow normal growth. Patient compliance requires education and careful monitoring, with reassurance and frequent follow-up either by the physician or by a diabetic day-care center.

If diet alone is unable to control the symptoms or normalize the serum glucose levels to an adequate level, hypoglycemic agents should be used. Insulin therapy is indicated in patients persistently hyperglycemic despite adequate diet and exercise, in all hyperglycemic pregnant women, and in patients in diabetic ketoacidosis. An intermediate-acting insulin (lente or NPH) is initially used, and about half of insulin-dependent diabetics can be controlled on one dose daily. Others, especially type I diabetics, require the addition of short-acting insulin in the morning, and they may further require twice daily (or even more frequent) injections of intermediate and short-acting insulin. The recent introduction of insulin infusion pumps may further improve control in selected diabetics. Insulin is used to normalize serum glucose levels; however, it is necessary to minimize or avoid its complications (hypoglycemia, allergy, lipoatrophy, lipohypertrophy, and immunologic resistance).

Commercially available insulins are regular, semilente, lente, ultralente, NPH, protamine zinc, and globin. NPH and protamine zinc have the action extended by binding of the molecule to protamine. The lente insulins have extended time action based on crystalline size. Globin insulin is bound to the protein globin. Insulin is obtained from cattle or pigs. The relative compositions of these two species is variable, but both are present in ordinary insulin preparations. Improved purity insulin, termed *single peak insulin*, has resulted from decreasing the proinsulin content of these preparations.

Insulin is absorbed directly into the blood stream, after intramuscular or subcutaneous injections. Only regular insulin can be injected intravenously, due to the presence of particulate matter in all other insulins. Exercise of a limb may result in accelerated absorption of insulin from the injection site. The presence of lipodystrophy apparently does not influence the rate of insulin absorption. About 1 percent of patients may develop local allergic reactions due to the development of an IgE antibody, which usually disappears with continued therapy. Occasionally this may require desensitization or the addition of a glucocorticoid to the insulin mixture. More generalized allergic reactions may occur due to the development of an IgG antibody, and desensitization to insulin is the treatment of choice. Some patients may develop insulin insensitivity after several months, when they develop antibodies directed toward either the injectable insulins or the contaminants of the insulin preparation (proinsulin, protamine, or zinc.) Monocomponent pork insulin is the least antigenic insulin, but allergic reactions, including anaphylaxis, have occured with this preparation. A completely nonantigenic insulin has yet to be developed. Patients with insulin sensitivity may first be tried on pure pork insulin, then monocomponent insulin, sulphated insulins, or high concentration (500 units) CZI; in severe cases patients may need the addition of glucocorticoids. Human insulin may soon be available.

Oral hypoglycemic agents decrease the serum glucose concentrations. Sulfonylureas produce their major action by increasing the sensitivity of the beta cells, and have recently been shown to increase the number of insulin receptors. The biguanides appear to decrease the gastrointestinal absorption of glucose, alter glucose metabolism in the peripheral tissues and the liver, and possibly alter peripheral receptors.

The major indication for the oral hypoglycemic agents is to treat patients with ketosis-resistant diabetes (type II) when the symptoms themselves cannot be controlled with diet. The use of oral hypoglycemic drugs is somewhat controversial, in view of a major multicenter study that indicated enhanced rate of cardiovascular deaths in patients taking these medications compared to the placebo-treated groups. Although this single study should not be taken as definitive evidence against the use of these oral agents, their use should be selective, depending on the clinical situation. The major role of these drugs is as an adjunct to diet, and they should not be used as a substitute for adequate dietary therapy.

The assay for glycosylated hemoglobin (HbA_{1c}) provides an index of diabetic control. Since hemoglobin is glycosylated during periods of high glucose concentration, and the erythrocytes circulate for about 100 days, the test reflects control during the past 3 months. The glycosylated hemoglobin assay is useful especially in type I diabetics with widely fluctuating glucose levels.

Diabetic Ketoacidosis and Hyperosmolar Coma

Decreased consciousness in a diabetic may be related to any other nonmetabolic cause of coma, but specific consideration should be given to ketoacidosis, hyperosmolality, hypoglycemia, and lactic acidosis. Some physicians treat a comatose diabetic with intravenous glucose as a trial of therapy, before establishing the correct diagnosis. This approach is unnecessary, since Dextrostix testing is available in most emergency settings and allows a gross assessment of the level of the blood glucose. Intravenous glucose administration may cause phlebitis or hyperglycemia, and may even precipitate hyperkalemia. True hypoglycemia, on the other hand, should be treated either with intravenous glucose or with intramuscular glucagon. Glucagon is of no value in patients in a state of starvation or who have liver disease.

The patient with ketoacidosis usually requires insulin and correction of water and sodium deficits. Because water losses usually exceed sodium losses, hypotonic saline is used, unless the patient shows signs of deficient circulating fluid volume. Gastric suction may be necessary to relieve gastric dilatation and to decrease the danger of aspiration. In patients with normal renal function, specific correction of the acidosis is usually not necessary, since insulin administration almost immediately decreases ketone production. Rapid reversal of acidosis may be hazardous, since the CSF pH may become acidotic due to diffusion of CO_2, but not bicarbonate, into the CSF. Hyperkalemia is characteristic, and usually responds to insulin administration and correction of the acidosis; after several hours, however, hypoglycemia and hypokalemia may develop. Hypoglycemia is usually avoided by adding 5 percent glucose to the intravenous fluid whenever the plasma glucose drops below 250 mg/dl. Since insulin increases the entry of potassium into cells, the serum potassium falls to the normal range, and addition of potassium to the intravenous fluid (10 to 20 mEq/hour) is necessary. Total body phosphates are also decreased in this state; therefore, the ideal potassium supplement is potassium dihydrogen phosphate.

The initial method of insulin administration to diabetics in ketoacidosis has been highly variable. An effective approach is to administer a bolus intravenous injection of 10 units of regular insulin, followed by a continuous intravenous infusion of about 0.1 units of insulin per kg per hour. Regular monitoring of the patient's clinical status should include the following parameters:

1. Blood pressure
2. Pulse rate
3. Jugular venous pressure
4. Urine output
5. Level of consciousness
6. Plasma glucose
7. The anion gap
8. Serum electrolytes
9. Renal function
10. Hematocrit

These should be charted on a flow sheet. Whatever initial decisions have been made regarding the type and amount of intravenous fluid, the route and amount of insulin, the amount of potassium replacement, and other factors, all may be modified on the basis of the clinical and biochemical response to the therapy. The patient's clinical picture should be reviewed every half hour for the first several hours. As soon as the patient's level of consciousness is adequate, if nausea is not present, oral fluids may be given. If a urinary catheter was initially utilized, this should be removed as soon as the patient is able to void. A search for an underlying precipitating cause, especially an infectious process, should be undertaken at the time of presentation and reassessed at a later time if no initial factor was identified.

The *hyperosmolar syndrome* consists of hyperglycemia resulting in hyperosmolarity with decreased consciousness, without any ketogenesis or serum pH alterations. The severe hyperglycemia usually results in glycosuria with decreased effective circulating fluid volume. The precipitating cause may be infection, other major stress, or drugs that decrease insulin action. The principle of therapy is restoration of fluid volume. Insulin is usually given cautiously, and the hyperglycemia is corrected slowly in an attempt to avoid frank hypoglycemia. Plasma osmolality should be decreased slowly to prevent cerebral edema as a complication. Because these are usually elderly patients, careful monitoring of the venous pressure may be necessary with the restoration of fluid volume.

HYPOGLYCEMIA

To understand the problem and approach to the patient with hypoglycemia (Table 13.11), it is mandatory to understand the basis of carbohydrate metabolism. In normal feeding, dietary carbohydrates are absorbed mainly as glucose. This stimulates insulin secretion into the portal vein, which acts on the liver and then on the peripheral tissues. The net response is to promote glucose uptake by muscle and

---

Table 13.11 **Causes of Hypoglycemia**

1. Hypoglycemia in the fed state (following meals)
   - A. Alimentary—tachyalimentation, previous surgery
   - B. Diabetes mellitus
   - C. Deficiency of counterregulatory hormones
   - D. "Reactive" or "functional"
2. Hypoglycemia in the fasting state
   - A. Inadequate hepatic glucose release
     - Parenchymal hepatic disease
     - Alcohol ingestion in the fasting state
     - Congenital glycogen storage disease
   - B. Insulin excess
     - Insulinoma
     - Exogenous insulin
     - Sulfonylurea ingestion
   - C. Counter regulatory hormone deficiency
     - Growth hormone deficiency
     - Glucocorticoid deficiency
   - D. Extrapancreatic tumors (non insulin secreting)

---

by adipose tissue cells. The hepatic effects are to promote glycogen storage and to inhibit gluconeogenesis. Since the gut absorption of glucose has a finite limit, the serum glucose will fall, resulting in decreased insulin secretion and, at a later time, the release of glucagon and growth hormone. Usually there is an asymptomatic "lag" phase, in which the serum glucose falls below the level prior to glucose ingestion, before the release of counterregulatory hormones and the inhibition of insulin brings the plasma glucose back to the pre-fed level. A random serum glucose measurement about 3 hours after eating may show a level within the "hypoglycemic range," but the patient may show no associated symptoms. If the serum glucose does fall even lower, there is a release of other counterregulatory hormones, such as glucocorticoids and catecholamines; the latter may produce symptoms of postprandial hypoglycemia. These counterregulatory hormones stimulate glycogenolysis and fatty-acid and glycerol mobilization, which allow the serum glucose to return to normal.

Postprandial Hypoglycemias

Hypoglycemic disorders that occur in the postprandial state are usually due to excessive glucose utilization, or to deficiency in the counter regulatory hormones.

In early diabetes mellitus delayed release of insulin may result in excessive levels at the time gut absorption has ceased; this results in a rapid fall of serum glucose and symptoms of hypoglycemia about 4 hours after eating. Patients with alimentary hypoglycemia have increased gut motility, with rapid gastric emptying from previous gastrectomy, other gut surgery, or from unknown idiopathic causes. This results in rapid absorption of glucose and rise in serum glucose levels, resulting in a rapid increased secretion of insulin. Since gut absorption then takes less time, the increased insulin causes a rapid fall in serum glucose, producing symptoms of hypoglycemia about 2 hours postprandially. In some patients, deficiency of counter regulatory hormones may result in failure of the serum glucose to return to normal after the "lag" phase, with symptoms of hypoglycemia at 3 or 4 hours postprandially. The most common postprandial hypoglycemia is "reactive" or idiopathic hypoglycemia. The pathogenesis is unknown, and appears to be an intermittent problem. To make this diagnosis, the patient's symptoms should coincide with the lowest part of the glucose tolerance curve at the "lag" phase, and symptoms produced during the OGTT should reproduce symptoms the patient has noticed. In this manner, the physiologic "lag" phase will not be overinterpreted as symptomatic hypoglycemia, when the symptoms are actually functional, psychoneurotic, or anxiety related.

The treatment of postprandial hypoglycemia is designed to minimize excessive flux of serum glucose in response to eating. Several small meals a day with relatively low carbohydrate content may be utilized, but not all patients respond to this. Simple sugars which are rapidly absorbable should be eliminated. Gastric emptying and intestinal motility may be decreased by anticholinergic drugs that inhibit vagal activity. For patients with associated psychoneurotic features, psychotherapy should accompany any form of therapy.

Fasting Hypoglycemia

Hypoglycemia in the fasting state is a totally different and usually more serious metabolic disorder than in the postprandial state. Most of the organic forms of hypoglycemia occur in the fasting state. When exogenous nutrients are not being ingested, the serum glucose levels are maintained by endogenous glucose production. To allow endogenous production of glucose in the fasting state, there must be adequate hepatic function with the ability to break down glycogen, the appropriate counterregulatory hormones must be present, and appropriate substrates for glucose production and inhibition of basal insulin secretion must be available.

Liver abnormalities due to either acquired liver disease or congenital glycogen storage disease also result in the patient's inability to maintain a normal serum glucose in the fasting state. Alcohol ingestion may produce hypoglycemia in the fasting state, as it appears to inhibit hepatic gluconeogenesis.

The counterregulatory hormones stimulate glycogenolysis (glucagon and epinephrine), provide precursors for glucose production, and induce enzyme activity for gluconeogenesis (cortisol and growth hormone); further, these hormones stimulate the release of free fatty acids and resultant ketones, which may be used as alternate fuel sources. Thus, deficiency of any one of these hormones may present with the inability to maintain a fasting serum glucose, with resultant fasting hypoglycemia.

Extrapancreatic tumors usually fibrosarcomas, or mesenchymal tumors, may also rarely produce fasting hypoglycemia. The mechanism of hypoglycemia is not clear, but may be due to secretion of nonsuppressible insulin-like activity or interference with normal intermediary metabolism. These tumors are massive in size and are usually clinically quite evident.

Increased effective insulin action due to insulin secretion from a beta cell tumor or due to iatrogenic insulin or oral hypoglycemia drugs will result in fasting hypoglycemia. The inappropriate secretion of insulin in the fasting state results in inhibition of hepatic gluconeogenesis, inhibition of peripheral release of precursors for gluconeogenesis and promotion of increased peripheral utilization of glucose. The diagnosis of an insulinoma depends on the finding of an inappropriately elevated insulin level compared with the concomitant serum glucose level. This may be obtained during the time of symptoms, after an overnight or prolonged fast (up to 72 hours), or before and after exercise after a fast (failure to suppress the hormone indicates hypersecretion). In the fasting person depleted of hepatic glycogen, the serum glucose may actually increase with exercise due to release of lactate from muscle metabolism, which the liver may then convert to glucose. The patient with nonsuppressible insulin secretion will not be able to utilize this mechanism, and therefore the serum glucose will actually fall during the exercise.

Clinical Manifestations

The signs and symptoms of hypoglycemia are related to the increased autonomic nervous system activity (tachycardia, anxiety, tremulousness, diaphoresis), as well as to decreased central nervous system function (headache, mental confusion, visual disturbances, and finally, changes of consciousness). If hypoglycemia progresses, the neurologic changes may include focal neurologic signs, seizures, bradycardia, hypothermia, and coma with absent corneal reflexes and fixed dilated pupils. The symptoms and signs depend on the rate, degree, and duration of fall of serum glucose.

Laboratory Diagnosis

The diagnostic approach to a patient with symptoms suggestive of hypoglycemia is, first, to determine whether the symptoms are related to the fed state (postprandial) or to the fasting state. To determine whether or not hypoglycemia is responsible for the symptoms, it is ideal to obtain a serum glucose determination during the particular episode, recognizing that low serum glucose levels may occur naturally in the course of changes in glucose flux throughout the day. If the symptoms are related to food ingestion, then the 5-hour glucose tolerance test is useful to document provocation of symptoms at the lowest level of OGTT. If the symptoms occur during fasting, then measuring simultaneous serum glucose and serum insulin levels after an overnight fast, especially before and after one-half hour of exercise, is a useful screening test. An insulin to glucose ratio of 0.25 is suspicious, and a ratio of 0.50 is almost diagnostic of insulin-induced hypoglycemia. Once hypoglycemia is documented, then the underlying cause should be specifically sought. If an insulinoma is suspected but cannot be proven by insulin and glucose levels after short fasts, long fasts, or after exercise, an insulin suppression test may be used. Administration of insulin to produce hypoglycemia allows measurement of the C-peptide (endogenous insulin) to indicate any suppressibility. Similarly, the administration of fish insulin (not measured by human radioimmunoassays) will produce hypoglycemia, and the endogenous insulin levels may be monitored by the usual fasts.

A patient self-administering insulin (surreptitious insulin administration) may be detected by the absence of C-peptide in the serum, in spite of measureable insulin. This indicates the injection of exogenous insulin, which is separated from C-peptide, quite unlike what occurs with endogenous insulin secretion. Such patients need psychiatric therapy.

Treatment

The treatment of an insulinoma is surgical removal of the tumor. Prior to surgery an elevated serum β-HCG suggests the cause of the hypoglycemia is an islet cell carcinoma. If this cannot be totally removed, then drug therapy is necessary, along with cancer chemotherapy. Drugs that impair beta cell function and reduce hypoglycemia include thiazides, diazoxide, and phenylhydantoin.

METABOLIC BONE DISEASE AND DISORDERS OF CALCIUM

BONE

Bone consists of a matrix (collagen trabeculae, cells, and mucopolysaccharide) impregnated with mineral crystals. Unmineralized matrix is referred to as osteoid. Collagen is a fibrous protein rich in hydroxyproline, which provides the environment for precipitation of calcium salts to form bone. The mineral crystals mainly consist of calcium phosphate but also contain magnesium, sodium, chloride, fluoride, and strontium ions. Fluoride appears to stabilize hydroxyapatite crystal (the calcium-phosphate form in

bone). Bone is analogous to reinforced concrete, with water and mineral (cement) providing compression strength, reinforced by collagen trabeculae (rods) providing tensile strength.

The first formed immature bone is called woven bone, which is metabolically active but lacks the strength of mature (lamellar) bone. Compact cortical bone consists of solid mineralized matrix with vascular channels mainly located in the shafts of long bones (about 80 percent of the skeleton). Spongy or trabecular bone consists of spicules of bone, located in the metaphyses of long bones and the vertebrae. Most of the compact bone is organized into longitudinal haversian systems, which contain a central canal ringed by lacunae containing osteocytes. The mature osteocytes are surrounded by fluid, which equilibrates with plasma in the blood vessels in the haversian canals and thus with the extracellular fluid.

Osteoclasts are multinucleated cells that continuously resorb bone (mineral and matrix), their main function being continuous bone remodeling. Following bone resorption new bone is formed along stress lines; this new bone provides easily mobilizable calcium. Parathyroid hormone (PTH) stimulates the low basal osteoclast activity. Most pathologic states of excessive bone resorption involve osteoclasts, for example, myeloma tumor cells producing an osteoclast-activating factor.

Osteoblasts arise from osteoprogenitor cells, and have the function of osteoid formation via production and secretion of collagen and glycosaminoglycans. The main stimulus to osteoblast modulation and activity is mechanical stress on bone.

The osteoid osteocyte is an entrapped osteoblast and has the primary function of mineralization of newly formed osteoid. It appears to secrete vesicles, which concentrate calcium-phosphate, and which are then deposited on bone collagen. Alkaline phosphatase is secreted by this cell and has some role in encouraging calcium-phosphate precipitation. Vitamin D is essential for normal mineralization of osteoid.

The mature osteocyte has a primary function in regulating extracellular fluid concentration of calcium ion via osteocytic osteolysis. The serum calcium concentrations may be maintained at normal levels, in minute-to-minute regulation, depending on PTH stimulation of osteocytic osteolysis by the mature osteocyte.

BONE GROWTH

Bone growth occurs by two processes:

1. Intramembranous bone formation: growth of bone from connective tissue without a prior state of

cartilage formation, as in the skull, and in all new bone formation after epiphyseal closure

2. Endochondral bone formation: growth of bone from ossification of cartilage, as in long bones. This involves replication of cartilage cells at the epiphyseal plates, which are then calcified, and the calcified cells undergo osteoclastic resorption followed by obsteoblastic new bone formation.

Growth of the skeleton depends on adequate secretion of growth hormone, somatomedin, and thyroid hormone. There is a spurt of growth at puberty associated with increased sex steroids, which also promote epiphyseal fusion in long bones. Chronic illness and malnutrition in childhood may result in defective bone growth and may cause dwarfism.

Skeletal Homeostatis

In general bone formation and resorption are coupled (Fig. 13.4). As osteoclasts continuously resorb bone at low basal levels (increased by PTH and vitamin D), the mechanical stress of the remaining bone is relatively increased and acts as the stimulus for osteoblastic bone formation. Subsequent mineralization requires adequate vitamin D, calcium, and phosphate concentrations. When bone resorption is greater than bone formation, there is a general decrease in bone mass, which is more evident in the trabecular bone.

Trabecular bone loss appears to involve loss of whole trabeculae, whereas cortical bone loss produces increasing spaces in the compact portion. Corticosteroids primarily decrease bone formation (antianabolic action on protein), while excessive thyroid increases bone resorption to a greater extent than bone formation. Growth hormone, androgens, and estrogens may increase bone formation but also increase bone resorption.

CALCIUM, PHOSPHATE, AND MAGNESIUM HOMEOSTASIS

Mineral Metabolism

Calcium

Besides contributing to the skeleton, calcium serves as a key component of cell membranes, controlling their permeability and their electric potential. It acts as a coupler between stimulus and secretion in endocrine glands, and is an essential factor in blood coagulation and in modulating the activity of various enzymes. Small amounts of calcium are lost from the body by cellular desquamation, and calcium that is absorbed in excess of body requirements is excreted by the kidney.

Calcium in the plasma is partly bound to proteins (mainly albumin) and partly ionized; the remainder is complexed to anions. Only the ionized form of calcium is biologically active, and unfortunately, most measurements of serum calcium are of total calcium. PTH is the primary regulator of extracellular fluid concentrations of ionized calcium. Vitamin D increases calcium and phosphate absorption from the gut and promotes its deposition in bone. In contrast, increased serum phosphate concentrations will decrease calcium levels in the serum by precipitating calcium and phosphate in bone or other tissues.

Phosphate

Phosphate is mainly present in the bone, but is also present in other tissues as cell membrane phospholipids, nucleic acids, and high energy bond compounds for intracellular metabolism. Phosphate absorption is largely passively coupled to calcium absorption; absorption is increased by vitamin D and decreased with chelating agents such as antacids.

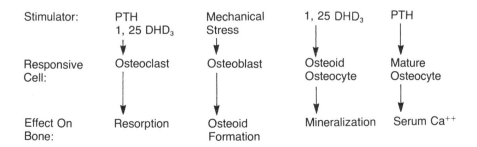

Stimulator:	PTH 1, 25 DHD$_3$	Mechanical Stress	1, 25 DHD$_3$	PTH
Responsive Cell:	Osteoclast	Osteoblast	Osteoid Osteocyte	Mature Osteocyte
Effect On Bone:	Resorption	Osteoid Formation	Mineralization	Serum Ca^{++}

Fig. 13.4 Skeletal Homeostasis and Calcium Homeostasis

Plasma phosphate exists as ionized, complexed, and protein bound. The ionized phosphate is in two forms, depending on the hydrogen ion concentration. Extracellular phosphate levels are modulated by serum calcium and by the renal and bone effects of PTH.

Magnesium

Magnesium is contained mainly in the bone, but also in the muscle. It is important in neuromuscular excitability and enzyme activity.

Hormones Involved in Mineral Homeostasis

Parathyroid Hormone

The four parathyroid glands are situated close to the posterior surface of the thyroid lobes. PTH maintains a normal serum calcium by mobilizing calcium from bone and conserving calcium excretion in the kidneys. PTH promotes the rapid mobilization of calcium from the extracellular fluid surrounding the osteocyte into the general circulation, and promotes the delayed but sustained mobilization of bone calcium during bone resorption by osteoclasts. In the kidney, calcium reabsorption is stimulated in the distal tubule, phosphate reabsorption is inhibited in both the proximal and distal tubules, and bicarbonate reabsorption is inhibited in the proximal tubule. The third major action of PTH on the kidney is the 1-hydroxylation of the 25-hydroxycholecalciferol to form the most active vitamin D metabolite. PTH and vitamin D act synergistically on bone, and when one is absent the other is much less effective.

Calcitonin

Calcitonin is produced by the thyroid parafollicular cells in response to an elevated serum calcium level, but secretion is also stimulated by gut hormones such as gastrin. Calcitonin promotes calcium incorporation into bone by inhibiting osteocytic and osteoclastic osteolysis and by decreasing calcium efflux from cells. Calcitonin promotes phosphate excretion and augments urinary secretion of sodium, potassium, calcium and magnesium. The importance of calcitonin as a major regulator of calcium metabolism is in doubt. There is no known deficiency state of calcitonin in man, and it may merely be a vestigial hormone.

Clinically, calcitonin is important in three ways: a) medullary carcinoma of the thyroid appears to be a cancer of the calcitonin producing cells of the thyroid, and measurement of serum calcitonin either basally or after stimulation with Pentagastrin may be used to detect pre-clinical forms of this disease. Since this cancer is commonly found as part of an inherited syndrome, one can use the calcitonin assay to screen family members when a case of the disease is discovered.

b) serum levels of calcitonin have been found to be elevated in some patients with non-thyroidal malignancies, such as carcinoma of the lung and breast. It therefore may act as a tumor marker.

c) calcitonin is used clinically to treat Paget's disease of the bone and can be used to manage some cases of hypercalcemia.

Vitamin D

The term vitamin D defines a group of sterols, now considered to be a hormone system because it includes chemical transformation in one organ (kidney) to give it specific biological activity in other organs (bone and intestine). Vitamin D_3 (cholecalciferol), derived from the diet and ultraviolet light conversion of 7-dehydrocholesterol in the skin, is stored in the fat and in the liver where it is converted to 25 hydroxy D_3. Patients with low phosphate concentrations or hypocalcemia develop a rise in PTH. This facilitates 1-hydroxylation of 25-hydroxy D_3 in the kidney to form 1, 25-dihydroxy D_3, the most active form of vitamin D. In the presence of hypercalcemia or hyperphosphatemia the formation of 24, 25-dihydroxy D_3 is favored, which is basically an inactivation of vitamin D. Vitamin D apparently exerts its biologic effects in a manner similar to that of the steroid hormones. The observed biologic effects include calcium and phosphate transport in the gut and mobilization of calcium from the bone. Vitamin D is also necessary for normal bone mineralization, and normal muscle formation. In the kidney it may promote reabsorption of phosphate. Even though the most active metabolite 1, 25-dihydroxy D_3 is the most important form, other forms such as the precursor 25-hydroxy D_3 or even 24,25-dihydroxy D_3 may have some important roles.

Other Hormones

Growth hormone mediates its action through the production of somatomedins (primarily in the liver), which stimulate osteoblastic activity and collagen production. Excessive growth hormone results in gigantism, while inadequate growth hormone results in short stature. Glucocorticoids in normal amounts are essential for skeletal growth, but in increased amounts they promote bone loss, via impaired generation of somatomedins, interference with vitamin D metabolism, and interference with intestinal calcium absorption. Sex steroids appear to inhibit bone resorption, and at puberty they produce epiphyseal closure. If secreted in increased amounts prior to puberty, they will result in shorter stature. Loss of sex steroids in the elderly population may contribute to the formation of osteopenia. Insulin appears to potentiate skeletal development, and insulin deficiency (diabetes) may have associated osteopenia. Thyroid hormone is necessary for bone formation and resorption; an excessive amount may result in osteopenia, while a deficient amount in childhood may result in short stature.

Other factors appear to affect mineral metabolism, such as prostaglandins (PGE_2), which stimulate bone resorption, and may be the underlying cause of hypercalcemia produced by certain malignancies. Osteoclast-activating factors also stimulate bone resorption and may result in hypercalcemia associated with multiple myeloma.

Hypocalcemia

Decreased ionized calcium results in an increased neuromuscular excitability (tetany, muscle spasm, laryngospasm, paresthesiae, and seizures). The development of tetany is related to the rapidity of onset of hypocalcemia rather than to its severity. Latent tetany is elicited in hypocalcemic subjects by tapping on the facial nerve and eliciting a twitch of the perioral muscles (Chvostek's sign) which also may be present in some normocalcemic individuals. Inflating the blood pressure cuff above systolic pressure for 2 minutes may cause transient ischemia resulting in carpal spasm (Trousseau's sign). Tetany has also been described due to hypokalemia, hypomagnesemia, and hyperventilation with alkalemia. Acute alkalemia may cause tetany due to increased binding of calcium with protein, which is pH dependent, resulting in decreased ionized calcium. The most common cause in developed countries is the hyperventilation syndrome. The causes of hypocalcemia are listed in Table 13.12.

Hypoparathyroidism produces hypocalcemia and hyperphosphatemia. Metastatic calcification occurs in the basal ganglia for unknown reasons. Ectodermal defects are common, such as cataracts, dry skin, sparse hair, brittle nails, underdeveloped teeth, and proneness to chronic monilia infection. Causes include surgical removal, or idiopathic hypoparathyroidism, which is associated with other autoimmune endocrine deficiencies in other organs. *Pseudohypoparathyroidism* results in resistance to PTH action, whereby injected PTH does not increase plasma calcium, decrease plasma phosphate, or increase the excretion of urinary cyclic AMP. The most likely cause is absence of PTH receptors. Clinical manifestations are similar to those of hypoparathyroidism, with the addition of some congenital defects, the most common being shortened metacarpals (4th and 5th), short stature, and round facies. Pseudopseudohypoparathyroidism presents with the skeletal deformities similar to pseudohypoparathyroidism, but without any of the biochemical aberrations or any abnormality in PTH secretion or action.

Clinical Assessment

1. History: The symptoms of hypocalcemia (paresthesiae, cramps, tetany, seizures), history of neck surgery, history of malabsorption or GI surgery, family history of possible multiple endocrine deficiency syndrome, and longstanding therapy with anticonvulsant drugs, all are useful clues.

2. Physical examination. The signs of pseudohypoparathyroidism, signs of hypocalcemia, neck scar, or skeletal changes compatible with rickets (bone pain, muscle weakness, Milkman line, bowing of legs) may be found on physical examination.

3. Laboratory investigation. Electrolytes including serum magnesium, renal function, and stool fat, should be assessed. Serum phosphate is elevated in hypoparathyroidism and renal failure, and low in osteomalacia, and serum PTH is elevated in osteomalacia and pseudohypoparathyroidism, and low in primary hypoparathyroidism.

4. Bone roentgenography. Signs of osteomalacia, short metacarpals, basal ganglia calcification, changes in keeping with secondary hyperparathyroidism may be identified.

Table 13.12 **Causes of Hypocalcemia**

Hypoparathyroidism
Pseudohypoparathyroidism
Elevated Phosphate (Uremia)
Hypomagnesemia
Vitamin D deficiency
    Genetic, dietary
    Malabsorption, anticonvulsant drugs
Acute pancreatitis
Factitious (hypoalbuminemia) Nephrotic syndrome, liver disease

Treatment

Treatment depends on the underlying cause, and may require administration of one or more of calcium, vitamin D, or phosphate; or removal of the cause, for example, discontinuing anticonvulsant drugs.

Hypercalcemia

Unsuspected hypercalcemia is now frequently detected by automated multianalyzers. The cause may be spurious, or may relate to increased intake and/or absorption of calcium, increased protein binding, or increased bone resorption (Table 13.13). Spurious hypercalcemia may occur due to venous stasis, or assay error. However, if red cells are not quickly separated after blood sampling, then phosphate leakage may result in a false lowering of serum calcium. Increased calcium absorption may occur after markedly excessive calcium intake, particularly if combined with absorbable antacids or vitamin D excess, or in sarcoidosis. Total serum calcium may be increased due to increased binding to serum proteins, primarily albumin, as may occur in dehydration. Excessive bone resorption may be due to endocrine causes (hyperparathyroidism), malignancy (bone metastases, tumor release of prostaglandins, ectopic production of PTH or PTH-like substance, or osteoclast activating factor), and immobilization when superimposed on states of rapid bone turnover (such as fractures in a growing child or a competitive athlete). Hypercalcemia in a patient with Paget's disease is likely due to associated hyperparathyroidism or immobilization. Hypercalcemia may also occur in the recovery phase of acute tubular necrosis with associated rhabdomyolysis.

Clinical Manifestations

Clinical manifestations of hypercalcemia are related to the GI, renal, neurologic, and cardiovascular systems. Nonspecific GI symptoms such as anorexia, nausea, vomiting, and constipation observed in hypercalcemic states may be due to altered GI motility. The increased incidence of peptic ulcer disease may be due to increased gastrin and HCl secretion, while pancreatic enzyme activation may result in pancreatitis. Impaired renal tubular response to ADH results in polyuria, polydypsia, and nocturia. Metastatic calcification may occur, particularly in the kidney (nephrocalcinosis); the latter may progress to renal fail-

Table 13.13   Causes of Hypercalcemia

Idiopathic
Increased Serum Albumin
    Dehydration
Increased Bone Resorption
    Hyperparathyroidism
    Malignancy
    Immobilization
Increased Calcium Absorption
    Milk-alkali syndrome
    Vitamin A, D toxicity
    Sarcoidosis
Others
    Hyperthyroidism
    Adrenal insufficiency

ure, and hypercalciuria may give rise to urinary calculi. Calcium may be deposited in the lateral aspect of the cornea (band keratopathy), which is clinically distinguished from an arcus senilis by the location of the latter at the superior and inferior limbus. Severe hypercalcemia may result in mental confusion, somnolence, and coma. Proximal muscle weakness and muscle aching with hyporeflexia may be predominant features, especially with hyperparathyroidism. Severe hypercalcemia, especially of rapid onset, is a medical emergency that may produce coma, renal failure, and cardiac arrhythmias. Further, hypercalcemia may potentiate digitalis toxicity.

Hyperparathyroidism   Excessive PTH secretion may be due to primary hyperparathyroidism (adenomas, hyperplasia, or carcinomas), secondary hyperparathyroidism due to a hypocalcemic stimulus, or so-called tertiary hyperparathyroidism due to excess PTH secretion resulting from previous longstanding secondary hyperparathyroidism. Ectopic hyperparathyroidism may occur from nonparathyroid neoplasms, the most common of which is squamous carcinoma of the lung or kidney. Excessive PTH action results in increased osteolysis, resulting in generalized osteoporosis, especially in the distal ends of the clavicles, vertebrae, and phalanges. The phalanges may show subperiosteal erosion and resorption of the terminal tufts. Excessive osteoclast hyperplasia may give rise to cystic bone erosions, which become linked with fibrous tissue (osteitis fibrosa cystica). The lamina dura of the teeth may be radiologically absent, and the patient may have bone pain and fractures due to skeletal demineralization. Primary hyperparathyroidism most commonly results from a single parathyroid adenoma in the neck, and less commonly, from an adenoma in the mediastinum. The next most common cause is parathyroid hyperplasia involving all glands. This may result as part of the multiple endocrine neoplasia (MEN) syndrome, type I or type II, and occasionally parathyroid hyperplasia or adenomas may occur on a familial basis separate from the MEN syndrome. Familial hyperparathyroidism must be differentiated from familial benign hypocalciuric hypercalcemia, which appears to be an impaired renal ability to excrete calcium, resulting in hypercalcemia but very few, if any, of the long-term complications associated with hyperparathyroidism.

The patient with hyperparathyroidism almost invariably shows an increased serum calcium; in 50 percent of cases there is a decreased serum phosphate, and an increased serum chloride is frequent. The alkaline phosphatase may be normal or elevated depending on the severity of bone disease. Roentgenograms may demonstrate generalized demineralization, with small bone cysts, subperiosteal phalangeal reabsorption, and renal calculi. The tubular reabsorption of phosphate is decreased. This test cannot be done in the presence of decreased renal function (creatinine clearance less than 30). Serum PTH assays are useful if available, and selective parathyroid vein catheterization may be used to localize the site of excess PTH secretion in those patients with previous negative surgical explorations. An increased 24-hour urinary cyclic AMP may serve as an indicator of PTH action in the kidneys. If primary hyperparathyroidism is ultimately diagnosed, then the possibility of the MEN syndrome should also be considered.

Approach to the Patient with Hypercalcemia

Even in unsuspected hypercalcemia a thorough clinical review often reveals very important diagnostic clues.

History The presence of hypercalcemia may be indicated by polyuria, polydypsia, and weakness. Diet and drug history should reflect the possibility of milk-alkali syndrome or vitamin D intoxication, therapy with thiazide diuretics, or the presence of immobilization. Symptoms that suggest malignancy, such as weight loss, cigarette smoking, cough, or others may be elicited.

Physical Examination The physical examination may uncover signs of metastatic clacification (such as band keratopathy), proximal muscle weakness, or hypertension, in keeping with primary hyperparathyroidism. Sarcoidosis may be suggested by lymphadenopathy, or pulmonary or skin lesions. A hematologic malignancy may be suspected because of localized bone tenderness, ecchymoses, or bleeding.

Laboratory Diagnosis Aside from the hypercalcemia, the serum phosphate may be low in hyperparathyroidism or some malignancies, and elevated in renal failure, vitamin D intoxication or some malignancies. An elevated serum alkaline phosphatase indicates bone or liver involvement. Hyperparathyroidism is often associated with a metabolic acidosis with a relatively low bicarbonate level and an elevated chloride level; this gives rise to an elevated chloride to phosphate ratio. A marked increase in serum globulins, especially if associated with increased uric acid, may suggest myeloma. Serum PTH is elevated in primary or ectopic hyperparathyroidism and low or normal in nonparathyroid hypercalcemia. In the absence of a serum PTH assay, the tubular reabsorption of phosphate may be a helpful measurement. A steroid suppression test is helpful in the differentiation of primary hyperparathyroidism from certain other forms of hypercalcemia. Steroid suppression of hypercalcemia is observed in vitamin D intoxication, sarcoidosis, and milk-alkali syndrome, whereas nonsuppression is characteristic of malignancy and hyperparathyroidism. A chest roentgenogram may demonstrate a hitherto occult lung malignancy, or sarcoidosis, and an IVP may detect a hypernephroma. The search for metastatic malignancy may require a skeletal survey and bone scan.

Treatment of Hypercalcemia

Treatment depends on the underlying cause. Specific measures may be instituted, such as mobilization, discontinuing oral intake of the causative agent, treating thyroid or adrenal disease, or surgery for primary hyperparathyroidism. Patients acutely symptomatic (especially if the serum calcium is greater than 14 mg/dl) should be considered as having a life-threatening emergency. The most important urgent treatment involves the immediate initiation of intravenous saline in large doses to restore blood volume and to initiate a calcium diuresis. This may, however, be ineffective or dangerous in the presence of cardiac or renal failure. Furosemide diuresis further enhances calcium excretion but requires fluid and potassium replacement. Hypophosphatemia should be corrected, because it aggravates the hypercalcemia by increasing calcium absorption and stimulating bone breakdown. Oral phosphate is useful in restoring normal serum calcium and phosphate.

More definitive forms of therapy include the following:

1. Mithramycin inhibits osteoclastic activity—an effect that lasts for several days—but may be toxic to platelets, liver, and kidney.

2. Salmon calcitonin blocks osteoclast activity, is safer than mithramycin, but is less effective. The only problem is allergy.

3. Glucocorticoids block intestinal calcium absorption and reduce bone turnover rates. They are particularly effective in treating hypercalcemia due to vitamin D toxicity, some hematologic malignancies, and sarcoidosis.

4. Diphosphonates block osteoclast activity.

5. Prostaglandin antagonists may be utilized in some malignancy-induced hypercalcemia thought to be prostaglandin mediated.

The treatment of chronic hypercalcemia includes a low dairy diet, increased sodium intake (if possible), and oral phosphate. Oral phosphate potentially may produce metastatic calcification, but generally this is not clinically apparent, and it is probable that the calcium is deposited in the skeleton. Renal function should be monitored carefully.

Hypophosphatemia

Manifestations of phosphate depletion relate to decreased cellular metabolic activity (enzyme activation) and energy production. Lethargy, anorexia, malaise, irritability, muscle weakness, and coma may ultimately lead to death in cardiorespiratory failure. Chronic phosphate depletion may result in osteomalacia or rickets. Hypophosphatemia may result from decreased intake (such as in alcoholism), malabsorption due to small bowel disease or excessive antacid administration, increased renal excretion (hyperparathyroidism and renal tubular disorders), and increased utilization such as the nutritional recovery syndrome of diabetic ketoacidosis.

Hyperphosphatemia

The most important effect of hyperphosphatemia is to reduce the extracellular fluid concentration of ionized calcium by promoting increased calcium-phosphate deposition in bones and other tissues. Metastatic calcifications most commonly occur in renal failure, and may result in nephrocalcinosis, pancreatic calcification, conjunctival and corneal calcification, arthritis from pseudogout, and chondrocalcinosis. Hyperphosphatemia resulting from excessive intake is rare. It may result from excessive cellular breakdown, such as an acute leukemic crisis. The most common mechanism is decreased excretion due to renal failure or, less commonly, hypoparathyroidism.

Hypomagnesemia

The major manifestation of hypomagnesemia is increased neuromuscular excitability producing myoclonus, choreoathetosis, tetany, and convulsions. Hypomagnesemia may result from a decreased intake (such as parenteral alimentation or alcoholism) or increased loss in the gut due to diarrhea or vomiting.

Hypermagnesemia

Hypermagnesemia may produce neuromuscular paralysis by a decreased sensitivity of the motor end-plate to acetylcholine. Absent deep tendon reflexes, hypotension, and finally respiratory and cardiac arrest may occur. Hypermagnesemia may result from increased intake of magnesium sulfate, with associated renal failure.

METABOLIC BONE DISEASE

Metabolic bone disease implies a defect in bone formation and/or bone resorption, and refers to a generalized affliction of the skeleton.

Osteoporosis

Osteoporosis is defined as decreased bone mass or decreased amount of normally mineralized bone. The bone is less dense on radiographs because of loss of bone (matrix and mineral), which can be confirmed by histologic examination. Decreased bone mass results from decreased bone formation and/or increased bone resorption. Decreased bone formation implies decreased matrix (osteoid) production, which may occur due to decreased stimulus to the osteoblasts (decreased mechanical stress on bone), decreased availability of substrate (mainly protein, as in malnutrition or hypercortisolemia), or defective osteoblasts (such as the genetic defect osteogenesis imperfecta). Decreased bone mass due to increased bone resorption may be due to (1) abnormal cellular invasion of bone (multiple myeloma, mastocytosis, histiocytosis, metastatic malignancy, or other factors), which directly erodes bone or produces prostaglandins that increase release of osteoclast-activating factors; or (2) may be due to an increase in PTH action. Increased PTH action may be due to an absolute increase in PTH (primary or secondary hyperparathyroidism) or to increased effectiveness of PTH on bone (decreased estrogen). Secondary hyperparathyroidism due to decreased serum levels of ionized calcium (decreased intake, decreased absorption, increased demand, increased renal loss) in the presence of adequate amounts of active vitamin D will cause osteoporosis; but if there is also deficient vitamin D, this will result in osteomalacia. Osteoporosis is referred to as primary (no recognizable etiology) or secondary.

Primary or Idiopathic Osteoporosis

Four common hypotheses attempt to explain the cause.

1. Lifelong subnormal mechanical stress to bone resulting in decreased skeletal mass. The primary stimulus for osteoblastic bone formation is mechanical stress on bones (ambulatory weight-bearing). The bone remains approximately constant from puberty to age 35 years.

2. Normal aging processes result in decreased bone formation, so that bone resorption after age 35 exceeds bone formation. This loss of bone mass will be accelerated if aging is accompanied by further diminished stress on bone. Menopause therefore contributes to normal change of life (aging) and there is evidence that hypoestrogenism further decreases bone formation. Osteoporosis is much more prevalent at a young age in white, small-framed females who have not "stressed their bones."

3. Chronic low calcium absorption. In North America the average daily dietary intake of calcium approximates 650 mg, while the phosphate (meat) intake approximates 1600 mg. The high phosphate to calcium ratio in the diet results in calcium-phosphate complexes in the bowel and decreases the net amount of calcium absorbed. Intestinal lactase deficiency syndrome may lead to milk avoidance, further aggrevating the low calcium to phosphate ratio. A small negative calcium balance over many years may gradually deplete skeletal calcium.

4. Chronic low grade secondary hyperparathyroidism. Minimally decreased calcium absorption will increase PTH secretion, which continues osteolysis at an accelerated rate, compared with the normal rate. It is possible that serum PTH increases with age.

The clinical symptoms of osteoporosis vary from asymptomatic (diagnosis made on incidental roentgenograms) to symptomatic fractures (vertebral, femoral neck, or forearm) with minimal trauma. The sites of the fractures are at the maximal stress points for bending or compression. Radiographic evidence of osteoporosis is first recognized in primarily trabecular bones (vertebrae), even though the total skeletal calcium is less than half of normal by this time.

The serum calcium, phosphorus, and alkaline phosphatase levels, as well as other laboratory parameters, are within the normal range. Histologic sections on bone biopsies show the decreased bone mass, while the amount of unmineralized osteoid (in terms of the decreased bone mass) is frequently increased from normal, and a minimal degree of osteomalacia may also be present. Quantitative histologic techniques and bone densitometry (noninvasive) provide more precise quantitation of bone mass.

The most effective treatment of primary osteoporosis is prevention, including ambulatory weight-bearing to ensure bones are stressed, and an adequate calcium and phosphate diet. For established primary osteoporosis, ambulatory weight-bearing and an adequate calcium intake are essential. Two grams of oral calcium per day and occasionally vitamin D may be utilized in small doses (only in association with calcium supplements, since vitamin D can cause bone resorption). If no significant clinical improvement is noted, or if the disorder is progressive, attempts to stimulate bone formation with fluoride along with calcium and vitamin D may be justified. Fluoride used alone may result in osteomalacia. Estrogens may be effective in increasing bone resistance to PTH-induced osteolysis. They may also have a significant long-term beneficial effect in preserving bone mass, and should definitely be given to a woman with premature ovarian failure. Recent studies have shown positive bone sparing and bone forming effects of estrogen therapy in hypogonadal and postmenopausal women.

Secondary Osteoporosis

The causes of secondary osteoporosis may be physiologic during chronic immobilization, or may be due to drug administration (chronic glucocorticoid therapy, chronic heparin therapy), endocrine disorders (Cushing's syndrome, hyperthyroidism, premature hypogonadism, hyperparathyroidism, diabetes mellitus), nutritional causes (severe calcium deficiency, scurvy, alcoholism), malignancy (multiple myeloma, multiple bone metastases), and hereditary disorders (homocystinuria, osteogenesis imperfecta). The diagnosis and treatment of secondary osteoporosis are directed toward the causative factors.

Osteomalacia and Rickets

In osteomalacia and rickets there is lack of compressive strength, so that the bones tend to bend and show partial cracks at stress points (pseudofractures), which are often bilateral. The bones may be tender due to expanding osteoid, and the muscles may be weak if there is low phosphate, resulting in a chronic waddling gait. Osteomalacia occurs in mature bone, while rickets is primarily a disorder of the chondroosseous linear growth areas. Both conditions are characterized by a relative excess of unmineralized bone (osteoid). The proximal myopathy may be more symptomatic than the bone disease. Osteomalacia may present with low back pain. Rickets results in swelling on the bone ends (metaphyses) especially in the radius and costochondral junction, giving rise to parasternal rachitic rosary. Bone deformity results in decreased stature and kyphosis, compression of the pelvis, and bossing of the frontal and parietal bones. In addition, the features of osteomalacia or proximal muscle weakness and bone tenderness occur. If the serum calcium is low, the manifestations of hypocalcemia may be present. The alkaline phosphatase levels in the serum are elevated in osteomalacia due to increased stress per unit of mineralized bone, resulting in increased osteoid production. Radiographically, generalized decreased bone density and biconcave vertebral bodies may be present. Looser zones are almost pathognomonic of osteomalacia, and consist of linear decalcification along the course of large blood vessels, usually distributed in the scapulae, pelvis, and proximal long bones. If hypocalcemia is present, then bone changes of secondary hyperparathyroidism may occur. Definitive diagnosis of osteomalacia depends on the demonstration of excess amounts of osteoid tissue on bone biopsy.

Decreased vitamin D action   results in decreased calcium absorption from the gut, secondary hyperparathyroidism, and resultant decreased serum phosphate. The hyperparathyroidism restores the serum calcium level at the expense of increasing osteolysis. This form of osteomalacia is responsive to vitamin D treatment (vitamin D-dependent rickets). Mechanisms of reduced vitamin D action are as follows:

1. Simple dietary vitamin D deficiency is uncommon in North America due to adequate food and exposure of the skin to sunlight. The diagnosis is clinically apparent. The treatment consists of small oral doses of vitamin D.

2. GI malabsorption syndromes result from disorders of fat absorption (decreased fat soluble vitamin D absorption). (See Chapter 12.)

3. Anticonvulsants such as phenylhydantoin and phenobarbital may decrease available 25-hydroxy D_3 by increasing hepatic metabolism of inactive metabolites. This will result in a decrease of calcium absorption from the gut. Some authorities advocate routine supplementation with calcium or vitamin D during anticonvulsant therapy.

4. Severe liver disease may result in decreased conversion of vitamin D to 25-hydroxy D_3.

5. Familial vitamin D-dependent rickets is due to a deficiency of the 1-hydroxylase, with resultant decreased conversion of 25-hydroxy D_3 to 1,24-dihydroxy D_3.

6. Renal osteodystrophy. Chronic renal failure is associated with decreased 1,25-dihydroxy D_3 production. This will produce all of the usual findings of osteomalacia (but with an elevated serum phosphate level) and evidence of renal insufficiency. Treatment consists of large doses of vitamin D or small doses of 1,25-dihydroxy D_3; serum phosphate levels can be reduced by decreasing phosphate absorption with the use of antacids to bind dietary phosphate.

7. Target tissue resistance to 1,25-dihydroxy D_3 may occur in uremia, and may also result from other mechanisms, such as with anticonvulsant drugs. Some patients have been described with primary end organ resistance to 1,25-dihydroxy D_3.

Phosphate deficiency   may cause impaired mineralization of bone with normal serum calcium and PTH.

1. Hypophosphatemic states may occur due to starvation or intravenous alimentation without added phosphate.

2. Renal phosphaturic syndromes are the most common cause. Familial hypophosphatemic rickets, "phosphate diabetes," and vitamin D-resistant rickets all show decreased tubular reabsorption of phosphate, and may be associated with concomitant decreased gut absorption of phosphate. This is the most common variety of rickets in the developed countries.

Excess renal phosphate loss may also occur in a variety of the Fanconi's syndrome or in renal tubular acidosis. This diagnosis is established by the presence of hypophosphatemia together with aminoacidurias or glycosuria, low serum bicarbonate, and high urine pH. Rarely, some benign tumors such as hemangiocytomas may produce a phosphaturic substance, which is not yet identified, and may present with hypophosphatemic osteomalacia. Treatment is surgical removal of the tumor.

Hypophosphatasia, a deficiency of alkaline phosphatase, is a rare cause of osteomalacia. It resembles rickets but, in contrast with that condition, shows dental abnormalities and excretion of normal quantities of inorganic pyrophosphate in the urine. The alkaline phosphatase is low in plasma and bone but normal in other nonskeletal tissues.

Osteopetrosis (Albers-Schönberg Disease)

Osteopetrosis is a rare inherited disorder characterized by abnormally dense bone that is structurally weak and liable to fracture. Anemia resulting from obliteration of the marrow space, and cranial nerve palsies resulting from foraminal overgrowth of bone may occur. The severe form presents in childhood, while the adult form, which is more benign, is characterized by short stature, bone deformities, and an increased tendency of bones to fracture. Routine biochemical studies, including serum calcium, phosphorus, and alkaline phosphatase, are normal. A similar clinical picture may be produced with chronic overdose of strontium or fluoride. There is no treatment available for osteopetrosis.

Paget's Disease (Osteitis Deformans)

Paget's disease is a common disease of unknown etiology in which there is excessive and abnormal remodeling of bone, usually localized but occasionally widespread. Excessive areas of active bone resorption of both trabecular and compact bone, associated with marked vascular tissue proliferation and fibrosis, is followed by the irregular deposition of immature woven bone, in which the pattern of collagen fibers is disorganized. The disease manifestations may vary from asymptomatic to debilitating. The most common bones affected are the pelvis, the femur, the skull, the tibia, and the vertebrae. Radiologically, various degrees of rarefaction and osteosclerosis coexist, representing excessive bone resorption and formation. The involved bones are usually expanded. Deformity and fracture of the long bones, kyphosis, and skull enlargement may result. An increased incidence of osteosarcoma may occur, in about 1 percent of cases. Neurologic complications may result from compressive spinal fractures, platybasia leading to brain-stem damage or increased intracranial pressure, or cranial neuropathies (such as deafness) resulting from foraminal impingement. The increased blood flow to bone may result in high output cardiac failure. The serum calcium and phosphate levels are usually normal, but the alkaline phosphatase level (reflecting bone formation) and the urine hydroxyproline level (reflecting bone collagen resorption) may be markedly elevated, depending on the severity of the disease. Although metastatic carcinomas from the prostate or breast may be osteosclerotic and appear radiographically similar to Paget's disease, they do not expand the bone as does Paget's disease. The majority of bone lesions are detectable by routine skeletal radiography and by bone scanning. The bone scan usually demonstrates the symptomatic lesions.

In mild or localized disease, no specific treatment is indicated. In more generalized and active disease immobilization should be avoided, and bone resorption may be inhibited with mithramycin, calcitonin, or diphosphonates. The serum alkaline phosphatase and urinary hydroxyproline may be used as indices of the activity of the disease, and therefore may be used as markers to assess treatment. If the patient must be immobilized due to illness or fracture, there will be increased bone resorption that is not balanced by bone formation. Hypercalcemia may develop, and may be severe enough to require therapy.

REFERENCES

1. Carlson, H.E.: Gynecomastia. N. Eng. J. Med. 303:795–798, 1980.
2. Gold, M.:The Cushing syndromes: changing views of diagnosis and treatment. Ann. Int. Med. 90:829–844, 1979.
3. Juan, D.: Hypocalcemia: differential diagnosis and management. Arch. Int. Med. 139:1166–1171, 1979.
4. Kidd, A., Okita, N., Row, V.V., Volpe, R.: Immunologic Aspects of Graves' and Hashimoto's Diseases. Metabolism 29:80–99, 1980.
5. Kreisberg, R.A.: Diabetic Ketoacidosis: new concepts and trends in pathogenesis and treatment. Ann. Int. Med. 88:681–695, 1978.
6. Levy, I.: Hyperlipoproteinemia and its management. J. Cardiovasc. Med. 5:435–452, 1980.
7. Maroulis, B.: Evaluation of hirsutism and hyperandrogenemia. Fertility and Sterility 36:273–302, 1981.
8. Morley, J.E.: The endocrinology of opiates and opioid peptides. Metabolism 30:195–209, 1981.
9. Nordin, B.E.C., Peacock, M., Aaron, J., et al.:Osteoporosis and osteomalacia. Clin. Endocrinol. Metabol. 9:177–205, 1980.
10. Odell, W.D., Swerdloff, R.S.: Abnormalities of gonadal function in men. Clin. Endocrinol. 8:149–180, 1978.
11. Pollet, R.J., Levey, G.S.: Principles of membrane receptor physiology and their application to clinical medicine. Ann. Int. Med. 92:663–680, 1980.
12. Walsh, J.H., et al.: Gastrointestinal hormones in clinical disease: recent developments. Ann. Int. Med. 90:817–828, 1979.
13. Weinberger, M.H., et al: Primary aldosteronism. Ann. Int. Med. 90:386–395, 1979.
14. Yen, S.S.C.: The polycystic ovary syndrome. Clin. Endocrinol. 12:177–208, 1980.
15. Verhoeven, G.F.M., Wilson, J.D.: The syndromes of primary hormone resistance. Metabolism 28:253–289, 1979.
16. Zervas, N.T., Martin, J.B.: Management of hormone-secreting pituitary adenomas. N. Engl. J. Med. 302:210–214, 1980.

14

Neurologic Disorders

Robert G. Lee, M.D. and Werner J. Becker, M.D.

The diagnosis and the treatment of disorders affecting the nervous system require a clinical approach that differs in several respects from that used for patients with diseases affecting other body systems. From a functional viewpoint, the nervous system includes not only the central nervous system (brain and spinal cord) but also the cranial nerves, spinal nerve roots and peripheral nerves, skeletal muscle, special sense organs subserving vision and hearing, and the various components of the autonomic nervous system. Symptoms of neurologic disease range all the way from disturbances of consciousness and higher intellectual function to localized muscle wasting and weakness or sensory loss due to a lesion affecting a single peripheral nerve.

Because of the complexity of the nervous system, the wide variety of symptoms and signs that occur as a result of the disorders, and the exacting nature of the neurologic examination, disorders affecting the nervous system are often considered the exclusive domain of the neurologic specialist. This attitude is reinforced by many textbooks of neurology that describe a vast number of obscure syndromes, often identified by confusing eponyms. However, by observing a few general principles and using a systematic clinical approach, the family physician or general internist should be able to identify and treat most of the common disorders affecting the human nervous system.

Perhaps more than any other medical specialty, neurology represents the direct clinical application of the basic sciences, particularly neuroanatomy and neurophysiology. Recent advances in these areas as well as in neuropharmacology and neurochemistry have contributed greatly to our understanding of the nervous system, and are beginning to have a major impact on clinical neurology. The development of new diagnostic techniques, notably computed tomography, has greatly increased the accuracy of neurologic diagnosis. Despite these advances, the traditional clinical approach and the general principles for dealing with a patient with a neurologic disorder have not changed.

GENERAL APPROACH TO A PATIENT WITH A NEUROLOGIC PROBLEM

As with any clinical problem, the starting point is a detailed history and careful evaluation of the patient's symptoms, followed by a systematic examination of the nervous system. The physician should then analyse the clinical data in an attempt to localize the site of involvement within the nervous system. A number of different disease processes may present with similar signs and symptoms when the same areas of the nervous system are involved. Further, an isolated sign such as localized muscle weakness can result from lesions at a variety of different locations. The importance of this initial step of establishing an anatomic diagnosis cannot be overemphasized. Too often it is neglected, and diagnostic errors occur as a result of jumping to immediate conclusions that the patient has a brain tumor or has suffered a stroke. Only after an attempt has been made to localize the lesion on clinical grounds should consideration be given to the nature of the underlying pathologic process.

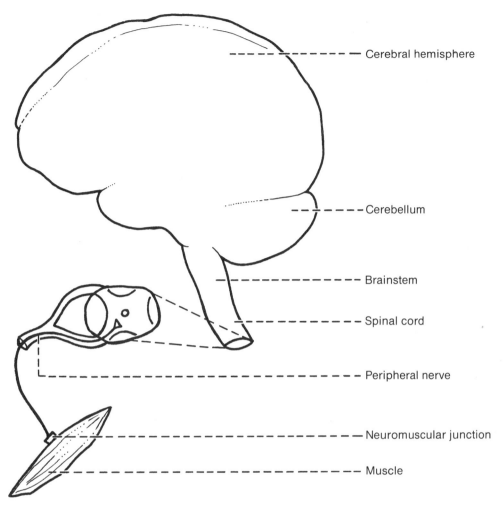

Cerebral hemisphere

Cerebellum

Brainstem

Spinal cord

Peripheral nerve

Neuromuscular junction

Muscle

Fig. 14.1 Major divisions of the nervous system from cerebral hemispheres to peripheral end-organ

In approaching the patient with a suspected neurologic problem, the physician should ask the following questions:

1. Do the symptoms and signs suggest the presence of a lesion involving the nervous system? Many patients present with symptoms such as headaches, dizziness, or numbness that cannot be attributed to any specific nervous system pathology.

2. Where is the lesion located? Can the symptoms and signs be accounted for by a single focal lesion, or is there evidence of diffuse involvement or disease affecting multiple sites in the nervous system?

3. What pathologic conditions are capable of producing a lesion at this site, and which of these is the most likely cause of the patient's symptoms and signs?

4. Why does a lesion at this site produce these clinical abnormalities? In what way are normal physiologic mechanisms altered?

Anatomic localization should be directed initially at defining the site of the lesion in broad terms to identify which of the major divisions of the nervous system is involved (Fig. 14.1). Do the clinical findings suggest a lesion in one cerebral hemisphere, in the brainstem, or in the spinal cord? Or, is the abnormality outside the central nervous system, involving nerve roots, peripheral nerves, or skeletal muscle? Once the general area of involvement has been identified, the findings can be reassessed to reach a more precise anatomic diagnosis indicating which lobe of the cerebral hemisphere is involved or which pathways in the spinal cord or brainstem are not functioning.

A simple example will illustrate how this approach

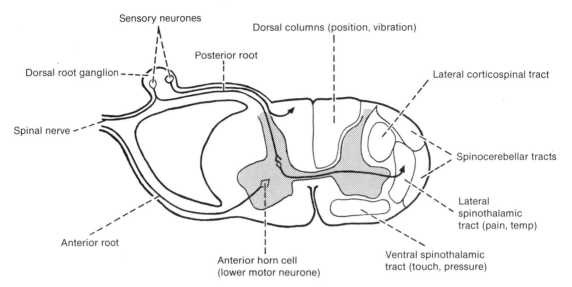

Fig. 14.2 Cross section of the spinal cord, showing the more important ascending and descending tracts and anterior and posterior nerve roots

can be useful. In a patient with weakness of one leg, the cause could be located anywhere along motor pathways from the cerebral cortex to the lumbar spinal cord, or the problem could be in the peripheral nerves or skeletal muscle. Other signs associated with the weakness help identify the level of involvement. If, in addition to weakness, there is muscle wasting, hypotonia, and diminished reflexes, the cause most likely lies somewhere in the peripheral nervous system. If there is hyperreflexia, increased tone, and an extensor plantar response, then the lesion must be above the level of the anterior horn cells, although it still could be anywhere between the motor cortex and spinal cord. If there is weakness accompanied by the "upper motor neuron" signs listed above, plus evidence of a 3rd nerve palsy on the opposite side, then there is a high probability of a focal lesion in the midbrain. This is the only site within the nervous system where a single lesion can involve both the 3rd nerve and descending motor pathways (Fig. 14.2).

Once it has been established that there is a lesion within the nervous system and its site has been located, then consideration should be given to the nature of the pathologic process. The clinical history is often very helpful at this stage. For example, consider a 65-year-old man who presents with aphasia, right hemiplegia, and a right homonymous hemianopia. These findings clearly indicate the presence of a focal lesion in the left cerebral hemisphere, but they do not help identify the pathologic process. If the history reveals that the patient has hypertension but has otherwise been well and suddenly collapsed unable to speak or move the right side of his body, it is most

probable that he has a vascular lesion—either a cerebral infarct or an intracerebral hemorrhage. If, however, we obtain a history of slowly progressive right-sided weakness and speech disturbance over the previous 6 weeks, accompanied by headaches and increasing drowsiness, then it is much more likely that the patient has a brain tumor.

THE NEUROLOGIC HISTORY

The general principles of history taking for neurologic problems are the same as for disorders affecting other systems, and do not require detailed elaboration here. However, there are a few special problems that should be considered. Terms such as dizziness, weakness, or numbness may have various meanings for different individuals. The physician should attempt to clarify exactly what the patient is experiencing when he uses these terms to describe his symptoms. Many neurologic illnesses are associated with alterations of consciousness or disturbances of language function or mentation that make it impossible for the patient to give an adequate description of his illness. In these situations it is essential to obtain additional historical data from a reliable third-party source. This is particularly true of patients with syncope or epileptic seizures, who often are totally amnesic for events occurring during an attack. Similarly, the work-up of a patient with dementia or asphasia is not complete without a description of the evolution of the patient's symptoms, provided by a relative or close friend.

THE NEUROLOGIC EXAMINATION

The neurologic examination is regarded by some as a laborious, time-consuming exercise requiring 30 minutes or more of the examiner's time. This may be true for some patients with complex problems and multiple neurologic signs. However, in a cooperative patient, an adequate evaluation of the nervous system should not add more than a few minutes to the total time required for a complete general physical examination.

A complete examination of the nervous system should evaluate the following components:

1. Mental status
2. Speech and language function
3. Cranial nerves
4. Motor function
5. Reflexes
6. Sensation
7. Stance and gait

Much is learned about mental status and language function while the history is being obtained from the patient, and detailed assessment of these functions is required only when the history or preliminary examination points to abnormalities in these areas. Cranial nerve examination should include visualization of the optic fundi and testing of visual fields by confrontation, assessment of visual and auditory acuity, testing of pupillary reflexes, and examination of eye movements. Corneal reflexes and facial sensation should be tested, any facial weakness or asymmetry should be noted, and movement of the pharynx and tongue should be observed. Assessment of olfactory function is occasionally useful.

Examination of the motor system should include inspection for any evidence of muscle wasting or involuntary movements. Muscle tone and strength should be documented in major muscle groups. Motor control and coordination are evaluated with maneuvers such as the finger-nose test, heel-shin test, and the ability of the patient to perform rapid alternating movements and fine finger movements.

Examination of reflexes is an important part of the neurologic examination. Tendon jerks, plantar responses, and abdominal reflexes should be elicited in all patients. Other reflexes such as the jaw jerk, grasp reflex, and sucking reflex should be tested in special circumstances.

The sensory examination can be difficult and tedious for both the examiner and the patient. However, in most patients relatively little time is required to test light touch and pinprick sense, position and vibration sense in the fingers and toes, and possibly one test such as stereognosis or two-point discrimination to assess higher discriminatory sense.

A great deal can be learned by observing the patient walk, since disturbances of gait are often an early sign of dysfunction at a number of different sites in the nervous system. In addition to observing the patient's normal walking gait, the examiner should assess balance by doing the Romberg test and having the patient perform tandem gait or heel-toe walking.

The techniques for performing the various parts of the neurologic examination are described in much greater detail in the references noted for this section (see References, end of chapter).

LABORATORY INVESTIGATION

The clinician has a large armamentarium of laboratory tests available to help him or her arrive at a specific diagnosis once the clinical data have been analyzed to establish an anatomic diagnosis, and a list of the most probable disease entites responsible for the patient's signs and symptoms has been compiled. The indications for these tests and the type of information they can provide will be discussed in detail in subsequent sections, while only a brief overview is given here.

The number of investigations and the order in which they are carried out will obviously vary according to the clinical problem. In a patient with a suspected intracranial problem, skull radiographs and an electroencephalogram are often carried out as preliminary screening tests. The EEG is essential for evaluating seizure disorders, but it may also provide useful information in patients with metabolic or toxic encephalopathies or focal structural lesions of the brain. It should be noted that the EEG and radiologic investigations such as computed tomography (CT scan) complement each other. The EEG assesses brain *function*, or electrophysiology, while the radiologic studies provide information concerning *structure*. During the short time since its development, the CT scan has become the single most valuable tool for demonstrating structural lesions within the brain. However, the cost and availability of this test is such that it cannot be used for routine screening purposes and should be reserved for cases in which there is a fairly high probability of an intracranial lesion. The radioisotope brain scan is still useful in certain situations. Angiography is a valuable and often essential procedure for investigating patients with cerebrovascular disorders. Pneumoencephalography and ventriculography are still indicated in some special situations, but have largely been supplanted by the CT scan.

Investigation of patients with suspected spinal cord or nerve root disorders begins with plain radiographs of the spine at the levels indicated by the clinical findings. If there is a strong suspicion of an intraspinal lesion, the next step is usually a myelogram. Spinal CT scanning may also be helpful.

Examination of cerebrospinal fluid may provide useful information concerning a number of neurologic disorders. The examination should include measurement of CSF pressure, a description of the gross appearance of the fluid, a cell count, and determination of CSF protein and sugar levels. If infection is suspected, a Gram stain, a culture, and a sensitivity test should be carried out. The presence of abnormal proteins in demyelinating diseases and related disorders may be suggested by elevation of the IgG fraction or the presence of oligoclonal protein banding. CSF examination is essential in cases of suspected meningitis and may be indicated if the clinical information suggests intracranial hemorrhage, although the presence of subarachnoid or intracerebral blood can usually be identified with a CT scan. CSF examination is also valuable in demyelinating disorders. However, the use of lumbar puncture as a screening test, to look for elevation of CSF protein as an indication of something wrong in the nervous system, should be discouraged.

Electromyography and nerve conduction studies are used to evaluate disorders affecting the peripheral nervous system. Elevation of serum enzymes such as creatine kinase, transaminase, and aldolase may point to a primary problem affecting skeletal muscle. In these cases, additional useful information is often provided by a muscle biopsy.

CLINICAL LOCALIZATION OF NEUROLOGIC DISORDERS

The starting point in neurologic diagnosis is the anatomic localization of the problem. In accordance with this principle, we shall begin with a discussion of the major signs and symptoms associated with focal disease at various levels of the nervous system. Problems such as weakness or sensory loss can occur as a result of lesions at many different sites in the nervous system. Fortunately, there is a tendency for neurologic signs and symptoms to be grouped into characteristic patterns or syndromes that should alert the physician to suspect a focal pathologic process at a specific site within the nervous system.

In this section we shall describe the clinical features associated with focal disorders affecting the major compartments of the central and peripheral nervous systems. Although the emphasis will be on the iden-

tification of focal lesions, it should be noted that some disease processes affect the nervous system diffusely or produce lesions at multiple sites. As we proceed through the nervous system, starting at the periphery and gradually working to higher levels of the central nervous system, we shall occasionally digress to discuss the differential diagnosis of important clinical problems that can occur as a result of lesions at several different sites.

Following this anatomically oriented introduction, subsequent sections will deal with specific disease entites and major pathologic processes.

CLINICAL MANIFESTATIONS OF NEUROMUSCULAR DISORDERS

Disorders affecting the motor unit produce a number of characteristic syndromes, most of which can be readily distinguished from central nervous system disorders. The term "motor unit" is used here to refer to anterior horn cells or motor neurons, their axons within the nerve roots and peripheral nerves, as well as neuromuscular junctions and skeletal muscle fibers. The major symptom common to most of these disorders is *muscle weakness*. The pattern or distribution of weakness and the presence of certain associated signs and symptoms help localize the site of involvement within the motor unit. As an initial step, the clinician should attempt to determine whether the problem is "myopathic" weakness due to a primary disorder of skeletal muscle, or "neurogenic" weakness resulting from a disorder affecting the motor nerve supply to muscle.

Skeletal Muscle

Most myopathic disorders have a predilection for involvement of proximal muscle groups, particularly muscles of the shoulder girdle and pelvic girdle and the flexors of the neck and trunk. Usually there is relative sparing of distal muscle, although a few rare myopathies represent exceptions to this general rule.

Patients with disorders such as muscular dystrophy or polymyositis have difficulty climbing stairs or getting up from a low chair. Weakness of the pelvic girdle and trunk muscles results in a characteristic waddling gait, often accompanied by exaggerated lumbar lordosis. Because of the shoulder girdle weakness, these patients have difficulty lifting heavy objects or reaching above their head to remove objects from a shelf.

In the early stages of a myopathy, muscle wasting is not nearly so prominent as in most neurogenic disorders, and tendon reflexes are usually preserved. Muscle tone is either normal or slightly reduced, and there are no sensory signs or symptoms. In the later stages of muscle diseases, considerable loss of muscle bulk may occur. Paradoxical enlargement or pseudohypertrophy of some muscle groups, such as the gastrocnemii, is a common finding in Duchenne type muscular dystrophy.

Some myopathies may be accompanied by specific clinical features in addition to weakness. Myotonia, or abnormally slow relaxation of muscles following contraction, occurs in myotonic dystrophy and a few other disorders. Prolonged contraction can be elicited on examination by tapping certain areas, such as the thenar eminence or the tongue with a reflex hammer. Cramps and contractures following exercise are a feature of some diseases involving a disturbance of carbohydrate or fat metabolism in muscle. Other disorders may be manifested by recurrent acute attacks of muscle weakness, accompanied by actual necrosis of skeletal muscle. Myoglobin released from the muscles is excreted through the kidneys, and produces a characteristic darkish-colored urine.

Neuromuscular Junction

Myasthenia gravis, like most of the primary disorders of skeletal muscle, tends to involve proximal limb muscles in a symmetric manner. The important clue to diagnosis in this disorder is fatigability. When muscle strength is tested, initially there may be only mild weakness, but with repeated or sustained contraction there is a definite increase in weakness, with subsequent return of strength following a period of rest. A diagnosis of myasthenia gravis is also suggested by involvement of ocular and bulbar muscles, producing symptoms such as diplopia, ptosis, dysarthria, and dysphagia. Fatigability can also be demonstrated in these muscle groups. Increasing ptosis of the upper lids becomes apparent during prolonged upward gaze, and progressive weakness of the muscles of articulation can be demonstrated by having the patient count or read aloud.

Nerve Roots and Peripheral Nerves

Diffuse Involvement

The symptoms of peripheral neuropathy include weakness, numbness, tingling, and, in some cases, burning discomfort. Neuropathies may selectively involve motor or sensory fibers, but in most cases there is mixed involvement of both types of fibers.

The presence of sensory signs and symptoms is an important point that favors involvement of peripheral nerves, rather than involvement of skeletal muscle, neuromuscular junction, or anterior horn cells.

The muscle weakness is most prominent in distal muscle groups and is usually associated with obvious wasting. Because of involvement of either the afferent or efferent components of the spinal reflex arc, tendon reflexes are diminished or absent. Sensory changes also involve the distal parts of the extremities, producing a characteristic "glove and stocking" pattern of sensory loss. The process may involve all sensory modalities, or there may be selective involvement of superficial sense (touch, pain, and temperature) or of deep sense (position and vibration).

Focal Involvement

Disorders affecting a single nerve or nerve root are characterized by localized muscle wasting and weakness and diminished reflexes in muscles innervated by that nerve, and impaired sensation in a pattern that corresponds to the area of innervation by a single nerve or nerve root. Pain is a common feature of nerve root disorders, and has a tendency to radiate into the area that is innervated by the involved root. Accurate diagnosis of these syndromes depends on a good working knowledge of the muscles that are controlled and the areas of the skin that are innervated by each of the major peripheral nerves and by the spinal nerve roots.

Anterior Horn Cells

Since poliomyelitis has become a rare disorder, the most commonly encountered disorder affecting anterior horn cells or spinal motor neurons is amyotrophic lateral sclerosis (motor neuron disease). In contrast to most polyneuropathies, the weakness resulting from anterior horn cell disease is usually asymmetric, particularly in the early stages. Muscle wasting is a prominent feature. Fasciculations or localized twitchings due to spontaneous discharges of individual motor units are also prominent and may preceed the onset of weakness. Although fasciculations do occur in healthy individuals and in patients with peripheral nerve or root pathology, they are much more prominent and widespread in anterior horn cell disease.

The occurrence of some signs of upper motor neuron dysfunction, such as hyperreflexia or Babinski responses, combined with obvious signs of lower motor neuron disease, is a characteristic feature of many cases of amyotrophic lateral sclerosis. The absence of any evidence of sensory involvement is another feature that helps distinguish these disorders from diseases affecting roots or peripheral nerves.

CLINICAL MANIFESTATIONS OF SPINAL CORD DISEASES

The spinal cord is a common site for pathology in a number of different disorders affecting the nervous system. The clinical findings that suggest involvement of the spinal cord are *weakness* affecting both lower extremities, accompanied by signs of upper motor neuron dysfunction, *sensory loss* affecting the legs and often the lower part of the trunk, and bladder dysfunction. If the lesion involves the cervical cord, weakness and sensory changes will also be apparent in the upper extremities. The absence of cranial nerve signs and other features suggesting pathology above the cervical level helps further to localize the disease process to the spinal cord.

Some knowledge of the anatomy of the spinal cord and the location of the major motor and sensory pathways is essential before one can accurately localize lesions involving the spinal cord. The clinically important structures are best seen by examining a cross section of the cord (Fig. 14.2). Descending motor pathways, particularly the corticospinal tract, are located within the lateral columns of white matter. Since the corticospinal tracts have already crossed at the level of the lower medulla, motor pathways in the lateral columns of the cord are concerned with movement of the limbs on the same side of the body. Other motor pathways such as the reticulospinal and vestibulospinal tracts descend in the anterior columns. These include both crossed and uncrossed fibers.

Sensory pathways follow two major routes once they enter the spinal cord. Fibers that subserve pain and temperature sense originate from neurons in the dorsal horn of the grey matter, cross through the central portion of the cord, and ascend in the lateral spinothalamic tract. Other fibers representing the central projections of neurons whose cell bodies are in the dorsal root ganglia enter the dorsal columns on the same side and ascend to the nuclei located at the upper end of the dorsal columns. Although recent experimental studies have raised some questions concerning the traditionally accepted role of the dorsal columns, it is still generally assumed that position and vibration sense are subserved by these pathways. Touch or pressure sense is represented in both the dorsal columns and the spinothalamic tracts. The other major pathways that should be noted in Figure 14.2 are the dorsal and ventral spinocerebellar tracts located superficially in the lateral columns.

Upper Motor Neuron Versus Lower Motor Neuron Dysfunction

The features that help identify weakness due to disorders of the lower motor neuron have already been discussed. These include prominent muscle wasting, reduced muscle tone or flaccidity, and diminished or absent tendon reflexes. Several important clinical findings help distinguish motor dysfunction resulting from lesions affecting motor pathways above the level of the anterior horn cells. Extensor plantar or Babinski responses are present, and there are signs of reflex hyperexcitability, including spasticity, increased tendon jerks, and clonus. Some degree of muscle atrophy may occur as a result of disuse, but this is not nearly so striking as the wasting in lower motor neuron dysfunction. These clinical signs are, of course, not specific for spinal cord lesions but can occur with involvement of motor pathways in the cerebral hemispheres or brainstem.

Many clinicians still refer to Babinski responses, increased tendon jerks, spasticity, and clonus as "pyramidal signs." This terminology is inaccurate, and its use should be discouraged. Animals studies indicate that a restricted lesion involving only the pyramidal tract results in a Babinski response and some loss of strength and control in distal muscle groups of the extremities. However, muscle tone and tendon reflexes are not increased, and clonus is not present. These abnormalities most likely occur as a result of involvement of descending pathways other than the corticospinal tract. It is important, therefore, to realize that the terms *upper motor neuron* and *pyramidal tract* are not synonymous. The pyramidal tract is only one of several upper motor neuron pathways.

Evidence of reflex hyperexcitability is often not present immediately following acute spinal cord injury. Initially the limbs are flaccid and tendon reflexes are reduced or absent. This state is referred to as spinal shock. After a variable period of time, reflex activity returns, muscle tone becomes increased, and clonus may be elicited.

On sensory examination the clue to the presence of a spinal lesion is the demonstration of a *sensory level*. Often this is located over the thorax or abdomen, areas that may be neglected during a routine sensory examination. A careful examination for sensory changes over the trunk is an important part of the investigation of a patient with a suspected spinal cord lesion. Sensory loss below the level of the lesion may involve all modalities, or there may be selective impairment of either pain and temperature sense or position and vibration sense. The sensory level for pain and temperature does not always correspond to the level of the lesion affecting the spinal cord. Because sensory fibers may ascend several segments above their point of origin before crossing to join the spinothalamic tract, the level below which pain and temperature sense is impaired may be several segments below the actual site of pathology. The phenomenon of sacral sparing occurs with some spinal cord disorders. Pain and temperature sense may be totally lost over many segments below the level of the lesion, but preserved over the sacral dermatomes on the buttocks and posterior thighs.

Other signs in addition to a sensory level may help localize the level of a lesion involving the lower thoracic cord. With a lesion around the T10 level, there will be weakness of the lower abdominal muscles with preservation of strength in the upper abdominal muscles. This results in upward deviation of the umbilicus when the patient tenses the abdominal muscles to raise his head or attempts to sit up. This is known as Beevor's sign. Abdominal reflexes may also be helpful. With a lesion at the T10 level, the upper abdominal reflexes will be preserved while the lower abdominal reflexes are absent.

Since normal bladder control is mediated by descending fibers in the lateral columns, bladder dysfunction is common in spinal cord disease. With acute cord lesions, the patient develops urinary retention and a flaccid bladder that may become markedly distended. Chronic cord lesions are accompanied by signs and symptoms of a spastic bladder. Bladder capacity is reduced, and symptoms such as frequency, hesitancy, or urgency of micturition are common. Incontinence may occur as a result of automatic reflex emptying of the bladder.

Specific Spinal Cord Syndromes

Acute or Subacute Spinal Cord Compression

Neoplastic or inflammatory processes in the extradural space can result in rapidly progressive loss of motor and sensory function in the lower extremities, accompanied by evidence of bladder dysfunction. Since the spinal cord can tolerate mechanical compression and the resulting ischemia for only a limited time, this situation should be considered a medical emergency. A myelogram should be performed without delay, and if a compressive lesion is demonstrated surgical decompression should be carried out.

Brown-Séquard Syndrome

Brown-Séquard syndrome is a classic neurologic syndrome that occurs as a result of hemisection of the spinal cord. Pure hemisection of the cord is a rare phenomenon, but may occur as a result of penetrating injuries by a knife or bullet. More commonly, a partial Brown-Séquard syndrome occurs when the cord is compressed from one side by an extradural mass lesion. The clinical findings include weakness, with signs of upper motor neuron dysfunction in the extremities on the same side as the lesion and reduced pain and temperature sense on the opposite side. If the dorsal columns are involved, there is reduced position and vibration sense on the same side. In addition, there may be ipsilateral incoordination of the extremities due to the combination of impaired proprioception and involvement of spinocerebellar pathways.

The Syndrome of a Central Cord Lesion

Another characteristic clinical picture occurs with a lesion involving the central part of the spinal cord. Syringomyelia is the classic example, but similar clinical findings may occur with intramedullary cord tumors, or sometimes following trauma to the spinal cord, particularly if spinal cord function has already been partially compromised by narrowing of the spinal canal due to spondylosis.

The first pathways to be involved are the crossing sensory fibers subserving pain and temperature sense. Therefore, the patient loses pain and temperature sense bilaterally, but, at least initially, has retained touch, position, and vibration sense. These lesions are often located in the cervical region and extend over several segments. The pattern of sensory loss may resemble a cloak or shawl, with loss of sensation over the shoulders, upper extremities, and upper thoracic dermatomes, and preserved sensation below this level. This so-called suspended sensory loss, together with the dissociation of pain-temperature sense and position-vibration sense, is strong evidence in favor of a central cord lesion.

Lateral expansion of the lesion from the center of the cord may lead to involvement of the anterior horns of the grey matter. This can result in a lower motor neuron pattern of weakness and wasting in muscles innervated by the involved spinal segments. Frequently this is most apparent in the intrinsic muscles of the hand. Further expansion into the lateral columns may involve descending motor pathways and produce signs of upper motor neuron dysfunction in the lower extremities.

Vascular Lesions of the Spinal Cord

Certain features of the blood supply of the cord help explain the clinical findings that occur as a result of spinal cord ischemia. The cord is supplied by a single midline anterior spinal artery and a pair of posterior spinal arteries, which originate (upper end) from the vertebral arteries. This blood supply is supplemented by a variable number of segmental arteries arising from the descending aorta and entering the spinal cord through the intervertebral foramina. The most important of these is the artery of Adamkiewicz, which is usually present on the left side between the T10 and L3 levels. If this artery is occluded by artheroma or damaged during surgical procedures performed on the abdominal aorta, there is a high risk of spinal cord infarction. Spinal cord circulation is most likely to be compromised in a "watershed zone" in the midthoracic region where the descending blood supply from the vertebral arteries meets the ascending supply from the lower segmental arteries.

The anterior spinal artery supplies the anterior two thirds of the spinal cord, including the anterior and lateral columns. The posterior one third of the cord, consisting mainly of the dorsal columns, is supplied by the posterior spinal arteries. Therefore, occlusion of the anterior spinal artery results in paraplegia and loss of pain and temperature sense below the level of the lesion, with sparing of position and vibration sense.

CLINICAL MANIFESTATIONS OF DISORDERS AFFECTING THE BRAINSTEM AND CRANIAL NERVES

The brainstem is an extremely complex and compact part of the central nervous system. It includes three major divisions—the midbrain or mesencephalon, the pons, and the medulla oblongata. Within the brainstem are the nuclei of cranial nerves 3–12. The emerging roots of these cranial nerves are a prominent feature of the external anatomy of the brainstem. The central core of the upper brainstem contains the reticular activating system, an extremely important area concerned with maintenance of normal consciousness. The brainstem also contains a number of "long tracts" that provide functional connections between the cerebral hemispheres and the spinal cord. These include several important descending motor pathways. Some, such as the corticospinal tract, merely pass through the brainstem; others, such as the reticulospinal and vestibulospinal tracts originate from nuclei within the brainstem.

The major ascending sensory pathways, the spinothalamic tract and the medial lemniscus, also pass through the brainstem en route to the thalamus and higher sensory centers.

Some familiarity with the anatomy of this region is required to enable one to appreciate the significance of signs and symptoms occuring as a result of brainstem lesions. Fortunately, it is not necessary for the clinician to be able to identify all the nuclei and tracts in the brainstem that are described in textbooks of neuroanatomy. A working knowledge of the location of cranial nerve nuclei and major motor and sensory pathways at three different levels in the brainstem—the midbrain, the midpons, and the upper medulla—should be sufficient to permit an understanding of the anatomical basis for most of the commonly encountered clinical syndromes associated with brainstem dysfunction. Cross sections of the brainstem at these three levels are illustrated in Figures 14.3, 14.4, 14.5.

With the large number of nuclei and pathways located in the brainstem, it is not suprising that the clinical features of brainstem dysfunction are complex and variable. The signs and symptoms that suggest the possibility of a lesion in the brainstem are as follows:

1. Alterations of consciousness
2. Cranial nerve palsies
3. Disturbances of eye movement control (for example, gaze palsies, diplopia, and nystagmus)
4. Vertigo
5. Dysarthria and dysphagia
6. Ataxia and incoordination
7. "Long tract" signs, that is, motor and sensory deficits in trunk and extremities
8. Disturbances in control of respiration, blood pressure, and heart rate

Few of these signs and symptoms, when they occur in isolation, are specific for pathology within the brainstem. It is the overall pattern or combination of several signs and symptoms that allows the clinician to predict with reasonable certainty whether a lesion is present in the brainstem. For example, the combination of cranial nerve palsies on one side and motor or sensory deficits involving the contralateral extremities, is highly suggestive of a focal disorder in the brainstem. Inspection of Figure 14.3 indicates that a fairly restricted lesion in the ventral part of the midbrain can result in an ipsilateral 3rd nerve palsy and contralateral hemiparesis due to involvement of motor pathways in the cerebral peduncle. Because long tracts are in close proximity to each other in the brainstem, it is not uncommon to observe bilateral motor and sensory deficits in the extremities.

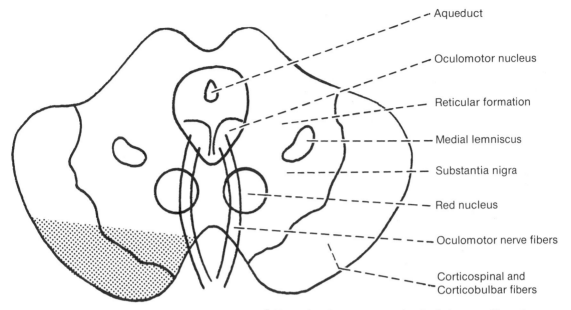

Fig. 14.3 Cross-section of the brainstem at the midbrain level. Damage to the shaded area will result in an ipsilateral 3rd nerve palsy and contralateral hemiparesis

Lateral Medullary Syndrome

The lateral medullary syndrome of Wallenberg is a classic example of a localized brainstem lesion producing multiple signs and symptoms. This usually occurs as a result of infarction in the territory supplied by the posterior inferior cerebellar artery. This may result from occlusion of this vessel or of its parent vessel, the veterbral artery. The area of involvement is indicated by shading in Figure 14.5; identification of the anatomic structures in this area permits the clinician to predict all the signs and symptoms that may occur with this syndrome.

These include vertigo, nystagmus, ataxia, dysar-

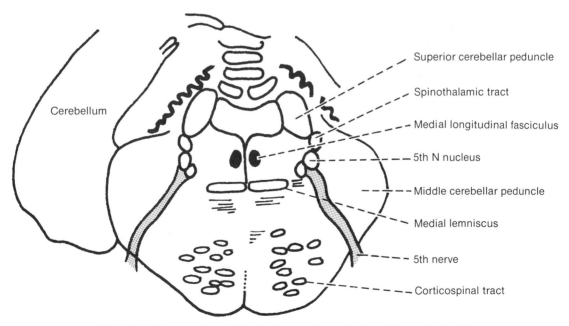

Fig. 14.4 Cross section of the brainstem through the mid-pontine level

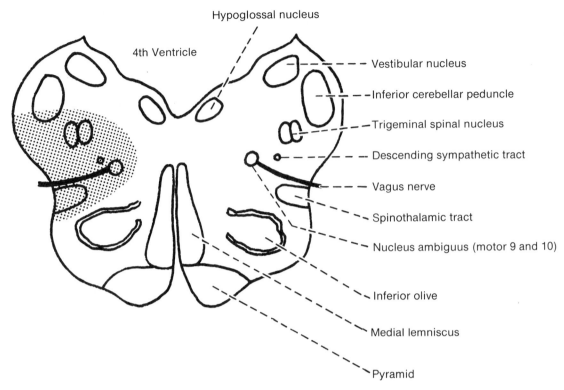

Fig. 14.5 Cross section of the brainstem through the upper medulla. The shaded area indicates the area damaged in the lateral medullary syndrome

thria, dysphagia, and weakness of muscles of the palate, pharynx, and vocal cord on the same side as the lesion. In addition, there is usually an ipsilateral Horner's syndrome, a diminished corneal reflex and reduced pain and temperature sense over the face on the same side as the lesion, and diminished pain and temperature sense on the contralateral side of the body below the trigeminal distribution. In addition, there is usually a cerebellar type of incoordination involving the ipsilateral extremities. There is really only one site in the central nervous system where a single lesion can produce this entire constellation of signs and symptoms. The anatomic basis for these clinical findings is outlined in Table 14.1.

In localizing lesions of the brainstem, it is also important to note which structures are not involved. In the lateral medullary syndrome there are usually no signs of corticospinal tract involvement or impairment of position and vibration sense, since the pathways that subserve these functions are located in the medial portion of the medulla. Familiarity with the major anatomic features of the brainstem should enable the clinician to localize with reasonable accuracy lesions occuring at other sites in the brainstem.

Table 14.1   **Lateral Medullary Syndrome—Anatomical Basis for the Major Clinical Features**

Signs and Symptoms	Structure Involved
Vertigo, nystagmus, ataxia	Vestibular nucleus and its connections
Dysarthria, dysphagia, vocal cord paresis	Nucleus ambiguus (10th nerve motor nucleus for striated muscle)
Ipsilateral Horner's syndrome	Descending sympathetic tract
Diminished corneal reflex, reduced pain and temperature sense over ipsilateral face	Descending tract and nucleus of trigeminal nerve
Reduced pain and temperature sense over contralateral side of body	Spinothalamic tract
Incoordination of ipsilateral extremities	Inferior cerebellar peduncle, cerebellar hemisphere

Cranial Nerve Palsies

Lesions that result in cranial nerve palsies may occur within the brainstem, outside the brainstem but within the subarachnoid space, or along the peripheral course of the cranial nerves as they emerge from the skull. The anatomic relationships of the cranial nerves are shown in Figure 14.6. The combination of cranial nerve palsies, long tract signs, and other symptoms such as vertigo or altered consciousness suggests that the problem lies within the brainstem itself. Asymmetric involvement of multiple cranial nerves suggests a more diffuse process outside the brainstem in the posterior fossa. This can result from inflammatory processes, such as chronic granulomatous meningitis due to tuberculosis or fungal infections. Diffuse infiltration of the meninges with metastatic carcinoma can produce a similar clinical picture.

Several clinically important syndromes involving cranial nerves are associated with specific lesions in the posterior fossa. One of these is the cerebellopontine angle syndrome. The most common lesion that occurs at this site is an acoustic neuroma, a benign tumor originating from Schwann cells of the 8th cranial nerve (see Fig. 14.24). Other lesions that occur at this site are meningiomas and cholesteatomas. The initial symptoms are usually tinnitus and loss of hearing. Involvement of the vestibular portion of the 8th cranial nerve results in mild disequilibrium and nystagmus. As the tumor enlarges and compresses adjacent structures, the 5th and 7th cranial nerves may be involved, with resulting ipsilateral diminished corneal reflex, decreased facial pain and temperature sense, and facial weakness. Further enlargement may lead to involvement of the cerebellar peduncles and incoordination of the ipsilateral extremities.

Another specific syndrome involving cranial nerves is the *jugular foramen syndrome*. This occurs as a result of a tumor of the jugular bulb, a glomus jugulare tumor. This involves cranial nerves 9, 10,

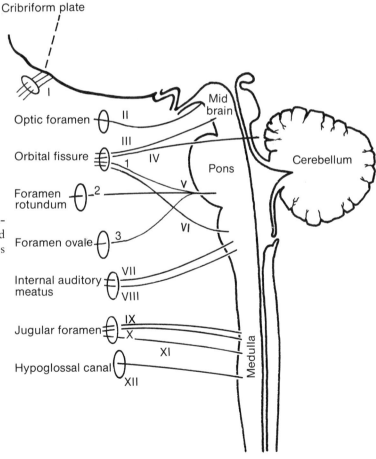

Fig. 14.6 Diagramatic representation of brain site-of-origin and foramina-of-exit of cranial nerves 1 through 12

and 11 as they exit from the skull through the jugular foramen. The resulting signs and symptoms include dysphagia, hoarseness, and diminished gag reflex, and weakness of the sternomastoid and trapezius muscles on the side of the lesion. Other cranial nerves including 7, 8, and 12 may become involved as the tumor enlarges.

Disturbances of Ocular Motility

Diplopia, nystagmus, and other disturbances of eye movement control are important localizing findings in many patients with neurologic disorders. Lesions responsible for these disorders frequently involve the brainstem and cranial nerves, but to appreciate the contribution of brainstem structures it is necessary to review briefly the entire system concerned with eye movement control.

Voluntary horizontal eye movements are initiated from cortical centers located in the frontal and occipital lobes. The frontal eye field is located anterior to the motor strip and is concerned with rapid or saccadic eye movements. The occipital center is responsible for smooth pursuit movements that are utilized to follow a moving target. Fibers from the frontal eye field project to a center for conjugate lateral gaze in the paramedian pontine reticular formation, in close proximity to the vestibular nucleus and the 6th nerve nucleus. Normal horizontal eye movements require coordination of activity of the lateral rectus for one eye and the medial rectus for the other eye. This is accomplished by the medial longitudinal fasciculus, a pathway located close to the midline of the brainstem connecting the pontine center for conjugate gaze and the 6th nerve nucleus on one side with the contralateral 3rd nerve nucleus. This pathway also receives input from the vestibular system.

The system that controls vertical eye movement is less well understood, but includes projections from the cortical centers to the pretectal area in the upper dorsal midbrain. From this site, fibers project to neurons in the 3rd and 4th cranial nerve nuclei, which control muscles involved in vertical gaze. A focal lesion involving the dorsal midbrain and pretectal area is manifested by paralysis of upward gaze (Parinaud's syndrome). This may be the presenting symptom of a tumor involving the pineal gland.

Eye movement disorders can be subdivided into three categories: *supranuclear, internuclear,* and *infranuclear.* In some respects this is analogous to the distinction between upper motor neuron disorders and lower motor neuron disorders affecting motor function in the extremities. Involvement of the supranuclear components of the ocular motor system is characterized by *gaze palsies.* These affect movement of both eyes in a particular direction. For example, a lesion involving the frontal eye field of the right cerebral hemisphere interferes with conjugate gaze to the opposite side, that is, to the left. A brainstem lesion involving the pontine center for conjugate lateral gaze is manifested by inability to look to the same side, that is, a lesion on the left side of the pons interferes with gaze to the left. The unopposed action of the contralateral pontine gaze center may result in tonic deviation of the eyes away from the side of the brainstem lesion.

Infranuclear eye movement disorders result from involvement of cranial nerves 3, 4, and 6 either within the brainstem or along the peripheral course of the nerves. These result in varying degrees of ophthalmoplegia, which affects the muscles of only one eye and results in diplopia.

The third category of eye movement disorders is *internuclear ophthalmoplegia,* which occurs as a result of a lesion involving the medial longitudinal fasciculus. This is a common site for demyelinating plaques in multiple sclerosis. Frequently these produce bilateral medial longitudinal fasciculus lesions. Ischemic lesions in the brainstem may produce unilateral internuclear ophthalmoplegia. Interruption of this connection between the 6th and 3rd nerve nuclei results in disconjugate eye movements. When the patient attempts to look to one side, the adducting eye fails to turn in. The patient is able to abduct the opposite eye but has difficulty maintaining it in an abducted position, and coarse jerky nystagmus occurs in this eye. Because different pathways are involved in activating the medial recti during convergence, the patient is usually able to adduct both eyes when he attempts to focus on a near object.

Isolated palsies involving cranial nerves 3, 4, and 6 occur fairly commonly, and are usually easily recognized. The 3rd nerve innervates four of the six extraocular muscles—the superior, medial, and inferior rectus, and the inferior oblique. Consequently, with a 3rd nerve palsy there is difficulty in turning the eye up, in, and down. Ptosis is usually present as well, since the 3rd nerve provides partial innervation of the levator palpebrae. Pupillary abnormalities occur as a result of involvement of the parasympathetic component of the 3rd nerve. The pupil becomes dilated and fails to contrict in response to light.

A 6th nerve palsy is associated with paralysis of the lateral rectus and inability to abduct the eye. Commonly the eye is partially adducted due to the unopposed tonic action of the medial rectus.

Fourth nerve palsies can be more difficult to identify. The 4th nerve innervates the superior oblique, which acts in conjunction with the inferior rectus to depress the eye. The superior oblique is the major depressor when the eye is in a partially adducted position. Therefore, patients with 4th nerve palsies experience maximum diplopia when they attempt to look down and in.

Complete palsies of these nerves are not difficult to identify. However, even minimal misalignment of the eyes will result in diplopia, and the paretic muscle responsible for this may not be readily identified on initial inspection of eye movements. Placing a red glass over one eye helps separate the images from the two eyes and allows the patient to identify which image is originating from which eye. Two simple rules help the examiner to identify the muscle or nerve responsible for the diplopia. First, the greatest separation of the images occurs when the patient attempts to look in the direction in which the weak muscle normally exerts its major action. Second, the image from the lagging eye is projected further in the direction of gaze. Thus, a patient with paresis of the right medial rectus experiences diplopia when he attempts to look to the left. The image from the right eye is perceived to be further to the left than the image from the left eye.

It should be noted that diplopia does not always indicate an isolated lesion affecting a single cranial nerve. Myasthenia gravis or certain myopathic disorders may cause weakness of multiple extraocular muscles and can produce fluctuating and sometimes confusing patterns of ophthalmoplegia.

Nystagmus

Nystagmus is a common and important clinical sign that may occur in association with lesions involving the vestibular system, the brainstem, or parts of the cerebellum. It is defined as an involuntary rhythmic oscillation of the eyes. In most cases there is a slow phase in one direction alternating with a rapid jerk of the eyes in the opposite direction. This is referred to as *jerk nystagmus*. By convention, the direction of the nystagmus is identified by the direction of the fast component. A less common form of nystagmus is *pendular nystagmus*, in which the eyes move with equal velocity in the two directions. This occurs with certain types of congenital nystagmus.

Nystagmus is not always indicative of nervous system dysfunction. Physiologic, or end-point, nystagmus may occur in normal subjects when they are required to maintain conjugate deviation of the eyes in an extreme lateral position. Stimulation of the vestibular system by rotation or caloric testing will also produce nystagmus in normal individuals. Optokinetic nystagmus is also a normal phenomenon that can be elicited by having a subject observe a moving pattern of alternating dark and light strips.

A number of different forms of pathologic nystagmus have been described, and several confusing and complex classifications have been proposed. It is not always possible to relate nystagmus to a lesion at any one specific site. However, a few simple observations during the clinical examination will help the physician determine which of the major categories of pathologic nystagmus he or she is observing. First, it should be noted whether the nystagmus is of the pendular or jerk type. The direction of the fast component should be identified, and the examiner should determine whether the nystagmus is horizontal, rotatory, or vertical. Are both eyes involved to the same degree, or are the movements disconjugate? In what direction of gaze does the nystagmus occur? Is it present in only one direction, or does it persist in the midposition with the subject looking straight ahead? Does visual fixation suppress or attenuate the nystagmus? Does the nystagmus occur only when the subject moves or assumes certain positions?

With this type of information it should be possible to differentiate between four major categories of pathologic nystagmus. These are as follows:

1. Vestibular nystagmus
2. Gaze paretic nystagmus
3. Positional nystagmus
4. Congenital nystagmus

Vestibular Nystagmus

Vestibular nystagmus occurs as a result of a unilateral lesion involving the peripheral or central components of the vestibular system. The loss of tonic vestibular input from one side causes the eyes to drift conjugately toward the side of the lesion. The fast component is away from the side of the lesion, and the amplitude of the nystagmus is increased by looking in the direction of the fast component. Nystagmus due to peripheral vestibular lesions is suppressed by visual fixation. This is less likely to occur with central vestibular disorders.

Gaze Paretic Nystagmus

Gaze paretic nystagmus, by contrast, is accentuated by fixation. The fast component is always in the direction of gaze, and the patient has difficulty maintaining tonic deviation of the eyes in any direction away from the midposition. This kind of nystagmus occurs with structural lesions at several sites in the brainstem and cerebellum. It is a common sign in patients with multiple sclerosis. It may also be produced by various drugs such as phenytoin, barbiturates, or diazepam. Asymmetric gaze paretic nystagmus usually indicates a structural lesion involving the brainstem or cerebellum, and in most cases the fast component is directed toward the side of the lesion.

Positional Nystagmus

Positional nystagmus characteristically occurs when the patient moves or turns quickly or when his head is placed in a certain position. It may be associated with lesions involving either the peripheral or central components of the vestibular system. A standard test used to elicit positional nystagmus involves moving the subject from a sitting posture to a supine position with his head extended over the end of the examining table and rotated to either the right or left. With peripheral disorders involving the labyrinth, there is usually a short latency before the nystagmus appears, the nystagmus tends to fade away as the position is maintained, and may be associated with marked subjective vertigo. Positional nystagmus of central (brainstem) origin appears almost immediately with movement, persists as long as the provocative position is maintained, and is associated with less vertigo.

Congenital Nystagmus

Congenital nystagmus occurs in various forms. It may have pendular characteristics but can switch to jerk-type nystagmus with gaze away from the midposition. It is almost always horizontal, and the frequency is often faster than what is seen with other forms of pathologic nystagmus. If it is pronounced, it can seriously interfere with visual acuity.

Vertigo

Vertigo is a hallucination of movement. Most commonly it consists of a feeling of rotation, either of the individual or of his surroundings. However, other illusions of movement such as a feeling of falling forward or being pushed or pulled to one side may occur with certain forms of vertigo.

Vertigo, as defined above, usually indicates a disturbance of function in the vestibular system, either in its peripheral components (labyrinth and 8th

nerve) or in the vestibular nuclei and their central connections in the brainstem. Under normal conditions there is a balanced input from the labyrinthine receptors to the central nervous system. Rotation causes movement of fluid in the semicircular canals, which alters the balanced input and signals that movement has occurred. Damage to the labyrinth or 8th nerve also creates an imbalance in the imput from the two sides, thus providing the central nervous system with false information concerning movement.

Dizziness is a term patients may use to describe a wide variety of symptoms including vertigo. It is important to determine whether they are experiencing real vertigo or other less specific symptoms such as lightheadness, faintness, or giddiness that can occur in association with many factors, such as postural hypotension, cardiac arrhythmias, anxiety, or hyperventilation.

The common causes of vertigo are listed below:

1. Peripheral Vestibular Disorders
   A. Meniere's disease
   B. Labyrinthitis
   C. Vestibular neuronitis
   D. Benign positional vertigo
   E. Toxic labyrinthitis
2. Central Vestibular Disorders
   A. Brainstem ischemia, that is, vertebrobasilar insufficiency
   B. Multiple sclerosis
   C. Brainstem tumors

Note that 8th-nerve tumors such as acoustic neuromas are not included in the above list. Although acute episodic vertigo may occasionally occur with this type of lesion, it is far more common for these patients to experience a vague sense of disequilibrium. Rarely, vertigo may occur with a disturbance affecting the cortical representation of the vestibular system in the superior temporal lobe. Occasionally seizure disorders originating in this area may be accompanied by vertigo.

In attempting to localize the site of a lesion producing vertigo, the physician should make careful note of other symptoms and signs occuring in association with the vertigo. Nausea, vomiting, ataxia, and nystagmus are commonly associated with most forms of vertigo, and their presence does not usually help distinguish between disorders affecting the peripheral and central components of the vestibular system. However, if the vertigo is accompanied by auditory symptoms such as tinnitus or hearing loss, it is most likely that the disturbance is in the periphery. For example, Meniere's disease is characterized by recurrent attacks of vertigo accompanied by tinnitus, reduced hearing, and a feeling of fullness or pressure in one ear.

The occurrence of other symptoms of brainstem dysfunction, such as diplopia, dysarthria, dysphagia, or altered consciousness, strongly suggests that the vertigo is due to central causes.

Facial Palsy

The facial nerve can be involved by a number of disease processes either within the pons or posterior fossa or in the facial canal, which runs within the petrous bone. By far the most common disorder encountered is Bell's palsy, an inflammatory disorder of uncertain etiology in which there may be considerable swelling of the nerve within the facial canal.

The initial approach to a patient presenting with facial weakness should be to determine whether the weakness is due to an upper motor neuron disorder or lower motor neuron disorder. With lower motor neuron facial palsies, the weakness involves both the upper and lower facial muscles. Often the patient is unable to voluntarily close the eye on the affected side. With upper motor neuron facial weakness there is relative sparing of the muscles of the upper half of the face, that is, the frontalis and orbicularis oculi.

The explanation for this is that the motor neurons controlling these muscles receive input from the motor cortex of both cerebral hemispheres, whereas motor neurons controlling the lower facial muscles receive synaptic input only from the contralateral motor cortex.

There are several other signs that may occur in association with a lower motor neuron facial palsy. These can be related to the sensory and autonomic fibers that travel along with the motor fibers in the facial nerve. Pain in or behind the ear is common during the acute stage of Bell's palsy. A small sensory branch of the facial nerve innervates part of the external auditory canal. The facial nerve also innervates the stapedius muscle, and weakness or paralysis of this muscle results in hyperacusis, another common symptom in the early stages of Bell's palsy. Taste sense over the anterior two thirds of the tongue is subserved by another branch of the facial nerve, the chorda tympani, and unilateral loss of taste in this area is a common feature with lower motor neuron facial palsies. Another autonomic branch of the facial nerve innervates the lacrimal glands, and decreased lacrimation may occur with facial palsies.

Bulbar and Pseudobulbar Palsy

The term *bulbar palsy* refers to weakness of muscles innervated by the lower cranial nerves whose nuclei are located in the medulla or "bulb." These include cranial nerves 9, 10, and 12. The major symptoms of bulbar palsy are dysarthria and dysphagia. Examination reveals reduced movement of the palate on phonation. If the lesion is unilateral, the palate will fail to elevate on the involved side. In addition, there will be reduction of the gag reflex and weakness of the tongue with deviation toward the side of the lesion when it is protruded. Atrophy and fasciculation of the tongue may also be observed. There is also an upper motor neuron syndrome which may interfere with control of these muscles and cause dysarthria and dysphagia. This is referred to as *pseudobulbar palsy*. The motor neurons that innervate these muscles, like those controlling the upper facial muscles, receive inputs from both cerebral hemispheres. Therefore, pseudobulbar palsy occurs only when there are bilateral lesions affecting the corticobulbar pathways. The four main features of pseudobulbar palsy are dysarthria, dysphagia, a hyperactive jaw jerk, and peculiar emotional lability. Emotional lability presumably occurs because brainstem mechanisms concerned with emotional expression are released from normal inhibitory influences from higher centers. The term "emotional incontinence" is sometimes used to describe this feature. The dysarthria of pseudobulbar palsy has a characteristic tight spastic quality and the speech sounds quite different from the slurred speech of a lower motor neuron bulbar palsy.

CLINICAL MANIFESTATIONS OF CEREBELLAR DYSFUNCTION

The cerebellum plays a major role in integrating motor function and controlling the sequence and timing of activation of different muscles during complex movements. Inputs to the cerebellum come from three main sources:

1. The cerebral cortex via cortico-ponto-cerebellar pathways
2. Muscle, joint, and cutaneous receptors in the extremities via the spinocerebellar tracts and dorsal columns
3. The vestibular nuclei and other nuclei within the brainstem

A large part of the output from the cerebellum is directed back to the motor cortex via the superior cerebellar peduncle and the ventrolateral thalamus. Other efferent fibers from the cerebellum project to various brainstem nuclei, including the lateral vestibular nucleus.

It has been proposed that the cerebellum receives information concerning motor commands originating from the cerebral cortex, compares this information with feedback signals from the moving extremity, and then generates appropriate error correction signals that are relayed back to the motor cortex. There is some experimental evidence to support this view, but much remains to be learned about the exact role of the cerebellum in the normal control of movement. Despite this, the clinical signs associated with cerebellar dysfunction have been well recognized for many years. These are summarized in Table 14.2. Two relatively distinct syndromes can be identified. One occurs with lesions affecting the vermis or midline cerebellar structures; the other is associated with more laterally positioned lesions in the cerebellar hemispheres.

Midline Cerebellar Syndrome

Disturbance of posture and gait are the hallmarks of a midline cerebellar lesion. The patient walks with a broad based staggering gait. He usually has great difficulty performing heel-toe walking or tandem gait. He may not be able to maintain equilibrium when he stands with his feet together. However, this deficit is usually not much worsened by closing the eyes, a feature which distinguishes cerebellar ataxia from ataxia due to loss of proprioceptive sensory feedback. Often there may be marked ataxia of gait with a lesion in the vermis, with little or no evidence of incoordination of individual extremities. Several disease processes affect the cerebellar vermis in a fairly selective manner. Alcoholic cerebellar degeneration exerts its major effects in this area. The vermis is also a common site for deposits of metastatic carcinoma.

Lateral Hemisphere Syndrome

Lesions involving the cerebellar hemispheres, particularly if they include the deep nuclei such as the dentate, result in a characteristic pattern of motor deficits affecting the arm and the leg on the same side as the lesion. Most of these are manifestations of errors in motor programming, that is, errors in the trajectory, velocity, and force of movement. When the patient attempts to move an extremity toward a target as during the finger-nose or heel-shin test, he may overshoot or undershoot the mark and have to make some terminal corrective movements. This is termed *dysmetria*. In addition, there is evidence of decomposition of movement: complex movements requiring coordinated activity in several different mus-

Table 14.2 **Signs and Symptoms of Cerebellar Dysfunction**

1. Midline Syndrome
    A. Ataxia of gait
2. Lateral hemisphere syndrome
    A. Hypotonia
    B. Limb incoordination
        Dysmetria
        Decomposition of movement
        Slowing of rapid alternating movements
    C. Intention tremor
    D. Pendular reflexes
3. Other Features
    A. Dysarthria
    B. Nystagmus
    C. Vertigo
    D. Nausea and vomiting

cle groups lose their normal smoothness and precision. Rapid alternating movements become slow and irregular (dysdiadochokinesis). In some cases a rhythmic intention tremor develops during target directed movements. This is more likely to be associated with a lesion in the outflow pathway in the superior cerebellar peduncle rather than with one in the cerebellar hemisphere itself.

Hypotonia is another feature of a cerebellar hemisphere lesion. Additional signs associated with this are pendular tendon reflexes and a rebound phenomenon or impaired "check"—a tendency to overshoot when a strong contraction is suddenly released.

It should be noted that these signs do not always indicate a lesion within the cerebellum itself. Ataxia of gait and incoordination of extremities can occur with lesions involving the spinocerebellar tracts in the spinal cord or cerebellar connections in the brainstem. Limb incoordination and slowing of rapid alternating movements can occur with lesions disrupting proprioceptive feedback either at the spinal cord level or in the somatosensory cortex. Also, the motor dysfunction that occurs with lesions affecting precentral cortex or parts of the basal ganglia may at times superficially resemble cerebellar dysfunction.

Several other signs of cerebellar dysfunction do not clearly fit into either the midline or lateral hemisphere syndrome. One of these is dysarthria. Speech becomes slurred and often has an explosive or staccato quality. In some respects this is analogous to the decomposition of movement that occurs with movements involving an arm or a leg. Nystagmus and various other disturbances of eye movement control, commonly occur with cerebellar lesions. Also, since the flocculonodular lobe of the cerebellum actually represents an extension of the vestibular system, symptoms such as vertigo, nausea, and vomiting may occur with pathology at this site.

CLINICAL MANIFESTATIONS OF BASAL GANGLIA DYSFUNCTION

The term *basal ganglia* refers to a cluster of nuclei located deep within the cerebral hemispheres and the upper brainstem. These include the substantia nigra, striatum (caudate and putamen), globus pallidus, subthalamic nucleus, and certain nuclei of the thalamus, particularly the ventrolateral-ventroanterior complex. The basal ganglia and their connections are sometimes referred to as the "extrapyramidal" motor system. However, this is an imprecise term that theoretically could include the cerebellum and all other components of the motor system except the pyramidal or corticospinal tract.

The main components of the basal ganglia and their interconnections are illustrated in Figure 14.7 and 14.8. As is the case with the cerebellum, there are extensive interconnections between the basal ganglia and the cerebral cortex, particularly with those areas concerned with control of movement. The major outflow of the basal ganglia occurs through the globus pallidus. Information from the globus pallidus is relayed through the ventrolateral thalamus to the motor cortex, from which multiple projections extend back to the caudate and putamen.

The clinical features of basal ganglia disorders are summarized in Table 14.3. Two distinct patterns of motor dysfunction occur. One is characterized by slowing or lack of movements (bradykinesia) and increased muscle tone. Parkinson's disease is a classic example of this type of disorder. The other syndrome is in many respects the exact opposite, and is accom-

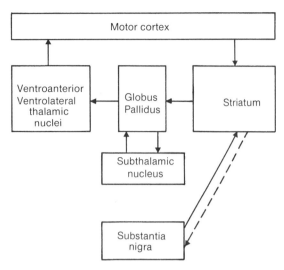

Fig. 14.8 Interconnections of the basal ganglia and cerebral cortex

panied by various types of excessive involuntary movement. Huntington's chorea is an example of a disorder in this category.

Recent advances in neurochemistry and neuropharmacology have made it possible to correlate these syndromes with specific neurotransmitter imbalances. In Parkinson's disease there is degeneration of dopaminergic neurons in the substantia nigra, with a resulting decrease in dopamine levels in the striatum. The clinical picture of bradykinesia, or reduced movement, can be considered to represent a *dopamine deficiency syndrome*. It is interesting to note that drugs such as phenothiazines that block dopamine receptors can produce a clinical syndrome very similar to parkinsonism.

The biochemical basis for Huntington's chorea is not yet fully understood, but there is evidence for a deficiency of acetylcholine and γ-aminobutyric acid in the striatum. These neurotransmitters normally function to counterbalance the effects of dopamine, so one could postulate that the abnormal involuntary movements occurring in Huntington's chorea are a

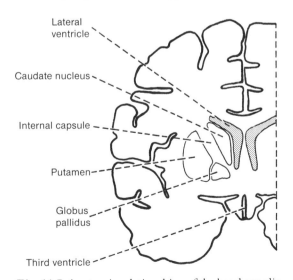

Fig. 14.7 Anatomic relationships of the basal ganglia and cerebral hemisphere

Table 14.3 **Signs and Symptoms of Basal Ganglia Dysfunction**

1. Reduced Movement
   A. Bradykinesia
   B. Rigidity
2. Excess Movement
   A. Resting tremor
   B. Chorea
   C. Athetosis
   D. Dystonia
   E. Hemiballismus

manifestation of a *relative excess of dopamine*. This view is supported by observations that parkinsonian patients treated with dopaminergic drugs may develop a variety of choreiform and dystonic movements if too much medication is administered.

Let us now consider the individual signs in greater detail. *Bradykinesia* literally means slow movement. Included under this general term are many of the features that are considered characteristic of Parkinson's disease. There is a general lack of spontaneous movement and an immobility of facial expression. All movements are slow and deliberate. Patients may have difficulty getting out of a car or chair and have trouble turning in bed. The gait is slow and shuffling, and associated movements such as arm swinging are reduced or absent.

The rigidity associated with basal ganglia disease differs in several respects from the other major category of increased muscle tone, spasticity. Rigidity has a plastic or "lead-pipe" quality, and remains constant throughout the full range of movement. The clasp-knife phenomenon is not present. Rigidity may be associated with a cogwheel phenomenon, a jerky increase in resistance that feels similar to pulling a lever over a rachet.

Chorea, athetosis, dystonia, and hemiballismus are not always clinically distinct signs, and may represent a continuous spectrum of excess involuntary movements. *Chorea* consists of rapid irregular jerky movements that can involve any part of the body, although the distal extremities are more likely to be affected. Facial grimacing and involuntary movements of the tongue are common. *Athetosis* is manifested by slower, writhing, purposeless movements. It is seen most commonly in certain forms of cerebral palsy. *Dystonia* refers to more persistent abnormal postures that are maintained for a period of time. The trunk and proximal limb muscles may be more involved than distal muscles. *Hemiballismus* consists of sudden violent flinging movements, often involving an entire extremity. The lesion responsible for hemiballismus is located in or very close to the subthalamic nucleus.

Tremor

The tremor of parkinsonism is something of a paradox, since most of the other features of the disease are manifestations of reduced movement. Tremor can occur in association with a number of other disorders, not all of which are manifestations of basal ganglia dysfunction. A simple classification of tremor follows:

1. Physiologic tremor
2. Pathologic tremor
   A. Resting tremor (parkinsonian tremor)
   B. Postural tremor (essential tremor, heredofamilial tremor, senile tremor)
   C. Intention tremor

Physiologic tremor is a rapid fine tremor occurring at a frequency of around 10 Hz. It is best seen in the outstretched hands. It is accentuated by factors such as fatigue, anxiety, and hyperthyroidism. Essential tremor is similar in many respects. It also is most apparent when muscles are contracted to maintain a fixed posture. The frequency may be similar to that of physiologic tremor or slightly slower. The head and trunk may be involved in addition to the extremities. The anatomic basis for essential tremor is unknown.

Parkinsonian tremor characteristically occurs when the limb is at rest and is at least partially suppressed by initiation of voluntary movement. The frequency is in the 4 to 7 Hz range. It tends to involve distal muscle groups and may have a pill-rolling quality.

Intention tremor has already been mentioned with cerebellar syndromes. It consists of rhythmic oscillations that occur during a target-directed voluntary movement. It is believed to occur as a result of a lesion involving the dentate nucleus or the outflow pathway from the cerebellum in the superior cerebellar peduncle.

DISORDERS OF THE CEREBRAL HEMISPHERES

Diffuse Involvement

Although the emphasis up to this point has been on the identification of focal lesions within the nervous system, it should be recognized that some disorders affect the entire brain without pathology being localized to one side or to any specific site. The general term *diffuse encephalopathy* can be used to refer to these conditions. Some of them are acute and rapidly progressive, while others are chronic or static and progress at only a slow rate.

Acute Encephalopathies

Alterations of consciousness and disturbances of mentation are the main features of an acute encephalopathy. The level of consciousness may vary from drowsiness and mild confusion to stupor or deep coma. In addition to alterations in consciousness, agitation, mood changes, hallucinations, and hyperactive irrational behavior often accompany acute encephalopathies. These features are collectively referred to as delirium. The classic example is delirium tremens associated with alcohol withdrawal, but similar clinical features may occur with acute meningitis or encephalitis, or in association with some metabolic or toxic encephalopathies.

Epileptic seizures may also accompany some of the acute diffuse encephalopathies. In some of these disorders the progressive deterioration in level of consciousness may be accompanied by other signs suggesting increased intracranial pressure, such as headache, vomiting, and papilledema.

Chronic Encephalopathies

Chronic disease processes that affect the cerebral hemispheres diffusely are most commonly characterized by the clinical syndrome of dementia. There is progressive deterioration of higher intellectual functions, such as memory, orientation, ability to think abstractly and make judgements, and grasp of general knowledge. The most common example of a disorder in this group is Alzheimer's disease. Usually consciousness is maintained, at least until the later stages of the illness. The problem of dementia and the disorders that cause it are discussed in greater detail in the section entitled Dementia.

Syndromes Associated with Focal Lesions of the Cerebral Hemispheres

Frontal Lobe Syndromes

Functions represented in the frontal lobes include movement of the contralateral side of the body and expressive language function. Large areas of the frontal lobes have as yet poorly defined or unknown functions. Many of the so-called silent areas of the cerebral cortex are located in the frontal lobe. It is, therefore, not uncommon for a slowly expanding tumor in the frontal lobes to attain considerable size before it produces obvious signs and symptoms.

There is evidence that the frontal lobes are concerned with many aspects of higher intellectual function. It is not surprising, therefore, that dementia is a common feature with frontal lobe pathology. In some cases this may be indistinguishable from the dementia that is associated with diffuse processes affecting the cerebral hemispheres. However, often there are additional features that help point to focal pathology in the frontal lobes. Flattening of affect and apparent lack of concern may be associated with the other features of dementia. Some patients with frontal lobe lesions exhibit a bizzare jocularity, with a tendency to incorporate many jokes and puns in their conversation. This has been described in the German literature as *witzelsucht*.

Certain pathologic reflexes are reliable indicators of frontal lobe pathology. These include the grasp reflex and the sucking or rooting reflex. It is interesting to note that these, along with Babinski response, are present in normal infants but disappear during the first year of life. Their reappearance with frontal lobe lesions suggests that mechanisms that normally inhibit them have been disrupted. Other reflexes, such as the palmomental reflex (localized contraction of the mentalis muscle in response to scratching the palm of the hand) and the "snout" or "pouting" reflex, may appear with frontal lobe lesions but have less specific localizing value than the grasp and sucking reflex.

Lesions affecting the more posterior part of the frontal lobe including the precentral gyrus are associated with varying degrees of hemiparesis involving the contralateral side of the body. If the lesion is anterior to the motor strip (area 4) but involves premotor areas (areas 6 and 8), weakness may not be a prominent feature but defects in control and coordination of movement may be present.

If the dominant frontal lobe is involved, particularly Broca's area, disorders of speech will be present. Most commonly these will take the form of expressive dysphasia, in which the patient is able to understand spoken and written language but is unable to speak or speaks in a slow hesitant (nonfluent) manner.

Less common manifestations of frontal lobe disease include disturbances of bladder and bowel function due to involvement of the paracentral lobule on the medial surface of the hemisphere. An uncommon but clinically important sign of some lesions affecting the base of the frontal lobes is anosmia, due to involvement of the olfactory tracts. This may be the earliest sign of an olfactory groove meningioma growing between the basal portions of the two frontal lobes.

Disturbances affecting the frontal eye field (area 8) produce valuable localizing signs. Normally this area is concerned with conjugate deviation of the eyes to the opposite side. Focal seizures originating in or near this area may begin with turning of the head and eyes to the opposite side (adversive seizures). Destructive lesions may result in tonic deviation of the eyes toward the side of the lesion, although it should be noted that this phenomenon may also occur with unilateral occipital lobe lesions.

Temporal Lobe Syndromes

The temporal lobe contains the cortical centers for auditory and vestibular function, although disturbances of these functions are relatively rare with cortical lesions. However, the area concerned with receptive language function (Wernicke's area), is located close to the cortical center for audition in the superior temporal gyrus of the dominant hemisphere. Dysphasia is a common symptom of temporal lobe pathology, and is discussed in more detail in a later section.

The white matter of the temporal lobes includes the lower half of the optic radiation. Fibers projecting from the lateral geniculate body to the visual cortex, loop around the temporal horn of the lateral ventricle (Meyer's loop). Pathologic changes in this area are associated with a contralateral homonymous field defect involving the upper quadrants of the visual fields.

Seizures are one of the most common manifestations of temporal lobe pathology, particularly with involvement of the mesial temporal lobe components of the limbic system, the hippocampus and amygdala. Seizures originating in the temporal lobe are accompanied by a variety of disturbances of consciousness, emotion, perception, and cognitive function and fall into the category of complex partial seizures (see Epilepsy).

The temporal lobes are concerned with some aspects of memory and learning. Recent memory and the acquisition of new information is a function of the limbic system, which includes the hippocampi and their connections via the fornix to the mamillary bodies and dorsomedian thalamus. Bilateral lesions affecting this system result in a syndrome in which the individual is no longer able to acquire and retain new information and may resort to confabulation as a compensatory measure (Korsakoff's syndrome). This can occur as a result of injury or disease affecting the hippocampi, although this is a relatively rare situation. A more common site for lesions causing Korsakoff's syndrome, particularly in chronic alcoholics, is in the mamillary bodies or thalamus (see Dementia).

Parietal Lobe Syndromes

A number of complex functions are represented in the parietal lobe. The most anterior portion of the parietal lobe, the postcentral gyrus, contains the cortical receiving area for somatic sensation. The more posterior parts of the parietal lobes have in the past been considered to be "association cortex." Newer information suggests that these areas play an important part in the integration of sensory input, both visual and somatic, with motor output.

The deeper white matter of the parietal lobes contains the superior portion of the optic radiation, which transmits information from the upper half of each retina to the visual cortex. Lesions involving these pathways result in a visual field defect that usually affects the contralateral inferior quadrant of the visual field for both eyes.

Focal lesions involving the postcentral gyrus or immediately adjacent cortex or the related subcortical white matter produce a characteristic disturbance of sensation known as "cortical sensory loss." Elementary sensations such as touch, pain, temperature, and vibration are relatively spared. However, higher discriminatory sensations including joint position sense, two-point discrimination, and the ability to localize sensory stimuli are impaired. In addition, there may be astereognosis, that is, the inability to identify objects placed in the hand, and graphesthesia, the inability to identify numbers or letters traced on the extremities contralateral to the side of the lesion.

The differences in functional specialization of the two cerebral hemispheres become apparent when one studies the effects of lesions involving the more posterior portions of the parietal lobes. Focal disorders affecting the dominant parietal lobe, particularly the region of the angular and supramarginal gyri at the posterior end of the Sylvian fissure, produce an interesting combination of symptoms that include agraphia, acalculia, right-left disorientation, and finger agnosia (inability to name or identify individual fingers). When all of these symptoms occur together, the clinical picture is referred to as Gerstmann's syndrome.

The nondominant parietal lobe is the area where the brain stores maps. These include the spatial representation for parts of the body as well as for extrapersonal space. Focal lesions in this area result in disturbances of body image and spatial disorientation.

Varying degrees of unilateral neglect and sensory inattention occur in patients with lesions affecting the nondominant parietal lobe. In its simplest form this may consist merely of sensory inattention or extinction. When simultaneous bilateral sensory stimuli are applied, the patient fails to perceive the stimulus on the affected side. With more extensive involvement, the phenomenon of anosognosia may be present. The patient is unaware of a hemiparesis or may even deny that there is any deficit even when it is pointed out to him. In the most extreme form, in which cortical representation of the contralateral extremities has been completely destroyed, the patient may deny that an arm or leg even belongs to him.

Dressing apraxia is another unusual symptom that occurs with nondominant parietal lobe lesions. The patient may have great difficulty organizing his clothing to get properly dressed, or he may fail to dress one side of his body.

Constructional apraxia is another manifestation of the spatial disorientation that occurs with nondominant parietal lobe dysfunction. The patient is unable to copy simple geometric designs. When asked to draw an object such as a face or a bicycle, parts are misplaced or not completed. A standard test often used is to ask the patient to insert the numbers at appropriate places on a clock face. Spatial disorientation is also manifested by a tendency for these patients to become lost in familiar surroundings. They have difficulty drawing a floor plan of their home or a simple map of their neighborhood.

Occipital Lobe Syndromes

The major functions of the occipital lobe are concerned with vision. Pathologic processes involving the primary visual cortex located on the medial surface of the occipital lobe produce a contralateral homonymous hemianopia. This area is supplied by the posterior cerebral artery, and occlusion of this vessel is a common cause of occipital lobe infarction and resulting hemianopia. More anteriorly placed occipital lobe lesions that involve visual association areas may produce inattention or extinction in the visual field on one side rather than an absolute field defect. Visual agnosia may also occur with lesions involving the visual association areas. In this disorder the patient is unable to identify objects by sight, despite the fact that visual pathways and primary visual cortex are intact.

Table 14.4   Assessment of Dysphasia

1. Spontaneous Speech
    A. Fluent or nonfluent
    B. Paraphasias
    C. Word-finding difficulty
    D. Circumlocution
    E. Grammatical errors
2. Comprehension
3. Naming
4. Repetition
5. Reading
    A. Out loud
    B. For comprehension
6. Writing

Bilateral dysfunction of the visual cortex, which sometimes occurs as a result of thrombotic or embolic lesions at the upper end of the basilar artery, results in a syndrome of cortical blindness. The presence of normal pupillary reactions in this situation indicates that visual pathways to the lateral geniculate body are intact. Peculiar changes in affect may accompany cortical blindness. In some cases, the patient may deny or be unaware that he is blind.

CLINICAL MANIFESTATIONS OF LANGUAGE DISORDERS

Definition

Dysphasia is an impairment of previously intact language abilities secondary to brain damage. The patient may be unable either to appreciate the symbolic meaning of words, or to produce them. In many cases both defects are present. Dysphasia results from focal lesions of the dominant cerebral hemisphere, which is usually the left hemisphere, and must be differentiated from the following entities:

1. Dysarthria is a disturbance of articulation resulting from interference with motor mechanisms controlling tongue, palate, or facial muscles.

2. Dysphonia is an inability to produce sound normally, and results from laryngeal dysfunction.

3. Global confusional states result from diffuse cerebral hemisphere dysfunction. Although the resemblance is only superficial, dysphasic patients are often considered confused.

Clinical Approach

The clinical examination of the dysphasic patient is summarized in Table 14.4.

The patient's speech, either spontaneous or in response to questions, should be assessed. Patients with fluent dysphasia will speak in phases and sentences, and normal speech rhythms and melody are relatively preserved. Their speech is, however, often remarkably devoid of meaning, with many circumlocutory phrases. They never get to the point, "beat around the bush," and produce very few meaningful nouns and verbs. Paraphasias (use of the wrong word or wrong sound within a word) are common. Patients with all types of fluent dyphasia have difficulty in naming objects.

Patients with nonfluent dysphasia have sparse slow effortful speech with abnormal rhythm (telegraphic speech). Sentences are often incomplete, but, in contrast to fluent dysphasia, patients are often able to convey substantial amounts of information.

Comprehension can be tested by giving the patient verbal commands to carry out. The patient's ability to find appropriate words can be tested by asking him to name objects in the room. More subtle deficits can often by unmasked by requesting the name of parts of objects (for example, the teeth of a comb or the crystal of a watch).

Asking the patient to repeat phrases after the examiner tests repetition ability. Poorer speech production on repetition than during spontaneous speaking is significant.

Classification

The major types of dysphasia with their principle clinical features are shown in Table 14.5.

Broca's dysphasia (expressive dysphasia) results from brain lesions in Broca's area (anterior speech area) immediately anterior to the motor strip (Fig. 14.9). Hemiparesis is usually present because of associated damage to the adjacent motor strip.

Wernicke's dysphasia (receptive dysphasia) results from damage to Wernicke's area (posterior speech area) in the superior temporal lobe. The cardinal feature of damage to this area is an inability to comprehend both spoken and written language. Global dysphasia results from destruction of both anterior and posterior speech areas, usually from middle cerebral artery occlusion.

Conduction dysphasia results from lesions between the two major speech areas, which damage the interconnections between the two areas. These patients show relatively good language comprehension, but are strikingly unable to repeat sentences and phrases after the examiner. Spontaneous speech pro-

Table 14.5 **Classification of Dysphasia**

Type	Comprehension	Repetition
Nonfluent		
Broca's	Good	Poor
Global	Absent	Absent
Fluent		
Wernicke's	Poor	Poor
Conduction	Good	Poor
Anomic	Good	Good
Isolation	Absent	Good

duction shows paraphasias, and circumlocution is prominent. Isolation dysphasia results when anterior and posterior speech areas are separated from the rest of the brain by infarction in the border zones between the major cerebral arteries. This usually results from hypotension.

Anomic dysphasia is characterized by great difficulty in naming and word-finding in the presence of fair to good comprehension and good ability to repeat. The responsible lesion is usually near the angular gyrus of the parietal lobe.

Dysphasia almost invariably results from focal cerebral lesions, usually infarction or tumor. Anomic dysphasia is at times an exception to this rule, and may result from more diffuse brain disturbances.

Not all patients with dysphasia fit precisely into the categories discussed. Most, however, can be classified according to their predominent language disturbance, and the responsible lesion can usually be localized to the anterior speech area, the posterior speech area, or both.

Apraxia

Apraxia is a related disorder of higher brain function in which the patient is unable to carry out a motor activity in the presence of intact motor and

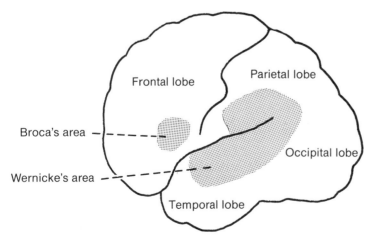

Fig. 14.9 Lateral view, left cerebral hemisphere, showing major speech areas

sensory systems, comprehension, and alertness, despite a desire to cooperate. Ideomotor apraxia is the most common form, and results from lesions that disconnect the posterior speech area from the motor control areas of the limb or facial muscles to be used in the test. These patients are unable to carry out, in response to a verbal command, a motor activity that can be easily performed spontaneously.

NEUROMUSCULAR DISORDERS

MUSCLE DISORDERS

Clinical Manifestations

Disordered muscle function in myopathy is due to primary disease of muscle and not secondary to peripheral nerve or CNS disease. Patients with myopathy present with weakness, which often has a definite topographic distribution and involves some muscles more than others. Proximal weakness with relative sparing of distal muscles is common. Deep tendon reflexes remain present until weakness is very severe. Muscle wasting may be prominent in the late stages. The major categories of muscle disorders are shown in Table 14.6.

Laboratory Investigation

In addition to general tests, the laboratory investigation of muscle disease involves serum creatine kinase (CK) determinations, electromyography (EMG), and muscle biopsy. Serum CK levels are elevated in diseases causing muscle necrosis, and are particularly high in Duchenne type muscular dystrophy and polymyositis. CK levels are normal or, at

Table 14.6 Neuromuscular Disorders

1. Muscle Disorders
    A. Muscular dystrophies
    B. Congenital myopathies
    C. Periodic paralysis
    D. Polymyositis
    E. Myopathy secondary to systemic disease
2. Neuromuscular Junction Disorders
    A. Myasthenia gravis
    B. Myasthenia syndrome
    C. Botulism
3. Peripheral neuropathy
    A. Mononeuropathy
    B. Multiple mononeuropathy
    C. Symmetrical sensorimotor polyneuropathy
    D. Autonomic neuropathy
4. Anterior Horn Cell disorders
    A. Motor neuron disease

Table 14.7 Muscular Dystrophies

1. Duchenne
2. Becker
3. Facioscapulohumeral
4. Myotonic
5. Other (Limb girdle and others)

most, mildly elevated with chronic weakness due to neuropathy or CNS disease. Serum CK levels can be markedly elevated in normal individuals after severe exercise and are also markedly elevated in hypothyroidism.

EMG demonstrates electrical activity, recorded on an oscilloscope from a needle electrode placed in muscle. Differentiation can usually be made between weakness related to myopathy and weakness resulting from other causes. Motor unit potentials, which reflect the summated electrical activity of muscle fibers in a single motor unit, tend to be small and of short duration in myopathy because diseased individual muscle fibers have dropped out. During minimal effort, the EMG will show activation of more motor units than normal (hyperrecruitment).

Muscle biopsy involves removal of a small fragment of muscle for histologic and histochemical studies. Primary muscle disease can usually be differentiated from other causes of weakness and, in addition, the specific type of muscle disease present can frequently be identified.

Muscular Dystrophies

The muscular dystrophies comprise a group of inherited myopathies that cause slowly progressive weakness. The more common muscular dystrophies are shown in Table 14.7.

Duchenne Type Muscular Dystrophy

Duchenne type muscular dystrophy is one of the most common and severe. It is inherited as an X-linked recessive trait and occurs only in males. Affected children walk at approximately the usual time, but may be awkward. Parents frequently notice nothing amiss until age 5 or 6 years when the child starts school. Progressive weakness follows, and walking is usually no longer possible by age 12 years. Patients have difficulty climbing stairs or getting up off the floor because weakness develops early in the pelvic girdle muscles. Pseudohypertrophy of the calf muscles is frequent.

A positive family history is usually present in patients with Duchenne type muscular dystrophy, but a family history may be absent, because 30 percent of all cases of X-linked muscular dystrophy are the result of new mutations in genetically normal mothers. Females who have a dystrophic son and either a dystrophic brother or maternal uncle are definite carriers of the genes. One half of the sons of these mothers will be affected. Sisters and other female relatives of dystrophic males are possible carriers. It may be difficult to determine for certain if such females are carriers or not. Serum CK levels are elevated in approximately 70 percent of carrier females, but a normal CK level does not rule out the carrier state. EMG studies and muscle biopsy may yield additional information.

In patients with Duchenne type muscular dystrophy, including younger siblings with the disease who are not yet symptomatic, serum CK levels are elevated to 5 to 10 times normal. EMG studies show myopathic changes, and muscle biopsy will show muscle necrosis, phagocytosis, an increase in connective tissue, fatty infiltration, and muscle regeneration. No treatment is currently available for Duchenne type muscular dystrophy other than physiotherapy, mechanical aids, and orthopedic procedures. Early diagnosis and genetic counseling of parents and other family members is of paramount importance.

Approximately 10 percent of cases of X-linked muscular dystrophy have a more benign course (Becker muscular dystrophy). In these families, affected patients usually have onset of weakness after age 7 years, and become wheelchair bound only after adulthood has been reached.

Facioscapulohumeral Dystrophy

Facioscapulohumeral dystrophy has a distinctive pattern of muscle involvement with marked weakness of the pectoral girdle, winging of the scapula, and facial weakness. Muscles of the pelvic girdle are not involved until later in the disease. Onset is usually between 7 and 25 years of age. Some patients are very mildly affected, while others show much more severe involvement. Inheritance is autosomal dominant.

Myotonic Muscular Dystrophy

Myotonic muscular dystrophy is an autosomal dominant dystrophy that often does not become apparent until adulthood. Weakness first involves the hands, arms, and feet dorsiflexors. Facial, oropharyngeal, and abdominal weakness is common and wasting of the sternocleidomastoid temporalis, and masseter muscles is usually striking. Deep tendon reflexes are lost early.

Voluntary myotonia is usually present, and is best demonstrated by asking the patient to tightly grip the examiner's hands for several seconds. The patient will be unable to open his hand quickly. Percussion myotonia is also usually present, as demonstrated by percussion of the forearm muscles and tongue. A quick contraction in response to percussion is normal, but in myotonic dystrophy the contraction remains for several seconds or longer. Myotonia results from a muscle cell membrane abnormality. Voluntary or percussion activation of muscles results in repetitive muscle fiber action potentials and the resulting "after contraction" prevents normal rapid muscle relaxation. Myotonia is also seen in myotonia congenita, paramyotonia congenita, and hyperkalemic periodic paralysis.

Myotonic dystrophy is associated with a large number of other features presumably related in some way to the underlying genetic abnormality. These include frontal baldness in men, cataracts and other ocular abnormalities, EKG abnormalities, impairment of smooth muscle function, testicular atrophy, low basal metabolic rate, abnormal glucose tolerance and reduced serum levels of IgG.

Progression of weakness in myotonic dystrophy is generally slow, and patients remain active into late adulthood. Marked weakness occasionally develops in infancy and early childhood. Mental deficiency is common in those cases with early onset. Many adults with the disease show apathy and lack of initiative.

Congenital Myopathies

These include a large number of muscle disorders with early onset of nonprogressive muscular weakness. Hypotonia, weakness, and feeding difficulty may be apparent at birth. Specific diagnosis usually requires a muscle biopsy. Central core disease, nemaline myopathy, and various mitochondrial myopathies are all examples of congenital myopathies.

Periodic Paralysis

A number of syndromes result in episodic weakness. The most common of these, hypokalemic periodic paralysis, has autosomal dominant inheritance. Penetrance is low in females, so the majority of clinically affected patients are males. Major attacks of weakness usually come on in the morning. Weakness is more marked in proximal muscles, and patients are frequently unable to get out of bed during an attack. Attacks may be precipitated by exertion and high carbohydrate meals, and usually last a number of hours. During these paralytic episodes, there is excessive entry of potassium into muscle, and serum potassium tends to be low.

Hyperkalemic and normokalemic forms of inherited periodic paralysis also occur. Periodic paralysis with intermittent weakness also occurs in thyrotoxicosis, and is relieved by treatment of the thyroid disease.

Polymyositis and Dermatomyositis

Polymyositis is an inflammatory myopathy with muscle damage resulting from autoimmune attack.

Clinical Manifestations

Polymyositis usually presents with slowly progressive proximal muscle weakness. Muscles may be painful and tender. Dysphagia occurs in 60 percent of patients, but diplopia is rare.

Patients with dermatomyositis present with muscle weakness similar to that in polymyositis, but have skin involvement as well. (see Chapter 18).

Laboratory Investigation

Serum CK levels are elevated in polymyositis, often to over 10 times normal.

Electromyography shows myopathic changes with hyperrecruitment of small amplitude, short duration muscle action potentials on voluntary effort. Numerous fibrillation potentials are also usually present because partial necrosis of muscle fibers will often separate muscle fiber segments from the endplate region.

Muscle biopsy shows inflammation, muscle fiber necrosis, phagocytosis, and evidence of muscle fiber regeneration (Fig. 14.10)

Treatment

Polymyositis usually progresses to severe weakness. Most patients respond to steroid therapy. Prednisone in high doses (100 mg daily) is given until weakness is resolving and CK levels return to normal. Prednisone dose is then gradually tapered, but maintenance therapy may be necessary for years.

Immunosupressive agents (methotrexate or aza-

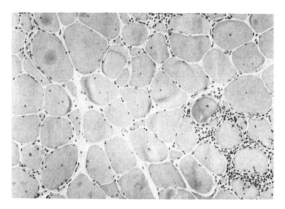

Fig. 14.10 Muscle biopsy from a patient with polymyositis, showing increased variation in muscle fiber diameter and internal nuclei, and a prominent inflammatory infiltrate (lower right corner)

thioprine) are often effective in patients refractory to steroids.

Underlying tumors should be searched for in elderly patients. Occasionally, tumor removal will be followed by remission of the polymyositis (see Chapter 18).

Myopathy Secondary to Systemic Disease

Myopathy with muscle weakness and wasting can occur in a number of endocrine disorders.

Both hyperthyroidism and hypothyroidism can be associated with marked proximal muscle weakness and wasting, which resolves upon treatment of the thyroid disorder. In addition, hyperthyroidism is associated with myasthenia gravis and periodic paralysis. Patients with hypothyroidism have elevated serum CK levels whether or not clinical myopathy is present.

Proximal limb weakness and wasting is common in patients with Cushing's syndrome, and also occurs with long-term steroid therapy. Serum CK levels are usually normal. Muscle biopsy shows selective atrophy of type 2 muscle fibers.

Hyperparathyroidism may also cause a myopathy with proximal limb weakness. Myalgias are often prominent. Treatment of the hyperparathyroidism reverses the weakness.

NEUROMUSCULAR JUNCTION DISORDERS

Disorders affecting the neuromuscular junction are shown in Table 14.6. The most important of these is myasthenia gravis.

Myasthenia Gravis

Pathophysiology

The neuromuscular junction consists of a nerve terminal, an intervening synaptic cleft, and the postsynaptic muscle cell membrane (Fig. 14.11). The nerve terminal contains vesicles of acetylcholine (ACh), which are released with the arrival of a nerve action potential. The released ACh combines with the postsynaptic acetylcholine receptors (AChR) and allows sodium Na$^+$ ions to enter the muscle cell. The released ACh is active only briefly as it is rapidly destroyed by acetylcholinesterase in the synaptic cleft. Threshold depolarization in the postsynaptic membrane results in a muscle cell membrane action potential and muscle fiber contraction.

Normal neuromuscular transmission depends on a sufficient number of "hits" between ACh molecules and the AChRs. In myasthenia gravis, antibodies directed at AChRs damage the postsynaptic region of the neuromuscular junction. AChRs are greatly reduced in number and the number of ACh-receptor combinations resulting from one nerve action potential may be insufficient to reach threshold postsynaptic depolarization.

In the normal neuromuscular junction there is a slight reduction in the amount of ACh released per nerve action potential with repetitive firing of the nerve axon. This reduction is normally of no consequence because a large safety factor exists. In myasthenia gravis, the decreased amount of ACh released with later nerve impulses is often insufficient to produce threshold depolarization in the postsynaptic membrane. Neuromuscular transmission thus fails with continuing activity, and weakness results (fatigability). With rest, effective neuromuscular transmission is restored.

Clinical Manifestations

Myasthenia gravis may occur at any age. The course of the disease is variable, and exacerbations followed by partial remissions may occur.

The usual presentation of myasthenia gravis is fluctuating weakness, which is often worse towards the end of the day (see Clinical Localization of Neurologic Disorders). Involvement of cranial nerve innervated muscles is common, and results in diplopia, ptosis, dysarthria, and dysphagia. Extraocular muscle weakness that does not follow the distribution of individual cranial nerves should always suggest myasthenia gravis.

Diagnosis

If the history and physical examination suggest myasthenia gravis, the edrophonium (Tensilon) test is useful in confirming the diagnosis. Edrophonium, an acetylcholinesterase inhibitor, slows destruction of ACh and improves neuromuscular transmission

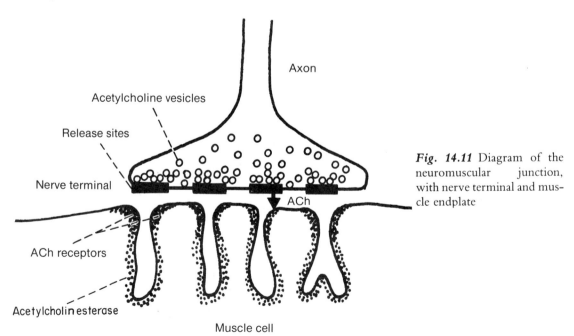

Fig. 14.11 Diagram of the neuromuscular junction, with nerve terminal and muscle endplate

in myasthenia gravis. The patient's strength in weakened muscle groups is evaluated as objectively as possible. The length of time that upward gaze can be maintained is often used. Increasing dysarthria can be quantitated by how far the patient is able to count before slurred speech occurs. The number of arm raises or deep knee bends the patient can do is easily quantitated, and the vital capacity of the lungs is measured. The patient is then given 2 mg of edrophonium intravenously, followed by a further 8 mg if no untoward reaction occurs. His strength is then reevaluated. In myasthenia gravis the improvement with edrophonium is often dramatic. If the response is equivocal, the edrophonium test may be done blindly with a control injection of saline.

Electrodiagnostic neuromuscular transmission tests are often helpful. With repetitive nerve stimulation at rates of 3 per second, many myasthenics will show a decrement in the amplitude of the evoked compound muscle action potential. Serum AChR antibodies can be demonstrated in 85 percent of patients with myasthenia gravis. A positive result is diagnostically helpful, but a negative result does not exclude the disease.

Patients with myasthenia gravis should also have a chest roentgenogram with oblique views, since 15 percent of patients have thymomas. Other autoimmune disorders are common in myasthenia gravis; thyroid antibodies, rheumatoid factor, antinuclear antibody, and immunoglobulins should all be assessed. Pulmonary function tests are also important in severe myasthenic patients.

Treatment

Anticholinesterase medications improve the strength of myasthenic patients, but usually weakness cannot be abolished completely. Pyridostigmine bromide (Mestinon) is the most useful of these because of its relatively long duration of action. Steroid therapy may be useful. Increased muscle weakness can occur with high dose steroid therapy, but can usually be avoided by increasing the dose more slowly. After several months, dosage is usually changed to an alternate day regimen. Immunosupressive drugs such as azathioprine (lmuran) are also effective in some patients who are refractory to steroid therapy.

Thymectomy should be done in myasthenics with thymoma to prevent local tumor spread. Eighty-five percent of patients without thymoma will also benefit from thymectomy, and for this reason thymectomy should be considered in all younger myasthenic patients. Improvement after thymectomy may take

from 1 to 10 years to occur. In some cases, thymectomy will eventually eliminate the need for continuing medical treatment.

In the acutely ill myasthenic patient with severe muscle weakness, plasmapheresis with removal of the AChR antibody will confer short-term benefit. This may obviate the need for mechanical ventilation in some patients, or shorten the length of respirator therapy.

Other Disorders of Neuromuscular Transmission

In botulism, the neurotoxin blocks neuromuscular transmission by preventing release of acetylcholine from motor nerve terminals. A somewhat similar mechanism is present in the Eaton-Lambert syndrome (myasthenic syndrome). This syndrome is usually associated with small cell lung carcinomas. Weakness is present, but cranial nerve innervated muscles are usually spared. Neuromuscular transmission improves with repetitive activity, so that hand grip may become obviously stronger with repetitive attempts. Neuromuscular transmission studies show an increase in the amplitude of the compound muscle action potential with rapid repetitive stimulation. These findings are the converse of those seen in myasthenia gravis. Guanidine improves muscle weakness in myasthenic syndrome. Tick paralysis does not affect the neuromuscular junction but rather appears to block conduction in the motor nerve terminals.

PERIPHERAL NEUROPATHY

Both the nerve axons and their myelin sheaths must be intact for normal function of the peripheral nervous system. Many different pathologic processes can affect the peripheral nervous system and produce neuropathy. Some neuropathies involve primarily damage to the myelin sheath. Others affect the nerve axons directly, and the myelin sheath degenerates secondarily to axonal dysfunction. Still other neuropathies appear to affect both axon and myelin sheath independently.

The main categories of neuropathy are shown in Table 14.6. The clinical features of neuropathy are discussed in the section entitled Clinical Localization of Neurologic Disorders. The history and physical examination will usually allow classification of the patient's neuropathy as either a mononeuropathy or polyneuropathy.

Mononeuropathies

Sensory and motor dysfunction limited to the distribution of a single peripheral nerve or nerve root indicate a mononeuropathy. The common mononeuropathies are listed in Table 14.8.

Carpal Tunnel Syndrome

Carpal tunnel syndrome is common and often bilateral. Symptoms usually begin in the dominant hand and consist primarily of numbness and tingling in the median nerve distribution. Pain is often prominent in the hand and may radiate up the arm as far as the shoulder. The patient is frequently awakened at night by his symptoms, and this rather characteristic feature helps differentiate carpal tunnel syndrome from other causes of hand numbness. Although symptoms result from compression of the median nerve at the carpal tunnel, patients frequently state that all fingers are involved.

Nerve conduction studies are diagnostic. Surgical decompression of the median nerve at the wrist is the treatment of choice. Most patients have no obvious predisposing cause, but hypothyroidism, acromegaly, amyloidosis, diabetes, rheumatoid arthritis, and occupational factors may all predispose a patient to carpal tunnel syndrome.

Ulnar Neuropathy

The ulnar nerve is easily damaged by repeated trauma in its precarious course around the elbow. Excessive leaning on the elbow is the most common cause. Bony abnormalities in the elbow region and any diffuse peripheral neuropathy can be predisposing factors. Some patients have entrapment of the nerve at the cubital tunnel just below the elbow.

Patients complain of numbness in the fourth and fifth digits. In more severe cases weakness and wasting of the hypothenar and interosseous muscles of the hand are present.

Nerve condition studies are diagnostic. Many mild

Table 14.8 Common Mononeuropathies

Carpal Tunnel Syndrome
Ulnar Neuropathy
Radial Nerve Palsy
Peroneal Nerve Palsy
Meralgia paresthetica
3rd Cranial Nerve Palsy
Bell's Palsy
Femoral Neuropathy
Nerve Root Compression Syndromes

cases are satisfactorily treated by avoiding pressure on the elbow. In patients with progressive or severe ulnar neuropathy, or with predisposing bony abnormalities at the elbow, surgical transposition of the nerve to the front of the elbow may be necessary.

Radial Nerve Palsy

The radial nerve is frequently injured by external compression at the spiral groove of the humerus. This is seen most commonly in patients who have slept in unusual positions or on hard surfaces after heavy alcohol drinking. The patient presents with paralysis of wrist and finger extension. The tricep is usually spared and all tendon reflexes are normal. These findings help differentiate radial nerve palsy from lower cervical nerve root compression syndromes.

Recovery eventually occurs with no specific therapy. EMG studies can help determine prognosis. If nerve compression has been mild, conduction block will be present as the result of segmental demyelination at the point of compression, but axonal degeneration will not occur. These patients recover in 1 to 2 months. If fibrillation potentials are present in the extensor muscles of the forearm, axonal degeneration has occurred, and recovery will take many months. Axonal regrowth from the point of compression occurs at a rate of approximately 1 mm per day.

A posterior interosseus nerve palsy will cause weakness of finger extension, but wrist extension will remain strong. The nerve may require surgical decompression.

Peroneal Nerve Palsy

Peroneal nerve palsy presents with weakness of ankle and toe extension and weakness of foot eversion. Peroneal nerve palsy usually results from compression of the peroneal nerve at the fibular head due to crossing the legs or lying on a hard surface. Foot inversion is intact in peroneal nerve palsy, and helps to distinguish it from compression of the fifth lumbar nerve root.

Nerve conduction studies are diagnostic. Therapy consists of avoiding further pressure on the nerve, and a foot brace if necessary to aid in walking.

Meralgia Paresthetica

Entrapment of the lateral femoral cutaneous nerve presents with numbness and tingling in the lateral thigh. There is no associated weakness. Symptoms usually are precipitated by pregnancy or obesity, and usually disappear with resolution of the precipitating factor.

3rd Cranial Nerve Palsy

Isolated 3rd cranial nerve palsy is caused by expanding posterior communicating artery aneurysm, transtentorial herniation, diabetes, and ophthalmoplegic migraine (see Headache).

In diabetic 3rd nerve palsy, the appropriate extraocular movements are affected (see Clinical Localization of Neurologic Disorders), but pupillary reactions are often preserved. With other 3rd nerve palsies, pupillary reaction to light is usually involved early.

Ptosis resulting from 3rd nerve palsy is usually associated with a dilated unreactive pupil and allows easy differentiation from ptosis due to Horner's syndrome.

Bell's Palsy

Isolated facial nerve involvement causes a lower motorneurone type of facial weakness with paralysis of both the upper and lower parts of the face (see Clinical Localization of Neurologic Disorders). The absence of other signs of brainstem involvement is helpful in diagnosis. The ear should be carefully examined, since the facial nerve may be involved by cholesteatoma. Other cranial nerves should also be carefully examined for evidence of involvement.

Approximately 85 percent of patients with Bell's palsy recover over weeks or months, with only minor residual weakness and an acceptable cosmetic result. A small minority have little or no recovery of facial nerve function. A short course of steroid therapy, beginning with 50 mg of prednisone daily and rapid tapering of dosage over 8 days, may reduce the number of unsatisfactory recoveries, if steroids can be started within 72 hours after onset of symptoms. Prednisone therapy will also rapidly relieve the retroauricular pain experienced by many patients with Bell's palsy.

Femoral Neuropathy

Mononeuropathy of the femoral nerve occurs most commonly in diabetes. Anticoagulant induced hemorrhage in the fascial planes surrounding the femoral nerve can also lead to femoral nerve palsy and may require urgent decompression. The main clinical features of femoral neuropathy are weakness of knee extension and loss of the knee reflex.

Nerve Root Compression Syndromes

Nerve root compression may result from many causes. Intervertebral disc protrusions are the most common cause. Radicular pain, often exacerbated by movement, coughing, or straining, is usually the most prominent symptom. Numbness and weakness in the distribution of the affected nerve root are common in more severe nerve root compressions.

Compression of S1 nerve root by herniated L5-S1 disc is the most common nerve root compression syndrome. Characteristically, there is pain on straight leg raising and reduction or loss of the ankle jerk. Sensory loss over the S1 distribution, particularly over the lateral border of the foot may be present. Weakness of foot plantar flexion is present in severe cases only.

Conservative therapy with bed rest and analgesia is indicated if pain and numbness are the only symptoms. Improvement will generally occur. If significant weakness is present, urgent surgical decompression of the nerve root is indicated or weakness may remain permanently. Intractable pain with failed conservative treatment is another indication for surgery. Myelography or spinal CT scanning prior to surgery is necessary to demonstrate the compressing lesion.

Multiple Mononeuropathy

Symptomatic involvement of two or more nerve trunks results in multiple mononeuropathy or mononeuritis multiplex. Nerve ischemia with microinfarction is a common cause, and usually results from diabetes or vasculitis. Brachial or lumbosacral plexus involvement from injury, diabetes (diabetic amyotrophy), or infiltrating tumor also fall within this classification.

Clinical symptoms and signs can usually be referred to the distribution of several peripheral nerve trunks. Nerve conduction studies help to confirm the diagnosis. The therapy is directed to the underlying disease.

Symmetrical Sensorimotor Polyneuropathy

The symmetric sensorimotor polyneuropathies involve multiple nerves simultaneously (Table 14.9).

Table 14.9 **Symmetrical Sensorimotor Polyneuropathy**

Acute
    Guillain-Barré syndrome
Chronic
    Metabolic
        Diabetes
        Uremia
        Porphyria
    Deficiency states
        Alcoholism
        Vitamin B_{12} deficiency
    Genetic
        Charcot-Marie-Tooth disease
    Toxic
        Lead and other metals
        Drug-induced (vincristine, nitrofurantoin)
        Organic compounds (N-hexane)
    Paraproteinemia and Amyloidosis
    Connective Tissue Disease
    Carcinoma
    Unknown

Acute Sensorimotor Polyneuropathy

Acute paralysis from peripheral neuropathy developing over days occurs in porphyria, diphtheria, and some toxic neuropathies. The vast majority of these cases, however, result from acute inflammatory polyradiculoneuropathy, also referred to as acute idiopathic polyneuritis or Guillain-Barré syndrome (GBS).

Pathophysiology The etiology of GBS is unknown. GBS is preceded by an acute respiratory or gastrointestinal infection in approximately 50 percent of cases. Surgery, cancer, immunization, and systemic lupus erythematosus apparently can precipitate GBS.

Pathologically, GBS is characterized by multiple focal areas of peripheral nerve myelin destruction. This myelin destruction results from autoimmune attack by lymphocytes sensitized to basic myelin protein. Experimentally, a similar neuropathy can be produced in animals by injection of peripheral nerve myelin basic protein.

Clinical Manifestations GBS usually presents with rapidly progressive muscular weakness most marked in the legs. Eventually, the face may be involved and even total external ophthalmoplegia may occur. Sensory abnormalities are usually less marked, but tingling paresthesiae are common. Deep tendon reflexes are lost early in the course of illness. Plantar responses remain downgoing, consciousness is preserved, and evidence of CNS involvement is rare.

Usually symptoms and signs progress gradually for several days or weeks. The patient's condition then remains stationary for several weeks, and finally gradual improvement occurs. The prognosis for eventual recovery is excellent, provided that mechanical ventilation and good supportive care is available for patients who become weak enough to require respiratory assistance.

GBS must be differentiated from other causes of acute weakness. The sensory symptoms and areflexia differentiate GBS from rapidly progressive polymyositis and myasthenia gravis. Absence of upgoing plantar responses and other signs of CNS involvement aid in differentiation from spinal cord disease.

Laboratory Investigation CSF examination usually shows elevated protein levels without pleocytosis. In the first few days of illness, however, CSF protein may be normal. Up to 50 lymphocytes per cubic mm are present in CSF in approximately 10 percent of cases.

Nerve conduction studies may confirm the diagnosis of neuropathy, but peripheral nerve conduction velocity may be normal if nerve damage is mainly at the nerve root level.

Treatment Milder cases require little in the way of treatment, but patients should be observed closely until recovery is occurring.

Respiratory function must be carefully monitored in more severe cases. This is best done by serial measurements of vital capacity. Blood gases are not reliable for this purpose, as they may remain normal until sudden respiratory insufficiency occurs. Further, the patient may appear quite comfortable until the final minutes of respiratory decompensation. Patients should be transferred to an intensive care unit if vital capacity falls to 50 percent of predicted levels, and endotrachial intubation is usually done if vital capacity falls below 25 to 30 percent. Patients may require mechanical ventilation for several weeks (see Chapter 15).

Patients with severe paralysis should be given subcutaneous herapin therapy to prevent venous thrombosis and pulmonary embolism. Autonomic disturbances are common in GBS, with both hypotension and hypertension. These require careful management. Steroid therapy should not be given since it does not hasten neurologic recovery and simply produces added risks. Careful nursing care is essential to avoid pressure sores. Physiotherapy is needed to prevent joint contractures.

Chronic Sensorimotor Polyneuropathy

Pathophysiology Chronic progressive nerve injury resulting in chronic symmetrical sensorimotor polyneuropathy may result from numerous causes. In most instances, the mechanism by which the disease or toxin produces nerve damage is unknown. Usually, neurons with longer axons are more susceptible to toxic influence or metabolic derangement. As a result, symptoms and signs usually appear first in the distal extremities and then gradually progress to involve more proximal areas.

Clinical Manifestations Chronic sensorimotor polyneuropathy usually presents with numbness in the feet (see Clinical Localization of Neurologic Disorders). As progression occurs, the legs and hands also become symptomatic. Motor involvement, with weakness and wasting, likewise begins distally. Deep tendon reflexes are lost early in neuropathy, particularly at the ankles. Some neuropathies, notably vitamin B_{12} deficiency, may be accompanied by spinal cord lesions with hyperreflexia and extensor plantars.

On examination of the patient, distal sensory loss may be apparent. Hyperpathia or hyperesthesia may be present. With hyperpathia, a tactile or other stimulus is perceived as markedly painful. With hyperesthesia, light stimuli may be perceived as abnormally intense, but sensation threshold is still elevated.

Mild neuropathies are frequently asymptomatic, and are discovered on routine examination. This is often the case with mild diabetic neuropathy, alcoholic neuropathy, and hereditary neuropathies. Charcot-Marie-Tooth disease is an autosomal dominant hereditary neuropathy that is often discovered as an incidental finding. In more severe cases, the patient presents with weakness and wasting of the distal legs. The peroneal muscles are affected early, with weakness of ankle and toe extension. Pes cavus is common.

Some neuropathies, particularly alcoholic, diabetic, and amyloid neuropathies, may be accompanied by severe pain in the affected areas, particularly the feet.

Differential Diagnosis and Laboratory Investigation The diagnosis of chronic sensorimotor polyneuropathy is usually easily established from clinical examination and nerve conduction studies. The underlying etiology is often much more difficult to determine. In fact, even with modern diagnostic techniques, no specific etiology can be demonstrated in many patients. Many of these likely have hereditary neuropathies.

Table 14.9 lists the major causes of chronic sensorimotor polyneuropathy, and Table 14.10 outlines a diagnostic approach to determine the underlying etiology. Laboratory investigations that may be helpful are shown. The physician must be guided by the clinical situation, and not all of the tests listed will be done on every patient.

Alcoholism is a common cause of neuropathy. Associated dietary deficiencies particularly of thiamine are probably more important than the alcohol itself.

Table 14.10 **Evaluation of Chronic Symmetric Sensorimotor Polyneuropathy**

History
  Toxin exposure
  Drugs
  Diabetes
  Diet and alcohol
  Cancer
  Recurrent abdominal pain
  Family history of neurologic disorder
Physical Examination
  Diabetes
  Renal disease
  Liver disease
  Collagen disease
Laboratory Investigation
  Fasting blood sugar and glucose tolerance test
  BUN
  Serum B_{12}
  Serum protein electrophoresis
  Rheumatoid factor
  Antinuclear antibodies
  Serum lead, mercury
  Chest film and intravenous pyelogram
  Rectal, nerve biopsy
  Nerve conduction studies and EMG

A history of recurrent abdominal pain may suggest acute intermittent porphyria, a rare cause of neuropathy.

Immunoglobulin abnormalities can result in neuropathy. Neuropathy is common in multiple myeloma. Monoclonal gammopathies are also associated with neuropathy, and many of these patients appear to have antibodies directed against peripheral nerves. Systemic lupus erythematosus, rheumatoid arthritis, and scleroderma are all associated with neuropathy, presumably through an autoimmune mechanism. Some malignancies, notably small cell lung carcinomas, also produce neuropathy through remote effects of the neoplasm by mechanisms not understood.

CSF examination can be useful in some cases. Chronic progressive and recurrent inflammatory polyneuropathies related to GBS produce CSF protein elevations. Rectal and nerve biopsy can be helpful in detecting amyloid infiltration in patients with amyloidosis.

Nerve conduction studies can help in confirming the presence of polyneuropathy, but are less useful in determining etiology. Both sensory and motor conduction velocities can be determined in multiple nerves. In neuropathy with demyelination, nerve conduction velocities will be markedly reduced. Neuropathies with primarily axonal involvement will show relatively normal nerve conduction velocity, but nerve action potentials may be absent distally in severely affected nerves. In nerve entrapment syndromes, the site of nerve compression can often be shown by focal conduction slowing which results from segmental demyelination at the point of compression.

Treatment   The treatment of chronic sensorimotor polyneuropathy is directed to the underlying disorder when this can be determined. Physiotherapy and maintenance of good general health are helpful adjuncts. Care must be taken to avoid injury to anesthetic feet and hands. Patients with painful peripheral neuropathies usually respond poorly to analgesics, but may be helped by combination therapy with amitriptyline and fluphenazine.

Autonomic Neuropathy

Autonomic neuropathy with postural hypotension, impotence, and bladder disturbances may be prominent in patients with chronic sensorimotor polyneuropathy. Neuropathy secondary to diabetes, paraproteinemia, and amyloidosis are particularly likely to have marked autonomic involvement.

Occasionally, autonomic neuropathy may be present in isolation. This occurs in diabetes, chronic postganglionic autonomic insufficiency, and acute or subacute pan-dysautonomia.

Treatment of these disorders is primarily that of postural hypotension. A mineralocorticoid (Florinef) is useful in expanding plasma volume. Ergonovine may be used to reduce venous compliance. Support garments aid by preventing venous pooling in the legs.

ANTERIOR HORN CELL DISORDERS

Anterior horn cell disorders comprise a group of syndromes in which the primary pathology is idiopathic degeneration of the anterior horn cells of the spinal cord, often in association with upper motor neuron degeneration. Because both upper and lower motor neurons are frequently involved, the term motor neuron disease is frequently used for these disorders. The cause of these syndromes is unknown.

Werdnig-Hoffman Disease

Werdnig-Hoffman disease is a genetic disorder of infancy. Weakness and hypotonia are usually obvious before the age of 6 months. Progressive anterior horn cell loss occurs, with death usually following before 2 years of age.

Kugelberg-Welander Disease

Kugelberg-Welander disease begins in adolescence and is slowly progressive. In contrast to amyotrophic lateral sclerosis, the weakness is mainly proximal.

Amyotrophic Lateral Sclerosis

Amyotrophic lateral sclerosis usually presents between the ages of 40 and 70 years with muscle weakness and fasciculation. Cases are usually sporadic, but approximately 10 percent are familial.

Weakness usually begins distally, is often asymmetric, and progresses inexorably. Pharyngeal muscles are frequently involved. Muscle wasting from denervation secondary to anterior horn cell loss is prominent, but many patients also show evidence of upper motor neuron involvement, with hyperreflexia, upgoing plantars, and pseudobulbar palsy. Muscle fasciculations are often present and are particularly well seen in the tongue, which is often atrophic. Sensory symptoms are absent.

The mean survival is about 3 years, with death usually resulting from respiratory complications (see Chapter 15). Prominent involvement of pharygeal muscles with dysarthria and dysphagia early in the disease (progressive bulbar palsy) indicates a poorer prognosis.

Investigation

Serum CK levels are normal or only mildly elevated to less than 2 times normal.

Electromyography shows a reduction in the number of motor units recruited on voluntary effort and motor unit potentials are often very large because collateral sprouting from surviving axons results in giant motor units. Fibrillation potentials indicating denervation are often prominent in rapidly progressing cases. Motor nerve conduction velocities are usually normal because surviving axons conduct at normal velocity. Sensory conduction velocities are also normal.

Muscle biopsy is not usually necessary for diagnosis. It will show denervated muscle fibers and evidence of reinnervation in the form of fiber-type grouping.

Differentiation of motor neuron disease from cervical spondylosis with myelopathy is occasionally difficult. Cervical spine radiographs are helpful, and myelography may occasionally be necessary.

No treatment is currently available for these disorders.

BASAL GANGLIA AND RELATED DISORDERS

Involuntary movements are prominent in a number of neurologic disorders, as shown in Table 14.11. Although basal ganglia lesions are prominent in many of these disorders, many show more widespread CNS pathology. Some, like myoclonus, result from lesions elsewhere in the nervous system. In still others the pathology is unknown. The clinical features of basal ganglia dysfunction are listed in Table 14.3.

PARKINSONISM

Etiology

Many etiologies can give rise to parkinsonism. These include encephalitis, manganese poisoning, carbon monoxide poisoning, and phenothiazine and butyrophenone medications. Aside from antipsychotic medications, by far the most common cause

Table 14.11 **Disorders with Involuntary Movements**

Parkinsonism
    Idiopathic (Parkinson's disease)
    Drug-induced
    Others
Chorea
    Huntington's chorea
    Sydenham's chorea
    Senile
    Cerebral infarction
    Chorea gravidarum
    Drug-induced
Athetosis
    Cerebral palsy
Dystonia
    Dystonia musculorum deformans
        Generalized
        Segmental
    Wilson's disease
    Drug-induced
Hemiballismus
    Cerebral infarction
    Brain tumor
Others
    Tardive dyskinesia
    Benign essential tremor
    Myoclonus
    Hemifacial spasm

today is idiopathic degeneration of the dopaminergic neuronal systems of the basal ganglia (Parkinson's disease).

The most constant pathologic changes found in patients with Parkinson's disease are severe cell loss and depigmentation in the substantia nigra. The dopaminergic neurons of the substantia nigra are particularly affected, and dopamine levels are far below normal in the substantia nigra and striatum. This degenerative process continues throughout life in patients with idiopathic Parkinson's disease, leading to gradually increasing severity of symptoms and signs.

Dopaminergic neurons from the substantia nigra project to the striatum. Normal motor function is dependent upon a balance between cholinergic and dopaminergic neuronal systems in the striatum. Loss of the dopaminergic input to the striatum in Parkinson's disease presumably contributes to the clinical features.

CNS degenerative changes are not always limited to the basal ganglia, and dementia is more common in patients with Parkinson's disease than in age-matched controls. Some degree of parkinsonism is common in patients with Alzheimer's disease and senile dementia.

Some patients with parkinsonism have well-defined degenerations of other neuronal systems. In progressive supranuclear palsy, vertical and horizontal gaze palsies are present in addition to rigidity and bradykinesia. Shy-Drager syndrome manifests a combination of parkinsonism with severe autonomic insufficiency and postural hypotension. Degenerative changes are prominent in CNS autonomic neuronal systems, particularly in the intermediolateral columns of the spinal cord.

Drug-induced parkinsonism results from dopamine receptor blockade in the striatum by phenothiazines and haloperidol. This receptor blockade, like dopaminergic neuronal degeneration, results in an imbalance in striatal neuronal systems.

Clinical Manifestations

The cardinal features of parkinsonism are bradykinesia, rigidity, and resting tremor. Their relative prominence varies from patient to patient, and some patients do not show all three features. In addition, patients with parkinsonism show poor postural reflexes and lose their balance easily. They tend toward a flexed posture, and walk with a small-stepped gait. Because of poor postural reflexes, they may tend to go faster and faster (festinating gait) and be unable to stop until they reach an obstruction.

An immobile mask-like face is typical, and patients may drool saliva because of poor automatic swallowing. The voice typically becomes low pitched and monotonous, and handwriting is often particularly impaired with tightly bunched small letters (micrographia).

Treatment

Dihydroxyphenylalanine (L-dopa) has revolutionized the treatment of Parkinson's disease. Although patients have a brain dopamine deficiency, dopamine itself cannot be administered because it fails to cross the blood brain barrier. L-dopa, the precursor of dopamine, can be given orally and will enter the brain. There it is converted to dopamine and will to some extent reverse the symptoms and signs of Parkinson's disease.

L-dopa is also converted to dopamine elsewhere in the body, and this leads to drug side effects, particularly nausea and vomiting. Because of this, L-dopa is now usually administered in combination with an L-dopa decarboxylase inhibitor (Sinemet, Prolopa), which will inhibit peripheral conversion of dopamine but will not enter the brain. With the drug combination, nausea is unusual.

L-dopa should be started in small doses and built up gradually, particularly in elderly patients. The final maintenance dose ranges from 500 mg to 1,500 mg of L-dopa in combination with the enzyme inhibitor. The patient response will determine the maintenance dose. The appearance of involuntary movements (dyskinesia) is the most common dose-limiting side effect. These movements usually affect the face with involuntary grimacing or pursing of the lips. Movements affecting other parts of the body also occur. Hallucinations, vivid nightmares, and psychosis may also result from L-dopa therapy.

Because of progressive basal ganglia degeneration, therapy generally becomes less effective with time. Marked oscillations of motor ability may occur (on-off effect). Anticholinergic drugs (benztropine, trihexyphenidyl) and amantadine given in addition to L-dopa may benefit some patients. Bromocriptine, a dopamine receptor agonist, may also improve symptom control. Surgery, with stereotactic placement of lesions in the ventrolateral nucleus of the thalamus, is still occasionally resorted to. It is effective mainly in relieving tremor.

Anticholinergic drugs are the most effective treatment for parkinsonism secondary to phenothiazines and haloperidol.

CHOREA

Chorea consists of rapid irregular movements that usually involve the distal extremities. The pathogenesis of these movements is not fully understood, but excessive or unopposed basal ganglia dopaminergic activity may be responsible. In this sense, some of the choreas are the opposite of Parkinson's disease.

Clinically, chorea is often best observed in mild cases by asking the patient to extend his arms with the hands pronated, and observing for involuntary movements of the fingers and wrists.

Huntington's chorea is an autosomal dominant inherited disorder with progressive chorea and dementia (see Dementia). Onset of chorea is usually in adult life, and mean age at death is 55 years.

Sydenham's, or postinfectious, chorea usually occurs in children, often in association with rheumatic fever. Streptococcal infections are the major cause. Pathologically, widespread vasculitic lesions are usually present throughout the brain. The chorea tends to be self-limited, and eventually resolves.

Senile chorea refers to chorea occurring in the elderly without intellectual deterioration or family history of Huntington's chorea.

Chorea may appear for the first time in pregnancy or with oral contraceptive use. It resolves with delivery or oral contraceptive discontinuation.

Chorea also rarely appears as a result of cerebral infarction.

Chorea usually responds to some extent to phenothiazine or haloperidol therapy. These drugs block dopamine receptors and presumably reduce the imbalance between cholinergic and dopaminergic activity in the striatum. It must be remembered, however, that these drugs can also produce abnormal involuntary movements in some patients.

DYSTONIA

Dystonic movements are relatively slow, sustained, powerful, involuntary movements.

Dystonia Musculorum Deformans

The biochemical or anatomic mechanisms giving rise to dystonia are unknown. Genetic factors are important in many of these patients.

A severe hereditary autosomal recessive form of dystonia occurs in families of Jewish background. Symptoms usually begin in childhood. Initial localized dystonic symptoms and signs frequently progress over years to generalized dystonia and severe disability.

An autosomal dominant inherited dystonia without ethnic predilection has also been described. These patients tend to have milder symptoms and signs that frequently begin in adulthood, and may remain localized to a portion of the body. Similar sporadic cases of dystonia also occur without positive family history.

Torticollis is one of the most common localized or segmental dystonias. In these patients, the head is spasmodically and involuntarily deviated to one side because of abnormal contraction of the sternocleidomastoid and other neck muscles. The patient cannot control these neck movements, but early in the course of torticollis, maneuvers like touching the chin or leaning the head back against the wall may temporarily stop the spasms. Dystonia may remain limited to the neck, or progression may occur with appearance of dystonic symptoms elsewhere. Patients with torticollis are often erroneously considered to be hysterical.

Dystonia may also present with localized involvement of the arm, leg, or other parts of the body. Writers cramp, particularly if associated with awkwardness of all fine movements of the hand, is frequently a form of localized dystonia.

Treatment of dystonia is unsatisfactory. Phenothiazines, haloperidol, L-dopa, and tetrabenazine have all been reported to help some patients. Torticollis is also treated surgically by producing spinal root section or stereotactic thalamic lesions.

Wilson's Disease

Wilson's disease should always be ruled out in patients presenting with dystonia, because early treatment is essential (see Dementia).

Drug-Induced Dystonia

Phenothiazines, haloperidol, and related drugs can produce transient dystonic syndromes. These drugs include prochlorperazine (Stemetil), a commonly used antiemetic. Patients often present with uncontrollable upward deviation of the eyes (oculogyric crisis), or may have more generalized involuntary muscle contraction. Because of the bizarre nature of the symptoms, patients are frequently considered hysterical. The offending drug should be discontinued, and benztropine (Cogentin) should be given intravenously.

HEMIBALLISMUS

Hemiballismus consists of violent involuntary movements involving one half of the body. The arm is usually most severely involved. Hemiballismus results from damage to the subthalamic nucleus, usually by infarction, hemorrhage, or tumor.

The violent movements must be reduced to prevent exhaustion, and this is usually best accompanied with chlorpromazine or haloperidol. Large doses are often required.

TARDIVE DYSKINESIA

Tardive dyskinesia manifests involuntary movements, usually affecting the lips, the tongue, and the face. They result from dopamine receptor alterations in the basal ganglia secondary to long-term phenothiazine therapy. The offending drug should be discontinued with the appearance of tardive dyskinesias. Even with drug discontinuation, the dyskinesias may remain permanently. Reserpine, tetrabenazine, and clonazepam may be of help in reducing the involuntary movements, but are often ineffective.

BENIGN ESSENTIAL TREMOR

Benign essential tremor is usually an autosomal-dominant inherited disorder, although a family history is lacking in some patients. Patients show a postural tremor that may be very marked, which involves the arms and often the head. Emotional stress exacerbates the tremor. Alcohol characteristically relieves it temporarily.

Patients with benign essential tumor have a good prognosis. Other neurologic symptoms and signs are absent, and benign essential tremor should not be confused with Parkinson's disease or other degenerative diseases. Hyperthyroidism can also cause a marked postural tremor and may need to be ruled out.

Beta-adrenergic blocking drugs (propranolol) are the treatment of choice, and they satisfactorily control tremor in most cases.

MYOCLONUS

Myoclonus consists of brief involuntary irregular muscle jerking. Numerous conditions can give rise to myoclonus. Indeed, few myoclonic jerks on awakening or falling asleep are a normal phenomenon.

Segmental myoclonus involves a single limb or the face, and may occur with a variety of CNS lesions.

Multifocal myoclonus with irregular muscle twitching occurring in many muscle groups suggests a metabolic encephalopathy, most commonly uremia.

Generalized myoclonus with repetitive rapid jerking involving much of the body occurs in patients with anoxic encephalopathy after cardiac arrest. These myoclonic jerks may at times be evoked by tactile or auditory stimuli.

Myoclonus also occurs in a number of epileptic syndromes. It is prominent in subacute sclerosing panencephalitis and Creutzfeldt-Jacob disease.

HEMIFACIAL SPASM

Hemifacial spasm is characterized by repetitive paroxysms of unilateral facial twitching. It is caused by facial nerve dysfunction. This may be either idiopathic or secondary to compressive tumors or aberrant vascular loops in the posterior fossa. Ephaptic (axon to axon) transmission in the facial nerve secondary to demyelination may be responsible.

CEREBELLAR AND SPINOCEREBELLAR DISORDERS

Gait ataxia and limb incoordination are the major manifestations of cerebellar disease (see Table 14.2).

Lesions producing symptoms and signs of cerebellar dysfunction are not always in the cerebellum itself, but may involve instead the efferent and afferent connections of the cerebellum in the brainstem and spinal cord. Disorders affecting the cerebellum and its connections are shown in Table 14.12.

Table 14.12   Causes of Cerebellar Dysfunction

Alcoholism
Drug Intoxication
Multiple Sclerosis
Tumor
    Primary cerebellar
    Metastatic to cerebellum
    Paraneoplastic syndrome
Cerebellar Hemorrhage and Infarction
Cerebellar Abscess
Encephalitis
CNS Toxins
Genetic Syndromes
    Friedreich's ataxia
    Olivopontocerebellar ataxia
    Ataxia telangiectasia
    Others

DIFFERENTIAL DIAGNOSIS

A number of disorders in addition to cerebellar disorders can result in gait disturbance, and to a lesser degree, limb incoordination. Interference with joint-position sense from posterior column lesions or peripheral neuropathy results in a severe gait disturbance. Pernicious anemia with myelopathy and Guillain-Barré syndrome may present in this way. Marked gait disturbance may also be present in patients with vertigo from labyrinthine disorders. Frontal lobe lesions and severe hydrocephalus can also result in gait disturbance.

In patients with cerebellar disease, the rate of progression of symptoms and signs is diagnostically helpful. Acute onset suggests cerebellar hemorrhage or infarction. Wernicke's encephalopathy with ataxia may also present acutely. A subacute onset suggests drug intoxication, postinfectious encephalomyelitis with cerebellar involvement, multiple sclerosis, cerebellar abscess, or metastatic tumor. A slower progression of symptoms and signs suggests primary cerebellar tumor. Gradual progression of disability over years occurs in many inherited cerebellar and spinocerebellar degenerations.

Evidence for involvement of other CNS neuronal systems may be diagnostically helpful. Many of the inherited spinocerebellar degenerations involve the corticospinal tract. Multiple sclerosis can involve any portion of the CNS, including the optic nerves.

ETIOLOGY OF CEREBELLAR DYSFUNCTION

Alcoholism

Alcoholism can lead to acute ataxia from intoxication. Wernicke's encephalopathy causes ataxia in association with other symptoms and signs (see Dementia). Alcoholism can also result in a more slowly progressive chronic cerebellar degeneration. In alcoholic degeneration of the cerebellum, the anterior vermis is usually involved out of proportion to other parts of the cerebellum, resulting in a marked gait disturbance with relatively little limb ataxia.

Drug Intoxication

Toxic serum levels of phenytoin are a frequent cause of ataxia and nystagmus. This diagnosis can be rapidly confirmed with serum drug level measurements.

Barbiturates and many other sedatives can cause

ataxia as well, but, unlike phenytoin, sedation is also usually prominent.

Multiple Sclerosis

Ataxia of limbs and gait is common in multiple sclerosis (see Demyelinating Disorders).

Tumor

Primary cerebellar tumors occur at all ages, but are most common in childhood (see Central Nervous System Neoplasms). If midline, these lesions may produce severe gait ataxia with very little associated limb coordination. Cerebellar metastatic tumors from a variety of primary sources are common in the elderly. As in childhood, vomiting and other symptoms of increased intracranial pressure are common in addition to ataxia.

Lung tumors, particularly small cell carcinomas, may cause a paraneoplastic cerebellar degeneration through remote effects of the tumor on the cerebellum. Ataxia occurs in these patients without any metastatic tumor tissue in the cerebellum itself. A similar syndrome occurs in childhood with neuroblastoma.

Cerebellar Hemorrhage and Infarction

These lesions produce acute ataxia, usually in association with vomiting and obtundation. Urgent surgical removal is essential (see Cerebrovascular Disorders).

Cerebellar Abscess

Cerebellar abscess presents with ataxia, headache, and increased intracranial pressure. It occurs most commonly with chronic otitis media (see Central Nervous System Infections).

Encephalitis

Postinfectious demyelinating syndromes may present with clinical involvement restricted to the cerebellum (see Demyelinating Disorders). These usually occur in childhood and are self-limited. Direct viral invasion of the cerebellum is less common. Differentiation from posterior fossa tumors is essential.

Toxins

Several organic toxins can result in marked, and at times irreversible, cerebellar damage. Cerebellar ataxia from this cause occurs in glue sniffers using toluene-containing glues.

Hereditary Syndromes

Numerous genetic syndromes cause ataxia through degeneration of the cerebellum and or its brainstem and spinal cord tracts. Some of these syndromes affect a number of other neuronal systems as well.

Friedreich's Ataxia

Friedreich's ataxia is one of the most common hereditary ataxias. Pathologic changes are mainly in the spinal cord, with degeneration of the posterior columns, spinocerebellar tracts, and later the corticospinal tracts. The large primary sensory neurons in the dorsal root ganglia are severely affected with resultant marked large sensory nerve fiber loss in posterior nerve roots and peripheral nerves. As in many metabolic degenerations, neurons with the longest axons are affected earliest and most severely. As a result, clinical findings are usually most marked in the feet and the lower limbs.

Disease onset is usually between the ages of 7 and 28 years. Progressive unsteadiness of gait is the main symptom. As might be expected from the pathologic lesions, joint position sense in the toes is lost early, and areflexia is present. Plantar responses are extensor. Pes cavus and kyphoscoliosis are common. Cardiomyopathy also occurs, and many patients die from cardiac complications.

No effective treatment is available.

Olivopontocerebellar Ataxia

Olivopontocerebellar ataxia is characterized by progressive degeneration of the inferior olive and pontine nuclei. Some cerebellar cortical degeneration may also be present, but the spinal cord is spared.

Onset is usually in adulthood, with slow progression. Ataxia of gait, incoordination of the extremities, and dysarthria are the most prominent clinical manifestations.

Ataxia Telangiectasia

This rare autosomal recessive disorder presents in childhood with ataxia, oculocutaneous telangiectasias, immunoglobulin deficiency (IgA), and recurrent sinopulmonary infections.

DISORDERS OF CONSCIOUSNESS

COMA

Normal conscious behavior can be subdivided into two categories: content of consciousness and state of arousal. The content of consciousness is tested by the mental status examination, and discussed in the section entitled Dementia. The level of arousal can be quantitated by the patient's reactivity to stimuli, and whether he appears awake or unconscious.

Pathophysiology

The reticular formation of the midbrain and upper pons projects diffusely through the thalamus to the cerebral hemispheres. Activation of the cerebral hemispheres by the reticular formation is necessary for maintenance of a normal alert state. Transection of the brainstem through the upper midbrain results in permanent coma.

Coma in man is produced by three basic mechanisms:

1. The reticular activating system in the brainstem can be compromised through compression or distortion. Mass lesions of cerebral hemispheres and cerebellum produce coma in this way.

2. Function of the cerebral hemispheres may be diffusely and bilaterally impaired by metabolic and toxic disturbances. Focal cortical lesions will not produce coma unless they are associated with enough mass effect to distort the brainstem.

3. Focal lesions involving the midbrain and upper pons directly will produce coma by interfering with the reticular activating system.

Cerebral Herniation Syndromes

The herniation syndromes are the mechanisms whereby supratentorial mass lesions produce impairment of consciousness. Increasing brainstem distortion gradually leads to increasing impairment of consciousness.

Central Herniation Syndrome   The central herniation syndrome usually occurs with frontal, parietal, and occipital masses, or with extracerebral lesions over the brain convexity, such as subdural hematoma.

The first sign that a supratentorial mass lesion is impairing diencephalic function is a reduction in alertness. With increasing enlargement of the mass, either by continued bleeding or increasing edema, stupor and then coma will follow as diencephalic and midbrain compression and displacement occur. Pupils often become small but remain reactive to light, and Cheyne-Stokes respirations are common as diencephalic compromise occurs. The eyes may be at rest, but will show a brisk response to the oculocephalic maneuver. Alternatively, roving eye movements may be present. Both plantar responses frequently become extensor. At this stage, the whole process can be reserved by emergency surgical decompression. If expansion of the mass continues, the midbrain eventually becomes compromised by displacement and secondary hemorrhage. The initially small pupils dilate to midposition and become fixed and unresponsive to light. The oculocephalic and oculovestibular responses become dysconjugate as the 3rd nerve nucleus is destroyed. Decerebrate posturing occurs, and tachypnea may develop. Once secondary midbrain hemorrhage occurs, the damage is irreversible.

In the central herniation syndrome, the pupils remain in equal size throughout, and become fixed to light only when it is too late to reverse the damage done. This contrasts with the uncal herniation syndrome.

Uncal Herniation Syndrome   Uncal herniation usually results from masses in the temporal lobe and middle cranial fossa. The uncus and hippocampal gyrus are pushed toward the midline and through the tentorial opening. The 3rd nerve may thus be compressed before any significant diencephalon or midbrain compression occurs. The pupils become unequal in size, and the larger pupil reacts only sluggishly to light or becomes totally unreactive. Impairment of consciousness develops simultaneously or slightly later. Impairment of extraocular movements usually follows rapidly.

The dilating unreactive pupil is a critical danger sign, since midbrain compression by the herniating uncus can develop very rapidly. Deep coma and irreversible midbrain damage occurs within minutes to a few hours. This rapid progression occurs because the midbrain is compressed directly by the herniating temporal lobe; the diencephalic stage of the central herniation syndrome has been bypassed. Immediate therapy is essential.

Definitions

A continuum of levels of consciousness obviously exists from normal consciousness to deep coma. These may be categorized as follows:

1. Normal consciousness
2. Clouding of consciousness and obtundation. These patients appear drowsy and frequently misinterpret sensory stimuli. As clouding of consciousness deepens, the patient becomes disoriented with respect to time and place (confused). Thinking is slow and incoherent, but such patients may carry on a simple conversation. Occassionally they become hyperexcitable and agitated.
3. Stupor. Patients with stupor may open their eyes and look at the examiner when stimulated repeatedly. They may moan and verbalize in response to pain, but responses to spoken commands are either absent or very slow. In the deeper stages of stupor, patients may be unresponsive to verbal stimuli, but can still accurately localize noxious stimuli with purposeful defensive movements.
4. Coma. This is a state of "unarousable unresponsiveness." These patients do not localize noxious stimuli and do not speak.

Normal sleep is a complex physiologic process involving well-defined electroencephalographic stages. The various stages of sleep result from interaction between the cerebral cortex and the raphe nuclei, the locus ceruleus, and other brainstem structures. Sleeping individuals present a physiologic state very different from that of the patient with coma, who will show none of the complex electroencephalographic activity characteristic of the lighter stages of sleep. Normal sleep requires an intact cerebral cortex and brainstem.

Delirium is an abnormal mental state with disorientation, fear, misperception of sensory stimuli, and frequently visual hallucinations. Some patients may be agitated when in the state described above as clouding of consciousness, and this may be a transient stage in the development of coma due to cerebral mass lesion. The great majority of delirious states, however, are due to diffuse metabolic disturbances of cerebral function, such as alcohol or barbiturate withdrawal. Delirium may also occur after head injury while the patient is recovering from an unconscious state.

Akinetic mutism describes a condition in which the patient appears alert but shows no evidence of mental activity. Spontaneous motor activity is lacking, and these patients vocalize very little if at all. Akinetic mutism is seen in patients with large deep bilateral frontal lobe lesions. Small lesions interrupting the paramedian reticular formation of the posterior diencephalon and severe communicating hydrocephalus may also result in this syndrome. A somewhat similar state, the vegetative state, is seen in patients with severe head injury or anoxic encephalopathy resulting from cardiac arrest or other causes. After an initial period of coma, usually lasting several weeks, sleep-wake cycles return. The eyes open in response to stimuli, the patient appears awake, but he does not obey commands or show purposeful motor activity. Many of these patients have diffuse cerebral cortical damage.

The patient with *locked-in syndrome* is unable to move arms or legs due to corticospinal tract dysfunction, and is unable to speak because of damage to corticobulbar tracts. These patients usually have a lesion in the ventral pons or midbrain, but remain fully conscious because the reticular formation in the dorsal brainstem is preserved. Vertical eye movements are present, but horizontal eye movements are absent. These patients have normal intellectual function and can be diagnosed by observing vertical eye movements in response to commands. It is important to recognize these patients, because sensory pathways through the dorsal brainstem may be more or less intact and they may well understand all that is said at the bedside. They should be kept as comfortable as possible, and all procedures must be carefully explained to them.

Differential Diagnosis

The causes of coma are legion, but may be classified into four major categories, as shown in Table 14.13.

By far the most common supratentorial mass le-

Table 14.13   **Etiology of Coma**

Supratentorial Mass Lesions
    Intracerebral hemorrhage
    Subdural hematoma
    Brain tumor and abscess
    Cerebral infarct with edema
Subtentorial Lesions
    Brainstem infarct
    Brainstem hemorrhage
    Cerebellar hemorrhage
Diffuse brain disturbances
    Drug overdose
    Metabolic encephalopathy
    Anoxic-ischemic encephalopathy
    Meningitis and encephalitis
    Subarachnoid hemorrhage
    Head injury and concussion
    Epileptic seizure (Postictal state)
Psychiatric Problems

sions causing coma are intracerebral hemorrhage and subdural hematoma. Intracerebral hemorrhage is usually associated with a history of hypertension. Subdural hematoma is frequently associated with head trauma, but the trauma may have been so slight that it is easily forgotten by family or friends. Other mass lesions such as brain tumor or brain abscess are less common causes of coma.

The most common subtentorial lesions causing coma are brainstem infarction and pontine hemorrhage. Cerebellar hemorrhage and cerebellar infarction with edema are less common, and produce coma by brainstem compression.

Overall, diffuse brain disturbances are by far the most common cause of coma. Of these, drug overdoses are the most common. Metabolic encephalopathies also cause diffuse impairment of brain function; these include hepatic encephalopathy, uremia, diabetic ketoacidosis, hypoglycemia, hyponatremia, hypothyroidism, hypercalcemia, hyperosmolar states, hypercapnea, and others. Anoxic-ischemic encephalopathy secondary to cardiac arrest is another important cause of coma. Meningitis may present as coma, and must be considered early, because urgent antibiotic therapy is mandatory. An unwitnessed epileptic seizure may present as coma in the postictal state. Coma from this cause usually lasts at most a few hours, although confusion may persist for as long as 24 hours. Subarachnoid hemorrhage and encephalitis are additional important causes. Head injury with concussion is usually obvious. Exceptions occur, however, particulary in alcoholics and drug users; signs of trauma should be carefully looked for.

Psychiatric disturbances (exclusive of drug overdose) cause only a small number of cases. Disturbances of this kind include conversion reactions, catatonic stupor, and depression.

Clinical Examination

The clinical approach to the comatose patient is summarized in Table 14.14. When faced with a patient in coma, the clinician should immediately consider four points:

1. Is the airway clear?
2. If an adequate airway is present or has been established, are the patient's respirations adequate to prevent cerebral hypoxia?
3. Is the blood pressure adequate to prevent organ damage?
4. If the cause of the patient's coma is not immediately obvious, is hypoglycemia a possibility?

Table 14.14 **Clinical Assessment of the Patient in Coma**

Emergency Evaluation
Airway
Breathing
Blood pressure
Hypoglycemia
Level of Consciousness
Clouding
Stupor
Coma
General Examination
Fever
Stiff neck
Signs of trauma
Liver disease
Diabetes
Cardiac disease
Pulmonary disease
Neurologic Examination
Fundi
Pupils
Extraocular movements
Oculocephalic and oculovestibular reflexes
Lateralizing motor signs
Pattern of respiration
Collateral History

It is pointless to make an accurate diagnosis of coma after a thorough and lengthy examination only to find that irreversible brain damage from hypoxia, hypotension, or hypoglycemia has occurred. Hypoglycemia is frequently overlooked. It is particularly common in diabetics on insulin, but it may occur in alcoholics, or result from overdose of insulin or oral hypoglycemic agents. An immediate bedside Dextrostix determination is helpful. If any doubt exists, blood should be drawn immediately for blood sugar determinations, and 50 ml of 50 percent dextrose and water should be administered intravenously without waiting for the result. Such glucose administration will not harm any patient in coma regardless of the cause.

Once the clinician is satisfied as to the above four considerations, he or she should quickly gauge the patient's level of consciousness so that further improvement or deterioration can be noted. Does the patient respond to voice, or to pain only? Various painful stimuli may be used. Severe pressure on the supraorbital nerves at the upper rim of the orbit is helpful; a grimace is the usual response. If asymmetric, the grimace may give evidence for a focal cerebral lesion with hemiparesis. Pressure applied over the sternum or to Achilles tendon are also commonly used. Probably the most useful painful stimulus is a strong pinch administered separately to the skin of each axilla.

It is best to describe the patient and his level of

responsiveness rather than simply to state that he is in stupor or coma. The patient's response should be characterized as follows:

1. Moaning or verbalization in response to pain
2. Purposeful response to pain. In these instances, the patient will move an arm to try and push or pull the examiner's hand away.
3. Nonspecific movements or reflex withdrawal movements only
4. Decorticate posturing in response to pain
5. Decerebrate posturing in response to pain
6. No response to pain

Asymmetry between the two sides in response to pain may indicate a hemiparesis. The various non-purposeful responses to pain imply progressively deeper levels of coma, with finally no response to pain at all. It should be noted that reflex withdrawal movements of the limbs in response to pain should not be considered purposeful, since such movements may be produced by an intact spinal cord alone.

The general physical examination may give important clues. Cyanosis and evidence of chronic obstructive lung disease may suggest CO_2 narcosis. Hepatomegaly, spider nevi, and fetor hepaticus indicate liver failure. Hypertension and anemia may suggest renal failure. Fever and a stiff neck are found in meningitis and subarachnoid hemorrhage. Neck stiffness may, however, occasionally be absent in these two disorders. Scalp or facial bruises, Battle sign (discoloration and bogginess over the mastoid indicating basilar skull fracture), and bleeding from the ear, all indicate head trauma, possibly with subdural hematoma.

A detailed neurologic examination should then be done to look for evidence of focal signs and a possible correctable mass lesion. Papilledema indicates raised intracranial pressure of at least 6 to 12 hours duration, and suggests an intracranial mass lesion. Optic disc swelling may also be seen in patients with hypertensive encephalopathy. Fresh rounded (subhyaloid) retinal hemorrhages suggest subarachnoid hemorrhage. Diabetic retinopathy suggests either hypoglycemia or diabetic ketoacidosis.

Pupillary size and reaction to light must be carefully assessed. In most metabolic encephalopathies, pupils tend to be small, and the pupillary reaction to light is preserved until very late in the progression of coma. Exceptions to this are atropine and glutethimide overdose. The presence of a unilateral large and sluggishly reactive pupil indicates transtentorial herniation with pressure on the ipsilateral 3rd nerve. This situation constitutes an emergency, as a subdural hemorrhage is a common cause of this syndrome, and is potentially treatable. An intracerebral hemorrhage may cause a similar picture, as may a ruptured posterior communicating artery aneurysm. Pupils with no reaction to light bilaterally may indicate bilateral 3rd nerve palsy or midbrain damage related to transtentorial herniation, midbrain infarction, or severe diffuse brain ischemia secondary to cardiac arrest. With third nerve compression, pupils are fixed and dilated. With midbrain destruction, sympathetic pathways as well as the third nerve are destroyed, and pupils are fixed in midposition. Terminally, due to systemic adrenalin release, they may also become widely dilated. Small (pinpoint) pupils that are still reactive to light indicate pontine hemorrhage or narcotic overdose. In pontine hemorrhage, the cholinergic (pupilloconstrictor) innervation to the iris through the 3rd nerve remains intact, whereas the sympathetic pathways (pupillodilator) that descend in the brainstem are destroyed.

Full roving horizontal eye movements in the comatose patient indicate a structurally intact brainstem. The oculocephalic reflex (doll's-head eye phenomenon) is useful for testing the integrity of brainstem structures. When the head is rapidly rotated to the right by the examiner, the eyes in a lightly comatose patient immediately move conjugately to the left (that is, in a direction opposite the direction of head rotation). By turning the head to the right, the left, and up and down, the examiner can test the integrity of the semicircular canals, the 8th nerve, the 3rd, 4th, and 6th cranial nerves and their brainstem nuclei, and the median longitudinal fasciculus. In addition, the pontine horizontal gaze centers and the midbrain tectum must be intact if horizontal and vertical oculocephalic responses are present. Structural brainstem lesions will disrupt this reflex, or result in dysconjugate eye movements. The oculocephalic reflex will be intact in most patients with metabolic encephalopathy and drug overdose. Phenytoin intoxication may, however, disrupt the reflex early. The reflex will also be absent in very deep coma due to any cause.

The oculovestibular reflex (caloric response) tests essentially the same structures as the oculocephalic reflex, but a more powerful stimulus can be administered; thus, this reflex may be present when the oculocephalic reflex has been nonspecifically depressed by deep coma. After careful inspection of the eardrum to ensure that it is intact, and to ensure that the external auditory canal is not blocked by cerumen, the ear is carefully irrigated with icewater. Approximately 120 cc should be used before the oculovestibular reflex is considered totally absent. The ears should be irrigated separately, approximately 5 minutes apart. In the conscious patient or patient with coma of psychiatric origin, nystagmus will develop, with the fast component away from the irrigated ear. The patient may complain of vertigo and vomit. In the more deeply comatose patient, no nystagmus will occur, but the eye will drift to the side of the irrigated ear. No response to icewater irrigation implies absence of labyrinthine function (due to previous Meniere's disease, streptomycin toxicity, or other injury); 8th nerve destruction secondary to acoustic neuroma, basilar skull fracture or meningitis; or brainstem destruction by infarct, hemorrhage, or compression. Extreme depression of brainstem function by drugs is also a possibility, but in this situation respirations are also depressed. Phenytoin overdose is an exception and can at times abolish the oculovestibular reflex in the absence of coma.

Ocular bobbing with rapid conjugate downward deviation of the eyes and a slow return to midposition suggests a pontine lesion, usually pontine hemorrhage.

More sustained downward eye deviation indicates a lesion compressing the midbrain tectum, such as thalamic hemorrhage. Patients with obtundation, ataxia, nystagmus, and other disturbances of extraocular movement may have a cerebellar hemorrhage with secondary brainstem compression. Vomiting is usually prominent in these patients.

Motor examination is useful mainly in indicating a lateralized or focal brain lesion. Reduced spontaneous movements, or reduced movements in response to pain on one side of the body relative to the other indicates a structural brain lesion. An asymmetry in muscle tone, or deep tendon reflexes again indicates a hemiparesis, as does a unilateral extensor plantar response. Raising one arm at a time and letting it fall is frequently a convincing way to demonstrate reduced muscle tone and hemiparesis contralateral to the cerebral lesion in patients with light coma. A hemiparesis in the comatose patient usually implies a cerebral hemorrhage, cerebral tumor, or a subdural hematoma. However, a chronic subdural hematoma can occasionally cause coma without producing any lateralizing signs. Focal neurologic signs may occasionally occur in patients with metabolic encephalopathies such as hepatic encephalopathy, but they will be transient and fluctuating. Repeated examination at short intervals is helpful in these circumstances.

Bilateral extensor plantar responses indicate bilateral corticospinal tract lesions, and may be due to a pontine hemorrhage or transtentorial herniation. They are, however, also compatible with a marked metabolic encephalopathy. Bilateral decorticate posturing (flexion of arms and extension of legs) or decerebration (extension of both arms and legs, frequently with internal rotation of the arms) in response to pain are useful in indicating which levels of the central nervous system are still functioning. Bilateral decerebration, coma of sudden onset, and pinpoint pupils usually indicate pontine hemorrhage.

The patient's breathing pattern may offer important clues. Hyperventilation suggests metabolic acidosis due to salicylates, diabetes, other toxins, or hepatic encephalopathy. Hyperventilation in the more deeply comatose patient may also result from pulmonary disease. Pulmonary edema may be the direct result of brainstem injury.

Cheyne-Stokes respiration is a waxing and waning pattern of respiration with periods of hyperpnea regularly alternating with apnea. This pattern occurs in patients with bilateral cerebral hemisphere dysfunction due to bilateral structural lesions or diffuse metabolic depression. The appearance of Cheyne-Stokes respirations may indicate incipient transtentorial herniation.

The pathophysiology of Cheyne-Stokes respirations is as follows. In the presence of bilateral hemisphere lesions, brainstem respiratory centers produce an exaggerated ventilatory response to carbon dioxide stimulation of chemoreceptors. This results in the hyperpneic phase of Cheyne-Stokes respiration. When the blood carbon dioxide level drops below the point where it stimulates the respiratory centers, breathing stops, and in the presence of bilateral cerebral lesions will not start (posthyperventilation apnea) until the carbon dioxide level again rises. Thus, cycles of hyperpnea alternating with apnea continue indefinitely. In patients with cerebral lesions, the appearance of Cheyne-Stokes respirations is greatly potentiated by hypoxemia, a prolonged circulation time, and pulmonary congestion.

Apneustic breathing with a pause at full inspiration, and ataxic breathing with a completely irregular respiratory pattern indicate damage to the lower pons and medulla oblongata.

The importance of the history in the evaluation of the comatose patient cannot be overemphasized. While by definition the comatose patient cannot give a useful history, data from witnesses, relatives, friends, and ambulance personnel can be very helpful. As the physician begins his emergency assessment he should immediately despatch nurses, colleagues, or whoever is available to find or contact people who may be able to provide helpful information. Did the coma begin suddenly and catastrophically, or did it develop gradually over hours or days? A sudden onset suggests intracerebral hemorrhage, brainstem infarction or hemorrhage, subarachnoid hemorrhage, or cardiac arrest; subdural hematoma only causes sudden onset of coma when head trauma is severe and obvious. Slowly progressive evolution over hours and days suggests subdural hematoma, meningitis, or metabolic encephalopathy. Is the patient diabetic or does he have other significant systemic disease such as hypertension or heart disease? Is he alcoholic? Was he depressed, taking sedatives or antidepressants, and are all his prescribed pills accounted for? Empty, recently prescribed pill bottles brought in from the patient's residence can rapidly provide a plausible cause for the patient's coma, and if compatible with the clinical findings can make extensive investigation unnecessary.

Laboratory Investigations

All patients in coma should have a white blood count, determinations of hemoglobin, blood sugar, BUN, serum sodium, potassium, chloride, and calcium, and measurements of blood gases and pH.

Liver function tests including prothrombin time and serum ammonia may be indicated. Many endogenous toxins probably contribute to the coma of hepatic encephalopathy, and the serum ammonia does not always correlate well with the level of unconsciousness.

In suspected drug overdose, a large number of drugs including tricyclic compounds, barbiturates, salicylates, acetaminophen, phenytoin, and narcotics can be screened for, depending on the laboratory facilities available. Salicylates and phenobarbital can be easily quantitated, and the significance of the drug's presence assessed. Others, such as the tricyclic compounds, are detected by the drug screen but not easily quantitated, so the significance of a positive screen should be evaluated carefully. A patient with an intracerebral hemorrhage may be on amitriptyline for depression, and thus will have a potentially misleading but positive drug screen for tricyclic compounds.

If an intracranial mass lesion is suspected, the skull roentgenogram may be helpful, but the CT scan is the best way of confirming or ruling out an intracerebral hemorrhage, subdural hematoma, or brain tumor. Cerebral angiography can also demonstrate these lesions, but is more invasive and time consuming. With progressing depth of coma and incipient transtentorial herniation, it is mandatory that these investigations be carried out without delay.

If meningitis is a possibility, lumbar puncture should be carried out immediately. Lumbar puncture is contraindicated in the presence of an intracranial mass lesion, as it may speed the development of transtentorial herniation. The patient may not show signs of progressive transtentorial herniation until several hours after lumbar puncture, because leakage of CSF continues from the dural tear made by the needle. Lumbar puncture is usually safe in the absence of papilledema and lateralizing neurologic signs. If meningitis is a strong possibility, it is important not to allow radiologic procedures to unduly delay examination of cerebrospinal fluid and initiation of therapy.

With clinically obvious subarachnoid hemorrhage, a lumbar puncture is not indicated, and most neurologists and neurosurgeons would proceed directly with a CT scan to demonstrate subarachnoid blood, and a four-vessel angiogram to demonstrate the aneurysm.

Treatment

The first imperative in the treatment of coma is to ensure adequate oxygenation of the patient. Endotracheal intubation and mechanical ventilation must be initiated immediately if respirations are inadequate. If blood pressure is inadequate and hypovolemia appears likely, rapid administration of fluids is essential. Other causes of hypotension, such as myocardial infarction or arrhythmia, should be considered. Immediate administration of 50 ml of 50 percent dextrose is mandatory if hypoglycemia is a possibility. Valuable time should not be wasted awaiting blood glucose results from the laboratory. Blood should be drawn prior to glucose administration to confirm the diagnosis, as the patient's clinical response to glucose administration may be slow, equivocal, or absent if hypoglycemia has been prolonged. Adrenal insufficiency should be suspected in patients with hypotension, hypoglycemia, and an elevated serum potassium.

If narcotic overdose is suggested by history, by needle marks on the patient's skin, or by small constricted pupils, a therapeutic trial of naloxone (Narcan) can be helpful in confirming or countering this suspicion. Naloxone in sufficient dose will quickly arouse the patient with narcotic induced coma. The effect is short lived, however, as the half-life of naloxone is usually much less than that of the narcotic that is causing coma. The patient may thus quickly lapse into coma again, and possible respiratory insufficiency. Naloxone may also precipitate an acute withdrawal syndrome in narcotic addicts.

One to 2 mg of physostigmine may reverse the catatonic psychosis of patients with tricyclic overdose (see Chapter 1, Drug Abuse).

Drug overdose requires gastric lavage and charocal instillation to bind unabsorbed drug. Gastric lavage is indicated even though many hours may have elapsed since the drug was ingested. With a large overdose gastric emptying may be greatly delayed, and large amounts of ingested drug can still be removed after many hours. Aspiration of gastric contents must be avoided during passage of the stomach tube, by tilting the bed head down; prior endotracheal intubation is necessary if coma is deep enough to suppress the cough reflex.

Salicylate overdose should be suspected if gross hyperventilation is present. Salicylate blood levels over 50 mg per dl may indicate a severe degree of poisoning.

Insulin overdose requires special consideration. With massive insulin overdose, the half-life of insulin can be greatly prolonged. The patient may require careful observation and large amounts of intravenous glucose for several days.

Diabetic ketoacidosis and hyperglycemic hyperosmolar nonketotic coma are discussed in detail in Chapter 13, under Diabetes Mellitus. Hypercalcemia is also discussed in Chapter 13.

Hepatic encephalopathy is treated by emptying the gastrointestinal tract of blood if a gastrointestinal bleed has occurred. This is best accomplished with repeated enemas. Lactulose is administered by nasogastric tube, to reduce the absorbtion of ammonia. Lactulose is hydrolyzed by bacterial action in the colon and produces an acidic diarrhea. Ammonia (NH^3) in the gut is converted to the less-readily-absorbed ammonium ion (NH^4). If the hepatic encephalopathy has been precipitated by an infection, this must be vigorously treated.

Renal failure can be effectively treated by peritoneal dialysis or hemodialysis. Coma related to hypothyroidism (myxedema coma) should be treated by intravenous levothyroxine and hydrocortisone.

If meningitis is a serious consideration, appropriate antibiotic therapy must be started early. If the spinal fluid is cloudy or if bacterial meningitis is a strong clinical possibility, antibiotic therapy should be started immediately after lumbar puncture, before the results of CSF analysis are received from the laboratory.

Careful observation of the patient is important, as the clinical condition of the patient in coma may change very rapidly. In drug overdose, respiratory insufficency may develop suddenly.

Patients with expanding intracranial mass lesions develop progressively deeper coma as transtentorial herniation occurs. If an operable mass lesion is suspected and the patient is deteriorating, emergency CT scanning to identify the responsible lesion and neurosurgical intervention are necessary. Most intracranial mass lesions can be successfully decompressed surgically if the diagnosis is made before irreversible brainstem damage from cerebral herniation occurs. Deep intracerebral hematomas are an expection. Cerebellar hematomas and swollen cerebellar infarcts, however, can be surgically decompressed with good results.

Measures to Reduce Cerebral Edema

Mannitol produces an osmotic gradient between cerebral tissue and the circulating blood. Water will leave the brain, thereby reducing intracranial pressure. The volume of normal brain tissue where the blood brain barrier is still intact will be reduced, but mannitol will not reduce the size of a cerebral hematoma or tumor. It may buy enough time to allow for successful emergency investigation and treatment. It will, however, relieve intracranial pressure only temporarily. Two-hundred and fifty to 500 ml of 20 percent mannitol given rapidly intravenously may reduce intracranial pressure enough to delay irreversible transtentorial herniation by 30 minutes to several hours. A urinary catheter should be inserted as a massive diuresis usually follows mannitol administration.

Dexamethasone (Decadron) should be started, even though cerebral edema will not be reduced immediately. An initial dose of 10 mg is usually used, followed by 4 to 6 mg every 6 hours.

Fluid restriction is also useful in reducing cerebral edema, and overhydration with excessive intravenous fluids should be avoided.

General measures in the treatment of coma should include careful nursing to avoid bedsores. The patient should be carefully positioned to avoid brachial plexus injury, ulnar neuropathy, and peroneal nerve palsy due to compression. The corneas should be kept moist by means of ointment or methyl cellulose eye drops, and the eyes should be kept closed by tape if necessary. Antacids by nasogastric tube or cimetidine intravenously are useful in preventing acute gastrointestinal hemorrhage associated with stress.

The management of coma requires detailed clinical knowledge and sound judgement. The following two case histories illustrate some of the pitfalls that may be encountered in managing these patients.

Case 14.1

A 28-year-old female suddenly developed severe right-sided headache during sexual intercourse. Headache and vomiting persisted, and so an hour

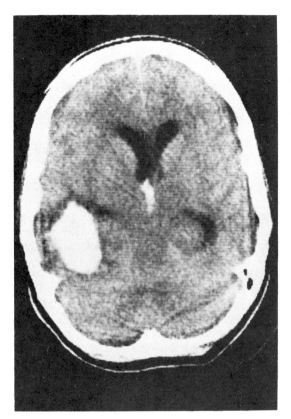

Fig. 14.12 Brain CT scan of Case 14.1, showing fatal right temporal lobe intracerebral hematoma

later, at 2:00 AM she was brought to the local emergency department in a small town. She was alert, and no focal neurologic signs were noted. She was held for observation.

At 6:00 AM she was still oriented, but becoming increasingly drowsy. At this point, it was decided to transfer her to a larger center, but the urgency of the situation was not fully appreciated. Although the local hospital was only a three-hour ambulance ride from a neurologic-neurosurgical unit, she did not arrive there until 5:00 PM. On arrival she had fixed dilated pupils, bilateral decerebrate posturing in response to pain, and deep coma. She required intubation for failing respirations shortly after arrival. Intravenous mannitol did not change her clinical status. Head CT scan showed a large superficial intracerebral right temporal hematoma (Fig. 14.12). Several days later she was declared brain dead and respiratory support was discontinued.

This patient illustrates the importance of drowsiness and increasing obtundation in the patient with sudden headache and suspected intracranial mass lesion.

Increasing drowsiness suggests diencephalic compromise and onset of the central herniation syndrome.

Time may be of the essence, and the patient may need to be treated or transported to a treatment center rapidly. If further deterioration occurs with increasing depth of coma as indicated by reaction to pain and other stimuli, mannitol intravenously may provide several more hours time in which to arrange neurosurgical intervention. In this patient, mannitol in the ambulance might have allowed a more favorable result. Although most intracerebral hematomas are not operable, this patient with a relatively superficial intracerebral hematoma in the nondominant hemisphere might have had a good result from surgery.

Case 14.2

A 55-year-old known alcoholic was admitted to the emergency department in a stuporous state. Although his eyes were open, he would not respond to commands, and would react to pain only with purposeful defensive movements. He was afebrile and had no neck stiffness.

In view of his alcoholism, a diagnosis of subdural hematoma was considered despite the lack of focal neurologic signs. Meningitis was also considered a possibility. An immediate head CT scan was done to rule out a subdural hematoma, which would contraindicate a lumbar puncture. The scan was normal, and was immediately followed by lumbar puncture. This showed grossly purulent cerebrospinal fluid and penicillin G, 24 million units daily, was started in divided doses every 2 hours. CSF cell count was 4,000 with 95 percent neutrophils. CSF glucose was 5 mg /100 ml, and CSF protein was 200 mg /100 ml. Gram stain showed gram-positive diplococci and diagnosis of pneumococcal meningitis was made.

Chest roentgenogram showed an infiltration suggestive of pneumonia. Final diagnosis was pneumococcal pneumonia, and meningitis.

Thiamine and antibiotic therapy resulted in recovery from the meningitis, but the patient was left with a Korsakoff's psychosis. Irreversible thalamic damage had presumably occurred secondary to thiamine deficiency prior to entering hospital.

As this patient illustrates, the debilitated, stuporous, or comatose patient with meningitis may not demonstrate stiff neck and fever. Careful clinical judgment must be exercised, and all clinical features must be taken into account.

SYNCOPE

Definition

Syncope means "cutting short." The term is used for episodes of transient loss of consciousness not due to epileptic seizure.

Pathophysiology

Syncope usually results from a sudden impairment of brain metabolism brought about by a hypotensive reduction in cerebral blood flow. The brain is extremely active, metabolically, and is very sensitive to ischemia. Total cerebral blood flow is normally maintained at a constant level despite wide fluctuations in arterial blood pressure. As a result of this autoregulation, cerebral blood flow will not decline unless arterial blood pressure falls below 60 mm Hg mean arterial pressure. This is equivalent to a blood pressure of 80/50. Actual fainting or syncope occurs at some point below this.

Cerebral ischemia affects first the cortex and the basal ganglia, which are highly sensitive to hypoxia, and then several seconds later affects the hypothalamus and midbrain. The initial phases of syncope are due to diffuse cerebral hypoxia rather than to hypoxia of the reticular activating system in the midbrain.

When the cerebral hemispheres are sufficiently ischemic, the bulbopontine reticular formation is liberated from the inhibitory control of higher centers. At this point, neuronal discharge from the reticular formation frequently results in a brief tonic contraction of body muscles and a few generalized clonic movements. There are rarely more than one or two clonic movements, and these are not the result of an epileptic cortical discharge. In addition, the reticular formation discharge tends to increase vascular tone. This, together with assumption of a horizontal posture as the patient falls, increases venous return to the heart and serves again to raise the blood pressure.

Patients with syncope frequently have their eyes turned up as they lose consciousness. This ocular revulsion is not a convulsive phenomenon, but simply due to loss of consciousness.

Differential Diagnosis

Whether the patient has had a syncopal attack or an epileptic seizure must first be determined. Several points in the clinical history help make this distinction. The history is critical, and if necessary bystand-ers or witnesses should be contacted. Those bringing the patients in should not be allowed to leave until a collateral history has been taken. The following distinctions are useful in differential diagnosis:

1. Epileptic seizures occur in any body position, whereas syncope usually occurs in the upright or sitting posture. Cardiac arrhythmias are exceptions to this.

2. With epilepsy, the patient frequently experiences a sudden loss of consciousness without warning, and may fall so suddenly that he sustains significant injury. Most patients with syncope have a more gradual loss of consciousness and therefore usually do not hurt themselves. Cardiac arrhythmias, particulary with asystole, again are an exception, and may result in very sudden falls with injury.

3. Patients with tonic-clonic seizures generally have no warning of their impending loss of consciousness. Partial seizures may have an aura suggesting a focal cerebral epileptic discharge. Patients with many types of syncope, particularly vasovagal syncope, frequently have definite premonitory symptoms of nausea, perspiration, and weakness.

4. Convulsive movements are usually much more prominent in an epileptic seizure.

5. The epileptic is generally unconscious for at least several minutes. Syncopal attacks usually last only seconds, but occasionally can last longer.

6. Patients with seizures usually show postictal confusion which can be very severe. Postictal confusion is very mild or lacking in syncope, but may be present with prolonged syncope.

If a diagnosis of syncope is made, the underlying etiology must be determined. The various causes of syncope are shown in Table 14.15. The rapidity of loss of consciousness, and also the speed of recovery, can be important clues. A very sudden loss of consciousness without warning suggests a seizure. However, syncope secondary to orthostatic (postural) hypotension, vertebrobasilar insufficiency, carotid sinus hypersensitivity, and cardiac arrhythmia may result in sudden loss of consciousness. These patients will also recover mental function very quickly once consciousness has been regained. Usually there will be other clues. The patient with orthostatic hypotension will have attacks of syncope only when arising from a supine or a sitting position. The patient with vertebrobasilar insufficiency is usually elderly and may have evidence of widespread atherosclerosis. These attacks are usually initiated by standing up or by head turning. Blood pressure measurements may be significantly different between the two arms. The patient with carotid sinus syncope may have attacks while wearing tight collars, while shaving, or

Table 14.15   **Causes of Syncope**

Hypotension (Insufficient Blood to Brain)
1. Inadequate Vasoconstriction
    A. Vasovagal attacks
    B. Postural hypotension
2. Mechanical Reduction of Venous Return
    A. Valsalva maneuver
    B. Cough
    C. Micturition
    D. Atrial myxoma
3. Hypovolemia
4. Cardiac Arrhythmias
    A. Atrioventricular block (Stokes–Adams attacks)
    B. Sick sinus syndrome
    C. Episodic ventricular fibrillation or tachycardia
    D. Carotid sinus syncope
    E. Glossopharyngeal neuralgia
5. Other Causes of Reduced Cardiac Output
    A. Cardiac tamponade
    B. Myocardial infarction
    C. Aortic stenosis
    D. Pulmonary stenosis
    E. Pulmonary hypertension and embolism
Abnormalities of Blood
1. Hypoxemia
2. Anemia
3. Hypoglycemia
4. Reduced PCO_2 (Hyperventilation attack)
Cerebral causes
1. Vertebrobasilar Insufficiency
2. Hypertensive Encephalopathy
3. Colloid Cyst of Third Ventricle
4. Emotional Disturbances (Hysterical seizures, anxiety attacks, and others)

sometimes while laughing. The patient with cardiac arrhythmia may have cardiac conduction abnormalities on the electrocardiogram. However, a normal electrocardiogram does not rule these out, and prolonged cardiac monitoring may be necessary.

Syncopal attacks of slow onset and also with a slow resolution suggest syncope secondary to hyperventilation or hypoglycemia.

Precipitation of syncopal attacks by emotional stress, warm surroundings, pain, the sight of blood, or emotional shock suggests a vasovagal attack. There is usually a short premonitory phase of nausea, perspiration, palpitation, weakness, and confusion before loss of consciousness. Patients frequently describe their vision as going dark before they lose consciousness. Patients usually are young and otherwise healthy. Patients with migraine or family history of migraine appear particularly prone to this syndrome. Once the supine posture is reached, the patient regains consciousness rapidly with no postictal confusion. Observers frequently mention that the patient appeared very pale just prior to loss of consciousness; the pulse rate is slow. The mechanisms of a vasovagal attack are somewhat different from most other types of syncope. Whereas in or-

thostatic hypotension there is a failure of sympathetic vasoconstrictor mechanisms to maintain blood pressure in the upright posture, during a vasovagal attack there is, in addition, a sudden activation of the parasympathetic nervous system with vagal mediated cardiac slowing and active vasodilation in skeletal muscles. This tremendous drop in peripheral vascular resistance results in profound hypotension and fainting.

Vasovagal attacks and syncope secondary to orthostatic hypotension are by far the most common causes of syncope. Orthostatic hypotension may result from a number of causes. The patient may have an autonomic neuropathy related to diabetes. Many other peripheral neuropathies, particularly those resulting from paraproteinemias and amyloidosis, have involvement of the autonomic nervous system. On the other hand, the patient may be taking medication such as antihypertensives, tricyclic antidepressants, or phenothiazines, all of which interfere with autonomic nervous system function and result in orthostatic hypotension. Orthostatic hypotension is also common in patients with adrenal insufficiency, dehydration, and hypovolemia from any cause.

Syncope occurring with exertion should always alert the physician to the possibility of aortic stenosis (see Chapter 16).

Laboratory Investigation

Frequently, very little laboratory investigation is required. A careful history and physical examination done by a clinician familiar with the various types of syncope results in an accurate diagnosis in most cases. Many laboratory tests can be of value and must be tailored to assess the most likely causes (Table 14.15). Electrocardiography and prolonged ambulatory cardiac monitoring are necessary in patients with suspected cardiac arrhythmias. If epilepsy is a consideration, the EEG is helpful.

It must be stressed that syncope is due to global cerebral ischemia, and is very rarely the result of an embolic transient ischemic attack. Hemodynamically significant stenosis in the vertebrobasilar circulation may cause syncope (vertebrobasilar insufficiency), but such lesions are usually not accessible to surgery. Cerebral angiography is rarely indicated in the patient with syncope.

Treatment

Most patients require only reassurance that their infrequent attacks are not of a serious nature. This is particularly true of vasovagal attacks. Instructions to lie down or to put the head down immediately on feeling faint are often helpful. Patients who faint when getting up quickly should be advised to get up slowly. The family of the patient prone to syncope should be told to immediately place the patient flat or in the head-down position when unconsciousness occurs. At no time should he be held in a sitting or standing posture during syncope, as this will prolong cerebral ischemia and prevent recovery. Where a significant underlying disease is found, specific treatment may be required. Patients with cardiac brady-arrhythmias may require a pacemaker. Patients with cough syncope may benefit from intensive therapy of their pulmonary disease. Volume expansion with mineralocorticoid therapy (Florinef) may benefit patients with severe postural hypotension.

NARCOLEPSY

The narcoleptic tetrad consists of sleep attacks, cataplexy, hypnogogic hallucinations, and sleep paralysis.

Narcolepsy is a sleep disorder in which the patient has an irresistible need to sleep a number of times during the day. Prior to falling asleep, there is a build-up of drowsiness, and after a brief nap of 10 to 15 minutes, the patient usually awakens feeling refreshed.

Narcolepsy is associated with cataplexy in approximately 70 percent of cases. Cataplexy consists of a sudden loss of muscle tone that is precipitated by emotions such as laughter, elation, or anger. At such times, the patient may suddenly collapse and fall to the ground, remaining fully conscious throughout. These attacks may be brought on by meeting an old friend, winning at a game, or a variety of other situations. Many of these attacks may be more minor in nature, and simply cause the patient's head to fall forward or the jaw to drop open. The attacks last only a few minutes.

Sleep paralysis occurs in approximately 50 percent of patients with narcolepsy. The patient is awake but unable to move just prior to falling asleep or upon awakening. Vivid hallucinations may also occur upon awakening or falling asleep, and are present in approximately 25 percent of patients with narcolepsy.

Although the exact mechanisms of these sleep disorders are unknown, they most likely are a disorder of brainstem structures involved in REM (rapid eye movement) sleep. During REM sleep, muscle hypotonia similar to that seen in cataplexy occurs, but the patient is normally asleep during this time. Sleep paralysis may have a similar explanation, and the hypnogogic hallucinations are reminiscent of dreams occurring during REM sleep.

Patients with sleep attacks and cataplexy frequently demonstrate a REM period occurring within 15 minutes of sleep onset, if an EEG recording is done during sleep. Such REM sleep periods do not occur so soon after sleep commences in normal adults.

Narcolepsy and cataplexy usually begin in adolescence or young adulthood. A family history is common, and males are more often affected than females.

Narcolepsy responds best to methylphenidate (Ritalin). If methylphenidate fails, amphetamines will usually control these symptoms, but they have more severe side effects.

It is important to realize that cataplexy will not respond to methylphenidate or amphetamines, and that it is best treated with imipramine (Tofranil) in a dose of 75 to 125 mg/day. Methylphenidate and imipramine may be used together in patients with both narcolepsy and cataplexy. Patients with narcolepsy usually have well-defined intermittent attacks of sleepiness during the day, and the diagnosis is fairly obvious clinically. At times, however, these patients also complain of more prolonged and diffuse daytime drowsiness. In patients complaining of excessive daytime sleepiness, a number of other diagnoses should be considered. These include hypothyroidism, amphetamine withdrawal, sleep apnea, and chronic idiopathic hypersomnia. (Kleine-Levin syndrome). The patient with sleep apnea has daytime sleepiness because of grossly disturbed nocturnal sleep. During sleep, these patients either cease to make respiratory effort, or have obstruction of the upper airway (see Chapter 15).

The Kleine-Levin syndrome is a rare condition of unknown etiology affecting primarily males who experience episodic somnolence and excessive eating (megaphagia).

EPILEPSY

Few conditions in medicine are as dramatic as an epileptic seizure. In a generalized tonic-clonic seizure, the patient is instantaneously thrown from a state of complete normality to one of violent unconsciousness. Mercifully he remains completely amnesic for the event on recovery. The time of the next seizure cannot be predicted. Epilepsy, meaning "to seize upon" or to "lay hold of," comes from the future tense of the Greek verb, which indicates the uncertainty of the patient's future.

DEFINITION

Epilepsy is a condition characterized by recurrent seizures. A convulsion or seizure is due to an excessive discharge of cerebral neurons. Approximately 1 in 20 individuals has a seizure during his lifetime. Between 0.5 and 1 percent of the general population have recurrent seizures.

PATHOPHYSIOLOGY

The exact origin of the abnormal neuronal discharges that underlie a clinical convulsion are not fully understood. Neurons might be hyperexcitable because of cell membrane abnormalities, or because of synaptic abnormalities. In some seizure types, epileptic discharges arise focally in a small abnormal area of the cerebral cortex. Such discharges may occur around brain tumors, or in areas of cortical gliosis secondary to previous injury. Similar epileptic neuronal discharges can be produced in animals by applying penicillin or other substances to a small area of the cerebral cortex.

A balance normally exists between excitatory and inhibitory processes, and allows for normal cerebral cortical function. In an epileptic focus, inhibitory mechanisms at times appear to fail. Microelectrode studies have shown that the resting membrane potential of neurons in an epileptic focus is normal. Intermittently, striking long-lasting depolarizations of the neuronal cell membrane occur. These are called paroxysmal depolarization shifts (PDS), and except for their size and duration they resemble normal excitatory postsynaptic potentials (EPSP). Similar to the normal EPSP, PDS can be evoked by afferent volleys of excitatory nerve impulses.

During the PDS, large numbers of action potentials are generated in the neuronal axon, as threshold depolarization is exceeded. If this excessive neural activity remains localized to the epileptic focus, the patient may remain asymptomatic. However, at other times, the neuronal discharges may spread far and wide through the brain and give rise to clinical seizure activity. Failure of inhibitory mechanisms may be the factor that allows occasional spread of the seizure discharge.

Some epileptic seizure discharges appear to begin simultaneously in all parts of the cerebral cortex. The pathophysiology of these seizures is poorly understood. They may begin in the thalamus and spread to all areas of the cerebral cortex, or they may result from diffuse cortical hyperexcitability.

The electroencephalogram (EEG) is a recording made from electrodes placed on the patient's scalp. It records the voltage changes that occur over various parts of the brain surface over time. During a seizure, abnormal rapid high voltage discharges are recorded, reflecting the excessive neuronal activity in the brain.

CLASSIFICATION

A distinction should be made between the classification of the epilepsies and the classification of epileptic seizures. Classification of epilepsy type is based not only on the seizure type, but also on other criteria, such as family history, age at onset, etiology, and the presence or absence of neurologic or psychologic evidence of brain damage. Classification of seizure type, on the other hand, is based on the clinical and EEG features of the seizures themselves, regardless of etiology.

A patient with one type of epilepsy may have several different kinds of seizures. Thus, patients with primary generalized epilepsy may have both absence (petit mal) and tonic-clonic (grand mal) seizures. Patients with partial epilepsy may have both partial seizures with complex symptomatology and, occasionally, partial seizures that become secondarily generalized.

The International Classification of the Epilepsies is shown in Table 14.16 in abbreviated form. The primary distinction in this classification is between the generalized epilepsies, in which the neuronal discharges appear to begin in all parts of the cerebral cortex simultaneously, and the partial epilepsies, in which the abnormal neuronal discharges begin in a localized area of the cortex, but may spread from there.

A second major distinction is made between those patients whose epilepsy has no apparent underlying cause, except perhaps a genetic predisposition, and those in whom seizures are attributable to cerebral or systemic disease. Primary generalized epilepsy has no apparent underlying cause, although a positive family history is common, and genetic factors may be important. Secondary generalized epilepsy includes patients with generalized seizures who have detectable cerebral pathology. It is assumed that all cases of partial epilepsy are due to some type of cerebral damage.

***Table 14.16* Classification of Epilepsy**

Generalized Epilepsies
Primary generalized epilepsies
Secondary generalized epilepsies
Partial (Focal) Epilepsies

Table 14.17 shows the International Classification of Epileptic Seizures. The primary distinction in this classification is between partial seizures and generalized seizures. In partial seizures, the first clinical changes indicate activation of anatomic or functional systems of neurons limited to part of a single hemisphere. EEG changes in these seizures are restricted to scalp regions over the area of cortex implicated clinically, at least at seizure onset.

Generalized seizures do not include any focal symptoms or signs. The EEG changes are from the start bilateral and symmetric over the two hemispheres.

CLINICAL MANIFESTATIONS

Partial Seizures

Partial seizures with elementary symptomatology, like all partial seizures, reflect the function of the cerebral cortical areas through which the seizure discharge passes. In the classical jacksonian seizure, the seizure discharge begins in a portion of the motor cortex, and spreads to adjacent cortical structures. These patients may, for example, develop twitching in the facial muscles on one side, and then show spread of motor activity to the hand and arm, and finally to the leg. This reflects the spread of seizure

Table 14.17 **Classification of Epileptic Seizures**

Partial Seizures (Seizures Beginning Locally)
  Partial Seizures with Elementary Symptomatology (Generally Without Impairment of Consciousness)
    With motor symptoms (includes Jacksonian seizures)
    With special sensory or somatosensory symptoms
    With autonomic symptoms
    Compound forms
  Partial Seizures with Complex Symptomatology (Generally with Some Impairment of Consciousness)
    With impairment of consciousness only
    With cognitive symptomatology
    With affective symptomatology
    With psychosensory symptomatology
    With psychomotor symptomatology (automatism)
    Compound forms
  Partial Seizures Secondarily Generalized
Generalized Seizures (Bilaterally Symmetric and without Focal Onset)
    Absences (petit mal)
    Bilateral massive epileptic myoclonus
    Infantile spasms
    Clonic seizures
    Tonic seizures
    Tonic-clonic seizures (grand mal)
    Atonic seizures
    Akinetic seizures
Unclassified Seizures (Due to Incomplete Data)

activity from the area of motor cortex controlling the face, to the remainder of the motor cortex of that hemisphere. The patient may remain completely conscious and alert throughout such a seizure.

If seizure discharges spread through the sensory cortex, the patient will experience numbness or tingling instead of muscle twitching. Some patients may experience both motor activity and sensory symptoms, indicating more wide spread seizure activity, and these would be known as compound forms. *Autonomic symptoms* such as pupil dilatation, sweating, and salivation may also occur. Flashing lights and other unformed visual hallucinations may also occur in partial seizures with elementary symptomatology.

Partial seizures with complex symptomatology may also take a number of forms. These seizure discharges involve cortical association areas, resulting in more complex symptoms. The patient may show only mild impairment of consciousness, and may continue walking or other activity. However, they may not respond when spoken to, and may show other evidence of impaired awareness of their surroundings.

The term *cognitive symptomatology* refers to a diverse group of complex mental states that alter the entire content of a patient's consciousness, and have been called "dreamy states" by some. These include the *deja vu* phenomenon, wherein the patient develops an overwhelming feeling that a given situation has happened before.

Affective symptomatology refers to partial seizures in which the patient experiences a strong emotional state as part of his seizure. By far the most common of these emotional states is fear.

Psychosensory symptomatology refers to hallucinations occurring as part of a seizure. These may be visual or auditory, and occasionally compound hallucinations involving several sensory modalities may occur. The visual hallucinations in complex partial seizures consist of formed images. Olfactory hallucinations usually take the form of a strange unpleasant smell which the patient can describe only incompletely. No matter how vivid or complex the patient's hallucinations may be, the patient afterwards always realizes that the hallucination was an experience imposed on him, and not a part of his surrounding reality.

Psychomotor symptomatology includes lip smacking, swallowing, compulsive patting or rubbing of body parts, fumbling with clothing and other similar activities occurring during a seizure. These automatic activities are often referred to as automatisms.

Partial seizures with complex symptomatology are characterized by motor and psychic behavior that is inappropriate for the time and place. The patient is often amnesic for events occurring during the seizure, but consciousness is not totally lost, and some capacity to react to the environment is still present. Many patients, however, will have some memory of their seizure, particularly for those symptoms occurring near its onset. Hallucinations, for example, can often be described in detail after the seizure. Patients amnesic for most of their seizure may experience an aura that warns them that a seizure is coming. This aura is produced by a focal epileptic discharge, and is simply the initial part of the seizure. The nature of the aura depends on where in the brain the patient's seizure originates.

Patients may have frequent partial seizures wherein the seizure discharge remains localized to a small portion of the cortex. Some of these seizures, however, may become secondarily generalized. The seizure discharge probably spreads to subcortical structures and from there quickly spreads to involve the whole cerebral cortex. The following case is an example of this.

Case 14.3

A young man had frequent attacks of a sudden feeling that he was in a dream and that he had done before what he was doing at that moment. This dreamy feeling was then quickly followed by a weird, strange smell. The episode was all over in a matter of seconds and those around him would observe nothing amiss. Occasionally, however, these attacks were followed by sudden loss of consciousness, convulsive movements of all limbs, and urinary incontinence. Following these latter attacks, he was confused for at least several hours.

This patient experienced partial seizures with complex symptomatology of a compound form, that is, his seizure included both cognitive symptomatology and psychosensory symptomatology. In addition, much less frequently, he experienced partial seizures with secondary generalization.

Generalized Seizures

Absences (petit mal) occur mostly in children. They are uncommon after the age of 20 years. Classically, there is a fixed vacuous stare without any other sign of a seizure. If the patient is reading or talking aloud, he will suddenly stop for several seconds and then will resume at the point where he left off. He is frequently unaware that anything has hap-

pened. If spoken to during an attack, the patient will not respond. Fluttering of the eyelids or mild clonic rhythmic movements of the upper extremity may occur in some prolonged absence attacks.

Tonic-clonic seizures (grand mal) may have a very brief period of dizziness, confusion, or a sense of rising epigastric distress prior to seizure onset. An occasional patient will cry out. He usually has no memory of this cry afterwards. Most patients have no warning symptoms whatsoever. Loss of consciousness occurs rapidly and is followed by the tonic phase, which consists of strong forceful contractions of all muscles. The tonic phase may last from a few seconds to several minutes, and the patient becomes cyanotic during this time. He then enters the clonic phase with brisk intermittent clonic movements of all limbs. Incontinence of urine may occur. The postictal state then follows. The patient initially remains unconscious, and then passes through a period of confusion before gradually returning to a normal mental state.

Many patients with absence seizures also have tonic-clonic seizures, or develop them later in life.

Bilateral massive epileptic myoclonus consists of single or multiple myoclonic jerks involving both sides of the body simultaneously. If the legs are involved, the patient may be thrown to the ground. These seizures may occur in association with absence seizures and tonic-clonic seizures in patients with primary generalized epilepsy. They are common in patients with diffuse cerebral disease and secondary generalized epilepsy. They are particularly prominent in patients with subacute sclerosing panencephalitis.

The remaining generalized seizure types listed in the classification are seen mainly in patients with diffuse cerebral damage. Clonic seizures and tonic seizures are similar to tonic-clonic seizures except that either the tonic or the clonic phase is missing. In atonic seizures, there is loss of postural tone and the patient slumps or falls. Akinetic seizures consist of an arrest of movement without particular loss of tone.

Infantile spasms are a peculiar seizure form that usually begins in the first year of life and is almost always associated with brain damage.

DIFFERENTIAL DIAGNOSIS OF SEIZURES

Generalized tonic-clonic seizures must be differentiated from syncope (see Disorders of Consciousness). The patient with syncope lasting longer than 10 seconds may occasionally have a few clonic movements of the limbs, and if the bladder is full he may pass urine. This may cause diagnostic confusion. A significant injury during the episode, tongue biting, strong motor activity, incontinence, and postictal confusion all suggest seizure as opposed to syncope. Absence seizures must be differentiated from day dreaming and normal periods of inattention. Collateral history from the mother and teacher are often most important, as is the EEG. An attack may frequently be precipitated in the office by hyperventilation. Asking the patient to count while he hyperventilates will help to show the seizure, as he will temporarily stop counting during the attack.

Partial seizures are of such varied form, that complete description of all types is impossible. The most common error is to not even consider the diagnosis of partial seizure when seeing a patient with transient episodes of bizarre behavior, hallucination, or peculiar lapses of consciousness. Amnesia for events occurring during the episode points to a diagnosis of epilepsy, although as already mentioned some patients do recollect some events occuring during the partial seizure. Differentiation from psychosis usually is not difficult in most patients, because they are mentally normal between the relatively short attacks. A careful history is usually sufficient to differentiate seizures from acute anxiety attacks and hyperventilation.

In children, differentiation of absence seizures from partial complex seizures with impairment of consciousness only, may be difficult. Absence seizures usually have a duration of less than 10 seconds, frequently occur many times a day, have no aura, and no postictal confusion. Partial seizures usually have a longer duration, occur at most several times a day, frequently have an aura, and almost invariably have postictal confusion. Automatisms suggest partial seizures. The EEG, if abnormal, is diagnostic.

The reflex epilepsies are seizures triggered by a definite stimulus, such as flashing lights, television, geometric patterns, music, reading, and other stimuli.

Some seizure-like attacks are psychiatric in origin. Hysterical seizures (pseudoseizures) should be suspected when the seizure pattern does not conform to recognized seizure types, or when seizures occur only at opportune moments. Usually the patient is unaware of the psychologic nature of his attacks, and is oblivious to any connection between his seizures and his life situation. These patients frequently show a *la belle indifference* attitude to their seizure problem. Tongue biting and incontinence are generally absent, although there are exceptions to this. The seizures may be prolonged and bizarre. There is usually no postictal confusion, and there may be obvious secondary gain. Pseudoseizures are most common in the epileptic who also has genuine epileptic seizures. This makes the situation very difficult to sort out. As has been described, partial complex seizures can take a great variety of forms. Except in very obvious cases, the diagnosis of pseudoseizure should be one of exclusion, and made only with great caution.

ETIOLOGY

The etiology of primary generalized epilepsy is unknown, but genetic factors appear to play a significant role. In patients with primary generalized epilepsy, 12 percent of siblings will have seizures. Perinatal trauma is thought to be an important factor in the etiology of epileptic seizures, particularly partial seizures. During molding of the head at birth, significant mesial temporal lobe herniation through the tentorial notch is thought to occur, resulting in brain tissue injury and later gliosis. These areas of damage, although small, may become epileptic foci and cause seizures that may not begin until many years after birth.

Head trauma at any time in life may similarly result in focal areas of brain injury and gliosis. Overall, among patients admitted to hospital after head injury, 5 percent develop epilepsy (defined as one or more seizures occurring more than 1 week after injury). The risk of developing epilepsy is much higher if the injury is complicated by intracranial hematoma or depressed skull fracture, or if seizures occur in the first week following injury. Fifty percent of patients who will develop epilepsy do so in the first year after injury. A significant number of patients will develop epilepsy more than 10 years after injury. Only 40 percent of seizures developing after head injury show focal features clinically. The remainder appear generalized, although a focal origin with rapid generalization is not ruled out, and may be demonstrated by the EEG.

Epilepsy may be the first clinical manifestation of a brain tumor. In children with seizures, very few have brain tumors. With advancing age this proportion increases so that in patients developing seizures for the first time between the ages of 20 and 30, approximately 3 percent will have a brain tumor. In patients presenting with their first seizure between the ages of 50 and 60 years, approximately 15 percent will harbor a brain tumor.

Prior central nervous system infection, prolonged febrile seizure, cerebrovascular accident, and developmental abnormalities may all lead to later epilepsy. Many metabolic disorders including hyponatremia, hypoglycemia, and uremia may result in seizures. Correction of the underlying metabolic abnormality will terminate the seizure disorder. Alcohol and barbiturate withdrawal are a common cause of generalized seizures. Seizures from alcohol withdrawal (rum fits) usually occur between 7 and 48 hours after the patients stops drinking. Alcohol withdrawal seizures are an entity distinct from delirium treatments, which usually begins 48 to 72 hours after drinking has ceased. Although a cluster of seizures may occur, alcohol withdrawal seizures are generally short and self-limited (see Chapter 1).

EVALUATION OF THE PATIENT PRESENTING WITH SEIZURES

Clinical Examination

The patient presenting with seizures should be carefully evaluated. The underlying etiology should be determined if possible as specific therapy may be required. Careful classification of the patient's epilepsy and seizure type will also be helpful, as this will help determine prognosis and choice of drug therapy. The history should include a description of the patient's attacks from friends or relatives. In particular, localizing factors suggesting focal cerebral pathology should be watched for. These include convulsive movements beginning on one side of the body, consistent turning of the head and eyes to one side at seizure onset, and postictal neurologic deficits (Todd's paralysis).

The patient's age at onset should be established, and seizure frequency determined. Inquiry should be made regarding significant past head injury, abnormal birth history, nervous system infection, and family history for seizures.

Physical examination may indicate localizing neurologic signs suggestive of brain tumor or other types of focal brain damage. An asymmetry of the skull or extremities suggests damage to one cerebral hemisphere prenatally or at birth, cafe au lait spots on the skin suggest neurofibromatosis (von Recklinghausen's disease).

Laboratory Investigation

All patients with a possible seizure should have an EEG. An abnormal EEG will confirm the clinical diagnosis. It will also help to classify the patient's seizure type.

The EEG may be the only investigation necessary. For example, a 6-year-old girl with typical absence attacks who is otherwise completely normal most likely has primary generalized epilepsy. If the EEG shows short generalized 3 Hz spike and wave bursts and normal background rhythms, this diagnosis is confirmed, and no further investigation is necessary.

Most patients will not have a seizure during the EEG recording, but the interseizure (interictal) EEG may still be of great value. In patients with primary generalized epilepsy and absence (petit mal) seizures, the interictal EEG shows spike and wave bursts in approximately 80 percent of cases. In patients with partial seizures with psychomotor symptomatology, approximately one third will show interictal focal epileptic abnormalities on the EEG. A sleep EEG will increase the rate of abnormal findings to approximately one half. Prolonged EEG recordings and the use of special sphenoidal electrodes will further increase the percentage of patients showing abnormalities. However, the initial routine EEG will be normal in approximately 65 percent of patients with partial epilepsy.

An epileptic abnormality on the EEG does not necessarily mean that the patient has had or is going to have seizures. For example, if EEGs are done on all siblings of patients with primary generalized epilepsy and absence seizures, 40 percent will show an epileptic abnormality very similar to that seen in the patient with clinical seizures. However, of these siblings, only 25 percent with the EEG abnormality will have clinical seizures. Those individuals with the EEG abnormality only and without clinical seizures should not be treated with anticonvulsant medication.

Skull roentgenograms and a radioisotope brain scan or brain CT scan are indicated in most patients presenting with their first seizure in adulthood. The main reason for doing these tests is to rule out a brain tumor. The likelihood of finding a tumor depends largely on the patient's age at the time of his first seizure. The presence of a focal abnormality on neurologic examination increases the likelihood of brain tumor.

Patients being evaluated for their first seizure should have determinations of blood sugar, BUN, and serum electrolytes including a serum calcium. The majority of patients presenting with their first seizure in adulthood will show no abnormality on investigation. These patients may still be classified as to type of epilepsy and seizure on the basis of clinical findings and laboratory investigations. Most of these patients presumably have their seizures as a result of genetic factors, occult perinatal trauma (birth injury), or old head trauma.

TREATMENT

General Principles

In most patients, epilepsy is a chronic disorder, and the treatment period will extend over many years. A good physician-patient relationship is invaluable and will encourage the patient to comply with therapy. Failure of patients to take medications as directed is one of the most common causes of treatment failure.

General management of the patient includes attention to social factors, education and reassurance of the patient and his relatives, job counseling, and counseling regarding the operation of a motor vehicle. In general, patients are encouraged to lead as normal a life as possible. Patients should not swim alone. Showering may be preferable to bathing, as patients with uncontrolled seizures have been known to drown in the bathtub. Most major cities have epilepsy associations that can assist the patient and his physician in many ways.

Drug Therapy

General Principles

A decision must be made whether or not to initiate drug therapy in the adult presenting with a first tonic-clonic seizure and normal investigations. The decision to treat is based primarily on the risk of further seizures. Available evidence would suggest that, of adults experiencing a single tonic-clonic seizure without obvious cause, a significant percentage, possibly even 50 percent or more, will not have further seizures. If the initial seizure was precipitated by obvious stress, for example severe sleep deprivation or emotional stress, the incidence of patients going on to further seizures is even lower.

The decision to institute long-term anticonvulsant therapy should be made by the physician in consultation with the patient. Many physicians recommend placing the patient on long-term anticonvulsant therapy after a single tonic-clonic seizure, whereas others, particularly if the EEG is normal, would withhold therapy until a second seizure has occurred. The patient's occupation, social situation, and need to operate a motor vehicle are significant factors.

Most patients are started on anticonvulsants after their first definite seizure.

In childhood, the seizure threshold rises somewhat with increasing age. For this reason, tapering of anticonvulsant therapy is often indicated after a child has been free of seizures for several years, particularly if the EEG is normal. Once adulthood is reached, there is little further change in seizure threshold with age, and less justification for tapering anticonvulsant therapy. Seizures in adults are likely to recur when medication is stopped.

The absence seizures of primary generalized epilepsy usually have ceased by age 20, making further therapy unnecessary in most patients.

The majority of epileptic patients achieve good seizure control on anticonvulsant drug therapy. Surgical excision of the epileptic focus in the cerebral cortex is indicated in a small minority of patients. Surgery is usually reserved for patients with intractable seizures that cannot be controlled medically. Only patients with partial epilepsy are candiates for surgery, and the seizure focus must be in an area of the brain that can be excised without causing prohibitive functional deficits.

Anticonvulsant Drug Choice

For absence seizures, the drugs of choice are ethosuximide and valproic acid. Valproic acid has the advantage of also suppressing tonic-clonic seizures, while ethosuximide is ineffective for tonic-clonic seizures. Nevertheless, ethosuximide is still considered the drug of choice for patients with primary generalized epilepsy and absence seizures alone by many authorities.

In patients with tonic-clonic seizures, phenytoin, phenobarbital, primidone, and carbamazepine, are probably equally effective. Controlled drug trials, particularly with the older drugs, are limited. Phenytoin is considered the drug of choice for such seizures in adults by many because it is nonsedating (in contrast to phenobarbital), and is generally better tolerated than primidone. Carbamazepine is considered the drug of choice by many for partial seizures, but the other three major anticonvulsant drugs listed above, particularly phenytoin, are also useful in these patients. Valproic acid is effective against both tonic-clonic and partial seizures, and at times may obtain seizure control where other drugs have failed. The most important factor in effective therapy is not which drug is chosen, but proper use of the drug selected based on a sound knowledge of its pharmacology.

The best practice is to use one drug alone to its limit (the achievement of good therapeutic drug levels as measured in the laboratory), before considering the addition of a second drug. Combinations of more than three drugs are rarely indicated, and usually increase toxicity rather than improving seizure control. The great majority of patients should be on only one to two drugs. In patients with tonic-clonic seizures not completely controlled on phenytoin, phenobarbital or carbamazepine should be added.

Anticonvulsant therapy is not usually necessary for alcohol withdrawal seizures (see Chapter 1).

Treatment of Status Epilepticus

Status epilepticus is defined as a continuous convulsion lasting longer than 1/2 hour, or a series of 2 or more convulsions occurring without intervening recovery of consciousness. The treatment of tonic-clonic status epilepticus is a medical emergency. A clear airway should be established and anticonvulsant therapy initiated immediately. It should be emphasized that most tonic-clonic convulsions are short and self-limited, lasting only several minutes. Intravenous diazepam is not indicated in such patients, as it has potential side effects and may complicate further observation of the patient's neurologic status. If the seizure persists beyond several minutes (the postictal confusional period should not be considered as part of the seizure for this purpose), intravenous therapy as discussed for status epilepticus should be given.

Status epilepticus should be treated with intravenous diazepam (Valium) 10 mg given over 2 minutes. The major side effect of intravenous diazepam is respiratory depression and obtundation. The patient should be observed carefully and respiration assisted mechanically if necessary. Diazepam, 10 mg given intravenously, will quickly stop most epileptic seizures. However, plasma levels of diazepam fall rapidly as the drug is redistributed throughout the body, and seizure protection is largely gone in 20 minutes. During this time interval therapeutic levels of phenytoin should be established to protect the patient against seizure recurrence. To achieve therapeutic levels of phenytoin quickly, a loading dose of 12 to 15 mg/kg must be given intravenously. Phenytoin should not be given faster than 50 mg/min, to avoid side effects such as cardiac arrhythmias and hypotension. Hypotension during intravenous administration of phenytoin is frequent, particularly in older fragile patients. Blood pressure should be monitored frequently, and the infusion rate slowed if hypotension occurs. The full loading dose can ultimately still be given in most patients.

Intravenous phenytoin alone is effective in the therapy of status epilepticus. This method of treatment might be considered where subsequent observation of the patient's level of consciousness is important, as for example after a head injury. Phenytoin tends to precipitate rapidly in acidic solutions, and therefore should be given in saline rather than dextrose solutions. Phenobarbital and paraldehyde can also be used in the treatment of status epilepticus. Phenobarbital given in the large doses required has the disadvantage of producing marked sedation and respiratory depression.

The patient should be cooled if the temperature goes over 38.5° C. Blood gases and electrolytes should be assessed and abnormalities treated. Bicarbonate therapy should be used cautiously, since acidosis is to some extent protective in preventing seizures.

Approximately half of patients presenting with status epilepticus have had no previous seizures, and suffer from head injury, brain tumor, cerebrovascular accident, CNS infection, or drug withdrawal. The remaining are known epileptics who have either stopped their anticonvulsants or have a nonspecific infection, such as an acute viral illness. If patients are known to be on maintenance phenytoin therapy, the intravenous loading dose of phenytoin may be reduced somewhat. Even if the patient has therapeutic phenytoin levels prior to being given the usual loading dose, significant complications are unusual, although respiratory depression may occur. Nystagmus, ataxia, and somnolence from phenytoin toxicity may be present for a brief period. A blood sample taken prior to phenytoin loading can be very useful in these patients. Subtherapeutic phenytoin levels suggest that ineffective drug therapy or poor patient compliance was the cause of the patient's status epilepticus.

Patients with absence status (petit mal status) seizures are generally conscious, but appear dazed and confused, and may have some fluttering of the eyelids. They are best treated with intravenous diazepam followed by maintenance drug therapy for absence seizures.

Focal status (epilepsia partialis continuans) consists of continuous twitching of a localized body part lasting for hours, days, or even longer periods. Patients with partial complex seizures, may also present in status epilepticus (psychomotor status). They appear confused, may show automatisms, but are generally at least partially responsive to their environment and breathing adequately. Like absence status and focal status, these patients should be treated promptly, but they do not represent a medical emergency. Initial therapy for focal and psychomotor status epilepticus should be intravenous phenytoin followed by maintenance therapy.

Epilepsy and Pregnancy

Seizure tendency becomes somewhat worse in one half of epileptics during pregnancy. An almost equal number are unchanged, while a small minority have some amelioration of their seizure disorder. Phenytoin, phenobarbital, and primidone appear significantly and approximately equally teratogenic, with an increased incidence of cleft palate and congenital heart defects. A fetal hydantoin syndrome with dysmorphic craniofacial features has also been described. Little data is available on the safety of the new anticonvulsants during pregnancy, and this remains to be established. The incidence of spina bifida in the newborn may be increased by maternal valproic acid therapy during pregnancy.

The risk of malformation is not high enough to

discourage pregnancy in most epileptics, but certain precautions should be followed. All epileptics on medication should be advised to consult with their physician prior to becoming pregnant. At that time the need for anticonvulsant drugs should be reassessed, and the number of drugs reduced if possible. If a trial of drug withdrawal is advisable, this should be done prior to and not during pregnancy, as tonic-clonic convulsions are dangerous to the fetus. If drug treatment is necessary, blood levels should be monitored. Dosage requirements may change during pregnancy, and this may result either in recurrent seizures, or in toxic drug levels with increased risk of teratogenicity.

Anticonvulsant Drugs

Phenytoin The usual maintenance dose of phenytoin in adults is 300 mg/day. The drug has a plasma half-life of approximately 24 hours, and need be given only once or twice a day. Probably 100 mg in the morning and 200 mg at bedtime is ideal. There are differences in absorption between Dilantin and other generic phenytoin formulations, so if the patient is switched from one brand of phenytoin to another, it may be wise to check serum levels.

The rate of phenytoin metabolism varies greatly from individual to individual. It is useful to measure serum phenytoin concentrations after initiating therapy. On a standard dose of 300 mg/day, a significant number of individuals will be subtherapeutic, and a small additional number will be toxic. These measurements should not be made until the patient has been on maintenance therapy for at least 5 days, as it takes approximately 5 drug half-lives before serum concentrations reach a stable level.

Phenytoin should never be given intramuscularly, because it is very poorly absorbed by this route. The therapeutic range for phenytoin and other anticonvulsants is shown in Table 14.18. As phenytoin serum levels increase, nystagmus appears at approximately 20 μg/ml, ataxia at 30 μg/ml, and lethargy at 40 μg/ml. The patient should be warned that im-

balance and clumsiness may indicate phenytoin toxicity.

Skin rashes from drug hypersensitivity occur, usually within the first 10 days of therapy, and require discontinuation of the drug. Numerous other side effects can occur, and include gingival hyperplasia, hirsutism, acne, and osteomalacia.

Phenobarbital In adults, phenobarbital is used mainly as a second drug, particularly with phenytoin. Many patients will show intolerable sedation in the upper half of the therapeutic range, although tolerance usually develops to some extent with time. Phenobarbital has many of the same side effects as phenytoin. The half-life is long, and it need be given only once or twice a day. The average daily adult dose is 90 to 120 mg.

Carbamazepine Carbamazepine therapy must be started with small doses, approximately 200 to 400 mg/day, or most patients will experience intolerable side effects. The dose is then built up gradually to the usual maintenance dose of 600 to 1,000 mg daily. The half-life of the drug is short, so it should be given in divided doses 3 to 4 times daily. Initial side effects on starting therapy include diplopia, blurred vision, drowsiness, dizziness, and nausea, but these can usually be avoided if the dose is built up slowly. Patients with cardiac disease may develop arrhythmias. An allergic skin rash requires discontinuation of the drug. Transient leukopenia is frequently seen on initiation of therapy. This usually resolves on continuing therapy, but does require reduction in dose or cessation of therapy if the total white blood cell count falls below 3,500, or if the granulocyte count falls below 25 percent of the total white blood cell count.

Valproic Acid This drug also is better tolerated if the dose is built up slowly. Hepatic toxicity has been reported, and liver function tests should be performed prior to starting therapy and every 2 months thereafter.

Valproic acid blocks phenobarbital metabolism. If given to patients already on phenobarbital, phenobarbital blood levels will rise markedly, and should be monitored carefully. The phenobarbital dose frequently must be reduced by as much as 50 percent.

Table 14.18 Anticonvulsant Serum Levels

Drug	Therapeutic Range (μg/ml)
Phenytoin	10–20
Phenobarbital	15–40
Primidone	8–12
Carbamazepine	6–12
Valproic Acid	50–100
Ethosuximide	40–120

DEMENTIA

DEFINITION

Dementia is a mental state characterized by the loss of previously acquired intellectual function. Although many patients with dementia have a slowly progressive and irreversible deterioration of intellectual function, our definition does not necessarily imply irreversibility. The patient with mental deterioration from hypothyroidism is considered demented, even though this may be reversible with treatment. Serious head injury may result in nonprogressive dementia of sudden onset.

A distinction should be made between dementia and delirium. Delirium is an acute confusional state that is transient in nature, and usually characterized by gross disorientation, illusions, visual hallucinations, agitation, and autonomic overactivity. Delirium is usually due to an acute toxic or metabolic encephalopathy.

Dementia implies a diffuse disorder of cerebral function. This term should not be used for clearly focal brain disorders such as dysphasia or apraxia. However, relatively small cerebral lesions, if bilateral, may result in dementia. Wernicke-Korsakoff syndrome and the lacunar state are examples of this.

PATHOPHYSIOLOGY

The anatomic and physiologic basis of higher intellectual function is poorly understood. Thus, precise description of the pathophysiology of dementia is impossible.

Considerable information is available on the neuroanatomic basis of memory. The limbic system including the hippocampus and several thalamic structures (medial dorsal nuclei and mamillary bodies) appear necessary for the formation and/or recall of new memories. A patient with bilateral hippocampal lesions or with bilateral lesions in the medial dorsal nuclei of the thalamus is unable to form new memories, even though he may otherwise appear intellectually quite normal. Such patients will never learn the name of a new friend or a new address. Yet, they may recall events of 20 years ago, as these appear to be stored diffusely in the cerebral cortex and are accessible without the intervention of the hippocampus. They may also have a normal digit span, as this function appears to depend on the cortical areas involved in the modality tested (for example, speech areas for verbal immediate recall).

Patients with diffuse cortical degeneration from Alzheimer's disease frequently have a disproportionate deficit in recent memory early in their course. This probably occurs because the cerebral degeneration tends to be most marked in the hippocampus.

Most patients with dementia have diffuse cerebral cortical damage. In Huntington's chorea, diffuse cortical neuronal loss is present in addition to the basal ganglia changes. In progressive supranuclear palsy (Steele-Richardson-Olszewski syndrome), however, mild dementia occurs with pathologic changes in the basal ganglia and brainstem, but without significant cortical or white matter lesions.

The brain normally atrophies with age. Average brain weight in males at age 80 is 1,200 grams, compared to 1,400 grams in the young adult. After the age of 30, it is said an individual loses 100,000 neurons each day. Although probably inaccurate, these figures indicate that one may lose millions of neurons without significant change in intellectual ability. In fact, the correlation of CT scan-demonstrated brain atrophy and intellectual function is far from perfect, and many individuals retain good intellectual function in the presence of considerable brain atrophy.

CLINICAL ASSESSMENT

The intellectual changes occurring in dementia can be assessed by the mental status examination. This should include the items listed in Table 14.19.

The patient must be sufficiently alert for a reliable mental status examination. Assessment of language function should detect the patient with dysphasia. Evaluation of mood or affect is important. Many depressed patients give a superficial impression of dementia due to lack of interest and poor concentration. Prominent delusions, paranoia and hallucinations suggest schizophrenia.

Memory assessment deserves special emphasis. Immediate memory is tested by digit span. The patient repeats a series of digits after the examiner. Most patients can repeat at least seven digits forward, and completion of this test indicates that the patient understands what is expected and has sufficient alertness to cooperate. Digit span will be normal in most patients until dementia is well advanced. Recent memory is tested by asking the patient to remember three objects (for example, a color, a number, and a name). The exercise is rehearsed until the patient has learned the objects and has repeated them several times. The

Table 14.19 **Mental Status Examination**

Level of Consciousness
General Appearance and Behavior
Orientation
Language
Mood
Memory (Immediate, Recent, and Remote)
Thought Content (Delusions, Paranoia)
Perceptual Disturbances (Illusions, Hallucinations)
Intellectual Function
General information
Calculation
Proverbs and similarities
Judgment
Insight

patient is then distracted by discussion of some other topic. The three objects are then no longer retained by immediate memory, but must be recalled through recent memory mechanisms. His ability to recall the three objects can then be tested at varying intervals of time. Recent memory is grossly deficient in patients with bilateral hippocampal lesions and in Wernicke-Korsakoff syndrome. Recent memory also is affected relatively early in most cortical degenerations. Remote memory is assessed by the individual's ability to recall events of past years.

Subtraction of serial seven's from 100 is a test of both concentration and calculation ability. Interpretation of simple proverbs such as, "Don't cry over spilled milk," tests the patient's ability for abstract thought. In similarity testing, the patient is asked to describe, for example, how a car is like an airplane. The correct response is that both are modes of transportation, and responses such as, "Both have wheels," indicate a problem with abstract thought.

Judgement is often tested by asking the patient how he would find a friend whose address he did not know in a strange city. Most patients will reply that they would look in the phone book. Inability to give such a straightforward response, in our society, implies a deficit in intellectual functioning.

Some patients with early dementia are frustrated by their intellectual deficits and may become hostile when the examiner attempts to assess their mental status. These patients should be shown sympathy, and if necessary their intellectual function should be assessed by indirect means during casual conversation. Patients with more advanced dementia frequently have little insight into their problem. They may even deny any problem with intellectual function and be unwilling to cooperate with suggested investigations.

A careful mental status examination will usually determine the presence or absence of dementia. In milder cases, however, it must be remembered that the patient's family may be much more sensitive than the physician to minor changes in his mental function. Psychologic testing may be of benefit in difficult cases, and may also be of help in differentiating depression from true dementia.

Evaluation of dementia includes a careful history and physical examination. A history of cold intolerance and hoarse voice may suggest hypothyroidism. Choreic movements suggest Huntington's chorea, and myoclonic jerks indicate Creutzfeldt-Jakob disease. A hemiparesis suggests chronic subdural hematoma or slowly growing intracranial tumor. Gait disturbance and urinary incontinence are typical of normal pressure hydrocephalus.

DIFFERENTIAL DIAGNOSIS

The causes of dementia are numerous. The most important etiologies are listed in Table 14.20.

The majority of patients presenting with dementia have cerebral atrophy of unknown cause and are classified either as Alzheimer's disease (see below) if they are younger than 65 years of age, or as senile dementia if they are older than 65 years. Vascular disease causes fewer than 15 percent of cases of dementia. Other relatively common causes of dementia include intracranial space-occupying masses and alcoholism.

In patients initially thought to be demented, but in whom other diagnoses are eventually found, depression and drug toxicity are prominent.

With present knowledge, dementia can be successfully treated and reversed in the conditions listed in Table 14.21.

Table 14.20 **Etiology of Dementia**

1. CNS Degeneration
   Alzheimer's disease
   Senile dementia
   Huntington's chorea
2. Metabolic Disorders
   Hypothyroidism
   Hypercalcemia
   Hypoglycemia
   Hypoxia
   Uremia
   Wilson's disease
   Dialysis dementia
   Liver disease
3. Deficiency Diseases
   Wernicke-Korsakoff syndrome
   Pernicious anemia
4. Mass Lesions
   Brain tumor
   Subdural hematoma
   Brain abscess
5. Vascular Diseases
   Atherosclerosis
   Hypertensive vascular disease
   Bilateral carotid occlusive disease
6. Infectious Disease
   Meningitis and encephalitis
   Subacute sclerosing panencephalitis
   Progressive multifocal leukoencephalopathy
   Creutzfeldt-Jakob disease
   Syphilis
7. Traumatic Brain Injury
   Head injury with brain damage
   Punch-drunk syndrome
8. Toxic Disorders
   Metals and organic compounds
   Carbon monoxide
9. Miscellaneous
   Multiple sclerosis
   Normal pressure hydrocephalus

Table 14.21   **Reversible Dementia**

Hypothyroidism
Hypercalcemia
Wilson's Disease (Early)
Wernicke-Korsakoff Syndrome (Early)
Vitamin B_{12} Deficiency (Early)
Drugs, Toxins
Some Systemic Metabolic disorders (Hepatic Encephalopathy and Others)
Brain Tumor
Subdural Hematoma
Chronic Meningitis (Cryptococcus)
Normal Pressure Hydrocephalus

Early diagnosis is essential if dementia is to be reversed in some of these. In particular, Wernicke-Korsakoff syndrome is a medical emergency, and thiamine must be administered as soon as possible.

LABORATORY INVESTIGATION

The laboratory investigation is used to establish a specific etiology where possible and to detect those patients with reversible dementing syndromes.

The history and physical examination may indicate a specific cause for the patient's dementia. If the cause is not obvious, a number of routine investigations should be done in all patients. These include hemoglobin, white blood count, BUN, blood sugar, serum sodium, potassium, chloride, calcium, thyroxin, VDRL, liver function tests, chest roentgenogram, skull roentgenogram, and electroencephalogram (EEG).

Serum vitamin B_{12} is also frequently measured as dementia due to vitamin B_{12} deficiency without hematologic or spinal cord involvement has on rare occasions been reported.

Lumbar puncture is not usually helpful in the investigation of dementia, but rare cases of chronic meningitis, such as cryptococcal meningitis, have been reported to cause dementia without clearcut symptoms or signs of meningitis.

A radioisotope brain scan detects many intracranial tumors and over 90 percent of chronic subdural hematomas. Brain CT scan is considerably superior and will show virtually all brain tumors and chronic subdural hematomas large enough to cause dementia (Fig. 14.13). In addition, brain CT scan will demonstrate the ventricular enlargement of normal pressure hydrocephalus, and indicate the degree of brain atrophy present in patients with Alzheimer's disease or senile dementia. All patients with presenile dementia (dementia before age 65 years) should have a brain CT scan. In older patients, who are more likely to have senile dementia, the necessity for CT scanning must be determined on an individual basis (Fig. 14.14 and 14.15).

Other useful investigations include radioisotope cisternography, cerebral angiography, and special biochemical tests. The indications for these will be discussed in a later section.

TREATMENT

Specific therapy is available for only a minority of patients with dementia. This therapy depends on the underlying cause. Thyroxin will gradually reverse the dementia of hypothyroidism if onset has occured in adult life. Untreated neonatal hypothyroidism results in irreversible mental retardation (cretinism). Genetic counseling is important for the families of patients with hereditary dementias such as Huntington's chorea.

For the majority of patients with dementia, no specific therapy can be offered, but general measures

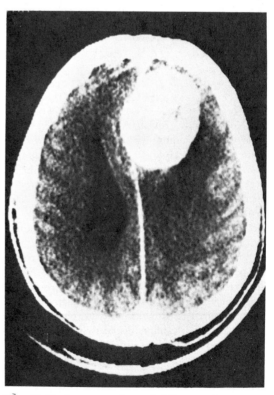

Fig. 14.13 Contrast enhanced CT scan of a 52-year-old man presenting with dementia. The large frontal meningioma shown here as a white lesion was successfully removed surgically. Marked improvement of mental function followed

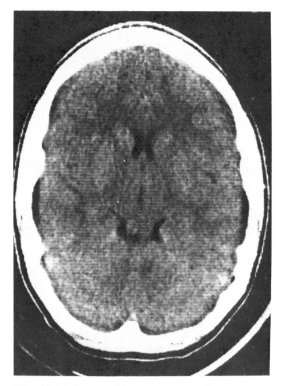

Fig. 14.14 A normal brain CT scan of a 14-year-old girl. Note small size of ventricles and lack of prominence of sulci

the patient is no longer capable of responsible judgement. The physician can also aid the family in making contact with the appropriate community social service agencies.

SENILE DEMENTIA

Senile dementia is characterized by diffuse cortical degeneration with brain atrophy. The pathologic changes in the brain are often less marked but otherwise identical to those found in Alzheimer's disease. The distinction between senile dementia and Alzheimer's disease is therefore somewhat arbitrary. The two likely represent the same disease process.

Microscopically, the degenerated cortex contains multiple argyrophilic senile plaques. These are clumps of degenerated axons and dendrites. Neuronal cell bodies containing skeins of twisted neurofibrils (neurofibrillary tangles) are also prominent. Granulovacuolar neuronal degeneration is the third characteristic change.

It is of interest that similar pathologic changes, although usually much less marked, are also seen in the brains of elderly people without dementia.

may considerably alleviate the burden carried by the patient and his family. Treatment of associated systemic diseases, such as chronic infections, malnutrition, and diabetes, may significantly improve the patient's level of function. Cautious drug therapy of depression and psychosis is helpful. Reducing the patient's need for lost functions by structuring the environment is useful. Quiet and familiar surroundings are best for these patients. Simple measures like hanging signs in the various rooms of a house telling the patient where he is may also be helpful. Many demented patients become agitated and considerably worse in unfamiliar surroundings and in the dark. Leaving a light on at night in the hospital room can help a patient with failing mental abilities orient himself and prevent agitation and confusion. Holidays in unfamiliar places are generally not advisable for patients with failing mental function.

Intellectual deterioration in a loved one, together with the resulting changes in personality and behavior, is probably one of the most profound tragedies of life. The family frequently requires considerable support. The physician can help to ease the burden by careful discussion with the family. The family may require assistance in obtaining legal advice when

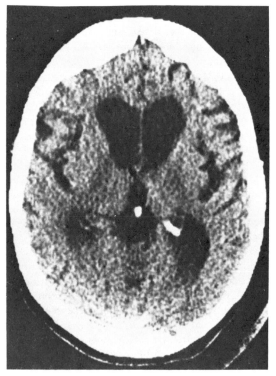

Fig. 14.15 Brain CT scan of a 75-year-old patient with senile dementia. Cerebral ventricles are grossly enlarged, and brain sulci are very prominent secondary to brain atrophy

ALZHEIMER'S DISEASE

Alzheimer's disease, in its presenile and senile form, is by far the most common cause of dementia. The progression of Alzheimer's disease in younger patients is usually more rapid, and in the occasional rapidly progressing case, severe dementia may develop over several months. Brain atrophy is often most marked in the frontal and occipital lobes.

The initial symptoms of Alzheimer's disease may suggest a psychogenic illness, with anxiety, depression, and restlessness. Memory disturbances soon follow, and eventually all intellectual functions are affected. Because of poor insight and judgement, patients soon are unable to handle their business and social affairs.

Only nonspecific supportive therapy is available. The patient usually dies 5 to 10 years after the onset of illness, from respiratory infections.

Pick's disease is a less common cause of presenile dementia. Clinically it is indistinguishable from Alzheimer's disease, but pathologically Pick's disease is characterized by brain atrophy most marked in frontal and temporal lobes. Neuronal cell loss, extensive gliosis, and intracellular argyrophilic inclusion bodies are the main pathologic features.

HUNTINGTON'S CHOREA

Huntington's chorea is inherited as an autosomal dominant trait. Choreic movements are usually the first manifestations of the disease and may affect the face, trunk, or extremities. Mental changes usually become evident somewhat later, but may develop simultaneously or even precede the movement disorder. Most patients become symptomatic during or after the fourth decade.

Pathologically, there is striking atrophy and neuronal loss in the caudate nucleus and to a lesser degree in the remainder of the basal ganglia. Neuronal cell loss is also diffusely present in the cerebral cortex. Marked atrophy of the caudate nucleus on CT scan strongly suggests the diagnosis.

Disease progression is slow, and survival for 15 years after illness onset is common.

WILSON'S DISEASE

Wilson's disease shows autosomal recessive inheritance. An abnormality in copper excretion is present and results in toxic accumulation of copper in liver, brain, and other organs.

The primary neurologic manifestation of Wilson's disease is a movement disorder manifesting tremor, dystonia, chorea, and dysarthria. Dementia is usually mild early in the illness.

The Kayser-Fleischer ring, a green or golden copper deposit around the peripheral cornea, is characteristic of this disorder. It is always present on slit lamp examination when neurologic disturbances are present in Wilson's disease.

Patients with Wilson's disease may present in childhood or adult life. The diagnosis is confirmed by a serum ceruloplasmin concentration below 20 mg/dl and the presence of either the Kayser-Fleischer ring, or a liver biopsy copper concentration greater than 250 µg/g dry weight. Occasional patients with Wilson's disease have a serum ceruloplasmin level greater than 20 mg/dl, and more sophisticated tests can be done if the diagnosis appears clinically likely. Urine excretion of copper in most patients with Wilson's disease is over 100 µg/day.

Early diagnosis is essential, as life-long penicillamine treatment can prevent the appearance of new neurologic symptoms. Symptoms already present may be reversed if treatment is started early.

WERNICKE-KORSAKOFF SYNDROME

Wernicke's encephalopathy is a neurologic disorder of acute onset characterized by oculomotor disturbances, gait ataxia, and a global confusional state. Korsakoff's psychosis is an abnormal mental state in which recent memory is affected out of proportion to other cognitive functions. The two conditions may be regarded as facets of the same disease related to alcohol abuse (see Chapter 1).

It is imperative that all alcoholics with evidence of encephalopathy be given immediate parenteral thiamine when initially examined. A delay of several hours may result in less complete recovery from encephalopathy. Intravenous glucose administration without concomitant thiamine therapy worsens the prognosis.

CEREBROVASCULAR DISEASE AND DEMENTIA

Several distinctive clinical features are usually present in dementia resulting from vascular disease, and these aid in differential diagnosis.

Patients with multiple cerebral infarctions (multi-infarct dementia) from atherosclerosis or thromboembolic disease may lose large amounts of cerebral tissue. In addition to focal symptoms and signs, these patients may show dementia with a global loss of intellectual function. These patients usually have a stepwise progression, with each stroke adding to their disability, they lack the smooth progressive debility characteristic of Alzheimer's disease or senile dementia.

The lacunar state results from degeneration of small arteries secondary to hypertension. Multiple small infarcts (lacunes) deep in the cerebral hemispheres and internal capsules bilaterally result in dementia. These patients also usually show stepwise progression of symptoms and have dysphagia, dysarthria, brisk tendon reflexes, and extensor plantar responses secondary to corticobulbar and corticospinal tract involvement.

Occlusion of one or both carotid arteries by atheroma is occasionally cited as a cause of dementia in individual case reports. In some of these patients, focal neurologic signs have not been prominent. The implication is that vascular surgery, either carotid endarterectomy or middle cerebral-superfical temporal artery bypass, might be helpful in these patients. Experience would indicate that such patients are unusual, but cerebral angiography may occasionally be indicated in patients with dementia.

NORMAL PRESSURE HYDROCEPHALUS

In normal pressure hydrocephalus (NPH), obliteration of CSF pathways over the convexity of the brain by inflammation or fibrosis interferes with CSF absorption. This inflammation may be idiopathic or secondary to previous subarachnoid hemorrhage, head trauma, or meningitis. The ventricles enlarge, and CSF absorption eventually occurs transependymally through the ventricular wall. A new equilibrium develops, and the ventricles remain large, but CSF pressure is often within normal limits. Prolonged CSF pressure monitoring will, however, reveal CSF pressure abnormalities in many of these patients.

Patients often show a triad of dementia. gait disorder, and urinary incontinence. The urinary incontinence and gait disturbance tend to occur earlier and are more prominent in NPH than in dementia from other causes.

Brain CT scan will show large cerebral ventricles without significant cortical atrophy. This is in contrast to Alzheimer's disease, where diffuse brain atrophy results in large cerebral ventricles and widened brain sulci. A radioisotope cisternogram is indicated if the clinical examination and brain CT scan support NPH. A radioisotope in colloidal form is injected into the lumbar subarachnoid space and carried up the CSF pathways to the head. Normally, the isotope will pass over the cerebral hemispheres to the superior sagittal sinus where it is absorbed into the blood stream. In patients with normal pressure hydrocephalus, the isotope will not progress over the brain convexities and will instead enter the ventricles and remain there for an abnormally long period of time.

A ventriculoatrial or ventriculoperitoneal CSF shunt may reverse dementia from NPH. An accurate diagnosis must be made, for patients with Alzheimer's disease do not respond to CSF shunting. The morbitity of the surgery is considerable in these elderly patients, and shunting should not be done unless the diagnosis of NPH seems firmly established.

Unfortunately, only 50 percent of patients with NPH respond to CSF shunting. The response rate is slightly higher in patients with NPH secondary to known causes than in patients with idiopathic NPH.

CREUTZFELDT-JAKOB DISEASE

Dementia from Creutzfeld-Jakob disease usually becomes apparent between 40 and 60 years of age. Rapid progression is common, and disease duration is usually measured in months. In addition to dementia, bizarre behavior, visual distortions, hallucinations, and ataxia are often prominent. Myoclonic jerks are characteristic, and in the presence of dementia they should always suggest Creutzfeld-Jakob disease. Muscular atrophy from anterior horn cell degeneration also occurs. The EEG usually shows periodic EEG complexes within 10 weeks of disease onset, and is frequently diagnostic.

Creutzfeld-Jakob disease is caused by a slow virus infection. Particular care must be taken in handling blood, spinal fluid, and autopsy material from patients with this disease. Human to human transmission has occurred via corneal transplantation.

No effective therapy presently exists for this disease.

SUBACUTE SCLEROSING PANENCEPHALITIS

Subacute sclerosing panencephalitis (SSPE) usually affects young children. Eighty percent of cases occur before age 11 years, with boys affected 5 times as frequently as girls. The onset is usually insidious, with personality change and decline in school performance. Myoclonic seizures typically occur, and are difficult to control. Cortical blindless is common, and the patient becomes bedridden within 1 year of onset with severe intellectual deterioration.

The etiology of this devastating disease is persistent brain infection with measles virus. The EEG is diagnostic and shows periodic complexes. CSF lgG levels are very high, and consist mainly of measles antibody.

Antiviral agents are being tried in this disorder, but no effective therapy is yet available.

HEADACHE

Headaches are common, and are the result of benign disorders in the vast majority of patients. In a small number of patients, however, headache is caused by serious underlying disease. For this reason, every headache patient must be carefully assessed. A thorough knowledge of the various headache syndromes is essential for successful management.

PATHOPHYSIOLOGY

Pain-Sensitive Structures

Headache arises from intracranial and extracranial pain-sensitive structures. The brain itself, the veins and arteries over the brain convexities, and most of the dura are not sensitive to pain. The major intracranial pain-sensitive structures include:

1. The middle meningeal artery and other dural arteries
2. The major intracranial arteries at the base of the brain
3. The dural sinuses and major cerebral veins
4. The nerve roots of cranial nerves 5, 9, and 10
5. The upper 3 cervical nerve roots

Extracranial pain-sensitive structures are also important in the generation of headache, and include the skin, scalp blood vessels, and the muscles of the head and neck.

Headache Mechanisms

Headache results from involvement of pain-sensitive structures by one of several mechanisms. Traction on a sensitive blood vessel or cranial nerve root results in traction headache. Subdural hematoma, brain tumors, and other mass lesions can cause headache by this mechanism. Dilatation of cerebral and extracranial arteries by drugs, fever, or other causes results in vascular headache. Sustained contraction of scalp and neck muscles results in muscle contraction headache.

Pain Referral Patterns

The ophthalmic division of the trigeminal nerve supplies the entire supratentorial portion of the cranial cavity. Pain generated in this area is referred to the cutaneous distribution of the ophthalmic division, particularly to the forehead and eyes.

The posterior fossa is innervated largely by the upper three cervical nerves, and pain arising here is referred to the occipital region and back of the neck.

ETIOLOGY

Headache can result from numerous causes. The classification of headache shown in Table 14.22 is based on headache mechanisms, and allows for simple grouping of the major types.

Migraine

Migraine headaches result from paroxysmal vascular instability. For unknown reasons, these patients periodically experience vasoconstriction, followed by vasodilation in the cerebral and scalp arteries. The neurologic symptoms that make up the aura of clas-

Table 14.22 **Headache**

1. Vascular
    A. Migrainous
        Classic
        Common
        Cluster
    B. Nonmigrainous
        Drug-induced
        Fever
        Hypoxia
        Hypercapnia
        Ischemia
        Hypertension
        Postictal
2. Muscle Contraction Headache
3. Traction
    A. Tumors
    B. Hematomas
    C. Brain abscess
    D. Post–lumbar puncture
4. Inflammatory
    A. Intracranial
        Meningitis
        Subarachnoid hemorrhage
    B. Extracranial
        Temporal arteritis
5. Others
    Sinus and dental
    Ocular and otic
    Neuralgias
    Delusional

sical migraine result from brain ischemia during the vasoconstriction phase. The head pain results from the vasodilation that follows, and from sterile inflammation of the arterial wall that accompanies the vasodilation.

The etiology of these events is not known. A CNS disorder of vasomotor control may be responsible. Many vasoactive amines including serotonin and histamine have been implicated in the pathogenesis of migraine. Hereditary factors appear important.

Classic Migraine

Headaches in classic migraine are often preceded by an aura. Visual auras are the most common, and usually consist of bright scintillations, wavy lines, and fortification spectra. Another common aura consists of tingling of one hand and the lower face on the same side. The tingling may appear simultaneously in the two areas, but often takes several minutes or more to spread from one area to the other. This slow march is typical of migraine, and is unlike the rapid spread of symptoms with transient ischemic attacks or focal seizure.

The aura usually lasts approximately 20 minutes and then disappears as the headache starts, although the relationship of aura to headache is not always typical. The headache is throbbing, severe, often unilateral, and lasts several hours. The aura may occur without the headache, and the headache may at times come on without the aura in a given patient.

Most classic migraine sufferers have numerous headache attacks with neurologic auras without complication. Rarely, a patient may suffer a permanent neurologic deficit. In ophthalmoplegic migraine, a permanent 3rd nerve palsy develops. The 3rd nerve is damaged by pressure from adjacent edematous dilated cerebral arteries. Ophthalmoplegic migraine must be differentiated from posterior communicating artery aneurysm. Permanent hemiplegia results on rare occasions from cerebral hemisphere ischemia during the vasoconstriction phase of migraine.

Common Migraine

Over 80 percent of migraine sufferers have common migraine. Auras, if present, consist of fatigue, psychic disturbances, diarrhea, or other autonomic symptoms. Frequently no aura is present. The headache may be unilateral, but bilateral headache is common. The pain is usually throbbing in nature, and may be very severe. Headache usually lasts for hours,

and occasionally for days. Nausea and vomiting is common.

Cluster Headache

Cluster headache occurs primarily in men. This is in contrast to other forms of migraine, which are more common in women. Characteristically, the patient experiences short attacks of severe unilateral head pain concentrated around the temporal region or the eye. An individual attack usually lasts 30 minutes to several hours, and the patient may have many attacks in a day. Nocturnal attacks are common. Redness and tearing of the ipsilateral eye is often present during attacks.

The patient typically has many attacks during a period of several weeks or months (a cluster), and then is free of headache for months or years until another cluster occurs.

Nonmigrainous Vascular Headaches

Many other vascular headache syndromes exist. Nitroglycerin induced headache results from sudden vasodilation of cerebral arteries. Headache associated with hangovers, fever, and postictal states all belong in this category.

Although many patients with hypertension have no headache related to their hypertension, some patients have morning occipital headaches that disappear after a few hours. These headaches often resolve after successful treatment of hypertension. Acute generalized throbbing headaches occur in hypertensive crisis and hypertensive encephalopathy.

Vascular headaches also occur in some patients with cerebral ischemia, probably related to dilatation of collateral blood vessels.

Muscle Contraction Headache

Sustained muscle contraction in scalp and neck muscles may cause head pain as a result of metabolites from the contracting muscle or muscle ischemia. Muscle contraction headaches are approximately as common as migraine, and account for 45 percent of headache problems.

Acute muscle contraction headaches are characterized by frontal, occipital or generalized dull aching head pain lasting several hours. They are often triggered by emotional or physical stress.

Chronic muscle contraction headaches are usually described by the patient as a constant dull head pain that is frontooccipital, band-like, or occipital. Pain may involve the neck and upper shoulder area. Frequently the pain is present all day every day for weeks or months. The pain does not usually keep the patient awake at night, but concomitant depression may interfere with sleep. Nausea and vomiting are unusual.

Post traumatic muscle contraction headaches begin after minor or major head trauma. Dull aching head pain is present for most or all of the patient's waking hours for months or even years.

An underlying depression is very common in chronic muscle contraction headache. Why depression should result in chronic scalp and neck muscle contraction in some individuals is not clear. Other symptoms of depression such as frequent crying, anorexia, and sleep disturbances may be prominent.

Traction Headache

Increased intracranial pressure (ICP) usually causes a very characteristic headache with generalized head pain, nocturnal or early morning wakening, and vomiting. This headache description should always suggest an intracranial mass lesion. Posterior fossa lesions with obstructive hydrocephalus in particular tend to cause this headache syndrome.

Smaller brain tumors without increased ICP may also cause headache. These headaches may be rather nondescript, intermittent, and may respond to simple analgesics.

Chronic subdural hematoma may cause severe headaches that initially are unilateral but later become generalized. The headaches usually start immediately after the injury as the hematoma applies traction to neighboring cerebral veins.

Headache is frequent after lumbar puncture. Continued leakage of CSF from the needle puncture site leads to distortion of pain-sensitive intracranial structures. These headaches are rapidly relieved by lying down, but soon resume if the patient sits or stands.

Inflammatory Headache

Intracranial

Bacterial and viral meningitis usually are accompanied by severe headache if the patient is sufficiently alert. Photophobia and pain on head and eye movement is common. Pain may extend down the back.

Subarachnoid hemorrhage usually causes a severe headache of sudden or even explosive onset. The head pain is generalized, with a particularly strong occipital component. The headache lasts for at least several days. Unless previous subarachnoid bleeding has occurred, the headache is usually described as the worst the patient has ever experienced and unlike previous headaches. Headache with onset during exertion or sexual intercourse are particularly suspicious for subarachnoid hemorrhage. The patient is often drowsy and signs of meningeal irritation are usually but not invariably present.

Extracranial

The headache of temporal arteritis is usually persistent, severe, and frequently has a burning quality. Extreme scalp tenderness is characteristic of temporal arteritis although scalp tenderness also occurs in migraine and muscle contraction headache. The headache of temporal arteritis is usually progressive in severity. Jaw claudication, transient episodes of monocular blindness, diplopia, and generalized muscular pain (polymyalgia rheumatica), all are suggestive of temporal arteritis. The superficial temporal artery or other scalp arteries may be thickened and tender. Early diagnosis is essential for treatment to prevent permanent visual loss (see Chapter 18).

Temporal arteritis is rare in patients younger than 50 years of age, and increases in incidence with increasing age.

Other Headache Types

Numerous other headache types exist. Ocular conditions such as acute glaucoma may cause head pain. Headaches resulting from sinusitis usually have a prominent facial component, and tenderness is often present over the inflamed sinus.

Trigeminal neuralgia usually produces pain limited to one or more divisions of one trigeminal nerve. Sudden paroxysms of severe lancinating pain are characteristic, separated by relatively pain-free intervals. Frequently, touching the face, swallowing, or eating will trigger the pain. Trigeminal neuraligia may be caused by tumors and multiple sclerosis, but is usually idiopathic. Compression of the trigeminal nerve by tumor usually results in more constant pain, and sensory loss. In idiopathic trigeminal neuralgia, sensory loss is absent.

Delusional headaches are the only headache type with no peripheral pain mechanisms. Patients often have obvious mental disorders. The headache may be described in very dramatic terms and usually does not fit other headache categories. The location of the head pain may have symbolic significance for the patient.

CLINICAL APPROACH

The key to successful headache management is a careful description of the patient's pain. Its nature and location should be outlined and the frequency and length of individual attacks determined. Auras, other associated symptoms, precipitating factors, and relieving factors should all be asked for. Similar headache attacks going back many years are a good indication that the headaches are of a benign nature. A detailed personal, family, and social history are often required.

If the patient fits one of the classic headache syndromes of migraine or muscle contraction headache and no ominous physical findings are present to suggest serious intracranial pathology, laboratory investigation may be kept to a minimum. Good patient follow-up will further reduce the chances of missing serious organic disease. Atypical headaches may require further investigation. Onset of a new headache later in life, with gradual progression in severity, should always suggest organic pathology. Headaches that are consistently localized to one side of the head with every attack also suggest an intracranial lesion. Although often unilateral, migraine headaches usually do eventually involve both sides of the head at different times.

The patient should be carefully examined for papilledema, focal neurologic signs, and meningismus. If any of these are present, further investigation is essential.

Differentiation of migraine and muscle contraction headache is not usually difficult. Headache features aiding in this differentiation are shown in Table 14.23. Some patients have features of both headache types and a number of patients have both. It must then be determined which headache is the major problem, and treatment must be instituted accordingly.

INVESTIGATION

The routine use of expensive radiologic procedures to screen for possible intracranial lesions in most pa-

tients with headache should be discouraged, because the yield of positive findings is extremely low.

The investigation of headache is essentially that of the suspected underlying disease. If increased ICP or a mass lesion is suspected, a skull roentgenogram may show demineralization of the sella turcica or a shifted pineal gland, but many intracranial lesions will be missed. A brain CT scan will exclude virtually all mass lesions large enough to cause headache. An isotope brain scan will also demonstrate most intracranial tumors or chronic subdural hematomas. The investigation of subarachnoid hemorrhage is discussed in the section entitled Cerebrovascular Disorders; meningitis is discussed in the section entitled Central Nervous System Infections.

The sedimentation rate is generally elevated in suspected temporal arteritis, and may lead to biopsy (see Chapter 18).

Many systemic illnesses, for example anemia, can exacerbate a patient's headache. Investigations in this regard should again be guided by the patient's symptoms and signs.

TREATMENT

Effective headache treatment depends on an accurate diagnosis. This section will deal primarily with migraine and muscle contraction headache. The therapy of possible underlying lesions such as brain tumors and hematomas is discussed in other sections.

Migraine

General Measures.

A careful history often reveals trigger factors. The patient may be able to avoid these and reduce the frequency of his headaches. Birth control pills should be discontinued if they exacerbate migraine headaches. Many other medications, including indomethacin, reserpine, hydralazine, and nitroglycerine

Table 14.23 **Differential Diagnosis: Migraine versus Muscle Contraction**

Migraine	Muscle Contraction
Onset under 30 years	Frequently later
Pain Often Unilateral	Bilateral
Throbbing Initially	Steady Pain
Usually Lasts Hours	Often Lasts Days
Severe Pain	Moderate Pain
Aura Common	No Aura
Nausea and Vomiting Common	No Nausea
Scalp Tenderness Common	Scalp Tenderness Common

can exacerbate migraine headaches, and the need for these should be reassessed.

A good physician-patient relationship and reassurance that the headaches are of a benign nature may help reduce headache.

Pharmacologic Therapy

A decision must be made whether to employ symptomatic or prophylactic therapy. If headache attacks are severe and occur at least weekly, or are prolonged for days, prophylaxis is usually the best course.

Symptomatic Therapy Simple analgesics in moderate dosage are at times effective. In children, this is usually the only medication required. In adults, ergotamine preparations are usually necessary. These may be given orally. If headaches are accompanied by vomiting, rectal administration is preferable.

Sensitivity to ergotamine varies greatly from patient to patient. Vomiting is the most common dose-limiting side effect of ergotamine. Individual tolerance is best determined during a headache-free interval. The proper dosage will relieve headache but not cause nausea; the whole dose should be taken immediately at headache onset.

Serious toxicity from ergotamine used in proper dosage is rare. Tingling, coldness of the digits, and intermittent claudication are serious danger signs that require reduction in dosage or drug discontinuation.

Prophylactic Therapy A number of drugs will reduce the frequency of migraine attacks. Pizotyline, amitriptyline, propranolol, ergonovine and methysergide are effective in some patients and should be tried in approximately the order listed. It is impossible to predict which medication will work best in a given patient. Once an effective drug has been found, it is usually continued for approximately 4 months and then tapered to assess continuing need. In this way, over 90 percent of migraine patients with frequent headaches can be effectively managed.

Cluster Headaches

Ergotamine suppositories, ergotamine tartrate aerosol, intramuscular ergonovine and inhalations of 100 percent oxygen have all been reported as effective for individual cluster headache attacks.

The headache clusters themselves may be shortened by prophylactic medication including methysergide, propranolol, prednisone and lithium.

Muscle Contraction Headache

Acute muscle contraction headaches respond to analgesics, hot baths, or alcohol.

Treatment of chronic muscle contraction headache can be very difficult, and requires an ongoing supportive physician-patient relationship. Analgesics, relaxation therapy, and psychotherapy may be helpful, but most patients eventually require long-term drug treatment. The most effective medication is amitriptyline, which is frequently effective whether or not depression appears to be present. The usual dosage is 50 to 100 mg given in a single dose at bedtime. Higher doses may at times be necessary. If headaches are relieved, the amitriptyline should be tapered after 4 months. The medication can be reinstituted if headache recurs.

Temporal Arteritis

See Chapter 18.

Trigeminal Neuralgia

Carbamazepine 600 to 1,000 mg/day is effective in most patients. Treatment should be gradually discontinued after several months, since the trigeminal neuralgia may have gone into remission by that time. Phenytoin and clonazepam may benefit some patients not responsive to carbamazepine. If drugs are ineffective or cannot be tolerated, neurosurgical section of the trigeminal nerve root or stereotactic lesioning of the root is often effective.

CEREBROVASCULAR DISORDERS

Cerebrovascular disorders are the third ranking cause of death in North America after coronary heart disease and cancer. Although the complications of cerebrovascular disease occur mainly in the older population, 20 percent of the patients involved are under age 65 years. The incidence of stroke in the general population rises from approximately 0.5 percent per year between the ages of 55 and 64 years, to 2 percent per year between the ages of 75 and 84. The term "stroke" is applied to a number of clinical syndromes resulting from cerebrovascular disease. The hallmark of all these syndromes is the sudden onset of symptoms and signs.

The major categories of cerebrovascular disease are shown in Table 14.24.

Table 14.24   **Categories of Cerebrovascular Disease**

Disease Process		Relative Incidence (Percent)
Occlusive Cerebrovascular Disease		
Ischemic brain infarction		70
Thrombotic	30	
Embolic (from heart and proximal arteries)	25	
Lacunar	15	
Transient ischemic attacks only		10
Intracerebral Hemorrhage		10
Subarachnoid Hemorrhage (Aneurysm, Arteriovenous malformation)		10

OCCLUSIVE CEREBROVASCULAR DISEASE

Clinical Manifestations

Because of its high metabolic rate, the brain is highly vulnerable to ischemia. Should impairment of circulation be sufficient to result in tissue necrosis and infarction, the resulting neurologic deficit is often permanent, since the neurones of the central nervous system do not regenerate. As one part of the central nervous system usually cannot compensate for the lost function of another, recovery of function after a large cerebral infarct is frequently limited. The signs and symptoms that may result from cerebral infarction are as varied as the functions of the brain itself. Atheromatous involvement of the cerebral arteries, often with superimposed thrombosis on the atheromatous plaque, is the underlying cause.

Atheroma may involve any part of the cerebral arterial circulation (Figs. 14.16 and 14.17), but is most common in the larger vessels, with a striking predilection for involvement around the bifurcation

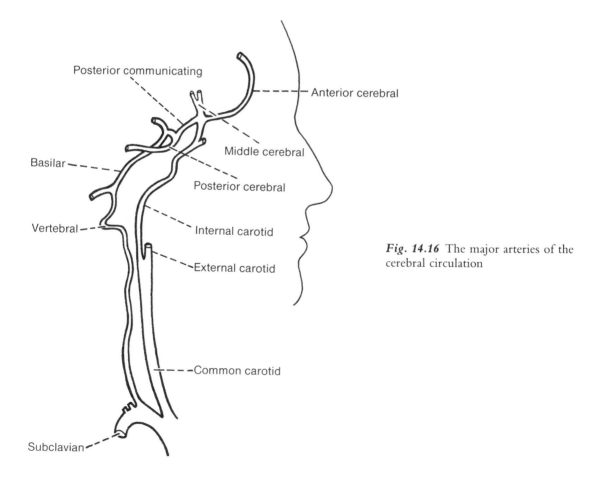

Fig. 14.16 The major arteries of the cerebral circulation

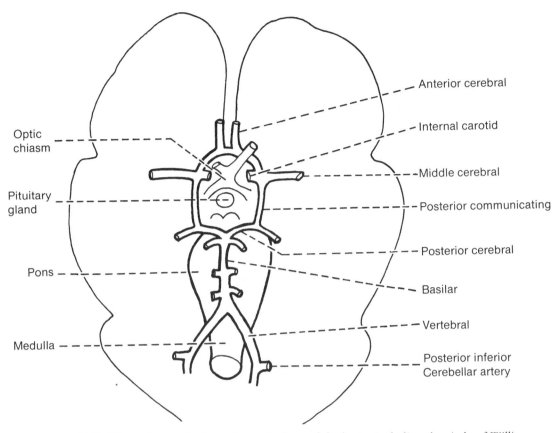

Fig. 14.17 The major cerebral arteries at the base of the brain, including the circle of Willis

of the common carotid artery. Atheromatous involvement of the more distal cerebral vessels beyond the middle cerebral artery bifurcation, or of other vessels of similar size, is unusual except in the presence of hypertension. Occlusion in these smaller arteries is usually due to emboli that have originated more proximally in the cerebral arteries, the extracranial vessels or the heart. Occlusion of the middle cerebral artery itself is more commonly due to emboli from the heart or carotid bifurcation than to local atheroma. Alternatively, occlusion of the proximal internal carotid artery at the bifurcation is more commonly the result of local atheroma, with or without superimposed thrombosis.

Transient Ischemic Attacks

Approximately 30 percent of patients with cerebral infarction have had prior transient ischemic attacks (TIAs). A TIA is defined as a transient focal neurologic disturbance of vascular origin that lasts for less than 24 hours and leaves no permanent residual deficits. Usually the symptom lasts for only seconds or minutes.

The symptoms of a TIA depend on the area of brain affected. A typical TIA involving the middle cerebral artery territory might consist of transient hemiparesis, possibly associated with numbness and tingling. Transient dysphasia is common in TIAs affecting the dominant hemisphere. Episodes of monocular loss of vision (amaurosis fugax) suggest ischemia in the distribution of the ophthalmic artery. Like TIAs involving the middle cerebral artery distribution, these may occur in association with a stenotic lesion at the carotid bifurcation. TIAs in the vertebrobasilar territory may be accompanied by a variety of symptoms including diplopia, dysarthria, vertigo, or facial numbness.

Platelet emboli arising from atheromatous plaques in more proximal vessels are thought to give rise to most TIAs. Platelet-fibrin clots may form on atheromatous plaques, particularly if they become ulcerated. Periodically, fragments of these clots break off and are carried into the distal cerebral circulation where they cause transient occlusion of small vessels; these occlusions later break up, and circulation is restored. Less commonly, TIAs may result from hemodynamic factors. For example, transient hypotension occurring in a patient with severe stenosis of a major cerebral vessel may result in focal cerebral ischemia and TIA.

Symptoms resembling TIAs may occur with other disorders, including classic migraine, partial (focal) seizures, and hypoglycemia. Rarely, a brain tumor may present with transient focal neurologic symptoms, probably on the basis of partial seizures. The focal nature of TIAs should be stressed. Symptoms of global cerebral ischemia such as syncope are rarely due to embolic TIA (Table 14.15).

TIAs are important because they may be a warning sign of an impending major stroke. The risk of cerebral infarction following an initial TIA is approximately 6 percent during the first month; over a 5 year period 25 percent of patients will develop cerebral infarction. In patients who have no history of TIA, the risk of cerebral infarction is less than 2 percent per year, even in the oldest age groups. The investigation and management of a patient presenting with an initial TIA should therefore be carried out with some urgency.

Cerebral Infarction

The neurologic deficit of cerebral infarction is usually of sudden onset. This feature helps distinguish these patients from those with brain tumors where the deficit is usually slowly progressive. The onset of cerebral infarction may occasionally be stuttering or step-wise (stroke in evolution, or progressing stroke).

The location of the brain infarct may be inferred from the patient's symptoms and signs following the principles outlined in the section entitled Clinical Localization of Neurologic Disorders. The most common stroke syndrome is probably that resulting from infarction in the territory of one middle cerebral artery, with hemiplegia and unilateral sensory loss. Dysphasia will be present if the lesion is in the dominant hemisphere. The actual extent of the infarct will depend on the availability of collateral circulation to the area involved, and therefore the severity of the resulting symptoms and signs can be quite variable from individual to individual. This syndrome can result from either internal carotid or middle cerebral artery occlusion. A homonymous hemianopia without other clinical signs usually results from occlusion of the posterior cerebral artery. Complete or partial homonymous hemianopia may also result from occlusion of the middle cerebral artery. Occlusion of the anterior cerebral artery usually results in hemiplegia, with the weakness more marked in the leg than in the arm and the face. In contrast, middle cerebral artery occlusion usually causes hemiplegia, with paralysis more marked in the arm and the lower face.

Lacunar Infarction

Lacunar infarcts are small infarcts lying deep in the basal ganglia, thalamus, or white matter of the cerebral hemispheres and brainstem. They are found primarily in patients with hypertension, and are due to segmental occlusion of very small penetrating arteries as a result of hyaline degeneration of the arterial wall. A number of distinctive lacunar syndromes have been described. Pure motor hemiparesis due to internal capsule or basis pontis lesions occurs without any associated sensory symptoms or signs. Pure sensory stroke from a small thalamic infarct results in sensory loss without any motor dysfunction. Multiple bilateral lacunar infarcts can cause pseudobulbar palsy and dementia. Lacunar infarcts are frequently small, and patients often show considerable recovery of function. Unlike patients with TIAs or small cerebral infarcts resulting from thromboembolic phenomena related to carotid stenosis, the patient with a small lacunar infarct is not at immediate risk for massive cerebral infarction.

In addition to lacunar infarction, patients with hypertension may develop small areas of infarction deep in the cerebral hemispheres, resulting from atheromatous involvement of smaller arterial branches and penetrating arteries. Hypertension is also complicated by accelerated atheromatous changes in larger arteries at the usual sites, such as the carotid bifurcation.

Cerebral Embolism

Cerebral embolism may result in occlusion of the cerebral arteries. A common source for emboli is the heart, although such emboli may also arise from atheromatous plaques in the proximal carotid arteries and the aorta.

Patients with mitral stenosis and atrial fibrillation are at particularly high risk for cerebral emboli, with a risk approximately 18 times that of age-matched controls. Other cardiac conditions predisposing to cerebral emboli and infarction are atrial fibrillation of any cause, recent myocardial infarction with mural thrombus, atrial myxoma, mitral valve prolapse, and endocarditis.

Investigation and Treatment

The medical and surgical therapy of cerebral infarction and TIAs is controversial. More data from properly controlled clinical trials is desperately needed to place stroke therapy on a sound scientific basis. In all patients, the decisions regarding investigation and treatment must take into account the patient's age, general medical health, and existing neurologic disability.

Little can be done to reduce the amount of brain damage in acute cerebral infarction, because brain tissue is usually irreversibly damaged within minutes of circulatory interruption. Good supportive medical care and rehabilitation once the patient has stabilized are important in improving the outcome. It is essential that patients at risk for further ischemic episodes are identified, and measures taken to reduce that risk where possible.

TIA and Completed Infarction with Minor Residual

The patient with TIA involving the carotid distribution should be urgently admitted to hospital for investigation. Some authors recommend early heparin anticoagulation for such patients, but there is not universal agreement on this issue. If anticoagulation is considered, a brain CT scan should be done, if available, prior to anticoagulation, as it may be clinically impossible to differentiate a cerebral infarction with minor residual deficit from a small intracerebral hemorrhage. If the TIA has cleared completely with no remaining neurologic symptoms or signs, a cerebral hemorrhage is even less likely, but a CT scan prior to anticoagulation is advisable because tumors and other cerebral lesions may occasionally present with transient symptoms resembling TIA.

A carotid bruit on clinical examination may indicate an internal carotid artery stenosis, but such bruits are frequently absent in patients with severe stenosis, or if present may arise from the external carotid artery. Noninvasive techniques such as doppler ultrasonography of periorbital vessels, oculoplethysmography, ophthalmodynamometry, and B-scans of the carotid bifurcation can be useful in screening patients prior to angiography. However, noninvasive tests have a significant number of false positives and false negatives.

Patients with TIAs in the carotid distribution should be considered for carotid angiography (Fig. 14.18), and for surgical removal of a carotid stenosis if one is found. Carotid angiography is not indicated

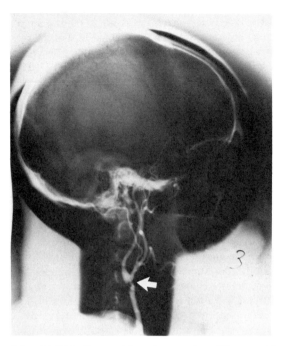

Fig. 14.18 Left carotid angiogram in a 58-year-old man with TIAs. The arrow indicates a 90 percent left internal carotid artery stenosis at the carotid bifurcation

if associated illness or advanced age of the patient is such that he or she is not a surgical candidate.

The risks of angiography and surgery are significant, and vary greatly from center to center. When a specialized team with extensive experience in carotid surgery is available, these risks can be as low as 1 to 2 percent morbidity and mortality in carefully selected patients. In patients with stable angina, recent myocardial infarction, congestive heart failure, chronic obstructive lung disease, or who are neurologically unstable, the operative morbidity and mortality may go as high as 10 percent. All such high-risk patients should be carefully evaluated prior to angiography and surgery, and many may be better off with more conservative medical therapy. Surgery is usually only considered if a carotid stenosis of 60 percent or greater is found. Such lesions may serve as a source for emboli or may progress to become hemodynamically significant obstructions. With lesser degrees of stenosis, medical therapy is usually employed to prevent thrombosis and embolization. Occasionally surgery is employed for deeply ulcerated but nonstenosing plaques.

Two modes of medical therapy are available. According to controlled trials, acetylsalicylic acid (ASA) will reduce the risk of subsequent stroke in male patients with TIAs by approximately 48 percent. Its efficacy in females is less certain. The optimal dose has not yet been established, but the dosage used in these trials was 325 mg 4 times a day. The usefulness of other antiplatelet drugs has not been established.

There is some evidence that coumadin anticoagulants reduce the risk of subsequent cerebral infarction in patients with TIA. However, the risk of hemorrhagic complications, including intracranial hemorrhage, is significant in these patients, particularly after the first few months, with long-term anticoagulation. Because of these risks, some authors advocate its use for several months after the first TIA, followed by ASA therapy.

Patients with TIAs in the vertebrobasilar circulation rarely have lesions amenable to surgical intervention, and these patients should be treated medically from the start without angiography. If symptoms are not controlled by medical therapy, or if there is reason to suspect a hemodynamically significant carotid stenosis in addition to vertebrobasilar disease, such patients may occasionally benefit from carotid surgery in an attempt to improve collateral circulation to the posterior fossa. Most of the vertebrobasilar arterial system is not accessible to surgical intervention. Bypass surgery can be performed when atheromatous lesions are present at the origin of the vertebral artery or in the subclavian artery itself.

Patients with carotid distribution TIAs and complete internal carotid artery occlusion or with occlusion or stenosis of the middle cerebral artery may be helped by extracranial-intracranial bypass surgery. In this procedure an attempt is made to improve blood flow in the middle cerebral vascular bed by anastomosing the superficial temporal artery to a branch of the middle cerebral artery.

Cerebral Infarction (Completed Stroke)

Patients with cerebral infarction with deficits persisting for more than 24 hours but who have only minor residual symptoms and signs are best treated in a manner similar to TIAs. The risk in these patients for recurrent stroke is only slightly less than that for patients with TIA. Patients with lacunar infarction are exceptions to this rule, and will not benefit from angiography or surgery, however, these patients need careful control of hypertension.

Patients with major cerebral infarction (Fig. 14.19) seldom benefit from angiography, surgery, or anticoagulation, since the brain tissue at risk has been largely destroyed. Conservative therapy with good supportive care, gradual ambulation, and vigorous

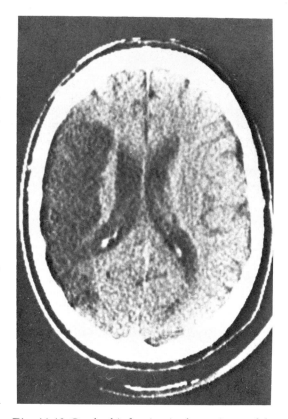

Fig. 14.19 Cerebral infarction in the territory of the right middle cerebral artery. This brain CT scan was done 3 months after sudden onset of left hemiplegia. The large lucent (dark) area lateral to the right lateral ventricle indicates the area of infarction

long-term physiotherapy and rehabilitation constitute the treatment of choice.

Progressing Cerebral Infarction (Stroke in Evolution)

In a minority of cases, cerebral infarction appears to evolve in a stepwise fashion over hours or days. This may result from progressive stepwise closure of a cerebral artery from thrombosis, or possibly repeated episodes of embolization from a carotid or vertebral artery plaque. Anticoagulation may be of benefit in these patients.

Cerebral Embolism

Emboli from the heart are common causes of cerebral infarction, and a careful clinical cardiac assessment is essential in all patients with cerebral infarction.

Echocardiography can confirm the presence of suspected valve lesions or vegetations that may act as sources of emboli. The electrocardiogram will confirm the presence of recent myocardial infarction or atrial fibrillation. Anticoagulation is indicated in patients with TIA or cerebral infarction due to cardiac emboli. This therapy will not change the extent of cerebral infarction already present, but is given to prevent further emboli. In the patient with an already established cerebral infarction, controversy exists as to when heparin therapy should be started. Some authors recommend early anticoagulation to prevent further emboli. Others will wait for a variable period of time because of the risk of anticoagulant-induced hemorrhage into the cerebral infarct. In patients with cerebral infarction and subacute bacterial endocarditis, anticoagulation is not advisable because of the risk of hemorrhage.

Stroke Prevention

Prevention of cerebral infarction would be the ideal treatment. Careful hypertension management is the most important measure available for stroke prevention at the present time. Cerebral infarction also correlates to some extent with obesity, smoking, and serum cholesterol levels, but these correlations are not as strong or clear cut as they are in coronary heart disease.

INTRACEREBRAL HEMORRHAGE

Etiology

Intracerebral hemorrhage is relatively common. Hypertensive patients are at much greater risk for intracerebral hemorrhage, probably because of degenerative changes in small penetrating cerebral arteries. Intracerebral hemorrhage may also occur secondary to anticoagulant therapy, blood dyscrasia, head trauma, arteriovenous malformation, and brain tumor. Subacute bacterial endocarditis may lead to intracerebral hemorrhage through rupture of a mycotic aneurysm. Ruptured berry aneurysm usually leads to subarachnoid hemorrhage alone, but hemorrhage into the adjacent brain parenchyma may occur.

Intracerebral hemorrhage secondary to hypertension tends to occur in the basal ganglia–internal capsule region, the thalamus, the cerebellum, and the pons. Hemorrhage elsewhere in the brain may also occur, but in these cases other etiologies should be suspected.

Clinical Manifestations

Like cerebral infarction, hemorrhage into the brain parenchyma presents with focal neurologic deficits. Significant drowsiness or coma early in the patient's course suggests intracerebral hemorrhage rather than cerebral infarction (see Disorders of Consciousness).

Most intracerebral hemorrhages have a sudden, often catastrophic onset. Unlike subdural hematoma, a history of trauma is usually absent. In patients found stuporous or comatose, however, the differential diagnosis can be clinically difficult. Patients with chronic subdural hematoma may not give a history of head trauma, but usually present with an insidious, slowly progressive course unlike the course of intracerebral hemorrhage.

Basal ganglia hemorrhages usually present with abrupt hemiplegia, sensory loss, and hemianopia. Dysphasia is present with dominant hemisphere hematomas. Transient loss of conjugate gaze to the side away from the lesion is common.

Thalamic hemorrhage produces hemiplegia, usually associated with profound sensory loss, and early obtundation with frequent progression to coma. Loss of upward gaze with downward deviation of the eyes is common due to pressure on the midbrain tectum.

Massive cerebellar hemorrhage presents rapidly with coma, brain stem signs, and death. In more slowly progressing or less massive cerebellar hemorrhage, vomiting is prominent, and consciousness may be lost gradually. Ataxia, particularly truncal ataxia, is common, and conjugate ocular gaze palsy, nystagmus, and dysarthria are frequently present. In contrast, motor power and sensory function tend to be relatively preserved.

Pontine hemorrhage usually presents with sudden catastrophic loss of consciousness, vomiting, bilateral decerebration, and extensor plantar responses. Pupils are constricted (pinpoint) but retain their reaction to light. Ocular bobbing may be present.

Investigation and Treatment

The diagnosis of intracerebral hemorrhage can be rapidly confirmed or ruled out by CT scan. Fresh blood is more radioopaque than brain or CSF, and is clearly visible on CT scan if present in any significant amount (Fig. 14.20). Skull roengenograms may show a displaced pineal gland. Lumbar puncture is not recommended as a diagnostic measure, and may precipitate fatal transtentorial or tonsillar brain herniation if a hematoma of significant size is present.

The prognosis of patients with basal ganglia and

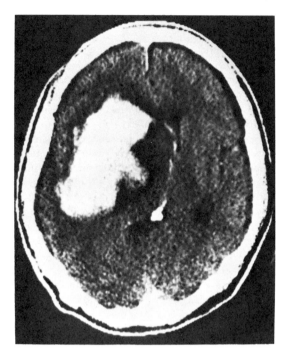

Fig. 14.20 Nonenhanced CT scan showing a massive intracerebral hemorrhage (large white area) in a 73-year-old man with sudden left hemiplegia and progressive obtundation. Onset of symptoms occurred 8 hours prior to CT scan

thalamic hemorrhage is poor, but depends primarily on the size of the hemorrhage. Patients who become comatose within 24 hours have a mortality rate approaching 80 percent. In patients still conscious at 24 hours, the mortality is approximately 30 percent. Nevertheless, many patients with smaller intracerebral hemorrhages do very well.

The therapy of intracerebral hemorrhage includes corticosteroid therapy to prevent cerebral edema, antihypertensive treatment if necessary, and avoidance of overhydration. Early surgical evacuation of the hematoma may have a place in more superficially located hemorrhages, particularly in the nondominant cerebral hemisphere. The results of surgery have been disappointing in deeper intracerebral hemorrhage, and it is seldom indicated in these patients.

Cerebellar hematomas should be promptly evacuated surgically. Once coma supervenes, irreversible brain stem damage usually occurs secondary to compression by the hematoma, and the prognosis is very poor. Patients still conscious on admission may deteriorate rapidly, so diagnostic measures and surgery should be carried out without delay.

The prognosis of patients with pontine hemorrhage is extremely grave, and no effective therapy is available.

SUBARACHNOID HEMMORRHAGE

Etiology

Ruptured berry (saccular) aneurysm is the most common cause of subarachnoid hemorrhage (SAH) between the ages of 20 and 70 years. Prior to this age, SAH is more frequently the result of bleeding from an arteriovenous malformation. No etiology can be documented in approximately 20 percent of patients with SAH, although hypertensive vascular disease may account for some of these. SAH is common in head trauma, and, rarely, may also occur as a complication of brain tumor.

Berry aneurysms are balloon-like expansions of the arterial wall attached to the parent vessel by a narrow neck. They occur at cerebral arterial bifurcations, probably due to defects in the arterial media that occur at these points. Hypertension, atheroma, and increasing age all apparently contribute to aneurysm formation. Approximately 30 percent of aneuryms occur in the anterior communicating artery region, and an equal number at the internal carotid–posterior communicating artery junction. Aneurysms at the first bifurcation of the middle cerebral artery make up most of the remainder. A smaller number occur elsewhere on the internal carotid artery, and approximately 5 percent of intracranial aneurysms occur in the posterior fossa.

Clinical Manifestations

Severe headache of sudden onset is the usual presentation of ruptured aneurysm with SAH. The headache usually becomes rapidly generalized, with the occipital component often particularly severe. The headache is in most cases distinctive and unlike the patients previous headaches. Sudden headaches beginning during marked exertion and sexual intercourse should always arouse suspicion that a SAH has occured.

The patient often appears ill, and may become irritable or obtunded and confused. With severe SAH, coma may occur at bleed onset and death may follow within minutes or hours.

Neck stiffness and other signs of meningial irritation are usually present on examination, although initially these may be very mild. Subhyaloid fundal hemorrhages appear within hours in some patients. Focal neurologic signs are generally absent, unless bleeding has ruptured into the brain parenchyma, or severe vascular spasm is present. Aneurysms at the internal carotid–posterior communicating artery junction are exceptions to this rule, and sometimes

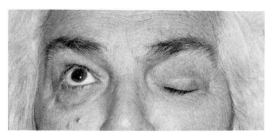

Fig. 14.21 Sixty-two–year–old female with left posterior communicating artery aneurysm and left 3rd nerve palsy. She is unable to open her left eye. The left pupil is dilated and unreactive to light

cause a 3rd nerve palsy because the aneurysm is immediately adjacent to the 3rd cranial nerve. Indeed, expansion of these aneurysms may at times cause unilateral periorbital headache and 3rd nerve palsy days or even weeks prior to rupture. This combination of symptoms and signs should lead to early diagnosis and surgery prior to the bleeding (Figs. 14.21 and 14.22). Smaller or "sentinel" hemorrhages occasionally occur with aneurysm at any site prior to the first major bleed. These patients present with severe generalized headache of sudden onset, which usually lasts at least several days. If the diagnosis is made at this stage, surgery can usually be carried out with good results.

The natural history of ruptured cerebral aneurysm is formidable. If patients survive the first hemorrhage, approximately 25 percent will have a recurrent SAH within 2 weeks, and many of these will be fatal.

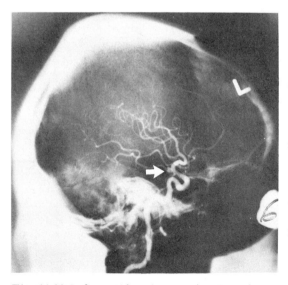

Fig. 14.22 Left carotid angiogram showing a berry aneurysm (arrow) at the posterior communicating artery (same patient as Fig. 14.21)

When patients survive long enough after their first SAH to undergo angiography, 50 percent will die from rebleeding within 6 months if untreated. Vascular spasm frequently comes on within a few days of hemorrhage and may result in cerebral infarction. Communicating hydrocephalus with confusion and dementia may occur within several weeks of bleeding due to blood breakdown products and subarachnoid space fibrosis that block CSF absorbtion. The syndrome of normal pressure hydrocephalus with dementia may also occur in a more insidious fashion at a later time.

Investigation and Treatment

The patient with suspected SAH should be immediately admitted to hospital. If the clinical presentation is typical, cerebral angiography should be done early to demonstrate the aneurysm and to establish a definite diagnosis. A CT scan demonstrates the subarachnoid blood in many cases, but may be negative if the amount of bleeding is slight. Lumbar puncture is not recommended in clinically obvious cases. However, in patients with unusual headache in whom SAH is possible but unlikely, lumbar puncture is useful in proving or ruling out this diagnosis. If bloody CSF is thought to be the result of traumatic lumbar puncture, the CSF should be centrifuged and the supernatant examined. The supernatant will be clear in traumatic tap but xanthochromic if SAH has been present for 6 hours or more.

The treatment of berry aneurysm is surgical. Rebleeding is prevented by placing a clip over the neck of the aneurysm and isolating it from the circulation. In the stuporous or comatose patient, however, the morbidity and mortality of surgery is prohibitive, and the patient must be treated medically until his condition improves. Unfortunately bleeding may recur in the waiting period, with disastrous results.

The timing of surgery in patients arriving at the hospital in good condition with only headache and neck stiffness is controversial. Surgery is frequently delayed for 1 to 2 weeks after SAH, as early surgery may potentiate vascular spasm and attendant complications. Some neurosurgeons, however, do operate early on patients arriving at the hospital in good condition, thus circumventing the danger of rebleeding. Advances in neurosurgery, particularly microsurgical techniques and the use of the operating microscope, have greatly improved the outlook in ruptured aneurysm. Operative mortality is now less than 5 percent if the patient is in good condition at the time of surgery.

While waiting for surgery, arterial hypertension

should be carefully controlled. Stool softeners should be given to avoid constipation and straining. Steroids are frequently given to reduce cerebral edema, and strict bed rest is enforced. Antifibrinolytic drugs such as E-aminocaproic acid are used in some centers to reduce the risk of rebleeding from the aneurysm, but the effectiveness of this therapy is unproven.

SAH resulting from arteriovenous malformation (AVM) has an appreciably lower mortality and recurrence rate than that resulting from ruptured aneurysm. If surgically accessible, the AVM may be removed, but frequently this is impossible.

The treatment of SAH from other causes is that of the underlying disease.

CENTRAL NERVOUS SYSTEM NEOPLASMS

INTRACRANIAL TUMORS

Intracranial tumors occur with sufficient frequency to present an important problem in the differential diagnosis of neurologic illness. Approximately two percent of all autopsies show brain tumors.

The major types and their relative frequency of occurrence are shown in Table 14.25.

Clinical Manifestations

Brain tumors produce symptoms by two major mechanisms. First, they compress or destroy brain tissue in their immediate vicinity. Second, they may cause increased intracranial pressure. This may result

Table 14.25 **Intracranial Tumors**

Tumor Type		Percentage of Total
Primary Brain Tumors		50
Glioblastoma and astrocytoma	20	
Oligodendroglioma	3	
Ependymoma	3	
Medulloblastoma	2	
Meningioma	8	
Acoustic neuroma	4	
Pituitary adenoma	4	
Others (craniopharyngioma, epidermoids, pinealoma, and others)	6	
Metastatic Tumors		50
Lung	20	
Breast	10	
GI Tract	5	
Kidney	5	
Others (Melanoma, thyroid, testicular, and others)	10	

Table 14.26 **Main Presentations of Intracranial Tumors**

Focal Neurologic Symptoms and Signs
Mental Changes
Increased Intracranial Pressure
Seizures
Headache
Endocrine Disorders

directly from tumor bulk and edema, or may occur because of interference with CSF circulation.

The major presenting symptoms and signs of brain tumors are listed in Table 14.26.

Focal Neurologic Symptoms and Signs

Neurologic symptoms resulting from brain tumors are usually of gradual onset and slowly progressive. This is in contrast to most stroke syndromes. The nature of the focal symptoms and signs will depend on the area of brain involved.

Hemiparesis with or without sensory changes is a common manifestation of cerebral hemisphere tumors. Aphasia may be present with tumors of the dominant hemisphere.

Visual field defects commonly result from brain tumors. Occipital lobe tumors cause a contralateral homonymous hemianopia. Temporal lobe tumors interfere with the optic radiations and cause a homonymous upper quadrant visual field loss ("pie in the sky" defect). Pituitary tumors and craniopharyngiomas frequently compress the optic chiasm, and can cause a variety of visual field defects. The most common is a bitemporal hemianopia resulting from damage to the crossing chiasmal fibers from each nasal retina. Visual loss is present in the temporal field of each eye. If the patient is examined with both eyes open, one eye will cover for the other, and the visual loss will be missed.

Optic nerve gliomas and meningiomas cause progressive visual loss in one eye. These gliomas occur most commonly in children and in von Recklinghausen's disease (neurofibromatosis). Optic nerve meningiomas are more common in adults.

Tumors in the pineal region compressing the midbrain can produce loss of upward gaze and loss of pupillary reaction to light (Parinaud's syndrome). Tumors in this region include pinealoma, germinoma, teratoma, and glioma.

Focal signs may be produced by tumor involvement of cranial nerves. Olfactory groove meningiomas produce anosmia through destruction of the olfactory nerves. Sphenoid ridge meningiomas may cause unilateral blindness, disturbances of extraocular movements and ipsilateral forehead numbness through involvement of cranial nerves 2 to 6. Unilateral exophthalmos may also occur. Brainstem gliomas can produce multiple cranial nerve palsies and long-tract signs, because they involve the medulla and pons. Acoustic neuromas arising from the 8th cranial nerve produce unilateral hearing loss and chronic imbalance and dizziness. Cranial nerves 5 and 7 may be involved as the tumor enlarges.

Mental Changes

Mental changes from brain tumors may range from apathy and dementia to witzelsucht (forced joking and punning). They are particularly prominent with frontal and temporal lobe tumors, and are insidious in onset and slowly progressive.

Increased Intracranial Pressure

Large supratentorial gliomas, meningiomas, and metastatic lesions produce increased intracranial pressure (ICP) by the space-occupying effects of tumor bulk and surrounding edema. Increased ICP can also result from obstruction to CSF flow through the ventricular system (obstructive hydrocephalus) (Fig. 14.23). Meningeal spread of carcinoma and lymphoma interferes with CSF absorption by obliterating the subarachnoid space and arachnoid granulations. This results in communicating hydrocephalus and increased ICP.

Patients with increased ICP frequently have generalized headache. These headaches may however be quite intermittent. Nocturnal or early morning wakening with vomiting is highly suggestive of increased ICP, although migraine at times may also cause nocturnal headache.

Unilateral or bilateral 6th nerve palsy may occur in increased ICP of any cause. This nerve has a long intracranial course and may become stretched or injured, with resulting weakness of eye abduction and diplopia. Third nerve palsy may be present if transtentorial herniation occurs. Repeated transient clouding of vision occurs in some patients with chronically increased ICP and papilledema. This likely results from optic nerve ischemia.

With increasing ICP, drowsiness and coma eventually occur from transtentorial herniation. Transient episodes of loss of consciousness may occur related to surges in ICP. These are particularly common in patients with 3rd ventricular colloid cysts, but may occur in increased ICP of any cause. Papilledema is frequently present but may be absent in some patients despite chronically increased ICP.

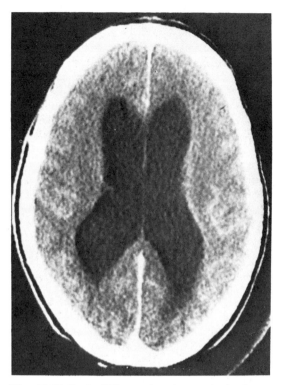

Fig. 14.23 Brain CT scan showing marked enlargement of both lateral ventricles secondary to aqueduct obstruction by midbrain tumor. This 52-year-old man presented with headache and transient loss of consciousness

Intracranial tumors, subdural hematomas, and other mass lesions are the most common cause of subacute and chronically elevated ICP. Hypertensive encephalopathy presents with headache, confusion, and bilateral optic disc swelling, and must be considered in the differential diagnosis. Benign intracranial hypertension (pseudotumor cerebri or meningeal hydrops) also presents with chronic headache and papilledema. It occurs mainly in children and obese young women. This diagnosis is one of exclusion, and intracranial mass must be ruled out by radiologic investigation. Lumbar puncture will show normal CSF under increased pressure. Treatment consist of steroids and repeated lumbar punctures, and most patients gradually recover. Occasionally, progressive visual impairment will necessitate surgical decompression to prevent blindness.

Seizures

A seizure is the initial symptom in 15 percent of brain tumors. The younger the patient at the time of his first seizure, the less likely he is to have a brain tumor. Tumors will be found in less than 1 percent of children presenting with seizures. Although many of these seizures clinically have a focal onset, many appear clinically generalized, probably reflecting rapid spread of epileptic activity from its focus of origin.

Even on careful examination, not all of these patients will be found to have focal neurologic signs. Slow-growing low-grade temporal lobe gliomas may apparently produce seizures for as long as 20 years without producing other symptoms.

Syncope can occur in patients with increased ICP, and is presumably due to sudden surges in ICP. Drop attacks also occur, in which the patient falls to the ground with loss of muscle tone and strength in his legs, but does not lose consciousness.

Headache

Headache is the initial symptom in approximately 20 percent of brain tumors. Brain tumor should be suspected in patients with headaches of recent onset that are progressing in severity. Presence of headache exclusively on one side of the head during all attacks, or nocturnal and early morning headache with vomiting, should arouse suspicion. Localized headaches result from disturbance of pain-sensitive structures; generalized headache with vomiting results from increased ICP. Posterior fossa tumors generally produce occipital headache until increased ICP occurs, at which point the headache becomes generalized.

Although these guidelines can be helpful, many patients with headaches resulting from brain tumor have rather nondescript headaches that are intermittent, not severe, and that respond to simple analgesics. For this reason, every patient presenting with headache deserves a careful history and neurologic examination. The presence of focal neurologic deficits or evidence of ICP should lead to further investigation (see Headache).

Endocrine Disorders

Thirty percent of pituitary adenomas have no detectable hormone secretion and present with visual field changes, headache, or hypopituitarism resulting from compression of the remainder of the gland by the tumor.

Sixty percent of pituitary adenomas cause increased serum prolactin levels, due to either direct secretion by the tumor or interference with normal hypothalamic inhibition. Women may have amenorrhea and galactorrhea. Men may show decreased libido and hypogonadism. A smaller proportion of pituitary adenomas secrete growth hormone and may present with acromegaly. A further minority secrete ACTH and present with Cushing's disease (see Chapter 13).

Pituitary apoplexy is a particularly dramatic presentation of pituitary adenoma. This hemorrhagic infarction of the pituitary adenoma and the resulting edema results in severe headache, visual field loss, oculomotor palsies, stiff neck, and bloody CSF. Pituitary apoplexy is a medical emergency. Steroid treatment is usually adequate, but neurosurgical decompression is occasionally necessary.

Laboratory Investigation

The skull roentgenogram may show abnormal calcification in the tumor in craniopharyngioma, oligodendroglioma, and meningioma. Hyperostosis involving the inner table of the skull is frequently present in meningioma. If the pineal gland is calcified, a pineal shift may suggest a mass lesion in one cerebral hemisphere. The sella turcica may show demineralization of cortical bone, suggesting increased ICP. Enlargement of the sella turcica suggests pituitary adenoma. An enlarged sella turcica may also be due to the empty sella syndrome (see Chapter 13).

A chest roentgenogram may show a primary lung tumor or multiple metastatic lesions. Both indicate that the intracranial lesion is likely a metastatic tumor.

Lumbar puncture is contraindicated in most patients with brain tumor. An exception is the patient with meningeal carcinomatosis, for which CSF cytology is diagnostic.

The isotope brain scan will detect many intracranial tumors. While the blood-brain barrier prevents the circulating radioisotope from entering normal brain, this barrier is no longer intact in many tumors, and radioisotope will accumulate in the tumor. The tumor is demonstrated as an area of increased radioisotope uptake in meningiomas, cerebral metastasis, and malignant gliomas. Other less vascular tumors such as low-grade astrocytomas and epidermoid cysts are frequently missed.

The head CT scan is now the investigation of choice. The injection of contrast material just prior to CT scan enhances the density of vascular structures, including many brain tumors, and makes their detection easy (Fig. 14.24). Even isodense tumors that do not enhance are usually visible because of displacement of normal intracranial structures such as the ventricular system. Demonstration of small brainstem tumors remains difficult, but CT scan resolution is continually improving.

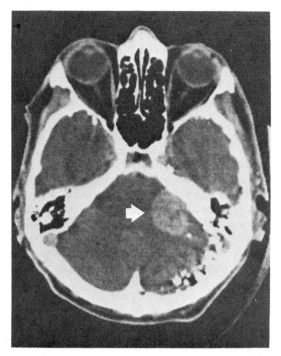

Fig. 14.24 Contrast-enhanced brain CT scan showing an acoustic neuroma (arrow) in a 60-year-old man with hearing loss in the left ear

Angiography has been largely replaced by the CT scan for brain tumor detection. Angiography is still sometimes used to show the vascular supply of tumors prior to surgery.

If the CT scan appearance suggests metastatic brain tumor, lung, breast, and kidney are the most likely primary sites.

The patient with a single CT scan brain lesion suggestive of metastatic tumor may require craniotomy for definitive diagnosis if no primary tumor is evident. Multiple intracranial lesions are highly suggestive of metastatic tumor, and craniotomy is usually not indicated.

Treatment

The mass effect of brain tumors frequently is due in part to surrounding edema. Steroid therapy will reduce this edema and ICP, and also may produce significant improvement in focal symptoms such as hemiparesis or dysphasia. Measures to reduce cerebral edema are discussed in a preceding section under Coma, Treatment.

Meningiomas, acoustic neuromas, and other benign tumors can frequently be completely removed. Even in histologically benign tumors, however,

complete removal may be impossible if the tumor involves vital CNS structures. Improved neurosurgical techniques, including use of the operating microscope, are allowing better removal of benign tumors in difficult locations.

Astrocytomas usually show no clear demarcation between the tumor and normal brain, and tend to infiltrate widely. Cure is seldom possible, but partial removal will reduce ICP and provide tissue for diagnosis. Cystic cerebellar astrocytoma of childhood can frequently be cured by surgery.

Radiation therapy is of benefit in most intracranial tumors that cannot be totally removed. Steroids are given to reduce cerebral edema during radiotherapy. Patients with cerebral metastasis are usually treated with radiotherapy alone. Chemotherapy is of value in certain instances, but the blood-brain barrier makes chemotherapy of CNS tumors difficult.

The prognosis of most patients with malignant brain tumors, including glioblastoma and metastatic lesions, is still very poor, and is measured in months despite all available therapies. Hopefully, further advances in therapy will improve the outlook for these patients.

MENINGEAL CARCINOMATOSIS

Meningeal carcinomatosis (carcinomatous meningitis) refers to widespread meningeal involvement with sheaths of tumor cells. Both intracranial and spinal meninges may be involved. Patients may present with mental changes, headache, and obtundation due to increased ICP. Others present with multiple cranial nerve palsies. Spinal nerve roots may also be involved, with limb weakness and areflexia. After an intracranial mass lesion has been ruled out, lumbar puncture should be done. CSF usually shows a lymphocytic pleocytosis and a reduced glucose level. CSF protein levels are often elevated. Repeated lumbar punctures and CSF cytologic examinations may be necessary to demonstrate malignant cells. The primary tumor is usually a lung carcinoma or malignant lymphoma.

SPINAL CORD TUMORS

Spinal cord tumors account for 15 percent of primary central nervous system tumors. The majority are benign and amenable to surgical therapy if the diagnosis is made before irreversible damage from spinal cord compression has occurred.

Intramedullary tumors lie within the spinal cord substance. Intradural and extradural tumors lie outside the spinal cord. Most metastatic lesions are extradural, whereas the majority of primary spinal cord tumors are intradural or intramedullary (Table 14.25).

Clinical Manifestations

Radicular pain aggravated by coughing and straining is frequently the initial symptom in spinal cord tumor. Localized pain in the back is also commonly present. Characteristically, the pain becomes worse in the supine position and frequently wakens the patient at night. This feature should alert the physician to the possibility of spinal cord tumor, since the pain associated with many other spinal disorders is relieved by lying down.

As the tumor enlarges, the patient develops weakness and/or numbness below the level of the lesion, and gait disturbance. Urinary retention, urgency, and incontinence are all common features.

Tumors in the cervical region may cause wasting and weakness of the hands due to segmental involvement of nerve roots and anterior horn cells, and long-tract signs in the legs by compression of the descending corticospinal tract fibers. Above the level of the cauda equina, tumors may cause hyperreflexia, weakness, ankle clonus, sensory loss, and upgoing plantar responses. All modalities of sensation may be lost in a radicular distribution at the level of the lesion. A sensory level to pinprick on the trunk helps to identify the level of the tumor, although the tumor may actually lie several segments above. Tumors compressing the cauda equina will cause hyporeflexia and flaccid paralysis of the legs.

Schwannoma

Schwannomas are the most common primary spinal cord tumors and account for 30 percent of cases. Because they arise from the nerve root, radicular pain and segmental weakness is often present initially. Tumor enlargement eventually results in spinal cord or cauda equina compression. Schwannomas may grow through the intervertebral foramen and lie partly in the spinal canal and partly in the chest or abdomen. A similar tumor, the neurofibroma, is common in von Recklinghausen's disease, and frequently occurs at multiple sites.

Meningioma

Meningiomas occur most commonly in the thoracic region and make up 25 percent of primary spinal cord tumors. They are most common in middle-aged

women. These tumors usually cause a slowly progressive paraparesis, with spasticity, urinary urgency, and sensory loss.

Glioma

Astrocytomas are the most common intramedullary tumors of the spinal cord. These tumors usually present with back pain and slowly progressing paraparesis or quadriparesis. Although they are generally histologically benign and compatible with long survival, complete surgical removal is impossible.

Ependymomas occur most commonly in middle-aged men. The most common site is on the filum terminale, where they tend to compress the cauda equina and cause flaccid weakness of the legs. Pain radiating into the legs is a common mode of presentation.

Metastatic Tumors

Tumors metastasizing to the spinal cord may arise from many sources. The more important ones are listed in order of frequency in Table 14.27. Many of them also involve the vertebral bodies. Pain is frequently the first clinical manifestation, followed by paraplegia. These tumors often cause a very rapid neurologic deterioration, and paraplegia may develop over several days.

Differential Diagnosis

Spinal cord tumors must be differentiated from a number of other spinal cord lesions.

Pyogenic abscess may cause spinal cord compression. Pyogenic abscesses are rare, and usually are associated with fever and extreme spinal vertebral tenderness.

Herniated intervertebral discs typically present with cervical or lumbar radicular symptoms, but large disc protrusions may occasionally cause spinal cord or cauda equina compression. Discs usually involve the lower cervical nerve roots, the 5th lumbar

Table 14.27 **Spinal Cord Tumors**

Primary	Metastatic
Schwannoma	Lung
Meningioma	Breast
Glioma	Lymphoma
Astrocytoma	Prostate
Ependymoma	Kidney
Others	

nerve root, or the 1st sacral root. The vast majority involve only one nerve root. Symptoms due to discs tend to improve over time, whereas those related to spinal cord tumors progress.

Spinal cord infarction is uncommon. Symptoms are usually of sudden onset, and occur mainly in elderly patients and diabetics. Aortic aneurysm surgery, dissecting aneurysm, and vasculitis may also result in infarction. Lesions tend to involve the midthoracic spinal cord. The posterior columns may be spared because of collateral circulation.

Cervical spondylosis with secondary cervical myelopathy is relatively common. Cervical nerve roots and anterior horn cells may be involved at the cervical level, resulting in areflexia and weakness in the arms. The legs show weakness, hyperreflexia, and spasticity, and sensory changes may be present. This disorder usually occurs in the elderly, and is common in patients with severe rheumatoid arthritis.

Demyelinating disease, including transverse myelitis and multiple sclerosis, can cause paraparesis and quadriparesis, and may mimmic a spinal cord tumor. Multiple sclerosis in particular can cause a chronic progressive myelopathy. Evidence for other central nervous system lesions in addition to the spinal cord lesion are common in multiple sclerosis.

Pernicious anemia causes a chronic progressive myelopathy (subacute combined degeneration) with involvement of both posterior columns and corticospinal tracts. Loss of joint position sense and vibration sense in the feet is usually marked. A peripheral neuropathy, also resulting from the vitamin B_{12} deficiency, is often present as well. This may result in absent ankle reflexes despite the corticospinal tract involvement.

Syringomyelia, a cavity in the substance of the spinal cord, may be difficult to differentiate from an intramedullary spinal cord tumor. Some spinal cord tumors, notably astrocytomas, may have a syrinx in association with them. Otherwise, syringomyelia may be associated with previous trauma, Arnold-Chiari malformation, or possibly degenerative changes. Syringomyelia is most common in the cervical spinal cord.

Investigation

The investigation of suspected spinal cord tumor is primarily radiologic. Plain spine roentgenograms may show bone destruction by metastatic cancer and suggests metastatic tumor as a cause of spinal cord compression. Severe degenerative changes in the cervical spine suggests myelopathy from cervical spondylosis. Lumbar disc space narrowing may result from a herniated intervertebral disc.

Myelography remains the definitive investigation for diagnosis of spinal cord tumor and herniated intervertebral disc (Fig. 14.25). Myelography also frequently shows changes in syringomyelia, but is usually normal in multiple sclerosis and transverse myelitis.

Spinal CT scanning is less invasive than myelography and can show intervertebral disc protrusions and spinal cord tumors. As experience with this technique grows and scanner resolution improves, CT scanning is certain to become even more useful.

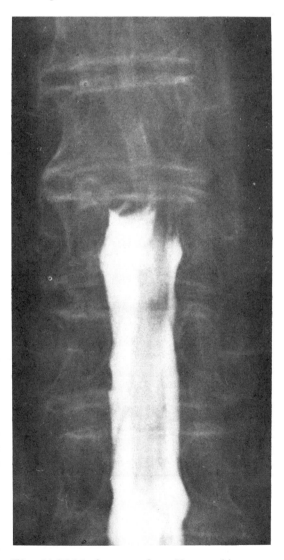

Fig. 14.25 Myelogram of an 82-year-old woman presenting with paraparesis and lower limb numbness. The patient is tilted head down, but the flow of dye is completely obstructed at the T9 level. A concave filling defect produced by the obstructing intradural meningioma is evident at the top of the dye column

Treatment

The treatment of most spinal cord tumors is surgical. Early diagnosis is essential for a good result. With metastatic tumors, progression of paraplegia may be rapid, and investigation and treatment must be carried out without delay to relieve spinal cord compression. Once the patient is fully paraplegic, recovery is unlikely after surgery.

Steroid therapy and urgent radiotherapy satisfactorily decompress the spinal cord in some patients with compression from metastatic cancer. This may be the treatment of choice, particularly in the very old or ill patient with known metastatic disease.

DEMYELINATING DISORDERS

Several diseases affect primarily the myelin sheath. Central nervous system (CNS) myelin produced by the oligodendroglial cell differs significantly from Schwann cell-produced peripheral nerve myelin. It is not surprising therefore, that some diseases affect primarily one or the other. In Guillain-Barré syndrome only peripheral nerve myelin is injured by autoimmune attack (see Neuromuscular Disorders). In multiple sclerosis (MS), primarily CNS myelin is affected.

Multiple sclerosis, acute disseminated encephalomyelitis, and progressive multifocal leukoencephalopathy will be discussed in this section. Hereditary leukoencephalopathies, which present primarily in childhood, will not be discussed here. Demyelinating disorders are classified in Table 14.28.

MULTIPLE SCLEROSIS

Few diseases compare in tragedy to rapidly progressing multiple sclerosis (MS). Nevertheless, many patients with MS suffer little disability even after many years. The unpredictability of the disease is only one of the many enigmas of MS.

Table 14.28 Demyelinating Disorders

1. Multiple Sclerosis
2. Post Infectious
      Acute disseminated encephalomyelitis
3. Infections
      Progressive multifocal leukoencephalopathy
4. Metabolic
      Vitamin B_{12} deficiency
      Central pontine myelinolysis
      Marchiafava-Bignami disease

Etiology and Pathology

The etiology of MS is unknown. Destruction of CNS myelin in MS appears due to antibody-mediated autoimmune attack. The cause of this immune injury remains unknown, and although an underlying viral etiology has been postulated for MS, this remains unproven. Various immunologic abnormalities, including defects in lymphocyte suppressor-cell activity, have been found in MS patients, but the significance of these abnormalities remains uncertain. It is clear, however, that many MS patients have clones of plasma cells in the CNS, producing monoclonal IgG antibodies that presumably are directed against myelin antigens. It is unknown what initially triggers this antibody production, and it is equally unclear what factors cause the remissions and exacerbations of MS.

The MS plaque is a focal area of myelin destruction. Oligodendroglial cells in the lesion are destroyed, but the axons in the lesions are largely spared. In contrast to the peripheral nervous system, remyelination in the CNS is very limited. Thus, the destroyed myelin in the MS plaque is never adequately restored. Despite this, many patients suffering an acute exacerbation of MS recover considerably from the symptoms experienced during the acute attack. Some of this recovery may result from resolution of the initial inflammation and edema present in the MS plaque. In addition, nerve action potential conduction through the demyelinated area may eventually be restored by means other than remyelination. After an initial period of conduction block, there is evidence that continuous nerve action potential conduction similar to that seen in normal unmyelinated fibers may eventually be established in demyelinated large nerve axons. Although relatively slow, such nerve action potential conduction might account for some recovery of function.

Epidemiology

MS has a striking geographical distribution, and is far more common in temperate zones than in the tropics. High incidence areas include southern Canada, the northern United States, and western Europe from Switzerland northward. In such areas, the disease prevalence approaches 60 cases per one hundred thousand people. Less marked but similar high-risk zones exist in the southern hemisphere.

The risk of developing MS is apparently determined by place of residence prior to age 15 years. Should the individual move from one risk zone to another after 15 years of age, he takes his old risk with him regardless of future places of residence. This has suggested to some that a viral infection usually contracted in childhood may determine later risk of developing MS.

MS has a far higher prevalence among relatives of MS patients than in the general population. In siblings and parents of MS patients, the disease occurs approximately 20 times as frequently as in the general population. The disease prevalence in first cousins of MS patients is at least 5 times that in the general population, and certain HLA types are more common in MS patients. When one twin is affected, the risk of the other twin developing MS is approximately 30 percent in monozygotic twins, but only 15 percent in dizygotic twins. This would suggest that genetic factors are important in the etiology of MS. Environmental factors common to a family setting, however, would also explain some of the data.

MS is 1.4 times more common in women than in men. Most patients experience onset of symptoms between the ages of 20 and 40 years, but a small percentage of cases have onset before age 10 years or after age 50 years.

Clinical Manifestations

The clinical presentation of MS depends on the location of the first symptomatic plaque. The majority of patients present with weakness, paresthesiae, or disturbances of vision. Less common presenting symptoms are ataxia, vertigo, bladder dysfunction, and mental changes. A period of fatigue and malaise frequently precedes the first neurologic symptom, and such nonspecific symptoms may be prominent throughout the subsequent course of the disease.

Acute optic neuritis is a common mode of presentation. The patient experiences visual loss that usually progresses over hours or days, and may be mild or severe. Usually only one eye is affected, but occasionally both eyes are simultaneously involved. Central vision is affected more than peripheral vision, usually with marked reduction in visual acuity. Pain on eye movement due to optic nerve inflammation is common and diagnostically helpful. The visual loss usually remains unchanged for several days or weeks, and then gradually improves. Many patients regain normal or near normal vision, but a small minority show little recovery of vision. If the area of demyelination and inflammation in the optic nerve is near the optic disc, fundoscopy shows optic disc swelling (papillitis). Unlike papilledema from increased intracranial pressure, papillitis is usually present in one eye only—an important aid in diag-

nosis. If the optic lesion is further back in the optic nerve (retrobulbar neuritis), the patient's clinical presentation is similar, but fundoscopy is normal ("the patient sees nothing and the physician sees nothing").

Follow-up studies indicate that within 10 to 15 years after their first attack of optic neuritis, approximately 50 percent of patients manifest other CNS lesions compatible with multiple sclerosis. Optic neuritis then may be a first manifestation of MS, may occur later in the course of MS, or may be an isolated event in a patient who will never have further CNS symptoms.

Brainstem and cerebellar involvement in MS is common. This may result in a variety of symptoms, including dysarthria, dysphagia, vertigo, facial weakness or numbness, ataxia, and trigeminal neuralgia. Probably the most common brainstem manifestation of MS is diplopia because of interference with brainstem oculomotor mechanisms. A bilateral internuclear ophthalmoplegia is particularly suggestive of MS (see Clinical Localization of Neurologic Disorders).

Spinal cord lesions in MS commonly produce weakness and paresthesiae, although these symptoms may also result from lesions at other levels of the CNS. Spinal cord involvement may take several forms. In acute transverse myelitis, the patient usually presents with rapidly progressing numbness and tingling in the legs, which progresses to involve the entire body below a certain level. A sensory level is usually present in the thoracic or cervical area, and indicates the level of spinal cord involvement. Associated weakness may be mild or marked. A demyelinating lesion involving sensory and motor white-matter tracts is responsible for the symptoms and signs. Eventual recovery ranges from poor to virtually complete. Approximately 15 percent of patients with acute transverse myelitis go on to develop MS. In the remaining patients, the spinal cord demyelination would appear due to postinfectious demyelination (encephalomyelitis).

Some patients with MS have multiple episodes of more restricted numbness and weakness involving limbs and trunk, related to smaller spinal cord demyelinating lesions. Still others develop a progressive demyelinating myelopathy with slowly increasing weakness and sensory changes.

Mental changes are rarely the presenting manifestation, but are common as the disease progresses. An inappropriate euphoria is present in some patients. Patients with longstanding or rapidly progressing disease may show dementia, and even coma can occur.

The course of patients with MS is extremely variable. Most patients have a remitting and relapsing course, with partial or complete recovery after each attack. Others, particularly those with onset of MS in the older age range, suffer a progressive disease course from the very start. Patients with a remitting and relapsing course may change to a progressive course at any time.

The eventual prognosis of multiple sclerosis in the individual patient cannot be predicted. As a group, approximately 25 percent are markedly disabled after 10 years. However, these figures are probably biased, since mildly affected patients are less likely to be entered into a clinical series. Patients presenting with optic neuritis and with paresthesiae seem to have a better prognosis than patients presenting with weakness or ataxia.

In patients presenting with a CNS symptom suggestive of MS, careful inquiry regarding past neurologic symptoms is important, particularly as disease exacerbations may be separated by many years. These past symptoms may have been relatively minor, and the patient frequently does not volunteer the information unless asked. A careful search for evidence of other CNS lesions on physical examination is important. A pale optic disc indicates past optic neuritis. Hyperreflexia, upgoing plantars, ataxia, and other signs all may indicate additional CNS lesions, some of which may have been asymptomatic.

The diagnosis of MS can at present be proven only by brain biopsy or autopsy. Through careful clinical assessment, however, the clinician can determine the likelihood of MS in a patient presenting with appropriate symptoms. Clinically, definite MS is present in patients with a remitting and relapsing history with two or more episodes, and with evidence of two or more separate CNS lesions. Lesions must be predominantly in white matter. Age of onset should be between 10 and 50 years, and signs and symptoms should have been present for at least 1 year. The diagnosis is also partially one of exclusion, and any better diagnosis must not be apparent.

Further categories of probable and possible MS have been defined for patients in whom MS appears likely, but who do not satisfy the above criteria. Categories prefixed by the term *progressive* have been proposed for patients without relapses and remissions.

Multiple sclerosis produces focal CNS lesions, and, at least initially, can mimic a number of other conditions including brain and spinal cord tumor. Onset of symptoms in an MS relapse is not usually as sudden as in stroke, but occasionally differential diagnosis can be difficult. Slowly progressive spinocerebellar degenerations can also at times resemble progressive MS. Several disorders other than MS can produce a remitting and relapsing course, with multiple CNS lesions. Behcet's disease falls in this category. Uveitis and ulcers of the buccal and vaginal mucosa characteristic of Behcet's disease aid in differential diagnosis. Lupus erythematosus, polyarteritis nodosa, and other forms of vasculitis with CNS involvement may at times mimic MS.

Laboratory Investigation

The laboratory investigation may contribute in two ways. CSF analysis and various evoked response tests may help to confirm the clinical impression of multiple sclerosis, while brain CT scan and myelography help to exclude other possible CNS lesions such as brain and spinal cord tumors.

The CSF may be normal, but frequently it shows a number of abnormalities. A mild mononuclear CSF pleocytosis is present in approximately 30 percent of patients, and a similar number show an elevation of CSF total protein. CSF gammaglobulin (IgG) levels are elevated in approximately 70 percent, and CSF oligoclonal IgG bands are found in over 90 percent. Such CSF IgG elevations and oligoclonal bands are also found in a number of other CNS diseases, including neurosyphilis, subacute sclerosing panencephalitis, and other CNS infections. Taken in light of the total clinical picture, however, the CSF examination can be very useful.

Evoked response studies assess conduction velocity in CNS white-matter tracts. A sensory stimulus in any modality is applied to the patient repetitively, and the electrical response of the brain is recorded with the aid of computer averaging techniques. By measuring the evoked response latency (time from stimulus presentation to brain electrical response), an indication of conduction velocity is obtained in the white-matter pathway being assessed. As might be expected, patients with MS frequently show slowing of CNS conduction velocity, presumably related to MS plaques in the pathways tested. The most useful evoked response test in MS at the present time is the visual evoked response to pattern reversal stimulation. Visual evoked response usually remains permanently abnormal in eyes with previous optic neuritis, and therefore may help to confirm a previous vague history of optic neuritis. Further, it demonstrates optic nerve lesions in a significant proportion of MS patients who have never had previous visual symptoms and who have a normal clinical eye examination. The auditory brainstem evoked response and the somatosensory evoked response can similarly indicate asymptomatic and symptomatic lesions. Thus, evoked responses may indicate additional unsuspected CNS lesions in patients with possible MS, and thereby help to confirm diagnosis.

In addition to excluding other CNS diseases, the brain CT scan may show multiple cerebral white-matter lesions in patients with MS. Only the larger MS plaques are shown. These may occur anywhere in cerebral white matter, but have a predilection for the periventricular regions.

Treatment

No satisfactory treatment presently exists for MS. ACTH and steroids may hasten symptomatic resolution of the acute attack by reducing inflammation and edema. They do not appear to affect disability remaining after the attack, and do not change the long-term prognosis.

Immunosuppressives such as azathioprine are used for rapidly progressing severe MS. There is evidence that supports their use, but definitive controlled studies are not yet available.

Most therapy available in MS is symptomatic in nature. Although most patients should be informed of the diagnosis as soon as it is reasonably certain, it is important to convey an optimistic outlook. In general, it is best if the patient continues with his usual activities and occupation as long as possible.

Diplopia may make reading difficult, and an eye patch may make a large difference to the patient's well being.

Patients may find they function better in a cooler environment as residual MS symptoms tend to be worse with slight increases in body temperature. Increased body temperature reduces the safety factor of nerve action potential transmission, and marginally conducting fibers may undergo conduction block.

Physiotherapy is helpful in reducing motor disability, relieving spasticity, and preventing flexion contractures. Gait training may improve walking. Various appliances including canes, and braces for foot drop, may be helpful. Walkers are useful for more advanced gait disability. Wheelchairs when necessary must be properly fitted. Ramps, handrails, and various supporting bars placed in the home can be of great usefulness. Disabling spasticity and painful or bothersome flexor spasms are best treated with lioresal (Baclofen). Dantrolene (Dantrium) is used when lioresal cannot be tolerated. Diazepam (Valium) at bedtime can be very useful for flexor spasms occurring at night. The effectiveness of these agents is limited because they may increase weakness, and many MS patients depend on increased muscle tone in the legs to support them while standing or transferring.

The most common bladder disturbance occurring in MS is urinary urgency and frequency. These pa-tients have a hyperactive detrusor reflex due to lesions in white-matter spinal cord tracts. Reducing bladder tone with the anticholinergic drug propantheline (Probanthine) can be very useful. The drug can be taken regularly, or only before social outings. The minimal effective dose is best. Standard dosages are 15 mg 3 times a day with 30 mg at bedtime.

Bladder atony due to sacral cord white-matter lesions can be treated with bethanechol (Urecholine), or intermittent self-catheterization. A cystometrogram will help to define the type of bladder disturbance present.

Trigeminal neuralgia is common in patients with MS, and relates to brainstem plaques in the trigeminal nerve root entry zone or its central connections and nuclei. The therapy of choice is carbamazepine (Tegretol).

MS patients may also require drug therapy and counseling for emotional reactions to their disease. Although it is true that at present the progression of the patient's disease cannot be significantly altered, this should not discourage physicians from doing all they can to help the MS patient with his problems.

ACUTE DISSEMINATED ENCEPHALOMYELITIS

Acute neurologic symptoms suggesting CNS disturbances occasionally follow acute viral illnesses and immunizations. Similar syndromes occur spontaneously, possibly triggered by inapparent viral infections. The term *encephalomyelitis*, indicating both brain and spinal cord involvement, is used for these syndromes, although this term is also applied by some to illnesses characterized by direct viral invasion of the CNS. The etiology of the postinfectious and postimmunization syndromes discussed here is an immune attack on CNS myelin. Perivenous demyelination is prominent in the pathology of these syndromes, and both white- and grey-matter lesions are present. As both small vessels and myelin appear to be damaged, *postinfectious* and *postimmunization vasculomyelinopathy* may be better terms for these conditions, and are used by some authors.

Approximately 1 in 1,000 cases of measles is complicated by a disseminated encephalomyelitis fitting this category. A similar post infectious encephalomyelitis occurs in rebella, chickenpox, mumps, pertussis, and other infections. Similar syndromes follow rabies vaccination, smallpox vaccination, measles immunization, and possibly others.

The onset is sudden, and occurs within several weeks after the preceding illness or vaccination. In measles encephalomyelitis, onset may precede the rash. Usually there is rapid progression for several days, then stabilization for several days or weeks, followed by recovery. Recurrences are rare. The mortality in measles encephalomyelitis is approximately 12 percent.

Clinical symptoms and signs depend on whether involvement of the CNS is truly disseminated, and on which parts of the CNS are involved in cases with only localized involvement. Lethargy, coma, optic neuritis, ataxia, focal brainstem syndromes, and transverse myelitis have all been described. Some patients with optic neuritis who do not progress to multiple sclerosis may be examples of a localized postinfectious encephalomyelitis.

Approximately 80 percent of patients with acute transverse myelitis are thought to have localized acute postinfectious or postimmunization encephalomyelitis. The remainder have multiple sclerosis.

Corticosteroids appear to improve acute disseminated encephalomyelitis, and although still controversial, should probably be used in most cases.

PROGRESSIVE MULTIFOCAL LEUKOENCEPHALOPATHY

Progressive multifocal leukoencephalopathy is due to a common, normally harmless virus that causes severe CNS disease under conditions of impaired host immunity. The disease is uncommon and occurs primarily in patients with lymphoma, leukemia, or carcinoma, or in patients on immunosuppressive therapy. Multiple areas of myelin distruction are present in the CNS, and intranuclear inclusion bodies containing polyoma virus particles are present in oligodendroglial cells. Clinically, symptoms and signs suggest multiple asymmetric lesions of the brain and, at times, spinal cord. Hemiplegia, aphasia, hemianopia, and organic mental changes are common. CT scanning may show multiple brain white-matter lesions. CSF is usually normal.

Isolated reports of successful treatment with cytosine arabinoside or adenine arabinoside have been made, but efficacy has not been clearly established.

VITAMIN B_{12} DEFICIENCY (PERNICIOUS ANEMIA)

Pernicious anemia, with inability to absorb vitamin B_{12}, can damage all parts of the nervous system. Neurologic involvement may occasionally precede development of anemia.

Myelopathy with posterior column and corticospinal tract involvement presents with tingling in the hands and feet, and gait ataxia from sensory loss. Romberg's sign is present, and joint position sense and vibration sense in the feet are lost early. Hyperreflexia is common due to corticospinal tract damage.

Vitamin B_{12} deficiency also causes a peripheral neuropathy. Frequently myelopathy and peripheral neuropathy are present in the same patient. In patients with peripheral neuropathy, reflexes may be reduced or absent.

Dementia resulting from vitamin B_{12} deficiency is rare, but may occur in association with the other neurologic manifestations or, rarely, in isolation.

Immediate therapy with parenteral vitamin B_{12} is essential, because established neurologic symptoms and signs may reverse only incompletely after therapy.

CENTRAL PONTINE MYELINOLYSIS

Central pontine myelinolysis is uncommon, and occurs primarily in malnourished alcoholics. It has been reported in nonalcoholics, particularly in association with hyponatremia. Clinically, symptoms usually evolve over several days, with the patient developing quadriplegia, pseudobulbar palsy, and locked-in syndrome. Pathologically, a large area of demyelination is present in the ventral pons, with relative preservation of axons.

MARCHIAFAVA-BIGNAMI DISEASE

This rare disease occurs in alcoholics, and is characterized by symmetric demyelination in the corpus callosum. The clinical presentation is diverse, and includes intellectual deterioration, emotional disorders, aphasia, tremor, rigidity, and paralysis. Some recovery is possible if abstinence from alcohol is achieved.

CENTRAL NERVOUS SYSTEM INFECTIONS

Central nervous system infections are among the most lethal infectious diseases. Rapid diagnosis and immediate therapy are essential, particularly in bacterial meningitis and brain abscess.

CNS infections can be classified according to site of involvement and etiologic agent as shown in Table 14.29.

Table 14.29 Central Nervous System Infections

Meningitis
  Acute bacterial
  Tuberculous
  Viral
  Fungal
  Others
Brain abscess
  Bacterial
  Fungal
Encephalitis
  Herpes simplex
  Slow virus
  Others

MENINGITIS

Meningitis is an infection or inflammation within the subarachnoid space.

Bacterial Meningitis

Bacteria usually reach the meninges through the blood stream. Middle ear and sinus infections, ruptured brain abscess, skull fractures, neurosurgical incisions, and congenital neuroectodermal defects are less common routes of invasion. Once the CSF is involved, there is rapid dissemination of infection throughout the subarachnoid space.

Hemophilus influenzae, Streptococcus pneumoniae (pneumococcus) and *Neisseria meningitides* (meningococcus) account for over 85 percent of cases of acute bacterial meningitis.

H. influenzae is the major cause of meningitis in childhood between the ages of 1 month and 5 years. It may occasionally cause meningitis in young adults, and usually follows an upper respiratory tract infection or otitis media.

Meningococcus is the most common cause of meningitis between the ages of 5 and 25 years. Meningococcal meningitis may occur in epidemics. It is characterized by rapid progression and is accompanied by a rash in approximately 50 percent of cases. The rash may be morbilliform, petechial, or purpuric. Circulatory collapse may occur and, rarely, adrenal failure secondary to adrenal hemorrhage (Waterhouse-Friderichsen syndrome).

Pneumococcal meningitis occurs in all age groups, but mainly in patients under the age of 6 and over the age of 25. It is the most common cause of meningitis in the middle-aged and the elderly. It is frequently preceded by bronchitis, pneumonia, otitis media, and sinusitis. Predisposing factors for pneumococcal meningitis include alcoholism, sickle cell disease, basal skull fracture, bacterial endocarditis, and previous splenectomy.

Escherichia coli and staphylococcal meningitis occur mainly in the neonate and the elderly. Staphylococcal meningitis also occurs at any age as a complication of penetrating head trauma and neurosurgical procedures.

Listeria monocytogenes, Pseudomonas organisms, and a variety of other bacteria also occasionally cause meningitis, particularly in immunosuppressed patients and patients with cancer.

Clinical Features

In addition to the cardinal features of fever, headache, and neck stiffness, acute bacterial meningitis may be complicated by seizures, focal neurologic signs, and increased intracranial pressure. There may be confusion and delirium followed by progressive deterioration of consciousness to stupor and coma. Fever and neck stiffness may be minimal in elderly patients and alcoholics.

Laboratory Investigation

If there is a strong clinical suspicion of bacterial meningitis, lumber puncture should be performed immediately. If the clinical examination shows papilledema or lateralizing neurologic signs, it may be preferable to obtain a CT scan to rule out a brain abscess prior to a lumbar puncture. However, CSF examination and initiation of appropriate antibiotic therapy should not be unduly delayed. A delay of even a few hours in starting therapy may significantly affect the outcome.

The CSF pressure is usually elevated above 180 mm H_2O. The fluid may be grossly cloudy and purulent (Table 14.30). Microscopic examination reveals over 1,000 WBC/mm^3, and often much larger

Table 14.30 CSF Changes in Meningitis

	Acute Bacterial	Tuberculous	Viral
White Blood Cells	Polymorphonuclear cells	Lymphocytes	Lymphocytes
Protein	Elevated	Elevated	Normal or Elevated
Glucose	Depressed	Depressed	Normal

numbers are present. Usually over 90 percent of these cells are polymorphonuclear leukocytes. The initial CSF examination reveals grossly clear fluid with a cell count of less than 100 WBC/mm^3 in a small percentage of patients with bacterial meningitis. The characteristic CSF changes of acute bacterial meningitis may be masked if the patient has been treated prior to lumbar puncture with antibiotics for a presumed upper respiratory infection.

CSF protein is usually elevated and often over 100 mg/dl.

CSF glucose is low, usually less than 40 mg/dl, and in many cases less than 10 mg/dl. It is important to obtain a blood sugar determination at the time of lumbar puncture in cases of suspected bacterial meningitis. CSF glucose values less than 40 percent of the blood glucose values support a diagnosis of bacterial meningitis unless the blood sugar is unusually high.

An immediate Gram stain of the CSF should be done; often this reveals the causative organism. Gram-positive diplococci indicate pneumococcus; pleomorphic coccobacilli indicate *H. influenzae*.

CSF cultures are positive in 80 percent of cases. They are frequently negative in partially treated bacterial meningitis. Detection of bacterial antigen in the CSF by countercurrent immunoelectrophoresis may be helpful in such cases. Blood cultures should be done as well, and are positive in 50 percent of patients with bacterial meningitis. Leukocytosis is an almost invariable finding, except in the old or debilitated.

Treatment

Appropriate antibiotic therapy should be started immediately after lumbar puncture. The choice of antibiotics depends on the causative organism or the age of the patient if the causative organism is not known.

Initial Therapy   In adults, if the organism is not immediately identified on Gram stain, treatment should be commenced with intravenous penicillin G, 24 million units/day in 6 or 12 divided doses. This is the best therapy for pneumococcal and meningococcal meningitis. If there is reason to suspect staphylococcus, a penicillinase-resistant penicillin should be added (cloxacillin, methicillin, or nafcillin).

In the younger adult who may have *H. influenzae*, or in other patients in whom a gram-negative organism is suspected, chloramphenicol, 4 to 6 g/day in 4 divided doses, should be given in addition to penicillin G. Ampicillin 12 g/day is preferred as an alternative to chloramphenicol, once the *H. influenzae* strain is proven susceptible to ampicillin. Chlor-

amphenicol penetrates the blood-brain barrier extremely well, in contrast to most other antibiotics effective against gram-negative bacteria.

Specific Therapy   When CSF culture and sensitivity results are available, treatment should be continued with the most appropriate antibiotic. For staphylococcal meningitis, oxacillin, cloxacillin, or nafcillin, 12 to 16 g/day, is used. If the organism proves penicillin sensitive, therapy should be changed to penicillin G.

In patients with penicillin allergy, vancomycin may be used for suspected staphylococcal meningitis; however, experience with this drug is limited. Cephalosporins penetrate the blood-brain barrier very poorly, and their usefulness in meningitis is limited. Chloramphenicol is useful in patients with penicillin allergy. Two new cephalosporins, Cefotaxime and Moxalactam, appear promising for the treatment of gram-negative meningitis. See Table 7.4, Chapter 7.

For pseudomonas, ticarcillin should be given with tobramycin, because the two drugs act synergistically against this organism.

The duration of therapy for pneumococcal, meningococcal, and *H. influenzae* meningitis should be at least 10 days. Treatment should continue for at least 7 days after the patient becomes afebrile. For other organisms, therapy may need to be continued for 3 weeks or longer. All therapy should be intravenous. CSF should be reexamined shortly after antibiotics are stopped.

For infections with less sensitive organisms, particularly gram-negative organisms, minimum inhibitory concentrations should be determined for the organism cultured and used to guide antibiotic therapy.

Childhood Meningitis   For meningitis in children under the age of 5 years *H. influenzae* must be strongly suspected, and drug doses determined by body size.

Treatment of Contacts   Treatment of the patient's contacts is necessary only for meningococcal meningitis. Family, household members, and others in intimate contact with the patient for prolonged periods should be treated. School classmates need not be treated. Therapy for adult contacts should be sulfadiazine, 1 gram twice a day for 2 days, if the organisms are sulfadiazine sensitive. If the meningococci are resistant to sulfadiazine, or if their sensitivity is unknown, rifampin, 600 mg twice a day for 2 days, should be used. All treatment courses are 2 days in length. Smaller doses should be used in infants and children.

General Treatment Measures   Hospitalized patients with meningococcal meningitis should be isolated until they have been on antibiotic therapy for 24 hours. After this point they are no longer infective. Isolation is not necessary for other types of meningitis.

Overhydration due to excessive intravenous fluids should be avoided, as this may contribute to cerebral edema. Seizures may require anticonvulsant therapy. The syndrome of inappropriate antidiuretic hormone secretion may develop in meningitis, and lead to hyponatremia. Fluid restriction is usually adequate therapy.

In patients with recurrent bacterial meningitis, an anatomic defect may be responsible. Frontal bone cribriform plate fracture and congenital fistulas from skin to subarachnoid space in the occipital or sacral region should be carefully looked for.

TUBERCULOUS MENINGITIS

In regions where the incidence of tuberculosis is low, tuberculous meningitis occurs mainly in adults, and results from reactivation of dormant infections.

The presenting signs and symptoms are headache, irritability, fever, and neck stiffness. The illness is more protracted than acute bacterial meningitis, and symptoms may be present for several weeks before the diagnosis is considered. Confusion, disorientation and other mental changes are often prominent features. Multiple cranial nerve palsies may occur due to involvement of the basal meninges.

CSF shows a lymphocytic pleocytosis with 100 to 1,000 WBC/mm^3. Protein concentrations are elevated, and glucose concentrations are reduced. Attempts should be made to demonstrate the organisms in the CSF by acid-fast stains. However, positive results are obtained in only 20 percent of cases. Demonstration of active tuberculosis elsewhere in the body strongly supports the diagnosis of tuberculous meningitis in a patient with appropriate CSF findings.

Patients often need antituberculous therapy prior to definite confirmation of the diagnosis by culture. Treatment should not be delayed, because a delay will worsen the prognosis if tuberculous meningitis is present. Isoniazid and rifampin both cross the blood-brain barrier, and are the treatment of choice. Streptomycin may also be used, but it crosses the blood brain barrier poorly.

FUNGAL MENINGITIS

Cryptococcus neoformans is the most common cause of fungal meningitis. Although it may occur in previously healthy individuals, about 50 percent of patients with cryptococcus meningitis have a predisposing illness or are receiving immunosuppressive therapy. The clinical picture is that of a chronic meningitis with headache, evidence of meningeal irritation, and mental changes. India ink stains of CSF reveal cryptococci in 40 percent of cases. Cultures are positive in less than 50 percent of cases. CSF cryptococcal antigen can be detected in over 85 percent of cases, and determination of serum antigens is also useful.

Histoplasmosis, blastomycosis, coccidiodomycosis, and aspergillosis are less common causes of fungal meningitis.

The treatment of choice for fungal meningitis is administration of amphotericin B and fluorocytosine.

VIRAL MENINGITIS

Viral meningitis (aseptic meningitis) may be caused by numerous viruses, but echovirus, coxsackievirus, mumps, and lymphocytic choriomeningitis probably account for the majority of cases. Polio is now a rare cause of viral meningitis in the developed countries with immunized populations.

The patient presents with headache and mild to moderate fever. On examination, neck stiffness is common but may be mild. Significant obtundation or focal signs are unusual.

CSF examination shows a lymphocytic pleocytosis with normal or elevated protein and normal glucose. The normal CSF glucose is important, because this CSF pattern accompanied by a low CSF glucose suggests tuberculous meningitis. A low CSF glucose occasionally does occur in mumps meningitis. In the first 24 hours of infection, neutrophils may predominate in the CSF in viral meningitis, and differentiation from early bacterial meningitis may be difficult.

Other conditions that may cause difficulty in differential diagnosis are partially treated cases of bacterial meningitis, cryptococcal meningitis, and meningitis due to unusual organisms such as *Listeria monocytogenes* in immune compromised patients.

Patients with viral meningitis require no specific treatment and recover in several days. Brief hospitalization is often advisable so the patient can be observed for other diagnostic possibilities.

BRAIN ABSCESS

Etiology

Brain abscesses result from contiguous spread of infection from middle ear, mastoid, or frontal sinus; by hematogenous spread from distant septic foci, such as lung abscess, bronchiectasis, osteomyelitis, and skin infection; or from penetrating head injuries. Patients with a right-to-left shunt, as in congenital heart disease or pulmonary arteriovenous fistula, are at increased risk for brain abscess.

In the adult, anaerobic lung abscess may precede bacterial brain abscess. Streptococci, usually anaerobic or microaerophilic, are associated with other anaerobes, particularly *Bacteroides* species. A variety of gram negative rods including *E. coli, Enterobacter, Klebsiella,* and *Proteus* species may cause brain abscess, particularly in association with chronic ear infection. Staphylococci also produce brain abscess, usually in conjunction with septicemia arising from skin and bone infection or with penetrating head injuries. Fungal brain abscess usually occurs in association with lowered resistance from systemic illness or immunosuppression.

Clinical Manifestations

Brain abscesses usually present as a mass lesion with focal neurologic signs, and with symptoms of increased intracranial pressure. The focal signs depend on the site of the lesion. Headache, fever, and vomiting may be present. Neck stiffness is not common, and obvious signs of infection may be absent. Evidence of septic foci elsewhere should increase suspicion of brain abscess, as should the presence of other predisposing factors such as immunosuppression.

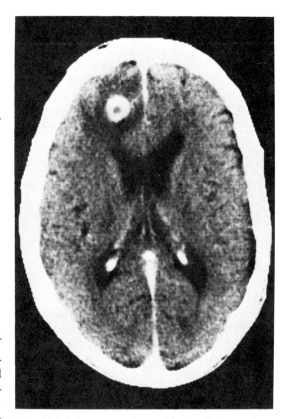

Fig. 14.26 Contrast enhanced brain CT scan showing a *Nocardia* brain abscess. A typical ring shadow showing a vascular capsule around a necrotic center is present

Laboratory Investigation

Peripheral leukocytosis is common, but fever and leukocytosis may be lacking once the abscess is encapsulated.

Lumbar puncture is usually contraindicated because of the intracranial mass lesion. If it is done, a pleocytosis with both lymphocytes and neutrophils is usually present. Total cell count is usually less than 400 WBC's/mm^3. CSF protein is normal or elevated, and CSF glucose is normal. CSF cultures are usually negative. Blood cultures are more useful, and should be done in all patients with brain abscess before initiating therapy.

All patients with suspected brain abscess should have a skull and chest roentgenogram to search for possible sources of infection, such as frontal sinusitis, mastoid infections, and lung abscess.

A radioisotope brain scan will demonstrate most brain abscesses. A brain CT scan will provide more precise information regarding the size and location, how much edema is present, and whether the capsule has formed (Fig. 14.26).

Treatment

If the brain abscess is diagnosed early before a definite capsule has formed (cerebritis), medical therapy alone may be sufficient to irradicate the infection. These patients must be observed closely, because deterioration secondary to an enlarging intracranial mass may be precipitous and require emergency neurosurgical intervention. If seizures occur, they should be treated with anticonvulsant therapy.

Most patients will have an encapsulated abscess, and require surgical drainage or excision as well as antibiotic therapy. Unless the patient presents with increased intracranial pressure and rapid deterioration, treatment should consist of antibiotic therapy followed by elective surgical excision. Abscess contents should be cultured both aerobically and anaerobically, and fungal organisms should be searched for.

Brain abscess with no apparent predisposing infection should be treated with chloramphenicol 6 to 8 g/day in combination with penicillin G, 24 million units/day. Chloramphenicol penetrates the brain parenchyma better than any other antibiotic, and reaches higher concentrations in the abscess. If the patient is immunosuppressed or leukopenic, gentamicin and carbenicillin should be added, since gram-negative bacteria are then frequently present in the abscess.

In patients with chronic ear infection, recent neurosurgery or head trauma, a penicillinase resistant penicillin and gentamicin should be added to chloramphenicol since staphylococci and gram-negative bacteria are frequently present. Fusidic acid may be useful in staphylococcal brain abscess. Antibiotics should be continued parenterally for at least 6 weeks.

Fungal brain abscesses should be treated with amphoteracin B, usually in combination with fluorocytosine.

ENCEPHALITIS

Viral encephalitis results from viral invasion of the CNS. Numerous viruses may cause encephalitis or meningoencephalitis. These include various arthropod-borne viruses that may cause epidemics of encephalitis. Examples of these are western and eastern equine encephalitis. Direct viral invasion of the CNS should be distinguished from the postinfectious syndrome of acute disseminated encephalomyelitis, which is discussed in the section entitled Demyelinating Disorders. Slow virus disorders including Creutzfeldt-Jakob disease and subacute sclerosing panencephalitis are discussed in the section entitled Dementia. Progressive multifocal leukoencephalopathy, another CNS viral infection, is discussed in the section entitled Demyelinating Disorders.

The most common serious encephalitis encountered in medical practice is herpes simplex encephalitis. This will be the only type discussed in detail here.

Herpes Simplex Encephalitis

Etiology

Herpes simplex type I occasionally invades the central nervous system and produces encephalitis. Previous or recent herpes labialis may or may not have been present.

Clinical Manifestations

Patients of any age may be affected. Headache, nausea, and vomiting are frequently present for several days prior to diagnosis. Early neurologic manifestations include personality change, lethargy, con-

fusion, bizarre behavior, hallucinations, and seizures. Because of these mental changes, patients may initially be considered to have psychiatric problems. Fever and leukocytosis in such patients should always instigate a careful neurologic examination and consideration of encephalitis. Because of the predilection of the virus for the temporal lobes, focal signs may initially be subtle or absent. Seizures frequently give the first clear indication that encephalitis is present. Later, hemiparesis, aphasia, and coma are common, and indicate cerebral edema and ongoing brain necrosis.

Laboratory Investigation

If focal signs are prominent, a CT scan is indicated to rule out other mass lesions prior to lumbar puncture. CSF examination may be normal in herpes encephalitis, but usually a pleocytosis is present. CSF white blood cell counts range from only a few to several hundred WBC/mm^3, and both lymphocytes and neutrophils may be present. CSF protein is normal or elevated, glucose is usually normal but may be low.

The EEG is diffusely or focally abnormal in all cases, and useful in confirming the clinical suspicion of encephalitis. Periodic EEG complexes are present in some patients, and are strong evidence for encephalitis. The isotope brain scan and CT scan will show focal lesions once brain edema or necrosis is present.

If herpes encephalitis is clinically likely, a brain biopsy should be done. This is the only way to prove the diagnosis. Brain biopsy allows microscopic demonstration of intranuclear viral inclusion bodies typical of herpes, and isolation of the virus by culture.

Treatment

Early diagnosis is essential, as evidence is mounting that treatment with adenine arabinoside if started early before the onset of coma improves the prognosis (see Chapter 7, Table 7.5). Even with treatment, however, a substantial number of survivors are left with permanent neurologic deficits.

Overhydration from excessive intravenous fluids should be avoided, and seizures should be treated with anticonvulsants.

HEAD INJURY

The major complications of head injury are shown in Table 14.31.

Table 14.31 Complications of Head Injury

Concussion
Cerebral Edema with Brain Herniation
Brain Contusion and Laceration
    Focal neurologic deficits
    Intellectual impairment
    Posttraumatic epilepsy
Intracranial Hematoma
    Intracerebral
    Epidural
    Subdural
        Acute
        Chronic
Others
    Posttraumatic headache
    Memory impairment
    Dizziness

COMPLICATIONS OF HEAD INJURY

Concussion

Concussion refers to an acute loss of neurologic function following head injury. The brief loss of consciousness following many milder head injuries results from concussion. The patient is usually amnesic for a brief period of time before the head injury (retrograde amnesia) and for a short time afterward (anterograde amnesia).

Cerebral Edema

Progressive cerebral edema may occur after severe head injury, and lead to increased intracranial pressure (ICP), transtentorial herniation, and death. The amount of cerebral edema may increase for several days following head injury.

Brain Contusion

Brain contusion and laceration occur with more severe head injury, and may result in permanent focal neurologic damage. Widespread structural damage to the CNS can result in permanent intellectual impairment.

Epilepsy with recurrent seizures also occurs with increased frequency after head injury (see Epilepsy). Patients with acute intracranial hematomas from head injury have a subsequent 30 percent incidence of epilepsy. Depressed skull fractures, and seizures in the initial days after head injury, also increase risk of later epilepsy.

Intracranial Hematoma

Intracerebral hematomas are common with severe head injury and contribute to focal CNS damage.

Epidural hematomas result from arterial bleeding between the dura and the skull. Patients with fracture lines crossing the middle meningeal artery are at particular risk. Shortly after recovery from the initial period of unconsciousness, an expanding epidural hematoma may cause rapidly progressive coma and death. Alternatively, an epidural hematoma may cause rapidly deepening coma without an intervening lucid interval.

Acute subdural hematoma results from venous bleeding from torn dural sinuses or bridging veins. If bleeding is rapid, the presentation is similar to that of epidural hematoma, although progression is usually slower.

Chronic subdural hematomas may occur after relatively minor head trauma. The patient usually recovers from the head injury, which may or may not have caused initial unconsciousness. Weeks or months later progressive obtundation and dementia occur, with or without focal neurologic signs. Chronic subdural hematomas are particularly common in alcoholics, demented patients, and in patients on anticoagulants. The history of previous head injury may not be available because of its minor nature or the patient's mental state.

Other Complications

Patients with otherwise uncomplicated head injury may suffer from a number of posttraumatic syndromes. Dizziness may persist for a number of months, and probably results from injury to the labyrinth or posterior fossa structures. It usually clears eventually without treatment. Memory difficulties are common but they usually clear unless the head injury has been severe. Posttraumatic headache can be a significant problem and can last many months.

INVESTIGATION AND TREATMENT

The key to successful head-injury management is careful observation. Patients who have been unconscious should be observed closely, preferably in hospital, for 12 to 24 hours. Even head injury without unconsciousness may result in significant complications such as chronic subdural hematoma, and the patient and family should be warned to return if neurologic symptoms develop.

Observation of the patient includes hourly assessment of level of arousal, orientation, pupillary responses to light, extraocular movements, strength, and vital signs. Progressive deterioration in level of consciousness indicates an expanding intracranial hematoma or increasing cerebral edema (see Disorders of Consciousness). New focal neurologic signs also indicate an expanding intracranial hematoma. Changes in vital signs, particularly with bradycardia and widening pulse pressure, may indicate increasing intracranial pressure.

Sedation and mydriatics should be avoided because they may obscure important changes in the patient's condition. Seizures must be treated. Phenytoin is the drug of choice because it is nonsedating. Codeine is useful if analgesics must be given.

The patient should be positioned on his side to avoid aspiration. Measures to reduce cerebral edema should be instituted. These are discussed in the section on Coma, Treatment.

Skull roentgenograms are done in most patients who have been unconscious. Fratures indicate a severe head injury, and a shifted pineal gland suggests intracranial hematoma. However, it must be remembered that patients with normal skull films may still have suffered significant cerebral injury.

The CT scan is the single most useful procedure for demonstrating intracranial hematomas in patients with focal neurologic signs or progressive obtundation. Acute epidural and subdural hematomas are

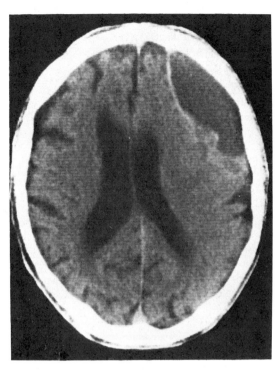

Fig. 14.28 Brain CT scan of a patient with a chronic left frontal subdural hematoma. Displacement of the frontal horn of the left lateral ventricle is present

readily visualized, since fresh blood is more radiopaque than brain tissue (Fig. 14.27). Emergency surgical evacuation of the hematoma is essential. Measures to reduce cerebral edema may reduce ICP temporarily while surgery is arranged (see Disorders of Consciousness).

Chronic subdural hematomas are also well demonstrated by CT scan, and are visualized as biconvex lucent lesions over the brain surface (Fig. 14.28). Except for very small hematomas, surgical removal is again the treatment of choice.

The possibility of a significant cervical spine injury should always be considered, particularly if the patient is unconscious. If such an injury is considered, the head and neck should be immobilized and cervical spine roentgenograms obtained.

PSYCHIATRIC DISORDERS

Disorders of thought, emotion, and life adjustment may be a result of mild and transient life stresses or may relate to underlying severe abnormalities of mental function. The spectrum of normal function merges with the abnormal. In some individuals, the criteria for a psychiatric disorder can be clearly identified and appropriate treatment can be considered.

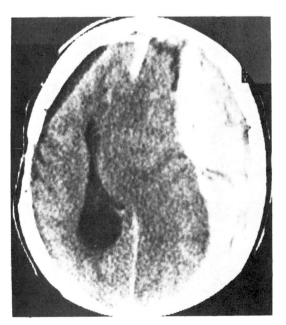

Fig. 14.27 Brain CT scan of a patient with an acute left subdural hematoma following head injury. Lateral ventricles are displaced to the right

A comprehensive approach to psychiatry is beyond the scope of this text. Three major aspects will be discussed, as they relate to medical illness:

1. A classification of psychiatric disease
2. An overview of psychiatric emergencies
3. Psychiatric problems frequently encountered in hospitalized patients.

CLASSIFICATION OF PSYCHIATRIC DISORDERS

Table 14.32 indicates the major categories of psychiatric disease. For further information, the reader should consult *The Diagnostic Statistical Manual of Mental Disorders*, referenced at the end of this chapter. This recent publication represents the best synthesis of diagnostic criteria currently available, and presents a detailed discussion of each condition.

Organic Mental Disorders

These include behavioral disturbances caused by or associated with impairment of brain tissue function. Symptoms are due to deterioration of cerebral function, and to psychologic reactions associated with the loss of function. Entirely different physical illnesses affecting the brain can at times lead to identical behavioral disturbances. Dementia and delirium are the two major syndromes resulting from organic brain disease (see Disorders of Consciousness). In addition, organic hallucinosis may occur in alcohol and drug withdrawal states. Other abnormal behavioral states may arise due to organic disease, for example, the apathetic personality of the patient with bilateral frontal lobe lesions.

Management consists of treating the underlying disease where possible, and symptomatic therapy of behavioral disturbances. Special attention must be given to the use of medications in these patients. The fragile demented elderly patient requires smaller doses of antidepressants, and may suffer more from drug side effects. If agitation is a problem, it is often better to use low doses of phenothiazines such as thioridazine (Mellaril), rather than benzodiazepines or barbiturates, which tend to be long acting and may exacerbate the patient's confusion.

Table 14.32 Psychiatric Disorders

Organic Mental Disorders
Schizophrenic Disorders
Affective Disorders
Anxiety-Based Disorders
Personality Disorders

Schizophrenic Disorders

Schizophrenia occurs with approximately equal prevalence in all cultures. Approximately 0.5 percent of the population is affected. The main features of this group of disorders are abnormalities in thought content, mood, and behavior. Schizophrenia can be subdivided into catatonic, paranoid, and other types. Schizophrenics are usually alert; memory and orientation are preserved. These features help distinguish schizophrenics from patients with organic mental syndromes in which confusion, disorientation, and amnesia are prominent manifestations. The four fundamental symptoms of schizophrenia are the following:

1. An associative disturbance (thinking becomes bizarre and illogical)
2. Autism (the patient is preoccupied with ideas derived from fantasies and reality testing is impaired)
3. Affective incongruity (mood is often inconsistent or exaggerated, flat, or blunted)
4. Ambivalence (contradictory feelings and attitudes are abnormally intense).

Common manifestations of thought disorder in schizophrenia are muteness, thought blocking, neologism, verbigerations, difficulties with abstract thought, and difficulty in screening out irrelevant material. Hallucinations, delusions, illusions, and ideas of reference may be prominent.

Transient reactive psychoses that show somewhat similar symptomatology may be seen from time to time.

The etiology of schizophrenia is unknown, but a relative overactivity of dopaminergic systems in the brain has been postulated. This is supported by the fact that many drugs effective in the treatment of schizophrenia are dopamine-receptor blocking agents.

Treatment is primarily pharmacologic, with phenothiazines or related drugs proving most effective. Hospitalization may be necessary during acute exacerbations of the disease, but with long-term phenothiazine therapy and social support systems, most of these patients can now be treated as outpatients with only intermittent hospitalization.

Affective Disorders

In the affective disorders, alterations of mood, both depression and mania (bipolar), are prominent. Primary depression occurs *de novo*, unrelated to another psychiatric disorder or physical illness. It is characterized by varying degrees of psychomotor and vegetative dysfunction, hopelessness, and feelings of worthlessness and guilt. Secondary depression may occur in the course of life stresses, often associated with anxiety neurosis or medical illness. Symptoms of depression include lowered self-esteem, guilt feelings, loss of energy, and loss of interest. Vegetative changes, likely reflecting hypothalamic dysfunction, include anorexia, unintentional weight loss, insomnia, and reduced libido. Poor concentration is often complained of, and either psychomotor retardation or agitation may be present. Thoughts of death and suicide are common. Mania is at the opposite pole from depression; it is characterized by elevated mood, motor overactivity, pressure of speech, flight of ideas, hallucinations and delusions, and impaired judgment and insight. Diagnosis of a bipolar illness requires a history of hypomania or mania in the patient or a close family member. Patients with manic episodes are termed *bipolar 1*. Patients with both manic and depressive episodes are termed *bipolar 2*. A unipolar illness has depressive episodes only. Patients with mania frequently have a positive family history, and genetic factors may be important. Patients with depression only are less likely to have a positive family history. Patients with mania and depression appear to have disturbances in catecholamine and indoleamine neuronal systems. Tricyclic antidepressants and monamine oxidase inhibitors used in treatment of depression tend to elevate CNS levels of these neurotransmitters.

Lithium will induce remission of mania and also some biologically based depressions. It is useful in prophylaxis of bipolar affective disorders. Brain cells of patients responsive to lithium therapy appear to have membrane defects and accumulate lithium more than cells of nonresponsive patients or normal controls. Lithium serum levels must be monitored and maintained in the therapeutic range. Symptoms and signs of lithium toxicity include confusion, obtundation, tremulousness, myoclonus, muscle twitching, and ataxia. Clinical signs of lithium intoxication occasionally can occur with lithium blood levels within the usual therapeutic range, particularly when the patient is also taking other medications. Tricyclic antidepressants are useful in the treatment of acute depression, and as prophylaxis to prevent cyclic recurrences. Use of electroconvulsive therapy and monamine oxidase inhibitors is at present limited, but these agents are still occasionally helpful.

Anxiety-Based Disorders

Anxiety is an unpleasant sensation similar to fear, but does not have an external object, or is greatly out of proportion to any external threat. In its milder form, it can be called apprehension, and in its most severe form, panic. The anxiety-based disorders generally have onset in adult life. A period wherein anxiety itself is the main symptom may precede other symptoms. Disability is usually relatively mild.

These disorders are subdivided into a number of subtypes. Phobic disorders include agoraphobia, claustrophobia, and others. Somatoform disorders include somatization, conversion disorders, psychogenic pain, and hypochondriasis. Dissociative disorders such as fugue states, multiple personality states, and depersonalization are also classified here, as are obsessive compulsive disorders. The etiology of all of these disorders is unknown. Conflicts over sexuality, dependency, and aggression have figured prominently in theories of etiology. In some patients anxiety leads to the hyperventilation syndrome (see Chapter 15), chest pain mimicking coronary artery disease (see Chapter 16), headaches, indigestion, inability to concentrate, and drug abuse. The underlying emotional state may only become apparent after extensive unrewarding search for organic disease. Specific features of anxiety should be identified, for example, agitation, changes in behavior or performance, insomnia, and fear.

Treatments are multiple, and consist of psychotherapy, including, in severe disorders, psychoanalysis, group psychotherapy, desensitization and aversion techniques, assertion training, and behavior modification techniques.

Personality Disorders

These disorders are behavioral aberrations acquired early in life and are relatively chronic. They can present with varying degrees of severity. Among these disorders are paranoid, schizoid, histrionic, compulsive, dependent, passive aggressive, and borderline personality disorders.

Particular mention must be made of the psychopathic or antisocial personality disorder. These individuals appear unable to relate in a meaningful way to other people or to empathize with them. They do not experience anxiety while planning or performing acts that would produce anxiety in normal individuals. They are impulsive, often aggressive, and seem unable to learn from experience or to postpone gratification.

Because of these characteristics, psychopaths frequently run afoul of the law. Eventually, after 30 years of age, many psychopaths become less aggressive. They then tend to be inadequate individuals with chronic unemployment and transient social relationships. The etiology of psychopathy is unknown, although both constitutional factors and environmental factors have been postulated to be important.

Suicide

Suicide is considered acceptable in some societies. In North America and Western Europe, the vast majority of patients who commit suicide appear to be suffering from a psychiatric illness. Patients with fatal or incurable physical illnesses account for only a small proportion of suicides.

When a patient has attempted suicide or appears at risk for suicide, it is necessary to judge the actual risk, since this has implications for management.

Several guidelines are helpful. Most patients who commit suicide are depressed. A severe depression with somatic complaints and vegetative symptoms (insomnia and the like) increases the risk of suicide. Hopelessness expressed by the patient and a history of prior suicide attempts further increases the risk. The patient should be asked directly whether he is preoccupied with thoughts of death and suicide, and whether he has made any plans to kill himself. If he has a logical and well thought out plan, the risk is increased. Suicidal risk is increased in the single, widowed, or divorced person. Males have a higher risk of successfully completing suicide than females. If the patient has just attempted suicide, the seriousness of the present attempt indicates the risk of further attempts. Evidence of careful planning and premeditation indicates serious risk, as does being alone at the time of the suicide attempt. Over 6 percent of patients with a serious attempt will successfully commit suicide within 5 years. This is more than double the rate after nonserious attempts. The presence of adequate social support systems for the patient reduces the risk.

Suicidal risk can also be high in hallucinating schizophrenics and in acutely delerious patients. Alcoholism may cause depression and increases the risk of suicide.

Management of suicidal patients consists primarily of careful observation. Patients should be hospitalized if they

1. are over 45 years of age and have just made their first suicide attempt;
2. have just survived a violent near-lethal premeditated attempt;
3. took precautions to avoid being rescued;
4. attempted suicide and have psychosis or lack of social support; or
5. survived the suicide attempt but refuse help.

With present medical practice, approximately 65 percent of patients are sent home from emergency departments the same day of the suicide attempt. Ninety-nine percent of these patients are alive at the end of 1 year. Once the patient with a suicide attempt is admitted to hospital, further suicide attempts in hospital are unusual, except in the young schizophrenic patient and the middle-aged severely depressed patient. These patients should be watched very carefully. The first 3 months after discharge are also very high-risk periods for these patients.

Patients admitted for nonpsychiatric conditions make up the majority of in-hospital suicides in general hospitals. These patients frequently have emotional stresses in addition to their physical illness, and a loss of emotional support. Others have an acute organic brain syndrome with confusion. Patients with chronic renal failure on dialysis have a particularly high risk of suicide; perhaps as many as 5 percent of such patients dying of suicide.

Treatment of the patient who becomes suicidal in hospital consists of removing all potentially dangerous objects from the room and effectively locking the window. Careful observation is most important, with someone remaining with the patient at all times if the risk is considered serious. The patient should be given the emotional support and attention he needs, and given control over his situation insofar as is medically possible.

The Violent Patient

Psychotic patients and patients in delirious states such as alcohol withdrawal can occasionally become violent. Individuals with this potential as indicated by past history should be treated with appropriate medications to prevent a violent outbreak. The presence of a friend or relative, in addition to a special hospital attendant, is often useful in handling these situations.

When a patient becomes obstreperous or threatens violence, and must be physically subdued, the best policy is to muster a sufficient number of attendants quickly in order to achieve this. Attempting to subdue such patients without sufficient manpower can be disastrous. For these agitated patients, chlorpromazine 50 to 100 mg or haloperidol 5 mg given intramuscularly every 1 to 3 hours is usually effective. Occasionally larger doses may be called for. Body restraints are necessary at times, but may precipitate or increase agitation. Establishing verbal contact with the violent patient and encouraging him to talk freely about his current feelings may defuse the situation and allow successful administration of medication.

Panic States

These are most commonly caused by anxiety disorders. Acute schizophrenic psychosis, hallucinogens (bad trip), amphetamine intoxication, and delirium are less common causes. Patients with anxiety disorders will usually respond to sympathy and reassurance, and discuss their feelings with the physician. The psychotic patient is less likely to do so.

Management must be individualized. Phenothiazines are useful in psychotic patients. For panic states associated with hallucinogenic substances, support and reassurance (talking the person down) is the treatment of choice. This is usually effective if done by a friend of the patient. Constant supervision in a quiet lighted room is important. If sedation is necessary, diazepam, short-acting barbiturates, or chloral hydrate are the best agents to use. Patients with anxiety disorders may require long-term support and careful management. If medication is needed, low doses of tricyclic antidepressant drugs (imipramine) is often best. Alcohol withdrawal is treated as outlined in Chapter 1.

PROBLEMS ARISING IN HOSPITALIZED PATIENTS

The Demanding Patient

Demanding patients create problems on hospital wards because they request or feel entitled to more services than the staff deems appropriate. A number of underlying disorders may result in demanding patients. The patient may be an obsessive compulsive perfectionist who finds it difficult to cope with reality, that is, the hospital ward environment. In other cases, excessive demands by the patient are a compensation for the helplessness that the patient feels as a result of his illness. Passive-aggressive individuals may also become a problem because of demanding behavior, and in these patients this may reflect hostility to other patients and hospital staff.

In managing these patients, it is important that the staff discuss in detail with the patient what is reasonable, and hopefully a suitable compromise can be made. It is always better to confront such patients in a reasonable but firm manner rather than to let their demands continue until the staff becomes so angry that compromise is impossible. Limits should be set, and in many cases the patient will accept these. The staff should recognize the anger aroused in themselves by such patients, and should act in a positive manner to resolve the situation rather than simply avoid the patient.

Sign-Out Against Medical Advice

Many patients who threaten to sign themselves out are dissuaded from doing so when they speak with a reasonable physician who will act as their advocate. Rather than a sudden spontaneous act, the patient's threat to sign himself out is usually the result of a series of incidents between the patient and the hospital staff. The patient usually feels he has been mistreated, misunderstood, or that his case has been mismanaged. The best course of action is to find an individual, preferably a physician, who can discuss the situation with the patient, and assure the patient that he has an ally. Patients are usually relieved at being able to remain in hospital, once it appears that a resolution of their perceived problem is in sight. If the problem cannot be resolved, an overnight pass frequently helps if this is medically possible. This gives the patient a sense of control, and may resolve the situation.

The individual with organic brain disease who is having difficulty coping with a strange hospital setting may develop panic and anxiety, and be difficult to deal with by the above methods. Round-the-clock attendance by a family member and careful explanations by the hospital staff usually resolve this situation.

REFERENCES

Clinical Approach to Neurologic Problems

1. DeMyer W.: Technique of the Neurologic Examination. New York, McGraw-Hill, 1969.
2. Mayo Clinic and Mayo Foundation: Clinical Examinations in Neurology. Philadelphia, W.B. Saunders, 1976.

Clinical Localization of Neurologic Disorders

3. Baloh, R.W., Honrubia, V.: Clinical Neurophysiology of the Vestibular System. Philadelphia, F.A. Davis, 1979.
4. Brodal, A.: Neurological Anatomy. New York, Oxford University Press, 1981.
5. Geschwind, N.: Aphasia. N. Engl. J. Med. 284:654, 1971.
6. Glaser, J.S.: Neuro-ophthalmology. Hagerstown, Maryland, Harper & Row, 1978.
7. Kertesz, A.: Aphasia and Associated Disorders. New York, Grune & Stratton, 1979.
8. Dyck, P.J., Thomas, P.K., Lambert, E.H.: Peripheral Neuropathy. Philadelphia, W.B. Saunders, 1975.
9. Eldrige, R., Fahn, S.: Dystonia. Advances in Neurology. Vol 14. New York, Raven Press, 1976.
10. Gilman, S., Bloedel, J.R., Lechtenberg, R.: Disorders of the Cerebellum. Philadelphia, F.A. Davis, 1981.

Disorders of Consciousness

11. Plum, F., Posner, J.B.: The Diagnosis of Stupor and Coma. Philadelphia, F.A. Davis, 1980.

Epilepsy

12. Eadie, M.J., Tyrer, J.H.: Anticonvulsant Therapy. 2nd ed. Edinburgh, Churchhill Livingstone, 1980.
13. Jennett, B.: Epilepsy After Non-Missile Head Injuries. Chicago, Year Book Med. Pub., 1975.
14. Richens, A.: Drug Treatment of Epilepsy. Chicago, Year Book Med. Pub., 1976.

Dementia

15. Strub, R.L., Black, F.W.: The Mental Status Examination in Neurology. Philadelphia, F.A. Davis, 1977.
16. Victor, M., Adams, R.D., Collins, G.H.: The Wernicke-Korsakoff Syndrome. Philadelphia, F.A. Davis, 1971.
17. Wells, C.E.: Dementia. 2nd ed. Philadelphia, FA Davis, 1977.

Headache

18. Dalessio, D.J.: Wolff's Headache and Other Head Pain. 4th ed. New York, Oxford University Press, 1980.
19. Lance, W.J.: Mechanism and Management of Headache. 3rd ed. London, Butterworths, 1978.
20. Raskin, N.H., Appenzeller O: Headache. In: Smith L.H., (ed.) Major Problems In Internal Medicine, vol XIX. Philadelphia, WB Saunders, 1980.
21. Sacks, O.W.: Migraine. Berkeley, University of California Press, 1970.

Cerebrovascular Disorders

22. Easton, J.D., Sherman, D.G.: Management of Cerebral Embolism of Cardiac Origin. Stroke 11:433, 1980.
23. Russell, R.W.R.: Cerebral Arterial Disease. Edinburgh, Churchill Livingston, 1976.
24. Sandok, B.A., Furlan, A.J., Whisnant, J.P., et al: Guidelines for the Management of transient ischemic attacks. Mayo. Clin. Proc. 53:665, 1978.
25. The Canadian Cooperative Study Group: A randomized trial of aspirin and sulfinpyrazone in threatened stroke. N. Engl. J. Med., 299:53, 1978.

Central Nervous System Neoplasms

26. Weiss, L., Gilbert, H.A., Posner, J.B.: Brain Metastasis. Boston, G.K. Hall, 1980.

Demyelinating Disorders

27. McAlpine, D., Lumsden, C.E., Acheson, E.D.: Multiple Sclerosis: A Reappraisal. Edinburgh, Churchill Livingstone, 1972.

Psychiatric Disorders

28. Diagnostic and Statistical Manual of Mental Disorders. 3rd ed. American Psychiatric Association, 1980.
29. Hackett, T.P., Cassem, N.H., eds: Handbook of General Hospital Psychiatry. Saint Louis, C.V. Mosby, 1978.
30. Liebowitz, M.R., Klein, D.F.: Differential diagnosis and treatment of panic attacks and phobic states. Ann. Rev. Med, 32:583, 1981.

15

The Respiratory System

Clarence A. Guenter, M.D.

Many clinical respiratory problems occur predictably in certain age groups, in epidemics, or on the basis of environmental factors. Examples include the neonatal respiratory distress syndrome, which is a major cause of morbidity and mortality in premature infants, and acute viral respiratory tract infections, which are very common in children 6 months to 6 years of age. The socioeconomically deprived frequently suffer more severe disease as a result of malnourishment, overcrowding, and high rates of transmission of infection. In the undeveloped countries, childhood mortality may range as high as 50 percent, with diarrheal diseases and respiratory infections as the major causes of death. A wide variety of illnesses occur sporadically throughout the subsequent years of life, with chronic bronchitis, emphysema, and lung cancer gaining prominence in the fifth and sixth decades.

Environmental factors can now be implicated in most common lung diseases. Infectious agents transmitted by airborne droplet nuclei, occupationally generated organic and inorganic dust, and cigarette smoke are the most common established causes. Host factors, such as immunity to infection, immunologic reactions to inhaled antigens and genetic predisposition, may be as important as duration and extent of exposure in determining the development or severity of these diseases.

The lungs are commonly involved secondarily as a result of injury, infection, or disease in other organ systems. Patients with septic shock, multiple organ system failure, extensive trauma, or postoperative complications of surgery performed on areas remote from the thorax commonly develop respiratory failure by mechanisms not clearly understood. Thromboembolic phenomena, whose major manifestations may appear in the respiratory system, generally result from venous thrombosis due to immobilization or vascular injury related to other diseases.

The challenge lies in identifying and treating the lung disease, as well as correcting abnormal gas exchange. The physician must frequently ask himself, "Might these symptoms be a result of respiratory failure?" or, "How will this lung problem affect oxygen and carbon dioxide transport in the blood?". Central nervous system dysfunction, cardiac dysfunction, or acid-base disturbances may be predominantly a result of respiratory problems in patients with severe or complex lung diseases.

SYMPTOMS AND SIGNS OF RESPIRATORY DISEASE

RESPIRATORY SYMPTOMS

Cough

Cough is a major lung defence mechanism. This reflex is stimulated by mechanical deformation or chemical irritation of irritant receptors in the mucosa of the larynx and tracheobronchial tree. Stimulation of the reflex results in an inspiratory phase, adduction of the vocal chords, and finally a forceful contraction of the abdominal and expiratory intercostal muscles, generating a high intrathoracic pressure that is followed by rapid opening of the glottis. The high intrapulmonary pressures result in rapid expiratory flow of air, which carries mucus through the larger bronchi, the trachea, and the laryngeal structures. Cough is a common symptom of acute or chronic irritation of the tracheobronchial tree. Mild respiratory tract infection such as the common cold, severe parenchymal disease such as pneumonia, or nonpulmonary problems such as cardiogenic pulmonary edema—all may present with cough as a prominent symptom.It is important to determine whether the cough is dry and nonproductive or is associated with expectoration. If productive, is the sputum white and mucoid, purulent, or blood containing? How much sputum is produced? The persistent, irritated nonproductive cough of a viral tracheobronchitis or pneumonia is commonly quite distinctive from the gurgling cough productive of purulent sputum associated with bacterial pneumonia or bronchiectasis. Cough associated with exposure to dust, cold air, or nocturnal cough may raise suspicion of bronchial asthma. Most patients with infectious diseases and cough are somewhat improved during sleep. The cough reflex can be suppressed by drugs, and may be diminished in neuromuscular diseases. Diminished sensitivity of the cough reflex predisposes to aspiration of foreign material, and neuromuscular weakness may impair the clearance effect of the cough reflex.

Dyspnea

Dyspnea, or shortness of breath, is a common complaint useful in directing the attention of the physician to disease of the respiratory or cardiovascular system. It is a complex symptom indicating a distressing sensation associated with breathing, but is interpreted differently by different patients and different physicians. Other feelings of discomfort in the chest, such as angina pectoris and pain caused by pleural or chest wall diseases, must be differentiated from dyspnea. Awareness of normal breathing or of normally increased ventilation during exercise must not be confused with dyspnea. Patients with the hyperventilation syndrome complain of dyspnea even though their arterial oxygen level is high and their carbon dioxide level is abnormally low. This is a neurotic misinterpretation. Individuals with severe hypoxemia at high altitude experience only mild dyspnea even when the reduced oxygen levels might be life-threatening. Conversely, patients with lung fibrosis may experience severe dyspnea when their arterial blood gases are near normal. Patients with respiratory muscle weakness commonly develop respiratory failure with only minimal dyspnea.

These facts demonstrate the complex pathophysiology that must enter into the interpretation of breathlessness; there is no uniformly satisfactory theory to explain the symptom. The most generally applicable theory suggests that dyspnea depends on awareness of respiratory movements and mechanical loading of the respiratory muscles and tendons. Thus, an inappropriate degree of breathing activity may be interpreted as an inappropriate load. It is generally useful to clarify what circumstances or activities cause dyspnea, to what extent the patient is incapacitated, and what factors are known to relieve the symptoms. The classification used by the New York Heart Association is a useful means of standardization, and is presented in Chapter 16.

Chest Pain

The major characteristics of chest pain associated with severe intrathoracic disease are discussed in Chapter 16. The central burning chest pain commonly associated with acute infectious tracheitis may occasionally be confused with ischemic heart pain. Aggravation by cough generally permits the correct diagnosis. Pleuritic chest pain is commonly sharp and clearly related to factors causing friction between pleural surfaces such as respiratory motion and cough; the most important diagnostic confusion is occasioned by pain that arises from intercostal muscles, ribs, or costochondral cartilages. These can readily be identified by palpable localized chest wall tenderness. The onset and duration of pain as well as associated symptoms are useful additional information.

Hemoptysis

It is most important, and often difficult, to ascertain whether the symptom of hemoptysis reflects blood coughed up from the tracheobronchial tree, or blood that may have been coughed from the posterior pharynx as a result of hematemesis or epistaxis. True hemoptysis is generally a serious symptom. Frank blood produced in a patient without known respiratory disease requires detailed investigation. Flecks of blood streaked sputum in a patient with pneumonia, known bronchiectasis, chronic bronchitis, or a severe viral tracheobronchitis generally warrants observation without specific evaluation. The most common causes of frank hemoptysis are lung cancer, pulmonary infarction, chronic tracheobronchial infection such as bronchiectasis, and very rarely, tuberculosis. Recurrent or progressive hemoptysis is an indication for examination of the larynx and tracheobronchial tree by bronchoscopy, if physical examination and chest roentgenogram have not identified the cause.

Table 15.1 Physical Findings in Pulmonary Disease

	Chest Movement During Breathing	Position of Trachea (Mediastinum)	Percussion Note	Transmitted Sounds		Adventitious Sounds
				Tactile Fremitus	Breath Sounds	
Atelectasis (Collapse)	→	T	dull	↑ or ↓ᵃ	↑ or ↓ᵇ	Crackles
Pleural Effusion	→	A	dull	→	→	? rub
Pneumothorax	→	A	resonant	→	←	—
Consolidation	→	N	dull	←	←	crackles
Bronchopneumonia	→N	N	dull	→ or ↑ᵇ	→ or ↑ᵇ	crackles, wheezes
Emphysema	N	N	resonant	→	↓	crackles, wheezes
Asthma	N	N	N	N	←	wheezes

ᵃ increased with peripheral lung collapse, decreased with lobar obstruction
ᵇ depends on associated bronchial obstruction
↓ Decreased
↑ Increased
N Normal
T Toward affected side
A Away from affected side

Wheezing

Wheezing represents whistling noises created by turbulence through bronchial tubes. Patients with bronchial asthma or chronic bronchitis are frequently aware of audible wheezing that may be more severe at times when symptoms are worse or when mucoid secretions accumulate in the tracheobronchial tree. Occasionally patients recognize that the wheeze is generated in one side of the chest, when a major bronchus is obstructed by a foreign body, tumor, or stenosis. When wheezing is present it can be confirmed by auscultation of the thorax. Wheezing was once considered the cardinal manifestation of bronchial asthma, but nocturnal breathlessness and cough are now recognized with at least equal frequency.

NONRESPIRATORY SYMPTOMS

Exercise Intolerance (Easy Fatigability)

Patients with severe respiratory failure commonly develop easy fatigability. They may describe this as weakness, lack of energy, or inability to perform previously accustomed activities. Most commonly, dyspnea is the presenting complaint, but fatigue may be a more prominent symptom, particularly in severely hypoxemic patients.

Headaches

Severe hypoxemia, with or without retention of carbon dioxide and respiratory acidosis, may result in headaches. These headaches are commonly more severe at night or early in the morning after rising. Current evidence regarding nocturnal hypoxemia suggests that severe dips in oxygen saturation during sleep may contribute to these symptoms. Patients with advanced respiratory failure may develop elevated cerebrospinal fluid pressure and papilledema. These symptoms are occasionally misinterpreted as manifestations of cerebral tumors (pseudotumor).

Confusion, Irritability

Patients with severe hypoxemia may develop a wide range of central nervous system signs including, first, poor judgment, then, confusion, and eventually coma. During the intermediate stages, marked irritability may be present, frequently associated with discoordinated ataxic movements. The mechanisms are not clearly established but improvement in blood gases generally results in amelioration of the symptoms.

Sleep Disorders

Insomnia is a common complaint in patients with respiratory disorders. Acute infections often result in cough, causing sleep disturbances. Obstruction of nasal passages, chronic bronchitis and emphysema, thoracic wall deformities, and a variety of other lung diseases have been associated with marked disturbances of sleep with periods of profound nocturnal hypoxemia. Excessive daytime somnolence is also a frequent clue to disordered breathing during sleep (see subsequent discussion under Disorders of Respiratory Control).

Edema

Patients with chronic respiratory failure commonly have edema of the lower extremities. Those with cor pulmonale may have edema due to right heart failure; however, it more commonly results from inactivity while patients are sitting upright; the partial occlusion of the dependent leg veins causes hydrostatically induced edema. When the edema is markedly asymmetric, the possibility of lower limb venous thrombosis must be considered.

PHYSICAL SIGNS IN PULMONARY DISEASE

Major clinical signs of lung disease relate to mechanical changes in the lungs and peripheral manifestations of abnormal gas exchange. The clinical features are discussed in relation to individual conditions. Table 15.1 illustrates comparative changes useful in identifying disease. Cyanosis is discussed later under Oxygen Transport; Clubbing, and Osteoarthropathy in the section entitled Lung Cancer.

LABORATORY DIAGNOSIS OF RESPIRATORY DISEASES

TESTS OF LUNG FUNCTION

Ventilatory Function

The best understood and most commonly used tests of lung function involve measurement of (1) the vital capacity (VC);(2) the timed vital capacity, with particular emphasis on the forced expiratory flow in the first second(FEV$_{1.0}$);(3) the maximum midexpiratory flow rate, or forced midexpiratory flow (FEF$_{25-75\%}$); and (4) the maximum voluntary ventilation (MVV). These are readily measured on any water-sealed spirometer, and the first three are readily measured on most electronic or simple bedside spirographs now available. The VC is a reasonable estimate of the overall inspiratory strength and the distensibility of the respiratory system. It is reduced as a result of poor effort, muscle weakness, skeletal disease of the chest wall, obesity, and lung disease resulting in low compliance. The VC is not a sensitive test for subtle or minimal disease. The FEV$_{1.0}$ is a measure of clinically significant obstruction to air flow, and is somewhat less sensitive than the FEF$_{25-75\%}$. The MVV is a sprint test of lung function, and may be abnormal with muscle weakness, poor effort, or as a result of restrictive or obstructive lung disease.

Abnormalities of ventilatory function identified on the spirogram are generally termed *obstructive* if the major abnormality is a reduced rate of expiratory air flow, and *restrictive* if the major abnormality is a reduced vital capacity. Many lung diseases have mixed abnormalities. The test must be performed with the physician or technician and the patient well informed and enthusiastic. A full effort will generally be demonstrated by highly reproducible curves, with results varying by no more than 5 to 7 percent. A minimum of three efforts should be recorded, and more if these are not reproducible.

While the spirogram is a relatively crude test of lung function, and cannot be counted on to pick up very early disease, it is generally abnormal in patients who have dyspnea due to lung disease.

The flow-volume loop is now preferred as a measure of ventilatory function, at least partly because it also allows assessment of inspiration. Inspiratory flow rates are reduced in upper airway obstruction, and appear to be abnormal in many patients with obstructive sleep apnea. The vital capacity, timed vital capacity, expiratory flow rates, and inspiratory flow rates, all can be calculated from the flow-volume loop.

Some very useful measures of ventilatory function are related to static lung volumes; these are the residual volume, the functional residual, and the total lung capacity. The residual volume is the component that cannot be measured by the normal spirogram or the flow-volume loop. The vital capacity may be reduced by obesity or lung fibrosis, in which these volumes are all reduced, or by emphysema, in which all volumes are above normal. These measurements require a well-standardized pulmonary function laboratory, but a good estimate may be obtained from routine chest roentgenograms. When the diaphragms remain elevated (10th posterior rib or above) during deep inspiration, the total lung capacity is probably reduced. When the diaphragms are below the 11th rib, and particularly if the upward convex curvature in the lateral view is flattened, the total lung capacity is probably increased.

More subtle abnormalities of ventilatory function can be identified by a measurement of the closing volume, an analysis of alveolar gas concentrations during slow expiration, and other tests of "small airways function." There is strong recent evidence that mild but definite abnormalities in peripheral airway function are demonstrable in cigarette smokers, workers exposed to grain dust, and persons exposed to other occupational pollutants. These changes may precede the development of more severe lung disease. While these more subtle abnormalities are of particular interest in research regarding pathogenesis and epidemiology of disease, they have little relevance to bedside assessment of symptomatic patients.

Gas Exchange in the Lungs

Gas transfer from the alveoli to the blood is generally assessed indirectly by measuring the effects on gas levels in the blood leaving the lungs. Such measures represent an overall average, and may not demonstrate the severity of abnormalities in small regions of lung.

Arterial oxygenation can be assessed by transcutaneous spectrophotometry using a commercially available oximeter. The results correlate well with arterial blood saturations, but the instrumentation is not commonly available, and it is costly. Most hospitals are equipped to analyze arterial blood gases. The use of blood gas analysis in assessing oxygen and carbon dioxide transport is discussed in the subsequent section entitled Abnormal Oxygen Transport and Respiratory Failure.

Other measures of gas exchange in the lung are available. The carbon monoxide diffusing capacity (D$_{LCO}$) is a measure of carbon monoxide diffusion and combination with hemoglobin. It is utilized because of its similarity to oxygen in transfer and hemoglobin binding. This is not purely a test of diffusion but rather a measure of gas transfer. The carbon monoxide diffusing capacity is reduced in diseases with reduced capillary surface area (pneumonectomy and emphysema), pulmonary vascular obstruction (pulmonary embolism), and diseases affecting alveolar wall and lung interstitium (pulmonary fibrosis and pulmonary edema). It is frequently abnormal in disease in patients who still have near-normal arterial blood gases at rest. There is a very wide range of normal values for the carbon monoxide diffusion capacity. Consequently, the test is more useful in follow-up of an individual patient to document the course of disease or the response to therapy, rather than in diagnosis.

Blood gas exchange varies greatly throughout the day with activity, with position, and during sleep. Complete assessment of the patient may require analysis of blood gas exchange under a wide variety of conditions.

Distribution of Ventilation and Perfusion

In patients with disease of an entire lobe of lung, physical examination generally demonstrates changes in percussion note or breath sounds (Table 15.1). A simple posteroanterior chest roentgenogram will reveal atelectasis, consolidation, or infarction. Similarly, a large pleural effusion or pneumothorax is readily recognized clinically. Partial dysfunction of a lung region or diffuse abnormalities may be more difficult to identify on physical examination. Radionuclide lung scans may be performed after inhaling the radioisotope by counting the radioactivity over multiple lung regions or photographing the entire lung field with an Anger camera. Segmental or lobar abnormalities in ventilation will be readily identified by the decreased radioactivity, and subsegmental areas will demonstrate a mottling effect. Computerized techniques permit detailed analysis of relatively small lung regions.

Assessment of regional perfusion to the lung is much more difficult. The stethoscope cannot discriminate an obstructed pulmonary artery in the same way that it can discriminate an obstructed airway. Injection of radionuclides into the venous system will result in distribution of the isotope to the pulmonary circulation. Generally, macroaggregates are tagged with the radioisotope, and they sequester in the lung capillaries. Consequently, radioactivity will be identified wherever there is lung perfusion, and it will concentrate in proportion to the blood flow through that region. Pneumonia, pleural effusion, bullous emphysema, and pulmonary embolism all result in localized abnormalities of perfusion. Generalized obstructive lung disease often results in a mottling defect. While a normal lung scan practically excludes thromboembolism, an abnormal lung scan is compatible with many diseases (see Chapter 4).

RADIOGRAPHIC INVESTIGATION

The chest roentgenogram is a first-line investigation in patients with many respiratory diseases. The posteroanterior exposure permits visualization of most of the bony thorax, the lateral margins of the mediastinum, and about 70 percent of the lung parenchyma. The trachea and major bronchi are commonly apparent. A lateral chest roentgenogram allows visualization of another 20 percent of lung field, including the retrocardiac area and the retrosternal area. Detailed approaches to interpreting the chest roentgenogram must be part of the expertise of every physician generalist.

Isotope imaging of lung perfusion and ventilation is particularly useful, as already discussed.

Tomographic views of the lung field permit sharper focus at different prescribed levels in the chest. Abnormalities in the hila, obscure infiltrates or masses, and evidence of calcification can be best clarified by tomographic views. Oblique views with overpenetration are helpful in the diagnosis of rib fractures. Lateral decubitus views will demonstrate subpulmonic and small pleural effusions. A film exposed during expiration will amplify a small pneumothorax, making it more readily identifiable. Ultrasound is useful in localizing loculated pleural effusions. Computed tomography (CT scan) is particularly helpful in mediastinal disease.

ELECTROCARDIOGRAPHY

The electrocardiogram may show abnormalities suggestive of pulmonary hypertension as indicated by right ventricular and right atrial changes (see Cor Pulmonale, Chapter 16).

ANALYSIS OF PLEURAL FLUID

Pleural effusions that are large enough to be radiographically demonstrable may require aspiration and analysis. These are discussed in detail in the section entitled Pleural Diseases.

SPUTUM ANALYSIS

Sputum expectorated from the lower respiratory tract is very useful in identifying infectious agents, and may be a suitable source of material for cytologic screening for tumors.

In general the sputum should be collected by the

physician to be sure that it represents a deep coughed specimen. The tenacious mucoid portion of sputum may be cultured for aerobic organisms, and should be Gram stained. The Gram stain preparation will permit an assessment of whether the material is predominantly saliva (with many squamous epithelial cells) or a lower respiratory tract sample. If there is a preponderance of one type of bacterial organism such as *Streptococcus pneumonia*, it may be highly suggestive of the etiology of infection. Microorganisms present within the polymorphonuclear leukocytes are more likely playing an important role in infection.

When patients with lung infection are unable to provide an adequate sputum specimen, when they have complex or resistant lung infections, or when anerobic infections are suspected, transtracheal aspiration of the airways may be necessary. Transtracheal aspirates are less contaminated by oral flora and yield a much higher proportion of etiologic organisms. Cultures for fungi, tuberculosis, and other agents may require special media.

Sputum to be used in cytologic screening for tumor is best collected in the morning. Patients with bronchogenic carcinoma, particularly the squamous cell type; have the highest positive yield.

BIOCHEMICAL TESTS

A wide range of biochemical abnormalities occurs in lung disease. Serum lactic dehydrogenase is often elevated in pulmonary infarction and diffuse lung fibrosis. Angiotension-converting enzyme is commonly increased in patients with active sarcoidosis. Lung tumors are frequently associated with metabolic and endocrine abnormalities. Each of these laboratory findings is discussed in relation to the pertinent diseases.

ABNORMAL OXYGEN TRANSPORT AND RESPIRATORY FAILURE

Cellular metabolism throughout the body depends on respiration. Delivery of oxygen to the cells organelles and removal of carbon dioxide from the cell are the final major functions of gas exchange in the lung. Gas exchange in the tissues is therefore dependent on several steps in the respiratory pathway:

1. Inspired gas concentrations
2. Alveolar ventilation in the lung
3. Oxygen binding to hemoglobin in the blood

4. Cardiac output
5. Regional perfusion to tissues
6. Tissue factors.

Reduced oxygen delivery to the cells is known as *tissue hypoxia*, and should not generally be referred to as *anoxia* unless there is a complete absence of blood flow. When tissue hypoxia is predominantly a result of diminished blood flow, it is commonly referred to as *ischemia*. Mild tissue hypoxia may result in subtle changes in organ function, such as impaired judgment or perception—the earliest changes in cerebral function. More advanced degrees of hypoxia may result in confusion, disorientation, coma, or actual cellular death. Since the body is capable of numerous adaptive responses, it is difficult to predict the specific organ and extent of injury that will result from a given level of hypoxia in a given patient. *Acute hypoxemia* in the previously healthy patient is best illustrated by the manifestations associated with rapid ascent to high altitude, as discussed below.

Alveolar ventilation is the major determinant of clinically important changes in carbon dioxide. Carbon dioxide removal from the cells, hemoglobin binding of carbon dioxide, and atmospheric gas concentrations are not limiting factors under most physiologic conditions.

Impaired removal of carbon dioxide results in respiratory acidosis. This results in the physiologic changes and clinical manifestations summarized in Table 15.2. Clinical manifestations are more common when the pH is reduced below 7.2. In contrast, patients with lung disease frequently are stimulated to hyperventilate, resulting in respiratory alkalosis. When the alkalemia reaches pH levels greater than 7.50 to 7.55, numerous manifestations may become apparent (Table 15.3).

CONDITIONS RESULTING IN REDUCED OXYGEN DELIVERY TO TISSUES

Altitude

Reducing the barometric pressure with ascent to altitude, air flights, or space travel results in a predictable reduction in barometric pressure (Fig. 15.1). The highest altitude that man has achieved without supplemental oxygen is the top of Mount Everest, which has an elevation 8,828 meters. The barometric pressure there is about 250 mm Hg. Most individuals have considerable difficulty with ascent above 4,000 meters elevation. The average effects of reduced inhaled partial pressure of oxygen resulting from increased altitude, are demonstrated in Figure 15.2. It

Table 15.2 **Respiratory Acidosis**

Physiological Effects	Clinical Manifestations
Central Nervous System	
Dilated cerebral vessels → increased cerebrospinal fluid pressure	Headache, dyspnea, somnolence, psychosis, papilledema, focal neurological signs, neuromuscular irritability (asterixis) may progress to frank coma
Depressed cortical function	
Respiratory center stimulation (medulla and carotid bodies)	Hyperventilation
Renal and Metabolic	
Transfer of H^+ into cells and K^+ out. Thus, early increased serum K^+, subsequent increased excretion of K^+	None significant
Excretion of Cl^- and reabsorption of bicarbonate	Elevated serum bicarbonate
Depressed glycolysis and cellular metabolism	
Reduced hemoglobin affinity for oxygen	
Cardiovascular	
Decreased myocardial contractility	Heart Failure
Increased or decreased irritability	Arrhythmias
Decreased responsiveness to catecholamines	
Systemic responsiveness to catecholamines	Systemic hypotension
Pulmonary vascular and bronchial smooth muscle contraction	Pulmonary hypertension

(From Guenter CA, ed: Pulmonary Medicine, 2nd ed. Philadelphia, JB Lippincott, 1982, with permission.)

is evident that the reduced levels of oxygen in the inspired air are transmitted through the respiratory pathway and finally cause reduced oxygen in the blood leaving the tissues (mixed venous blood). The adaptive response to the hypoxia of high altitude includes an increase in cardiac output, systemic vasodilitation, increased production of erythropoietin resulting in increased hemoglobin levels, and respiratory stimulation resulting in increased ventilation and respiratory alkalosis. The effects on cardiac output, ventilation, and hemoglobin levels clearly improve total oxygen delivery to tissues. Pulmonary

vasoconstriction results from the hypoxia, causing pulmonary hypertension.

At very low levels of altitude, no changes can be demonstrated in central nervous system function. At altitudes varying from 1,500 to 2,500 meters, there may be slight alterations in perception, impairment of judgment, and decreased efficiency of learning. These symptoms become more prominent at altitudes over 3,000 meters. Above these levels, headaches, nausea, listlessness, insomnia, and alterations in breathing pattern (Cheyne-Stokes respiration) are common. The symptoms are diminished if the ascent

Fig. 15.1 This graph demonstrates the effect of altitude on barometric pressure and partial pressure of oxygen. The partial pressure of oxygen is a fixed proportion (20.95 percent) of the total barometric pressure, and is plotted by the interrupted line. The atmospheric partial pressure of oxygen at sea level is approximately 160 mm Hg, and is reduced to half that value at 18,000 feet. It is in the range of 50 to 55 mm Hg at the top of Mount Everest, nearly 30,000 feet elevation. (From Guenter CA, ed: Pulmonary Medicine, 2nd ed., Philadelphia, JB Lippincott, 1982, with permission.)

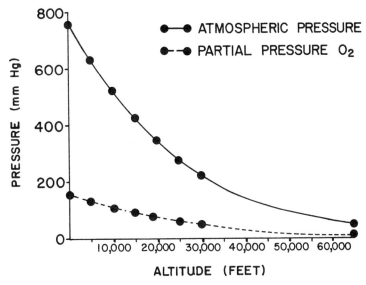

Table 15.3 **Respiratory Alkalosis**

Physiological Effects	Clinical Manifestations
Nervous System	
Decreased cerebral blood flow	Anxiety, numbness and tingling, seizures, light-headedness
Increased excitability	
Increased neuromuscular irritability	
Renal and Metabolic	
Chloride retention and bicarbonate excretion	Carpopedal spasm
Decreased ionized serum calcium and magnesium	Increased reflexes
Increased glycolysis and metabolic rate	Chvostek's Trousseau's signs
Increased production of lactic acid	
Increased catecholamine release	
Cardiovascular	
Systemic vasoconstriction	Palpitations
	Arrhythmias
Tachycardia	
Increased myocardial irritability	
Respiratory	
Bronchoconstriction	Dyspnea

(From Guenter CA, ed: Pulmonary Medicine, 2nd ed. Philadelphia, JB Lippincott, 1982, with permission.)

is gradual, and can be modified or prevented by pre-treatment with carbonic anhydrase inhibitors (for example, acetazolamide), which cause a metabolic acidosis, stimulate ventilation, and reduce hypoxemia. Above 4,000 meters elevation, retinal hemorrhages commonly accompany the severe headaches.

The clinical characteristics of acute altitude illness are listed in Table 15.4. High-altitude pulmonary edema may occur at as low as 2,400 meters elevation, but generally does not occur at altitudes under 3,000 meters. Patients develop cough, dyspnea, and occasionally life-threatening clinical pulmonary edema. The symptoms are only relieved by immediate removal to low altitudes, or oxygen therapy.

Anemia, Abnormal Hemoglobins

In persons with normal hemoglobin, 1.34 ml of oxygen will bind with each gram of hemoglobin. Since there are commonly 15 g of hemoglobin, this will result in approximately 20 ml of oxygen bound per dl. Reduced hemoglobin levels are common in disease, and are readily documented clinically. The decrease in oxygen content in the blood in anemia is directly proportional to the level of hemoglobin. It is more difficult to recognize hemoglobin that has abnormal binding characteristics.

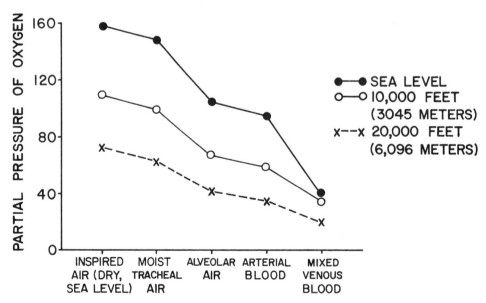

Fig. 15.2 The effect of altitude on partial pressures of oxygen in the respiratory pathway is shown here. Average values at sea level, at 10,000 feet, and at 20,000 feet elevation are graphed. Since each individual will adapt somewhat differently, this represents an average response. Many adaptive mechanisms blunt the effect of high altitude on tissue oxygen or mixed venous blood oxygen. Increased ventilation, increased cardiac output, polycythemia, and shifts in oxyhemoglobin affinity all are utilized to improve the tissue PO$_2$. (From Guenter CA, ed: Pulmonary Medicine, 2nd ed., Philadelphia, JB Lippincott, 1982, with permission.)

Table 15.4   **Clinical Characteristics of Acute Altitude Illness**

Acute mountain sickness	
Headache	Chest discomfort
Nausea	Peripheral edema
Vertigo	Retinal hemorrhages
Insomnia	Weakness
High-altitude pulmonary edema	
Dyspnea	Tachypnea
Cough	Cyanosis
Sputum	Lung crackles
	Chest roentgenogram infiltrates
High-altitude cerebral edema	
Severe headache	Papilledema
Vomiting	Coma
Ataxia	Extensor plantar responses
Abnormal behavior	
Hallucinations	Varied focal neurological deficits

(From Guenter CA, ed: Pulmonary Medicine, 2nd ed. Philadelphia, JB Lippincott, 1982, with permission.)

Carboxyhemoglobin, which results from increased environmental carbon monoxide, is common in patients who smoke cigarettes or who inhale high concentrations of automobile exhaust fumes, and in fire fighters and victims of fires. Carbon monoxide has a very high affinity for hemoglobin (more than 200 times the oxygen-binding capacity), but it is rapidly removed from the body when the atmospheric levels are reduced. Cigarette smokers have levels of carbon monoxide that depend on the number of cigarettes smoked and the pattern of inhalation. In general, one package per day smokers have 3 to 5 percent carboxyhemoglobin; two package per day smokers have 5 to 8 percent carboxyhemoglobin; and three package per day smokers have more than 10 percent carboxyhemoglobin. We have demonstrated, however, that inhalation of three cigarettes in a slow deliberate fashion can raise the carboxyhemoglobin levels to 6 percent in a previous nonsmoker.

Carboxyhemoglobin levels greater than 3 percent have been shown to cause minor changes in psychomotor function, increased levels of hemoglobin, and increased symptoms in patients with disease. Patients with angina develop pain at lower work loads; patients with intermittent claudication in the legs develop pain with reduced leg exercise; and patients with obstructive lung disease, who may also be hypoxemic due to low arterial oxygen pressures, have reduced exercise tolerance. Severe headaches and confusion develop in patients with more than 20 percent carboxyhemoglobin, and life-threatening coma and tissue injury occur at levels greater than 40 percent carboxyhemoglobin.

If the patient is ventilating normally, replacing air with 100 percent inhaled oxygen quickly washes out the body's carbon monoxide. The time required to reduce the carboxyhemoglobin 50 percent is approximately 250 minutes when breathing air, and 40 minutes when breathing 100 percent oxygen. If ventilation is suppressed due to drugs or carbon monoxide toxicity, artificial ventilation should be instituted. Hyperbaric oxygen is highly desirable, but it rarely can be obtained within the time required. Mild carboxyhemoglobin toxicity generally resolves with complete recovery. Severely elevated levels may be associated with permanent neurologic sequelae, cardiac or skeletal muscle injury with myoglobulinuria, and hepatic damage.

Many other variants of hemoglobin may affect oxygen transport. Fetal hemoglobin has exceptionally high binding to oxygen, but it is rapidly replaced by adult hemoglobin in the first months of life. Hemoglobin Chesapeake and other forms have increased affinity for oxygen, and usually result in little if any impairment of oxygen delivery to tissues. Hemoglobin Kansas and other forms have reduced affinity for oxygen, and commonly result in polycythemia (see Chapter 17).

Pulmonary Disease, Arterial Hypoxemia

The most common cause of reduced oxygen transport in clinical practice relates to abormal pulmonary function. Disorders of the respiratory pump may result in alveolar hypoventilation as outlined below. Hypoventilation results in build up of CO_2 in the lungs and, therefore, reduced alveolar oxygen. If ventilation is normal, gas exchange in the lungs may be impaired as a result of ventilation perfusion imbalance, physiologic or anatomic right-to-left shunts, or impaired diffusion.

The simplest test for impaired lung transport of oxygen is measurement of the arterial blood gases. The arterial PCO_2 will immediately identify whether the patient is ventilating normally, has hyperventilation, or has hypoventilation. The alveolar-arterial oxygen gradient provides data regarding oxygen transport across the lungs, and can be calculated from the following formula:

$$\text{Alveolar-Arterial Gradient} = P_AO_2 - P_aO_2$$

$$\text{where } P_AO_2 = PIO_2 - \frac{PaCO_2}{0.8}$$

$$0.8 = \text{correction factor for metabolic Respiratory Quotient}$$

A = Alveolar; I = Inspired; a = Arterial.

The normal alveolar-arterial oxygen gradient increases on average from 5 mm Hg at age 15 years to about 20 mm Hg at age 70 years, with an average level of 10 mm Hg. Levels of 20 mm Hg or more are clearly abnormal. Measurements should be made during exercise, recumbency, or sleep if clinically indicated. Most often, a high alveolo-arterial gradient indicates ventilation-perfusion imbalance; some areas are perfused but not ventilated proportionately.

While the alveolar-arterial oxygen gradient indicates the severity of impairment of oxygen transfer within the lung, the implications for oxygen delivery to the tissues are more dependent on the level of he-

moglobin and the oxyhemoglobin saturation. The student may wish to recall the oxyhemoglobin dissociation curve (Fig. 15.3), several specific points on the curve should be borne in mind. An arterial PO_2 greater than 90 mm Hg is associated with a 95 percent saturation. An arterial PO_2 of 40 mm Hg is associated with approximately 70 percent saturation (mixed venous blood). An arterial PO_2 of 26 mm Hg is associated with 50 percent saturation (sometimes referred to as P_{50}). Hypothermia, alkalemia, and administration of large amounts of stored blood shift the curve to the left, thus increasing oxygen affinity and raising the oxygen saturation for the same level

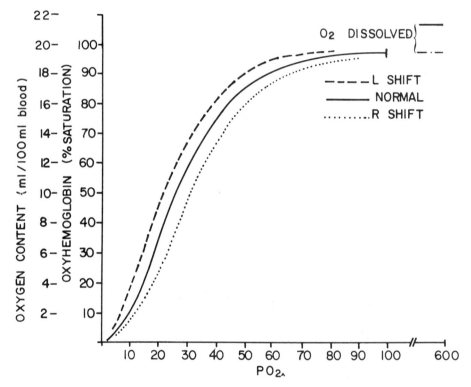

Fig. 15.3 The oxyhemoglobin dissociation curve. The oxygen content and saturation increase in proportion to the PO_2. When the hemoglobin is 95 percent saturated (PO_2 greater than 80 mm Hg) further increases in PO_2 produce small increases in oxygen content. Increasing the PO_2 from 100 to 600 mm Hg results in a small additional increase in oxygen content (about 1.8ml/100 ml, almost all in dissolved form). As the PO_2 is reduced from arterial blood values (80 to 100 mm Hg) to mixed venous values (about 40 mm Hg), the saturation is reduced from 97 percent to 70 percent. This permits a high oxygen content in the venous blood in spite of a relatively low extracting partial pressure at the tissue level. Factors that shift the curve to the right facilitate the unloading of oxygen, and factors that shift the curve to the left facilitate the loading of oxygen. For example, normal blood provides an oxygen content of 15 ml/100 ml of blood with a PO_2 of 40 mm Hg; the curve shifted 5 mm to the right provides 15 ml of oxygen at a PO_2 of 46 mm Hg; the curve shifted 5 mm to the left provides 15 ml of oxygen at a PO_2 of 36 mm Hg. (From Guenter CA, ed: Pulmonary Medicine, 2nd ed., Philadelphia, JB Lippincott, 1982, with permission.)

of PO_2. Acidemia, fever, and high phosphate levels shift the curve to the right and result in lower oxygen saturation levels for the same PO_2.

In otherwise normal persons, cyanosis appears when sufficient desaturation of hemoglobin takes place. This may be a result of reduced arterial saturation (central cyanosis) or increased extraction at the capillary level (peripheral cyanosis). In general, it is difficult to recognize cyanosis clinically when the arterial PO_2 is greater than 55 mm Hg. In the presence of polycythemia, however, a mildly reduced arterial PO_2 may be associated with cyanosis. Methemoglobin, sulfhemoglobin, and hemoglobinopathies with decreased oxygen affinity (for example, hemoglobin Kansas) all may result in cyanosis with normal levels of arterial PO_2. Other causes of pigmentation such as argyria (silver toxicity) and hemochromatosis may result in pigmentation simulating cyanosis.

Reduced Tissue Perfusion

Measurement of cardiac output at rest and during stress such as exercise provides an estimate of the total blood flow. In general, the cardiac output increases under conditions of arterial hypoxemia and anemia; however, many patients with respiratory disease have reduced cardiac output due to pulmonary hypertension and right heart failure. Further, aging patients commonly have associated heart disease with left ventricular dysfunction due to hypertension or coronary artery disease. The combined effects of arterial hypoxemia and reduced perfusion are difficult to quantitate at the bedside. Similarly, reduced organ blood flow due to atherosclerotic vascular disease may be difficult to assess. Consequently, the clinician rarely has quantitative estimates of oxygen supply to a specific organ in the patient unless a research-quality laboratory is available.

RESPIRATORY FAILURE

There is no clearcut definition of respiratory failure. Any lung condition in which exercise tolerance is limited by dyspnea or fatigue is evidence of respiratory failure. However, by common practice we only diagnose respiratory failure in patients who have major problems with gas exchange in the lungs; arterial hypoxemia with or without hypercapnia. The impact on the patient depends largely on the rate at which respiratory failure develops. A sudden illness resulting in an arterial PO_2 of less than 50 mm Hg may be associated with considerable dyspnea and

limitation of activity. Conversely, chronic lung disease with blood gases in the same range may be tolerated relatively well.

Acute Respiratory Failure

Patients with the various respiratory disorders discussed below may present with acute disturbances in gas exchange. Many clinicians like to distinguish these patient groups for therapeutic reasons. Hypoxemia with a normal or low arterial PCO_2 is termed *hypoxemic respiratory failure; elevated PCO_2 is termed ventilatory failure.*

Hypoxemic Respiratory Failure

Patients with hypoxemic failure usually have a strong respiratory drive with respiratory rates exceeding 25 breaths/min, an intact neuromuscular system, and adequate matching of lung ventilation and perfusion to permit carbon dioxide removal. The hypoxemia is generally a result of extensive regional lung disease or diffuse disease causing profound imbalance of ventilation in relation to perfusion. Mild to moderate bronchial asthma, pulmonary edema, pneumonia, acute atelectasis, and pulmonary embolism all result in hypoxemic respiratory failure.

Patients with severe hypoxemic respiratory failure should have corrective measures implemented and arterial blood gases reanalyzed within 20 to 30 minutes to ensure adequate improvement. Arterial PO_2 levels below 20 mm Hg are rarely compatible with survival past minutes to hours. Levels below 30 mm Hg must be considered life-threatening. Levels in the 30 to 50 range should be treated urgently, and, unless the patient has been chronically in this range, the objective should be to improve the arterial PO_2 to above 60 mm Hg.

Adult Respiratory Distress Syndrome (ARDS)   This term has been used for patients with a wide variety of diseases causing diffuse alveolar damage and hypoxemic respiratory failure. These patients typically have bilateral disease, diffuse roentgenographic infiltrates in the lungs, reduced lung compliance with low lung volumes, and very high alveolar-arterial oxygen gradients. The patients characteristically have rapid shallow respiration. Synonyms in other books include *white wet lung, shock lung, noncardiogenic pulmonary edema, capillary leak,* and *low-pressure pulmonary edema.* The specific causes of this condition and the approaches to therapy are discussed in the section entitled Pulmonary Edema.

Table 15.5 **Selection of Device for Oxygen Administration to Hypoxemic Patients**

Method of Administration	Approximate Inhaled Oxygen Concentration (%)	Patient Best Suited
Room air	21	Normal
Low-range oxygen Low-flow (1–2 L/min): mask or nasal cannula	25–30	Patients with chronic respiratory disease whose PCO_2 rises when given oxygen
Venturi mask	24, 28, 32	
Medium-range oxygen Medium flow (4–6 L/min): mask or nasal cannula	35–45	Most patients with moderate hypoxemia due to a variety of causes
High-range oxygen High-flow (10–15 L/min): mask with reservoir bag	70–90	Patients with severe hypoxemia not corrected by medium range oxygen
Endotracheal tube	Any concentration to 100	
Endotracheal tube and respirator	Any concentration to 100	
Endotracheal tube and respirator with positive end-expiratory pressure	Any concentration, frequently permits reduction to safe levels of inhaled oxygen	Patients who require greater than 60% of inhaled oxygen

(From Guenter CA, ed: Pulmonary Medicine, 2nd ed. Philadelphia, JB Lippincott, 1982, with permission.)

Principles of Management of Hypoxemic Respiratory Failure Patients with mild to moderate arterial hypoxemia (PO_2 greater than 50 mm Hg) and a documented and treatable lung disease, such as an episode of bronchial asthma, respiratory tract infection, or pulmonary embolism, can generally be managed by supplemental inhaled oxygen for a few days and treatment of the underlying cause. Patients with more severe hypoxemia in whom the diagnosis is not obvious require immediate detailed diagnostic evaluation. It must always be borne in mind that measures utilized to improve arterial oxygen pressures are only helpful if the underlying disease is treated or is healing. The following modalities to improve gas exchange must be considered in every patient with hypoxemic respiratory failure of unknown cause:

1. Measures to improve uniform distribution of inhaled air. Careful appraisal is essential regarding the appropriateness of bronchodilators, chest physiotherapy to improve mucous drainage, or tracheobronchial suction. In many patients distribution of ventilation will be improved by having the patient remain sitting upright or semirecumbent. This permits improved diaphragm function and reduces the development of dependent lung edema. Frequent repositioning from side to side is useful. Other measures to improve the functional residual capacity, such as frequent deep breathing, may be helpful. With severe hypoxemic respiratory failure, the use of artificial ventilation, occasionally including positive end-expiratory pressure to increase the lung functional residual capacity, may be life-saving.

2. Measures to reduce lung edema. Fluid balance, appropriate use of diuretics, and assessment of cardiovascular function must be considered.

3. Measures to prevent thromboembolism. In appropriately predisposed patients, thromboembolism may be an accompanying cause if not the major cause of lung injury. Anticoagulant therapy with heparin must always be considered.

4. Identification and treatment of infection. Viral, bacterial, rickettsial, fungal, and parasitic infections may all cause widespread lung injury with hypoxemia.

5. Attention to associated mechanisms of lung injury. Aspiration of gastric and oropharyngeal contents, thromboembolism, intravenous fluid overload, nosocomial infection, and prolonged recumbency all contribute to impaired lung function in hospitalized and ill patients.

Initial treatment is directed toward the underlying cause and toward correction of the arterial hypoxemia. Antibiotics, bronchodilators, diuretics, efforts to increase the functional residual capacity, and airway care emphasizing cough or tracheal suction may all be necessary. Supplemental oxygen should be provided simultaneously, as required. Mechanisms to provide sequential increases in inspired oxygen concentrations are outlined in Table 15.5

Endotracheal intubation and the use of artificial ventilation may be lifesaving, but should be undertaken with caution in view of their attendant complications.

Ventilatory Failure

Patients with acute elevations in PCO_2 above 50 mm Hg have *ventilatory failure* and are always considered to have severe respiratory failure. Every effort must be made to understand the underlying cause. Central nervous system depression, acute airway obstruction, exacerbations of airways disease in patients with previous lung disease, or systemic illness in patients with marginal ventilatory reserve are common precipitating factors. It is noteworthy that patients with acute pulmonary edema or episodes of bronchospasm due to bronchial asthma generally develop hypoxemia with hyperventilation. When these patients have a PCO_2 in the normal or slightly elevated range, it generally indicates a severe problem requiring aggressive treatment. Carbon dioxide elimination is generally improved by treatment of the underlying cause. Bronchodilators, antibiotics, diuretics, correction of electrolyte abnormalities, removal of sedation, or airway care should be given as appropriate. Artificial ventilation may be necessary for patients with respiratory failure and coma, patients with neuromuscular disease, or patients in whom the respiratory failure deteriorates in spite of aggressive conservative management.

Chronic Respiratory Failure

Patients with chronic lung disease may tolerate derangements in blood gases reasonably well at levels that ordinarily cause incapacitating illness in acute disease. It is important to document arterial blood gases and ventilatory function from time to time in follow-up of these patients in order to identify deterioration, or to document improvement in response to therapy. Chronic respiratory failure is often associated with pulmonary hypertension, right ventricular failure, and polycythemia. The clinical characteristics and management of chronic respiratory failure are discussed in detail in the section entitled Obstructive Lung Diseases.

DISORDERS OF THE RESPIRATORY PUMP

The breathing apparatus consists of a large and delicately engineered bellows (thorax) surrounding the intricately constructed gas exchange apparatus (lungs). This bellows changes its volume by the action of muscle groups controlled by the central nervous system. At rest and during sleep, the respiratory rhythm is predominantly controlled by complex neurologic networks originating in the brain stem. These determine respiratory rate as well as duration of inspiration and expiration. Speaking, singing, sighing, defecating, and many other activities are associated with modulation of breathing rhythm. Sleep may also be associated with striking changes in breathing patterns, some of which appear to be physiologic and others of which clearly represent disorders.

DISORDERS OF RESPIRATORY CONTROL

The Neural Control System

Hyperventilation

Hyperventilation indicated by a low PCO_2 is characteristic of patients with mild to moderate pulmonary disease who usually have some hypoxemia. The hyperventilation is not usually entirely corrected by administration of oxygen and probably involves nonchemical receptors within the lungs. Numerous other clinical circumstances, including the use of medications, are associated with hyperventilation. These are listed below.

Causes of Hyperventilation
Chemoreceptor stimulation
    Arterial hypoxemia
    Metabolic acidosis
    Hypotension
Stimulation of pulmonary receptors
    Pneumonia
    Pulmonary embolism
    Asthma
    Pulmonary edema
    Pulmonary fibrosis
Drugs
    Theophylline
    Catecholamines
    Salicylates
    Progesterone
Anxiety neurosis (hyperventilation syndrome)
"Central neurogenic hyperventilation" of head
    injury
Associated with Cheyne-Stokes breathing
Hepatic failure
Fever

Central neurogenic hyperventilation occurs in patients with extensive neurologic damage due to head injuries or intracranial bleeding. While such patients frequently improve if hypoxemia is corrected, they commonly continue to hyperventilate to some degree, and occasionally to the extent that respiratory alkalemia causes other adverse effects.

The *hyperventilation syndrome* is generally considered to be a response to anxiety, and is most commonly seen in young patients under unusual stress. Such patients frequently have a history of other psychosomatic complaints, and in many instances attacks occur during periods of depression. Marked increase in rate and depth of breathing with a respiratory alkalosis in the absence of lung disease, are the hallmarks of the condition. Numbness and tingling in the fingers and toes or around the mouth, myalgia, carpopedal spasm, and, occasionally, generalized tetany occur. Palpitations, tachycardia, and sharp twinges of chest pain are common. Occasionally the symptoms are indistinguishable from angina pectoris, and nonspecific ST and T wave changes may be present on the electrocardiogram. In symptomatic patients, arterial blood gases will generally reveal a PCO_2 of less than 20 mm Hg and a pH greater than 7.50. Treatment consists of patient education, reassurance, and rebreathing from a reservoir such as a paper bag until the alveolar and arterial carbon dioxide levels are restored toward normal and symptoms are reduced. Occasionally the hyperventilation syndrome is difficult to distinguish from pulmonary embolism, bronchial asthma, or ischemic chest pain, without more sophisticated diagnostic procedures.

Cheyne-Stokes Breathing

Some patients breath with an irregular pattern, with the amplitude of individual breaths waxing and waning over a 30- to 60-second period. Occasionally there may be a pause or apneic spell following a cycle during which respiration is built up gradually to a peak rate and depth followed by a gradual decline. Periodic breathing is most commonly found among patients with diffuse loss of cerebral-cortical function or patients with chronic heart failure. It may occasionally be found during the early stages of sleep, particularly in older subjects or normal individuals at high altitude. In itself, Cheyne-Stokes breathing has no significance beyond that of the neurologic or cardiac disorder, but in neurologic disease it implies a poor prognosis. Arterial blood gas analysis generally reveals a reduced arterial PCO_2 with a chronic respiratory alkalosis, and that this reduction is more severe just at the end of the high amplitude ventilation phase.

Ataxic and Apneustic Breathing

Ataxic breathing is completely irregular, with interspersed long and short pauses. Apneustic breathing is associated with pauses of 30 to 60 seconds, often occurring during inspiration. Both of these abnormal rhythms are associated with severe central nervous system disease.

Hiccough

A hiccough is a spasmodic inspiratory movement involving both diaphragm and intercostal muscles associated with transient closure of the glottis. This is a distressing and tiring symptom when persistent. It occurs mainly in male patients, for reasons unexplained. Although this may be a result of central nervous system disease involving the medulla, it is more frequently associated with disease in the upper abdomen, diaphragm, mediastinum, or heart, and is presumed to be due to irritation of the phrenic or vagus nerves. Transient episodes of hiccough occur in normal individuals. Persistent hiccough may require treatment. A wide range of useful remedies include stimulation of the pharynx with a nasal catheter, drugs such as phenothiazines, breath holding, or drinking cold water.

Primary Alveolar Hypoventilation

This syndrome may occur in infants, children, or adults. It is characterized by hypoxemia, hypercapnia, cyanosis, and polycythemia. Frequently pulmonary hypertension with cor pulmonale and clinical evidence of right ventricular failure is present. In severe cases thromboembolism and respiratory tract infection seem to be associated features. Many of these patients have a history of encephalitis. When tested, these patients have a blunted ventilatory response to carbon dioxide and an impaired ventilatory response to exercise. They are peculiarly susceptible to respiratory depression induced by sedatives and narcotics.

This diagnosis is usually reserved for patients with normal or near normal pulmonary function tests who have no clinical evidence of neuromuscular disease and no evidence of central nervous system–depressing drugs. The treatment includes management of any associated lung disease, avoidance of sedation, trial of respiratory stimulating drugs (theophylline, progesterone) or artificial electrical pacing of the phrenic nerve. Assessment of respiration during sleep is particularly important in these patients.

Causes of Hypoventilation
Lack of usual stimulus
    Metabolic alkalosis
    Hyperoxia
    Sleep
Reduced "respiratory center" activity
    Drugs, for example, sedatives, hypnotics, narcotics
        Local CNS damage, such as head injury or poliomyelitis

Myxedema
Idiopathic (primary) alveolar hypoventilation
Damage to descending tracts or peripheral nerves
Neuromuscular disease
Chest wall and pleural disease
  Kyphoscoliosis
  Flail chest
  Pneumothorax
Lung disease
  Obstruction of trachea, larynx, or bronchi
Inefficiency of gas exchange
  Increased dead space
  Decreased tidal volume

Breathing During Sleep

A good night's sleep is normally characterized by passing in and out of several electroencephalographically clearly defined sleep states. The first few hours are spent mainly in slow wave sleep, but as the night goes on this is interrupted by intervals of rapid eye movement (REM) sleep. During the latter phase there is rapid movement of the eyes, skeletal muscle tone falls, deep tendon reflexes are lost, dreams occur, and heart rate and breathing become irregular. Changes of tone in the respiratory muscles take place during these stages of sleep. During REM sleep the intercostal muscles become less active, and there is decreased activity in the pharyngeal and laryngeal muscles (including the genioglossus, which causes the tongue to protrude, and the posterior cricoarytenoid, which is the major abductor of the vocal chords). Without contraction of the latter muscles, the soft tissues of the upper airway tend to be sucked together with each inspiration, partly or completely obstructing the passage of air. When this occurs to a major extent, snoring is the result, and in extreme forms, *obstructive apnea*. During sleep several defense mechanisms are less effective. The cough and gag reflexes are depressed, mucociliary clearance is slowed, and arousal due to hypoxia, hypercapnia, increased work of breathing, or airway irritation is less likely. Since sleep generally occurs in the supine posture, there is a fall in functional residual capacity, resulting in mild hypoxemia; regurgitation of stomach contents is more likely, and gravity draws the tongue back into the pharynx. In addition, certain lung diseases, particularly bronchial asthma and left ventricular failure, are often exaggerated at night or in the supine posture.

Apneic spells, mild transient hypoxemia, and minor cardiac arrhythmias occur in a large portion of the population, particularly in males. Patients with excessive episodes of sleep apnea frequently complain of insomnia and demonstrate daytime somnolence. Such patients generally have more than 30, and frequently hundreds of, episodes of sleep apnea. Three types of apnea are commonly recognized: central, obstructive, and mixed. While the neurologic mechanisms are not entirely clear, clinical recognition depends on the activity of two groups of muscles; the inspiratory muscles (diaphragm and intercostals), and the upper airway muscles (cricoarytenoids, genioglossus, and pharyngeal). If the inspiratory muscles do not contract, there is no air flow. This is termed *central apnea*. If the inspiratory muscles contract but the upper airway muscles fail to do so, the pharynx is sucked closed and airflow is reduced or completely obstructed. This is known as *obstructive apnea*. Many patients, however, demonstrate both abnormalities at different times.

Obstructive sleep apnea appears to be the most common of these problems, clinically, with a male-to-female ratio of about 8 to 1. Most but not all patients are obese, and in these patients the abnormalities tend to be more severe with increasing degrees of obesity. The mean age of diagnosis is approximately 45 years. Patients are rarely aware that their problem arises from sleep, but a careful history often is highly suggestive. Loud snoring and abnormal muscular activity are almost always recognized by the spouse. More than half demonstrate intellectual deterioration, excess of daytime sleepiness, and personality change. It is noteworthy that these patients have a peculiarly severe and unpleasant form of snoring that often requires the spouse to make alternative sleeping arrangements. Impotence and decreased libido occur in one third to one half of these patients, and morning headaches are common. Monitoring of respiratory muscle activity commonly demonstrates hundreds of apneic spells per night, with up to 40 percent of the time spent with no air flow. Marked sinus arrhythmia occurs in synchrony with apnea, and occasionally periods of asystole, atrioventricular block, and multifocal premature ventricular contractions occur. Severe arterial hypoxemia is characteristic, and systemic hypertension generally occurs during apneic spells. While obesity is the most common accompanying abnormality, anatomic lesions of the upper airway, including nasal obstruction, enlarged tonsils, laryngeal stenosis, and acromegaly, all have been associated with increased incidence of obstructive apnea. The treatment consists of weight reduction where appropriate, relief of airway obstruction where present, and administration of drugs (medroxyprogesterone). The most successful treatment is to place a permanent tracheostomy to bypass the obstruction. Following tracheostomy most patients have a dramatic improvement in neuropsychiatric symptoms and cardiopulmonary signs of disease. This drastic form of treatment should be reserved for patients who have been very carefully evaluated and whose course can be followed by clear documentation of the results.

Central apnea occurs in patients with narcolepsy, previous bulbar poliomyelitis, and numerous other neurologic diseases. These patients frequently have depressed responses to carbon dioxide and hypoxemia while awake. These relatively uncommon patients can be managed by use of respiratory stimulant drugs, nocturnal ventilators, rocking beds, or phrenic nerve pacing. Patients treated with phrenic nerve pacing have been shown to frequently develop obstructive apnea, suggesting that the central nervous system control of the pharnygeal and inspiratory muscles is abnormal.

Nocturnal hypoxemia is common to a mild degree in normal individuals, and may be sufficiently prominent to be worrisome in patients with stable lung disease and arterial hypoxemia. When such individuals develop sleep apnea, periods of hypoxemia may be severe and associated with marked hypercapnia. Patients with clinical evidence of pulmonary hypertension, marked polycythemia, carbon dioxide retention, or symptoms of sleep disorders should be evaluated with respect to marked sleep hypoxemia. Treatment with supplemental oxygen frequently relieves evidence of pulmonary hypertension and cor pulmonale, improves central nervous system manifestations, and may reduce arrhythmias, but the duration of apneic spells is often increased and respiratory acidosis may be more severe. Consequently, treatment with oxygen must be initially monitored to assess the effects on alveolar ventilation. Drugs such as medroxyprogesterone and acetazolamide have been shown to improve nocturnal oxygen saturations in polycythemic hypoxemic patients in certain circumstances.

The Chemical Control System

Oxygen plays a significant role in stimulating ventilation through the carotid chemoreceptors, with increasing levels of stimulation down to arterial PO_2 levels as low as 20 to 25 mm Hg. In patients who are more severely hypoxemic, central nervous system depression overrides this effect, and ventilation is depressed as well. Carbon dioxide stimulates ventilation through the carotid chemoreceptors and the medullary chemoreceptors bathed in cerebrospinal fluid. Bilateral removal of the carotid bodies has been performed surgically in some patients and appears to result in reduced ventilation, with mild hypoxemia and a slight increase in carbon dioxide levels.

The carotid and medullary chemoreceptors are also sensitive to changes in hydrogen ion concentration. Decreasing levels of pH as seen in metabolic acidosis stimulate ventilation, causing hyperventilation. Increased levels of pH as seen in metabolic alkalosis result in depressed ventilation.

CHEST WALL DISORDERS

Neuromuscular Disease

Neuromuscular diseases predictably affect the most energy-dependent breathing maneuvers. There is a reduction of ability to inhale, which results in a reduced vital capacity and total lung capacity. Eventually the breathing pattern becomes rapid and shallow, and the functional residual capacity may be reduced. With the loss of deep inhalations, microatelectasis develops, and hypoxemia is common. If this condition persists, pulmonary hypertension with right ventricular failure may develop. In severe cases ventilation is sufficiently impaired to prevent elimination of carbon dioxide, resulting in respiratory acidosis. Patients with generalized neuromuscular disease may also have dysfunction of the larynx and swallowing mechanisms, making them prone to aspiration. They frequently have an ineffective cough. Inactivity resulting from weakness of the limbs may result in deep vein thrombosis and pulmonary embolism. Many forms of primary muscle disease are associated with myocardiopathy. Poliomyelitis, motor neuron disease, the muscular dystrophies (in the adult, particularly myotonic dystrophy), acute polyneuritis (Guillain-Barré syndrome), and myasthenia gravis represent the more commonly encountered causes of respiratory muscle weakness. Tetanus, which is common in underdeveloped countries, is exceedingly rare in the Western world. Botulism may cause respiratory muscle paralysis, and generally occurs in outbreaks related to inadequate food processing procedures.

Ineffective muscle activity may be localized to certain muscle groups. Patients with tetraplegia due to high cervical cord injuries may lose all intercostal muscle activity but retain diaphragm activity. Such patients have immediate reductions in vital capacity to less than half normal, with severe respiratory compromise. If they survive, diaphragm activity appears to become more efficient and the vital capacity improves to somewhat greater than half normal by the third to sixth week after injury.

Since the diaphragm is innervated through the 3rd to 5th cervical nerve roots, high cervical cord injuries are incompatible with spontaneous breathing. Bilateral diaphragm paralysis occurs rarely due to brain stem or cervical injury, surgical trauma to the phrenic nerves, or neuromuscular disease involving primarily the diaphragms. Unilateral paralysis of the diaphragm is relatively common, and occurs in relation to tumors impinging on the phrenic nerve (bronchogenic carcinoma and lymphoma), surgical trauma, and polyneuropathies. Unilateral diaphragm paralysis is associated with about 20 percent reduction in vital capacity but few respiratory symptoms, unless there is associated lung disease. Transient abnormalities of diaphragm function occur commonly in patients with abdominal disease. Subdiaphragmatic abscess is generally unilateral, and is associated with an elevated hemidiaphragm that is immobile. Upper abdominal surgery (cholecystectomy and gastrectomy) is generally associated with immediate inhibition of diaphragm activity during spontaneous ventilation. This apparently results in lung volume loss, basilar lung atelectasis, hypoxemia, and, perhaps, predisposition to lung infection. This is transient and generally improves within 3 to 5 days postoperatively. Patients with bilateral diaphragm paralysis or weakness demonstrate definitive clinical findings. During inspiration the chest cage is pulled upward and expands by the action of intercostal muscle contraction. Careful observation of the upper abdomen demonstrates that the anteroposterior abdominal diameter is decreased on inspiration, because the diaphragm and abdominal contents are also drawn upward by the negative intrathoracic pressure (paradoxical breathing). On expiration the thoracic diameter is decreased due to relaxation of the intercostal muscles, but the abdominal diameter is passively increased. Many patients with weak diaphragm function actually contract the abdominal musculature to increase the intraabdominal pressure during expiration. Such palpable contraction of the rectus abdominus during the expiratory phase of normal supine resting ventilation is clearly abnormal.

Obesity

The major health hazards of obesity are dealt with in Chapter 1. Patients with severe obesity develop a reduced compliance of the chest wall and, partially as a result of the abdominal pressure, push the diaphragm up and into the thorax. These changes result in a reduced vital capacity, reduced functional residual capacity, and the abnormalities are markedly increased in the supine position. Severely obese patients are characteristically hypoxemic and the hypoxemia is also worse in the supine position. Nocturnal hypoxemia is commonly severe. Obstructive sleep apnea and other symptoms associated with disordered sleep are relatively common. These patients are also predisposed to deep venous thrombosis and thromboembolic phenomena which contribute to the hypoxemia. Cyanosis, polycythemia, pulmonary hypertension and right ventricular failure may occur with severe obesity. The additional insults of cigarette smoking, or other associated lung disease are tolerated poorly.

A few obese patients develop chronic carbon dioxide retention and respiratory acidosis. These patients are particularly prone to developing pulmonary hypertension and cor pulmonale. These obese, somnolent, plethoric individuals have been likened to the "fat boy" in Dickens' novel and referred to as the Pickwickian Syndrome. Unfortunately the pathophysiology of this end stage respiratory failure is not clearly understood. Many of these patients have reduced ventilatory responsiveness to hypoxemia and carbon dioxide and episodes of sleep apnea. It is remarkable that most patients will have dramatic improvement in their cardiopulmonary function with a 7 to 10 kg weight loss.

Ankylosing Spondylitis

See Chapter 18.

Kyphoscoliosis

Kyphoscoliosis is a lateral curvature and rotation of the vertebral spine. Mild to moderate degrees of kyphoscoliosis are associated with no detectable change in lung function. Severe degrees of kyphoscoliosis (greater than a 60° deviation in direction of the spine) are associated with progressively increasing restriction of lung function. The vital capacity is reduced, ventilation of the lung on the concave side is reduced, and marked ventilation-perfusion imbalance occurs. These patients develop hypoxemia, are more prone to respiratory tract infections, and, in those with severe spinal deformity or associated lung disease, cor pulmonale is common. These patients are also more prone to sleep disorders and nocturnal hypoxemia. In advanced disease the respiratory failure may require treatment with long-term oxygen administration and nocturnal artificial ventilation.

Pregnancy and Ascites

Increased intraabdominal volume causes increased intraabdominal pressure and elevation of the diaphragm. This results in a reduced functional residual capacity that is aggravated in the supine position. Recumbent hypoxemia is common. Pregnancy is also associated with hyperventilation thought to be a result of hormonal effects of progesterone. Arterial PCO_2 is frequently in the low 30s (mm Hg).

Pectus Excavatum

The funnel chest deformity of the sternum and adjacent ribs is generally only of cosmetic significance. The posteriorly displaced sternum may cause lateral displacement of the heart with an apparent cardiomegaly on posteroanterior chest roentgenograms. A few instances of impaired cardiovascular performance have been reported in very severe cases. Surgical treatment for pectus excavatum is generally only justifiable on cosmetic grounds.

Pectus carinatum is a pigeon-breast deformity of the upper sternum and adjacent ribs with no attendant changes in lung function.

DIAGNOSIS OF THE PATIENT WITH DISEASE OF THE RESPIRATORY PUMP

The early clues to disorders of the respiratory pump depend entirely on careful history taking and thoughtful examination. Symptoms suggestive of nocturnal disorders may best be obtained from the spouse or other housemates. Unusually severe snoring, nocturnal muscle activity, personality changes, and daytime somnolence should warrant particular review. On examination, abnormal breathing patterns suggestive of intercostal or diaphragm weakness may be present. Obesity, marked kyphoscoliosis, ankylosing spondylitis, and other chest wall deformities are readily identified on examination. Definitive diagnosis of respiratory control abnormalities may require assessment of respiratory motion and blood gases during sleep, and assessment of ventilatory response to hypoxia, carbon dioxide, or exercise. Neuromuscular disease causing weakness of breathing efforts will result in reduced vital capacity and reduced ability to generate an inspiratory effort. Inspiratory muscle force can be easily measured by

having the patient make maximal inspiratory effort against a closed valve and measuring the pressure at the mouth. When breathing at residual volume, normal men can generate about 120 cm of water negative pressure and normal women can generate about 90 cm. Similarly, diaphragm activity can be measured by assessing the transdiaphragmatic pressure during breathing maneuvers, using an esophageal tube to indicate pleural pressure and a gastric tube to indicate abdominal pressure. When disease of the respiratory muscles is considered likely, such assessment must be carried out in a well equipped laboratory by personnel having experience in assessment of respiratory neuromuscular function.

ACUTE RESPIRATORY TRACT INFECTIONS

VIRAL INFECTION SYNDROMES

The range of common respiratory manifestations of viral infection is outlined in Table 15.6. These infections are transmitted by droplet nuclei from person to person, with a highly variable rate of infection dependent on host defense mechanisms and degree of contact. Close association and crowding appear to be important in potentiating the infections.

The Common Cold

This is the most common respiratory viral disease encountered by humans. The infections may be caused by many different viruses, but the presenting symptoms are remarkably similar from individual to individual. Variations peculiar to each individual may occur and, a given person tends to get the same combination of symptoms whatever the causative organism. The disease usually starts with a feeling of dryness and stuffiness in the upper respiratory tract affecting the nasopharynx. Hypersecretion of mucus and lacrimation are common. These fluids are generally clear and mucoid. Systemic symptoms including headache, malaise, and mild fever or chills may be present, but the disease process is usually over in 3 to 4 days. Examination of the mucus membranes of the upper respiratory tract reveal them to be hyperemic and edematous. Complications are rare, but in patients with chronic respiratory disease, secondary bacterial infection is more common.

There is no specific therapy. Symptomatic therapy generally includes antihistamines and salicylates. The popular interest in vitamin C as a preventive drug has some scientific evidence to support it, but the

Table 15.6 **Common Respiratory Syndromes and Their Etiologic Agents**

Pathogen	Child cold	Adult cold	Laryngotracheo bronchitis[a]	Flu	Adult pneumonia	Child pneumonia	Pleuritis, pericarditis
Respiratory virus							
Influenza A	+	−	+	+ +	+	+	−
Influenza B	+	−	+	+ +	+	+	−
Influenza C	+	+	−	−	−	+	−
Parainfluenza	+	+	+ +	+ +	−	+	−
R. S. Virus	+	+	+	+	−	+ +	−
Adenovirus	+ +	+	+	+ +	+	+	−
Rhinovirus	+	+ +	+	+	−	−	−
Coronavirus	−	+ +	−	+	−	−	−
Non-respiratory viruses affecting respiratory tract							
Coxsackie virus	+	+	+	+	−	−	+
Echo virus	+	+	+	+	−	−	+
Rubeola	+	+	+	+	+	+	−
Varicella	+	+	+	+	+	−	−
Nonviral agents							
Psittacosis (*Chlamydia psittaci*)	−	−	−	+	+ +	+	−
Rickettsia (*Coxiella burnetii*)	−	−	−	+	+ +	−	−
Mycoplasma (*M. pneumoniae*)	−	−	+	+	+ +	+	±

(From Guenter CA, ed: Pulmonary Medicine, 2nd ed. Philadelphia, JB Lippincott, 1982, with permission.)
[a] presents as croup in the child.
− Rare if ever.
+ Occasional.
+ + Prominent feature.

benefits are marginal at best. William Osler's recommendation may remain the best advice: "There is just one way to treat a cold, and that is with contempt." Antibiotics should be avoided unless there is evidence of secondary bacterial infection.

Many patients develop allergic rhinitis with symptoms comparable to those of a cold. Treatment of allergic rhinitis may be quite effective so it is well worth the physician's effort to attempt to make the distinction. Patients with allergic rhinitis commonly have seasonal "colds," some known allergies, and the nasal secretions generally contain large numbers of eosinophils. Further, it is not possible to identify a source case.

Pharyngitis

Viral pharnygitis results in sore throat and some difficulty in swallowing, and may be associated with mild headache, nasal stuffiness, and systemic symptoms. Erythema, swelling, and occasionally exudative mucoid patches of secretions in the pharynx are visible. Cervical lymph nodes may be enlarged and tender. It is often difficult to differentiate viral phar-

yngitis from infectious mononucleosis or the more serious streptococcal pharyngitis or pharyngeal diphtheria. Patients with viral infection tend to have minimal if any leucocytosis. Where there is any doubt, throat swabs should be cultured to identify bacterial organisms.

Acute Laryngotracheal Bronchitis

Hoarseness, loss of voice, and pain in the region of the upper trachea in a patient with a mild febrile illness and a persistent nonproductive cough are characteristic. The symptoms may last 7 to 10 days and be associated with chest wall pain resulting from the severe cough effort. If the sputum becomes purulent and fever increases, secondary bacterial infection must be considered.

Bronchiolitis

Viral infection of the small airways results in cough, wheezing, dyspnea, cyanosis, and labored breathing. This syndrome is most common in infants but is occasionally seen in adults.

Table 15.7   **Differentiation of Pneumonia Resulting from Infectious Agents**

| Clinical Features | Organisms | | | |
	Viral	Rickettsial	Mycoplasmal	Pyogenic Bacterial
Community history	Epidemic	Animal, bird contacts	Family illness	Not significant
Prodrome	Upper respiratory General malaise	General malaise	Upper respiratory General malaise	Occasional pharyngitis
Onset	Gradual	Gradual	Gradual	Sudden
Cough	Persistent Nonproductive	Persistent Nonproductive	Persistent Nonproductive	Persistent Purulent, bloody sputum
Chest pain	Uncommon	Uncommon	Uncommon	Common, pleuritic
Physical findings on chest examination	Minimal	Minimal	Crackles, rhonchi diffuse	Localized, well defined
Roentgenogram findings	Patchy, nonspecific	Patchy, nonspecific	Patchy, lower lobes, unilateral	Localized
Leukocyte count	Normal leucopenic Mildly elevated	Normal leucopenic Mildly elevated	Normal leucopenic Mildly elevated	Polymorphonuclear Leucocytosis
Sputum smear	Few leucocytes Epithelial debris	Few leucocytes Epithelial debris	Few leucocytes Occasionally leucocytes without bacteria	Numerous leucocytes Intracellular bacteria
Pleural fluid	Rare	Rare	Rare	Common, occasionally with empyema
Blood cultures	Negative	Negative	Negative	+10 to 40%
Serology	Definitive	Definitive	Definitive	Not helpful
Response to antimicrobials	None	Tetracycline or chloramphenicol	Tetracycline or erythromycin	Good. Requires identification of organism
Secondary bacterial infection	Common	Uncommon	Uncommon	Uncommon

(From Guenter CA, ed: Pulmonary Medicine. 2nd ed. Philadelphia, JB Lippincott, 1982, with permission.)

Viral Pneumonia

Viral penumonia is the most common cause of infective pneumonia up to the middle years life. It may be associated with conjunctivitis, laryngitis, tracheobronchitis, or bronchiolitis, but is generally only diagnosed if chest roentgenograms demonstrate infiltrates. Examination of the chest commonly reveals normal findings or minimal changes in breath sounds and mild dullness to percussion, with scattered inspiratory rales. Signs of lobar consolidation or pleural effusion are uncommon. A high fever, marked dyspnea, cyanosis on exertion, an irritating nonproductive cough, loss of appetite, headaches, and general malaise frequently accompany the illness. Viral pneumonia commonly occurs in epidemics. In the adult the most common agents are influenza, parainfluenza, and adenoviruses. Adenoviruses are particularly common in military recruits and students of residential schools. Occasionally rubella or varicella viruses may cause pneumonia, and in adults this tends to be relatively severe. The features differentiating viral pneumonia from mycoplasma and bacterial pneumonia are presented in Table 15.7.

Less Common Viral Syndromes

Herpangina is an acute illness characterized by pharyngeal discomfort, low grade fever, and small vesicles typically located on the anterior pillars of the tonsils and soft palate. Pleurodynia (Bornholm disease) is an acute epidemic illness most commonly caused by coxsackie virus B. The disease presents with fever, severe pleuritic chest pain, and often a small pleural effusion.

SPECIFIC VIRAL INFECTIONS

Influenza Virus

The influenza virus has been responsible for many of the world's major pandemics. Certain of these pandemics have been associated with extremely high mortality rates, with disastrous socioeconomic effects. In 1918 the mortality worldwide was estimated at more than a million. Although influenza C virus is relatively stable antigenically, influenza A and B are quite unstable, and hence it is possible to undergo more than one infection in a lifetime. Each year large

Table 15.8 **Clinical Patterns of Influenza and Its Respiratory Complications**

Presentation	Time of Onset	Groups at Special Risk	Prognosis
Bronchiolitis	Variable	Infants, COPD	Fair
Viral pneumonia			
Localized	Early	All	Good
Diffuse	Early	Underlying disease	Poor
Bacterial pneumonia			
Localized	Late	All	Good
Diffuse	Early	Underlying disease	Poor
Combined bacterial-viral pneumonia	Early	Underlying disease	Poor

(From Guenter CA, ed: Pulmonary Medicine. 2nd ed. Philadelphia, JB Lippincott, 1982, with permission.)

outbreaks occur in institutions, military camps, schools, or communities. Although influenza B is usually a milder illness than influenza A, it is associated with a greater incidence of postinfectious sequelae, especially Reye's syndrome. This complication consists of an encephalopathy resulting in coma and frequently death. The mechanism of the central nervous system manifestations has not been established.

Clinical Manifestations of Influenza Virus Infection

The illness arising from influenza virus infection is one of sudden onset, with headache, chills, muscle aches and pains, and fatigue. Respiratory symptoms are initially often lacking. The eyes may be tender, with lacrimation and photophobia. Several days later nasopharyngeal irritation becomes apparent, with rhinorrhea and sneezing. Fever with a temperature ranging to 41°C is common. The higher the temperature, the more severe the disease. Anorexia, thirst, and constipation are common. Within 5 to 7 days a persistent nonproductive cough develops. At this stage, a hemorrhagic tracheobronchitis is common. In the uncomplicated case, respiratory symptoms usually last 5 to 7 days; however, if the fever has not subsided by the fifth day one should reconsider the diagnosis or suspect a secondary bacterial infection. Viral pneumonia, bacterial tracheobronchitis, or superimposed bacterial pneumonia are important considerations (Table 15.8).

In patients with underlying lung, cardiovascular or renal disease, influenza virus infection inflicts a high mortality.

Laboratory Findings

The peripheral blood leukocyte count is commonly reduced, but may be elevated to 12,000 WBC/mm³. In the uncomplicated case, chest roentgenograms are normal, but abnormalities ranging from minor asymmetric infiltrates to diffuse bilateral infiltration may occur in severe viral pneumonia. Viral isolation may be possible in specimens obtained by tracheal suction or throat swabs taken in the early stage of illness. Complement fixing or hemaglutination-inhibiting antibodies can be detected in acute and convalescent sera. A fourfold rise in titer is diagnostic of recent influenza infection. Immunofluorescent staining of bronchial secretions may permit the diagnosis to be made very early, when these techniques are available.

Prevention and Therapy

Influenza epidemics can generally be prevented by current immunization practices. Since the antigenicity of the influenza virus is only known at the beginning of each season, the vaccine must be formulated in accordance with the experience that year. The vaccine of the previous year is generally ineffective (see Chapter 7).

In patients who have not been immunized but who are exposed to an epidemic, the antiviral agent amantadine should be prescribed. This drug is effective as a prophylactic agent, providing about 60 percent protection against clinical illness in exposed, susceptible populations. If treatment of symptomatic influenza with amantadine is begun within 24 hours of the onset of symptoms, the course of the illness is shortened and viral shedding is abbreviated. The usual adult dose of 100 mg twice daily causes marked side effects, consisting of insomnia, anxiety, and difficulty in thinking, in about 5 percent of people. The dose should be reduced in patients with renal insufficiency. Amantadine is effective against influenza A but not influenza B.

Treatment of influenzal pneumonia is symptomatic. Patients with asthma or other obstructive lung diseases may require vigorous bronchodilator therapy. Hypoxemia may be sufficient to require oxygen. Secondary pneumonia due to pneumococcal or staphylococcal infection is common, but should only be treated when the characteristic features of bacterial infection become clinically apparent.

Adenovirus

Pharyngitis, rhinitis, conjunctivitis, and adenopathy are common characteristics of adenoviral infections, which may cause pneumonia, particularly in young adults living in crowded quarters.

Rhinovirus

Rhinovirus is the most common cause of the common cold.

Rubeola Virus

Measles is predominantly an exanthematous disease causing severe systemic illness. Occasionally in childhood, and more commonly with increasing age, patients with measles infection develop severe viral pneumonia that is clinically similar to influenza pneumonia.

Varicella-Zoster Virus

The virus of chicken pox is only occasionally associated with penumonia. This may be severe in women in the child-bearing age, particularly pregnant women. The lung lesions may be associated with pleural effusions, hemoptysis, and chest pain indistinguishable from lung infarction. Once the diagnosis is established, the treatment is supportive, as for other causes of acute respiratory failure.

BACTERIAL INFECTION SYNDROMES

Sinusitis

Acute *sinusitis* is estimated to occur in up to 25 percent of adults at some time in their lives. Patients present with fever, headache, and, commonly, nasal discharge. The infection generally results from obstruction of drainage from the sinus. Transillumination or radiographic examination of the sinuses generally permits a diagnosis by demonstration of fluid levels. The most common organisms include *Streptococcus pneumoniae* and *Hemophilus influenzae*,

but anerobic organisms may also be present. Treatment includes specific antibiotics and measures to relieve obstruction. Topical vasoconstrictors may be of some benefit during the acute phase, to promote drainage.

Epiglottitis

Epiglottitis is most commonly due to *H. influenzae*, and may cause upper respiratory obstruction in young children. *Pharyngitis* may be caused by *Streptococcus pneumonia*, *Corynebacterium diphtheriae*, and other organisms. Streptococcal infection should be diagnosed in order to prevent the development of poststreptococcal complications such as rheumatic fever. In nonimmunized individuals diphtheria is an important consideration. Severe systemic illness with a tenacious fibrinoid white membrane in the pharynx is characteristic of diphtherial pharyngitis. Obstruction due to pharyngeal edema and slough, myocarditis, neuritis, and secondary infection are severe sequelae. The organism is responsive to penicillin and the course may be modified by early use of antitoxin.

Bronchitis

Purulent bronchitis develops particularly in individuals with preceding airways disease. Cough, purulent sputum, central chest pain associated with cough (probably due to tracheitis), and low-grade fever may be present. In patients with chronic lung disease, respiratory failure may result. The most common organisms are *Streptococcus pneumoniae* or *H. influenzae*; however, staphlococci, *Pseudomonas* organisms, and others may be important considerations, particularly in hospitalized patients or the chronically ill. Antibiotic therapy is indicated, although the response to therapy is commonly less dramatic than with pneumonia.

Acute Bacterial Pneumonia

Clinical Manifestations

An abrupt onset of severe illness characterized by cough, purulent or bloody sputum, tachypnea, tachycardia, fever, and commonly pleuritic chest pain is typical of bacterial pneumonia. Many patients have a history of a prodrome suggesting a previous upper respiratory tract infection. *Streptococcus pneumoniae* is the most common cause of bacterial pneumonia. Prior to widespread use of antibiotics, the disease generally followed a course in which the patient developed a complete edematous consolidation of a lobe. Clinically this was detectable by the presence of dullness and increased transmission of breath and spoken voice sounds through the lung tissue to the chest wall. Radiographically, the pneumonic density was restricted to the anatomical lobe involved. Other organisms that cause lobar pneumonia include *Klebsiella pneumoniae* and, rarely, *H. influenza*. The early use of antibiotics in developed countries appears to limit the natural progression of the infection. Patients now frequently have minimal infiltrate or patchy bronchopneumonia in one or more lobes, regardless of the organism.

Patients with bacterial pneumonia (Table 15.7) may have certain features that increase the likelihood of identifying specific organisms. A single large cavity with foul smelling sputum, with or without an associated pleural effusion, suggests anaerobic organisms. Multiple cavitary lesions throughout a lobe suggests necrotizing pneumonia due to gram-negative bacteria (*Klebsiella*, *E. coli*, *Pseudomonas*, and others) or *staphylococci*. While pneumonococcal bacterial pneumonia is responsible for more than 90 percent of spontaneous bacterial pneumonias in otherwise normal people, gram-negative bacteria legionella, staphylococci, and anaerobic infections play a much more prominent role in hospital-acquired pneumonias and in patients with chronic disability.

Laboratory Assessment

Laboratory assessment of patients with pneumococcal pneumonia reveals peripheral blood polymorphonuclear leukocytosis, many polymorphonuclear leukocytes in expectorated sputum, and occasionally intracellular bacterial organisms, which strongly suggests their likelihood as an etiologic agent. Careful sputum analysis is of utmost importance. If the patient is capable of expectorating sputum, the physician should select material most representative of lower respiratory tract secretions for Gram stain and culture. If the patient is unable to produce sputum, bronchoscopy with particular attention to avoidance of contamination by upper airway organisms, or transtracheal aspiration may be desirable. Most patients should have blood cultures taken, since bacteremia will confirm the offending organisms. Pleural effusions should be tapped to determine whether they are infected, and if so, they should be drained. Radiographic examination will demonstrate increased density in the lung fields; frequently this helps to determine whether localized clinical findings are due to airway secretions or to definite parenchymal disease. Bacterial antigens in blood and pleural fluid may permit immediate identification of the infecting organism by counterimmunoelectrophoresis. Patients are characteristically hypoxemic, but arterial blood gases will help assess the severity of respiratory failure.

Prevention and Treatment

Bacterial pneumonia is the most common infective cause of death and the fifth most common cause of death in the North American population. Patients at increased risk should receive preventive pneumococcal vaccine (see Chapter 7). Treatment with the appropriate antibiotics, supplemental fluids in dehydrated patients, oxygen, and early management of complications substantially reduces mortality. For *Streptococcus penumoniae*, parenteral penicillin is the antibiotic of choice and is recommended as 600,000 units aqueous penicillin G or procaine penicillin, at 12 hour intervals for 5 to 7 days, or at least for 72 hours after the patient becomes afebrile. Patients with the complications of endocarditis or meningitis should receive 10 to 12 million units intravenously daily. In patients who are allergic to penicillin, erythromycin or clindamycin are acceptable alternatives.

Bacteremia may be demonstrated in about 30 percent of patients and parapneumonic pleural effusions may be demonstrated in up to half of patients, but extrapulmonary spread of infection occurs infrequently.

ANAEROBIC INFECTIONS

The lower respiratory tract is chronically exposed to anaerobic organisms, which are normal flora in the upper respiratory tract. These include bacteroides, clostridia, anaerobic streptococci, and others. Individuals with episodes of unconsciousness due to seizures, alcoholism, or anesthetics are particularly prone to aspirating large volumes of upper airway secretions. Further, those patients with poor hygiene of gums and teeth are likely to have larger innocula of oropharyngeal contents.

Patients commonly present with an acute onset of afebrile illness with cough that several days later becomes productive of copious quantities of foul smelling purulent secretions. This may be associated with pleuritic pain and clinical evidence of pleural effusion. Occasionally such patients present primarily with central nervous system symptoms as a result of brain abscess.

Clinical and radiographic findings are those of a

large localized abscess (most commonly in the dependent lung zones), surrounding parenchymal infiltrate, and frequently pleural effusion.

Laboratory investigation demonstrates polymorphonuclear leukocytosis, polymorphonuclear predominance in sputum with a variety of microorganisms, and occasionally positive anaerobic blood cultures.

Most patients respond well to treatment with penicillin, but, rarely *Bacteroides fragilis* is present and may be resistant to this management. Two to 4 million units of penicillin are generally given in 4 divided doses per day for a prolonged period. Treatment should be continued until the process is clinically and radiographically stable—frequently 6 to 8 weeks or longer.

Patients with lung abscess must be carefully evaluated for the possibility of aspiration of a foreign body, and bronchoscopy may be indicated.

Lung Abscess

Lung abscess is a term applied to patients who have an acute febrile illness with radiographic evidence of necrosis and surrounding inflammation. A cavity, with or without a horizontal fluid level, and infiltrate around the entire circumference of the lesion are the hallmarks. Cavitary lesions most commonly occur with anaerobic lung infections, but multiple cavities of differing size are common in any of the necrotizing pneumonias. Apical cavities are more commonly due to tuberculosis. Septic lung infarction, fungal infections, bronchiectatic cysts, loculated hydropneumothorax, infected emphysematous bullae, and necrotizing vasculitis all may produce cavitary lesions.

INTERMEDIATE INFECTION SYNDROMES

Several organisms listed in Table 15.6 may be classified as bacteria although they present clinically with characteristics more like those of the viral pneumonic syndrome. These include the *Chlamydia* organisms that cause psittacosis, rickettsiae, and mycoplasma organisms—all of which are responsive to antibiotics. The presenting features are listed in Table 15.7. By far the most common of these is *Mycoplasma pneumoniae*, which has a predilection for patients in the second and third decades of life. In young adults, acute pneumonia occurs with approximately equal frequency due to influenza virus, *Mycoplasma pneumoniae*, or pneumococcus. Influenza virus and *Mycoplasma* can be cultured on special media and identified; however, serologic tests for rising antibody

titers are more generally used. A fourfold rise in antibodies is considered diagnostic. Mycoplasmal infection will cause elevated cold-agglutinin titers in 60 percent of patients.

Several organisms cause pneumonia less commonly but have a more serious prognosis. *Legionella pneumophilia* has occured in epidemics with a high attack rate. The clinical syndrome is that of high, unrelenting fever, relative bradycardia, hyponatremia, frequent gastrointestinal symptoms, nonproductive cough, and lack of organisms demonstrable on Gram stain of sputum. Myalgia, hematuria, abnormal liver-function tests, and toxic encephalopathy are frequently associated. Radiographically, fluffy rounded peripheral densities are characteristic. The course is improved by treatment with erythromycin 4 g/day parenterally.

INFECTIONS OF IMMUNOCOMPROMISED HOSTS

Many patients are predisposed to respiratory infections as a result of associated disease or primary immunologic deficiencies. Table 15.9 outlines the range of disturbances that may predispose to lung infection. Among adults, recurring bronchopulmonary infections are most often due to chronic pulmonary disease. Chronic bronchitis, cystic fibrosis, asthma, and the immotile cilia syndrome all impair mucociliary transport and presumably reduce bacterial clearance. Repetitive inoculation of the lung following aspiration of oropharyngeal contents is particularly likely in alcoholism and neuromuscular diseases. Splenectomy results in an increased risk of pneumococcal infections. Currently, reticuloendothelial malignancy and the impairment of host defence induced by antineoplastic drugs significantly predispose these patients to lung infection (see Chapters 6, 7). Few clinical features permit confident etiologic diagnosis of infections in compromised hosts. Table 15.10 outlines the range of causes for lung infiltrates that commonly must be considered in immunosuppressed patients and those with underlying reticuloendothelial malignancies. In these patients, peripheral blood leukocyte counts, serologic response to infection, clinical presentations, and radiographic features may be unhelpful; for this reason bronchoscopy with tissue aspiration, transbronchial biopsy, or open lung biopsy are more frequently necessary to establish a diagnosis. The therapeutic hazards of antifungal, antituberculous, or antiprotozoal therapy generally require a firm diagnosis prior to treatment.

Preventive therapy with trimethoprim-sulfame-

Table 15.9   Causes of Compromised Hosts

Primary Immunodeficiency States

Immunodeficiencies	Abnormalities of Inflammatory Response
B Cell function deficiencies	Humoral (complement deficiency, alternate pathway defects, e.g., sickle cell
T Cell function deficiencies	disease)
B & T Cell function deficiencies	Phagocyte function (neutropenia, defects in chemotaxis, defects in
	phagocytosis and intracellular killing)

Immunodeficiency States Associated with Other Diseases

Nonmalignant Disease	Malignant Disease	Drug-Induced
Diabetes mellitus	Leukemia	Leukopenia
Uremia	Hodgkin's disease	Impaired Phagocyte function
Rheumatoid arthritis	Multiple myeloma	Impaired B & T Cell function
Viral infection	Other forms of cancer	
Post surgical		
Malnutrition		

Nonimmune, Nonmalignant Diseases that Predispose to Recurrent Respiratory Infections

Lung Diseases	Other Cardiothoracic Diseases	Noncardiothoracic Diseases
Chronic bronchitis	Pulmonary edema	Alcoholism
Cystic fibrosis	Esophageal reflux and aspiration	Neuromuscular Disease with
Immotile cilia syndrome		aspiration
Asthma		Splenectomy

(See also Table 6.10, Chapter 6.)

thoxazole in patients who are immunosuppressed due to cancer chemotherapy, substantially reduces the incidence of clinical infection.

PARASITIC INFECTIONS

A wide variety of parasitic infections may affect the lung. *Trichinella spiralis*, the pork worm, may cause infection of respiratory muscles, with respiratory weakness. *Entamoeba histolytica*, the organism that causes intestinal amebiasis, may also cause pleuropulmonary disease. This generally occurs as a result of transdiaphragmatic rupture of a hepatic abscess into the pleural space or development of a bronchopleural fistula. These patients have cough, copious chocolate-colored sputum, and localized findings of lower lobe pneumonia or pleural effusion.

Discrete lung masses may result from echinococcal infections demonstrating thin-walled cystic lesions, which occasionally rupture into the bronchus or the pleural space. In North America these are most common in the far north, and humans are nearly always infected through handling dogs. In other areas of the world sheep, wolves, caribou, cattle, pigs, camels, or other humans may be the source. Table 15.11 summarizes the major clinical features and drugs of choice for more frequent parasitic infections involving the lungs.

Infections due to *Schistosoma* are a common cause of pulmonary hypertension in edemic regions, particularly Egypt, Northern Africa, Central Africa, and the Far East. Schistosomes are the most common cause of cor pulmonale in endemic regions.

Wherever water is purified and monitored for its purity, and standards for cooking meat and storage

Table 15.10   Causes of Roentgenographic Infiltrates in Compromised Hosts

Localized Infiltrates	Diffuse Infiltrates
Infection	Infection
Common bacterial agents	Common bacterial agents, especially in leukemia and severe neutropenia
L. pneumophilia and related organisms	Opportunistic fungi—Candida, Aspergillus
Pathogenic fungi	Viral—CMV, influenza, varicella-zoster
M. tuberculosis	Miliary tuberculosis
P. carinii	*P. carinii*
Other	Other
Pulmonary embolus	Malignancy—lymphangitic spread or multifocal
Lung hemorrhage	Leukoagglutinin reaction (transfusions)
Malignancy, especially cancer and lymphoma	Drug toxicity or hypersensitivity
Radiation pneumonitis	Sepsis

(From Guenter CA, ed: Pulmonary Medicine. 2nd ed. Philadelphia, JB Lippincott, 1982, with permission.)

Table 15.11   **Parasites That Affect the Respiratory System**

| Parasite | Major Presenting Features | | Drugs of Choice |
	Pulmonary	Nonpulmonary	
Protozoa			
Entamoeba histolytica	Pleural effusion, lung abscess	Hepatic disease, diarrhea	Diiodohydroxyquin, metronidazole
Pneumocystis carinii	Diffuse pneumonia	None	Trimethoprim-sulfamethoxazole, pentamidine
Helminths			
Schistosoma hematobium, mansoni, japonicum	Patchy infiltrates, pulmonary hypertension	Hepatic, gastrointestinal, genitourinary disease	Niridazole, stibophen, antimony sodium, domercapto-succinate
Cestodes (tapeworms)			
Echinococcus granulosis	Empyema, patchy infiltrates, hydatid cysts	Hepatic disease	Mebendazole
Nematodes (roundworms)			
Strongyloides stercoralis	Patchy infiltrates	Skin rash, pruritis, diarrhea, anemia, disseminated infestation	Thiobendazole
Trichinella spiralis	Chest pain, muscle tenderness	Muscle pain, diarrhea	Corticosteroids, thiobendazole

of food are maintained, parasitic infections of the lung are distinctly uncommon. Occasionally parasitic infections occur in the immunocompromised host even under these conditions.

CHRONIC LUNG INFECTIONS

MYCOBACTERIAL INFECTIONS

Pulmonary Tuberculosis

The death rate due to tuberculosis has decreased throughout the world, but the remarkable decline in the developed countries is largely a result of public health measures and antituberculous chemotherapy. It has been estimated that 30 percent of all deaths in the 17th century in London were caused by tuberculosis. At present this is reduced to about 1.0 per 100,000 population. In Western countries, the most common age of active tuberculosis has changed from childhood to 45 years and older. This represents a shift to predominantly reactivation forms of tuberculosis. Even in the developed countries certain segments of the population are at much greater risk for developing tuberculosis than others. The black populations in the United States, individuals living in crowded urban, low socioeconomic conditions, the Canadian native Indian, and the populations in penal institutions have a very much higher incidence of tuberculosis than the average population. Recent immigrants from countries with high rates of tuberculosis are now providing up to one third of the new

cases in North America even though they represent a very small portion of the total population.

Transmission of the Disease

Tuberculosis is an airborne infection spread by invisible droplet nuclie that are suspended in air. These nuclei are generated during talking, coughing, and sneezing. Because the particles are in the range of 1 to 10 microns in size, they remain suspended until inhaled, at which point they may impact along the walls of the bronchial tubes or terminal airways, become established, and reproduce. Larger particles that settle on surfaces in the environment are innocuous. Consequently fomites, books, bedding, or eating utensils are not involved in the spread of tuberculosis and require no special attention when caring for a patient with the disease. Ordinary hand washing removes organisms to which the physician or nurse may be exposed. Contamination can be prevented by simple measures to reduce the innoculum (such as directing the patient to cough through a mask or filter, having ultraviolet light and/or frequent air changes in the room, or having the nurse or physician wear a mask to reduce inhalation of droplet nuclei).

The most effective method for preventing transmission is to reduce the numbers of available bacteria by antituberculous chemotherapy. Soon after institution of antituberculous chemotherapy, even an active case of tuberculosis becomes noninfectious. The risk to the household contacts or family is reduced within days, and there is consequently no need to isolate these patients in the home or community. Occasional individuals with far advanced disease and/or resistant organisms may be better managed by respiratory isolation until the appropriate chemotherapy is clearly demonstrated to be effective.

Pathogenesis and Pathology

When an appropriate droplet nucleus reaches a susceptible site in the respiratory bronchiole or alveolus, multiplication begins. Macrophages migrate to the area and the organism is phagocytosed, but continues to multiply. Edema forms and fibrin deposition takes place. Polymorphonuclear cells may be attracted. This nonspecific inflammatory reaction occurs early and tubercle bacilli enter the lymphatic channels and are transmitted to regional lymph nodes. They may also spread hematogenously throughout the body. There is evidence that the bone marrow, liver, and spleen are almost always seeded, but infection is seldom established in these sites. In contrast, the regional lymph nodes, upper lung zones, renal parenchyma, epiphyseal lines, and cerebral cortex appear to be very hospitable sites for infection to become established. Acquired immunity develops soon, and further multiplication of the bacilli is controlled in the great majority of the initial lesions. Approximately 5 to 15 percent of patients initially infected with the tubercule bacillus develop clinical disease in the 5 years following infection, and another 3 to 5 percent develop disease during the remainder of their lifetime.

Cellular immunity develops about 2 to 10 weeks after the initial infection and results in inflammation and necrosis. This immunity may be demonstrated by the tuberculin skin test reaction. The tissue reaction produced during this phase is called *granulomatous inflammation*. The granuloma consists of a necrotic center with surrounding collagen, lymphocytes, fibroblasts, and new capillary formation. The necrotic area is termed *caseation necrosis* because of its thick, white, cheese-like material containing many destroyed bacilli. These necrotic areas may calcify, undergo resorption, fibrose, or, when enlarged, may empty into a bronchus, forming a cavity. The infection may spread along the bronchial tubes, extend directly to the pleura or pericardium, spread through the regional lymphatics, or spread hematogenously. Occasionally, particularly in children, swelling of the regional lymph nodes may cause obstruction of the bronchial tubes. Hematogenous spread results in innumerable tiny foci throughout the lungs and other organs. These present radiographically as milet-seed–sized nodules, popularly referred to as miliary tuberculosis. This represents the severest and most life-threatening form of disease.

Patterns of Infection

Initial or primary infection was previously seen predominantly in childhood. With the decreased rate of exposure to tuberculosis, it is now also commonly seen in adulthood. The initial infection is more common in the periphery of the middle or lower lung zones, presumably because they are exposed to more droplet nuclei. The regional lymph nodes are characteristically involved. There is limited hematogenous seeding, and this infrequently leads directly to clinical illness. Usually there is an interval of months to years or even decades before the disease is evident. Occasionally pleural effusions or erythema nodosum may be the presenting manifestation.

Reinfection tuberculosis occurs years or even decades after the initial infection. This is due to endogenous bacilli that begin to multiply, and which characteristically involve the upper lung zones.

The currently recommended classification of patients with respect to tuberculosis status is presented below.

Classification of Tuberculosis

0. No tuberculosis exposure, not infected (no history of exposure; reaction to tuberculin skin test not significant)

1. Tuberculosis exposure, no evidence of infection (history of exposure; reaction to tuberculin skin test not significant)

2. Tuberculous infection, no disease (significant reaction to tuberculin skin test; negative bacteriologic studies [if done], no clinical or roentgenographic evidence of tuberculosis)

3. Tuberculosis: Current disease (*M. tuberculosis* cultured [if done]; otherwise, both a significant reaction to tuberculin skin test and clinical or roentgenographic evidence of current disease)

> Location of disease
> > Pulmonary
> > Pleural
> > Lymphatic
> > Bone or joint
> > Genitourinary
> > Disseminated (miliary)
> > Meningeal
> > Peritoneal
> > Other

Bacteriologic status
 Positive by
  Microscopy only (date)
  Culture only (date)
  Microscopy and culture (date)
 Negative (date)
 Not done
Chemotherapy status
 On chemotherapy since (date)
 Chemotherapy terminated (date)
The following data are necessary in certain circumstances:
 Roentgenogram findings
 Normal
 Abnormal
 Cavitary or noncavitary
 Stable or worsening or improving
 Tuberculin skin-test reaction
 Significant
 Not significant

4. Tuberculosis: No current disease (history of previous episode[s] of tuberculosis, or abnormal stable roentgenographic findings in a person with a significant reaction to tuberculin skin test; negative bacteriologic studies [if done]; no clinical or roentgenographic evidence of current disease)

The extensive epidemiologic studies and public health measures instituted on an international scale for the prevention and treatment of tuberculosis have provided data permitting standardized therapeutic approaches that can be followed with considerable confidence.

Clinical Manifestations

Most patients presenting with tuberculosis have minimal if any symptoms. When present, very slowly progressive fatigue, lethargy, anorexia, weight loss, irregular menses, and low-grade fevers are the most common symptoms. The fevers classically occur in the afternoon and may be accompanied by defervescence and sweating at night. Initially these vague symptoms may be attributed to emotional stress or excessive work. Less commonly there is an acute onset with spiking temperatures, chills, myalgia and generalized weakness attributed to a flu like illness. There is an almost imperceptible onset of cough which may be nonproductive, or productive of mucoid sputum. Occasionally this is blood streaked. Dyspnea is uncommon except when accompanied by other cardiopulmonary disease or a large pleural effusion. Physical examination of the chest may be entirely normal, or consistent with broncho-pneumonia or pleural effusion.

The tuberculin skin test, as a measure of delayed hypersensitivity, is positive in about 90 percent of patients with active disease, and, if repeated in one or two weeks, will be positive in an additional small number of patients. A 10 mm or larger diameter for the indurated lesion is considered a true reaction, and cutaneous responses with a smaller diameter are classified as not significant. Some patients with tuberculosis have no reaction to tuberculin antigen, and false negatives may occur in individuals with recent viral infections, overwhelming febrile illness, lymphomas, or sarcoidosis, and in patients receiving adrenal corticosteroid therapy or immunosuppressant drugs.

Laboratory Assessment

Mild normochromic normocytic anemia is common after prolonged disease. The peripheral leukocyte count tends to be normal but an increased number of circulating monocytes may be present. Radiographic evaluation may demonstrate a wide variety of presentations. Apical, pleural, and cavitary disease with fibrotic streaking toward the hilar lymph nodes is the most common chronic change. On radiographic examination, a soft, fluffy infiltrate in the second interspace and prominent hilar lymph nodes compromise the most common lesion in initial infection. If healing takes place, a subpleural calcified lymph node and a calcified hilar lymph node are commonly the only residual findings (Ghon complex). Otherwise unexplained pleural effusion, atelectasis of a middle lobe due to obstruction by enlarged regional lymph nodes, apical fibrotic changes with retraction of the hilar lymph nodes and vessels, and miliary nodules may all be present. The nature of the radiographic change can raise the index of suspicion, but there are no diagnostic characteristics.

Sputum smears should be examined for acid-fast bacilli, or should be assessed for mycobacteria by fluorescent techniques. Morning sputum specimens should also be cultured, and the laboratory must be alerted so that the appropriate culture media are utilized.

Treatment of Tuberculosis

Preventive treatment is highly effective in household contacts of persons with active and untreated infectious disease. Children should receive isoniazid (INH) 10 mg/kg/day with a maximum of 300 mg/day. The tuberculin skin test should be repeated three months after exposure is terminated, and if the reaction is not significant INH can be discontinued. If the reaction is positive, INH is continued for as long as a 1 year. Young adults up to age 35 years should have similar treatment. An alternative means of preventing tuberculosis is vaccination of high-risk groups who are initially tuberculin–skin-test negative, with BCG (bacillus of Calmette and Guerin). The protection offered is modest, and probably not indicated for most individuals working in the developed countries, but it appears to provide significant protection particularly against tuberculous meningitis in the less developed countries.

Other high risk groups include the individual whose skin test reaction has converted (increased by at least 6 mm within 24 months from less than 10 mm in diameter), individuals with positive skin-test reactions who are receiving corticosteroids or cancer chemotherapy, and patients with hematologic or reticuloendothelial malignancies, silicosis, unstable diabetes, or gastrectomy. Such individuals should receive INH daily for 1 year; children, 10 mg/kg/day up to the adult dose of 300 mg/kg/day. In previously infected individuals age 35 years or older without the above risk factors, preventive therapy is not recommended at the present time.

Patients with active pulmonary tuberculosis should receive a prolonged, well-defined course of multiple drug therapy to prevent the emergence of resistant organisms and to ensure control of the disease without risk of subsequent reactivation. While two-drug therapy for at least 2 years has had the widest application, the high antibacterial action of current drugs indicates that 12 to 18 months of INH and rifampicin are generally adequate. Short course chemotherapy is gaining increasing popularity. INH and rifampicin given for 9 months, with either streptomycin or ethambutol for the first 2 months, shows great promise and is now in common use in some centers.

Patients with resistant organisms, poor compliance, or unusually extensive disease may require drug regimens tailored to their particular conditions.

Extrapulmonary Tuberculosis

Between 10 and 15 percent of patients with active tuberculosis present with extrapulmonary disease, and about half of those with extrapulmonary disease have no evidence of active lung disease.

Lymphatic tuberculosis most commonly involves the anterior and posterior cervical nodes, with supraclavicular, submandibular, axillary and other nodes being involved much less commonly. About half of the patients have evidence of tuberculosis in other sites including the lungs. The diagnosis generally requires proof of myobacteria on cultures from material obtained surgically. While mycobacterial lymphadenitis is almost invariably due to *M. tuberculosis* in adults, in children infection with other mycobacteria such as *M. scrofulaceum* is common.

Pleural tuberculosis is the next most common extrapulmonary form. The pleural fluid generally is straw colored exudate, with a protein of greater than 3g/dl and predominant lymphocytosis. The pleural fluid glucose is usually less than 50 percent of a concurrent blood sugar. While organisms are rarely identified in the fluid, multiple sample pleural biopsies will permit a tissue diagnosis in 65 to 75 percent of cases. Fluid and tissue cultures commonly grow mycobacteria.

Genitourinary tuberculosis commonly involves both kidneys, but is frequently first recognized because of asymptomatic hematuria or pyuria. Symptoms are more common when bladder involvement causes frequency or dysuria, or when epididymitis develops. An intravenous pyelogram may visualize abnormalities in the calyces, but fresh morning midstream urine specimens, cultured for mycobacteria, are the most reliable means of establishing the diagnosis. Smears of urine for acid fast bacteria are not done because of the false-positive results from saprophytic mycobacteria.

Bone and joint tuberculosis involves the spine in about 50 percent percent of cases, the hips in 15 percent, and the knees in 15 percent. Any joint, however, may be involved. Spinal tuberculosis most commonly results in limitation of motion and tenderness. Roentgenographically there is early disc space narrowing with subsequent destruction and collapse of vertebral bodies. Paraspinous abscesses may result in displacement of the posterior mediastinal line along the thoracic spine, or obscuring of the psoas shadow in the lumbar region. The diagnosis is established by aspiration of the abscess or biopsy.

Meningeal tuberculosis is uncommon, and is described in Chapter 14. Peritoneal tuberculosis is also uncommon and may result in abdominal pain, fever of unknown origin, and mild to moderate ascites with fluid characteristics similar to tuberculous pleural effusions. Bilateral adrenal tuberculosis may cause acute adrenal failure.

Miliary tuberculosis results from hematogenous spread, and is somewhat more common in immunosuppressed patients. As with many other forms of extrapulmonary tuberculosis, only about half of the patients have evidence of active pulmonary disease at the time of diagnosis. Fever, inanition, tachycardia, tachypnea, hepatomegaly, lymphadenopathy, signs of meningeal irritation, and splenomegaly are all common features. Disseminated multiple tiny nodules throughout the lung fields are the hallmark. Anemia, white blood counts ranging from leukopenia to leukemoid reactions, and electrolyte disturbances are common. Disseminated tuberculosis is frequently lethal unless antituberculous chemotherapy can be initiated soon enough to have full effects.

Extrapulmonary tuberculosis is generally treated with three drugs: isoniazide, rifampicin, and streptomycin.

ATYPICAL MYCOBACTERIA

A wide variety of other mycobacteria account for about 1 percent or, in some regions, up to 10 percent of patients with mycobacterial disease. *M. kansasii* occurs particularly in the Southern and Midwestern United States. *M. intracellulare* occurs in the Midwestern and Southeastern United States, as well as in several other countries. The mode of transmission of these organisms appears to be through soil, water, food, plants, and animals. Person-to-person spread has seldom been established. *M. bovis* is almost nonexistent in areas where tuberculosis control has been achieved in cattle and where milk is pasteurized.

Pulmonary infections with the atypical mycobacteria are more common in the presence of underlying pulmonary disease such as chronic obstructive pulmonary disease, pneumoconiosis, previous tuberculosis, and bronchiectasis. These other mycobacteria are generally recognized because *Mycobacterium tuberculosis* has not been identified on culture, and repeated cultures have consistently grown one or more of these organisms. Only *M. kansasii* responds in the same manner as disease due to *M. tuberculosis*. The others may be very resistant to chemotherapy, and treatment must be entirely individualized.

FUNGAL INFECTIONS

A variety of systemic fungal infections were discussed in Chapter 7. Although each of these may on occasion cause pulmonary infection, coccidioidomycosis, histoplasmosis, *Candida albicans*, and *Aspergillus* species are the most common. Coccidioidomycosis and *Candida albicans* are discussed in Chapter 7. Histoplasmosis and aspergillosis will be dealt with here.

Histoplasmosis

The organism *Histoplasma capsulatum* is inhaled, generally from soil or chicken or bat droppings mixed with soil. The droplet nuclei are deposited in the alveolar wall in much the same way that tuberculosis infection takes place, but unlike tuberculosis, person-to-person transmission does not occur.

The most common form of infection is subclinical or unrecognized in the acute phase. Subsequent demonstration of a positive histoplasmin skin test, with or without a radiographically demonstrable pulmonary nodule, or pleural calcification may be the only evidence. This infection is endemic, particularly along the St. Lawrence River valley, some areas along the Atlantic seaboard, the Mississippi, the Ohio, the Missouri, and the Tennessee River valleys, and these regions can be readily identified by the high incidence of positive histoplasmin skin tests.

Acute pulmonary disease presents with a dry hacking cough, fever, headache, anorexia, and myalgia. Examination of the chest may be normal or may reveal evidence of localized disease. Radiographic examination may demonstrate pneumonic infiltrate and hilar or mediastinal lymph node enlargement. In severe infection, bilateral infiltrates with severe hypoxemia may develop. The disease may progress to complete healing with no residuum, or may resolve into multiple nodular densities that progress to calcification during subsequent years. Conversely, chronic cavitary changes may take place that are indistinguishable from tuberculosis. Rarely, disseminated infection may involve the liver, the spleen, the bone marrow, and other organs.

The diagnosis may be suspected by the clinical presentation. Serology for compliment fixation becomes positive early after infection, and almost all affected patients have a positive serological test within 4 weeks of the onset of symptoms. Early in the disease, however, serology may be negative, and treatment decisions may be critical. The histoplasma skin test is very useful in epidemiologic studies but is commonly negative during the acute phase of the disease and may spuriously cause elevated serological titers. Therefore, it should not be performed as a diagnostic test in acute histoplasmosis. With acute, progressive disease, fiberoptic bronchoscopy for bronchial washings, brush specimens, and transbronchoscopic biopsy are recommended to obtain material for culture and histologic examination for the organism. Cultures require special media, and many laboratories are unsuccessful in growing the organism.

The vast majority of patients with histoplasmosis

do not require treatment, however, the severely ill and those with progressive disease or chronic cavitary disease require a full course of antifungal treatment. At present the drug of choice remains amphotericin B.

Aspergillosis

Aspergillus infections in the lung may present in varying patterns:

1. Mycetoma represents a slowly growing fungus ball, generally in a previous cavitary lesion of the lung. The fungal growth is innocuous unless recurrent hemoptysis or secondary infection occurs.

2. Bronchopulmonary allergic aspergillosis may give rise to asthma accompanied by eosinophilia, patchy and transient infiltrates, and thickened bronchial walls. When patients with asthma are relatively refractory to other forms of treatment, the possibility of chronic colonization by aspergillus, with hypersensitivity to the organism, should be considered. IgE levels commonly are markedly elevated. These patients may respond to systemic corticosteroid therapy.

3. Invasive pulmonary aspergillosis may occasionally cause localized nodular lesions, infiltrates, or cavities, particularly in patients who are seriously immunosuppressed.

4. Disseminated aspergillosis may present as a fulminant, systemic, multiorgan infectious illness with or without obvious lung disease. This form is rarely seen unless the last is severely immunocompromised.

Antifungal therapy is considered appropriate for invasive pulmonary or disseminated aspergillosis, but is generally not given for the other forms.

OBSTRUCTIVE LUNG DISEASE

THE SPECTRUM OF CHRONIC AIRWAY DISEASE

Patients with a variety of airway diseases may have similar symptoms. Cough, wheezing, sputum production, dyspnea and exercise intolerance are characteristic of each of the obstructive diseases. This frequently results in a superficial diagnosis of asthma in the patients with emphysema, or a diagnosis of chronic bronchitis in the patient with asthma. Detailed attention to onset, duration, precipitating factors, associated symptoms, family history, and char-

acter of the sputum often allows a clinical suspicion of one disease or the other. Subsequent laboratory evaluation should generally permit discrimination among these airway diseases; this is of utmost importance, since the therapeutic approach differs for each.

There is some recent evidence to support the hypothesis that recurrent viral infection in childhood may be associated with a higher incidence of increased airway reactivity (asthma) and eventually with a higher incidence of chronic bronchitis and perhaps emphysema. Some current studies suggest that childhood lung disease may either constitute a marker of the predisposed individual or result in structural alterations that subsequently predispose the patient to adult lung disease. The details of such a link remain to be established.

Asthma

Etiology and Pathogenesis

Asthma, a disease characterized by widespread increased responsiveness of the trachea and bronchi to various stimuli, is manifested by narrowing of the airways that changes in severity either spontaneously or as a result of therapy. One to 5 percent of adults and perhaps as many as 10 percent of children have these characteristics. In some individuals the precipitating factors are clearly related to exposure to extrinsic antigens, and the mechanisms can be attributed to a type I immune reaction (see Chapter 6). Antigen, and immune globulin E in the predisposed individual, trigger the release of mediators including histamine, slow-reacting substance of anaphylaxis (leukotriene), and other mediators that cause smooth muscle contraction and bronchoconstriction, increased secretion of bronchial mucus, and, in chronic forms, hypertrophy of mucosal glands and bronchial muscle. In these individuals clinical symptoms and physiologic abnormalities can be produced by exposure to the appropriate antigen. In other patients, nonspecific irritants including chemicals, dusts, or cold air may result in bronchoconstriction through mechanisms that are not well understood. These patients have "intrinsic" asthma.

Asthmatic reactions may be immediate in response to the appropriate stimulus, or delayed for 6 to 12 hours. The delayed reactions are often attributed to a type III immune mechanism (see Chapter 6).

The clinical circumstances in which asthma frequently occurs include the following:

Circumstances in Which Asthma Occurs

Acute exposure to antigen
Precipitated by drugs and diagnostic procedures
During the course of respiratory tract infection
After exposure to air pollution
In relation to occupational dusts or fumes
During coughing or laughing
Aggravated at night
Induced by exercise
In response to emotional stress
For no apparent reason in either atopic or nonatopic subjects

As many as 10 percent of asthmatics may have symptoms aggravated or precipitated by use of aspirin. The aspirin-sensitive patients commonly have nasal polyps. Other drugs that have been recognized to precipitate bronchospasm include indomethacin, phenylbutazone, aminopyrine, ibuprofen, food additives such as tartrazine, and a wide range of other medications currently being studied. Hypersensitivity reactions to any drug or radiographic dye may be associated with bronchospasm. Severe bronchospasm and cardiovascular collapse remain the most life-threatening features of an anaphylactic reaction.

Upper and lower respiratory tract infections often cause increased bronchospasm in patients with hyperreactive airways. Statistically, viral infections are much more common than bacterial infections in precipitating symptoms. During times of heavy urban air pollution and local air pollution within industries or factories, asthmatics are prone to more severe symptoms.

Innumerable occupations have been identified that are associated with increased bronchospasm. Farmers exposed to grain dust, synthetic rubber workers utilizing toulene diisocyanate (TDI), cotton workers, lumber workers (particularly those using cedar), and many others have been well studied. The patient presenting with asthma that is aggravated during the course of a day's work, or that is worse in the evening after a day's work but relieved when off work during a weekend or during vacation, should be considered for the possibility of occupational asthma.

In severe asthmatics, bronchoconstriction is generally worse at night and improved by midafternoon. This nocturnal dip in lung function is often associated with episodes of dypsnea and cough. The mechanism is not clear. In many patients exercise precipitates asthma. The severity of bronchoconstriction is related to the temperature of the air inhaled and to the minute ventilation. In most patients exercise-induced asthma can be abolished by inhaling warm humidified air. A precise mechanism for the bronchoconstriction is not established, but immunologic mediators or neural factors including increased vagal activity have been implicated. More than one mechanism may be important in particular individuals.

Clinical Manifestations

Patients with asthma characteristically present with symptoms of nocturnal cough, wheezing, dyspnea, and exercise intolerance. The symptoms are typically intermittent, interrupted by periods in which the patient is entirely free of symptoms. Commonly there is a history of "chest colds" consisting of prolonged cough and wheezing following acute respiratory tract infections. The symptoms may be clearly seasonal, may be related to known inhalants, or may be chronic and prolonged.

Physical examination demonstrates changes that vary according to the severity of the disease.

Mild Asthma   In the mildest forms, cough without any physical findings may be the only symptom. The diagnosis depends on demonstration of airways obstruction by flow volume loops or spirometry, a response to bronchodilators, or precipitation of obstruction by provocation tests.

Moderately Severe Asthma   These patients generally have mild resting tachypnea, slightly prolonged expiration, and, on auscultation of the thorax, scattered wheezes (rhonchi) throughout the lung fields bilaterally.

Severe Asthma   Patients with severe asthma are generally very anxious, with a respiratory rate exceeding 25 breaths per minute. Use of accessory muscles is prominent with intercostal indrawing. Careful measurement of blood pressure generally reveals a pulsus paradoxus of more than 10 mm Hg. Cyanosis may or may not be present. Auscultation of the thorax may reveal prominent wheezing, or even diminished breath sounds in those with severe limitation of air flow.

Sputum production is generally minimal during the acute attack, but the patient may cough up thick white mucoid material and occasionally bronchial casts.

Complications

Complications of asthma may be life-threatening. Severe bronchospasm may produce life-threatening hypoxemia with metabolic acidosis and arrhythmias. Pneumothorax and pneumomediastinum may occur during severe episodes, but are more common in those patients requiring intubation and artificial ventilation. The hazards of artificial ventilation are substantially increased in patients with asthma, presumably because of the high airway resistance. Large mucous plugs may accumulate, resulting in mucoid impaction with lobar atelectasis, or patchy areas of atelectasis demonstrable on chest radiographs. The mortality has been progressively decreasing in recent decades, and, in large centers, patients who arrive at the hospital after having experienced cardiorespiratory arrest with brain damage represent the most common examples of death secondary to asthma.

Laboratory Diagnosis

Hematologic and immunologic studies may be supportive but are of little help in establishing a diagnosis. Eosinophilia, when present, may suggest allergic causes. Elevated IgE levels support type I mediated immune mechanisms. In rare instances the association of eosinophilia, increased IgE levels, and intractable asthma may suggest allergic bronchopulmonary aspergillosis. Cultures for aspergilla may be helpful in these individuals. Sputum examination may reveal eosinophils, but it is more useful as a method to rule out bacterial infection.

The most helpful laboratory test is a measurement of expiratory flow rate. Patients with mild asthma may demonstrate minimal expiratory obstruction to flow that improves after inhaling of bronchodilator. Patients with moderate to severe asthma show striking reductions in expiratory flow that can be easily identified by the 1-sec vital capacity. If the 1-sec vital capacity is below 1.0 litre it indicates severe obstruction (in the adult), and the need for urgent intervention.

Arterial blood gas analysis is helpful in the severe asthmatics, to determine whether carbon dioxide retention is developing. Most asthmatics hyperventilate and will therefore have a low PCO_2 and a high pH. This respiratory alkalosis results in a shift in the oxyhemoglobin association curve to the left and a higher oxygen saturation than would otherwise be predicted for the characteristically low PO_2 (Fig. 15.3). Hypoxemia is uniform, presumably because of ventilation perfusion imbalance throughout the lungs. Only in severe bronchoconstriction does CO_2 retention begin. Therefore, a normal or elevated PCO_2 is an omnious finding, and it demands urgent intervention. In patients with increased PCO_2 and respiratory acidosis, the oxyhemoglobin dissociation curve shifts to the right; cyanosis is then more likely.

Therapy

Patients with mild asthma may require no treatment, particularly if their symptoms are insignificant. Patients with nocturnal cough frequently benefit from inhaled bronchodilators in the evening before retiring. Episodes of asthma related to exercise, excursions to the country, working in the garden, and other predictable events can often be prevented by prophylactic inhaled bronchodilators.

Moderate asthma acquires more aggressive therapy. Since asthmatic obstruction increases the patient's sensitivity to further obstruction (asthma is asthmagenic), the objective is complete or near complete reversal. Inhaled bronchodilators should be the mainstay of therapy. If symptoms are not controlled easily with demonstrated return of expiratory flow rates to normal or near normal, oral bronchodilators should be added. Systematic administration of the drugs should be followed by regular measurement of expiratory flow rates to ensure complete or near complete reversal of bronchospasm. The most common cause of treatment failure is poor compliance with medication regimens, or continued exposure to precipitating factors. The possibility of exposure to animal dander, house dust, or other organic dusts, occupational factors, or drugs that may precipitate asthma must be considered, and the precipitating factors eliminated. If all of these measures produce unsatisfactory results, inhaled sodium cromoglycate or inhaled corticosteroids should then be added to the regimen.

Patients with severe asthma require urgent treatment, which should be monitored for early response. The following criteria are important in establishing the urgency of treatment:

Criteria for Severity of Asthma
One-second vital capacity less than 25 percent of predicted value
Use of accessory muscles
Cyanosis
Tachypnea (respiratory rate greater than 25 breaths/min)
Pulsus paradoxus increased
Arterial hypoxemia and/or hypercapnia
Partial or minimal response to initial drug therapy
Previous severe attacks
Severe nocturnal episodes

Patients with severe asthma should immediately receive inhaled bronchodilators, intravenous bronchodilators, and intravenous corticosteroids. The 1-sec vital capacity should be measured and repeated

Table 15.12   Drugs Useful in Treating Bronchospasm

Drug	Route of Administration	Duration of Action (hours)	Major Side Effects
Sympathomimetics (Beta$_2$ selective)			
Isotharine	inhaled	3–4	
Orciprenaline	oral or inhaled	2–4	
Terbutaline	oral or inhaled	4	
Salbutamol	oral, inhaled, intravenous	4	
Feneteral	oral or inhaled	4–8	Tremor, tachycardia
Theophylline	oral or intravenous	6	Tachycardia, nausea, arrhythmias
Corticosteroids	oral or intravenous	6–24	Hypercorticolism
Drugs Useful in Preventing Bronchospasm			
Systematic bronchodilators	as above	6	none
Disodium cromoglycate	inhaled	6	Mucous membrane *Candida* infections
Inhaled beclamethazone	inhaled		

hourly until it demonstrates improvement to at least 50 percent of normal. Table 15.12 outlines drugs most useful in management of acute asthma.

Differential Diagnosis

Bronchial asthma must be distinguished from other diseases that may present with wheezing and cough. Pulmonary edema due to left ventricular failure or mitral valve disease may cause nocturnal cough, breathlessness, and wheezing. A thorough cardiovascular history and examination supplemented by an electrogram and chest x-ray will generally make this distinction. Recurrent infection in individuals with immunodeficiency diseases, or chronic bronchitis in the cigarette smoker, may produce symptoms with some intermittent characteristics. The most difficult problem occurs in patients with chronic asthma whose response to bronchodilators may not be as striking as that in patients with acute episodic asthma, and may be misinterpreted as representing stable chronic obstructive pulmonary disease.

Bronchiolitis

Infants tend to develop severe obstruction of the airways at the bronchiolar level commonly due to respiratory syncytial virus infection. In adults, an irreversible fibrosing disorder of small airways, bronchiolitis obliterans, may be a sequel to acute viral infection, but has also occurred as a complication of inhalation of irritant gases.

Chronic Bronchitis

Etiology and Pathogenesis

Chronic bronchitis is a diagnosis based on the medical history, and is defined as chronic productive cough of at least 3 month's duration on 2 successive years. The symptoms are associated with pathologic evidence of mucous hypersecretion, inflammatory changes in the bronchial walls, and bronchial wall edema. The most important predisposing cause is cigarette smoking, but many other factors may contribute to a predisposition to chronic bronchitis (Table 15.13). Immunoglobulin A deficiency, bronchial asthma, chronic exposure to irritant fumes or air pollution, and familial factors may all be significant.

Table 15.14 demonstrates the progression of symptoms and lung function abnormalities that occurs in a heavy cigarette smoker. The duration and severity of cough does not correlate with the severity of obstruction and lung function tests, but correlates generally with the number of cigarettes smoked and the duration of smoking (often expressed as pack-years).

Clinical Manifestations

The patient with chronic bronchitis generally presents with cough productive of white mucoid sputum. This may occasionally become purulent during episodes of acute bacterial infection, and may occasionally be blood streaked due to trauma to superficial mucosal vessels. The cough may or may not be associated with airways obstruction, but in the advanced stages there is commonly breathlessness and

Table 15.13   Cigarette Smoking

Adverse Effects of Cigarette Smoking
1. Depend on:
    A. Nature of device, that is, length of tube, temperature of smoke, presence of filters
    B. Art of the smoker (depth and amount of inhalation)
    C. Duration of smoking history (for example, pack-years)
2. Carboxyhemoglobin with increased angina and claudication
3. Overall life expectancy reduced.
4. Increased incidence of:
    A. Artherosclerotic vascular disease (2 to 3 times that of nonsmokers)
    B. Lung cancer (6 to 50 times as high as nonsmokers)
    C. Chronic obstructive lung disease (bronchitis and emphysema)
    D. Decreased size of newborn (smoking mothers)
    E. Lung disease in household companions
Contents of Cigarette Smoke (One Cigarette)
    500 milligrams: 5–10% moist particulate matter
                       12–15% carbon dioxide
                       3–6% carbon monoxide
Approximately 1,200 additional components (include nitrogen, oxygen, water, nicotine tar)

widespread ventilation perfusion imbalance resulting in hypoxemia. The patient may have noted frequent "chest colds," suggesting that lower respiratory tract infections are more common due to impaired mucocilliary clearance in the damaged mucosa. Physical examination may reveal cyanosis, occasional finger clubbing, use of accessory muscles of respiration, low level diaphragms bilaterally, and diffuse inspiratory crackles or wheezes. The auscultatory findings may improve or get worse after cough. When the patient reaches the stage of advanced obstructive disease, all of the features of severe airways obstruction, hyperinflation, and cor pulmonale discussed in the section entitled Emphysema, may be present.

In large studies of patients with chronic obstructive pulmonary disease, a subgroup of bronchitic patients has been recognized who have severe hypoxemia, alveolar hypoventilation, and, in the more advanced cases, cor pulmonale. These patients have type B chronic obstructive pulmonary disease; they have been referred to as "blue bloaters," in contrast to the "pink puffers" described in the section entitled Emphysema.

Patients with advanced chronic bronchitis frequently present with severe respiratory failure and right heart failure. Common precipitating events include respiratory tract infection, increased respiratory demands due to severe systemic infection, left ventricular failure due to associated cardiovascular disease, use of central nervous system depressant drugs, and occasionally pneumothorax. Each of these possible causes should be considered in every patient presenting with exacerbations of respiratory failure. The prognosis is highly variable. Many patients survive for 10 to 15 years after disabling chronic bronchitis first undergoes treatment, and others succumb early to an episode of acute respiratory failure.

Laboratory Assessment

The hemoglobin is frequently elevated as the result of polycythemia secondary to chronic hypoxemia. The arterial PO_2 is generally reduced due to widespread ventilation perfusion inequalities. In the early phases the arterial PCO_2 is reduced, but with progressive disease, hypercapnia and respiratory acidosis develop. The respiratory acidosis may be very severe during acute exacerbations. Lung function studies demonstrate reduced expiratory flow rates, which are minimally responsive to bronchodilator therapy. The chest roentgenogram may be normal or may demonstrate hyperinflation as discussed in the section entitled Emphysema, and there may be prominent bronchial markings throughout the lung fields as a result of bronchial wall thickening. The chest roentgenogram and the electrocardiogram may demonstrate right ventricular hypertrophy as discussed in Chapter 16, in the section entitled Pulmonary Heart Disease.

Treatment

The most important factor in the treatment of chronic bronchitis is ridding the patient of contact with irritants. In most instances this equates to ces-

Table 15.14   Natural History of Chronic Obstructive Pulmonary Disease (COPD)

Age 15 to 25	Age 25 to 35	Age 35 to 45	Age 45 to 55	Age 55 to 65
Smoking Asymptomatic	↓ Exercise tolerance Subtle function abnormalities	Productive cough ↓ $FEF_{25-75\%}$ ↓ $FEV_{1.0}$	Dyspnea on exertion Loss of time from work Frequent chest colds Hypoxemia Abnormal spirometry	Cor pulmonale Respiratry failure Severe disability Death

(From Guenter CA, ed: Pulmonary Medicine. 2nd ed. Philadelphia, JB Lippincott, 1982, with permission.)

sation of smoking. Unfortunately, as with alcoholism and obesity, smoking is frequently part of a behavioral pattern, and stopping requires exceptional motivation on the part of the patient. Pneumococcal and influenza vaccines should be administered in efforts to reduce respiratory tract infections. Patients with severe chronic bronchitis and obstructive disease require a systematic program to improve airway and cardiovascular function. Systematic inhaled and oral bronchodilator therapy are usually beneficial.

Every patient with chronic bronchitis and airway obstruction deserves bronchodilator therapy. Commonly a reversible component of the airway obstruction is present, and inhaled bronchodilators as well as oral theophylline may improve expiratory flow rates, oxygenation, and breathlessness. Further, theophylline may reduce pulmonary vascular resistance and improve right ventricular function. Patients with initial evidence of airway obstruction whose bronchial responsiveness is uncertain should all receive a course of corticosteroid therapy with careful monitoring to establish the degree of response. Significant numbers of presumed bronchitics may have a strong asthmatic component that is responsive to inhaled corticosteroids, but this is best determined by a carefully monitored 1-month trial of systemic corticosteroid therapy.

Patients with chronic hypoxemia may require supplemental oxygen. While hypoxemia is invariably worse at night, it may significantly limit exercise during the day. Recent studies indicate that 24-hr supplemental oxygen results in an improved life expectancy when compared with nocturnal oxygen supplementation alone. During acute episodes of respiratory failure and right heart failure it may be helpful to reduce the hemoglobin by phlebotomy.

Acute respiratory tract bacterial infection should be treated with appropriate antibiotics. Cultures from most patients will grow *Streptococcus pneumoniae* or *Hemophilus influenza*. The precise role of these organisms in precipitating acute respiratory failure, or in the chronic bronchial inflammation, has not been established.

Severe acute respiratory failure that is initially unresponsive to vigorous medical therapy may require intubation and mechanical ventilation.

Emphysema

Etiology and Pathogenesis

Emphysema is a common form of severe disabling obstructive lung disease. Males are affected 4 to 10 times as commonly as females. In most patients the etiology appears to be similar to that of chronic bron-

chitis, and, in fact, emphysema and chronic bronchitis are commonly present in the same patient. The emphysema consists of destructive changes in the lung parenchyma with coalescence of alveolar spaces to form larger, variably sized air spaces with much reduced alveolar surface areas. Two major types of emphysema occur: *centrilobular emphysema*, which involves the respiratory bronchiole and distal structures to form lobular destructive changes with a predilection for the upper lung zones, and *panlobular emphysema*, which is a more diffuse destructive process with a predilection for the lower lung zones. The emphysema associated with cigarette smoking is more frequently predominantly centrilobular. The emphysema associated with hereditary deficiency of protease inhibitors (α_1-protease inhibitor deficiency) is more commonly panlobular. Theories of pathogenesis have included recurrent infection with lung destructive changes, obstruction by the mucous causing increased tension on lung structures, chronic cough with increased forces on the lung, and many other causes. The most attractive hypothesis at present relates to the observation of familial antiprotease deficiency and associated emphysema. About 1 in 2,000 births in North America is associated with a genetic deficiency of α_1-globulin. These individuals have reduced capacity for inhibition of a variety of proteolytic enzymes. Experimental work suggests that elastase from polymorphonuclear leukocytes or alveolar macrophages is capable of destroying connective tissue, particularly elastin, in the lung when inhibitors are deficient. A wide variety of conditions in which protease enzymes may be increased at the tissue level, or inhibitors decreased, could therefore result in protease-antiprotease imbalance. It is clear, for example, that cigarette smoke may increase protease by attracting leukocytes and macrophages, and decrease inhibitor action by direct effect on the protein at the local tissue level. Consequently, cigarette smoke may promote emphysema through this mechanism. Destruction of peripheral lung parenchyma reduces the retractile properties of the lung (elasticity), permitting the lung to over expand. Further, the bronchi are normally distended because of the elastic traction on the bronchial walls. When this is reduced, they may become less patent during inspiration and actually collapse when peribronchial pressures are increased during expiration. Patients with emphysema, therefore, may have airway obstruction even in the absence of secretions, smooth muscle contraction, or bronchial muscle hypertrophy. The obstruction to expiratory flow results in regional disparities in filling and emptying of the lung, with hypoxemia arising because of widespread ventilation perfusion inequalities.

Clinical Manifestations

The signal symptom of emphysema is dyspnea on exertion. Unless there is associated chronic bronchitis or asthma, wheezing and cough are lacking. As the condition advances, obstruction to air flow may predispose to respiratory tract infection, and each infection may cause severe respiratory failure. The increasing lung destruction results in overinflation of the lungs, with characteristic depression of the diaphragm and decreased movement of the diaphragm on inspiration. In the advanced stages physical examination typically reveals an emphysemic habitus. This includes weight loss, mild cyanosis, pursed-lip breathing on exercise, and use of accessory muscles of respiration; on examination of the thorax the supraclavicular and infraclavicular fossae are deeper, and the entire thorax tends to move up and down as a unit. There is little reduction in thoracic volume on expiration. Percussion reveals a very resonant thorax, with low diaphragms that are below the usual level of the 10th rib posteriorly at normal end expiration. Total circumferential expansion of the thorax may be reduced below 5 cm when assessed by a vital capacity maneuver. Ausculation reveals reduced intensity of breath sounds, with inspiratory crackles (râles) commonly heard particularly in the lung bases. In patients with predominant upper lobe centrilobular emphysema the breath sounds may be most reduced in that region. Patients with predominant lower lobe panlobular emphysema frequently have distant breath sounds at the bases, with normal breath sounds over the upper lung zones.

Although cor pulmonale and right heart failure may occur late in the course of emphysema, both tend not to be as severe in the earlier stages, as seen in patients with chronic bronchitis. Secondary polycythemia is less marked, probably since hypoxemia is mild. Carbon dioxide retention generally occurs only in end-stage disease. Complications of emphysema include an increased risk of thromboembolism, secondary polycythemia, right heart failure, spontaneous pneumothorax, and severe bullous changes in which focal destructive lesions may expand to occupy a large portion of the thorax. In these patients, surrounding lung tissue may be predominantly compressed and nonfunctional.

Laboratory Assessment

The hemoglobin may be elevated, but rarely by more than 2 or 3 g/dl. Arterial blood gases characteristically demonstrate hypoxemia with PO_2 measurements ranging in the 50 to 70 mm Hg range at sea level. Throughout most of the course, mild hyperventilation will be present, but in advanced disease hypercapnia and respiratory acidosis develop. Ventilatory function tests reveal obstructive expiratory flow, with no improvement after bronchodilators. Further, this obstruction remains remarkably stable from visit to visit. The carbon monoxide diffusing capacity is generally reduced because of the reduced pulmonary capillary surface area. Measures of lung elasticity or lung compliance demonstrate an excessively distensible lung. Cardiovascular investigation demonstrates cor pulmonale (see Chapter 16).

The cause of emphysema may be suspected if the serum α_1-antiprotease is severely reduced.

Where chronic bronchitis and emphysema are combined, their relative contributions as causes of obstructive airway disease may be very difficult to ascertain. Where patients present with pure forms of one or the other, the diffusing capacity (reduced in emphysema) and measures of lung elasticity (elasticity lost in emphysema) may be most helpful.

Radiographic examination in advanced disease demonstrates hyperinflation, marked decrease in bronchovascular markings in the periphery of the lung, and prominent central pulmonary arteries. A firm diagnosis of emphysema is established if bullae are apparent on the chest film. Cardiomegaly is uncommon by standard criteria because the marked descent of the diaphragm results in a long, narrow cardiac silhouette. The marked increase in anteroposterior diameter may mask right ventricular enlargement.

Treatment

There is no known treatment for emphysema. At present experimental studies manipulating the protease-antiprotease system are underway. Treatment is directed toward improving symptoms, resolving associated disease, and reducing complications. These patients are ideal candidates for pneumococcal and infleunza vaccine. Bronchodilator therapy should be given in the hope that some reversible component of the airway obstruction may improve. Theophylline may improve pulmonary hypertension. Acute bronchitis should be treated as soon as symptoms develop. When hypoxemia becomes severe, long-term home oxygen may be desirable.

Exercise programs and, in particular, fitness exercises may be very useful in improving the level of the patient's performance. These programs do not generally alter lung function significantly but may substantially enhance the patient's capacity to undertake various tasks.

Surgical therapy for large localized bullae is occasionally helpful in highly selected patients.

Bronchiectasis

Etiology and Pathogenesis

Bronchiectasis was common prior to the widespread use of antibiotics. In earlier times, destructive pulmonary infections probably set up foci for further infection of the lung. In recent years bronchiectasis occurs in patients who have cystic fibrosis, deficiencies of immunity, and immotile cilia syndrome. Occasionally bronchiectasis develops distal to a localized endobronchial obstruction.

Chronic infection of the distal airways results in microabscesses, surrounding fibrosis, secondary inflammatory changes in the bronchial walls, and copious purulent secretions. As a result, the functional residual lung volume is reduced and airways become obstructed. The secretions interfere with distribution of air flow, and the resulting ventilation perfusion inequalities cause hypoxemia. The infection is generally chronic, but superinfection by new organisms or exacerbations of infection may result in recurrent pneumonia or febrile episodes due to exacerbations of localized disease.

Clinical Manifestations

Bronchiectatic patients characteristically present with recurrent episodes of respiratory tract infection accompanied by cough, copious purulent sputum, and variable degrees of breathlessness. If the infection is far advanced and has not been appropriately treated, finger clubbing may be present. When a single lobe is involved there is little impairment of lung function. Where more than one lobe is involved, ventilatory function is impaired, and breathlessness may become a prominent symptom. In advanced disease respiratory failure and right heart failure are common. In some patients recurrent hemoptysis is the major symptom. This may be massive in patients with extensive bronchiectasis wherein the bronchial circulation is providing high blood flow to the inflammatory tissues.

Cystic fibrosis occurs in about 1 out of 1,500 births in whites, and its incidence varies considerably among other races. This familial condition is inherited as an autosomal recessive, but the carrier cannot be identified by any known test. Cystic fibrosis may be diagnosed at birth because of meconium ileus, in childhood because of early childhood respiratory infections or failure to grow, or in later childhood or adolescence because of milder evidence of bronchiectasis. This great spectrum of clinical presentations must be borne in mind to ensure consideration of the diagnosis. Recurrent respiratory tract infections, bronchiectatic lung destruction, hemoptysis, or pneumothorax occur during the relentlessly progressive course of deterioration. Relatively few patients survive to the third and fourth decades. Death results from respiratory failure with cor pulmonale. Aggressive treatment of the bronchiectasis and nutritional problems improves survival.

Laboratory Assessment

It is important to establish the diagnosis is bronchiectasis, because the therapeutic program becomes one of life-long management. Patients with cystic fibrosis are diagnosed by elevated sweat chloride levels, and, when present, by the family history of other members affected and evidence of pancreatic or gonadal dysfunction. Patients with immunoglobulin deficiency should be recognized by serum immunoglobulin assays.

Patients with dextrocardia, associated recurrent sinusitis, or male infertility should be considered with respect to the immotile cilia syndrome. Bronchial or nasal mucosal biopsies with electron microscopic examination of the cilia may be diagnostic. If these underlying disorders causing generalized bronchiectasis are not present, bronchography may be indicated to establish a firm diagnosis and explore the extent of the disease. Occasionally, if all treatment measures fail, resection of localized disease may be indicated. Routine chest radiographs are occasionally suggestive of bronchiectasis, particularly when they demonstrate increased bronchial markings, recurrent infection, and cystic changes in the regions of infiltration. Patients with agammaglobulinemia and cystic fibrosis develop characteristic bilateral nodular and infiltrative disease, with multiple cavitary changes.

Ventilatory function studies are normal if one lobe is involved. With more than one lobe involved, restrictive and obstructive changes are characteristic. Arterial hypoxemia is common.

Treatment

Treatment consists of management of the underlying condition, and vigorous efforts to suppress infection. Sputum should be cultured to identify the dominant organisms. Bronchodilators, postural drainage, and chest physiotherapy in patients with copious sputum may be useful. These should all be administered on a systematic basis even after the acute evidence of infection has ceased. Antibiotic therapy should be administered until the sputum is nonpurulent and has diminished to the lowest achievable volume. Many patients benefit from systematic intermittent antibiotic therapy, for example, 7 to 10 days each month. Conceptually, this constitutes recurrent suppression of bacterial growth rather than prophylactic antibiotic therapy. Broad-spectrum antibiotics such as ampicillin, tetracycline, or sulfamethoxazole-trimethoprim are all suitable agents. Surgery is only considered in those patients in whom systematic and aggressive conservative therapy has failed, and who have predominantly localized disease.

Patients with cystic fibrosis may also require pancreatic enzyme replacement. Those with hypogammaglobulinemia may not absorb antibiotics. Therefore, in infections not responding to oral antibiotics, drug blood levels should be assessed.

PULMONARY VASCULAR DISEASE

PULMONARY EDEMA

Edema of the lung consists of increased water in the lung tissues. It may produce its effects predominantly because of interstitial fluid or alveolar fluid accumulation. A wide variety of conditions may result in focal fluid accumulation in the lung as occurs in pneumonia, pulmonary infarction, lung contusion, or localized aspiration of gastric contents. Clinically these conditions are generally considered separately, and the term *pulmonary edema* is reserved for those conditions that are thought to involve lung tissues in a more generalized manner. The physician may be confused, however, if regional hydrostatic changes in the lung or structural abnormalities of the lung are not considered in assessing patients with pulmonary edema. For example the patient with bullous emphysema will not develop edema in areas where blood flow has been disrupted due to the lung disease, such a patient may appear to have patchy pulmonary edema, which may be confused with more focal processes such as pneumonia.

The causes of pulmonary edema may be divided into two general categories: increased pulmonary capillary pressure and increased pulmonary capillary permeability.

Increased Pulmonary Capillary Pressure

Etiology and Pathogenesis

Left ventricular failure (due to any cause), mitral stenosis, and excess intravenous fluid administration are all common causes of elevated pulmonary capillary pressure that may result in increased transfer of fluids from the intravascular space to the surrounding tissues (Fig. 15.4). The increased loss of fluids from the intravascular bed probably results initially in a sharp increase in interstitial fluid delivered through the lymphatic system. Eventually the capacity of this system is exceeded, and the interstitial spaces swell. The perivascular and peribronchial tissues have lax connective tissue and are flooded first. At this stage impaired ventilation of distal lung units may result in hypoxemia and measurable abnormalities of air flow. Additional fluid loss from the vascular bed into the lung tissues may result in alveolar flooding.

Patients with head injuries, intracranial bleeding, or severe hypoxemia as occurs at high altitude may also develop pulmonary edema, and this is probably at least partly due to increased capillary pressure.

While cardiogenic pulmonary edema is only recognized acutely when pulmonary venous pressures rise above 18 to 21 mm Hg, it is almost always present when the pressures exceed 30 mm Hg. Patients with fluid overload frequently appear to develop lung edema at lower left atrial pressures; many of these patients have reduced plasma osmotic pressure due to hemodilution.

Clinical Manifestations

Tachypnea, tachycardia, breathlessness, anxiety, and eventually cyanosis are characteristic manifestations of pulmonary edema. When the pulmonary edema occurs at night due to redistribution of blood in patients with left ventricular failure, orthopnea is a prominent symptom.

Physical examination may demonstrate clinical findings of heart failure or mitral valve disease (see Chapter 16), and examination of the lungs may reveal evidence of pleural fluid, diffuse bilateral wheezes on auscultation, and inspiratory crackles, particularly marked in the dependent lung zones. It is noteworthy that upright patients generally have the crackles in the posterior bases of the lungs, whereas supine patients may have them throughout their posterior lung fields. Occasionally patients who have a strong preference for lying on one side or the other may have rales limited to the dependent side.

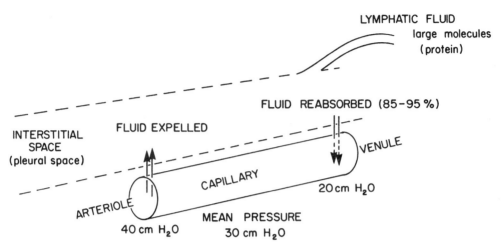

Fig. 15.4 This drawing illustrates the factors involved in fluid accumulation in body tissues. The same general mechanisms, dependent on Starling forces, are active with respect to the systemic interstitial space, the pulmonary interstitial space, or the pleural space. In the systemic artery the pressure at the level of the arteriole is about 40 cm H_2O and at the venule about 20 cm H_2O. The mean capillary pressure is about 30 cm H_2O. The oncotic pressure of osmotically active agents in the capillary is about 30 cm H_2O. Consequently water leaves the capillary at the arteriolar end due to hydrostatic pressure, but is reabsorbed at the venous end due to osmotic pressure. Some residual fluid is drained from the interstitial space through the lymphatic channels, which are also active in moving cells and large molecules which cannot be reabsorbed.

In the pulmonary blood vessels the pressure at the arteriole level is 15 to 20 cm H_2O and the pressure at the venule level is 5 to 10 cm H_2O. The key difference between these and the systemic vessels is the pressure in the interstitial space. Pleural space pressure is transmitted to the interstitial space and is subatmospheric. Consequently, the transcapillary pressure is quite similar to that in the systemic vascular bed.

Laboratory Assessment

Laboratory tests are utilized to assess the alterations in lung function and the evidence of increased lung water. Arterial blood gases demonstrate hypoxemia with a high alveolar arterial oxygen gradient and hyperventilation. In severe pulmonary edema, respiratory acidosis and occasionally metabolic acidosis may develop. The ventilatory function demonstrates a restrictive defect and evidence of obstruction of small airways. The chest radiograph demonstrates the following abnormalities with increasing levels of pulmonary venous pressure:

1. More prominent upper lobe blood vessels, reflecting dilatation of upper lobe pulmonary veins and redistribution of arterial blood flow

2. Perivascular haziness

3. Dilated subpleural peripheral lymphatics (Kerley's B-lines) and intralobar pleural fluid

4. Pleural effusions (more commonly on the right) and alveolar edema

The alveolar edema is frequently distributed in a bilateral perihilar pattern.

Treatment

The most important aspect of treatment is to identify and correct the underlying cause. In addition, removal of intravascular fluid reduces hydrostatic pressure. Intravenous diuretics should be given in severe cases, and oral diuretics in milder cases to ensure renal removal of excess fluid volume. Clinical improvement is often apparent within minutes of administration of furosemide, which is the intravenous drug of choice. Other measures such as correction of arrhythmias and administration of oxygen, systemic vasodilators, or, occasionally, mechanical ventilation may be life-saving. In very severe pulmonary edema phlebotomy or reduction of circulating blood volume by venous tourniquets on all limbs may be life-saving.

Increased Capillary Permeability

Etiology and Pathogenesis

Diffuse alveolar damage may result in fluid leakage from pulmonary capillaries into the interstitium and alveolar spaces. Many insults to the capillaries have been demonstrated experimentally to cause pulmonary edema. The precise mechanism or site of the lung injury has not been defined (see also Adult Respiratory Distress Syndrome and Acute Respiratory Failure). The following list summarizes the more commonly described clinical situations in which increased capillary permeability, or low-pressure pulmonary edema, occurs:

Causes of Low-Pressure Pulmonary Edema

Drugs—heroin, methadone, salicylates, oxygen toxicity

Sepsis—pneumonia, bacteremia

Trauma—lung contusion, fat embolism

Aspiration or inhalation of irritants—gastric acid, smoke, toxic chemicals, near drowning

Other disorders—cardiopulmonary bypass, paraquat poisoning, pancreatitis, uremia, multiple blood transfusions

Since the major defect is a breakdown of the capillary barrier, the edema fluid in the alveoli will have characteristics very similar to plasma. Frequently it is blood stained, and the protein concentration is characteristically high. Measurements of pulmonary venous pressure demonstrate normal or only modestly elevated levels. It is now clear that combined fluid overload and minor capillary permeability defects may result in severe pulmonary edema when it would not be expected (Fig. 15.5).

Clinical Manifestations

The most important clinical feature is the predisposing condition. Patients with one major predisposing condition have a significantly increased risk

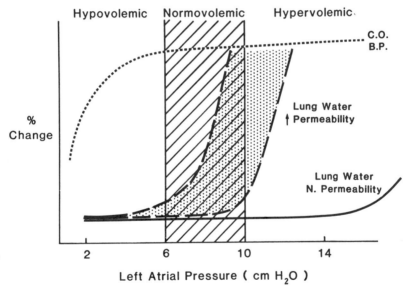

Fig. 15.5 This schematic drawing demonstrates the response of cardiac output and blood pressure to infused fluids. The dotted line illustrates the dramatic increase in cardiac output and blood pressure when severe hypovolemia is corrected. Further infusion of fluid beyond the low normovolemic range results in modest further increases in cardiac output and blood pressure. As the intravascular volume is replenished and then expanded, the left atrial pressure progressively increases through the normovolemic to the hypervolemic state. Lung water remains normal until left atrial pressures exceed 15 cm H_2O, and then it begins to accumulate in the lungs if further fluid is administered. In lungs with increased permeability, the lung water may increase dramatically if hydrostatic pressure is increased within the normovolemic range when left atrial pressure is relatively low (see stippled area between interrupted lines).

of developing increased-permeability lung edema. Patients with two or more predisposing conditions have a four- to six-fold increase in risk, as seen in patients with trauma and sepsis. The highest risk is within one to two days of onset of the predisposing condition.

Cough productive of edema fluid, tachypnea and tachycardia, breathlessness, and the clinical manifestations of lung edema described above may be present. Frequently, however, the underlying disease presents the overriding clinical manifestations.

Laboratory Assessment

Arterial hypoxemia with a high alveolar arterial oxygen gradient, and hyperventilation are characteristic in the early phases of this disorder. These patients may develop severe and life-threatening respiratory failure. When oxygenation deteriorates to the extent that they require mechanical ventilation and an inspired oxygen concentration greater than 50 percent, mortality within 7 to 14 days approaches 50 percent. When edema fluid is available through an endotracheal tube, it should be assayed for protein content to establish that high capillary permeability is the cause. In advanced degrees of lung edema, the vital capacity is severely reduced, and the functional residual capacity is reduced. This may be best demonstrated by the chest radiograph, which reveals bilateral high diaphragms and bilateral infiltrates; these may be quite symmetric or asymmetric, depending on the underlying mechanism.

Treatment

In most patients the definitive underlying cause cannot be identified or is untreatable. Consequently, supportive care and therapy aimed at maintaining the patient until healing occurs is all that is available. This consists of aggressive management of hypoxemic respiratory failure, attempts to reduce intravascular fluid volume to the lowest tolerated level (thereby reducing lung hydrostatic pressure), and measures to identify infectious complications early. Figure 15.5 illustrates the relationship between fluid administration and the development of lung water in patients with normal pulmonary capillaries and in patients with increased permeability. Patients with increased capillary permeability represent the greatest challenge in respiratory intensive care.

PULMONARY EMBOLISM

Thromboembolism

Venous thrombosis and thromboembolic lung disease are discussed in detail in Chapter 4.

Other Causes of Pulmonary Embolism

Septic pulmonary embolism may result from bacterial endocarditis or from septic phlebitis stemming from an area of infection such as appendicitis, pelvic inflammatory disease, or the site of intravenous drug abuse. Patients with septic embolism commonly develop multiple pulmonary infiltrates, often with cavitary infarction.

Amniotic fluid embolism may occur in women having unusually difficult labor or in women who have automobile accidents and severe compressive abdominal trauma in the third trimester of pregnancy. Patients characteristically develop severe low-pressure pulmonary edema as described above.

Air embolism is a major hazard of thoracic surgery and intravenous therpay. Further, it may occur after penetrating injuries of the veins, particularly in the thorax. Perhaps the most common cause in clinical medicine is the use of subclavian venipuncture to establish central venous lines in intensive care units or for parenteral nutrition. Once the air gains entry to the vascular system it passes through the right heart to the pulmonary circulation. Amounts ranging from 10 ml to 50 ml may cause an audible churning, crackling sound in the right heart and acute pulmonary hypertension. Amounts exceeding this may be associated with sudden death. Standard intravenous line insertion and care of intravenous administration sets requires thorough training and avoidance of air embolism.

Fat embolism occurs most commonly following multiple fractures of the long bones, the sternum, or the pelvis. About 12 to 72 hours after the fractures, or an aggressive manipulation of the fractures, the patient may develop petechiae (most commonly in the anterior axillary folds and conjunctiva), confusion, fever, hypoxemia, and bilateral pulmonary infiltrates. The most life-threatening and treatable aspect is hypoxemic respiratory failure (see Pulmonary Edema). Rigorous splinting and early definitive treatment of unstable fractures appears to have reduced the incidence of this complication. Corticosteroid treatment has been suggested, but is of uncertain benefit.

Tumors, and foreign bodies injected intravenously may also result in pulmonary embolism.

PULMONARY HYPERTENSION

The pulmonary vascular bed is much more distensible than the systemic vascular bed, and normal individuals only develop elevated pressures during moderate to severe exertion. Since the arterial pressure is low, the pulmonary artery pressure is much more sensitive to changes in the venous pressure than is the pressure in the systemic circulation. The following equation summarizes the interrelationships between pulmonary artery pressure, blood flow, and pulmonary venous pressure.

Pulmonary artery pressure

$$= \left\{ \begin{array}{ccc} \text{Pulmonary} & & \text{Pulmonary} \\ \text{vascular} & \times & \text{blood} \\ \text{resistance} & & \text{flow} \end{array} \right\} + \begin{array}{c} \text{Pulmonary} \\ \text{venous} \\ \text{pressure} \end{array}$$

Primary Pulmonary Hypertension

Primary pulmonary hypertension is a relatively rare condition that must be distinguished from other causes of pulmonary hypertension. It occurs predominantly in young adults, who generally present with dyspnea, easy fatigability, syncope, and, frequently, retrosternal chest pain. On physical examination they have evidence of right ventricular hypertrophy and right ventricular failure. There is no uniformly satisfactory treatment, but numerous reports of improvement with vasodilator drugs indicate that a trial of therapy is appropriate.

Secondary Pulmonary Hypertension

Hypoxemia due to altitude, or respiratory failure due to any cause is probably the most common cause of pulmonary hypertension. Patients with bronchitis, asthma, obesity, or emphysema may develop this variety of pulmonary hypertension. Those with emphysema have destructive capillary changes that add to the increased pulmonary vascular resistance. In those with advanced respiratory failure and respiratory acidosis the acidemia contributes to the pulmonary hypertension. Pulmonary thromboembolism causes pulmonary hypertension acutely, which may be sustained in patients with recurrent thromboembolism.

Connective tissue diseases with pulmonary vasculitis may result in primary vascular changes with pulmonary hypertension. Kyphoscoliosis with severe chest wall distortion may cause pulmonary hypertension as a result of respiratory failure. Congenital heart disease with a sustained high left-to-right shunt is associated with gradual structural changes in the pulmonary vascular bed causing pulmonary hypertension.

In all of these conditions, if the pulmonary hypertension is sustained, there is hypertrophy of the vascular smooth muscle, which further adds to obliteration of the vascular bed and to increased pulmonary vascular resistance. Treatment consists of correction of the underlying cause, relief of hypoxemia, and the management of right ventricular failure. The management of right ventricular failure is discussed in Chapter 16 in the section entitled Cor Pulmonale.

PULMONARY ARTERIOVENOUS FISTULAE

Arteriovenous malformations, or fistulas, may occur only in the lung, or may occur as a widespread disorder throughout the body. These patients may present with dyspnea, cyanosis, epistaxis, GI bleeding, clubbing of digits, and cutaneous or mucosal hemangiomas.

Characteristically, rounded densities are seen anywhere in the periphery of the lung fields. Most of these will be associated with a continuous murmur on auscultation.

PLEURAL DISEASE

PLEURITIC PAIN

The mechanisms of chest pain are discussed in detail in Chapter 16. Pleuritic pain is almost always unilateral and tends to be in the lower and lateral part of the chest. Occasionally it is referred to the shoulder or the abdomen. It is usually well localized, and is aggravated by deep breathing, coughing, or body movements. It may be distinguished from myocardial pain, which is generally central or substernal, or tracheobronchial pain, which is also substernal, related to cough, and often characterized by a burning quality. Pleuritic pain is caused by conditions that affect parietal pleura; the visceral pleura does not contain pain fibers.

It is of utmost importance to identify the cause of pleuritic pain if possible. A rib fracture results in exquisite localized tenderness over the region of the fracture and may be demonstrable radiographically on special rib views. Spontaneous pneumothorax, lung infections, pulmonary embolism with infarction, pleural neoplasm, and viral pleuritis (epidemic pleurodynia) are all associated with roentgenographic abnormalities. Other conditions such as herpes zoster, connective tissue diseases, and subdiaphragmatic abscess may not be recognized on the chest roentgenogram.

Occasionally pleuritic pain cannot be ascribed to any of the above causes, and may require symptomatic treatment until it resolves or until the underlying condition develops more fully.

Treatment consists of the use of analgesic or narcotic drugs. Indomethacin has been particularly useful. Occasionally the only successful analgesia is achieved by intercostal nerve block.

PNEUMOTHORAX

Etiology and Pathogenesis

Accumulation of gas in the pleural space may be spontaneous or secondary to lung injury. Spontaneous pneumothorax occurs commonly in young previously healthy adults, particularly males. Such primary spontaneous pneumothorax results from rupture of subpleural blebs into the pleural space. Most patients have entirely normal chest roentgenograms after recovery. Secondary spontaneous pneumothorax occurs with antecedent lung disease. Chronic obstructive pulmonary disease, diffuse parenchymal lung disease as in interstitial fibrosis, and necrotizing pneumonia are commonly associated with spontaneous pneumothorax.

On medical wards, pneumothorax most commonly occurs in patients on mechanical ventilation. This is particularly common in patients who require positive end-expiratory pressure (PEEP). Such patients may also develop pneumoperitoneum due to dissection of air through diaphragmatic orifices. Rupture of the esophagus is a rare but important cause of pneumothorax, generally it is left sided and associated with an effusion.

Clinical Manifestations

Patients generally present with dyspnea, pleuritic chest pain, and occasionally cough. The patient appears breathless, and the affected hemithorax appears larger than normal size (Table 15.1). During quiet breathing the affected hemithorax will show less respiratory excursion than the normal side; it will be more resonant to percussion, with decreased transmission of voice and breath sounds. The extent of abnormality depends on the size of the pneumothorax. Bilateral pneumothorax is fortunately rare since it is difficult to recognize on physical examination. Patients with severe obstructive lung disease may have hyperresonant lung fields that make side-to-side comparisons confusing.

The chest roentgenogram reveals a pleural lung margin that has collapsed away from the thoracic wall, and an air layer interposed between the lung tissue and the rib margin. This is most marked toward the top of the lung. Small pneumothoracies can be best demonstrated on expiration since the volume of the hemithorax becomes smaller and the proportion of air is larger.

Treatment

A small pneumothorax in an otherwise healthy individual causes no significant adverse effects, and may not require drainage. When the pneumothorax occupies 30 to 50 percent of the hemithorax, drainage is generally desirable. This can be performed by introducing a large intravenous catheter through the second intercostal interspace anteriorly (under local anesthesia), with underwater drainage. Alternatively, a thoracostomy tube may be inserted for drainage. Recurrent pneumothorax at a later date is common. When a pneumothorax has recurred on the same side on three occasions it is generally considered advisable to treat the patient by pleurodesis.

Tension pneumothorax is a life-threatening condition in which a valve mechanism allows continuing accumulation of pleural air without relief of the pressure. The mediastinum is shifted to the opposite side, venous pressure is frequently increased, and blood pressure and cardiac output are reduced. Severe dyspnea, and hypoxemia are present. If the patient's clinical status deteriorates rapidly, therapy must be started on the basis of the physical findings. A large-bore needle or thoracostomy tube should be inserted promptly; the diagnosis will be confirmed by the rush of air out of the chest.

PLEURAL EFFUSIONS

The parietal and visceral pleural surfaces are normally covered with a thin layer of fluid that reduces friction and facilitates motion during respiration. A small amount of pleural fluid may be demonstrated even in normal individuals when the thorax is opened, or on lateral decubitus roentgenograms.

Physiologic mechanisms result in fluid transfer from the parietal pleura into the pleural space and from the pleural space into the capillaries of the visceral pleura. The factors that can be predicted to affect fluid accumulation are similar to those that determine lung edema formation (see Fig. 15.4). An increase in capillary pressure due to increased systemic venous pressure or pulmonary venous pressure will result in increased hydrostatic forces. Reduced osmotic pressure due to low serum proteins will result in less fluid being reclaimed. Further, considerable evidence suggests that lympatic drainage of the lung may be impaired by disease in the lymph nodes, or by increased systemic venous pressure. This may contribute to fluid accumulation.

In addition to the changes in hydraulic and osmotic forces, changes in permeability of the pleural vessels may result in pleural effusions.

Etiology and Pathogenesis

Generalized disorders may present with unilateral, but commonly bilateral, effusions. These are generally due to hydraulic-osmotic factors, and the characteristics of the fluid demonstrate that they are transudates. Congestive heart failure, hypoalbuminemia, and hepatic disease with ascites are the common causes.

A wide range of diseases may predispose to pleural capillary injury, thereafter the fluid has the characteristics of an exudate. These include parapneumonic effusions, neoplasms, pulmonary infarction, connective tissue diseases (see Chapter 18), subdiaphragmatic inflammatory disease, postmyocardial infarction syndrome, and, rarely, myxedema.

Active infection of the pleural space may cause bacterial empyema.

Trauma, neoplasm, and pulmonary infarction are commonly associated with hemothorax. Lymphoma, other malignancies, and surgical trauma may occasionally result in disruption of the thoracic duct with chylothorax.

Clinical Manifestations

Patients with pleural disease and effusions may present with pleuritic pain, or with clinical manifestations due to the space occupied by the pleural fluid. A small pleural effusion may not cause any signs or symptoms. As the pleural effusion increases in size to involve at least one third of the hemithorax, dyspnea is a common symptom. Physical examination of the chest demonstrates decreased respiratory movement of the affected side; and with large effusions, physical examination demonstrates a shift of the mediastinum away from the affected side (Table 15.1). There is dullness to percussion below the level of the effusion, with decreased tactile fremitus and decreased breath sounds. Frequently a narrow band of increased tactile fremitus and breath sounds is demonstrable at the upper margin of the effusion, presumably as a result of peripheral lung compression.

The clinical findings of a pleural effusion are occasionally confused with those of lobar atelectasis, particularly if the bronchus is obstructed; but a shift in the mediastinum away from the side of the lesion should help differentiate these conditions. Consolidating pneumonia may cause dullness to percussion, but breath sounds and tactile fremitus are characteristically increased over the affected area.

Laboratory Assessment

Radiographic investigation is an integral part of establishing the diagnosis. With large pleural effusions, homogenous density is observed over the lower hemithorax, with a meniscus tracking up the lateral chest wall that confirms that the fluid is in the pleural space. Occasionally, particularly in the presence of underlying disease, lateral decubitus films may be necessary to demonstrate that the fluid moves within the pleural space.

Laboratory assessment is most helpful in exploring the etiology. In patients with heart failure, hypoalbuminemia, or marked ascites, thoracentesis is not necessary unless the fluid fails to clear after appropriate therapy of the underlying disease has been administered. When thoracentesis is performed in these conditions, the findings are characteristic of a transudate (Table 15.15). In patients without an obvious cause for pleural effusion, thoracentesis should be performed, and in most instances simultaneous needle pleural biopsy should be obtained. Routine analysis should include simultaneous measurement of serum and pleural fluid protein, LDH, glucose, and amylase. In addition, pleural fluid cell counts and differential white blood cell counts should be obtained.

Patients with purulent fluid should have Gram stains and cultures for aerobic and anaerobic organisms. Patients with sanguinous or bloody fluid should have examination for neoplastic cytology.

In spite of vigorous efforts to establish a diagnosis, 10 to 20 percent of pleural effusions in hospitalized patients remain unexplained. Unexplained pleural effusions should be assessed aggressively for the pos-

Table 15.15   **Pleural Fluid Characteristics**

Pleural Fluid Components	Transudate	Exudate	Empyema
Pleural Fluid/Serum Protein	< 0.5	> 0.5	> 0.5
Pleural Fluid/Serum LDH	< 0.6	> 0.6	> 0.6
Pleural Fluid pH	> 7.3	> 7.3[a]	< 7.3
Pleural Fluid, glucose	> 60 mg/dl	> 60 mg/dl[b]	< 20 mg/dl
Cells	few	> 500/mm^3 predom. lymphocytes	> 5,000/mm^3 predom. poly's

[a] pH is occasionally reduced in patients with neoplasms
[b] May be very low in rheumatoid arthritis

sibility of tuberculosis (see Mycobacterial Infections).

Treatment

Patients with severe dyspnea and large pleural effusions should have immediate aspiration to improve ventilation. Aspiration of large amounts of fluid may be associated with mediastinal shift and reexpansion pulmonary edema. It is generally recommended that approximately 1 liter or approximately half of one hemithorax be removed initially. The remainder of the fluid should be drained gradually over several days. Free flowing exudates and transudates may be drained by needle aspiration; however, purulent empyema and hemothorax usually requires a large-bore thoracostomy tube. Empyema and hemothorax should be drained as completely as possible to avoid subsequent development of fibrothorax.

Aside from relief of symptoms and prevention of subsequent pleural complications, treatment is primarily directed toward the underlying disease.

Patients with rapidly reaccumulating large pleural effusions due to neoplasm may benefit from chemical pleurodesis. The most popular method involves installation of tetracycline into a previously evacuated pleural space, followed by continuous suction for 24 to 48 hours to ensure adherence of the visceral and parietal pleurae.

FIBROTHORAX

Patients with previous empyema, pleural tuberculosis, or extensive lung trauma with poorly drained large hemothorax may develop a thick pleural fibrotic lesion that restricts lung expansion. This may result in a reduced vital capacity. Pleural thickening is readily demonstrated by chest roentgenograms.

DIFFUSE PARENCHYMAL LUNG DISEASE

GENERAL APPROACHES

Patients with chronic diffuse parenchymal lung disease may present with a wide variety of respiratory symptoms, or may be entirely asymptomatic but show major radiographic abnormalities. When confronted with this problem, the physician must begin with a comprehensive differential diagnosis. Textbooks of pulmonary medicine list several hundred potential causes. Since these can generally not be considered individually at the outset, a general approach to sorting these out by groups is most helpful. The key factors that permit the physician to be discriminating in diagnostic approaches are the following:

1. Associated disease
2. Environmental or occupational exposure
3. Rate of progression
4. Episodic or stable characteristics
5. Degree of functional impairment

Distinctive characteristics of various diseases are emphasized below. Cough, easy fatigability, and dyspnea that is particularly marked on exertion are common. Lung function studies demonstrate a reduced vital capacity (restrictive pattern) but flow rates are commonly well preserved, that is, the 1-sec vital capacity remains greater than 75 percent of the total vital capacity. Functional residual capacity may be reduced, as is the total lung capacity. Arterial blood gases frequently demonstrate hypoxemia with a high alveolar-arterial oxygen gradient, with a low PCO_2. The majority of these patients develop more severe hypoxemia during exercise.

DISEASE GROUPS

Table 15.16 outlines the major categories of diffuse parenchymal lung disease. A large variety of unusual

Table 15.16   Diffuse Parenchymal Lung Disease

1. Interstitial Pneumonia
2. Allergic Alveolitis
3. Sarcoidosis
4. Hemorrhagic syndromes
5. Pneumoconiosis
6. Connective Tissue Diseases
7. Drug Induced Lung Disease
8. Neoplasms

diseases including eosinophilic granuloma of lung, radiation pneumonitis, and amyloidosis are not included in these classifications.

Interstitial Pneumonias

Etiology and Pathogenesis

A wide variety of insults may result in a common lung injury typified by *idiopathic pulmonary fibrosis*, also known as *diffuse interstitial fibrosis* or *fibrosing alveolitis*. This may occur following the adult respiratory distress syndrome due to any cause, viral pneumonia, aspiration pneumonia, lung radiation, and numerous other events. The mechanism of lung injury is not clear, but recent studies demonstrate a prominent inflammatory reaction in the lungs with increased lymphocytes and polymorphonuclear leukocytes that can be demonstrated by bronchoalveolar lavage. The mechanisms of tissue injury have been postulated to be the same mechanisms responsible for injury in other types of inflammation reviewed in Chapter 18, Figure 18.4.

Clinical Manifestations

Patients with parenchymal lung disease typically present with a nonproductive cough and dyspnea on exertion, and on examination demonstrate elevated diaphragms bilaterally, indicating restrictive lung disease. Thoracic excursion is reduced on maximum inspiration, and commonly inspiratory crackles are heard, particularly in the lung bases. Clubbing and cyanosis are common.

Laboratory Assessment

Aside from the evidence of restrictive lung disease outlined above, evidence of an inflammatory alveolitis is the major finding. Increased inflammatory cells in alveolar lavage fluid, and evidence of inflam-

mation on isotope scanning are characteristic during the active phase of the disease. Once the acute phase has resolved (often months to years) stable restrictive disease is characteristic. Patients with new symptoms and evidence of disease, progressive disease as demonstrated by radiographic changes, or changes in lung function should be assessed by transbronchial or open lung biopsy to exclude other more treatable disease. Serial lung function tests most useful in detecting progression of disease include the chest radiograph, vital capacity, carbon monoxide diffusing capacity, and arterial blood gas response to a standardized exercise load.

Treatment

Patients with minimal or nonprogressive disease generally require no treatment. With documented deterioration of lung function high dose corticosteroid therapy is given on a trial basis for several months, with carefully monitoring of the response as described above. The need for continued corticosteroid therapy is determined by the degree of response demonstrated. Patients with active inflammatory changes shown on lung biopsy or in alveolar lavage fluid, generally have more likelihood of improvement on steroid therapy.

Allergic Alveolitis

Etiology and Pathogenesis

Numerous inhaled organic materials may produce allergic alveolitis. Moldy hay (farmer's lung), redwood sawdust (sequoiosis), and bird droppings (bird fanciers lung) represent a small number of the many well-described agents. It is probable that all four immunologic reactions are involved in various patients. In the early stages of the disease eosinophila, granuloma formation, and cellular interstitial infiltrates are characteristic, and are associated with evidence of bronchospasm. If the condition recurs, diffuse interstitial fibrosis may develop, resulting in severe, disabling restrictive lung disease.

Clinical Manifestations

The characteristic history includes fever, malaise, myalgia, arthralgia, and chest tightness developing 4 to 8 hours after exposure to the appropriate dust. A dry cough is characteristic. The patient is tachypneic, may be wheezing, and may have râles over the lower lobes. Spontaneous improvement generally occurs in 12 to 24 hours.

Laboratory Assessment

Peripheral blood eosinophilia and elevated immune globulin E levels may be present. Pulmonary function studies demonstrate combined restrictive and obstructive lung disease with a low carbon monoxide diffusing capacity. If appropriate antigens are available, precipitating antibodies are frequently demonstrable in the serum. The most common antigen in farmers lung is from *Thermophilic actinomycetes*. Skin test hypersensitivity may also be demonstrated.

Treatment

The most important factor is identification of the offending agent and removal from the environment. High-dose corticosteroid therapy (equivalent of 60 mg/day of prednisone) reduces systemic toxicity and appears to hasten resolution of the pulmonary lesion. Bronchodilators may be of benefit.

Sarcoidosis

Etiology and Pathogenesis

Sarcoidosis is one of the most studied lung diseases. It is a systemic disease characterized by granuloma formation with or without clinical manifestations of constitutional illness. Extensive efforts to establish an infectious etiology have been fruitless. While there are numerous immunologic disturbances associated with active disease, at present the cause remains unknown. The lung is the organ most commonly involved, and is affected in more than 95 percent of patients with the disease. Lymph nodes are involved in more than 75 percent; the spleen, the liver, the skin, the eyes, the joints, the nervous system, and the myocardium are involved with decreasing frequency. The granulomatous lymphadenopathy may result in paratracheal and bilateral hilar lymph node enlargement that commonly lasts for months and resolves spontaneously. In 10 to 20 percent of patients a more chronic form of the disease develops, characterized by extensive pulmonary granulomatous involvement progressing to diffuse fibrosis.

Clinical Manifestations

Most patients are recognized during a mild or inconsequential illness when routine chest roentgenography demonstrates hilar adenopathy. Occasionally systemic symptoms such as fever, arthralgia, and erythema nodosum may be present. In about one third of patients the chest roentgenogram demonstrates parenchymal infiltrates, and a smaller proportion of patients have hepatomegaly, splenomegaly, or subcutaneous nodules.

Laboratory Assessment

Serum proteins may demonstrate a polyclonal increase in gammaglobulin. Hypercalcemia is occasionally present, but hypercalciuria is more frequent. Pulmonary function studies may demonstrate restrictive disease and a reduced diffusing capacity in patients with severe parenchymal lung involvement. Serum angiotensin-converting enzyme is commonly elevated during the active phase of the disease, for reasons not understood. Alveolar lavage fluid demonstrates increased lymphocyte populations in the airways. A firm diagnosis depends on histologic evidence of noncaseating granulomas in the absence of specific granulomatous infections. Transbronchial lung biopsy generally provides the most accessible tissue. When lymphadenopathy or cutaneous nodules are present they should be biopsied instead.

Treatment

Patients with hilar adenopathy and no progressive disease should be followed for 6 months to 1 year, until evidence of regression of their disease. To ensure early detection of progressive lung disease they should be monitored by chest radiographs, lung function studies including the diffusing capacity, and exercise studies. The angiotensin-coverting enzyme may be a helpful index if it is elevated.

Evidence of progressive disease is generally interpreted as an indication for corticosteroid therapy. This is initiated with high-dose (equivalent of 60 mg/day of prednisone) corticosteroid therapy for at least 1 month; the dosage is gradually tapered while monitoring for evidence of active disease.

Other indications for corticosteroid therapy include hypercalcemia, myocardial sarcoid, evidence of central nervous system disease, and occular manifestations. While it has not been confirmed that corticosteroids prevent complications, there is common consensus that remissions may be induced by corticosteroid therapy.

Hemorrhagic Syndromes

Diffuse capillary vasculitis may be seen in idiopathic pulmonary hemosiderosis and in Goodpasture's syndrome. These patients develop hemoptysis and anemia associated with diffuse bilateral infiltrates. Those with Goodpasture's syndrome also have glomerulonephritis and demonstrable circulating antiglomerular basement membrane antibodies. These rare conditions may constitute medical emergencies. Plasmapheresis has been helpful in addition to the use of corticosteroids and immunosuppressive drugs.

Pneumoconiosis

Etiology and Pathogenesis

Lung injury as a result of inhalation of inorganic dust may provoke chronic proliferative and destructive lung lesions. Silicosis results from the inhalation of free silicone dioxide particles. These are fibrogenic, and may cause widespread whorled nodules throughout the lung fields, or progressive dense scarring of the upper lung zones known as *progressive massive fibrosis*. In most patients this is a result of hard rock mining, sand blasting, stone cutting, or other occupational exposure.

Asbestosis results from inhalation of asbestos fibers. Diffuse pulmonary fibrosis occurs. Biopsies or occasionally sputum may demonstrate the charactertistic feruginous body. Patients have generally been exposed through use of asbestos-containing insulation materials, particularly in relation to insulation, plumbing, shipyard, and demolition work. Vigorous occupational education regarding asbestos has reduced the incidence of this problem in recent years. Another complication of asbestos exposure is the development of neoplasms. Mesothelioma is most highly correlated, but gastric carcinoma and lung cancer are also increased.

Coal workers' pneumoconiosis is a controversial lung disease that occurs in coal miners, it is distinct in effect from silica. Multiple pinpoint nodules throughout the lung fields associated with symptoms of chronic bronchitis have been ascribed to the inhalation of coal dust. Disturbances in pulmonary function are restricted to minimal evidence of airways disease, unless associated cigarette smoking or other inorganic dust inhalation is combined.

Beryllium, talc, cadmium, and many other inorganic dusts are known to cause lung disease. Patients with a history of occupational exposure to any organic or inorganic dust must be considered for potential lung damage. The physician is urged to pursue the specific agent through reading of textbooks of occupational lung disease.

Clinical Manifestations

A few typical features may be helpful in leading the physician to a diagnosis of a specific pneumoconiosis. Hilar adenopathy is common early in berylliosis. Multiple small nodules on the chest roentgenogram are typical of silicosis. Basilar râles and clubbing are common in asbestosis.

Laboratory assessment may require lung biopsy if the occupational exposure is not clearly defined. Treatment consists of removal of the patient from the offending environment.

Connective Tissue Diseases

Etiology and Pathogenesis

The connective tissue diseases are discussed in detail in Chapter 18. Rheumatoid arthritis and the much more rare progressive systemic sclerosis (scleroderma) are the most common causes of diffuse parenchymal lung disease. Rheumatoid arthritis may also be associated with pleural effusion, and occasionally with parenchymal nodules, which may cavitate. The parenchymal lung disease may occasionally precede other organ involvement in the connective tissue diseases.

Drug-Induced Lung Disease

Table 15.17 itemizes lung diseases and the more common drugs that produce the particular patterns. A wide variety of additional drugs may cause lung

Table 15.17 **Drug-Induced Lung Diseases**

Disease Pattern	Drug or Agent
Diffuse Fibrosis	Antineoplastic drugs (for example, bleomycin) Nitrofurantoin
Pulmonary Edema	Narcotics, salicylates, nitrofurantoin
Pulmonary Infiltrates with Eosinophilia	Penicillin, sulfa drugs
Hilar Adenopathy or Widened Mediastinum	Diphenyl hydantoin

disease less commonly. It is of utmost importance to devote detailed exploration to the potential role of drugs as etiologic agents in patients presenting with parenchymal lung disease.

Neoplasms

Primary lung neoplasms generally cause lung masses or more extensive infiltration due to infection or obstruction of bronchi. Metastatic neoplasms may occasionally present as diffuse parenchymal disease due to widespread hematogenous metastases, or so-called lymphangitic spread. Broncho-alveolar carcinoma is a primary lung neoplasm that may present with bilateral diffuse infiltrates. These patients are frequently severely hypoxemic with restrictive lung disease, and have a very poor prognosis.

LUNG TUMORS

BRONCHOGENIC CARCINOMA

Etiology and Pathogenesis

Bronchogenic carcinoma is the tumor with the highest mortality rate in males in the Western world. It is second only to breast cancer as a cause of cancer deaths in females. The rate of increase in cancer deaths due to these tumors has accelerated dramatically during the past 20 years, and is thought to reflect the epidemic of cigarette smoking. Although urban air pollution and occupational exposure to uranium, asbestos, hematite, and other factors all contribute to the increased risk of lung cancer, by far the highest correlation is with cigarette smoking. The following cell types are commonly recognized:

1. Squamous cell carcinoma, 30 to 45 percent
2. Adenocarcinoma, 30 to 40 percent
3. Small cell undifferentiated carcinoma, 20 percent
4. Broncho-alveolar carcinoma, 10 percent

Patients over age 40 years and those with a history of heavy smoking or previous exposure to high-risk occupational hazards, should be considered particularly at risk.

Clinical Manifestations

Patients with bronchogenic carcinoma may present with a variety of features, depending on the location or spread of the tumor. Table 15.18 itemizes

Table 15.18   Common Presentations of Lung Cancer

Location	Clinical Features
Endobronchial Disease	Cough, hemoptysis, obstructive pneumonia, atelectasis
Apical Tumors	Brachial plexus compression, Horner's syndrome (Pancoast's tumor)
Metastatic Disease in the Thorax	
Pleural	Pleuritic pain, effusions
Mediastinal	Phrenic, recurrent laryngeal (L) palsy, superior vena cava obstruction, tracheal compression, dysphagia
Pericardial	Atrial arrhythmias, tamponade
Distant Metastasis	Bone pain, pathologic fractures, intracranial tumor, hepatomegaly, supraclavicular nodes, subcutaneous nodules

common presenting features. Aside from local effects related directly to tumor, systemic and metabolic features may be important.

Weakness, weight loss, fatigability, low-grade fever, and anemia are particularly common manifestations of lung tumors. These systemic features are poor prognostic indicators. Since these patients are generally chronic cigarette smokers, symptomatic obstructive lung disease is frequently associated.

Hypercalcemia may occur with bronchogenic carcinoma as a result of bony metastases, but may also be the result of parathyroid hormone–like secretion from squamous cell carcinoma. More commonly, hyponatremia may be associated with inappropriate secretion of ADH, and hypercortisolism may result from ACTH secretion by oat cell carcinoma. A myasthenic syndrome with marked muscle weakness and large muscle myopathies occurs frequently.

Clubbing of digits is seen in about 20 percent of patients, and is most commonly associated with bronchogenic carcinoma when accompanied by hypertrophic osteoarthropathy characterized by tender edematous thickening of the periosteum of the radius and ulna or tibia and fibula.

Laboratory Assessment

Patients with hilar or peripheral lung masses on chest radiographs and patients presenting with unexplained hemoptysis must be considered to have a malignant lung tumor until proven otherwise. Sputum cytology for neoplastic cells may be diagnostic. More commonly, bronchoscopy with brushing or biopsy of lesions is necessary. A firm histologic or cytologic diagnosis is necessary before treatment can be planned. Clinical evidence of metastatic disease in any of these organs requires aggressive documentation, since treatment will be determined by evidence of spread. In the absence of symptoms or physical findings suggesting metastatic disease, liver scans, bone scans, and computed tomography of the brain are not indicated.

Treatment

The first step in treatment is definitive staging of the tumor (see Chapter 5). Most large centers now enroll patients in standardized treatment protocols. In patients with no evidence of metastases or direct invasion of chest wall or mediastinum, surgical resection with the intent of cure is the treatment of choice, except with small cell undifferentiated (oat cell) carcinoma. If the patient has metastatic disease, local radiation therapy holds the greatest promise for control of symptoms due to intracranial tumor, bony metastases, vena cava obstruction, bronchial obstruction, or recurrent hemoptysis. Five-year survival in all patients with bronchogenic carcinoma is less than 10 percent. Patients with small cell undifferentiated carcinoma have a 90 percent one year mortality without treatment, but respond dramatically to combination chemotherapy and radiotherapy; numerous survivors are now living after two or more years.

Metastatic Carcinoma

Because of the large pulmonary vascular bed, numerous tumors metastasize preferentially to the lung. Tumors draining directly into the systemic venous system most commonly cause discrete lung metastases. These include carcinoma of the breast, kidney, and testicles. Gastrointestinal tract tumors commonly produce symptomatic hepatic metastases first. Pleural metastases are common, and occur particularly frequently from carcinoma of the breast. The diffuse widespread metastatic pattern known as "lymphangitic spread" results in severe dyspnea, hypoxemia, and rapidly progressive restrictive lung disease.

There is evidence that surgical resection of metastatic lesions may prolong life when certain tumors such as osteogenic sarcoma and hypernephroma are involved.

Table 15.19   Nonmalignant Lung Tumors

Very Common
  Granulomas
        histoplasmosis, tuberculosis, coccidioidomycosis
Common
  Lung abscesses before rupture into bronchus
  Slowly resolving pneumonia
  Pulmonary infarct
  Hamartoma
Less Common
  Bronchial adenoma
  Arteriovenous fistula
  Infected bullous lung lesion

Benign Tumors of the Lung

Lung nodules may result from lung infection, infarction, congential anomalies, or new growth. When the nodules are multiple, and when no overt primary is present to suggest metastatic carcinoma, granulomas due to tuberculous or fungal infection are generally the cause. Dense calcification, particularly when concentric, suggests an inflammatory cause.

The most useful characteristic in differentiating between benign and malignant masses is the rate of growth. When a patient presents with a lung mass with no other evidence of disease and no helpful historical information, it is important to consult any previous films. If the patient is over age 40 years, is a cigarette smoker, and shows radiographic features consistent with a malignant neoplasm, needle aspiration or surgical resection of the mass must be considered. If, however, the mass has been present previously, if there is evidence that it is not growing, if the patient is a nonsmoker and under age 40 years, or if "popcorn" calcification consistent with a hamartoma is present, observation may be appropriate. Table 15.19 lists common benign lung tumors.

LUNG DISEASE SECONDARY TO OTHER PROBLEMS

TRAUMA

Building construction that occurs at great heights, high-speed motor vehicle traffic, and recreational vehicles such as motorcycles and snowmobiles have all contributed to a high incidence of major trauma. More than 100,000 individuals in the United States and a proportionate number in Canada die each year due to trauma. Because these individuals are generally young, this represents the highest number of life-years lost due to premature death. Contrary to popular teaching, most thoracic trauma does not require surgical intervention. Pneumothorax and hemothorax may require chest tube drainage. Contusion of the lung requires oxygenation and supportive care as do other causes of respiratory failure. Patients with multiple rib fractures may require analgesia and vigorous chest physiotherapy. Early recognition of lung infection permits appropriate antibiotic treatment. Multiple rib fractures with an unstable chest wall may result in a "flail chest," characterized by paradoxical motion of a panel of the chest wall and hypoxemic respiratory failure. Mechanical ventilation may become necessary if underlying lung contusion or associated lung disease aggravates the respiratory failure. Occasionally rupture of the diaphragm causes herniation of abdominal contents into the thorax and results in respiratory failure. Laceration of the lung may cause hemoptysis, and a cavitary infiltrate on the chest roentgenogram. Persistent pneumothorax, or unresolving pneumonia following trauma should raise suspicion of a lacerated bronchus. Associated trauma to the myocardium may result in pericardial effusion or the changes of myocardial infarction.

Laceration of the aorta may cause widening of the mediastinum and bleeding (particularly into the left pleural space). Most patients die suddenly, but if they survive until a chest roentgenogram is available, these signs should alert the physician to early diagnosis and surgical treatment.

Emergency treatment is essential for tension pneumothorax, lacerated aorta, pericardial effusion with tamponade, hemothorax with persistent bleeding, or shock due to associated injuries.

Patients with major impact injuries should be immediately referred to a physician or surgeon experienced in detailed monitoring for and management of multiple organ injuries.

SURGERY

In most modern medical centers, the general anesthesia is perhaps the best monitored and supervised period of the patient's hospitalization. High standards of anesthesia demand adequate ventilation, oxygenation, airway control, and avoidance of aspiration. Certain operative procedures are associated with predictable deterioration of lung function and increased postoperative complications. Upper abdominal surgery such as gastrectomy and cholecystectomy results in a predictable deterioration in vital capacity by about 25 to 30 percent. Hypoxemia is characteristic, and these abnormalities return toward normal by 3 to 7 days postoperatively. Patients with marginal lung function prior to surgery may be at greater risk.

The hazards of pulmonary complications following surgery are related to the procedure performed, with declining risk as follows:

1. Pulmonary resection
2. Thoracic surgery without pulmonary resection (for example, coronary bypass)
3. Upper abdominal surgery
4. Lower abdominal surgery
5. Pelvic surgery
6. Surgery to extremities

The pulmonary complications include hypoxemia and reduced lung function, basilar atelectasis, pneumonia, thromboembolism, and, particularly with lung resection, pulmonary hypertension and arrhythmias.

The mechanisms for preventing thromboembolic disease are discussed in Chapter 4.

Patients particularly predisposed to postoperative infectious complications include those with recent upper respiratory viral infection, smokers, patients with demonstrable chronic obstructive lung disease, obese patients, and patients with immune deficiency disorders. Every patient being considered for an operative procedure should be assessed with respect to risks for postoperative complications. Elective procedures should be deferred until the risk factors are eliminated, if possible. Patients with airway disease should have treatment of infection, vigorous bronchodilator therapy, and aggressive postoperative physiotherapy and assessment of lung function.

ABDOMINAL DISEASE

When lower intrathoracic disease is not readily explained, the possibility of abdominal disease causing the lower thoracic problems should be considered. In severely ill patients, subdiaphragmatic abscess may result in elevated diaphragm, pulmonary infiltrate, and pleural effusion on the affected side.

Pancreatitis may be associated with bilaterally elevated diaphragms, pleural effusions (particularly on the left), and respiratory failure. Ascites may be associated with restricted motion of the diaphragm resulting in dyspnea and hypoxemia. Occasionally fluid will be transmitted to the pleural space, causing large and rapidly reoccurring pleural effusions.

REFERENCES

1. Fraser, R.G., Pare, J.A.P.: Diagnosis of Diseases of the Chest. 2nd ed. Philadelphia, W.B. Saunders, 1977.
2. Guenter, C.A., Welch, M.H., eds: Pulmonary Medicine. 2nd ed. Philadelphia, J.B. Lippincott, 1982.

3. Mattay, R.A., ed: Symposium on Chronic Obstructive Lung Diseases. Med. Clin. North Am. 65:457–701, 1981.

4. Petty, T.L.: Pulmonary Diagnostic Techniques. Philadelphia, Lea and Febiger, 1975.

5. Rinaldo, J.E., Rogers, R.M.: Adult respiratory distress syndrome. N. Eng. J. Med. 306:900, 1982.

6. U.S. Department of Health, Education and Welfare: Smoking and Health. A Report of the Surgeon General. PHS No. 79-50066, 1979.

7. Ziment, I: Respiratory Pharmacology and Therapeutics. Philadelphia, W.B. Saunders, 1978.

16

The Cardiovascular System

Joel S. Karliner, M.D., and Gabriel Gregoratos, M.D.

THE CARDIOVASCULAR HISTORY

One of the most important features of the assessment of the patient with suspected heart disease is the history, followed by a careful and detailed physical examination and an appropriate selection among various available noninvasive and invasive studies.

Chest Pain

A commonly difficult differential diagnosis encountered in clinical practice is that of chest pain. Even the most reliable patients may be unable to provide an adequate history, and even the most astute physician may have difficulty in ascertaining the nature of the chest pain by history alone. Nevertheless, the history is the single most important aspect of evaluating the nature and genesis of precordial discomfort. A careful analysis of factors that precipitate chest pain is essential since those characteristics are usually more specific than the intensity or character of the pain. A brief summary of some of the important considerations in the differential diagnosis of chest pain follows.

Angina Pectoris

By strict definition, angina pectoris simply means "pain in the chest," but by common usage it refers to pain that is precipitated by inadequate myocardial oxygen supply in relation to demand (i.e., ischemic pain). Thus, chest pain associated with coronary artery disease is classically produced by exertion and relieved by rest. Other precipitating conditions include heavy meals, emotional stress, sexual activity, walking in cold air, and tachyarrhythmias. Patients frequently describe the pain as a burning, pressing, or squeezing sensation. If it is severe the patient may spontaneously clench his fist over the middle of the chest (Levine sign). Often this pain may radiate to the shoulders, neck, jaws, arms or back (referred pain). Usually the left arm or hand is involved rather than the right; however, radiation is inconstant. Patients may also describe chest discomfort at rest. The pain may also occur in only one or more of the above described locations to which the discomfort usually radiates. Episodes of pain lasting 5 to 30 minutes, or which occur at rest (angina decubitus) are considered "unstable" or "intermediate" anginal syndromes. More prolonged pain should be considered as indicative of possible myocardial infarction. (See Coronary Disease Section.)

A useful therapeutic test is to prescribe sublingual nitroglycerin, which takes approximately 10 or more seconds to dissolve under the tongue, with onset of action approximately 45 to 60 seconds after dissolution. The peak action usually occurs about two minutes later and the total duration of action may be up to 10 minutes or more. Angina is usually relieved within three minutes after drug administration. Thus, patients whose pain or discomfort is relieved within a few seconds after administration of sublingual nitroglycerin or those who take a half hour or more for pain relief may not have true angina pectoris caused by coronary artery disease. However, any therapeutic test employing nitroglycerin only provides presumptive evidence for or against ischemic heart disease, since pain from other sources (e.g., esophageal spasm) may also be relieved by nitroglycerin.

Pericarditis

Pericarditis may produce chest pain simulating that of coronary disease. The stimulus for the pain presumably involves receptors in the parietal pericardium and in the adjacent pleura by the inflammatory process. Thus, the pain of pericarditis may be pleuritic, (i.e., it is exacerbated by such maneuvers as inspiration and coughing and is typically worsened by change in position).

Aortic Dissection

This pain usually begins in the chest and radiates to the back or into the abdominal or lumbar areas and may involve the legs, a symptom distinctly unusual for myocardial infarction. Although abdominal pain may be severe, rebound tenderness, spasm, and guarding of the abdominal wall usually are not present. The dissection can proceed proximal to the tear and produce aortic regurgitation. The pericardium extends to the base of the aorta, so aortic dissection may produce pericardial tamponade, generally a terminal event. If the aorta ruptures into the mediastinum, hemorhagic effusion and hemothorax may ensue, usually on the left. Dissection around major blood vessels may result in cerebrovascular occlusions, coronary occlusion, or marked discrepancies in the pulses of the arms or legs.

Pulmonary Infarction

Acute pulmonary thromboembolism without infarction usually does not produce chest discomfort. With massive pulmonary embolization, however, a reduction in cardiac output may lead to chest discomfort similar to that of angina pectoris. The pain associated with pulmonary infarction per se is usually pleuritic in nature (i.e., it is increased with inspiration, and is presumably related to inflammation of the parietal pleura). Pulmonary infarction can be recognized on the plain chest radiograph, usually as a wedge-shaped density in the lower lung field on either side. In addition, the physician should keep in mind predisposing factors such as obesity, history of phlebitis, pregnancy, malignancy, congestive cardiac failure, and immobility. The latter is especially important in elderly patients. Thus, the clinical setting

in which the chest pain occurs is often helpful in considering the differential diagnosis.

Pulmonary Arterial Hypertension

Patients with chronically elevated pulmonary artery pressure may complain of chest pain that resembles angina pectoris, but nitroglycerin is often ineffective. Exertional syncope may also occur, presumably as the result of low cardiac output. The pathogenesis of chest pain associated with pulmonary hypertension is uncertain. It has been suggested that an increase of right ventricular pressure within the wall of that chamber may compromise myocardial blood flow, resulting in ischemia and subsequent pain. Another possible cause is low cardiac output, resulting in reduced blood flow through the coronary arterial bed.

Anxiety

Perhaps the most common differential diagnostic problem in patients with chest pain is that of anxiety. The anxious patient not uncommonly complains of panprecordial discomfort. Anxious persons may also localize pain to the area "over the heart" (i.e., over the left precordium); this is an unusual location for classic angina pectoris. The pain in anxious patients usually does not radiate. Complaints of a "choking sensation" or "palpitations" lasting for half an hour to an hour or more are common. Such individuals also may hyperventilate and have acute or chronic emotional problems. However, it is obvious that patients with emotional problems and with anxiety may also develop heart disease and often the differential diagnosis is not entirely clear when the patient is first seen.

Barlow's Syndrome

Atypical chest discomfort may also occur in patients with the "click-murmur" syndrome associated with a billowing mitral leaflet. This syndrome is exceedingly common and is said to occur in approximately six percent of normal women and in a much smaller percentage of normal men. The chest discomfort may resemble that of the anxious patient and indeed a high incidence of "neurosis" has been described in these patients. The pain may last for hours or even days, is unrelieved by nitroglycerin, and usually is localized either to one area of the precordium or may radiate to many areas of the chest. However, it usually does not radiate to the arms, neck, or shoulders as does classical angina pectoris.

Pulmonary Disease

Generally speaking, acute inflammatory processes occurring in the lungs, such as viral or bacterial pneumonia, do not present a serious problem of differential diagnosis. The development of spontaneous pneumothorax, however, may present a more difficult problem. This event is accompanied by the sudden onset of pleuritic pain, on either side of the chest, frequently accompanied by dyspnea. Tension pneumothorax may be associated with a sensation of substernal pressure or choking.

Gastrointestinal Disease

Patients with reflux esophagitis commonly complain of dull squeezing lower precordial discomfort one-half hour to one hour after assuming a recumbent position. The discomfort may also occur after meals. It is usually relieved by assuming an upright position. Patients who awake with pain several hours after retiring should be suspected of having angina pectoris rather than reflux esophagitis.

The pain of peptic ulcer disease is characteristically midepigastric rather than substernal and is generally relieved by antacids. Typically it occurs between meals and is also relieved by eating. Acute events occurring in association with peptic ulcer disease, such as perforation and obstruction, may also mimic the discomfort of ischemic heart disease, but generally these lead to abdominal rather than chest findings. An association between gallbladder disease and coronary artery disease has been postulated; both may share a similar pathogenesis (i.e., elevated serum cholesterol). The pain of cholecystitis usually is in the right upper quadrant but occasionally radiates to the epigastrium as well as into the lower chest area. Again, precipitating factors are often helpful in differential diagnosis (i.e., relation to meals, nausea and vomiting, pleuritic chest pain on the right, often with radiation to the right shoulder). At times the differential diagnosis may be difficult and electrocardiographic changes may accompany acute attacks of cholecystitis. These usually represent repolarization abnormalities of uncertain pathogenesis; hyperventilation and dehydration may be factors. If the differential diagnosis is unclear, hospitalization may be required and then it may be necessary to obtain serial

electrocardiograms as well as serum enzyme determinations to exclude an acute myocardial infarction.

Both acute and chronic pancreatic disease may lead to precordial discomfort. The pain is usually epigastric and may radiate to the back; it is not uncommon for dissecting aneurysm to be considered in the differential diagnosis of acute pancreatitis. Serum enzyme determinations may be useful in helping to make the proper diagnosis. Pancreatitis frequently occurs in the setting of alcoholism, gallbladder disease or ulcer disease. Nevertheless, such patients may also have ischemic heart disease and when the pain of pancreatitis is acute, the electrocardiogram may also demonstrate changes consistent with ischemic heart disease.

Esophageal rupture is a catastrophic event which may cause chest pain mimicking that of myocardial ischemia or infarction.

Nonvascular Neuromuscular Disorders

Herniation of an intervertebral disc may cause nerve root compression and subsequent shoulder or arm pain, which may last for several hours and even days. In part the pain may be related to spasm in the muscle supplied by the nerve root. Pain due to compression of intervertebral discs is commonly aggravated by movement and by maneuvers that increase intraspinal pressure such as coughing, sneezing, or straining (Valsalva maneuver). Because the distribution of the pain may be in a dermatome similar to that associated with ischemic heart disease, the differential diagnosis may not be immediately apparent.

The thoracic outlet syndrome is caused by compression of vessels and nerves as they exit from the thoracic spine in the cervical region. Among the causes of this syndrome are a cervical rib, the scalenus anticus syndrome (anomalous insertion or hypertrophy of the anterior scalene muscle), or a large transverse process of one or the lower cervical vertebrae. Pain may involve the distribution of ulnar and median nerves on the affected side but can also extend to the shoulder and into the neck. Adson's maneuver, which may be helpful in diagnosing these conditions, is accomplished with the patient seated and the neck extended and the head turned to the side of the lesion. During subsequent deep inspiration, there is diminution or total loss of the radial pulse on the affected side.

Chest wall pain or "Tietze's syndrome" is associated with tenderness of the costochondral or costosternal joints. Discomfort of the xiphisternal joint may also mimic the pain of angina pectoris. The chest wall syndromes are frequently aggravated by movement, coughing, and deep breathing, can commonly be localized and reproduced by local pressure, and are often relieved by infiltration with a local anesthetic. Along with anxiety, chest wall pain is probably among the most common causes of chest discomfort. However, it is not uncommon for patients with acute myocardial infarction (for reasons that are unclear) to complain of chest wall discomfort. Generally speaking, reassurance and possibly mild analgesia are all that is necessary for patients with chest wall pain.

Fatigue

Patients with cardiovascular disease and incipient congestive cardiac failure or low cardiac output often complain of nonspecific symptoms, such as fatigue. Such individuals may complain of tiring easily, but there may be no overt findings on detailed physical examination. Because fatigue is such a nonspecific symptom, other causes, such as anemia, thyroid disease and depression, must be sought. Nevertheless, such a complaint may be the first clue to cardiac disease in a previously asymptomatic patient or may herald worsening of the patient's state in an individual with previously diagnosed heart disease.

Dyspnea

Along with fatigue, this is probably one of the most common symptoms reported by patients with heart disease. Initially, patients may complain of dyspnea on exertion and with worsening cardiac disease, complaints of orthopnea (dyspnea occurring in a recumbent position) and finally, paroxysmal nocturnal dyspnea (episodic breathlessness, usually occurring at night, that awakens the patient from sleep) are common. A less frequent symptom is trepopnea, which refers to breathlessness while lying on one side, usually on the left. Dyspnea on exertion may be quantitated in a semiobjective manner by describing the amount of exercise the patient must undergo in order to bring on symptoms of breathlessness. It is often useful to determine changes in a patient's status by asking him how many blocks he can walk, whether he can walk up hills or whether a given number of steps or flights of stairs causes shortness of breath. For some patients, it is useful to determine whether it is possible for the individual to make a bed without pausing. This task requires considerable exertion, and patients who cannot make a bed without stopping for a rest are often in New York Heart Association Clinical Class III (see below). Similarly, orthopnea is often "quantitated" by the number of pillows a person requires for sleep.

A useful functional classification as described by the New York Heart Association is a simple and valuable tool:

Functional Class I. Patients who have heart disease without limitation of physical activity. Ordinary activity does not cause symptoms.

Functional Class II. Patients with heart disease with slight limitation of physical activity. Ordinary physical activity causes fatigue, dyspnea, palpitation or angina pectoris.

Functional Class III. Patients with heart disease who have marked limitation of activity and experience symptoms with less than ordinary activity. They do not have symptoms at rest.

Functional Class IV. Patients who cannot engage in any physical activity without symptoms and may have symptoms at rest.

Like chest pain and fatigue, breathlessness may have a variety of causes other than heart disease. Among the most common of these is pulmonary disease, and it is often difficult to distinguish dyspnea due to lung disease from that due to cardiac dysfunction without a careful evaluation. Similarly, other conditions, such as obesity and a sedentary life style, may lead to dyspnea which is not due to cardiac disease.

Edema

Patients with both cardiac and noncardiac disease often complain of ankle swelling and pretibial edema, especially toward the end of the day. Such edema is usually not the result of cardiac disease unless there are other signs and symptoms of left and/or right-sided congestive cardiac failure. As an isolated symptom, pedal edema more often results from peripheral vascular disease, especially peripheral venous insufficiency. Alterations in serum proteins or other causes of edema should be sought in the absence of cardiac disease. However, the majority of patients with ankle swelling, especially edema that occurs at the end of the day, have no overt cardiac or noncardiac disease and require only reassurance.

Palpitations

Patients are often aware of "skipped beats," and the complaint of palpitations is a common one. By themselves, such complaints may range from an occasional premature ventricular beat to runs of supraventricular tachycardia and even ventricular tachycardia. It is sometimes helpful to ask the patient to reproduce the palpitations by tapping his fist on the table or against his thigh. In this way, it is occasionally possible to ascertain whether the individual is complaining merely of isolated premature beats or whether there may be sustained runs of tachycardia. However, the precise origin of premature beats and tachycardia usually can be ascertained only by direct observation, either in the hospital or more commonly by outpatient ambulatory monitoring.

Syncope

Syncope, either at rest or with exertion, may be the result of cardiac disease. In some instances, the patient complains only of "lightheadedness" or "graying-out spells." In all cases, more detailed information should be sought, especially with regard to neurological symptoms that may indicate either transient cerebral ischemic attacks and/or overt seizures. Syncope with exertion may be a cardinal sign of hemodynamically significant valvular aortic stenosis requiring urgent evaluation. Syncope at rest, which is due to cardiac disease, is most commonly the result of an arrhythmia, frequently bradycardia accompanying partial or complete heart block, and under these circumstances, careful rhythm monitoring is indicated.

OTHER ASPECTS OF THE HISTORY

Additional questions which should be asked of every patient include inquiry as to a previous history of systemic arterial hypertension or diabetes mellitus. A definite history of acute rheumatic fever should also be sought as should previous information regarding a cardiac murmur. The patient should be asked about recent weight gain or loss and whether there was hypertension or any other cardiovascular complication during pregnancy. A careful inquiry should be made regarding the patient's current medications, and, if any questions regarding medications arise, the patient should be asked to bring the medication to the physician's office for positive identification.

The family history may help to direct diagnostic approaches if ischemic heart disease, hypertension, or diabetes have been present at a young age.

THE CARDIOVASCULAR EXAMINATION

The thorough search for cardiovascular abnormalities requires the use of inspection, palpation, and auscultation. Special considerations in examining the cardiovascular system will be listed below, but it is assumed that the reader is familiar with the general principles of physical examination.

INSPECTION

General inspection of the patient may provide many clues to underlying heart disease. For example the detection of "mitral facies" (purplish pink nose and malar areas) suggests the presence of severe mitral stenosis. The appearance of a tall asthenic individual with a high arched palate should raise the possibility that the patient has Marfan's syndrome. If inspection of the precordium of a child or a young adult discloses prominence of the left hemithorax, the patient may be suffering from congenital heart disease, since cardiac enlargement present from early childhood will produce this skeletal abnormality. In the average size adult, the normal apical impulse is seen in the 5th interspace at or medial to the left midclavicular line. Displacement of the apical impulse inferiorly and/or laterally suggests cardiomegaly. The presence of other visible impulses should be sought: the impulse of a dyskinetic left ventricular segment following anterior myocardial infarction usually is seen medial to the apex beat; an impulse along the upper left sternal border may be due to a dilated pulmonary artery; or a systolic impulse along the upper right sternal border may be due to dilatation of the ascending aorta or (more likely) to an aortic aneurysm.

As the patient rests quietly with his torso at a 30 degree angle to the horizontal, careful inspection of the neck will disclose the height and configuration of the jugular venous pulse. Normally the height of the jugular venous pulse should not exceed a vertical distance of 10 cm from the mid right atrial level, which can be approximated by finding the intersection of the right fourth intercostal space and right midaxillary line. When the jugular venous pulse is visible, two distinct movements are present: the A and V waves. Timing of the A and V waves can be ascertained by simultaneous palpation of the contralateral carotid artery. The A wave slightly precedes the carotid pulse while the V wave generally coincides with the arterial pulse. In the normal individual the A wave exceeds the V wave in height and on inspiration the jugular venous pulse collapses.

Elevation of the jugular venous pulse above 10 cm occurs in the presence of right heart failure, tricuspid valve disease, and constrictive pericarditis. If the venous pressure is very high, the jugular venous pulse may be difficult to detect and the patient may have to sit upright to permit its visualization. Dominance of the V wave instead of the A wave usually occurs in the presence of large atrial septal defects with left to right shunt or severe tricuspid regurgitation.

Normally, prominent arterial pulsations are not present in the neck or above the clavicles. Visible arterial pulsations in the neck, the supraclavicular fossa, or the suprasternal notch usually result from an increase in arterial pulse pressure and occur in severe aortic insufficiency, hyperthyroidism, pregnancy, severe anemia, patent ductus arteriosus, and systemic arteriovenous fistula. Prominent arterial pulsations may be also due to dilatation and elongation of the aortic arch as seen in severe diastolic hypertension, coarctation of the aorta, and aneurysms of the ascending aorta.

Occasionally it may be difficult to distinguish arterial from venous pulsations in the neck, especially in patients with prominent systolic venous pulsations such as occur in atrial fibrillation and tricuspid regurgitation. In these circumstances the following maneuvers are helpful: Venous pulses can almost always be obliterated with mild to moderate pressure on the internal jugular vein at the base of the neck in the supraclavicular fossa. Arterial pulses cannot be abolished by this maneuver. Similarly, by changing the position of the patient the level of the venous pulsation will often change whereas arterial pulsations will remain the same. Finally, prominent systolic expansile pulsations which rise to the level of the angle of the mandible and cause the ear lobe to pulsate are almost always due to a systolic venous wave.

PALPATION

Palpation of the cardiovascular system should start with evaluation of the carotid pulses. A slowly rising small carotid pulse suggests the presence of severe aortic stenosis, especially if a palpable "shudder" is also detected. Conversely, a large volume rapidly rising, rapidly declining carotid arterial pulse suggests the presence of a runoff arterial lesion such as aortic insufficiency, patent ductus arteriosus, or systemic arteriovenous fistula. Comparison of right and left arm pulses is essential, as is comparison of the brachial and femoral pulses. In general, radial and femoral pulses should occur simultaneously; a significant delay in arrival of the femoral pulse (radiofemoral lag) suggests the presence of coarctation of the aorta. Femoral, popliteal, dorsalis pedis, and posterior tibial pulses should be palpated and graded as to volume or amplitude on a scale of one to four, especially if the patient is suspected of having peripheral vascular disease.

Palpation of the precordium is next in order and can provide the diagnosis in many patients. The presence of an apical "heave or thrust" (i.e., a sustained apical impulse) usually indicates left ventricular hyperterophy due to systolic overload of the left ventricle such as occurs in severe aortic stenosis or systemic hypertension. Conversely, a quick but diffuse apical impulse suggests volume overload of the left ventricle as seen in severe aortic insufficiency, patent ductus arteriosus, or systemic arteriovenous fistula. Right ventricular hypertrophy will usually produce a "lift" along the lower left sternal border or in the subxiphoid area. With severe pulmonary hypertension, pulmonic valve closure can be palpated as a discrete, sharp impulse along the upper left sternal border.

Palpation is also used to identify precordial thrills. A thrill is the palpatory equivalent of a loud murmur. In palpating for thrills the most sensitive part of the hand is the area overlying the heads of the metacarpals and not the finger tips. This portion of the hand should be placed at the apex along the left sternal border and along the upper right sternal border. Similarly, thrills should be sought in the suprasternal notch. Thrills must be categorized as systolic or diastolic; proper timing may be accomplished by the simultaneous palpation of the carotid arterial pulse with the other hand.

AUSCULTATION

The cardinal rule in listening for cardiovascular events over the precordium is for the examiner to listen with extreme care and concentration in an orderly, systematic, and comprehensive fashion. Furthermore, the examiner has to listen actively and not passively; by this we mean that the examiner must have fixed in his mind the portions of the cardiac cycle and the physiologic events occurring during the cardiac cycle and must listen specifically for the auscultatory events that abnormal physiology will produce. In order to initiate an orderly identification of cardiac cycles, it is often useful to proceed as follows: "Do I hear the first sound; is it accentuated, diminished, or split? Do I hear the second sound. . . ?" It is important to remember that one listens with the bell of his stethoscope applied lightly to the skin for medium and low frequency sounds and with the diaphragm of the stethoscope applied firmly to the skin for high frequency events. General auscultation should start in the second interspace along the upper right sternal border. Following a reverse S curve, the examiner should then listen along the upper left sternal border, the mid and lower left sternal border, and then gradually "inch" out to the apex. Auscultation then should be carried out in the left axilla, the interscapular area, the suprasternal notch, and over the carotid arteries. Pulmonary arterial bruits should be sought by listening over the axillae and over the entire thorax; systemic vascular bruits can be detected by listening over the abdomen and femoral arteries. Initially the patient should be examined in the recumbent position but also in a variety of other positions, of which the left lateral decubitus is the most important as it brings the heart in closer approximation to the chest wall; auscultation in this position will often reveal S3 and S4 gallops that were otherwise inaudible. Similarly, when one is listening for specific events the patient should be examined in the sitting, standing, or squatting position as mentioned below.

Certain specific events are best heard at specific locations on the precordium. For example, the murmur of mitral stenosis is invariably heard best directly over the apex beat with the patient in a partial left lateral decubitus position. Deviating even half an inch from the apex beat may cause one to lose the soft diastolic rumble of mild mitral stenosis. Curiously, however, the opening snap of mitral stenosis is heard best not directly over the apex beat but more medially, usually halfway between the apex impulse and the lower left sternal border and occasionally *at* the left sternal border. In the elderly adult, particularly one with increased anteroposterior chest diameter, the murmur of aortic stenosis is frequently heard only at the apex, and listening along the upper right sternal border (the "primary" aortic area) may be urewarding. Similarly, in the adult, the murmur of aortic insufficiency is almost always heard best along the lower left sternal border and not in the primary aortic area. In patients with severe chronic lung disease, heart sounds are frequently distant and murmurs and other auscultatory events may be totally missed unless one listens carefully over the xiphoid process and the upper epigastrium. Similarly, left sided S4 and S3 gallops frequently radiate well to the right supraclavicular fossa where they can be heard even though they may not be present on auscultation over the apex. If one encounters difficulty in distinguishing between the murmurs of mitral regurgitation and aortic stenosis, auscultation over such bony prominences as the acromium and the eighth cervical vertebra may be rewarding, since often the murmur of aortic stenosis will be heard there whereas the murmur of mitral insufficiency will not.

The observation of the effects of certain physiologic maneuvers or the administration of pharmacologic agents on auscultatory events can be of great help in specifically delineating the origin of sounds and murmurs and providing a definitive diagnosis. The commonly used interventions are respiration, the Valsalva maneuver, changes in position, sustained handgrip, and observation of post premature beat variations. The pharmacologic agents which may be utilized are amyl nitrite and phenylephrine. These maneuvers alter cardiac auscultatory events by evoking alterations in the cardiac volume, venous return, arterial pressure, heart rate, and cardiac output. A listing of the most common maneuvers employed and their effects on cardiac auscultatory events is presented in Table 16.1.

In addition to the effects listed, the Valsalva maneuver can be used to great advantage to distinguish events originating from the right and left heart. In general, during the straining phase of the Valsalva maneuver most sounds and murmurs become markedly attenuated. Following release of the strain, right

Table 16.1 **Physiologic and Pharmacologic Interventions as Aids to Auscultation**

Intervention	Increase	Decrease	No Change
1. Inspiration:	Physiologic splitting of S2, M of TS, TR, PR, RV S3, S4	M of MR, LV S3, S4	
2. Valsalva:	M of HOCM, LSM of FMV	M of AS, PS, MR, Venous hums	
3. Post PVC cycle:	M of AS, PS and HOCM		M of MR, TR
4. Squatting:	M of AR, MR, AS, PS	M of HOCM, ?LSM of FMV	
5. Amyl nitrite:	All SEMs, syst. A–V fistula, M of TS, TR, MS, LSM of FMV (duration) Pathologic S3, S4	M of AR, PDA, VSD with normal PVR, MR, TOF	
6. Phenylephrine:	M of VSD, MR, AR, PDA, A2–OS interval in MS	M of HOCM	
7. Sustained handgrip:	M of VSD, MR, AR, MS	M of AS, HOCM	

Abbreviation: S3 = third heart sound, S4 = fourth heart sound, A2 = aortic component of second sound, OS = opening snap, AS = aortic stenosis, AR = aortic regurgitation, MS = Mitral stenosis, MR = mitral regurgitation, PS = pulmonic stenosis, PVR = pulmonary vascular resistance, PR = pulmonic regurgitation, TS = tricuspid stenosis, TR = tricuspid regurgitation, M = murmur, SEMs = systolic ejection murmurs, LSM = late systolic murmur, FMV = floppy (billowing) mitral valve, VSD = ventricular septal defect, PDA = patent ductus arteriosus, TOF = tetralogy of Fallot, HOCM = hypertrophic obstructive cardiomyopathy (IHSS).

sided events will reappear within two to three cardiac cycles. Conversely left sided events do not reappear until at least four or five cardiac cycles have elapsed because of the pulmonary transit time.

NONINVASIVE DIAGNOSTIC TECHNIQUES

RESTING ELECTROCARDIOGRAM

A routine resting 12-lead electrocardiogram is indicated in all patients with proven or suspected cardiovascular disease. Such a record may also be useful in asymptomatic individuals as a "baseline" record. Because of contemporary mobility, it is often useful to provide the patient with a copy of his latest electrocardiogram. It is rarely necessary to order a routine electrocardiogram in a patient with known cardiac disease more than once yearly.

There are a number of pitfalls in recording the routine electrocardiogram. Careful attention should be given to electrode application to avoid electrical instability and interference. The electrocardiograph should be properly grounded, and careful attention should be given to standardization of each recording. When unusual or unexpected patterns appear on the standard 12-lead electrocardiogram, especially in the limb leads, evidence of lead reversal should be sought, the most common reversal being between the right arm and the left arm.

A report of the routine electrocardiogram should always include the following information: cardiac rate and rhythm; measurement of the PR, QRS and Q–T intervals; QRS axis in the frontal plane; identification of any abnormalities in the P wave, QRS complex, and T wave; and identification and characterization of any alterations in the S–T segment. Arrhythmias seen on a 12-lead electrocardiogram should be identified; it is often useful to record a "rhythm strip" with each resting electrocardiogram. Ambulatory electrocardiography and exercise electrocardiography are discussed below; specific abnormalities in the resulting electrocardiogram are discussed under each general category of cardiac disease.

VECTORCARDIOGRAM

The vectorcardiogram records the same information as the resting electrocardiogram, but displays the data in a different format (i.e., in the form of vector loops). These loops actually represent the projection of the instantaneous net cardiac spatial vector throughout the cardiac cycle on three anatomic planes. While vectorcardiography is not utilized in many centers, it is often useful to obtain a vectorcardiogram under certain specific circumstances. Among these are the identification of pre-excitation (Wolff-Parkinson-White syndrome); the identification of initial force abnormalities in patients with suspected myocardial infarction; and the measurement of QRS forces in patients with ventricular hypertrophy. In addition, the vectorcardiogram constitutes an important teaching tool which can illustrate many of the principles of scalar electrocardiography.

CHEST RADIOGRAPH

The chest radiograph should be a routine part of any diagnostic cardiac evaluation. It is a good indicator of overall cardiac size and may be helpful in the assessment of specific chamber or great vessel enlargement and in the assessment of pulmonary vascularity for the presence of venous congestion or alterations in pulmonary blood flow.

The prominent pulmonary vessels and interstitial edema seen with left ventricular failure are described in Chapter 15 in the section on Pulmonary Edema. By contrast, decreased pulmonary blood flow may occur in some congenital cardiac malformations, which are characterized by cyanosis accompanied by a right-to-left shunt.

Cardiac chamber size may be evaluated in both the frontal and lateral views. Usually the overall cardiac width is not more than half the transverse thoracic diameter (cardiothoracic ratio of less than 50%).

On the lateral roentgenogram, the retrosternal space, the lower third of which is normally occupied by cardiac tissue, may be partially "filled-in," indicating right ventricular enlargement. In the past, right and left anterior oblique views of the cardiac silhouette have been utilized for additional assessment of chamber enlargement, but these have been largely replaced by echocardiography.

Additional abnormalities to look for include calcification of the valves, thoracic aorta, coronary arteries, or pericardium; fluid accumulation in the fissures or in the costophrenic angles; or other abnormalities such as pulmonary infarction, pneumonia, pneumothorax, and abnormalities of the thoracic cage, such as the "straight back" syndrome.

EXERCISE ELECTROCARDIOGRAM

An exercise tolerance test should be performed when adequate information cannot be obtained by history, physical examination, and other noninvasive resting studies. This test may be especially useful in patients in whom the historical information is confusing, such as in individuals who complain of atypical chest pain or palpitations at low levels of exercise. Marked deviations of the S–T segment may occur in patients with critical left main coronary artery disease. Further, it may be useful to assess exercise tolerance in patients with various types of valvular heart disease (exclusive of advanced aortic valvular stenosis) in order to provide objective serial assessment of functional capacity so that planning of the time of operation may be aided. Exercise tolerance tests should not be used for routine screening in asymptomatic patients, save when sedentary older individuals wish to begin a strenuous exercise program.

The test should be carried out in the fasting state and the patient advised to wear comfortable clothing. Either a treadmill or an upright bicycle ergometer is used, and the electrocardiogram should be monitored continuously, preferably on an oscilloscope. The blood pressure should be taken throughout the test to insure that paradoxical hypotension does not occur. Control tracings should be taken in the supine and standing positions and after voluntary hyperventilation for 30 seconds.

Various protocols have been devised for the performance of the exercise electrocardiogram, but all of these aim to produce slow increments in myocardial oxygen demand with progressive physical activity. Based on nomograms, target heart rates can be identifed for patient groups by age and sex, but these obviously must be individualized depending on the reason for the test. Abnormalities that are sought include deviations of the S–T segment, supraventricular and ventricular arrhythmias, blood pressure response, and exercise tolerance. It is often useful for the physician to be present during the test so that if a patient complains of specific symptoms, these can be assessed. Deviations of the S–T segment greater than 1 mm below the baseline are generally considered to be evidence of coronary artery disease, and the magnitude of the deviation has been correlated with the severity and extent of coronary arterial narrowing. However, in many studies, it has been noted that the sensitivity and specificity of the treadmill test alone are relatively low and that these may be enhanced with the addition of radionuclide myocardial imaging.

A number of pitfalls should be recognized in the interpretation of exercise electrocardiography. Left ventricular hypertrophy, hypokalemia, and commonly used cardiovascular drugs such as digitalis and quinidine may invalidate the interpretation of the S–T segment response.

AMBULATORY ELECTROCARDIOGRAM

Ambulatory electrocardiography, commonly termed Holter monitoring after its inventor, has become an effective method for the assessment of ECG abnormalities not detected by the routine 12-lead recording. Ambulatory ECG monitoring is especially useful in patients who complain of "palpitations," lightheadedness, dizziness, syncope or for detection of arrhythmias after myocardial infarction. Correlation of arrhythmias (or their absence) with the patient's diary is often helpful in identifying the source of the presenting complaint. Continuous electrocardiographic monitoring provides the opportunity for the clinician to assess the frequency and potential severity of abnormal cardiac rhythms and to evaluate the efficacy of specific therapy. For initial recordings, 24-hour tapes seem to be preferable in order to establish any diurnal variation that may be present in a particular patient. Subsequent studies can be confined to 12 hours, or repeat 24-hour studies may be obtained, depending on the judgment of the clinician.

The treadmill exercise test may be useful on occasion for unmasking ventricular arrhythmias, especially in those individuals who have a specific history of exercise-induced ectopy; however, for practical purposes the ambulatory electrocardiogram seems to be the superior diagnostic test.

Recent advances in ambulatory electrocardiography include the ability to calibrate the recording so that ST-segment alterations can be quantitated. Using the ambulatory electrocardiogram, silent episodes of ST-segment depression can be detected. However, exercise tolerance tests remain the primary method for detecting changes in repolarization.

As with all diagnostic studies, ambulatory electrocardiography has a number of potential pitfalls. Obviously, ectopy may be sporadic and thus may not be detected during the time of recording or may be missed during rapid playback. Alterations may occur in both the speed of recording or playback, leading to erroneous diagnoses of both tachycardia and bradycardia. It is frequently difficult to distinguish P waves adequately on such tapes, and the specific nature of some arrhythmias may be hard to define.

ECHOCARDIOGRAM

Ultrasound evaluation of the heart is a very useful noninvasive approach for evaluation of the patient with known or suspected cardiac disease.

Information obtained from the M-mode echocardiogram includes measurements of left ventricular, left atrial, and sometimes right ventricular chamber size; assessment of the movement of the mitral, aortic, triscupid, and sometimes pulmonary valves; measurement of posterior left ventricular and interventricular septal wall thickness; and measurement of ejection phase indices of left ventricular performance. Valve motion and overall wall motion can be assessed using the two-dimensional approach and in the diagnosis of intracardiac masses, such as thrombi and tumors. The diagnosis of valvular vegetations in patients with endocarditis can also be more readily made using the two-dimensional method.

Echocardiography is useful in patients with coronary artery disease for the assessment of chamber size and wall motion. In patients with valvular heart disease, echocardiography offers the advantages of serial assessment of chamber size and valve motion.

An important use of M-mode echocardiography is in the diagnosis of pericardial effusion. The diagnosis of hypertrophic cardiomyopathy may be confirmed by echocardiography, and the presence or absence of mitral stenosis can be readily confirmed by this technique. In patients with congenital heart disease, two-dimensional echocardiography should be done routinely, especially prior to cardiac catheterization.

Echocardiography is subject to a variety of pitfalls. In many patients, especially in individuals with obstructive lung disease, adequate M-mode echocardiograms are difficult to obtain, and in many such patients two-dimensional studies may also be unsatisfactory. Careful attention must be paid to gain settings so that the pericardial space is assessed accurately. The echocardiogram must not be overinterpreted: for example, thickening of the interventricular septum in some individuals leading to an increase septal to posterior wall thickness ratio must not be overenthusiastically diagnosed as hypertrophic cardiomyopathy. Similarly, mitral valve prolapse, which is a very common condition, may be present in totally asymptomatic patients as an echocardiographic diagnosis.

RADIONUCLIDE TECHNIQUES

Assessment of Left Ventricular Function and Wall Motion

Both echocardiography and radionuclide angiography share the advantage that they do not induce measurable hemodynamic alterations. For determination of left ventricular function, the ejection fraction (EF) has been calculated in most studies. Nuclear imaging procedures used for the determination of left ventricular EF involve external monitoring of the cardiac blood pool with a gamma scintillation camera. Two general approaches have been employed.

The "First Pass" Approach

The first pass method refers to derivation of the EF from instantaneous count rates corresponding to the changes in left ventricular volume at end-systole and end-diastole. A variety of 99m Tc labeled radiopharmaceuticals may be used for this procedure. The radiopharmaceutical is rapidly injected into an antecubital or external jugular vein, and precordial activity is recorded during the first circulation through the heart using a gamma scintillation camera. The information is stored on magnetic tape. Both right and left ventricular EF can be computed from the cyclic fluctuations of the left ventricular time-activity curve by dividing the difference between count rates at end-diastole and at end-systole by the count rate at end-diastole.

The "Equilibrium" Approach

A second approach is to use radioactive substances that remain evenly distributed through the vascular space but remain confined to it ("blood pool"), including the cardiac chambers, thereby providing an opportunity to examine both ventricles simultaneously when "equilibrium" (complete mixing) has been reached. This ECG gated cardiac blood pool imaging or multigated acquisition imaging technique permits visualization of all four cardiac chambers simultaneously; however, varying degrees of superimposition of these structures occur, depending on the angle of view.

The radiopharmaceutical used for this procedure must remain evenly mixed within the vascular space. The types of material used include 99m Tc coupled to human serum albumin and in vivo labeling of the patient's own red blood cells with 99m Tc.

A physiologic marker, such as the electrocardiogram, is used to indicate the beginning and end of each cardiac cycle. The signal is used to start and stop the scintillation camera recording in order to assemble identically phased brief recording periods either continuously throughout successive cardiac cycles or for discrete periods at end-diastole and end-systole. This is necessary because insufficient counts are available during a single cardiac cycle. After recording, the left ventricular borders are traced either manually or by computer from the gated images.

Supine or upright bicycle exercise can be employed for evaluation of global and regional left ventricular function. Patients with coronary artery disease tend to exhibit a decline in EF during exercise, whereas normal individuals usually display an increase in this measure.

Assessment of the Myocardium

99m Technetium Pyrophosphate Scintigraphy

Although a number of agents have been used to image damaged myocardium, the one used most commonly has been 99m technetium pyrophosphate (PYP).

If a scintigram obtained between 12 and 24 hours after the onset of symptoms is negative, the study should be repeated between 36 and 72 hours after the acute event, because the temporal evolution of scintigraphic abnormalities may be quite variable. Whether this method provides greater diagnostic specificity and sensitivity than other conventionally employed methods in the diagnosis of acute myocardial infarction is uncertain. In the majority of clinical circumstances, the diagnosis of acute myocardial infarction can be made without the aid of scintigraphy and in many coronary care units, this procedure is not routinely used. However, where the abnormalities on the electrocardiogram and serum enzyme determinations are not diagnostic, the scintigram may be of some value.

Exercise Imaging with 201-Thallium

Considerable recent interest has centered around the use of this agent injected during exercise in order to enhance the sensitivity of the exercise tolerance test. The clinical use of cationic tracers is based on the principle that tracer uptake by myocardial cells is proportional to regional myocardial blood flow. Thus, at rest areas supplied by narrowed coronary vessels may exhibit normal tracer uptake but when the radiopharmaceutical is injected during exercise, the concentration is decreased in comparison to normally perfused areas. When tracer uptake is absent at rest and does not change during exercise, the presence of previous myocardial infarction or scar tissue of some other etiology is suggested, while a new perfusion defect appearing during exercise suggests an area of transient, reversible myocardial ischemia.

CONGESTIVE HEART FAILURE

DEFINITION

Congestive heart failure is an abnormal physiologic state caused by the inability of the heart to deliver sufficient blood to satisfy the metabolic requirements of the tissues. Under ordinary circumstances, the diagnosis of cardiac failure is based on a typical history of breathlessness, fatigue, reduced exercise tolerance, or symptoms suggestive of pulmonary edema or right ventricular failure. Specific findings on physical examination may indicate left or right ventricular failure, or both. Thus, the left ventricular impulse is often displaced; gallop rhythm with prominent third and fourth heart sounds and signs of pulmonary congestion may be present. Evidence of vascular blurring, dilatation of pulmonary veins, or parenchymal infiltrates on a chest radiograph are frequent but not invariable associated findings. In patients with pulmonary hypertension, a right ventricular lift, right ventricular gallop sounds, the murmur of tricuspid regurgitation, increased jugular venous pressure, hepatomegaly and peripheral edema may signal right heart failure.

PHYSIOLOGIC CONSIDERATIONS

Both heart size and left ventricular pressure are important determinants of myocardial wall tension, which in turn is probably the major influence on myocardial oxygen demand (Fig. 16.1). Although resting cardiac size has been conventionally related to "preload" and left ventricular pressure to "afterload" on the myocardium, these two measures are directly related to left ventricular wall tension and hence to myocardial oxygen demand. The law of LaPlace states that wall force or tension (T) is directly related to the product of intracavitary pressure (P) and radius (r); in addition, myocardial wall tension is inversely related to ventricular wall thickness (h): $T = P \times r/h$. Thus, an increased "preload" at a given level of ventricular systolic pressure will augment wall tension, and vice versa; while an increase in "afterload" at any level of end-diastolic dimension or volume will also tend to increase wall stress. These considerations become particularly important when assessing the value of vasodilator agents in patients with congestive cardiac failure (see below).

The heart rate exerts an independent influence on myocardial oxygen requirements, tachycardia causing an increase and bradycardia a decrease. Drugs which alter the inotropic state of the left ventricle also alter myocardial oxygen demand with agents that increase the inotropic state augmenting demand and drugs that decrease it diminishing demand. According to these considerations, any therapeutic intervention that diminishes heart size, left ventricular pressure, heart rate, and inotropic state will tend to decrease myocardial oxygen demand.

Determinants of Myocardial Oxygen Supply

Under ordinary circumstances, increases in myocardial oxygen demand, influenced by the factors discussed above, are met by an appropriate increase in myocardial oxygen supply (Fig. 16.1). The amount of oxygen supplied to the heart is directly related to coronary blood flow, the oxygen content of arterial blood, and the amount of oxygen extracted from the blood by the heart. Since the heart extracts a high and relatively fixed amount of oxygen from the blood flowing through the coronary circulation, augmentation of coronary flow is the major practical mechanism by which increased metabolic demands can be met.

Coronary blood flow is markedly diminished during systole because the vessels are compressed by the myocardium. This phenomenon is not of major sig-

nificance in the epicardial arteries, which extend primarily over the surface of the heart, as compared with the subendocardial vessels, which are compressed during systole. As a result of this compression, systolic flow is markedly diminished through these vessels and aortic diastolic pressure becomes a major influence on coronary blood flow. Indeed, in the presence of hypotension and frank cardiogenic shock, aortic diastolic pressure is probably the major determinant of coronary flow. Under ordinary circumstances, however, the absolute level of aortic diastolic pressure is not the sole hemodynamic determinant responsible for driving blood through the coronary circulation. Because the coronary vessels are exposed to intramyocardial pressure during diastole as well as systole, it is clear that the net driving force responsible for maintaining coronary flow during diastole must be the difference between aortic diastolic pressure and intramyocardial diastolic pressure. When left ventricular diastolic pressure is elevated, as it often is in congestive cardiac failure, there may be significant diminution of subendocardial blood flow. Therefore, it seems clear that reduction in diastolic pressure and cardiac size will also reduce myocardial wall tension, thereby reducing myocardial oxygen demand. Thus, appropriate treatment of congestive cardiac failure should reduce demand while at the same time increasing supply.

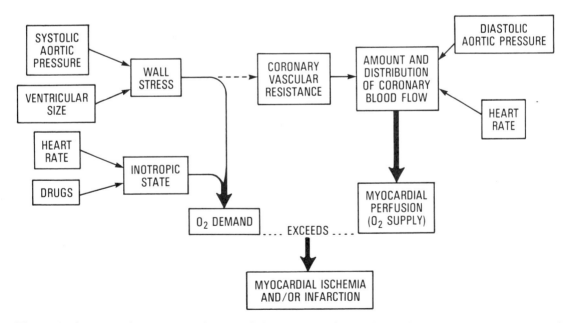

Fig. 16.1 The major determinants of myocardial oxygen supply and demand are shown. The treatment of congestive heart failure in acute myocardial infarction depends on a favorable balance of the factors shown above. (Karliner, J.S., Gregoratos, G. (eds.): Coronary Care. Churchill Livingstone, New York, 1981, with permission.)

Hemodynamic Observations

Studies of patients with congestive cardiac failure generally reveal that the cardiac output is depressed, although in some patients with "high output failure" due to thyrotoxicosis, anemia, or an arteriovenous communication, the cardiac output may be elevated. With the low output form of cardiac failure, the ejection fraction (ratio of stroke volume to end-diastolic volume) is generally reduced. The left ventricular end-diastolic pressure is usually increased and this pressure is transmitted to the left atrium and to the pulmonary capillaries, resulting in an increase in the pulmonary arterial wedge pressure. Pulmonary artery pressure may be increased, depending on the compliance characteristics of the pulmonary vascular bed and the duration and severity of the "left-sided" dysfunction. The pulmonary artery pressure and the pulmonary artery wedge pressure generally increase in response to exercise, and these findings account at least in part for exertional dyspnea. Accompanying the reduced cardiac output is a widened arteriovenous oxygen difference. The peripheral vascular resistance is often increased in patients with congestive cardiac failure. In general, the more severe the heart failure, the lower the systemic arterial pressure and cardiac output and the higher the peripheral vascular resistance.

TREATMENT

Digitalis

The beneficial effects of digitalis in patients with congestive cardiac failure result from direct stimulation of the contractile state of the myocardium; it augments the cardiac output and lowers the abnormally high left ventricular end-diastolic pressure. By contrast, some have argued that there is little evidence to substantiate the effects of chronic digoxin therapy in patients with congestive cardiac failure and have advocated abandoning its use under these circumstances entirely because of the high incidence of drug toxicity. This will remain a matter of controversy until additional well-controlled prospective studies can be performed to further substantiate the time-honored use of this drug in patients with chronic congestive cardiac failure.

The potentially beneficial effects of digitalis may also in part depend on initial heart size before administration. In the presence of cardiomegaly and left ventricular failure, digitalis may reduce myocardial oxygen demand, particularly due to a fall in end-diastolic volume, which in turn results in a decline in systolic wall tension (see LaPlace relationship

above). Thus, the increase in contractility produced by digitalis tends to increase myocardial oxygen demand but, in the dilated, failing heart which becomes smaller after glycoside administration, the concurrent reduction in wall tension presumably counteracts the oxygen cost of augmented contractility.

The physician must be thoroughly familiar with the specific digitalis preparation to be used. Under most circumstances, this preparation will be digoxin. The dose of drug depends on many factors, among the most important of which is renal function, since digoxin is cleared primarily by the kidneys. Glomerular filtration rate declines with age, and older patients may be more susceptible to digitalis intoxication. Thus, the estimation of serum digoxin level may be of great help in the management of such patients. However, complete reliance should not be placed on the measurement of the serum digoxin level, since serious arrhythmias due to digitalis intoxication may be present at levels below the usual "therapeutic range" which is considered in most laboratories to be in the neighborhood of 2 ng/ml. Digoxin dosage is easiest to manage in patients with atrial fibrillation, since reduction of the ventricular response to 60–80 beats per minute at rest is the ideal goal (See Chapter 10, Fig. 10.4).

The method of digitalis administration is dictated by the clinical situation. For example, in patients with rapid atrial fibrillation, full dosing within 12 hours may occasionally be indicated. For severe congestive cardiac failure, full dosing within 24–36 hours is usually the rule. Only in a monitored patient with sinus rhythm is more rapid administration indicated. For mild or borderline congestive cardiac failure, initial therapy with diuretics will usually be the treatment of choice (see below), and gradual treatment with digitalis over a period of several days is usually adequate. Experimental evidence indicates that even small amounts of digitalis may have a beneficial effect on a failing heart and, thus, "full digitalization" is not a prerequisite for hemodynamic improvement.

Digitalis Administration by the Intravenous or Intramuscular Route

The onset of action of intravenous digoxin is between 10 and 20 minutes; peak action occurs within two to three hours. The time required for disappearance of one-half of physiologic activity as well as the half-life determined chemically are approximately equivalent in this preparation, and in a patient without renal insufficiency averages 36 hours. In the patient who has not received a glycoside in the recent past, the initial intravenous dose is 0.75 mg followed by 0.25 mg every two to four hours. Ordinarily, 1.5 mg intravenously should not be exceeded during the first 24 hours. Complete excretion of the drug takes anywhere from three to six days and is delayed in patients with renal insufficiency. When renal failure, hypokalemia, or hypothyroidism is present, the initial dose should be reduced by 25 to 50 percent. In patients with acute myocardial infarction, it has been recommended that 1.5 mg be given in the first 36 hours. If the diagnosis of myocardial infarction is in doubt, intramuscular digoxin may lead to elevation of serum creatine kinase. Unless the determination of the specific isoenzyme of creatine kinase (MB–CK) is available, intramuscular digoxin as well as other intramuscular medications should be avoided in the patient with myocardial infarction.

Moderately Rapid Oral Therapy within 24–36 Hours

This method is appropriate for use in patients with rapid atrial fibrillation when the situation is not urgent but when it is necessary to control the ventricular response within a relatively brief period of time. In addition, this method is appropriate for patients with acute congestive cardiac failure in whom reasonably rapid treatment is desirable. In patients who have not previously received digitalis, an initial dose between 0.5 to 1.0 mg of digoxin may be given by mouth, followed by 0.25 mg orally every six to eight hours until a clinical response is achieved. The average range for the total oral "digitalizing" dose is between 1.5 to 3.0 mg given over several days.

Slow Oral Treatment

When therapy over a two to four-day period is desirable, a starting dose of 1.0 mg of digoxin followed by 0.25 to 0.5 mg every 12 hours for six doses may be given. When dosing over a period of five to eight days is desirable, it is possible to begin with a maintenance dose of digoxin of 0.25 mg or, less commonly, 0.5 mg daily. After one week, an adequate level of digitalis in the serum will be achieved even though a "digitalizing dose" was not given initially. Therefore, a loading dose is not necessary when slow oral dosing is the preferred method (See Chapter 10, Fig. 10.4).

Maintenance Dose

In general, a maintenance dose of 0.25 mg orally daily for digoxin is adequate for adults. Some patients may require a larger amount, especially those with atrial fibrillation in whom the ventricular response is the guide to therapy. Other patients may exhibit symptoms or signs of digoxin intoxication on a daily dose of 0.25 mg and a smaller dose such as 0.125 mg daily may be adequate. Other patients may require a combination of these doses on alternate days. In patients receiving oral quinidine, the level of serum digoxin may be raised. Since quinidine is often employed in patients with heart disease, special care should be taken to search for signs of digitalis intoxication in such patients, and under these circumstances, measurements of serum digoxin level appear to be indicated. Further, in older patients the renal clearance of quinidine itself may be reduced.

Recognition and Management of Digitalis Intoxication

Nausea and vomiting are common symptoms of digitalis toxicity and should not routinely be attributed to other causes in patients receiving the drug. Visual changes are uncommon but are a useful clue when present. Frequently the diagnosis of digitalis intoxication is an electrocardiographic one. A commonly missed sign of digitalis intoxication is the appearance of an atrioventricular junctional rhythm in patients with atrial fibrillation. The regularization of the cardiac rhythm in patients with atrial fibrillation should not be attributed to the reappearance of sinus rhythm, unless this is proved by an electrocardiogram. The presence of a regular rhythm ranging between 40 and 100 beats/minute in patients who have previously been in atrial fibrillation commonly represents a junctional rhythm and indicates atrioventricular dissociation. Although this rhythm in itself is usually not a dangerous one, the continued administration of digoxin may lead to more serious and even fatal arrhythmias.

Other arrhythmias that can be due to digitalis intoxication include paroxysmal atrial tachycardia with or without block; junctional and ventricular ectopic beats; ventricular tachycardia and ventricular fibrillation. However, all these arrhythmias, especially the ventricular ones, are common in many patients with cardiac disease, especially acute ischemic heart disease, and complicate the problem of the administration of digitalis in this setting. Other rhythms which can result from digitalis excess include sinus bradycardia and first, second, and third degree atrioventricular block. Repolarization abnormalities (ST and T wave changes) are common after digitalis administration and do not indicate the presence of intoxication.

In some patients, the margin between the dose of

glycoside required for an optimum therapeutic effect and for the development of toxicity is small. Hypokalemia, hypomagnesemia, hypothyroidism, renal insufficiency, and old age all lower the threshold to digitalis intoxication. The first step in the treatment of digitalis intoxication is discontinuation of the drug. The blood urea nitrogen, serum creatinine, serum potassium and, if possible, the serum magnesium and digoxin levels should be measured. Deficits of potassium and/or magnesium should be corrected as described below under Adverse Reactions to Diuretics.

The *mild arrhythmias*, including first degree A–V block, second degree block of the Wenckebach type, atrioventricular junctional rhythm with a ventricular response of 60–100 beats per minute, sinus bradycardia, occasional premature ventricular or junctional contractions, and paroxysmal atrial tachycardia with block with a ventricular response of less than 100 beats per minute require little therapy other than discontinuation of the drug. On the other hand, two or more premature ventricular contractions occurring in a row, brief bouts of ventricular tachycardia, and higher degrees of atrioventricular block require more vigorous treatment.

Intractable supraventricular and ventricular arrhythmias with ventricular rates exceeding 130 beats per minute may lead to circulatory collapse and/or pulmonary edema. When such arrhythmias are thought to be caused by digitalis intoxication, DC cardioversion may be utilized as a last resort if other measures, such as correction of electrolytes and the cautious administration of intravenous propranolol have failed. Low energies (10–15 joules) may be tried initially. Although such treatment is potentially hazardous, with ventricular fibrillation an ever present danger, it may be indicated in desperate situations. A temporary transvenous demand pacemaker is indicated when a digitalis-induced bradyarrhythmia is responsible for a low output state, if a trial of atropine has been unsuccessful. In the presence of acute ischemic heart disease, caution should be exercised since all these arrhythmias may be the result of infarction alone and unrelated to therapy with digoxin.

Diuretic Therapy

Pulmonary vascular congestion is commonly the result of an elevated left ventricular diastolic pressure. The hydrostatic pressure in the pulmonary vascular bed exceeds the plasma oncotic pressure and fluid accumulates initially in the peribronchial perialveolar lymphatic spaces and subsequently in the alveolar spaces themselves. The preferred initial approach to the therapy of congestive cardiac failure involves the use of intravenous or oral diuretics rather than the use of digitalis glycosides which may be added later. Diuretics act rapidly, causing volume loss and reduction in the pulmonary arterial wedge pressure and relief of dyspnea. The acute use of intravenous diuretic therapy, specifically furosemide, may lead to venous pooling due to venous dilatation within five minutes of drug administration, well before any diuretic effect can be documented.

Both furosemide and ethacrynic acid are known as the "loop diuretics." Although unrelated chemically, both of these agents are potent diuretics which interfere with sodium reabsorption throughout the nephron, but especially in the ascending limb of the loop of Henle (Fig. 16.2). They may be used both orally and intravenously, although for intravenous use, furosemide is the preferred agent because of occasional reports of deafness after intravenous ethacrynic acid. Occasionally patients with advanced heart failure respond only to the intravenous preparation, but after initial diuresis, oral therapy may achieve satisfactory results. The usual initial dose of furosemide should be 20 to 40 mg given intravenously, or 40 mg given orally. It is recommended that the initial dose of furosemide not exceed 240 mg and the initial dose of ethacrynic acid not exceed 250 mg, since higher doses are rarely more effective and adverse reactions may be more common (see below). Once the patient has responded to the initial dose of diuretic, subsequent doses may be given, based on dyspnea, tachycardia, and pulmonary rales or the level of the pulmonary capillary pressure and/or cardiac output, if these are being measured. Often patients will require a maintenance dose of anywhere between 20 and 120 mg of furosemide daily or subsequent therapy with one of the benzothiadiazide (thiazide) diuretics. These inhibit sodium reabsorption primarily in the proximal portion of the distal tubule and are effective compounds for oral therapy as well. Chlorothiazide and hydrochlorothiazide are similar in action and differ only in dosage. The dose of hydrochlorothiazide is between 50–100 mg daily, and for chlorothiazide between 500–1000 mg daily. Chlorthalidone is a longer acting agent and the usual dose is 100 mg/day. All the thiazide diuretics cause a modest increase in renal vascular resistance and depression of glomerular filtration rate and are relatively ineffective in patients with impaired renal function. Another diuretic which tends to cause potassium retention is triamterene. The sites of action and relative potencies of the diuretics are summarized in Table 16.2.

In some patients refractory to the above agents, spironolactone, which is an antagonist of the salt-

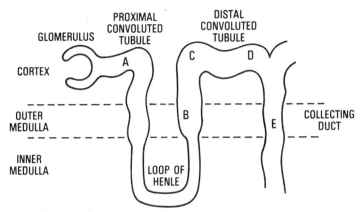

Fig. 16.2 The important sites for fluid and electrolyte transport within the nephron are shown in this schematic diagram. In this simplified construct, the important locations are: (A) Ordinarily 65–70% of sodium, chloride and bicarbonate reabsorption occurs in the proximal convoluted tubule. This ionic movement occurs with an equivalent transfer of water. (B) Another 10–15% of filtered sodium chloride is reabsorbed in the ascending limb of the loop of Henle. Water is generally not absorbed here, thus producing urinary dilution and accounting for the production of solute-free or "free" water. (C) At this site another 5–10% of filtered sodium is reabsorbed. Antidiuretic hormone (ADH) may act here. (D) (and possibly E) Here sodium, not exceeding 3% of the filtered load, is reabsorbed. In exchange, hydrogen and potassium ions are secreted from the renal tubular cells into the tubular lumen. Although this ionic transfer occurs independent of aldosterone, the exchange process is in general sensitive to and regulated by this hormone. (E) This site is also sensitive to antidiuretic hormone, and water absorption occurs when this substance is present. (From Puschett, J.B. Physiologic Basis for the use of new and older diuretics in congestive heart failure. J. Cardiovasc. Med., 2:119–134, 1977.)

retaining hormone aldosterone and which causes a reduction in the distal tubular exchange of sodium and potassium, may be added.

Adverse Reactions to Diuretics

Hypovolemia.   The locus of the major action of ethacrynic acid and furosemide is also the locus of the countercurrent multiplier apparatus that is the basic mechanism responsible for urinary concentration and dilution (i.e., the ascending limb of the loop of Henle) (Fig. 16.2). Normally this area is responsible for reabsorption of some 25 percent of the filtered load of sodium as compared to the residual 10 percent on which all the more distal reabsorptive mechanisms operate. Thus, when the filtered load of sodium is adequate, diuresis may be so massive as to produce a marked fall in pulmonary arterial pressure and left ventricular filling pressure and a reduction

in cardiac output. Subsequent to the diuresis, the kidney may then exhibit an appropriate response to the physiological stimulus of volume depletion, resulting in high urine osmolality and specific gravity, a very high concentration of creatinine and other nonreabsorbable solutes, and a low concentration of sodium. Renal blood flow and glomerular filtration rate are reduced, mediated in part by sympathetic nervous system activity and possibly, in part, by activation of the renin-angiotensin system. With a severe deficit, renal blood flow may be reduced to one-third of normal despite an adequately maintained arterial pressure. Afferent arteriolar constriction then occurs so that glomerular capillary hydrostatic pressure is inadequate to maintain filtration at normal levels. Thus, depressed renal function under these circumstances (prerenal azotemia) is a form of iatrogenic "renal ischemia," resulting from a reduction in renal blood flow but is not due to an inadequacy of metabolic function of the renal parenchymal cells.

Table 16.2   **Sites of Action and Relative Potency of Diuretics**

Agent	Major Site of Action Within the Nephron	Additional Site	Maximal Natruetic Effect (% of Filtered Load Excreted)
Thiazides	Distal tubule	Proximal tubule	5–8
Furosemide	Ascending loop of Henle	Proximal tubule	20–25
Ethacrynic acid	Ascending loop of Henle	Proximal tubule	20–25
Spironolactone	Distal tubule		2–3
Triamterene	Distal tubule		2–3
Amiloride	Distal tubule		2–3

(From Puschett, J.B.: Physiologic basis for the use of new and older diuretics in congestive heart failure. J. Cardiovasc. Med., 2:119–134, 1977.)

The combination of increased myocardial oxygen demand (tachycardia) and decreased coronary perfusion pressure (hypotension) resulting from excessive diuretic therapy may produce extension of myocardial ischemia. However, a carefully controlled diuresis resulting in a reduction in left ventricular filling pressure and volume may have a beneficial effect on cardiac output.

Hypokalemia and hypomagnesemia. The large amounts of sodium presented to aldosterone-sensitive sites of cation exchange in the distal nephron may induce large losses of potassium, with potentially serious consequences for inducing arrhythmias especially in the presence of digitalis. Potassium deficits should be corrected as rapidly as possible, but intravenous potassium chloride should not be given at a rate exceeding 15 mEq/hr, and the concentration of potassium should not exceed 40 mEq/L. For oral replacement therapy, between 20 and 80 mEq of K^+ are usually necessary, depending on renal function. Serum potassium levels should be monitored as the clinical situation indicates. Occasionally magnesium deficits may result from diuretic therapy. For intravenous magnesium replacement a 10 percent solution should be used: 40 ml of this preparation (3.25 mEq) may be given at a rate not exceeding 1.5 ml/minute.

When patients are changed to oral diuretic therapy, administration of the agent five days per week or on alternate days tends to help protect against serious potassium deficiency. Intake of food high in potassium and periodic monitoring of the serum potassium level are also indicated.

Additional side effects. Other adverse reactions which can occur following intravenous or oral diuretic therapy include excessive hyponatremia. Should this occur, water intake must be restricted to equal the estimated insensible loss (400–600 ml/day); diuretics are usually not effective until the electrolyte imbalance is corrected. Hypertonic saline should never be used in such a situation except when the serum sodium is exceedingly low (i.e., less than 100 mEq/L) and there is associated severe central nervous system disturbance and/or serious hypotension. Hyponatremia in nonedematous patients is usually the consequence of excessive diuretic therapy and salt restriction, both of which may have been used overenthusiastically. A less stringent diuretic regimen, with or without liberalization of dietary salt, is often sufficient to correct this imbalance.

Other occasional adverse reactions include a metabolic alkalosis which occurs in previously edematous patients who have received diuretic therapy. This is usually accompanied by the hyponatremia mentioned above and has been called a "contraction alkalosis" because of the volume depletion and potassium loss required to produce the alkalosis. Other less common adverse reactions include carbohydrate intolerance produced by furosemide or thiazides and the rare occurrence of nonketotic diabetic coma. Because of a fall in urea clearance caused by extracellular fluid volume depletion, hyperuricemia is common and acute gout can be precipitated in susceptible individuals.

Adverse reactions to the diuretics are summarized in Table 16.3.

MANAGEMENT OF ACUTE PULMONARY EDEMA

Under normal circumstances, the plasma oncotic pressure prevents the diffusion of fluids across the capillary membrane into the interstitial space. However, as congestive cardiac failure worsens, the capillary hydrostatic pressure increases and the plasma oncotic pressure is exceeded, resulting in transudation of fluid into the interstitial tissues and subsequently into the pulmonary alveoli themselves. In the

Table 16.3 **Adverse Reactions to Commonly Used Diuretics***

Reaction	Consequence
1. Hypovolemia	Tachycardia and hypotension with possible increase in ischemia
2. Hypokalemia	↑ in severity and duration of ventricular arrhythmias; precipitation of atrial, junctional or ventricular arrhythmias in digitalized patients
3. Hypomagnesemia	Same as hypokalemia
4. Hyponatremia	Central nervous system disturbances; possible adverse effect on ventricular arrhythmias
5. Metabolic alkalosis	Possible adverse effect on hypoxic myocardium; usually accompanied by hypokalemia, hypovolemia and hyponatremia
6. Worsening of carbohydrate tolerance	May cause fluid and electrolyte disturbances; nonketotic hyperosmolar coma rare
7. Hyperuricemia	Acute gout
8. Deafness (ethacrynic acid rare; furosemide exceedingly rare)	

* These reactions may occur as a result of all of the commonly employed diuretics except where indicated.
(Karliner, J. S., Gregoratos, G. (eds.): Coronary Care. Churchill Livingstone, New York, 1981.)

most severe instances, this can be seen as bubbling pink froth in the severely dyspneic patient. (See Pulmonary Edema, Chapter 15).

Therapeutic efforts must be directed at mobilization of the lung edema to improve gas exchange, and to improve oxygen delivery to the tissues. Inhaled oxygen should be provided and the arterial blood gases monitored to insure a set level of arterial pO_2. (See Respiratory Failure, Chapter 15.). Other measures should be instituted to improve cardiac function and decrease pulmonary venous pressure.

The proper management of pulmonary edema involves several of the approaches already discussed. Intravenous furosemide, 20–240 mg, is certainly a mainstay of treatment. In addition, morphine sulfate in doses of 5–15 mg intravenously may be exceedingly useful. It is advisable to begin with 5 mg intravenously, with increments of 2 mg every 5–15 minutes depending on the patient's response, to a maximum dose of 15 mg intravenously.

It has previously been taught that morphine produces a "pharmacologic phlebotomy," and that its major mechanism of action in reducing acute pulmonary edema resides in its ability to produce venous pooling resulting from acute venodilatation. However, it is more likely that morphine exerts its major action by inhibiting central sympathetic outflow, thereby reducing both peripheral vascular resistance and left ventricular contractility, resulting in a decrease in myocardial oxygen demand.

Additional measures to reduce venous return may be useful. When rotating tourniquets are used, the blood pressure cuff is blown up to 50–80 mmHg pressure on three limbs and rotated every five to 10 minutes. An alternative is to use a rubber tourniquet fastened tightly about the upper arms and thighs in three of the four extremities. Another neglected but often useful measure in the treatment of acute pulmonary edema is direct removal of blood from the circulation. Phlebotomy of 250–500 ml with monitoring of systemic arterial pressure can often produce dramatic relief.

With severe pulmonary edema, metabolic acidosis may be profound with an arterial pH of 7.1 or less and an increased anion gap (see Chapter 10). Under these circumstances, there is a base deficit, and the diagnosis of lactic acidosis may be made with confidence. The major goal of therapy is to improve left ventricular performance, and therapy with intravenous bicarbonate is not indicated; such solutions may cause acute and undesirable increases in plasma volume as well as a hyperosmolar state. Rapid change in blood pH to alkaline levels also may trigger cardiac arrhythmias, perhaps because of changes in serum potassium. Patients who develop such severe acidosis tend to hypoventilate and may require tracheal intubation and assisted ventilation.

Vasodilator Therapy

An important recent advance in the treatment of both acute and chronic congestive cardiac failure has been the introduction of vasodilator drugs. These agents, alone or in combination, reduce the afterload on the myocardium by reducing systemic arterial pressure and in some instances also reduce preload by causing peripheral venodilation. Both of these maneuvers will tend to produce a reduction in myocardial wall tension and, hence, in myocardial oxygen demand. The commonly used vasodilators and their mechanism of action are detailed in Table 16.4.

With acute congestive cardiac failure accompanied by mild to severe systemic arterial hypertension, intravenous nitroprusside at a dose of 0.2 to 5.0 $\mu g/kg/min$ appears to be a highly useful adjunct to

Table 16.4 **Major Actions of Vasodilating Agents Used in Afterload Reduction Therapy**

	Major Sites of Action	Chief Hemodynamic Effects			
		↓ PAW	↑ CO	↑ HR	↓ BP
Intravenous					
Sodium nitroprusside	A + V	+ +	+ +	0	+
Phentolamine	A + V	+ +	+ + +	↑	+
Nitroglycerin	V	+ + +	+	0	+
Oral					
Isosorbide dinitrate (ISO)	V	+ + +	+	0	+
Hydralazine (H)	A	±	+ + +	0	±
Prazosin	A + V	+ +	+ +	0	+
ISO + H	A + V	+ +	+ +	0	+
Captopril	A + V	+ + +	+	0	+ +

A = arterioles; V = veins; PAW = pulmonary artery wedge pressure; CO = cardiac output; HR = heart rate; BP = systemic blood pressure
(Modified from Karliner, J. S., Gregoratos, G. (eds.): Coronary Care. Churchill Livingstone, New York, 1981.)

therapy. The goal is to reduce the systemic arterial pressure and as a consequence to raise cardiac output. In the acute setting, it appears best to measure the pulmonary artery wedge pressure and the cardiac output serially, usually by thermodilution techniques, so as to judge the efficacy of therapy and to adjust the dose of the intravenous vasodilator. For chronic treatment, a variety of agents have been employed. Hydralazine in divided doses up to 300 mg daily is an effective arteriolar dilator. The alpha$_1$ blocking agent prazosin has effects on both the peripheral arteriolar and venous beds, resulting in combined arteriolar and venous dilatation. The dose of prazosin ranges from 3 mg daily up to as much as 20–25 mg daily. Refractoriness to the effects of this agent has been reported. Administration of organic nitrates, orally, sublingually, or cutaneously may provide effective combination therapy with either hydralazine or prazosin. The organic nitrates provide primarily venodilatation, thereby reducing the preload on the myocardium; the dose of isosorbide dinitrate may vary from 8 mg to 160 mg daily in divided doses, depending on patient tolerance and therapeutic response.

Recently, captopril, an oral angiotensin converting enzyme inhibitor, has been used to treat refractory congestive cardiac failure. The dose of this agent ranges from 12.5 to 100 mg three times daily, but treatment should be initiated cautiously as this drug may cause severe hypotension after the first one or two doses.

Vasodilator therapy should only be employed after other measures, including sodium restriction, control of systemic arterial hypertension, full therapeutic levels of digitalis, and adequate diuretic treatment. Patients who still have symptoms should be given a trial of oral vasodilator therapy. In some patients with advanced congestive cardiac failure, systemic arterial pressure may be quite low (e.g., 90–110 mmHg systolic). Even in such individuals, vasodilator therapy can be used cautiously, as experience has indicated that the reduction in systemic vascular resistance produced by arteriolar dilating agents results in an increase in cardiac output and mean arterial pressure is little altered.

The side effects of vasodilator therapy include headaches, nausea and vomiting produced by the organic nitrates; a peculiar initial hypotensive reaction to oral prazosin after the first dose, which is rare but which should be watched for carefully in all patients given this agent for the first time; and serological abnormalities such as a lupus-like syndrome which can be produced by prolonged treatment with oral hydralazine. Intravenous nitroprusside, if given over a prolonged period of time, can result in metabolism

of this agent from the thiocyanate to the cyanide form and can theoretically result in cyanide poisoning; fortunately, however, this complication is exceedingly rare. Intravenous nitroprusside can also result in the formation of methemoglobin.

Cautiously employed, both acutely and chronically, singly and in combination, these drugs have proved to be an important advance in the therapy of the more severe forms of acute and chronic congestive cardiac failure.

Additional Measures for the Treatment of Congestive Cardiac Failure

Although sodium restriction is highly desirable, clinical experience indicates that it is quite difficult for patients to adhere to very low sodium diets. Even with the availability of the newer diuretics, however, dietary control remains an important adjunct to the therapy of congestive heart failure and from the standpoint of patient education, it is useful to begin such treatment as soon as possible. In many patients, dietary indiscretion precipitates recurrent bouts of heart failure despite faithful adherence to medications such as digitalis and diuretics. Salt restriction to below 4 gm daily, which can be achieved by adding no extra salt to the meal, is usually advisable. Occasionally patients with advanced heart failure require a 1 gm/day salt regimen which necessitates limitation of salt in food preparation as well as elimination of many foods (for example, preprocessed meat and fish), but this is difficult for most patients to follow over prolonged periods of time. Another exceedingly important point in the control of congestive cardiac failure is the control of systemic arterial pressure. This, of course, is the goal of "afterload reduction." It is well to begin to educate the patient as soon as possible on the importance of controlling his or her arterial blood pressure.

CORONARY ARTERY DISEASE

RICK FACTORS

Coronary artery disease is most commonly the result of atherosclerotic narrowing of the coronary vessels. Its major symptomatic manifestations include angina pectoris, acute myocardial infarction, and sudden death due to ventricular arrhythmias. For the past several decades, epidemiological studies have established a number of "risk factors" for the development of coronary artery disease. These risk factors generally apply to populations studied (i.e., those in North America and Europe). Increased serum cholesterol, systemic hypertension, cigarette smoking, diabetes mellitus, and family history are the most important risk factors (see Chapter 2). Over the past few years, there has been an unexplained fall in the incidence of acute myocardial infarction in the United States, and it is postulated that this may be at least in part the result of attention to risk factors.

DIAGNOSIS

The cardinal symptom of coronary artery disease is precordial discomfort, The characterization of chest pain and its differential diagnosis are detailed in the section on history at the beginning of this chapter. It is well recognized that some patients have repeated bouts of acute myocardial ischemia demonstrable by ambulatory electrocardiography in the absence of symptoms. On the other hand, when the history is characteristic of angina pectoris, the resting electrocardiogram may be normal. When the ECG is abnormal, the following changes should be sought: significant (> 0.04 sec) Q waves in leads II, III, and aVF or in any of the precordial leads; accompanying repolarization abnormalities (S–T segment depression and/or T wave inversion); conduction abnormalities, such as left or right bundle branch block; and evidence of left ventricular hypertrophy. However, it is important to recognize that a wide variety of electrocardiographic changes in other conditions may resemble coronary disease. These are detailed in Table 16.5.

Physical examination in a patient with coronary artery disease may reveal evidence of systemic arterial hypertension. Often the cardiac examination is normal but a fourth heart sound may be either heard at rest or elicited by the handgrip maneuver. Often a murmur of mitral regurgitation due to papillary muscle dysfunction resulting from ischemia or previous myocardial infarction may be heard.

If the history is atypical, the resting electrocardiogram is normal and there is no previous history of acute myocardial infarction, further studies may be indicated to confirm the diagnosis. Such studies include an exercise test, radionuclide angiography for evaluation of left and right ventricular function, or [201]thallium scintigraphy for assessment of myocardial perfusion. In some patients, the diagnosis may only be established at the time of cardiac catheterization and coronary angiography (see below).

OFFICE MANAGEMENT

Office management of the patient with ischemic heart symptoms involves a number of therapeutic approaches. Cardinal among these is control of sys-

temic arterial hypertension. All patients should be instructed in the office in the use of sublingual nitroglycerin and a test tablet given to the patient so that he or she may identify any adverse reactions. Both the prophylactic and therapeutic use of sublingual nitroglycerin should be emphasized. The patient should take this medication before performing a task or physical exertion that will usually bring on an episode of typical precordial discomfort. It should be emphasized that nitroglycerin is not an addictive drug and frequent use does not lead to development of tolerance. For round-the-clock vasodilatation with organic nitrates, either oral, chewable, or sublingual isosorbide dinitrate may be used in doses ranging from 2.5 to 40 mg every six hours. The dose selection will depend upon patient response and tolerance. In some individuals, nitroglycerin paste may be used throughout the day or only at night as a substitution for isosorbide dinitrate. The dose of paste also depends on patient response and tolerance. The availability of cutaneous preparations that require only one daily application may help to simplify therapy.

Beta-adrenergic blocking agents, the prototype of which is propranolol, may be useful in the control of heart rate and blood pressure, both of which are major determinants of myocardial oxygen demand. For the treatment of ischemic heart disease, propranolol need only be given twice daily; in some patients, a beta$_1$ selective agent such as metoprolol may be useful, especially in individuals with obstructive lung disease or asthma. The dose of beta-blocking agents is highly variable, and it appears easiest to titrate such agents against the resting heart rate for a crude assessment of the degree of beta-adrenergic blockade. A resting heart rate between 50–60 beats per minute is a desirable goal. In many patients, a combination of organic nitrates and a beta-adrenergic blocking agent will prove useful. In some patients with heart failure, appropriately treated with digitalis and diuretics, angina pectoris may be further ameliorated by the use of additional specific vasodilator therapy with drugs such as prazosin (3–30 mg daily in divided doses), or hydralazine (30–200 mg daily in divided doses). Cardiac arrhythmias that lead to angina pectoris should be treated using appropriate antiarrhythmic drugs. As new therapeutic agents have become available, such as the calcium channel blockers (verapamil, nifedipine and diltiazem), their use in patients with stable angina pectoris has become more widespread. These agents are effective coronary artery and systemic arterial vasodilators but may also produce myocardial depression in some patients. They can be used in the presence of beta-adrenergic blockade. The combination of nifedipine and a beta-blocker appears to be particularly useful. However, verapamil in particular should not be used where atrioventricular conduction is impaired.

UNSTABLE ANGINA AND CORONARY ARTERY SPASM

Unstable angina represents the broad spectrum of symptomatic manifestations of myocardial ischemia intermediate in severity between stable, effort-induced angina and angina leading to inevitable myocardial infarction. It appears convenient to divide unstable angina into several clinical presentations:

1. Angina of recent onset, usually within the preceding month. This includes patients who develop angina within a month of documented myocardial infarction. One caveat pertains here, however: angina must begin sometime and one or two bouts of typical angina pectoris on exertion, which are relieved by rest, do not constitute unstable angina. It is the pattern and severity of angina which is the important factor.

2. Angina of effort with a change in pattern. This may be an increase in frequency, severity, or duration of previously stable effort angina or reduction in the stress required to precipitate pain. The pain may radiate to a new location or be accompanied for the first time by sweating or nausea. Organic nitrates and beta-adrenergic blockade may be less effective in relieving chest pain than had previously been the case.

3. A third pattern consists of angina that occurs at rest without apparent provocation. Some of these patients develop reversible S–T segment elevation or depression on the electrocardiogram taken during pain—a syndrome known as *variant angina*. This syndrome appears to result from a primary abnormality of coronary vasomotion in a major coronary artery, usually superimposed on an atheromatous narrowing. However, some patients have apparently spontaneous vasospasm without documented evidence of coronary artery narrowing.

Neither the clinical nor pathologic interface between unstable angina and acute myocardial infarction is clearly defined. Thus, differentiation of acute infarction from unstable angina is not always possible, even when sophisticated laboratory techniques are used. Some patients respond to an increase in the dose of a previously administered medication and additional measures to control systemic arterial pressure. Many patients with prolonged bouts of chest pain who do not exhibit acute myocardial infarction will require hospitalization and a "cooling-off period" accompanied by intensive medical therapy using the approach detailed above for outpatient management of angina pectoris. Many of these individuals require cardiac catheterization in order to define the anatomic extent of disease and to confirm, if possible, the occurrence of coronary arterial spasm. In patients with documented coronary artery spasm, the calcium antagonists, such as nifedipine, verapamil and diltiazem, seem to provide effective therapy, sometimes in conjunction with the organic nitrates.

INDICATIONS FOR CORONARY ANGIOGRAPHY AND CORONARY ARTERY BYPASS SURGERY

Opinions vary on the indications for coronary angiography in patients with ischemic heart disease. Most clinicians agree that patients whose symptoms are not well controlled by optimal medical therapy should undergo coronary arteriography with a view toward possible coronary artery bypass surgery. Younger individuals (under age 50) who develop manifestations of ischemic heart disease or who sustain a documented acute myocardial infarction are also candidates for coronary arteriography. As patients become older, there is less agreement as to the indications for this procedure and the spectrum of opinion ranges from those who would perform coronary arteriography in virtually all patients suspected of having ischemic heart disease to practitioners who recommend this procedure only when medical treatment has failed. Occasional patients require coronary angiography for pure diagnostic purposes; among these are individuals who complain of atypical chest pain in whom noninvasive diagnostic studies may be unrevealing or equivocal.

Aortocoronary bypass grafting for coronary artery disease has become a common form of treatment, and approximately 100,000 such operations are performed yearly in the United States alone. Randomized trials comparing surgical and nonsurgical treatment after preliminary coronary angiography involving patients with both stable and unstable angina pectoris have failed to show a reduction in mortality or infarction after bypass grafting, save for certain subsets of patients. Among these are individuals with left main coronary stenosis. However, nonrandomized trials in which the longevity of the operated patients is assessed using life table analysis have suggested that in patients with two and three vessel coronary disease longevity is indeed increased.

Operation appears clearly indicated in individuals who are refractory to medical therapy and in whom medication and/or symptoms prevent normal activity. The degree to which patients are able to tolerate symptoms of disease or side effects of medications varies greatly and as with every other major therapeutic decision, it is important to individualize recommendations. Patients with favorable coronary artery anatomy and well-preserved left ventricular function have the best outlook with regard to surgical morbidity and mortality. Advanced age, female sex, symptoms of congestive cardiac failure, left main coronary artery stenosis, impaired left ventricular function, and emergency surgery are associated with a higher operative mortality. It seems clear that operative mortality in coronary artery surgery has declined, but mortality figures reported from different institutions continue to vary (1.5 to 5 percent). This may be attributable to differences in experience of surgical teams, methods of anesthesia, or techniques of myocardial preservation as well as differences in the types of patients selected for surgery. Nevertheless, in appropriate selected patients, symptoms of angina pectoris can often be completely relieved and the individual returned to full activity with the ability to lead a productive life.

ACUTE MYOCARDIAL INFARCTION

Acute myocardial infarction is a major cause of adult mortality in industrialized western countries. This condition can be defined as deprivation of the blood supply to the heart (ischemia) for a period of time sufficient to produce structural damage and necrosis of the myocardium, often as the result of a coronary artery occlusion. Severe ischemic injury also may cause early electrophysiological disturbances that result in sudden death prior to the development of structural changes in the myocardium.

It has been suggested that coronary artery disease has reached epidemic proportions. For example, World Health Organization figures indicate that coronary artery disease accounts for one-third of all male deaths between the ages of 45 and 54 years in western countries. It accounts for death in about four out of every ten men when all age groups are considered. The advent of coronary care units has improved in-hospital mortality following acute myocardial infarction, especially in regard to deaths from arrhythmias. However, such units have had little impact on overall mortality, since over 60 percent of the deaths due to acute myocardial infarction occur early, outside of the hospital. Deaths due to heart failure or shock have become primarily responsible for in-hospital mortality. The social and economic costs associated with the loss of life and morbidity due to acute myocardial infarction in the working population remain an enormous problem.

CLINICAL PRESENTATION

The typical patient with acute myocardial infarction is a middle-aged or older male who complains of the sudden onset of severe, crushing, constricting, squeezing, or burning chest pain. Patients who have been suffering from angina pectoris frequently describe the pain of myocardial infarction as similar in quality but of much greater intensity. Typically, the pain is localized to the retrosternal region, but it may involve the anterior chest wall, both shoulders or arms, the neck, cheeks, lower teeth, or chin, the forearms or fingers, and the interscapular area. Occasionally the pain is epigastric and, especially when associated with nausea or vomiting, it may erroneously be ascribed to gastrointestinal causes. Often the pain of myocardial infarction is accompanied by sweating, dyspnea, pallor, and a sense of oppression or "impending doom." It commonly occurs at rest, lasts more than 30 minutes, and usually is not relieved by sublingual nitroglycerin.

There is little information on precipitating events which may immediately precede acute myocardial infarction. Some studies indicate that a high percentage of patients have prodromal symptoms or have visited a physician in the weeks prior to the acute event. However, the relation of acute myocardial infarction to physical exertion, emotional stress, new symptoms, or altered anginal patterns preceding the event has not been well defined.

Several patterns of onset of the clinical syndrome of acute myocardial infarction have been described:

1. The infarct is not preceded by symptoms and strikes the patient suddenly and unexpectedly.

2. A patient may suffer an attack of severe pain after ignoring several minor attacks in the hours or days preceding the infarction. Many patients visit a physician during this interval with complaints not necessarily referable to the cardiovascular system.

3. A patient may experience a series of attacks of "preinfarction" or "unstable" angina during several days or one to two weeks preceding the infarction.

4. A patient with chronic stable effort angina may suddenly develop the severe chest pain of acute infarction.

5. A patient with chronic stable effort angina may develop gradual acceleration of the anginal syndrome in a crescendo pattern culminating in myocardial infarction.

Acute myocardial infarction almost never occurs without some clinical evidence of left ventricular dysfunction which the careful observer can elicit at the bedside. The intensity of the first heart sound may be reduced; most patients exhibit an atrial gallop (S4), and a ventricular gallop (S3) is heard in about one-half of patients with acute myocardial infarction; its persistence may portend an ominous prognosis. Reduced intensity of the first heart sound tends to correlate with the associated decrease in left ventricular contractility, or it may result from papillary muscle dysfunction, with or without the accompanying murmur of mitral regurgitation. Rales may be present at the lung bases, and the clinical presentation sometimes is dominated by acute pulmonary edema, with or without shock. A fall in arterial blood pressure occurs commonly in myocardial infarction. Conversely, hypertension may be recorded in occasional patients, presumably as the result of the pain and anxiety accompanying the infarction.

Acute myocardial infarction may present in a variety of atypical clinical syndromes which often obscure the correct diagnosis:

1. The commonest unusual presentation of myocardial infarction is new onset or worsening of established congestive heart failure. Chest pain may or may not be present.

2. Atypical location or character of the pain is not infrequent; for example, localized elbow pain has been described as occurring with myocardial infarction.

3. Presentation with primarily central nervous system manifestations has been reported. A patient may present with a stroke, classic in all respects, as a result of embolization from a mural thrombus or of hypotension which may accompany a "silent" infarct.

4. Extreme anxiety and nervousness may be the predominant symptoms in occasional patients. These symptoms may be so severe that they completely obscure the chest pain of myocardial infarction.

5. Syncope may occasionally be the presenting symptom of myocardial infarction. Various mechanisms are responsible, but most often syncope is the result of an acute bradyarrhythmia or a hypotensive episode. Some patients who faint with the onset of acute infarction recover and do not recall pain at all.

6. Systemic arterial embolism may be the initial presentation of acute myocardial infarction.

7. Acute indigestion may be the presenting symptom, with the patient complaining of epigastric distress, nausea, vomiting, belching, and a sense of upper abdominal fullness.

8. Occasionally, acute myocardial infarction is totally "silent," with the patient recalling no symptoms, whereas the ECG shows evidence of subacute or chronic infarction. Silent infarcts have been reported to occur especially in the aged, in patients with diabetes mellitus, or during surgical operations under general anesthesia.

Atypical presentation (without chest pain) may occur in as many as 25 percent of patients with myocardial infarction. As a group, patients with atypical presentation exhibit (1) greater delay between onset of symptoms and establishment of the diagnosis of possible myocardial infarction, (2) higher values at hospital admission for heart rate, respiratory rate, temperature, and white blood count, and (3) greater in-hospital mortality. These differences are presumably due to delays in establishing the diagnosis and initiating appropriate therapy.

Many patients suffering from acute myocardial infarction die suddenly within minutes to two hours of the onset of symptoms. Thus, among males 50 years and younger, 60 percent of the deaths from acute myocardial infarction occur within one hour of the onset of symptoms, and the majority of patients with acute myocardial infarction die unattended at or near the place where they are stricken, before medical care arrives. Where mobile emergency care units are operating, early brady- and tachyarrhythmias are commonly diagnosed and ventricular fibrillation is the most common terminal event.

A variety of conditions may simulate the pain of acute myocardial infarction. Among the afflictions of the heart and lungs which should be considered are acute pulmonary embolism, acute pericarditis, spontaneous pneumothorax, dissecting aortic aneurysm and, rarely, mediastinal emphysema; dissecting aneurysm of the ascending aorta may involve the coronary ostia, producing secondary myocardial infarction. Among gastrointestinal conditions resembling the discomfort produced by myocardial infarction are those of acute "indigestion," esophagitis, hiatus hernia, cholecystitis, and pancreatitis.

LABORATORY DIAGNOSIS

During the first few days after acute myocardial infarction, mild fever, leukocytosis, and an elevated sedimentation rate are common but nonspecific findings. The crux of the diagnosis rests upon evolutionary changes in the electrocardiogram (ECG) and elevations in enzymes released into the serum as a result of myocardial cellular necrosis. In the presence of a convincing clinical history, the diagnosis of acute myocardial infarction is generally considered to be established if either: (1) there are typical ECG changes or (2) typical enzyme rises occur. In the absence of such a clinical history, both ECG and enzyme changes usually are required for a firm diagnosis. The use of radionuclide studies may further improve diagnostic accuracy.

Electrocardiographic Diagnosis

Electrocardiographic changes after coronary occlusion appear in three stages of increasing abnormality: ischemia, injury, and necrosis. In general, the stages of ischemia and injury are not accompanied by irreversible changes of the myocardial cell; however, the stage of necrosis implies irreversible damage to the myocardial fibers. Experimental occlusion of a coronary artery produces ECG changes which correlate in a general way with the severity and reversibility of the histologic changes in the myocardium. In naturally occurring myocardial infarction in humans, the three stages are not as discrete as in the experimental model, and they often occur more or less simultaneously on the ECG.

Ischemia leads to a local delay in the onset of repolarization and thereby to a prolongation of the QT interval with increased amplitude of the T wave. Depending upon whether the ischemic zone is subendocardial or subepicardial, leads overlying the involved area of the myocardium record upright or inverted T waves of increased amplitude and duration. These tall, broad T waves have been referred to as "hyperacute" T waves or as "T-terminale." Clinically, this initial stage of ischemia is transient, occurring only within the early minutes of an infarction, and it is therefore not commonly recorded on the ECG (Fig. 16.3).

The stage of myocardial *injury* is characterized by loss of the selective permeability of the injured cell membrane. This allows sodium ions to enter the cell as they move down the sodium concentration gradient with associated loss of intracellular potassium to the extracellular compartment. The net result of these ionic shifts is a decrease in the resting membrane potential of the cell (hypopolarization) which, in turn, causes a primary negative shift of the region of ECG between the T wave and the QRS (the TQ segment is displaced downward). The usual condensor-compensated ECG machine will then record the *negative* TQ shift as a *positive* ST segment shift, re-

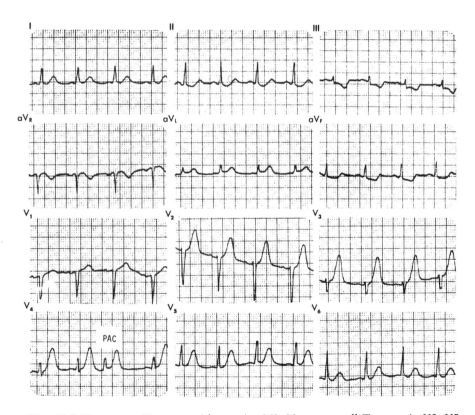

Fig. 16.3 Hyperacute T waves with anterior MI. Note very tall T waves in V2–V5, with slight ST segment elevation in aVL and reciprocal ST depression in leads II, III, aVF. Patient was complaining of severe chest pain and evolved an extensive anterior MI. PAC = premature atrial contraction. (Goldberger, A., Goldberger, E.: Clinical Electrocardiography, 2nd ed. C. V. Mosby, St. Louis, 1981, with permission.)

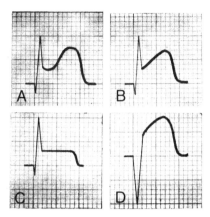

Fig. 16.4 ST segment elevation seen with acute infarction may have variable shapes, as shown in A to D. (Goldberger, A. Goldberger, E.: Clinical Electrocardiography, 2nd ed. The C V Mosby Company, St. Louis, 1979, with permission.)

sulting in the familiar pattern of an acute injury current (ST elevation) (Fig. 16.4). The theoretical basis of ST segment elevation is still a subject of discussion, and a variety of other explanations have been proposed.

Clinically, ST segment elevation appears in ECG leads that are related to the site of the infarct and it usually constitutes the first sign of a developing infarction. Reciprocal ST depression may be seen in leads reflecting the myocardial wall opposite those recording the acute injury pattern. The T wave is often obscured by the ST segment elevation, but if discernable, may show slight terminal inversion. This stage may last only a few hours, but persistent ST elevation is seen typically for several days and occasionally lasts several weeks. ST elevation in the right precordial leads (antero-septal myocardial infarction) tends to persist longer than the injury current recorded in the lateral precordial leads or the limb leads. Regression of the injury pattern heralds either recovery or, more commonly, necrosis of the involved myocardium. In the latter instances, return of ST segments toward the isoelectric line is accompanied by developing ECG signs of myocardial damage.

The stage of myocardial *necrosis* or infarction is characterized electrocardiographically by the development of abnormal Q waves in a lead or leads which normally do not record Q waves, and by reduction in QRS amplitude. In terms of the vector concept, the Q wave of infarction results from loss of the electrical forces in the necrotic myocardium with an associated reciprocal gain of forces oriented in the opposite direction. For example, infarction of the inferior (diaphragmatic) wall of the left ventricle results in loss of the initial forces oriented inferiorly (normally recorded as R waves in leads III and aVF) and, therefore, in the development of Q waves in leads III and aVF which now predominantly record potentials oriented *away* from the area of infarction (infarction vector). Clinically, the Q or QS complexes of infarction usually appear within several hours to a few days after onset of symptoms. Ordinarily, Q waves develop while the ST segment elevation is still prominent. With the onset of necrosis, the normal R wave is replaced by a QR or QS deflection. Changes in the initial force (development of Q waves) are not seen in infarctions that are nontransmural, but the amplitude of the R wave in appropriate leads may be diminished as muscle mass is lost. The QRS changes reflecting death of myocardial muscle may persist for months, for years, or indefinitely. With time they tend to become less prominent, especially those Q waves resulting from inferior myocardial infarction.

Clinically, it is useful to recognize a fourth electrocardiographic stage of myocardial infarction, the stage of evolution. During this stage, deep symmetrical T wave inversions appear in diagnostic leads, as the S–T segments return to the isoelectric baseline. These changes probably reflect ischemia of the myocardium surrounding the infarcted area that was present throughout the previous stages but masked by the current of injury. The abnormalities of the T waves due to transmural infarction may persist for months or years, or they may disappear to be replaced by "secondary" T wave abnormalities. The latter take the form of asymmetric and less deeply inverted T waves in diagnostic leads and are thought to reflect absence of significant repolarization potentials in the electrically inert site of healed myocardial infarction, with the result that opposing repolarization forces from normal ventricular myocardium rotate the T vector away from the infarcted region. Typical patterns are shown in Figures 16.5 and 16.6.

Localization of myocardial infarction by the ECG is useful, since both prognosis and incidence of complications differ in anterior and inferior infarctions. It must be kept in mind, however, that electrocardiographic localization is imprecise and dependent to a great extent on the distribution of the coronary arterial tree which normally may be quite variable. Furthermore, the specificity of ECG localization of

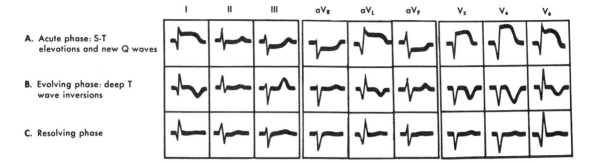

Fig. 16.5 Sequential changes with acute anterior wall MI. See text for details. (Goldberger, A., Goldberger, E.: Clinical Electrocardiography, 2nd ed. The C V Mosby Company, St Louis, 1981, with permission.)

an infarct diminishes in direct relation to the number of previous infarctions the patient has sustained.

It should be appreciated that multiple infarctions may occur and that areas of myocardial scarring frequently are present at autopsy which were not manifested by any ECG alterations. Once Q waves have appeared and the ST segments have returned to baseline, it may not be possible to assess the age of the infarct by the ECG pattern, since both acute and healed infarcts may exhibit the same alterations. Thus, serial ECGs are necessary in every case to arrive at a proper diagnosis.

A number of conditions may obscure or complicate the ECG diagnosis of acute myocardial infarction. Sometimes patients will seek medical advice because of chest pain, and only repolarization abnormalities (ST segment depression, T wave inversion) without Q waves will be found on the ECG. Under such circumstances, reliance must be placed on appropriate serum enzyme changes to substantiate the diagnosis of a subendocardial or nontransmural myocardial infarction. In the presence of left bundle branch block, the ECG diagnosis of acute myocardial

infarction is often difficult, but there are certain alterations which are helpful; these include the presence of upright T waves in the lateral precordial leads, T wave inversions in the anterior precordial leads, and the appearance of Q waves in leads V_5 and V_6. Right bundle branch block does not interfere with the development of abnormal initial forces (Q waves) after acute myocardial infarction. The Wolff-Parkinson-White syndrome may both mimic and mask the ECG pattern of acute myocardial infarction; however, if serial tracings are obtained during the acute clinical episode, suggestive repolarization changes may be recorded. Several conditions other than acute myocardial infarction can lead to the development of Q waves (Table 16.5).

Serum Enzyme Activity

Among the most useful enzyme activities measured is creatine kinase (CK). A variety of tissues contain CK, including heart, skeletal muscle, brain, lung and thyroid, and serum CK tends to rise in

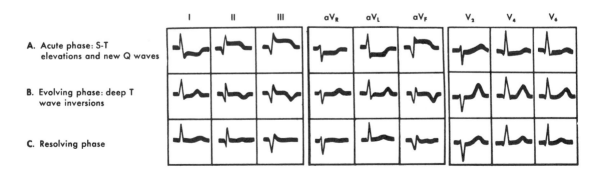

Fig. 16.6 Sequential changes with acute inferior wall MI. See text for details. (Goldberger, A, Goldberger, E: Clinical Electrocardiography, 2nd ed. C. V. Mosby, St. Louis, 1981, with permission.)

Table 16.5 **ECG Patterns Simulating Ischemic Myocardial Infarction**

Condition	ECG Findings	Comment
Conduction Disturbances		
1. Wolff-Parkinson-White syndrome	Tall R waves in right precordial leads or deep Q waves in leads II, III and AVF may mimic myocardial infarction	Q (delta) waves may disappear in the presence of a supraventricular tachycardia
2. Left anterior hemiblock	Small Q waves may appear in leads V_{1-3}	The Q waves may be transient, especially if the hemiblock is rate-dependent, or if the precordial leads are recorded one or two interspaces higher
3. Left bundle branch block	Q waves may be present in the right precordial leads	The initial forces tend to be anterior and to the left, producing right precordial Q waves. The same phenomenon occurs in left ventricular hypertrophy
Cardiomyopathies		
1. Specific		
a. Billowing mitral leaflet ("click-murmur" syndrome)	If present, Q waves are in II, III and aVF	Any cause of fibrosis may produce ECG changes that mimic myocardial infarction
b. Idiopathic hypertrophic subaortic stenosis	Q waves may be present in limb or precordial leads	Q waves due to septal hypertrophy
c. Duchenne's muscular dystrophy	Tall R waves in right precordial leads	
2. Nonspecific	Q waves and repolarization abnormalities are common	
Other		
Subarachnoid Hemorrhage	T-wave inversion in mid and lateral precordial leads	Mechanism unknown. Possibly central
3. Normal Variants		
a. Young, healthy males, especially blacks	"Early repolarization," including ST segment elevation in inferior, anterior and lateral leads	
b. Well-trained athletes	Tall R waves in right precordial leads; diffuse repolarization abnormalities	

shock from any cause, or after skeletal muscle trauma, including intramuscular injections, even in the absence of myocardial damage. Other noncardiac disorders in which CK may be elevated include muscular dystrophy, inflammatory disease of muscle, cerebral disease, alcohol intoxication, diabetes mellitus with and without ketosis, and convulsions. Serum CK contains three isoenzymes which can be separated by electrophoresis, MM (skeletal muscle), BB (brain), and MB, the isoenzyme which (in man) is virtually specific for cardiac muscle. About 15 percent of myocardial CK release is of the MB type, the remainder being largely MM. Methods for analysis of the cardiac-specific MB-CK are now routinely employed and have facilitated the diagnosis of acute myocardial infarction when the CK is elevated from other causes such as skeletal muscle trauma.

The CK usually begins to rise within four hours after the onset of symptoms of myocardial infarction, typically reaches a peak after 12 to 18 hours, and returns to normal in two to four days. Sampling every six hours for the first 24 to 36 hours after the onset of symptoms will identify the peak CK value in over 90 percent of instances.

Lactate dehydrogenase (LDH) also is abundant in a variety of tissues, including the liver, skeletal muscle, lung, kidney, red blood cells, heart, and lung, in decreasing order of activity. Serum samples are stable for days at room temperature. Peak elevation of the serum LDH usually occurs within 48 to 72 hours after acute myocardial infarction, later than the rise in CK, and it may remain elevated for many days. However, a high serum LDH level can be a nonspecific finding. Five LDH isoenzymes can be identified by methods now widely available, and an increase of the ratio LDH_1/LDH_2 is highly specific for acute myocardial infarction in the absence of hemolysis, renal cortical or cerebral infarction, and disseminated carcinoma. LDH isoenzymes have a long half-life and sampling once a day for LDH isoenzyme activity is sufficient.

A rise in the serum glutamic-oxaloacetic transaminase (GOT) was the first enzyme test to be employed. The GOT rises within 12 to 48 hours after the onset of myocardial necrosis and falls rapidly thereafter. It also is nonspecific and may be increased by skeletal muscle injury or hepatic damage.

For a definitive diagnosis of acute myocardial infarction, it is desirable to document a typical rise and fall in at least one of these serum enzymes.

Radiographic Findings

Distension of the upper lobe pulmonary veins occurs in up to 75 percent of patients with acute myocardial infarction. The appearance of the pulmonary vasculature at the time of adminission predicts the pulmonary arterial wedge pressure accurately in only about 40 percent of patients, overestimating the wedge pressure in 33 percent and underestimating it in 25 percent; but with serial chest films, the presence of pulmonary venous hypertension can be detected or excluded in about 60 percent of patients. A time-lag of many hours may occur after hemodynamic changes; the chest radiograph may remain normal despite a persistently elevated pulmonary arterial wedge pressure for as long as six to 24 hours. Serial radiographs confirm the frequent occurrence of left ventricular enlargement.

Noninvasive Assessment of Cardiac Function

With two-dimensional echocardiography, striking disorders of left ventricular wall motion have been observed within the first few hours after myocardial infarction. This technique can also be used to identify left ventricular thrombi and to diagnose ventricular septal rupture. Using radioisotope angiography, it has been found that the ejection fraction is reduced in the majority of patients with acute myocardial infarction.

Hemodynamic Findings

The central venous pressure, while useful as a measure of right ventricular filling pressure, provides an unreliable guide to the left ventricular filling pressure or pulmonary arterial (PA) wedge pressure. Thus, in patients with associated pulmonary disease the central venous pressure may be distinctly abnormal while the PA wedge pressure is normal, whereas the central venous pressure may exceed the wedge pressure in patients with right ventricular infarction. Often, the PA wedge pressure is substantially elevated in the presence of a normal central venous pressure.

The left ventricular end-diastolic pressure has been measured and is often elevated (>12 mmHg) after acute transmural myocardial infarction, even when clinical signs of left heart failure or shock are absent. The PA end-diastolic pressure correlates reasonably well with the mean left atrial and PA wedge pressures in the absence of tachycardia and pulmonary disease, although the left ventricular end-diastolic pressure may exceed these pressures. The PA wedge pressure is most commonly measured using a flow directed, balloon-tipped catheter whenever hemodynamic monitoring is necessary. The average levels of PA wedge pressure and the incidence of elevated PA wedge pressures found after acute myocardial infarction in various clinical categories of patients are summarized in Table 16.6.

When complete hemodynamic studies are available, various hemodynamic patterns associated with the clinical classes of patients can be identified (Table 16.6, Fig. 16.7). In uncomplicated patients (Class I), the blood pressure and cardiac output are normal or slightly diminished, and peripheral vascular resistance and central venous pressure usually are normal. With signs of mild congestive heart failure such as gallop rhythm and basilar rales (Class II), the cardiac index tends to drop, the blood pressure is maintained, and the PA wedge pressure is usually elevated. In general, the more severe the congestive heart failure, the lower the systemic arterial pressure and cardiac output, the higher the peripheral vascular resistance, and the more elevated the PA wedge pressure. Viewed in this context, cardiogenic shock (Class IV) forms the extreme end of the spectrum of

Table 16.6 **PA Wedge Pressure in Acute Myocardial Infarction**

Clinical Classification	Percent of Patients	Mean PA Wedge Pressure (mm Hg)		Percent Having Abnormal PA Wedge Pressure (>12 mm Hg)
		Average	Range	
Uncomplicated (I)	30	10	2–25	25
Mild LV failure (II)	45	15	5–25	65
Severe LV failure (III)	15	17	5–30	70
Cardiogenic shock (IV)	10	24	10–30	90

PA = Pulmonary arterial

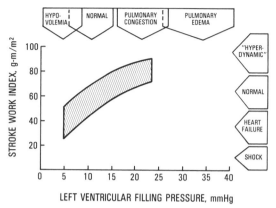

Fig. 16.7 The hemodynamic spectrum of cardiac function in acute myocardial infarction. In any given patient, the hemodynamic status can be assessed by using the function curve coordinates of filling pressure and left ventricular work depicted here. It should be recognized that the designations are only approximate and that considerable overlap probably occurs. (Modified after Heikkila, J.: Pump failure and haemodynamic subsets in acute myocardial infarction. Ann. Clin. Res. 9:112–123, 1977, with permission.)

impaired left ventricular performance after acute myocardial infarction. In the presence of shock, the cardiac index is extremely low, the wedge pressure usually is markedly elevated and the peripheral vascular resistance is high; rarely, shock occurs in the presence of a normal peripheral vascular resistance and shock with normal PA wedge and venous pressures indicates hypovolemia.

TREATMENT

Early Myocardial Infarction

Efforts to provide early treatment of arrhythmias and cardiopulmonary resuscitation within one or two hours after acute myocardial infarction have had increasing success. Early treatment of serious bradyarrhythmias by atropine, tachyarrhythmias by beta-adrenergic blocking agents, and ventricular tachycardia and fibrillation by lidocaine and electrical countershock have resulted in survival of many such patients.

Uncomplicated Myocardial Infarction

It has become standard practice in many countries to admit patients with acute myocardial infarction to an intensive coronary care unit. Because effective 24-hour electrocardiographic monitoring and prompt treatment can be achieved in such a setting, the death rate due to cardiac arrhythmias has been reduced. The patient without complications is usually observed in such a unit for 24 to 72 hours. Initial therapy is directed toward reassurance and relief of pain by intravenous administration of morphine or other opiates. In the coronary care unit, a vein is cannulated, and kept patent by means of a slow infusion of dextrose and water for administration of antiarrhythmic medication as necessary. The incidence of primary ventricular fibrillation decreases exponentially with time after acute myocardial infarction, and prophylactic administration of an antiarrhythmic agent such as lidocaine has been shown by some investigators to reduce the incidence of this complication. Such treatment may particularly be indicated in the early hours, since ventricular fibrillation is not necessarily preceded by warning ventricular ectopic beats.

Oxygen is usually administered. In patients who have an arterial oxygen saturation of 90 percent or above, oxygen administration may actually depress cardiac output, presumably by increasing systemic vascular resistance, but in patients with an arterial oxygen saturation of less than 90 percent, oxygen therapy appears beneficial. Oxygen administration does not appear to significantly reduce hyperventilation, which is probably the result of a change in pulmonary compliance.

Cautious early mobilization of patients with uncomplicated myocardial infarction is often carried out by the fourth to sixth day. Indeed, early mobilization and discharge within two weeks after hospitalization appears to have distinct medical, social, and economic advantages.

Some studies indicate that anticoagulation is advantageous in patients with acute myocardial infarction, but others suggest this treatment lacks direct benefit. While anticoagulation reduces the incidence of venous thrombosis and pulmonary embolism in patients requiring prolonged bed rest, use of a bedboard, elastic stockings, and early mobilization may accomplish the same effects without the risk of internal bleeding. There is no conclusive clinical evidence that anticoagulation reduces mortality or prevents complications in the usual patient with acute myocardial infarction. The indications for anticoagulants in the treatment of acute myocardial infarction are: (1) large infarction, (2) history of previous infarction, (3) congestive heart failure, (4) demonstration of left ventricular mural thrombi by ultrasound, and (5) complications requiring a prolonged period in bed. The use of small doses of subcutaneous heparin (5000 units two or three times daily) may be useful in patients requiring a long period of bed rest and is often employed routinely during the first week of treatment.

It has been proposed that reducing myocardial oxygen demands and increasing substrate delivery may reduce the size of a myocardial infarction in man. Whether or not such measures will prove useful in the clinical setting is under current investigation.

Ventricular Arrhythmias

Ventricular ectopic or premature contractions occur in almost all patients with acute myocardial infarction who undergo constant ECG monitoring. Ventricular fibrillation without prior arrhythmias (primary ventricular fibrillation) occurs with a frequency which decreases exponentially in the early hours after acute myocardial infarction. It has been suggested that indications for preventive antiarrhythmic therapy should be the appearance of more than five ventricular premature contractions per minute, three or more ventricular ectopic beats in a row (ventricular tachycardia), or isolated multifocal ventricular premature beats, all of which are associated with a higher incidence of ventricular tachycardia or ventricular fibrillation. An increased sinus rate also appears to be an important predisposing factor in patients who develop ventricular fibrillation. Some studies indicate that routine use of intravenous lidocaine for 48 hours may all but eliminate primary ventricular fibrillation.

Intravenous lidocaine is usually employed for the treatment of ventricular premature beats. The average plasma half-life of lidocaine in patients with normal hepatic function is 90 minutes; therefore, lidocaine is commonly administered as an intravenous bolus of 100 mg in order to rapidly achieve a therapeutic blood level, followed by a continuous intravenous infusion of 1–3 mg/min. Further salvos of ventricular premature contractions should be treated with 50 to 100 mg of lidocaine immediately. Refractoriness to lidocaine is unusual, but if this agent proves inadequate, procainamide should be added, in a dose of 100 to 250 mg intravenously. Procainamide may also be employed orally, but its short half-life requires use of 250 mg or more every three to four hours. Propranolol and other beta-adrenergic blocking drugs have been used successfully in the treatment of ventricular arrhythmias following acute myocardial infarction. Occasionally, diphenylhydantoin or bretylium tosylate intravenously may be tried when other drugs have failed.

When ventricular tachycardia is unresponsive to antiarrhythmic drugs, or when it produces serious hypotension, emergency electrical countershock is indicated, the defibrillator being set to deliver maximum energy (usually 400 joules). For electrical conversion of ventricular tachycardia, DC shock with synchronization to the R wave of the ECG is employed.

Whether or not patients treated with intravenous antiarrhythmic agents should be placed on oral antiarrhythmic agents such as quinidine during and after hospital discharge remains controversial. In some centers, patients are placed on quinidine sulfate 200 to 400 mg orally every six hours. The need for long-term antiarrhythmic therapy may later be assessed using ambulatory continuous ECG (Holter) monitoring or exercise testing one to three months after discharge from the hospital. Current evidence indicates that chronic use of beta-adrenergic blockers following myocardial infarction reduces the subsequent incidence of reinfarction and sudden death, at least during the first year.

Supraventricular Tachycardias

Sinus tachycardia is relatively common after acute myocardial infarction and requires no specific treatment, but rapid atrial tachycardia, atrial fibrillation, and accelerated junctional tachycardia generally require therapy. Digitalis frequently is useful in atrial fibrillation. Atrial and nodal tachycardias are frequently transient, and digitalis usually provides effective prophylaxis against their recurrence. Electrical conversion using R wave synchronized DC countershock may be required for persistent atrial tachycardia or atrial flutter, and should be followed by digitalis and quinidine.

Bradyarrhythmias and Heart Block

Sinus bradycardia and atrioventricular (A–V) dissociation are especially common after acute inferior or posterior myocardial infarction. Increased vagal tone as well as ischemia may be important in the pathogenesis of such dysrhythmias. Clinical observations in patients with mild bradycardia indicate that modest increments in heart rate produced by atropine (0.3 to 1.0 mg intravenously) can result in marked symptomatic improvement and increase of the systemic arterial pressure. However, routine use of atropine in patients with bradycardia and normal or elevated systemic arterial pressure is not warranted, and under some experimental conditions, atropine-induced tachycardia can enhance ischemic injury and increase the propensity to serious arrhythmias. Thus, the oxygen cost of too rapid a heart rate can exert a deleterious influence on the myocardium.

Second and third degree AV block unresponsive to atropine require insertion of a temporary transvenous pacemaker via an antecubital, brachiocephalic or femoral vein; usually adequate pacing can be achieved from the right ventricle and, with good technique, temporary catheter electrodes may function for as long as 10 to 14 days.

Recent comprehensive multicenter studies have helped to clarify the clinical significance of bundle branch block complicating acute myocardial infarction. In 432 patients with acute myocardial infarction complicated by bundle branch block (old or new), left bundle branch block was seen in 38 percent and right bundle branch block with left anterior fascicular block in 34 percent. "High degree AV block" (Mobitz Type II second degree AV block, or third degree AV block) occurred in 22 percent of these patients. The hospital mortality of patients with high degree AV block was increased over that of patients without this complication (31 vs. 2 percent, respectively) even in the absence of pulmonary edema and cardiogenic shock, with nearly all deaths due to the abrupt development of complete AV block. During the first year after infarction, patients with transient high degree AV block during hospitalization had a 28 percent incidence of sudden death or recurrent high degree AV block. Patients not paced had a higher incidence of sudden death or recurrent high-degree block than those who were paced (65 vs. 10 percent, respectively). On the basis of these studies, insertion of a temporary prophylactic pacemaker can tentatively be recommended in patients with acute myocardial infarction who have a substantial risk of progression to high degree of AV block, regardless of myocardial infarct location. These high-risk individuals include:

1. Patients with first degree AV block who also have either a new bundle branch block or bilateral bundle branch block, right bundle branch block plus left anterior fascicular block, or alternating bundle branch block (risk of progression 19–20 percent).

2. New bilateral bundle branch block without first degree AV block (risk of progression 31–38 percent).

Patients who survive high degree AV block during acute myocardial infarction should receive temporary pacing followed by consideration for implantation of a permanent pacemaker.

In patients who exhibit recurrent arrhythmias or conduction disturbances, monitoring in an intermediate care unit seems appropriate. Patients who develop right or left bundle branch block in association with anterior transmural myocardial infarction are especially prone to late in-hospital ventricular fibrillation and deserve long-term monitoring during recovery.

Pericarditis, Extension of Infarction and Postmyocardial Infarction Syndrome

An evanescent pericardial friction rub is common two to three days after acute myocardial infarction and may be associated with ST segment elevation on the electrocardiogram. Such ST segment elevations should be distinguished from extension of myocardial infarction by serial serum enzyme determinations. When a friction rub lasts more than 24 hours, consideration should be given to cessation of anticoagulant therapy if this has been previously instituted because of the danger of hemopericardium. A persistent pericardial friction rub occurring after a latent period (several days to two or more weeks), especially when accompanied by fever, arthralgias, pleural effusion, and pleuropericardial pain, should raise the suspicion of the *postmyocardial infarction syndrome*. This uncommon complication is thought to be an immune reaction to damaged cardiac tissues; it usually responds to aspirin, non-steroidal anti-inflammatory agents, or corticosteroids. Rarely this syndrome persists for months or even years after infarction.

Congestive Heart Failure

This complication occurs to a severe degree in about 15 percent of patients, although mild to moderate left ventricular failure is present in nearly 50 percent of patients (Table 16.6, Fig. 16.7). In this setting modest and variable benefit results from the cardiac glycosides. It appears that digitalis may become more effective as recovery ensues, although, with marked failure, early use may have some benefit. Alterations in renal hemodynamics commonly occur after acute myocardial infarction, and digitalis dosage should be modified appropriately in such patients. Bolus intravenous injections of rapidly acting glycosides may be hazardous, since digitalis administered in this fashion may raise the systemic arterial pressure acutely and compromise cardiac performance.

The usual criteria for diagnosis and treatment are detailed in the preceding section, Congestive Heart Failure, Treatment.

Cardiogenic Shock

This complication occurs in about seven to ten percent of patients (Table 16.6). Cardiogenic shock constitutes an extreme form of left ventricular "power failure" complicating acute myocardial infarction. Typically, there is a very low cardiac output, high pulmonary artery wedge pressure and elevated peripheral vascular resistance. The systemic systolic blood pressure is usually 90 mmHg or less (or 60 mmHg below the patient's usual systolic blood pressure); urinary flow is less than 20 ml/hr and there may be cool extremities and cerebral underperfusion. Hypovolemia should be carefully excluded before a diagnosis of cardiogenic shock is made. The venous pressure provides a clue, and a low central venous pressure (<7 mmHg) alone in the presence of shock after acute myocardial infarction constitutes an indication for the cautious use of plasma volume expanders. Pain, hypoxemia, electrolyte imbalance, and cardiac arrhythmias should be treated before the diagnosis of power failure is established. Most patients with cardiogenic shock have sustained widespread damage to the myocardium due to acute and/or recurrent myocardial infarction.

Hypovolemia should be excluded by recording an elevated pulmonary artery wedge pressure (>15 mmHg). Dopamine has been a useful agent in cardiogenic shock caused by acute myocardial infarction. It exerts a mild alpha-adrenergic agonist effect, causing vasoconstriction of peripheral capacitance and resistance vessels and a beta-adrenergic effect, causing a modest increase in cardiac rate and augmentation of myocardial contractility. It also causes nonadrenergically mediated dilation of renal and mesenteric vascular beds. The combination of dopamine with parenteral diuretic therapy may increase urine flow in some patients beyond that produced by either agent alone. An alternative agent that has also proved useful under these circumstances is dobutamine. Use of norepinephrine has not increased survival in patients with cardiogenic shock because of its marked peripheral and renal vasoconstrictor actions, the former effect causing an increased afterload on the myocardium, while the latter further compromises renal function. Isoproterenol generally should not be employed in the therapy of cardiogenic shock because of its propensity to augment heart rate and myocardial oxygen demands and to produce peripheral vasodilation.

Using the combination of dopamine or dobutamine and parenteral diuretic therapy, it has been possible to reduce acute mortality from 85 or 90 percent to 66 percent among patients with shock complicating acute myocardial infarction. An alternative approach is the use of the peripheral vasodilator sodium nitroprusside or nitroglycerin along with a pressor agent. Early mortality is reduced to about 60 percent with this mode of therapy, but long-term survival remains relatively poor with either medical approach.

In patients who are unresponsive to such measures, intraaortic balloon counterpulsation may be instituted. The use of aortic balloon counterpulsation alone has failed to alter survival figures greatly, but when followed by emergency coronary revascularization in selected patients there is improved prognosis. The number of long-term survivors remains disappointingly low with all approaches to the therapy of this condition.

Papillary Muscle Dysfunction and Rupture

Disordered function of the papillary muscles often follows acute myocardial infarction, occurring transiently in up to 60 percent of patients. In most patients, papillary muscle dysfunction is mild and leads to an apical late systolic murmur reflecting mitral regurgitation. There is a poor correlation between the intensity of the murmur and the degree of mitral regurgitation, especially when left ventricular function is severely depressed. Incompetence of the posterior mitral valve leaflet may be associated with a murmur which radiates to the base of the heart, simulating an aortic ejection murmur. The clinical course of papillary muscle dysfunction is quite variable, and in most cases the contractility of the left ventricle is a more important determinant of the outcome than the degree of papillary muscle dysfunction.

Rupture of the papillary muscle occurs in about one percent of patients with acute myocardial infarction. This catastrophic event is most common during the first week and is heralded by the rapid onset of acute pulmonary edema due to sudden left ventricular failure. The apical holosystolic murmur which occurs under such circumstances must be differentiated from the murmur produced by an equally serious event, rupture of the interventricular septum. Because the anterolateral papillary muscle has a more extensive collateral circulation, rupture of the posteromedial papillary muscle is four times more common. The clinical course is determined primarily by the site of rupture; if the entire trunk of a muscle ruptures, both mitral leaflets are deprived of support, there is massive mitral regurgitation, and death rapidly ensues. If a single head of the muscle ruptures, the degree of congestive cardiac failure is usually not as severe. Under these circumstances, if left ventricular performance is not severely depressed, mitral valve replacement may be life-saving, and 50 percent survival rates for one year have been reported after such operations.

Rupture of the Interventricular Septum

Ventricular septal rupture occurs in less than one percent of patients with acute myocardial infarction, usually being observed within the first week. Both anterior and inferior myocardial infarction can lead to interventricular septal rupture, and associated aneurysm formation in the anterior or inferior left ventricular wall is common. The magnitude of the left to right shunt usually is large and there is pulmonary arterial hypertension. A loud systolic murmur frequently is heard along the left sternal border, without axillary radiation, and a systolic thrill is palpable in 50 percent of patients. Cardiac catheterization or use of a balloon floatation catheter to demonstrate an oxygen step-up in the blood flowing through the right ventricle may be necessary to differentiate the findings from those of ruptured papillary muscle. Two-dimensional echocardiography or radionuclide angiography may be used to confirm the diagnosis noninvasively.

Because of the poor prognosis, operative closure of the ventricular septal defect usually is indicated. If possible, operation should be delayed from three to six weeks after the infarction to allow firm fibrous healing of the region, but successful early operative intervention (five to eight days after the appearance of the lesion) has also been reported. Regardless of the size of the defect, the major factor determining survival appears to be the extent and function of the surviving myocardium. A 50 percent survival rate one year after such operations has been reported.

Rupture of Heart and False Aneurysm

Rupture of the left ventricular free wall is found in about nine percent of autopsies after acute myocardial infarction; this complication usually occurs within two weeks. The anterior wall is most often involved, and rupture tends to be more common in patients with first infarctions. Cardiac rupture leading to hemopericardium results in shock and death due to cardiac tamponade.

Pathologic evidence suggests that in some instances there is slow leakage of blood into the pericardial space prior to complete rupture. This process occasionally culminates in the formation of a false ventricular aneurysm, which can be recognized by left ventriculography. This condition may be amenable to surgical therapy and successful operation for subacute cardiac rupture has been reported.

PROGNOSIS AFTER ACUTE MYOCARDIAL INFARCTION

About 60 percent of patients who expire after myocardial infarction die prior to hospitalization; the average 30-day mortality after hospitalization is about 20 percent, and overall 30-day mortality, therefore, averages about 45 percent. However, there is wide variation in mortality after hospital admission, which is dependent upon many factors. Prognostic indices have been developed based on weighted clinical scores for historical data, associated diseases, physical findings, left ventricular function, electrocardiographic abnormalities and rhythm disturbances. It also has been proposed that long-term (three-year) mortality can be related to age, heart size, degree of pulmonary congestion, and previous ischemia. In uncomplicated patients, without congestive heart failure (Class I) the 30-day mortality is about six percent; with mild congestive heart failure (Class II, pulmonary rales, third heart sound) mortality increases to 17 percent; with pulmonary edema (Class III) it rises to 38 percent; and with cardiogenic shock (Class IV) mortality is 80 to 90 percent. Low-level and submaximal exercise tolerance tests have been advocated as a means of identifying patients with a high risk of recurrence of ischemic symptoms—angina, recurrent infarction or sudden death—in the year after myocardial infarction.

REHABILITATION AFTER ACUTE MYOCARDIAL INFARCTION

Early mobilization and discharge from the hospital do not seem to alter the prognosis adversely in patients with uncomplicated acute myocardial infarction. After hospital discharge, convalescent or reconditioning centers, spas, and outpatient exercise programs have been employed with good results. Although the scope of such rehabilitation practices varies markedly, in some countries (such as Sweden, Germany, Yugoslavia, and Poland) well-equipped convalescent centers or spas offering structured physical activity and educational programs have been successful.

An important aim of such programs is the return of the patient to his usual job. In the United States, successful employment after myocardial infarction is more frequent in patients under age 50, who are in a favorable cardiac classification (New York Heart Association Class I or IIB), who have good motivation, and who have experienced a period of unemployment of less than one year. About 80 to 90 percent of patients with uncomplicated myocardial infarction return to work within six months, but successful vocational adjustment is not attained in the remaining patients. The reasons why patients without disability do not return to work include restrictions by the physician, psychosocial or personal factors, and nonmedical factors such as job opportunities, disability compensation, and community attitudes which favor restrictions for patients following myocardial infarction. A low percentage of patients return to work if there is residual cardiac disability.

Active participation in a reconditioning program can help to improve the quality of life following myocardial infarction. Exercise training also appears to alleviate psychological depression. Isotonic reconditioning exercises are most often employed, the intensity of such exercise usually being 60 to 80 percent of the individual's maximum aerobic capacity (or about 80 percent of maximum attainable heart rate). A significant reduction of the resting heart rate, lower systolic and diastolic arterial pressures, and a significant increase in physical working capacity have been reported in many patients who participate in such medically supervised programs. No conclusive data are available, however, on whether or not such physical conditioning modifies survival, reduces the risk of reinfarction, or enhances development of the coronary collateral circulation.

Advice concerning resumption of sexual activity is frequently sought. It has been reported that among long-married couples in which the male had suffered a previous acute myocardial infarction, the maximum heart rate attained during sexual activity averaged only 117 beats/minute for a relatively brief period. Thus, the demands of sexual activity may be equated with mild exercise, and normal (preinfarction) activity should be encouraged.

Education of the patient after myocardial infarction should involve "risk-factor" reduction, including treatment of hypertension, elimination of tobacco use, weight reduction, psychological stress reduction, and dietary programs, particularly in patients with hyperlipidemia. More research is needed concerning the role of personality, attitudes and behavior modifications in achieving successful rehabilitation.

ACUTE RHEUMATIC FEVER AND VALVULAR HEART DISEASE

Valvular heart disease and acute rheumatic fever are considered in the same section, since traditionally most instances of valvular heart disease in the adult were thought to be the result of rheumatic fever. This is no longer true, at least on the North American continent, as the incidence of acute rheumatic fever has been declining and other causes of valvular dysfunction have become more common.

ACUTE RHEUMATIC FEVER

Acute rheumatic fever is a multisystem inflammatory disease resulting from the complications of group A beta-hemolytic streptococcal infection. The revised Jones Criteria (Table 16.7) should be used for guidance in the diagnosis of rheumatic fever. The presence of two major criteria or of one major and two minor criteria suggests a high probability that the disease is present.

Etiology and Pathogenesis

The central role of a group A beta-hemolytic streptococcal infection in the causation of the initial and

Table 16.7 **Revised Jones Criteria for the Diagnosis of Acute Rheumatic Fever**

Major Manifestations:
    Carditis
    Polyarthritis
    Chorea
    Erythema marginatum
    Subcutaneous nodules
Minor Manifestations:
    A. Clinical
    Previous rheumatic fever or rheumatic heart disease
    Arthralgias
    Fever
    B. Laboratory
    Acute phase reactants (leukocytosis, elevated erythrocyte sedimentation rate, C-reactive protein)
    Prolongation of P–R interval
Plus: Supporting evidence of preceding streptococcal infection (Increased ASO or other antistreptococcal antibodies; positive throat culture for Group A streptococcus; recent scarlet fever)

recurrent attacks of acute rheumatic fever is based on the following evidence.

Clinical evidence. Approximately two thirds of patients with acute rheumatic fever will report an antecedent episode of acute pharyngitis.

Epidemiologic. Environmental, bacterial, and host factors that play a role in the development of acute rheumatic fever are also found to be closely related to the occurrence of streptococcal sore throat. These factors include the geographic latitude and altitude of residence, living conditions such as the presence of crowding, high humidity and poor socioeconomic factors.

Immunologic. Acute rheumatic fever will not occur in the absence of a streptoccal antibody response. Atlhough the antistreptolysin O titer will rise in only 80 percent of group A streptococcal infections, a streptococcal antibody response can be demonstrated if antihyaluronidase and antideoxyribonuclease B are measured.

Prophylactic. This is the most convincing evidence linking streptococcal infection to the genesis of acute rheumatic fever. Acute rheumatic fever will not develop in population groups receiving adequate chemoprohylaxis against streptococcal infections. This evidence was gathered by large scale studies in military recruits during and after World War II.

The precise manner in which group A beta hemolytic streptococci predispose to the development of acute rheumatic fever is still not known with certainty. There are several absolute requirements for the development of this disease. They include the presence of group A streptococci, the presence of a streptococcal antibody response, the persistence of streptococci in the pharynx for a period of time and location of the infection in the pharynx. It is known that streptococcal skin infections do not result in acute rheumatic fever. Similarly, acute rheumatic fever and acute poststreptococcal glomerulonephritis rarely if ever occur in the same patient. It has been demonstrated that skin strains of streptococci and the nephritogenic streptococci responsible for glomerulonephritis belong to different serotypes from the rheumatogenic strains and promote a different type of antibody response by the host (see Chapter 11, Poststreptococcal Glomerulonephritis).

The exact mechanism whereby group A beta hemolytic streptococci produce the inflammatory response known as acute rheumatic fever is also not well understood. Currently the mechanism accepted by most investigators in the field is autoimmunity. Multiple cross-reactive relations between group A streptococcus and human tissue antigens have been demonstrated. Autoantibodies to shared antigens have been demonstrated in sera of patients with acute rheumatic fever against cardiac, skeletal, and smooth muscle; heart valve fibroblasts; neurons in the basal ganglia; and a group A carbohydrate-related determinant in connective tissues. Circulating autoantibodies to these various antigens are present in much higher titers or occur more frequently in patients with acute rheumatic fever than in those with uncomplicated antecedent streptococcal infections. Although a direct relation between the presence of these autoantibodies and carditis has not been established, there is suggestive evidence that such autoantibodies react in vivo with the respective tissue to produce disease. This concept is supported by the presence of immune complex deposits in the myocardium.

Individual host factors are also thought to be of great importance in predisposing the patient to the development of acute rheumatic fever. In many instances there is a strong familial tendency towards the development of acute rheumatic fever in the absence of clear genetic factors predisposing to this disease. Similarly, it has been observed that the incidence of acute rheumatic fever at the time of streptococcal sore throat epidemics is approximately 20 times higher among those with a previous history of acute rheumatic fever. Whether this difference is the result of individual characteristics or results from modification of the individual's immune response following an initial attack of acute rheumatic fever is not clear.

Incidence

In instances of epidemic symptomatic streptococcal pharyngitis, the attack rate for acute rheumatic fever is approximately 3 percent. However, the attack rate will vary depending upon the clinical severity of the infection; in patients with less severe infection the attack rate may be 0.5 percent or even lower. Conversely, in the setting of epidemic streptococcal pharyngitis, the attack rate among those who have had a previous episode of acute rheumatic fever may be as high as 60 percent.

The incidence of acute rheumatic fever has declined precipitously on the North American continent during the past 30 years. Whether this decline is due to improvement in socioeconomic status with less crowding, improved public health measures, or prompt treatment of episodes of pharyngitis is not clear. There is evidence that the virulence of the rheumatogenic streptococcal strains may be declining and that there may be a dilution of the classical rheumatogenic strains by other strains less likely to cause acute rheumatic fever. Nevertheless, acute rheumatic fever remains highly prevelant in underdeveloped countries, particularly India, the Phillipines, and Southeast Asia.

Clinical Manifestations

Polyarthritis

The arthritis of acute rheumatic fever has been classically described as a migratory polyarthritis with sequential development of tenderness, redness, heat, and swelling of the affected joints. The knees and ankles are the joints affected most frequently, with involvement of the elbows, wrists and hips to a somewhat lesser extent. The small joints of the hands and feet and the shoulder joints are involved infrequently. The migratory and fleeting characteristic of rheumatic polyarthritis is seen much more commonly in children than in adults. In a recent report, the joint disease of adult patients with acute rheumatic fever was described as abrupt in onset, rapidly additive and eventually symmetrical with lower extremity large joint predominance in association with profoundly symptomatic tenosynovitis. No permanent joint deformities result from rheumatic polyarthritis, although in rare instances a chronic post rheumatic arthropathy has been described (Jaccoud's arthritis). The usual course of rheumatic polyarthritis is self-limited, with an average duration of 2 to 4 weeks. Some patients develop profound arthralgias and pain originating from large muscle groups or tendons adjacent to joints. Careful evaluation of the patient's joints in these cases discloses that there is no evidence of arthritis (i.e., there is no swelling, erythema or heat of the affected joint) and that the pain originates from adjacent muscles or tendons. This type of muscular and tendinous pains have on occasion been confused with the so called "growing pains" of children and adolescents. An inverse relationship has been described between the severity of poststreptococcal arthritis and poststreptococcal carditis in patients with acute rheumatic fever.

Carditis

Cardiac involvement in acute rheumatic fever includes the endocardium, myocardium, and pericardium. Myocardial involvement resulting in acute myocarditis is the least common cardiac manifestation. When patients with acute rheumatic fever develop congestive heart failure it is uniformly due to valvular involvement and not to myocarditis. The development of acute pericarditis usually indicates the presence of severe rheumatic carditis but on occasion a pericardial friction rub may be the major or

only clinical manifestation of acute rheumatic carditis. Cardiac involvement in general is unusual in adults unless the patient is experiencing a recurrent attack of acute rheumatic fever.

When the rheumatic process involves the cardiac valves and endocardium, valvular regurgitation is the initial common dysfunction. Mitral regurgitation is the most common lesion in acute rheumatic fever and is said to occur in approximately 70 percent of instances of acute rheumatic carditis. Combined aortic and mitral regurgitation is next in frequency with an incidence of approximately 23 percent, whereas isolated aortic regurgitation is distinctly uncommon and is said to occur in only 7 percent of patients.

Clinical manifestations of acute carditis include tachycardia and a soft or "muffled" first heart sound which most often is the result of a prolonged atrioventricular conduction time. When mitral regurgitation is severe, a palpable systolic apical thrill may be detected. The systolic murmur of mitral regurgitation is the most common auscultatory finding in acute rheumatic carditis. It is typically at least grade III/VI in intensity and holosystolic. The Carey-Coombs murmur that has been described in cases of acute rheumatic valvulitis is a soft, low pitched, early to middiastolic, short murmur heard best directly over the apex beat. It is probably of no special significance and in all likelihood represents increased diastolic flow across the mitral valve due to the mitral regurgitation. When aortic regurgitation is present, a high-pitched, blowing, early diastolic decrescendo murmur is best heard along the left sternal border at the third or fourth interspaces. A systolic ejection murmur audible at the base with radiation to the carotid arteries is most likely generated from ejection across the aortic valve and not due to aortic stenosis unless there is a preexisting aortic vulvular deformity. Similarly, the typical findings of mitral stenosis will not be found in the presence of acute rheumatic carditis unless there is preexisting chronic rheumatic mitral valve disease.

The electrocardiographic findings in acute rheumatic carditis are nonspecific. The most common is prolongation of the PR interval which is present in only one-third of patients with acute rheumatic fever and cannot be definitely related to other cardiac involvement or to the long-term cardiac prognosis. In all likelihood prolongation of the PR interval is not due to rheumatic myocarditis but rather to increased vagal tone, a common phenomenon, particularly in children and young adults who even under normal conditions may demonstrate prolongation of the PR interval.

When congestive heart failure complicates acute rheumatic carditis, its clinical manifestations are similar to those noted in adults with congestive heart failure from ischemic or valvular heart disease. However some differences exist: It is common for young patients with early cardiac failure to complain of dyspnea with no rales. Hepatic congestion occurs more commonly early and results in complaints of pain in the right upper quadrant or epigastrium. A dry nonproductive cough due to pulmonary congestion may be the first symptom of developing congestive heart failure and may be mistakenly attributed to an upper respiratory infection.

It is useful to classify acute rheumatic carditis as mild, moderate or severe because prognosis and treatment will vary depending upon the severity. Thus *mild* carditis is said to be present if the heart size is normal and only a grade II/VI mitral regurgitation murmur or a soft Carey-Coombs murmur are present. *Moderate* rheumatic carditis is said to be present if the cardiac auscultatory findings are more severe than above, more than one valvular lesion is appreciated, and congestive failure is not present. *Severe* carditis is diagnosed if cardiomegaly is present and signs and symptoms of congestive heart failure are also detected.

Sequelae are the rule with rheumatic carditis. Over 50 percent of patients with organic murmurs during an episode of acute rheumatic carditis will have residual heart disease. Of patients with severe carditis (as defined above), approximately 20 percent will die during the acute episode and almost all survivors will develop chronic rheumatic valvular heart disease.

Chorea

Chorea is almost never seen in adults. In childhood it is much more common in girls than in boys. Choreiform movements are purposeless, nonrepetitive, spasmodic movements which may involve any voluntary muscle group, including those of the face and tongue. Choreiform movements may be either partially controlled or exacerbated by voluntary effort. In severe cases the patient may be in constant involuntary motion and must be protected from injuring himself. This poststreptococcal type of chorea is usually self-limited and is commonly called chorea minor or Sydenham's chorea to distinguish it from the hereditary form, chorea major or Huntington's chorea.

Erythema Marginatum

This cutaneous manifestation of acute rheumatic fever is seen in only about 5 percent of patients. It is a flat or slightly raised nonpruritic rash, occurring on the trunk and thighs where circular or serpiginous shapes are usually formed. It is often an evanescent phenomenon and almost always coexists with chorea, arthritis, or carditis.

Subcutaneous Nodules

In approximately 5 percent of patients with acute rheumatic fever 1 to 2 cm firm, painless, colorless, small nodules develop near tendons or bony prominences of joints, particularly the elbows. These nodules are also a self-limited manifestation and are especially likely to develop with severe carditis.

Other Clinical Manifestations

Fever is common with no distinctive pattern. Epistaxis occurs in about 5 to 10 percent of patients, usually in association with carditis. Abdominal pain is a common complaint in children and is thought to be due either to hepatic congestion or to microvascular mesenteric involvement from the rheumatic process. A "rheumatic pneumonia" has been described consisting of patchy consolidation in the pulmonary parenchyma, as seen on a chest radiograph. It is thought that rheumatic pneumonia is not a distinct entity and in most instances can be explained on the basis of developing pulmonary edema or pulmonary infarction associated with congestive heart failure.

Differential Diagnosis

A variety of conditions must be considered in the differential diagnosis of acute rheumatic fever. When arthritis is the predominant clinical manifestation of rheumatic fever, such entities as juvenile rheumatoid arthritis, serum sickness, septic arthritis, collagen vascular diseases and postinfectious arthritis (Reiter's syndrome, Shigella, Salmonella, Yersinia) must be considered. Rheumatic myocarditis must be differentiated from idiopathic or viral myocarditis or pericarditis. Acute rheumatic endocarditis must be differentiated from the endocarditis of bacterial origin, especially since bacterial endocarditis may on occasion present with articular symptoms and the combination of fever, heart murmurs, and arthralgias.

Laboratory Findings

Leukocytosis with a mild to moderate left shift is a common finding in most cases of acute rheumatic fever. Elevated acute phase reactants such as the erythrocyte sedimentation rate and C-reactive protein are also seen in the majority of cases, as are elevated IGG and IGA immunoglobulins. Elevated antibody titers to streptococcal enzymes should be diligently sought, as discussed above. At least one of the following antibodies will be elevated in cases of documented acute rheumatic fever: anti-streptolysin O (ASO), anti-NADase, anti-DNAase B and antihyaluronidase. Titers against streptozyme, a concentrate of several extracellular streptococcal antigens, will be elevated in practically all patients with acute rheumatic fever.

Treatment

Once the diagnosis of acute rheumatic fever is established, an effort to eradicate streptococci from the pharynx is warranted even though these organisms may not be demonstrated by culture. A single intramuscular injection of 1.2 million units of benzathine penicillin is usually sufficient for this purpose. Patients allergic to penicillin may be treated effectively with oral erythromycin 250 mg four times daily for a period of ten days. Once streptococci are eradicated at the start of treatment, long-term prophylaxis against beta-hemolytic streptococcal infections must be initiated to prevent recurrent pharyngitis and rheumatic fever recurrences. The most effective regimen recommended is a monthly injection of 1.2 units of benzathine penicillin. However, oral regimens consisting of Penicillin G 250,000 units twice daily or sulfadiazine in a single 1 gram daily dose, are effective in preventing recurrent streptococcal pharyngitis in patients who faithfully take their medication. It is recommended that patients who have had carditis be maintained on antibiotic prophylaxis indefinitely. Patients without carditis are usually advised to continue prophylaxis for at least five years after the last acute attack or until they reach the age of 25 years.

Salicylate therapy is recommended for patients without carditis or with mild carditis, in doses which provide serum salicylate levels of 25 to 30 mg/dl. Also patients with moderate carditis of greater than three weeks' duration can probably be treated best with salicylates alone.

Although the use of corticosteroids in the treatment of acute rheumatic fever continues to be debated, most physicians agree that corticosteroids should be used in patients with severe carditis, patients with pericarditis, or patients with moderate carditis of less than three weeks' duration when first seen. Prednisone is usually administered in a dose of 2 mg/kg/day in four divided doses. Although corticosteroids are more potent antinflammatory agents than salicylates, they are more likely to be followed by a post-treatment rebound of the rheumatic process and have a higher incidence of side effects during prolonged therapy. Once the acute inflammatory process has been controlled by either salicylates or corticosteroids, treatment is usually continued until the sedimentation rate reaches normal levels and for several weeks thereafter. Salicylate therapy may be discontinued abruptly; administration of corticosteroids however, should be gradually tapered over a two-week period. An overlap course of salicylate therapy is usually added when corticosteroids are being tapered and should be continued for at least two weeks after steroid therapy has been discontinued in order to prevent poststeroid rebound.

General supportive measures include rest, although prolonged bedrest has been proven to be of little value and may, in fact, be psychologically detrimental if maintained for long periods of time. Patients with severe arthritis, uncontrolled chorea, and severe congestive heart failure will usually limit their activity on their own. Chorea is managed by preventing the patient from injuring himself by uncontrollable movements and especially by providing reassurance and strong psychological support to patients and families alike. Reassurance that the peculiar movements are due to a specific neurologic defect which is self-limited and will not leave any residual abnormality or intellectual impairment is of utmost importance.

Severe congestive heart failure is managed with the addition of diuretics and digitalis to the antiinflammatory therapy discussed above. In rare cases the rheumatic valvulitis is of such severity and extent that acute surgical replacement of an involved valve may be necessary.

AORTIC STENOSIS

Valvular aortic stenosis is found in approximately 25 percent of all adult patients with valvular heart disease. There is a 4 to 1 male to female ratio. Most patients over the age of 40 with valvular aortic stenosis have evidence of calcific deposits on the valvular tissues.

Etiology

The most common cause of valvular aortic stenosis is a congenitally bicuspid aortic valve. This is the most common congenital cardiovascular abnormality, estimated to occur in 1 to 2 percent of the population. There appears to be a genetic predisposition, with the incidence of bicuspid aortic valve rising to about 4 percent among offspring of at least one parent with this congenital abnormality.

Calcific aortic stenosis of the elderly is usually the end result of calcification of: (1) a bicuspid aortic valve, (2) a stenotic aortic valve due to the rheumatic inflammatory process, or (3) calcification of an otherwise entirely normal tricuspid aortic valve resulting from the normal "wear and tear" of aging. In general calcific aortic stenosis superimposed on an otherwise normal tricuspid aortic valve occurs in persons over the age of 70. On the other hand, calcific aortic stenosis superimposed on a congenitally bicuspid aortic valve or on a valve affected by the rheumatic process usually occurs earlier in life from age 50 on. However a significant age overlap exists.

Isolated aortic stenosis is almost never the result of rheumatic fever. In fact, it has been said that by definition aortic stenosis is not of rheumatic origin if the patient has a normal mitral valve.

Other forms of left ventricular outflow obstruction which may superficially mimic valvular aortic stenosis include hypertrophic obstructive cardiomyopathy (idiopathic hypertrophic subaortic stenosis), discrete congenital subvalvular aortic stenosis, and congenital supravalvular aortic stenosis. These lesions are discussed elsewhere in this chapter.

Pathophysiology and Natural History

The aortic valve deformity (whatever its cause) generally progresses in severity as the years go by. This occurs because of the abnormal blood flow pattern during ventricular ejection across the deformed aortic valve, which in turn produces further turbulence and trauma to the aortic valve, resulting in progressive thickening and eventually calcification of the valvular tissues.

The major hemodynamic alteration in valvular aortic stenosis is obstruction to left ventricular ejection resulting in the development of a systolic pressure gradient between the left ventricle and the aorta. This transvalvular pressure gradient progressively increases as the degree of valvular aortic stenosis increases with time. Left ventricular systolic pressure, therefore, progressively rises until left ventricular decompensation supervenes. The left ventricle adapts to the pressure load imposed on it by a stenotic aortic valve by developing concentric hypertrophy (increased wll thickness and increased muscle mass). Although early studies had suggested that the hypertrophied myocardium has impaired contractile properties, more recently the view has prevailed that

hypertrophy is actually beneficial, helping maintain peak ventricular wall stress in the normal range. Only in late stages of decompensated aortic stenosis is myocardial contractility impaired.

The severity of valvular aortic stenosis can be estimated by measuring the transvalvular pressure gradient as well as the flow during systole across the stenotic valve. In general, a mean transvalvular systolic gradient of 50 mmHg or more, or a calculated effective aortic valve orifice area of 0.7 cm^2 or less are thought to represent critical aortic stenosis.

The resting cardiac output is usually normal even in patients with critical aortic stenosis until such time as left ventricular failure develops. However subnormal increases of cardiac output can be expected in patients with severe aortic stenosis during exercise.

The concentrically hypertrophied left ventricle has diminished compliance properties. This results in an unusually forceful left atrial contraction pattern with the development of a large A wave in the left atrial pressure pulse or in the pulmonary artery wedge pressure pulse. As in other cases of increased ventricular stiffness, this vigorous atrial contraction is of great importance in maintaining normal left ventricular pump function, and its loss (as might occur in atrial fibrillation) frequently results in rapid aggravation of symptoms and significant reduction of cardiac output. Often patients remain asymptomatic for many years after the diagnosis of aortic stenosis has been made. Once symptoms develop, however, the clinical course is one of rapid deterioration. This downhill course is considerably more rapid in aortic stenosis than in aortic insufficiency, mitral insufficiency, or mitral stenosis. One study documented a 90 percent mortality rate in patients with valvular aortic stenosis within ten years after the diagnosis had been established. In another study the average survival was two years after the development of congestive heart failure, three years after the occurrence of syncope, and five years after the development of angina in patients with severe aortic stenosis.

Clinical Manifestations

In patients with isolated or predominant aortic stenosis, symptoms usually develop in the fourth or fifth decade. The three cardinal symptoms are dyspnea on exertion, syncope, and angina pectoris. Exertional dyspnea is the result of an increase in left ventricular diastolic pressure which in turn produces an increase in mean left atrial and pulmonary venous pressures. Exertional angina pectoris is identical in distribution and quality to the angina of coronary artery disease. However, in the setting of severe aortic stenosis, angina pectoris develops because of the imbalance between myocardial oxygen requirements and supply, even in the face of normal coronary arteries. The increased myocardial oxygen requirements are the result of the severe pressure load on the myocardium and the compensatory myocardial hypertrophy that is present. Syncope in severe aortic stenosis is usually exertional and is the result of a drop in systemic arterial pressure engendered by vasodilatation of the exercising muscles in the face of a fixed cardiac output. This may lead to a sudden ventricular dysrhythmia, which in turn produces a further drop in cardiac output.

When left ventricular decompensation develops in critical aortic stenosis, the resting cardiac output becomes markedly diminished and the systemic arterial pressure drops. The transvalvular pressure gradient also declines, resulting in a reduction in the intensity of the systolic ejection murmur.

The physical findings of valvular aortic stenosis are dramatic and well recognized. The blood pressure is usually in the normal range; severe systemic arterial hypertension is unusual in the face of hemodynamically significant aortic stenosis. The jugular venous pressure is usually normal, although the A wave may be somewhat accentuated. Palpation of the carotid arterial pulse reveals it to be of small volume, rising slowly with a delayed peak. A systolic thrill or "shudder" is frequently present.

Palpation of the precordium usually localizes the apex beat inferiorly and laterally to its normal position. Furthermore, the apical impulse is forceful, sustained, and outwardly thrusting because of the presence of left ventricular hypertrophy. In many cases a double apical impulse may be palpable, with the first component being a reflection of atrial systole and the second component of left ventricular systole. Although a systolic thrill is commonly palpable in the carotid arteries and the suprasternal notch, chest wall thrills may be difficult to appreciate in the elderly adult with a hyperinflated thorax. It may be necessary to examine the patient in full expiration and leaning forward in order to appreciate a systolic thrill along the upper right sternal border. A systolic chest wall thrill is commonly palpable in children and young adults with severe aortic stenosis. On auscultation, an early systolic ejection sound is frequently present in children and young adults with noncalcific valvular stenosis. However, with progressive increase in stiffness and calcification of the aortic valve, the ejection sound usually disappears in the older adult patient. Similarly, in severe calcific aortic stenosis the aortic component of the second sound may be absent and the second sound may appear single. When the aortic valve closure sound is preserved, paradoxical splitting of the second sound may be recognized. This occurs because of progressive prolongation of left ventricular ejection time, with aortic valve closure actually following instead of preceding pulmonic valve closure. Paradoxical splitting of the second sound is manifested by the presence of expiratory splitting with actual narrowing of the two components of the second sound during inspiration. The presence of an atrial diastolic gallop (S4) at the apex is commonly present in adults with severe aortic stenosis and results from left ventricular hypertrophy and increased ventricular wall stiffness. The atrial diastolic gallop does not signify the presence of left ventricular failure. However, the presence of an early diastolic gallop (S3) in adults with severe aortic stenosis usually signifies left ventricular failure and dilatation.

The murmur of valvular aortic stenosis is a harsh or rough systolic ejection murmur with a diamond configuration. In children and young adults the murmur is maximal at the base, usually the upper right sternal border, and radiates well to the suprasternal notch and both carotid arteries. In the elderly, however, the systolic ejection murmur is heard almost equally well at the apex and occasionally better at the apex than at the base of the heart. In this setting it may be confused with the murmur of mitral regurgitation even though the latter is a holosystolic high-pitched blowing murmur. The use of amyl nitrate and other maneuvers outlined in Table 16.1 can be very useful in differentiating these two murmurs.

The intensity of the murmur is of little help in determining the severity of aortic stenosis. Usually the murmur is quite loud (at least grade III/VI) and harsh or rasping in quality. However, the length of the murmur correlates in a rough way with the severity of valvular obstruction. The more severe the obstruction, the longer the murmur and the later its systolic peak.

Laboratory Findings

Electrocardiogram

In mild or moderate aortic stenosis the electrocardiogram is frequently normal. As the severity of the stenosis increases, however, and left ventricular hypertrophy progresses, the electrocardiogram becomes abnormal and exhibits signs of left ventricular hypertrophy. Precordial voltage is increased and in severe cases ST segment depression and T wave inversion (the so-called strain pattern) develop, especially in standard leads I and AVL and in the left precordial leads (Fig. 16.8). In elderly patients and

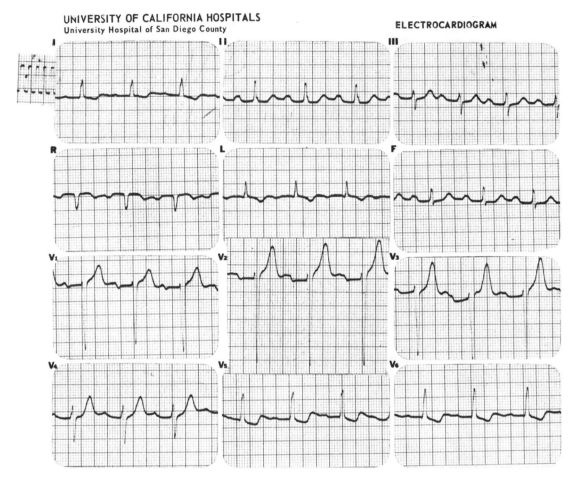

UNIVERSITY OF CALIFORNIA HOSPITALS
University Hospital of San Diego County

ELECTROCARDIOGRAM

Fig. 16.8 Electrocardiogram of a 43-year-old male with aortic stenosis. Left ventricular hypertrophy may be diagnosed from this tracing because of the prominent precordial QRS voltage, the flattened and depressed ST segments (systolic overload pattern) in the lateral leads and the presence of left atrial abnormality. First degree A–V block is also present.

in those with chronic obstructive pulmonary disease and hyperinflated lungs, the electrocardiographic signs of left ventricular hypertrophy may be blunted or obscured altogether. The rhythm is usually regular sinus, and atrial fibrillation is uncommon in patients with pure aortic stenosis. When present it should raise the question of coexisting mitral valve disease.

Chest Radiograph

The chest radiograph is helpful in confirming the diagnosis of valvular aortic stenosis but is generally not useful in estimating its severity. Overal cardiac size may be normal even in the face of severe aortic stenosis unless left ventricular decompensation has

occurred. Extreme degrees of left ventricular hypertrophy may be present, but the chest radiograph may show an overall normal cardiac size. However, in the posteroanterior projection the lower left cardiac border may be rounded with the apex of the cardiac silhouette pointing inferiorly—a sign of left ventricular hypertrophy. In the lateral projection the left ventricular silhouette may project posterior to the inferior vena cava shadow, indicating left ventricular enlargement. Localized poststenotic dilatation of the ascending aorta is present in the majority of cases of pure aortic stenosis and helps differentiate isolated stenosis from combined stenosis and regurgitation; in the latter case the aortic root is diffusely enlarged up to and including the aortic knob. In severe calcific aortic stenosis, the calcium deposits may on occasion be detected on the lateral chest radiograph. Optimal radiographic technique, however, is necessary to demonstrate these findings. Image intensification fluoroscopy is much more valuable than the plain radiograph in detecting calcium deposits in the aortic valve. A large amount of calcium in the region of the aortic valve has been shown consistently to correlate well with hemodynamically severe aortic stenosis.

Echocardiography

Echocardiography can aid substantially in estimating the severity of aortic stenosis if the echocardiogram is of sufficient quality to allow precise measurement of septal and posterior wall thickness; these measurements provide an objective assessment of left ventricular hypertrophy. In children with aortic stenosis, echocardiography allows reasonably accurate estimates of peak left ventricular pressure and therefore of the transvalvular pressure gradient. These estimates may be made by calculating the left ventricular mass/left ventricular volume and wall thickness/semiaxis ratios. In adults, however, these echocardiographic correlations are not as reliable. Increased reflectance from the aortic root suggests the presence of calcification, and when this occurs, image intensification fluoroscopy should be employed to confirm the presence of calcium.

Exercise Testing

The role of exercise testing in patients with aortic stenosis is not well defined. In general, because critical aortic stenosis can be associated with exertional syncope and death (probably as a result of exertional arrhythmias), most physicians prefer not to exercise patients with clinically suspected severe aortic stenosis. If symptoms need to be clarified or the patient's functional capacity must be ascertained objectively, invasive evaluation should first be carried out, with subsequent exercise testing to be undertaken only if the valvular stenosis has been found to be no more than moderately severe.

Cardiac Catheterization and Angiography

The definitive diagnosis and precise estimation of the severity of valvular aortic stenosis can only be made invasively by cardiac catheterization and angiocardiography. These studies should be carried out in all patients with clinically suspected severe aortic stenosis and especially if surgical treatment is con-

templated. Invasive studies are particularly important in patients with clinical signs of valvular aortic stenosis and angina pectoris in order to ascertain whether coronary artery disease coexists. Also, in patients with multivalvular disease the relative importance of each valvular lesion can often be exceedingly difficult to ascertain clinically and noninvasively and can only be estimated by cardiac catheterization.

In general, aortic stenosis is considered severe if the mean transvalvular pressure gradient equals or exceeds 50 mmHg or the effective aortic valve orifice area is less than 0.7 cm^2. Cardiac output must be measured carefully at the time of the measurement of the transvalvular pressure gradient. Patients with critical aortic stenosis and profound left ventricular failure may generate transvalvular pressure gradients of only 20 to 30 mmHg because of their extremely low cardiac output. Coronary arteriography should be an integral part of the catheterization study, since approximately 50 percent of patients with aortic stenosis and angina also have significant coexisting coronary artery disease.

Therapy

Symptomatic patients need to be treated for angina pectoris, syncope, or congestive heart failure. In general, nitroglyerin is effective for the treatment of angina due to aortic stenosis because by reducing left ventricular wall tension and systolic ejection time it favorably alters the ratio of myocardial oxygen demand and supply. The treatment of exertional syncope is largely preventive: patients should be advised to avoid exertion and all arrhythmias should be identified and corrected. Treatment of congestive heart failure in patients with valvular aortic stenosis consists of digitalis and diuretics. It is important to avoid excessive diuresis because the severely hypertrophied noncompliant left ventricle depends on an increased filling pressure to maintain end-diastolic fiber stretch and thereby adequate cardiac output. For the same reason, the use of vasodilator agents for afterload and/or preload reduction in these patients is fraught with danger and should be carried out with great caution. Severe congestive heart failure due to critical aortic stenosis constitutes a surgical emergency. The treatment of asymptomatic adult patients with severe aortic stenosis remains a difficult and unresolved problem. These patients risk sudden death, but this risk is low and surgery is not recommended if they are truly asymptomatic. All patients with aortic stenosis are at risk for the development of infective endocarditis and should receive prophylactic antibiotics for dental and surgical procedures.

Surgical Treatment

Patients with severe aortic stenosis who develop early symptoms of left ventricular decompensation, angina, or syncope are candidates for aortic valve surgery. Surgery should be carried out preferably before the development of overt congestive heart failure—which increases the risk of surgery considerably. In general, aortic valve replacement is almost always necessary for patients over the age of 40. In younger individuals and those with minimal or no aortic valve calcification, valvotomy may be successful. Advanced age is usually not a factor in considering surgery. Excellent results have been reported in patients over age 60, with hospital mortality for isolated aortic valve replacement of about 3 to 5 percent. These figures compare favorably with operative results in younger patients. Aortic valve replacement results in uniform improvement of symptoms. Even patients with profound symptomatic congestive heart failure respond well showing improved left ventricular ejection fraction and improved functional class postoperatively. It must be remembered, however, that patients undergoing operative replacement of their aortic valve exchange one disability for another. Prosthetic valves, although greatly improved during the past twenty years, remain imperfect.

AORTIC REGURGITATION

Etiology and Pathogenesis

Aortic insufficiency or regurgitation results from incompetence of the aortic valve, which allows regurgitation of a portion of the left ventricular stroke volume back into the left ventricle during diastole. In general, aortic valvular incompetence may be produced by aortic valve cusp defects or by dilatation of the aortic annulus.

Rheumatic and infective valvulitis are the common causes of aortic regurgitation due to cusp deformities. Congenital fenestrations of the aortic cusps, prolapse of an aortic cusp in association with a ventricular septal defect, valvular deformities associated with discrete membranous subaortic stenosis, and traumatic disruption of an aortic valve cusp are responsible for a small proportion of cases. Annular dilatation may develop following prolonged severe systemic hypertension, in Marfan's syndrome, or in rheumatoid spondylitis. Similarly, dissecting hematoma of the aortic root extending to the aortic annulus will often disrupt the integrity of the aortic valve and cause aortic regurgitation to develop.

The majority of patients with pure or predominant aortic regurgitation are males. However, if there is associated mitral valve disease, female patients predominate.

Pathophysiology and Natural History

Two distinct pathophysiologic syndromes of aortic regurgitation must be recognized: acute and chronic. In *chronic* regurgitation during diastole the left ventricle receives the right ventricular stroke output plus the regurgitant volume through the incompetent aortic valve. Therefore, left ventricular end-diastolic volume increases, resulting in increased myocardial fiber stretch and increased left ventricular stroke volume. Because the volume load develops gradually, the left ventricle and pericardium can accommodate the increased left ventricular diastolic volume, and a normal or near normal left ventricular end-diastolic pressure is maintained. The elevated left ventricular end-diastolic volume is the major compensating mechanism in aortic regurgitation, since it results in an increase of the left ventricular stroke volume. Aortic regurgitation is often well tolerated for many years, and symptoms of congestive heart failure do not develop until late in the course of the disease, when the left ventricle becomes markedly dilated and the left ventricular end-diastolic pressure rises. At this stage of the disease, left ventricular function deteriorates and the end-diastolic volume increases further without concomitant increases in aortic regurgitant volume or left ventricular stroke volume. Considerable hypertrophy of the left ventricular wall also occurs, and the hearts of patients with this lesion are among the largest encountered at autopsy.

In *acute* severe aortic regurgitation, on the other hand, the left ventricle has no time to dilate. Left ventricular diastolic pressure rises acutely, and this causes an acute rise in the left atrial pressure, which in turn results in early pulmonary edema.

Clinical Manifestations

The initial symptoms of chronic aortic regurgitation usually relate to an uncomfortable awareness of cardiac action due to the enlarged left ventricle and the high stroke volume. Palpitations and heart pounding may precede other symptoms for many years. As the cardiac reserve diminishes, exertional dyspnea is the first symptom to become evident and is followed by orthopnea, paroxysmal nocturnal dyspnea, excessive sweating, and angina pectoris.

The occurrence of angina pectoris in patients with chronic severe aortic regurgitation does not necessarily imply the presence of coronary artery disease. Angina due purely to severe aortic regurgitation occurs at rest as well as with exertion and is particularly frequent at night when it is commonly accompanied by severe diaphoresis. Anginal episodes may be particularly prolonged and their response to sublingual nitroglycerin is variable. As left ventricular failure progresses, symptoms of pulmonary and systemic congestion develop: orthopnea, dyspnea at rest, congestive hepatomegaly, peripheral edema, and ascites.

In *acute* severe aortic regurgitation, symptoms are almost entirely limited to those of pulmonary congestion. With massive acute aortic regurgitation patients may die in acute pulmonary edema. Lesser degrees of acute regurgitation produce severe dyspnea, hypoxia, and symptoms of poor peripheral perfusion.

The physical findings of *chronic* aortic regurgitation usually revolve around the presence of a large left ventricular stroke volume: wide pulse pressure and large volume arterial pulses. With so-called free aortic regurgitation, the patient's entire body often moves synchronously with cardiac action and a "bobbing" motion of the head with each systole may be seen (de Musset's sign). Systolic arterial pulsations often occur in the supra- and infraclavicular areas, the suprasternal notch, and along the sides of the neck. On palpation of large arteries, one appreciates a large volume pulse which rises and declines rapidly. Such a pulse has been called "water hammer" or Corrigan's pulse. Quincke's pulse consists of an alternating paling and flushing of the skin at the root of the nail while pressure is being applied to the tip of the nail and is thought to be due to capillary pulsations in severe aortic regurgitation.

The pulse pressure is uniformly widened with an elevation of the systolic pressure and diminution of the diastolic pressure. Measurement of the arterial diastolic pressure with a sphygmomanometer is often difficult in severe aortic insufficiency because systolic Korotkoff sounds may be audible over the large arteries even with the cuff completely deflated. Therefore, diastolic pressure in such cases should be taken at the time of "muffling" of the Korotkoff sounds ("phase IV"). This phase has been found to correspond quite well to the true intraarterial diastolic pressure. The level of the arterial diastolic pressure does not always corelate well with the severity of aortic regurgitation. As the disease progresses, and especially in *acute* aortic regurgitation, the left ventricular end-diastolic pressure becomes markedly elevated and therefore the arterial diastolic pressure

may be found in the 50 to 60 mmHg range as the two pressures equilibrate.

Inspection usually reveals a hyperactive precordium with the apex beat displaced laterally and inferiorly. On palpation, the apex beat is diffuse, larger than normal, hyperdynamic but not sustained. A diastolic thrill is often palpable along the left sternal border, and a systolic thrill may often be found in the suprasternal notch and the carotid arteries. The systolic thrill and associated systolic murmur are frequently due to high systolic flow across the aortic valve and do not necessarily imply the coexistence of aortic valvular stenosis. Palpation of the carotid arteries may reveal a systolic shudder or a bisferiens or bifid pulse.

On auscultation the first heart sound is soft and the aortic component of the second heart sound is usually normal. A third heart sound is commonly present and a systolic ejection sound and occasionally a fourth heart sound may also be heard. The murmur of aortic regurgitation is a high frequency, blowing, decrescendo diastolic murmur that is usually heard best in the adult along the mid and lower left sternal border. If the regurgitation is due to aortic root dilatation, the diastolic murmur may be louder along the right lower sternal border. The length of the murmur correlates generally with the severity of the aortic regurgitation: with mild aortic regurgitation the murmur is brief, usually lasting only through the first third or half of diastole. As the severity of the regurgitation increases, the murmur usually becomes longer and may become holodiastolic in patients with severe regurgitation. A systolic ejection murmur is usually present and heard best along the upper right sternal border. It is transmitted well to the suprasternal notch and to the carotid vessels and may be quite intense even in the absence of aortic stenosis.

An Austin-Flint murmur is often present in severe aortic insufficiency. This is a soft, rumbling, diastolic murmur usually heard best directly over the apex beat and probably is produced by partial, premature closure of the mitral valve by the regurgitant aortic jet. In patients with combined aortic and mitral valve disease, it is often difficult to determine whether an apical diastolic rumble represents an Austin-Flint murmur or the rumble of true mitral stenosis. As a rule, the rumble of organic mitral stenosis is usually longer than the Austin-Flint murmur and exhibits presystolic accentuation when sinus rhythm is present. The rumble of true mitral stenosis is often associated with a loud first heart sound and an opening snap. The administration of amyl nitrite helps greatly in distinguishing these two murmurs: an Austin-Flint rumble will diminish as the degree of aortic regurgitation decreases under the influence of amyl nitrite. Conversely, the rumble of organic mitral stenosis will often increase in intensity and duration during this maneuver. Auscultation over the femoral arteries will often reveal a to-and-fro murmur (Duroziez' sign) near where the vessel is mildly compressed.

The auscultatory features of acute aortic regurgitation may differ substantially from those of the chronic variety. Because of the rapid rise of left ventricular diastolic pressure, mitral valve closure occurs early, and as a result the intensity of the first heart sound is commonly diminished. For the same reason the Austin-Flint murmur in these cases is usually short and limited to mid-diastole. Arterial diastolic pressure is low but only mildly so because it is often supported by a markedly elevated left ventricular end-diastolic pressure. Arterial pulses may be collapsing but not as dramatically as in chronic aortic regurgitation. The diastolic murmur is often lower pitched and of shorter duration and frequently disappears in middiastole when pressures between the aorta and left ventricle may equilibrate.

Laboratory Findings

Electrocardiogram

Patients with mild aortic regurgitation may have a normal electrocardiogram. As the severity of the lesion increases, the electrocardiographic signs of left ventricular hypertrophy develop. In young patients with severe chronic aortic regurgitation, it is common for the electrocardiogram to demonstrate the so-called diastolic overload pattern. (Fig. 16.9). As left ventricular hypertrophy progresses, ST segment depression and T wave inversions usually develop in limb leads I and AVL and the lateral precordial leads. In acute severe aortic regurgitation the electrocardiogram is frequently normal.

Chest Radiograph

Left ventricular enlargement is almost always detectable in patients with chronic moderate or severe aortic regurgitation. The apex of the cardiac silhouette is displaced inferiorly and laterally on the frontal projection and may in fact extend below the left hemidiaphragm (Fig. 16.10A). Left ventricular enlargement may also be detected in the lateral projection, or more clearly in the left anterior oblique (Fig. 16.10B). In moderate and severe chronic aortic regurgitation, diffuse enlargement of the ascending aorta up to and including the aortic knob is usually seen.

In acute severe aortic regurgitation, the cardiac silhouette is often normal and the main radiographic findings are those of pulmonary congestion with evidence of interstitial or alveolar pulmonary edema.

Echocardiogram

Of all the noninvasive studies available, the echocardiogram provides the most quantitative evaluation of the severity of aortic regurgitation. The typical echocardiogram demonstrates fluttering of the anterior leaflet of the mitral valve because of the impact of the regurgitant jet on this structure and a hyperdynamically contracting left ventricle (Fig. 16.11). Measurements of ventricular volume, ejection fraction and wall thickness can be made from M-mode echocardiograms and may be quite useful in the long-term followup and management of patients with chronic aortic regurgitation. In acute aortic regurgitation, the M-mode echocardiogram may demonstrate premature mitral valve closure, which has prognostic implications. Two-dimensional sector echocardiography is useful in acute aortic regurgitation, as it often will demonstrate the presence of aortic valvular vegetations or a flail aortic cusp. Occasionally echocardiography helps make the diagnosis of aortic dissection by demonstrating a "double barrel" aortic root.

Cardiac Catheterization and Angiography

The main value of cardiac catheterization and angiocardiography in aortic regurgitation is in excluding or making the diagnosis of other valvular lesions or abnormalities of the aortic root and coronary arteries. The most common semiquantitative index of the severity of aortic regurgitation used clinically is the degree of opacification of the left ventricle following aortic root cineangiography. With severe aortic regurgitation, the left ventricle may be totally opacified and a left ventriculogram with analysis of ventricular function may be obtained from aortic root injection of contrast material.

Therapy

Severe chronic aortic regurgitation may be well tolerated for many years. Digitalis is helpful in maintaining normal function in volume loaded ventricles even in the absence of symptoms and is therefore recommended in patients with chronic severe aortic regurgitation and beginning left ventricular dilatation, even in the absence of symptoms of congestive

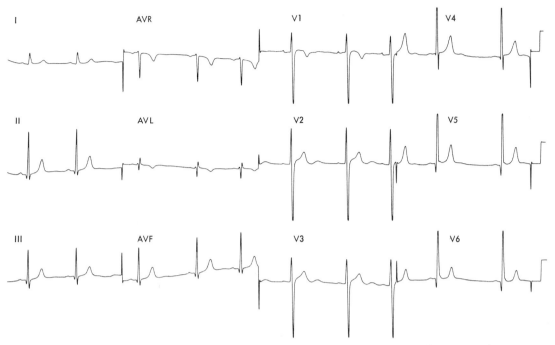

Fig. 16.9 Electrocardiogram of a 23-year-old male with aortic regurgitation. The tracing demonstrates findings of left ventricular hypertrophy with diastolic overload pattern: Prominent QRS voltage, deep Q waves in V5 and V6, prominently peaked T waves and J point ST elevation in lateral precordial leads.

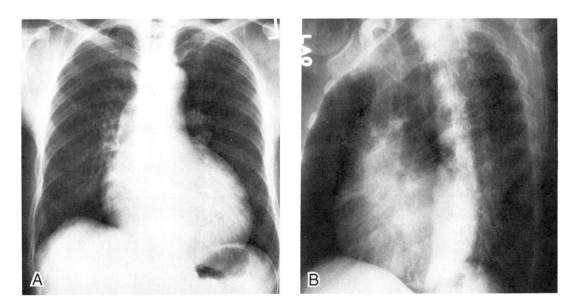

Fig. 16.10 Chest radiograph of a 62-year-old male with aortic regurgitation. (A) The posteroanterior projection shows cardiomegaly primarily due to left ventricular enlargement and a diffusely enlarged ascending aorta. (B) The 60° left anterior oblique projection confirms left ventricular enlargement since the left ventricle overlies the spine (normally, in this projection, the LV should clear the spine).

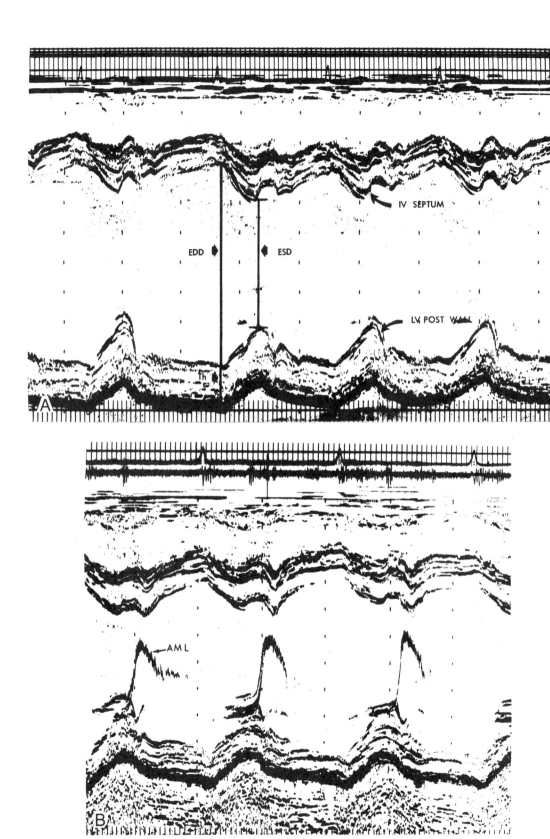

Fig. 16.11 M–mode echocardiogram of a 23-year-old male with aortic regurgitation. (A) The left ventricle is dilated (end diastolic dimension = 65 mm) but both the septum and the posterior wall contract vigorously. (B) The anterior leaflet of the mitral valve exhibits fine fluttering due to the impact of the regurgitant jet.

heart failure. When symptoms of congestive failure develop as a result of chronic severe aortic regurgitation, they usually respond well to treatment with digitalis, diuretics, and salt restriction. If angina is present, nitroglycerin and long-acting nitrate preparations should be tried. Cardiac arrhythmias and systemic infections are generally poorly tolerated in patients with severe aortic regurgitation and must be treated promptly and effectively. The management of acute aortic regurgitation will depend on the patient's hemodynamic status. With severe congestive heart failure, the usual emergency measures of oxygen administration, digitalis, and diuretics should be employed immediately. Vasodilator therapy for preload and afterload reduction can be most helpful in reducing acute pulmonary edema and improving forward cardiac output.

The question of when to intervene surgically in chronic severe aortic regurgitation constitutes a critical decision in managing these patients. Certainly, a patient who has developed severe left ventricular dilatation and signs and symptoms of left ventricular failure deserves aortic valve replacement. Emphasis has recently been directed toward replacing the aortic valve in cases of chronic severe aortic insufficiency even before symptoms of congestive heart failure have developed, because it has been shown that even in asymptomatic patients the left ventricle may undergo irreparable damage from the volume overload and dilatation. Serial echocardiograms have been advocated as the best way to follow asymptomatic patients with chronic severe aortic regurgitation. It must be kept in mind, however, that aortic valve replacement simply exchanges one disability (aortic regurgitation) for another (prosthetic valve).

In acute aortic regurgitation with associated congestive heart failure, early surgical intervention is generally indicated. The presence of large valvular vegetations has similarly been shown recently to correlate well with the subsequent need for surgical valvular replacement because of progressive hemodynamic deterioration.

The surgical results of aortic valve replacement in aortic regurgitation are generally good. Recent operative mortality has been between 10 and 15 percent. These mortality figures may be considerably lower if critically ill patients with infective endocarditis and acute congestive heart failure are excluded. Approximately 80 percent of those who survive the immediate postoperative period may be expected to become asymptomatic. Since preoperative left ventricular failure is associated with greater risk of post-operative left ventricular failure, even a mild degree of failure is an indication for early surgery in cases of chronic aortic regurgitation.

MITRAL STENOSIS

Etiology and Pathogenesis

Acquired mitral stenosis is almost always the result of rheumatic heart disease. A history of acute rheumatic fever can usually be obtained in 50 to 60 percent of adult patients with predominant or pure mitral stenosis. Rheumatic valvulitis heals by scarring, and this results in retraction and thickening of the mitral valve leaflets along with commissural fusion. The subvalvular chordae tendineae also fuse and shorten. These changes result in a reduction of the mitral valve orifice. The stenosis can be predominantly at the leaflet level due to commissural fusion or at the subvalvular level because of fusion of chordae tendineae which form a subvalvular "funnel." Both processes often coexist. Mitral stenosis is the most common chronic valvular deformity following acute rheumatic fever and occurs in approximately 40 to 50 percent of all patients with rheumatic heart disease. Females with pure or predominant mitral stenosis exceed males by a two-to-one ratio. Rarely, adult mitral stenosis may be the result of a congenital defect.

Pathophysiology

The major hemodynamic abnormality in mitral stenosis is elevation of left atrial pressure. As the mitral valve orifice area becomes progressively reduced from a normal value of approximately four to six square centimeters, progressive elevation of left atrial pressure is required to maintain a normal cardiac output. When the mitral valve orifice area approaches one square centimeter (severe mitral stenosis) a left atrial pressure of 22 to 25 mmHg is necessary to maintain a normal cardiac output. This elevation of left atrial pressure is reflected backward to the pulmonary veins and pulmonary capillaries and produces stiffness of the lungs, due to transudation of fluid across the capillary membranes. In pure mitral stenosis the left ventricular diastolic pressure is usually normal to low, and therefore a transmitral holodiastolic pressure gradient exists.

The level of left atrial pressure and the transvalvular gradient depend on heart rate and cardiac output. It is therefore common for patients with moderate to moderately severe mitral stenosis to be entirely asymptomatic at rest but to develop symptoms of pulmonary congestion with exertion (increased cardiac output) or during a bout of tachycardia. It is very common for the first episode of severe dyspnea to occur with a bout of atrial fibrillation. In this case left atrial pressure becomes elevated not only because of the shortening of diastole due to the rapid heart rate but also because of the loss of atrial contraction. In moderate mitral stenosis, pulmonary arterial pressure remains normal at rest although it may increase considerably with exertion.

With severe mitral stenosis pulmonary arterial hypertension develops as a result of three processes: (1) the passive retrograde transmission of the elevated left atrial pressure; (2) reflex constriction of the precapillary arterioles because of the left atrial and pulmonary venous hypertension; and (3) eventual obliterative changes of the pulmonary arterioles due to medial hypertrophy and intimal proliferation. Severe pulmonary hypertension eventually causes right ventricular failure and tricuspid and/or pulmonic valve regurgitation. An increase in pulmonary vascular resistance may be considered to be a protective mechanism to some extent, since it tends to prevent elevations of pulmonary capillary pressure and reduces the likelihood of pulmonary edema.

With moderate mitral stenosis the cardiac output may remain in the normal range at rest; however, it may fail to increase appropriately with exercise. In advanced cases the resting cardiac output is subnormal because of the severity of the stenotic process and right ventricular failure.

Clinical Manifestations

Patients with mild or moderate mitral stenosis may be entirely asymptomatic at rest and develop symptoms of dyspnea and fatigue only on marked exertion. As the severity of the stenotic process and the left atrial pressure level increase, exertional dyspnea develops even with minor forms of exercise. It is not uncommon for housewives with moderately severe mitral stenosis to be unable to perform such ordinary tasks as making a bed or sweeping a room without having to rest several times. Because of the slow progression of the disease, patients are often unaware of their exercise limitations as they gradually adapt to their illness. As the mitral stenosis becomes severe, symptoms of pulmonary congestion become more prominent. Orthopnea and paroxysmal nocturnal dyspnea are typical; palpitations may indicate episodes of paroxysmal atrial fibrillation. Hemoptysis is the result of ruptured bronchial mucosal venules; it is rarely severe and almost never life-threatening. It is more common in patients who do not have significant pulmonary arterial hypertension. As right ventricular failure develops, the symptoms of pulmonary congestion frequently diminish and are supplanted by symptoms of systemic venous congestion (i.e., right upper quadrant pain due to hepatic

congestion, ascites, and peripheral edema). The development of sustained atrial fibrillation frequently marks a turning point in the natural history of symptomatic mitral stenosis. From this point on, symptoms progress with increasing rapidity. Exercise tolerance is markedly diminished and pulmonary edema is a frequent occurrence. Furthermore, the development of chronic atrial fibrillation in association with severe mitral stenosis predisposes to the development of thrombi in the left atrium and especially the left atrial appendage. Such thrombi are frequently dislodged and embolize to the systemic circulation, most commonly the kidneys, spleen, brain and extremities and rarely the coronary arteries. The incidence of systemic embolization correlates with the presence of atrial fibrillation but not with the degree of mitral stenosis. It may even be as common in patients with mild mitral stenosis as in those with severe obstruction. Rarely, a large left atrial clot may suddenly obstruct the stenotic mitral valve and produce syncope, angina, and physical findings which vary with changes in body position. In this respect such a clot simulates the clinical manifestations of a left atrial myxoma.

Inspection of the patient with advanced mitral stenosis may reveal the presence of "mitral facies": there is a malar flush and the face appears blanched or blue. Peripheral cyanosis is also common in advanced cases due to significant reductions of cardiac output. If the patient is in sinus rhythm and pulmonary hypertension is present, the jugular veins will show an elevation of the venous pressure with a very prominent A wave due to vigorous right atrial contraction. If there is associated severe tricuspid regurgitation, the predominant jugular wave form is systolic (CV wave).

Palpation of the arterial pulse discloses an irregular irregularity if atrial fibrillation is present. The arterial pulse is usually small in amplitude due to the low cardiac output. Palpation of the precordium may disclose a left parasternal lift due to right ventricular hypertrophy. The apex beat is usually not displaced and is frequently indistinct. An apical diastolic thrill may be palpable in severe cases of mitral stenosis especially with the patient turned in the left lateral position. If severe pulmonary hypertension is present, a systolic impulse may be palpable along the upper left sternal border due to the enlarged main pulmonary artery and pulmonic valve closure may be palpable in this area.

The auscultatory findings of mitral stenosis are distinctive and pathognomonic. The first heart sound is usually accentuated and "snapping" in quality since mitral valve closure is delayed because of the high left atrial pressure. The opening snap of the mitral valve is best heard along the lower left sternal border and occasionally along the upper left sternal border. To differentiate an opening snap from a pulmonic valve closure sound, one should always carefully seek to determine whether the second sound is split in addition to the presence of the delayed opening snap. The timing of the opening snap is usually 60 to 120 msec after aortic valve closure. There is a rough correlation between the timing of the opening snap and the severity of mitral stenosis. As left atrial pressure rises with increasing severity of mitral valve obstruction, the opening snap will tend to occur earlier in diastole, perhaps 60 to 80 msec after aortic valve closure.

Following the opening snap is the characteristic low frequency, rumbling, diastolic murmur of mitral stenosis. This murmur is heard best at the apex during full expiration with the patient partially turned to the left lateral position, and with the bell of the stethoscope applied gently to the skin. The rumble is loudest at its onset immediately after the opening snap, tends to fade somewhat in late diastole and, if the patient is in sinus rhythm, becomes accentuated again in presystole and merges with the loud first heart sound. In cases of mild mitral stenosis the rumble may be very short and may be heard only in early diastole and presystole. In these cases mildly exercising the patient to increase the cardiac output may augment the intensity of the rumble as will the administration of amyl nitrite.

In patients with severely diminished cardiac output and especially in elderly patients with obstructive pulmonary disease and thoracic hyperinflation, the rumble of mitral stenosis may be missed if one does not seek it carefully. In general, one should always employ maneuvers such as vigorous coughing or exercise to augment the cardiac output if mitral stenosis is suspected and a murmur is not heard. Similarly, locating the precise point of the apex beat on the chest wall and auscultating directly at that point is of great importance in identifying the rumbling murmur of mitral stenosis.

Associated lesions commonly present include mitral insufficiency, aortic insufficiency, tricuspid insufficiency, pulmonic insufficiency, and, more rarely, tricuspid stenosis. The auscultatory findings of these lesions are discussed in their respective sections.

Laboratory Findings

Electrocardiogram

The common findings of left atrial abnormality include broad P waves in the limb leads (.12 seconds or more) and bifid P waves in V1. Atrial fibrillation is frequently present. The QRS complex may be normal even in patients with severe mitral stenosis. However, in the presence of significant pulmonary hypertension, mild right axis deviation to 90 or 100 degrees is commonly seen and RSR' complexes frequently occur in lead V1 as a consequence of late developing right ventricular hypertrophy (Fig. 16.12).

Chest Radiograph

The chest radiograph may be diagnostic in a large number of patients with mitral stenosis. There is straightening of the left heart border due to prominence of the main pulmonary artery segment and the left atrial appendage. These two structures fill the normally concave upper left border of the cardiac silhouette. The enlarged left atrium may be detected as a "double density" through the cardiac silhouette in the postanterior projection (Fig. 16.13). In the lateral projection the enlarged left atrium is present as a bulge on the posterior margin of the heart several centimeters above the level of the diaphragm and may be confirmed by posterior displacement of the barium filled esophagus. The overall cardiac size may be normal, but the presence of right ventricular enlargement causes a rounded appearance of the cardiac apex with the apex lifted up from the left hemidiaphragm. In the lateral projection, right ventricular enlargement manifests itself by filling of the retrosternal air space. Calcification of the mitral valve may also be seen in this view. As pulmonary venous hypertension progresses, the upper lobe vessels of the lungs become more prominent and conversely the lower lobe peripheral pulmonary vascular markings diminish. When the left atrial pressure exceeds 22 to 25 mmHg, Kerley B lines develop. These are fine, short, horizontal lines seen along the peripheral portions of the lower and mid lung fields and represent thickened interlobular septa and lymphatics due to chronic interstitial pulmonary edema.

Echocardiography

Both M-mode and two-dimensional echocardiography are very helpful in making the diagnosis of mitral stenosis. In approximately 85 percent of patients with mitral stenosis, the posterior mitral valve leaflet moves concordantly with the anterior mitral valve leaflet in an anterior direction during diastole. The mitral valve appears thickened and shows an increased intensity of echoes. If there is pulmonary hy-

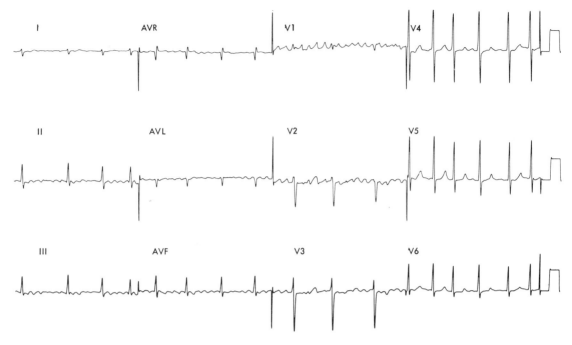

Fig. 16.12 Electrocardiogram of a 44-year-old male with mitral stenosis. Coarse atrial fibrillation is present. The frontal plane QRS axis is 90° (rightward deviation). QRS complexes in V1 are small and the persistence of S waves in V5 and V6 suggest the presence of right ventricular hypertrophy.

pertension, abnormalities of the pulmonic valve may be detected and the right ventricular dimensions may be increased. The left atrial size will also be increased in the majority of cases of mitral stenosis. Two-dimensional echocardiography will confirm the enlargement of the left atrium and right ventricle and demonstrate the thickened mitral valve, the subvalvular cordal thickening, and the restricted opening motion of the mitral valve in diastole. Echocardiography should be performed in all patients with the clinical diagnosis of mitral stenosis, as it will help differentiate the patient with mitral stenosis from the occasional patient with similar clinical findings due to a left atrial myxoma, cor triatriatum, or atrial septal defect.

Cardiac Catheterization and Angiocardiography

These techniques are helpful in quantitating the severity of mitral stenosis and excluding or quantitating associated valvular lesions. Hemodynamic measurements must include the pressure gradient across the valve and the cardiac output at rest and if possible in response to exercise. Left ventricular cineangiography should be performed in all instances to assess left ventricular systolic function, to evaluate the degree of subvalvular chordal and papillary muscle fusion, and to ascertain whether significant mitral insufficiency is also present. If a left atrial thrombus or tumor is suspected, left atriography should be performed either directly through a transseptal atrial puncture or, preferably, by injection of contrast material in the main pulmonary artery.

Therapy

Younger individuals with rheumatic mitral stenosis should receive penicillin prophylaxis against beta-hemolytic streptococcal infections and all patients with mitral stenosis should receive antibiotic prophylaxis at times of anticipated bacteremia.

When pulmonary congestive symptoms develop, if the patient is in sinus rhythm, digitalis is of no value. Initial congestive symptoms may be treated with reduction of levels of activity, sodium restriction, and diuretics. However, digitalis is of great importance when atrial fibrillation with a rapid ventricular response is present. In this setting, slowing the ventricular response by means of digitalis glycosides will often alleviate the majority of the conges-

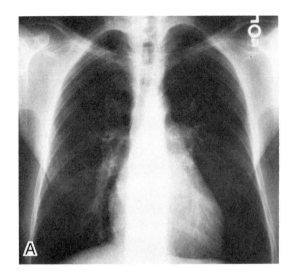

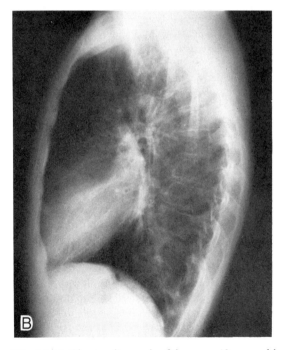

tive symptoms. In patients with pure mitral stenosis, if the heart rate can not be controlled with digitalis glycosides alone, the addition of a beta blocking drug (e.g., propranolol, metoprolol) will often be of substantial value. In patients with relatively recent onset atrial fibrillation, an attempt to revert the rhythm to sinus by means of electric cardioversion is warranted. In patients who have had atrial fibrillation for more than one year, in those with severe mitral stenosis, and in those with very large left atrial dimensions, sinus rhythm is usually not maintained. If cardioversion is successful, the addition of quinidine to the digitalis regimen may help maintain sinus rhythm and prevent recurrences of atrial fibrillation.

Patients with mitral stenosis and chronic atrial fibrillation should be treated with anticoagulant drugs to reduce the risk of systemic embolization. Anticoagulation for a period of 2 to 4 weeks should also be employed prior to cardioversion if the duration of atrial fibrillation is more than 48 hours.

Surgery in the form of either mitral valvotomy or mitral valve replacement is indicated in all symptomatic patients with calculated valve orifice areas below 1.5 cm^2. In general for patients below the age of 40 and those who have demonstrated a pliable mitral valve with no calcification and no associated or trivial mitral regurgitation, mitral valvotomy is preferred as it eliminates the complications of a mitral valve prosthesis. Final decision as to valvotomy versus valve replacement rests with the operating surgeon, since at the time of valvotomy extensive subvalvular chordal fusion may be found even though the mitral leaflets are relatively pliable. The surgical mortality for valvotomy is 2 to 3 percent and most patients show considerable improvement following operation. The risk of mitral valve replacement is in the 5 to 8 percent range. To this one should add the late morbidity and mortality due to the prosthetic valve. For these reasons, mitral valve replacement is recommended only for patients who are symptomatic on less than ordinary activity (New York Heart Association Class III).

Fig. 16.13 Chest radiograph of the same 43-year-old man with mitral stenosis. (A) The posteroanterior projection shows normal overall cardiac size. The left cardiac border is straightened (mitral configuration) due to prominence of the main pulmonary artery segment and of the left atrial appendage. The enlarged left atrium is seen as a circular "double density" through the cardiac shadow. The left main-stem bronchus is elevated because of the enlarged left atrium. (B) The lateral projection confirms the presence of left atrial enlargement (posterior displacement of the upper border of the cardiac silhouette).

MITRAL REGURGITATION AND MITRAL VALVE PROLAPSE

Etiology and Pathogenesis

In approximately 50 percent of patients, mitral regurgitation is produced by rheumatic valvulitis. In this setting it may be isolated or a manifestation of combined mitral stenosis and insufficiency. The same rheumatic process responsible for mitral stenosis also produces rigidity, deformity, and retraction of the valve leaflets with consequent mitral regurgitation. The classic "fish mouth" mitral valve is both stenotic and insufficient. The other 50 percent of patients have mitral regurgitation from nonrheumatic causes. These include congenital anomalies associated with endocardial cushion defects, spontaneous rupture of chordae tendineae, infective endocarditis with destructive lesions of the mitral leaflet, massive calcification of the mitral annulus, hypertrophic obstructive cardiomyopathy with distortion of the mitral valve, functional mitral regurgitation due to marked left ventricular dilatation, mitral valve prolapse and—most important—ischemic dysfunction of the papillary muscles and surrounding left ventricular myocardium. Mitral valve prolapse is the result of myxomatous degeneration of the mitral valve tissue with consequent redundancy and elongation of the leaflets and anchoring chordae tendineae (Barlow's syndrome).

Regardless of etiology, mitral regurgitation is a relentlessly progressive disease since enlargement of the left atrium tends to cause further dilatation of the mitral annulus and distortion of the posterior mitral leaflet, thereby increasing the valvular regurgitation. Also the commonly associated left ventricular dilatation results in progressively increasing valvular regurgitation which in turn causes increases in left atrial and left ventricular dimensions.

Pathophysiology

The pathophysiology and clinical manifestations of severe mitral regurgitation depend largely upon the compliance of the left atrium and pulmonary venous bed. *Acute mitral regurgitation* is associated with normal or actually reduced left atrial compliance. In this group there is little or no left atrial enlargement and remarkable elevations of left atrial pressure occur, commonly resulting in pulmonary edema. In the more chronic setting, patients with low left atrial compliance frequently develop marked increases of pulmonary vascular resistance and therefore pulmonary arterial hypertension. As in mitral stenosis, in this group of patients right ventricular failure is a common clinical manifestation. Sinus rhythm is usually maintained in patients with small left atria. On the other hand, patients with high left atrial compliance develop massive enlargement of the left atrium while maintaining normal or near normal left atrial pressure. The pulmonary artery pressure and pulmonary vascular resistance remain normal or only minimally elevated at rest in this group. Pulmonary

congestive symptoms are not a major manifestation because of the near normal levels of left atrial pressure. However, these patients are usually fatigued because of a chronically low cardiac output. In general, mitral regurgitation is of long standing in this group of patients, and atrial fibrillation is commonly present because of the markedly dilated and stretched left atrium.

Clinical Manifestations

As mentioned above, symptoms depend to a great extent upon the compliance of the left atrium. Sudden marked increases in left atrial pressure produce symptoms of pulmonary congestion (i.e., dyspnea, orthopnea, and paroxysmal nocturnal dyspnea). On the other hand, patients with only slight elevation of left atrial pressure and severe mitral regurgitation tend to have symptoms characteristic of low cardiac output (i.e., chronic fatigue, reduction in exercise tolerance, and exhaustion). Patients with severe pulmonary hypertension who develop right heart failure complain of symptoms of systemic congestion such as right upper quadrant pain, ascites, and peripheral edema.

Patients with *mitral valve prolapse* may also complain of palpitations due to associated atrial and ventricular ectopy and atypical precordial pain. The mechanism of pain in this syndrome has not been well documented, although it is thought that it may be due to localized ischemia of the papillary muscle and surrounding left ventricular myocardium produced by the increased tension placed upon these structures by the prolapsing mitral leaflet.

Blood pressure is usually normal even in the face of severe mitral regurgitation, although some widening of the pulse pressure may occur. The arterial pulse is usually normal; on occasion it may be brisk with rapid upstroke and decline. However, these changes never approach the magnitude of the pulse changes in aortic insufficiency. Inspection of the precordium frequently discloses the apex beat to be displaced laterally, and to be diffuse and hyperdynamic. This is confirmed by palpation. A systolic thrill is frequently present at the cardiac apex, and in rheumatic mitral regurgitation this thrill tends to radiate posteriorly toward the left axilla. A left parasternal systolic lift is frequently present, which may be due either to frank right ventricular hypertrophy or to lifting of the entire heart anteriorly by the enlarged left atrium as it is further enlarged during systole by the regurgitant jet.

On auscultation the first heart sound at the apex is usually diminished in intensity or actually absent.

An accentuated first heart sound at the apex is a useful sign in excluding severe isolated mitral regurgitation. The second sound usually splits normally. However, in severe mitral regurgitation the aortic valve may close prematurely, resulting in wide splitting of the second sound. A third heart sound at the apex is a common finding in patients with severe mitral regurgitation and it will often introduce a short diastolic rumble produced by the torrential early diastolic flow across the mitral valve. In the absence of mitral stenosis, this rumble is uniformly short and is not associated with a presystolic murmur. The characteristic auscultatory finding in patients with mitral regurgitation is an apical systolic murmur usually grade IV in intensity or louder. In patients with rheumatic mitral regurgitation, it is commonly holosystolic and radiates towards the left axilla. In patients with papillary muscle dysfunction, however, the murmur is usually mid- or late systolic and has a crescendo-decrescendo configuration. Similarly, the murmur of mitral valve prolapse is commonly initiated by a midsystolic click and has a crescendo configuration. The systolic murmur of nonrheumatic mitral regurgitation may radiate to the base of the heart instead of the left axilla, especially if it is due to prolapse of the posterior mitral leaflet or posterior papillary muscle dysfunction. In this setting and because such murmurs are not holosystolic, they may on occasion be confused with murmurs of aortic stenosis. In patients with ruptured chordae tendineae or fenestrations of a mitral leaflet, the systolic murmur may often have a musical or "cooing" quality. In acute mitral regurgitation, the apical systolic murmur is usually decrescendo and ends well before the second sound. A loud fourth heart sound is frequently heard in acute mitral regurgitation, and normal sinus rhythm is commonly maintained. These findings are in contrast to the findings of chronic regurgitation, in which case the rhythm is frequently atrial fibrillation and a fourth heart sound is distinctly uncommon, even when sinus rhythm is maintained.

Laboratory Findings

Electrocardiogram

The electrocardiogram in severe mitral regurgitation usually discloses signs of left atrial abnormality and left ventricular hypertrophy. The diastolic overload pattern of left ventricular hypertrophy is not as commonly seen in mitral as in aortic regurgitation. Patients with ischemic heart disease and mitral regurgitation often demonstrate the electrocardiographic signs of prior myocardial infarction or ischemic ST–T wave changes. In mitral valve prolapse, the electrocardiogram frequently demonstrates minor nonspecific ST–T wave changes over the lateral precordial leads. Atrial fibrillation is a common finding in chronic severe mitral regurgitation.

Chest Radiograph

The common radiographic findings in chronic severe mitral regurgitation are left atrial and left ventricular enlargement. Marked left atrial enlargement is characteristic of this lesion, and in severe cases the left atrium may be aneurysmally dilated and in fact form the right cardiac border on the posteroanterior projection. Extreme degrees of left atrial enlargement make the diagnosis of predominant mitral regurgitation secure. Although calcification of the mitral leaflets is common in mitral stenosis and combined mitral stenosis and regurgitation, it is distinctly unusual in patients with pure mitral insufficiency. A calcified mitral valve annulus may occasionally be seen in the lateral chest radiograph as an incomplete ellipse. In acute mitral regurgitation, both left atrial and left ventricular size may be normal, and the most striking radiographic findings are those of pulmonary venous hypertension and interstitial pulmonary edema.

Echocardiographic Findings

In chronic severe mitral regurgitation, the M-mode echocardiogram usually demonstrates increased left atrial dimensions and an enlarged left ventricle with increased end-diastolic and end-systolic dimensions. Ventricular function is usually well preserved until advanced stages of mitral regurgitation. In mitral valve prolapse, the characteristic echocardiographic pattern is that of mid or late systolic posterior displacement of one or both mitral leaflets. The abrupt posterior displacement of the mitral valve in midsystole usually coincides with the midsystolic click if one is present.

Cardiac Catheterization and Angiocardiography

These invasive procedures should be undertaken in all patients in whom surgical therapy is contemplated. Measurement of pulmonary artery pressure and pulmonary artery wedge pressure will provide a sensitive index of the hemodynamic compromise due to the mitral insufficiency. Catheterization of the left side of the heart with measurement of left ventricular end-diastolic pressure, selective left ventriculography, and coronary arteriography is mandatory to assess the degree of mitral regurgitation and left ventricular function. These hemodynamic studies are also helpful in diagnosing and assessing the severity of associated valvular lesions.

In patients critically ill with pulmonary edema due to acute severe mitral regurgitation, catheterization of the right side of the heart and measurement of the pulmonary artery wedge pressure are procedures that are useful in quantitating the severity of mitral regurgitation and in following the effects of therapy. In such cases, the pulmonary artery wedge pressure tracing will frequently demonstrate a large dominant systolic wave ("S" or "CV" wave) due to the transmission of the left ventricular systolic pressure through the noncompliant small left atrium to the pulmonary capillary bed.

Therapy

When patients with chronic severe mitral regurgitation develop symptoms of congestive heart failure, therapy is directed towards restriction of physical activity, restriction of salt intake, diuresis, and the administration of digitalis glycosides. Vasodilator therapy may also be of benefit. The same considerations apply to mitral regurgitation as discussed in the section on aortic insufficiency in terms of not allowing irreparable left ventricular dysfunction to take place prior to considering surgical treatment. The administration of digitalis glycosides in asymptomatic patients may retard the progression of left ventricular dilatation.

Treatment of mitral valve prolapse will depend upon its manifestations. If the major manifestation is an arrhythmia, the administration of the appropriate antiarrhythmic agent is warranted. In general both atrial and ventricular ectopy in patients with mitral valve prolapse are difficult to control. Beta blocking drugs such as propranolol or metoprolol should be tried first. Similarly, the atypical chest pain associated with mitral valve prolapse may be exceedingly difficult to control. In some cases propranolol may be of value and in others the administration of long-acting nitrates may help. Of utmost importance in this syndrome is strong and constant reassurance of the patient, since in the vast majority of cases, despite the presence of multiple symptoms, mitral valve prolapse tends to be a benign condition. All patients with mitral regurgitation are at an increased risk for the development of infective endocarditis. Antibiotic prophylaxis should therefore be administered at times of anticipated bacteremia.

Surgical therapy is directed toward reestablishing competence of the regurgitant mitral valve. Although on occasion plastic procedures and annuloplasty may be helpful in reducing the degree of mitral regurgitation, in the majority of cases surgical therapy implies mitral valve replacement. The surgical risk of this procedure is currently 5 to 10 percent, and depends to a great extent upon the degree of left ventricular dysfunction present as well as the underlying cause of mitral regurgitation. Patients with ischemic heart disease and severe mitral regurgitation present a higher risk than patients with severe mitral insufficiency due to mitral valve prolapse or rheumatic heart disease. The same considerations apply to mitral valve replacement in this lesion as were discussed with aortic regurgitation. The risk of surgery increases significantly in patients with overt congestive heart failure and poor left ventricular function. Furthermore, in such patients progressive myocardial failure may develop despite mitral valve replacement. It is therefore imperative that patients with chronic severe mitral regurgitation be followed carefully and mitral valve replacement be undertaken before marked deterioration of left ventricular function develops. The treatment of acute severe mitral regurgitation is almost always surgical. Pulmonary edema should be initially treated with diuretics and vasodilator agents so that the patient goes to surgery in the best possible state of compensation. The occasional case of rupture of a papillary muscle represents a catastrophic event and a true surgical emergency, since in such cases relief of pulmonary edema cannot be accomplished with any form of medical therapy.

TRICUSPID AND PULMONIC VALVE DISEASE

Tricuspid Stenosis

Etiology

Tricuspid stenosis is an uncommon lesion. Most cases are due to rheumatic valvulitis, and hemodynamically significant tricuspid stenosis is said to be present in 5 to 10 percent of patients with rheumatic mitral valve disease. Other rare causes of tricuspid stenosis include the carcinoid syndrome, endocardial fibroelastosis, endomyocardial fibrosis, and systemic lupus erythematosus.

Clinical Manifestations

The main symptoms of isolated tricuspid stenosis are those of systemic venous congestion with right upper quadrant discomfort due to hepatic congestion, peripheral edema, and ascites in severe cases. Symptoms of dyspnea are distinctly absent, since the lungs are "protected" by this lesion. When mitral and tricuspid stenosis coexist, mitral stenosis usually develops first; therefore, reduction of the symptoms of pulmonary congestion should raise the suspicion that tricuspid stenosis is developing.

Because of the elevated right atrial pressure, the jugular venous pressure is elevated to above 10 cm of water. Therefore jugular venous distention is often present and prominent A waves are seen in patients in sinus rhythm. The jugular venous V waves are not prominent (unless there is associated tricuspid regurgitation) and the Y descent that follows the V wave is usually slow and gradual because the stenotic tricuspid valve delays right atrial emptying during diastole.

In isolated tricuspid stenosis, the right ventricular and pulmonary arterial impulses are not palpable. The apex beat is not displaced and the precordium is generally quiet. On auscultation, the first heart sound is often reduplicated. A tricuspid opening snap may be heard along the lower left sternal border or the xiphoid process. A mid-diastolic low frequency rumble with presystolic accentuation heard best along the lower left sternal border or over the xiphoid process constitutes the auscultatory hallmark of tricuspid stenosis. The location of the murmur may be shifted leftward away from the left sternal border in cases of severe right atrial enlargement with rotation of the heart in a clockwise manner. An inspiratory increase in the intensity of the diastolic murmur (Carvallo's sign) is the only clinical finding that allows diagnosis of tricuspid stenosis with certainty. The increased right atrial filling combined with reduced right ventricular pressure during inspiration increases the transvalvular gradient and consequently diastolic blood flow and the intensity of the murmur.

Laboratory Findings

The electrocardiogram frequently shows signs of right atrial enlargement (i.e., tall, peaked P waves in limb leads II, III and aVF and in precordial lead V1). Usually P waves exceed 2.5 mm in height and are commonly associated with a prolonged PR interval. Signs of right ventricular hypertrophy are absent in isolated tricuspid stenosis and an electrocardiographic pattern unique for this lesion consists of small QRS complexes with an RSR' configuration in lead V1 associated with P waves of greater amplitude than the QRS complexes. The chest radiograph demonstrates rightward displacement of the right atrial border due to enlargement of this cham-

ber. The pulmonary arteries are not enlarged, and pulmonary vascular markings are normal or diminished. Echocardiography (especially two-dimensional studies) demonstrates reduced diastolic opening of the tricuspid valve in association with an enlarged right atrium.

Definitive diagnosis of tricuspid stenosis depends on the demonstration of a transvalvular diastolic pressure gradient between the right atrium and right ventricle.

Therapy

Since isolated tricuspid stenosis is unusual, treatment is commonly directed toward the coexisting and usually more severely stenotic mitral valve. The most important therapeutic tenet is to avoid missing this lesion so as not to allow a persistently stenotic tricuspid valve to interfere with the expected improvement following successful mitral or aortic valve surgery. Moderately severe grades of tricuspid stenosis may be corrected by tricuspid valvotomy at the time of mitral or aortic valve surgery.

Tricuspid Regurgitation

Etiology

The most common form of tricuspid regurgitation is functional regurgitation associated with right ventricular dilatation and failure from any cause. Infective endocarditis, on the other hand, is the most common cause of organic tricuspid regurgitation. Other causes of organic tricuspid regurgitation include the carcinoid syndrome and cardiac trauma.

Clinical Manifestations

The symptoms of tricuspid regurgitation are not distinctive and are usually overshadowed by the symptoms of coexisting mitral or aortic valve disease. Fatigue, decreased exercise tolerance, and dyspnea are probably related to low cardiac output. Peripheral edema and symptoms of hepatic congestion accompany severe tricuspid regurgitation.

The most important physical finding in tricuspid regurgitation is jugular venous distention with prominent systolic waves ("S" or "CV" waves). Functional tricuspid regurgitation usually aggravates existing clinical manifestations of right heart failure and accentuates jugular venous distention, ascites, pleural effusions, and peripheral edema. In this setting there may be a further increase in the jugular venous pressure on inspiration; however, this is not diagnostic for tricuspid regurgitation as it may be seen in any case of right heart failure. A systolic right ventricular lift is usually palpable along the lower left sternal border or in the subxiphoid region. A blowing holosystolic high frequency murmur is often heard in the same area. This murmur is uniformly accentuated during inspiration due to the increased systemic venous return. In severe cases of tricuspid regurgitation, systolic expansile pulsations of the liver may be detected.

Laboratory Findings

The electrocardiogram usually demonstrates atrial fibrillation. Right ventricular hypertrophy may be present in cases of functional tricuspid regurgitation associated with severe pulmonary hypertension. Patients with isolated tricuspid regurgitation will often demonstrate an RSR' pattern in V1, the so called "diastolic overload" pattern of right ventricular hypertrophy. The chest radiograph usually demonstrates cardiomegaly along with prominence of the right atrial border. In general, the cardiac silhouette will vary depending upon coexisting valvular abnormalities.

The echocardiogram may be useful in demonstrating right ventricular enlargement, paradoxic motion of the interventricular septum, and especially in identifying tricuspid leaflet vegetations or the flail tricuspid leaflet of a traumatically disrupted valve.

Cardiac catheterization and angiocardiography are of importance in establishing the diagnosis and quantitation of associated valvular lesions. In severe tricuspid regurgitation a characteristic "ventricularized" pressure pulse may be recorded in the right atrium.

Therapy

Treatment of severe tricuspid regurgitation associated with right heart failure consists initially of sodium restriction, rest, diuretics, and digitalis glycosides. If the tricuspid regurgitation is functional (i.e., secondary to severe pulmonary hypertension in a patient with mitral stenosis), the tricuspid valve should be inspected at the time of mitral valve surgery. If the valve appears intact and the tricuspid regurgitation is the result of tricuspid annular dilatation, simple annuloplasty in association with mitral valve surgery usually suffices.

Isolated tricuspid regurgitation is frequently well tolerated for many years. It is therefore customary to treat such patients conservatively with restricted activity, diuretics, and digitalis glycosides. If medical therapy fails, surgical therapy may be undertaken with plastic repair or replacement of the abnormal tricuspid valve.

Pulmonic Stenosis

Acquired pulmonic stenosis is extremely rare. It may be seen in the malignant carcinoid syndrome, rarely as a result of rheumatic valvulitis, or as a result of primary tumors of the pulmonic valve. On the other hand, congenital stenotic lesions of the pulmonary outflow tract are relatively common and are discussed in the section on Congenital Diseases.

The clinical manifestations of valvular pulmonic stenosis are easily recognized. A right ventricular lift along the left sternal border is usually palpable. A systolic thrill may be detected along the upper left sternal border. On auscultation a harsh or superficial systolic ejection murmur is heard maximally along the upper left sternal border and often radiates to both axillae along the pulmonary arteries. The pulmonic valve closure sound is usually attenuated, but when it is audible wide persistent splitting of the second sound is present. Treatment of severe pulmonic stenosis is usually surgical. Pulmonary valvotomy may be carried out with minimal surgical risk, and the published results have been generally good.

Pulmonic Insufficiency

Pulmonary valve insufficiency may be organic, due to deformity of the valve cusps or secondary to severe pulmonary hypertension. Causes of organic pulmonic insufficiency are congenital deformities, rarely rheumatic valvulitis, infective endocarditis, the carcinoid syndrome, syphilis, tuberculosis, and Marfan's syndrome. Insufficiency due to pulmonary hypertension is far more common and may result from pulmonary hypertension of any cause.

The murmur of organic pulmonic insufficiency is usually a medium frequency crescendo-descrescendo diastolic murmur that starts well after aortic valve closure and is heard best along the mid left sternal border. It often becomes accentuated in intensity during inspiration and early during the recovery phase of the Valsalva maneuver.

The murmur of pulmonic insufficiency due to severe pulmonary hypertension was first described by Graham Steell. It may be exceedingly difficult to differentiate this murmur from the murmur of aortic regurgitation. If both components of the second heart sound are audible, the pulmonic insufficiency murmur will be ushered in by pulmonic valve closure and not by aortic valve closure. However, this is a difficult auscultatory determination to make and phonocardiography is often required. The most practical way to differentiate aortic regurgitation from pulmonic regurgitation during cardiac catheterization is to perform an aortic root angiogram. If aortic regurgitation can be excluded, then the diastolic decrescendo murmur audible along the left sternal border may be ascribed to pulmonic regurgitation.

Treatment of pulmonic regurgitation generally revolves around therapy of the underlying or coexisting lesions. Relief of pulmonary hypertension will often result in disappearance of the pulmonic regurgitant murmur.

INFECTIVE ENDOCARDITIS

Infective endocarditis is a microbial infection of the heart valves, the endocardium adjacent to a congenital or acquired defect, or the endothelium of an aneurysm or an arteriovenous fistula. A large variety of microorganisms may be causative, and the infection may pursue either a prolonged or a fulminant course. In general, untreated endocarditis is fatal.

The clinical, microbiologic, and therapeutic features of this disease have undergone dramatic change during the past three decades. Patients with classic manifestations—fever, "changing murmurs," splenomegaly, signs of peripheral embolization, and multiple positive blood cultures—have become uncommon. Therefore the diagnosis of infective endocarditis must be considered not only in patients who are febrile and have a heart murmur but also in patients with unexplained anemia, glomerulonephritis, stroke, valvular heart disease with rapidly progressive symptoms, poorly controlled congestive heart failure, embolic occlusion of a major peripheral artery, multiple pulmonary emboli, saccular aneurysms, and in the postoperative cardiac patient who is not progressing satisfactorily. Similarly the distinction between "acute" and "subacute" endocarditis has lost much of its clinical significance.

The true incidence of infective endocarditis is not known. In several hospital series it has been listed as the admitting diagnosis in 0.2 to 5 patients per 1,000 hospital admissions. In general male to female ratios have been reported to range from 2:1 to 5:1 in various series. Similarly, the age distribution of this disease has changed during the past 30 years. Instead of primarily involving young adults as was documented

in the preantibiotic era, it currently affects elderly individuals, with a mean age close to 50. An increasing number of patients over the age of 60 years is being reported.

ETIOLOGY AND PATHOGENESIS

Streptococcus viridans continues as the most common causative organism of endocarditis. However, the incidence of *S. viridans* endocarditis has declined from 70 percent in the preantibiotic era to a current level of 40 to 50 percent of all cases. In part this is due to other streptococcal species replacing *S. viridans* as a cause of endocarditis. Both microaerophilic and anaerobic species are now being reported more commonly than in the past. Enterococci have been causing infective endocarditis with increasing frequency and are currently thought to be responsible for approximately 10 percent of all cases, particularly in women of childbearing age and elderly men. *Staphylococcus aureus* is responsible for approximately 25 percent of all cases of infective endocarditis today. This organism is responsible for more than 50 percent of the fulminant and rapidly progressive forms of endocarditis. *S. aureus* is the common causative organism of infective endocarditis in narcotic addicts using intravenous drugs, and it is also a common infective organism in endocarditis complicating open heart surgery. Coagulase negative *S. epidermidis* has been responsible for perhaps 10 percent of cases of infective endocarditis and is one of the most important pathogens in endocarditis complicating open heart surgery. A number of other microorganisms may be responsible for infections of the endocardium. Pneumococcal endocarditis has declined in frequency to less than 5 percent of all cases. When pneumococcal endocarditis develops, it frequently coexists with pneumococcal meningitis. Similarly the incidence of gonococcal endocarditis has declined to an occasional sporadic case. A variety of gramnegative bacilli are also responsible for infections of the endocardium; however, gram-negative bacillary endocarditis remains uncommon except as a complication of open heart surgery and in drug addicts. A variety of other microorganisms have been reported as responsible for sporadic cases of infective endocarditis. Fungal endocarditis is an unusual occurrence in the general population in the absence of predisposing factors. Infections due to various species of Candida, Aspergillus, and Histoplasma form the great majority of fungal endocarditis. The usual predisposing factors include prolonged antibiotic and/or glucocorticoid administration, preexisting bacterial infective endocarditis with antibiotic therapy, diabetes mellitus, intravenous glucose infusions, polyethylene catheter embolization, hyperalimentation, cardiac surgery, therapy with antineoplastic agents, and narcotic addiction.

Infective endocarditis occurs most often in patients with preexisting cardiac disease. In recently reported series, 72 percent of patients with infective endocarditis had evidence of a preexisting structural cardiac abnormality. Congenital and rheumatic heart disease were the two most common forms of preexisting structural heart disease. The presence of previous structural heart defects was significantly lower in endocarditis caused by *S. aureus* and *S. pneumoniae*.

Infective endocarditis most commonly involves the left side of the heart. The mitral valve is involved more often than the aortic valve and combined mitral and aortic valve involvement is quite common. Tricuspid and pulmonic valve endocarditis has been reported uncommonly. Similarly, simultaneous involvement of the right and left sides of the heart is uncommon, with a mean reported incidence of 1 percent. The highest mortality is seen in patients with multiple simultaneous valve infections, followed in order by aortic valve and mitral valve endocarditis. Among congenital cardiac defects, isolated aortic valvular stenosis is the defect most commonly associated with endocarditis, followed in order by ventricular septal defect, tetralogy of Fallot, hypertrophic obstructive cardiomyopathy, and atrial septal defect (uncommon).

In general, valvular insufficiency more commonly predisposes to the development of infective endocarditis than isolated valvular stenosis. Hemodynamic events are of paramount importance in the pathogenesis of the infection, as alterations in blood flow patterns can produce marked changes in the vascular endothelium. For example, infective endocarditis in patients with interventricular septal defects commonly involves the endocardium opposite the septal defect. Similarly, infection associated with patient ductus arteriosus develops on the pulmonary side of the ductus when the shunt is from the aorta to the pulmonary artery and on the aortic side of the ductus when the shunt is reversed.

Transient bacteremia which allows the deposition of microorganisms on the altered vascular endothelium is thought to be the initiating factor in most cases of infective endocarditis. Transient bacteremia may result from any infected focus on the body. It occurs in over two-thirds of patients following dental extraction and in many patients following tonsillectomy. Simple chewing of food may result in bacteremia in patients with gingival disease or dental infection. The deposition of fibrin and platelets at the site of the infection usually produces a vegetation.

Such vegetations commonly harbor microorganisms and are relatively impermeable to antibiotic agents; therefore, high doses of these agents are usually necessary in the treatment of endocarditis. Highly pathogenic organisms such as *S. aureus* or *S. pneumoniae* cause marked valvular tissue destruction, whereas less pathogenic organisms produce less tissue damage but are more prone to produce large polypoid vegetations which may embolize. Infection may extend from the edge of a valve leaflet to the subvalvular chordae tendineae, which may rupture, causing new or increased regurgitation. In aortic valve endocarditis, extension of the infection to the aortic valve annulus frequently produces valve ring abscesses with extravalvular extension of the infection.

The increasing use of parenteral illicit narcotic agents has been responsible for important changes in the frequency and clinical manifestations of infective endocarditis. It has been reported that the incidence of this disease among narcotic addicts is 30 times higher than in the general population. The most common organism in mainline heroin addicts is *S. aureus* and to a lesser extent *S. epidermidis*. In contrast, endocarditis among morphine or opium addicts is due to a variety of microorganisms including enterococci, *Pseudomonas aeruginosa*, *Enterobacter aerogenes*, *E. coli*, and Candida. Multipathogen infective endocarditis has been reported in parenteral drug users. Valves commonly involved in narcotic addicts are the aortic, tricuspid, and pulmonic valves, and both sides of the heart may be affected in some cases; when isolated tricuspid valve endocarditis is present, evidence of intravenous drug abuse should be sought.

PROSTHETIC VALVE ENDOCARDITIS

Infective endocarditis occurring within two months of prosthetic valve surgery (early) is usually due to gram-negative organisms, enterococci, or *S. aureus*. In late onset prosthetic valve endocarditis (more than two months after surgery), the most frequent microorganisms have been streptococci, especially viridans, gram-negative bacilli, and other miscellaneous microorganisms.

Prosthetic valve endocarditis presents a major therapeutic problem, since valve dysfunction secondary to the infection is the rule. Prosthetic valve detachment causing severe valvular regurgitation occurs in up to 80 percent of patients with an infected aortic valve prosthesis but only in approximately 30 percent of patients with an infected mitral valve prosthesis. Obstruction of the prosthetic valve by vegetations is more common in prosthetic mitral valves (70 percent) compared to only 7 percent of infected aortic prostheses. Early reports of endocarditis involving porcine heterografts suggest that this type of valve may be resistant to early postoperative bacteremias, is probably easier to sterilize than rigid prostheses, and, when infected, more durable than other tissue valves.

CLINICAL MANIFESTATIONS

Most patients with infective endocarditis present with nonspecific constitutional symptoms of insidious onset, including malaise, fatigability, fever, and weight loss. In some series the frequence of musculoskeletal symptoms (arthralgias, arthritis, low back pain, or myalgias) is as high as 44 percent.

Fever is the most frequent manifestation of infective endocarditis but is not invariably present. It is usually absent in the face of massive cerebral or subarachnoid hemorrhage due to embolism or rupture of a mycotic aneurysm, severe congestive heart failure, uremia, advanced age, and prior administration of antibiotic agents. Administration of suboptimal doses of antimicrobial agents is probably the most common cause for the absence of a febrile response.

Patients presenting with primarily central nervous system symptoms (stroke, delirium, and coma) have a significantly higher mortality rate when compared to patients without these symptoms.

Classically, a heart murmur has been thought to be the sine qua non for the diagnosis of infective endocarditis. However, as many as 15 percent with endocarditis may have no detectable murmurs at the time of initial examination. A murmur may appear first during therapy or not until some time after therapy has been completed, or it may fail to develop altogether. In one series cardiac murmurs were not detected in approximately one-third of individuals with acute endocarditis involving the left side of the heart. Similarly, two-thirds of patients with endocarditis involving the right side of the heart, especially the tricuspid valve, may have no detectable murmur initially.

Although the literature on infective endocarditis is replete with references to "changing murmurs" as part of the clinical picture, the concept needs to be reexamined and "change" defined. Many factors, other than valve destruction, may be responsible for changes in the characteristics of a cardiac murmur. For example, alterations in cardiac output, body temperature, or hematocrit may produce impressive changes in the intensity and other characteristics of a cardiac murmur completely independent of changes in valvular integrity. On the other hand, the *development* of a new *organic* regurgitant murmur or murmurs is virtually diagnostic of infective endocarditis if it occurs in the setting of acute sepsis. It is equally important to recognize that in the presence of infective endocarditis cardiac murmurs may be atypical. For example, the systolic murmur of tricuspid regurgitation (in the face of normal right ventricular pressure) need not be holosystolic and will certainly not be high frequency. Similarly, the diastolic murmur of aortic regurgitation may be relatively short because of early equilibration of aortic and left ventricular diastolic pressures and lower in frequency than the usual aortic diastolic blowing murmur.

Common cutaneous manifestations include petechiae which are seen in 20 to 40 percent of cases. They are frequently found on mucosal surfaces of the mouth, pharynx, or the conjunctivae. Small hemorrhages are often found in the retina; they may occasionally be flame-shaped and have pale centers (Roth spots). Splinter hemorrhages are linear hemorrhages found under the nails. They are nonspecific findings and are as likely to develop in response to trauma as to be due to infective endocarditis.

Tender subcutaneous purplish erythematous papules that develop in the pulp of the fingers have been called Osler's nodes and are thought to be highly suggestive of infective endocarditis, although they have been reported in systemic lupus erythematosus. They may occasionally necrotize and ulcerate. Janeway's lesions are larger erythematous nodular lesions that may develop on the palms of the hands or the soles of the feet. They are usually nontender and do not necrotize. Both of these lesions are distinctly uncommon, occurring perhaps in less than 10 percent of cases of subacute infective endocarditis and are even rarer in the more fulminant acute disease. Similarly, clubbing of the fingers has become a rarity probably because of the decreasing number of chronic or subacute cases.

Splenomegaly is common in the subacute or chronic form of the disease but distinctly unusual in the more acute cases. The spleen may be rarely tender, and occasionally a friction rub may be heard over it if a splenic infarct has taken place.

COMPLICATIONS OF INFECTIVE ENDOCARDITIS

Congestive Heart Failure

The most common complication of infective endocarditis is the development of congestive heart failure despite adequate treatment of the infectious process. Most often congestive heart failure is due to severe aortic regurgitation resulting from the perforation or destruction of aortic valve cusps. Congestive heart failure of recent onset carries a higher risk of death when compared to preexisting or aggravated congestive heart failure. Severe mitral regurgitation and combined mitral and aortic regurgitation are responsible for approximately one-third of cases of severe congestive heart failure. Patients with multiple valve involvement have the poorest prognosis (97 percent mortality in one recent series).

Extravalvular Complications

Many other cardiac complications, not involving the valves, contribute to the morbidity and mortality of infective endocarditis. These include myocardial infarction and myocardial abscess formation, sudden death caused by occlusion of a coronary ostium by a vegetation, extension of the infection through the myocardium resulting in the formation of fistulas, aneurysms, and perforations, and the development of atrio-ventricular block. Purulent pericarditis, with or without cardic tamponade, may result from rupture of an aortic ring abscess into the pericardial space.

Major Embolic Phenomena

After congestive heart failure, arterial emboli are the most frequent complications of infective endocarditis. The incidence of major emboli is estimated to be today between 15 and 35 percent of all cases of endocarditis. The most common sites of embolism are the coronary arteries, spleen, and kidneys. Splenic emboli are rarely detected during life but occur at necropsy in as many as 44 percent of cases. Splenic rupture is an uncommon sequel of embolism and infarction of the spleen and may be the first manifestation of infective endocarditis. Embolic occlusion of a large artery is uncommon, but when it occurs it suggests the large friable vegetations characteristic of fungal endocarditis.

Mycotic Aneurysms

Mycotic aneurysms are another major complication of infective endocarditis. They develop either as a response to embolic occlusion of the vasa vasorum or due to direct bacterial invasion of the arterial wall. They most frequently occur in the sinuses of Valsalva but have also been reported in cerebral arteries, pul-

monary arteries, celiac axis, ligated ductus arteriosus and at site of atherosclerotic disease in the aorta and its major branches. They are most frequent when relatively noninvasive oraganisms are involved and less common when the etiologic agent is *S. aureus*.

Neurologic Complications

A variety of neuropsychiatric syndromes occur in approximately 10 to 50 percent of patients with infective endocarditis. They include headache, lethargy, pyschosis, acute brain syndrome, cranial nerve palsies, seizures, and hemiplegia. Although major cerebrovascular accidents are an uncommon presentation for patients with infective endocarditis, the clinical adage "in hemiplegia in young adults always think of SBE" remains useful. Mycotic aneurysms of the cerebral arteries occur in 2 to 10 percent of patients with infective endocarditis. Patients usually remain asymptomatic until the aneurysm ruptures, but the development of a mycotic aneurysm may be accompanied by symptoms due to concomitant cerebral ischemia, meningoencephalitis, increased intracranial pressure, or cranial nerve palsies. Patients with mycotic cerebral aneurysms may exhibit asymptomatic cerebrospinal fluid pleocytosis. Such aneurysms may rupture as late as one to two years following bacteriologic cure.

Renal Complications

As a site of embolization the kidneys are second to the spleen. Although renal infarction is not commonly recognized during life, it has been found in 56 percent of patients with infective endocarditis at necropsy. Renal infarction has seldom been related to serious disturbances of renal function. Hematuria has been recorded in 37 to 93 percent of patients with infective endocarditis. The acute glomerulonephritis which occasionally develops as a complication of infective endocarditis is a form of immune complex disease, rather than of embolic origin.

Hematologic Complications

A normochromic, normocytic anemia occurs frequently. The combination of fever, anemia, petechiae, and splenomegaly should raise the possibility of infective endocarditis. A thrombotic thrombocytopenic purpura-like (TTP) syndrome can also be the presenting feature in some patients.

LABORATORY DIAGNOSIS

Microbiologic Studies

Isolation of the causative microorganism from the blood is an absolute requirement for the definitive diagnosis of any form of infective endocarditis. Blood cultures must be obtained before the initiation of antimicrobial treatment. Although it has been demonstrated that intravascular infections usually produce a continuous bacteremia, other studies have suggested that the bacteremia associated with infective endocarditis is qualitatively continuous but quantitatively discontinuous. Therefore, on occasion, many blood specimens may be drawn and still no positive cultures obtained. In general, however, three sets of blood cultures obtained over a 24 to 48 hour period will provide at least one positive culture in 95 percent of cases. Nevertheless, a number of series have documented infective endocarditis with persistently negative blood cultures in 10 to 15 percent of cases. Probably prior administration of antibiotic agents is the main reason for culture negative endocarditis. Another cause of culture-negative endocarditis is that some organisms require special microbiologic techniques for isolation.

Other Laboratory Studies

A normochromic, normocytic anemia may occur in up to 70 percent of cases. The white blood cell count may be elevated or normal. The erythrocyte sedimentation rate is elevated in up to 90 percent of cases; a normal sedimentation rate becomes an important negative finding when the diagnosis of infective endocarditis is considered. Rheumatoid factor is detected in one-third to one-half of patients with infective endocarditis, and the titer decreases with appropriate antimicrobial therapy. Intraleukocytic bacteria may be demonstrated in concentrates of venous blood in approximately 50 percent of patients with bacterial endocarditis, and may confirm the diagnosis of endocarditis in patients with negative blood cultures.

Electrocardiography

Patients with infective endocarditis demonstrate no specific abnormalities of the electrocardiogram. This is a useful laboratory test in detecting and following complications, such as the development of pericarditis or atrioventricular conduction abnormalities.

Chest Radiography

The chest radiograph does not demonstrate specific abnormalities as a result of infective endocarditis. It is, however, a most useful technique in evaluating the complications of the disease, especially the development of congestive heart failure. Many patients with acute left heart failure may demonstrate inconspicuous cardiac enlargement but impressive interstitial or alveolar pulmonary edema. In right-sided endocarditis (especially S. aureus endocarditis), the characteristic radiographic findings are those of septic pulmonary emboli, manifested as multiple, peripheral, cavitating densities.

Echocardiography

The identification of bacterial vegetations through two-dimensional echocardiography may be useful in the diagnosis of bacterial and nonbacterial endocarditis. Patients with echocardiographically demonstrable bacterial vegetations frequently require surgery for hemodynamic deterioration. It should be emphasized, however, that echocardiography does not differentiate between active and healed lesions. Premature mitral valve closure on the M-mode echocardiogram is an indicator of acute severe aortic regurgitation and may provide important prognostic information. In one series all patients with mitral valve closure preceding the onset of the QRS complex required surgical aortic valve replacement because of hemodynamic deterioration.

Cardiac Catheterization and Angiocardiography

When infective endocarditis results in congestive heart failure severe enough for surgery to be considered, cardiac catheterization and angiocardiography are frequently employed to define precisely the anatomic abnormalities and associated pathophysiologic state. These invasive procedures are of greatest value in multivalvular left heart lesions or when myocardial, pericardial, or pulmonary disease coexist and when it becomes necessary to accurately delineate associated extravalvular infection such as sinus of Valsalva aneurysms. Serious adverse reactions from these invasive procedures relate to dislodgement of vegetations with distal embolization and to further depression of the performance of an already failing left ventricle. Cardiac catheterization and cineangiography are probably contraindicated in patients with severe acute aortic regurgitation with rapidly progressive heart failure.

THERAPY

The most important contribution to patients with underlying structural abnormalities is prevention of infective endocarditis. This is discussed in detail in Chapter 7, Table 7.4. The specific congenital and valvular defects with greatest risk are summarized in the preceding section on etiology and pathogenesis.

In considering the treatment of infective endocarditis, it is useful to classify cases into two groups: uncomplicated (streptococcal endocarditis) and cases with complicated disease. Cases are classified as uncomplicated if they are caused by *Streptococcus viridans*, *Streptococcus bovis*, or *Streptococcus fecalis* with no evidence of hemodynamically significant valvular destruction. Generally, prognosis in this group is good, with a 90 to 97 percent bacteriologic cure rate. Organisms do not become resistant during therapy, and treatment regimens have been standardized for many years. Bacteriologic cure can usually be expected with four weeks of treatment. On the other hand, a case should be classified in the complicated group if the causative organism is a Staphylococcus, fungus, gram-negative bacterium or culture-negative. Similarly, patients with an intracardiac prosthesis, those allergic to indicated antibiotics, narcotic addicts, and pregnant women belong in this category. Finally, patients manifesting complications of heart failure, renal failure, distal embolization, mycotic aneurysm, intracerebral abscess, or aortic annular involvement also must be classified in the complicated group. Generally, the prognosis of the complicated group is uncertain, with a wide range (20 to 80 percent) of bacteriologic cure having been reported. The organism involved may become resistant during therapy and therapeutic regimens are not well standardized. Special sensitivity studies are often necessary as a guide to therapy and prolonged periods of treatment may be required. Cardiovascular surgery may often be necessary to achieve cure and/or treat complications.

Streptococcal Endocarditis

Streptococcus viridans and *Streptococcus bovis* are organisms that are usually highly sensitive to penicillin. Despite this high degree of sensitivity, streptomycin is frequently added to the regimen because of experimental evidence that has shown that the combination of penicillin and streptomycin is synergistic against penicillin-sensitive streptococci both in vitro and in vivo. Endocarditis due to this organism is usually treated with aqueous penicillin 1,000,000 units intravenously every 6 hours plus streptomycin 0.5 g intramuscularly twice a day for a period of two weeks. This course of therapy is followed by oral penicillin V 0.5 g four times daily for an additional two-week period.

Enterococcal Endocarditis

Streptococcus fecalis organisms are relatively resistant to penicillin or demonstrate intermediate sensitivity by disc testing. However, the combination of penicillin and streptomycin is most often effective because of the demonstrated synergism of these two agents against the enterococcus. Generally, aqueous penicillin is given in doses of 20 million units a day intravenously (in divided doses) combined with streptomycin 0.5 to 1 g intramuscularly twice daily for a period of four weeks. In a few cases a 6 week course of therapy may be required. Alternative regimens include the combination of penicillin and gentamicin, since 30 percent of enterococcal strains appear to be highly resistant to streptomycin in vitro. An alternative regimen utilizes ampicillin 8 to 12 g daily intravenously in divided doses plus gentamicin 3 mg/kg/day intravenously or intramuscularly for four weeks. Results of therapy have been equally good with both regimens.

Staphylococcus Aureus Endocarditis

Patients with infective endocarditis due to this organism are most commonly acutely ill and clearly fall in the complicated group. They must be treated for a minimum of four weeks in the hospital with parenteral therapy. Despite clear differences in protein binding, in vitro activity, and other pharmacodynamics, methicillin, nafcillin, and oxacillin have all proven to be equally effective in the treatment of staphylococcal endocarditis in the experimental animal and in clinical practice. These antibiotics should be administered in doses of 12 g daily (in divided doses) intravenously for a minimum of four weeks and occasionally for a period of 6 weeks, since large vegetations can be sterilized only with prolonged antimicrobial therapy. Cephalothin 12 g daily intravenously has also proven effective in the treatment of *S. aureus* endocarditis and is advocated by some. Similarly, a combination regimen of a semi-synthetic penicillin and gentamicin has been advocated in order to take advantage of the synergism between these two drugs.

Culture-Negative Infective Endocarditis

The usual patient with culture-negative infective endocarditis should be treated for enterococcal endocarditis as outlined above. Exceptions to this general rule are when infective endocarditis occurs in narcotic addicts, in the postoperative cardiac surgical patient, and when the clinical course is an acute fulminant one. In these three situations an antimicrobial agent directed against *Staphylococcus aureus* should be added to the antienterococcal regimen. The same general therapeutic rules apply prior to microbiologic identification of the infective agent.

Surgical Therapy

The indications for surgical intervention in infective endocarditis are congestive heart failure, persistent infection, a combination of congestive heart failure and persistent infection, dysfunction of a previously inserted prosthetic valve involved in the infectious process, and the development of life-threatening extravalvular complications. Congestive heart failure due to the development of acute aortic regurgitation is presently the leading cause of death from infective endocarditis. In this setting, the mortality with medical therapy alone is extremely high, and early aortic valve replacement has been undertaken with a 50 percent reduction in mortality.

Indications for early surgery and replacement of an infected aortic valve are: (1) Congestive heart failure which cannot be controlled by medical therapy. In these cases immediate surgery is indicated regardless of the activity of the infection. (2) Patients without congestive heart failure or with medically controllable failure should be treated with the standard four to six weeks of antimicrobial therapy. The decision regarding early valve replacement in this group should then be based on consideration of the hemodynamic severity of the aortic insufficiency as judged by physical findings and echocardiography, and on consideration of the anatomic aspects of the infection such as extravalvular extension.

MYOCARDIAL AND PERICARDIAL DISEASE

THE CARDIOMYOPATHIES

The term *cardiomyopathy* is employed to define cardiac disease manifested entirely or predominantly by symptoms of myocardial dysfunction. Ischemic, valvular, hypertensive, pulmonary, and congenital heart disease which may also affect the myocardium

are specifically excluded. Etiologically, it is customary to classify cardiomyopathies into a primary or idiopathic group and into a secondary group associated with specific systemic diseases or specific physical, chemical, and biologic agents. See Table 16.8 for a simplified physiologic and etiologic classification of the cardiomyopathies discussed below.

In this section we will discuss briefly the clinical manifestations of the three major pathophysiologic types of cardiomyopathy as well as certain specific entities common in western countries.

Congestive or Dilated Cardiomyopathy

Congestive cardiomyopathy is the most common pathophysiologic type of primary myocardial disease. Its cardinal clinical manifestations are those of left ventricular systolic dysfunction, since the left

Table 16.8   Classification of Cardiomyopathies

I. Pathophysiologic Classification
   A. Congestive (dilated)
   B. Restrictive
   C. Hypertrophic
     1. Obstructive (HOCM, ASH, IHSS)
     2. Non-obstructive
II. Etiologic Classification
   A. *Primary*
     1. Familial
     2. Peripartal
     3. Primarily endocardial involvement (endocardial fibroelastosis, parietal [Loeffler's] endocarditis)
     4. Idiopathic
   B. *Secondary*
     1. Connective tissue disorders: scleroderma, systemic lupus erythematosus, rheumatoid arthritis, rheumatic fever, ankylosing spondylitis, polymyositis
     2. Toxic agents: alcohol, cobalt, carbon monoxide, uremia, doxorubicin and other antineoplastic agents, x-irradiation
     3. Neuromuscular diseases: progressive muscular dystrophy, Friedreich's ataxia, myotonic muscular dystrophy
     4. Infections: viral (esp. Coxsackie B), bacterial, protozoal (toxoplasmosis, amebiasis, trypanosomiasis), parasitic (trichinosis), fungal (candida)
     5. Granulomatous: sarcoid
     6. Immunologic: serum sickness, amyloidosis
     7. Neoplastic infiltrative or metastatic disease: lymphoma, leukemia, melanoma
     8. Metabolic: hyper- and hypothyroidism, hyperparathyroidism, hemochromatosis, pheochromocytoma, acromegaly, diabetes mellitus
     9. Nutritional: beriberi, kwashiorkor
     10. Hematologic: sickle cell disease
     11. Post-traumatic: myocardial contusion

ventricle is much more commonly affected initially than the right ventricle. Thus, exertional dyspnea and a reduced exercise capacity are frequently the initial symptoms. They are followed by orthopnea, paroxysmal nocturnal dyspnea, and palpitations. Eventually, symptoms of right heart failure develop as well. Physical examination discloses an enlarged heart, distant heart sounds, the presence of ventricular (S3) and atrial (S4) diastolic gallops, and, if tachycardia is present, a summation gallop. Murmurs of mitral and/or tricuspid regurgitation are common. The arterial pulse pressure is narrow and the diastolic pressure may be elevated. The jugular venous pressure is frequently elevated when the right heart fails.

Electrocardiographic findings frequently include intraventricular conduction defects, most commonly left bundle branch block, diffuse ST–T wave changes or atrial fibrillation as well as low QRS voltage. Left ventricular hypertrophy patterns occur in a significant proportion of patients, as do findings of atrioventricular block and ventricular premature contractions. The chest radiograph commonly discloses marked enlargement of all four cardiac chambers. The echocardiogram usually shows dilated ventricular chambers, poorly contracting myocardium, and increased distance between the mitral valve and the interventricular septum.

Various degrees of pulmonary edema as well as pleural and/or pericardial effusions may be present. The natural history of idiopathic congestive cardiomyopathy is one of inexorable progressive decline, although many patients are only mildly symptomatic despite a marked reduction in the resting left ventricular ejection fraction. Severe congestive heart failure symptoms predominate, but death often occurs from an episode of acute thromboembolism (pulmonary or systemic) or from intractable ventricular arrhythmias. Treatment is difficult, since, in an advanced stage, congestive cardiomyopathy does not respond well to the usual diuretic and digitalis therapy of congestive heart failure. Vasodilator therapy may be used to advantage in this setting. Of course, if one is dealing with a secondary cardiomyopathy, treatment of the underlying systemic disease may be of help. Chronic anticoagulation has been employed in patients with a history of systemic or pulmonary emboli, atrial fibrillation, and low cardiac output.

Restrictive Cardiomyopathies

In this group of disorders the cardinal clinical manifestations are dominated by the abnormal physiology of "diastolic ventricular dysfunction." These are features of restriction to diastolic ventricular filling resulting primarily in elevation of pulmonary and systemic venous pressures. Although patients with congestive cardiomyopathy may often exhibit certain characteristics of restriction as well, it is useful to classify certain myopathies as primarily restrictive, since their initial presentation is that of diastolic rather than systolic ventricular dysfunction. Classically, primary amyloidosis, hemochromatosis, endocardial fibroelastosis, and parietal endocarditis are myopathies in which the restrictive characteristics predominate.

The clinical manifestations of restrictive cardiomyopathies include elevated systemic venous pressure, which in turn results in peripheral edema, symptoms of congestive hepatomegaly, and ascites. The jugular venous pressure is elevated on examination and prominent X and Y descents are often seen. The jugular venous pressure rises paradoxically on inspiration (Kussmaul's sign). There is moderate cardiomegaly, heart sounds are distant, and atrial and ventricular gallop sounds are common. Cardiac output may be maintained in the normal range early in the course of the disease but eventually declines. The electrocardiographic and radiographic features are not distinctive. The physical findings and, often, cardiac catheterization findings in restrictive cardiomyopathy may be indistinguishable from those of constrictive pericarditis. However, it is vitally important to make the correct diagnosis since constrictive pericarditis is a potentially curable disease.

Hypertrophic Cardiomyopathy

This entity is characterized by myocardial hypertrophy. Microscopically, the hypertrophied myocardial cells are thick, short, and often have large bizzare nuclei. Many muscle bundles are separated by clefts, contain increased amounts of connective tissue, and form distorted patterns. Depending upon the distribution of the hypertrophied myocardium, obstructive and nonobstructive forms of hypertrophic cardiomyopathy are recognized. Although these two forms may have somewhat different clinical presentation and prognosis, it is likely that they represent two different phases of the same disease. The major hemodynamic abnormality is poor diastolic compliance of the left ventricle and this appears to correlate best with the severity of the cardiomyopathy.

Patients with *obstructive hypertrophic cardiomyopathy* demonstrate a marked increase in upper ventricular septal muscle mass. This abnormality, in association with an anteriorly displaced anterior mitral valve leaflet, is responsible for the dynamic left ventricular outflow obstruction characteristic of this disorder. The obstruction occurs in the subaortic region and it is for this reason that this entity was originally referred to as idiopathic hypertrophic subaortic stenosis (IHSS). A small subgroup of patients with this disorder will exhibit predominant lower ventricular septal hypertrophy, which can produce a dynamic midventricular obstruction.

Patients with *nonobstructive hypertrophic cardiomyopathy* constitute approximately 10 to 20 percent of the total group. A more generalized increase in muscle mass characterizes this subgroup of patients, although the interventricular septum is invariably more hypertrophied than the posterior wall. Thus, this group also exhibits the abnormal septal to posterior wall thickness ratio that is the characteristic hallmark of hypertrophic cardiomyopathy.

Hypertrophic cardiomyopathy may be detected in asymptomatic patients, or patients may become symptomatic due to poor ventricular distensibility in the nonobstructive variety or they may develop symptoms secondary to a combination of poor ventricular distensibility and left ventricular outflow obstruction. The cardinal symptoms of hypertrophic obstructive cardiomyopathy are dyspnea, orthopnea, paroxysmal nocturnal dyspnea, and angina pectoris. Paradoxical splitting of the second heart sound may also be present. The hypertrophied left ventricle is often palpable as a heaving impulse at the apex. The apex beat is frequently bifid due to presystolic distention produced by atrial contraction. On auscultation a fourth heart sound can almost always be detected in the presence of regular sinus rhythm. Probably the most characteristic physical finding in this entity is the carotid pulse which invariably demonstrates a brisk upstroke and may be bifid or "bisferiens." A midsystolic murmur is often present at the lower left sternal border. Since the left ventricular outflow pressure gradient, which is responsible for the systolic murmur, is dynamic and variable from minute to minute depending upon the degree of myocardial contractility, ventricular filling, systemic arterial pressure and many other factors, the intensity of the murmur may also vary remarkably. A variety of maneuvers may be utilized to bring out the systolic murmur. These maneuvers are listed in the section on cardiac examination. Frequently there is associated mitral regurgitation in this condition because of the anterior displacement of the mitral valve apparatus. The coexistence of systolic outflow murmur and a mitral regurgitant murmur often presents a difficult diagnostic problem since these two murmurs respond in opposite fashion to many of the maneuvers employed.

The electrocardiogram is almost always abnormal, fulfilling criteria for left ventricular hypertrophy along with prolongation of the QRS duration. Abnormal Q waves are frequently seen, especially in the inferolateral leads. It is thought that these Q waves represent exaggerated septal activation forces and reflect the increased ventricular septal mass. The chest radiograph is not distinctive. Usually the overall cardiac size is normal, although signs of left atrial enlargement may be present along with evidence for pulmonary venous hypertension.

The most useful diagnostic study in hypertrophic cardiomyopathy is the echocardiogram. Asymmetric septal hypertrophy is almost always recorded with a ratio of septal to posterior wall thickness exceeding 1.5. In addition to increased thickness the interventricular septum contracts poorly and may be even totally akinetic. In contrast, posterior wall motion is excellent to exaggerated. The entire mitral valve apparatus is displaced anteriorly and is closer to the interventricular septum than normal. The diastolic slope of the mitral valve is diminished, reflecting the decreased filling rate of the left ventricle during diastole because of its reduced distensibility. During systole there is often abnormal anterior movement of the anterior mitral leaflet which may actually come into apposition with the septum. A typical echocardiogram is presented in Figure 16.14.

The natural history of hypertrophic obstructive cardiomyopathy is not well delineated. Once symptoms develop, if patients are not treated, a 3.5 percent per annum annual mortality rate has been reported. Sudden death is the most common mode of demise and accounts for approximately 50 percent of deaths. A major cardiac arrhythmia is probably responsible for most instances of sudden death. Treatment of hypertrophic obstructive cardiomyopathy will depend upon quantitation of the degree of systolic obstruction by cardiac catheterization. If a resting left ventricular outflow gradient of 50 mmHg or more is present, surgery in the form of septal myomectomy has been employed; patients with lesser degrees of resting pressure gradients or only with provocable outflow pressure gradients are probably best treated medically with beta blocking drugs (propranolol, metoprolol, etc.) or with the newer calcium blocking drugs (verapamil, nifedipine, etc.).

Arrhythmias in hypertrophic cardiomyopathy must be treated aggressively. Patients with reduced ventricular compliance respond particularly poorly to atrial fibrillation. Cardiac output may fall precipitously, and hypotension is common. Immediate electric DC cardioversion is indicated in this setting. Conversely, digitalis is not recommended unless cardioversion is not feasible. Parenteral verapamil may

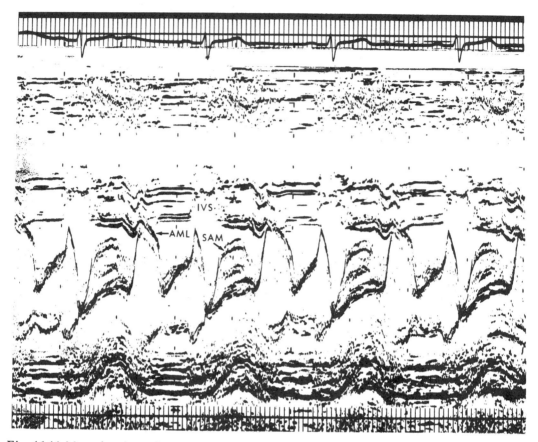

Fig. 16.14 M-mode echocardiogram of a 54-year-old male with hypertrophic obstructive cardiomyopathy. Note the thickened, poorly contracting septum (IVS). The entire mitral valve apparatus is displaced anteriorly. The anterior mitral leaflet E-F slope is diminished (AML). During systole the anterior leaflet of the valve moves abnormally anteriorly and almost touches the septum. (SAM = sytolic anterior motion).

well become a useful alternative to DC cardioversion.

Congestive symptoms are treated with diuretics. However, one must be careful not to overdiurese such patients, as they require higher than normal filling pressures for optimal diastolic function of the stiff left ventricle. Hypovolemia may contribute to reduced ventricular volume and dysfunction. Digitalis glycosides again are probably contraindicated because of their positive inotropic effect, which tends to increase the left ventricular outflow obstruction. Patients with hypertrophic cardiomyopathy and paroxysmal atrial fibrillation are particularly prone to thromboembolic complications; therefore, chronic anticoagulation should be employed. Because of the common coexistence of mitral valve abnormalities, patients with hypertrophic cardiomyopathy are at risk for the development of infective endocarditis.

Therefore antibiotic prophylaxis is indicated in these patients at times of anticipated bacteremia.

Peripartal Cardiomyopathy

This is a congestive cardiomyopathy that develops at any time from just prior to delivery to twenty weeks postpartum. Its cause is unknown, although antimyocardial antibodies have been implicated. Before diagnosing peripartal cardiomyopathy, it is important to exclude other myocardial diseases which present during pregnancy and may be aggravated by the stress of pregnancy, labor, and delivery. The typical patient with peripartal cardiomyopathy appears to be a malnourished young woman who is often black. The disease may result in death despite intensive treatment. Therapy is directed towards left ventricular failure with digitalis glycosides, diuretics, and vasodilator agents.

Alcoholic Cardiomyopathy

Alcohol is a direct myocardial toxin. Impaired left ventricular performance has been demonstrated following alcohol ingestion in both animals and humans. Furthermore, alcohol has been shown experimentally to change myocardial substrate utilization from carbohydrate to triglyceride and produce histologic evidence of myocardial cell injury. Classically the patient with alcoholic cardiomyopathy is a "binge drinker" who presents in florid congestive heart failure after having ingested large amounts of ethanol. Initially, the usual therapy for congestive heart failure and abstinence from alcohol will be successful in reversing this process. When myocardial damage becomes widespread and severe, response to treatment is poor. This entity must be separated from alcohol-induced beriberi heart disease, which is discussed below.

Cardiomyopathy Secondary to Antineoplastic Agents

This type of cardiomyopathy is recognized more and more frequently as cancer chemotherapy becomes more aggressive. Doxorubicin (Adriamycin) is the single most common agent responsible for this form of cardiomyopathy. Among patients receiving over 550 mg/m^2 surface area of this agent, 30 percent will develop a congestive cardiomyopathy. Concomitant radiotherapy to the mediastinum or administration of cyclophosphamide (Cytoxan) "sensitize" the myocardium to adriamycin, and congestive cardiomyopathy may develop at lower dose levels. Attempts to detect impending cardiotoxicity from this agent by noninvasive techniques prior to development of frank cardiomyopathy are not always reliable.

Cardiomyopathy of Neuromuscular Disorders

Patients with Friedreich's ataxia frequently show cardiomegaly and signs and symptoms of congestive heart failure. At necropsy cardiac abnormalities are found in almost 100 percent of patients with this disorder. Replacement of myocardial fibers with connective tissue along with evidence of extensive interstitial fibrosis are common pathologic findings.

Clinically, the picture is that of a congestive cardiomyopathy in association with a variety of cardiac arrhythmias.

Patients with progressive muscular dystrophy, and especially classic Duchenne's dystrophy, characteristically demonstrate abnormal electrocardiograms with evidence of tall R waves and increased R/S ratios in the right precordial leads in association with abnormal Q waves inferiorly. These electrocardiographic abnormalities are probably due to dystrophic myocardial changes the extent of which is genetically determined. Congestive heart failure develops frequently as a preterminal event and often follows years of cardiac stability during which the only evidence of cardiac disease is the abnormal electrocardiogram.

Cardiomyopathy of Hemochromatosis

Cardiomyopathy may develop in both idiopathic and secondary forms of hemochromatosis. In the secondary form, the incidence of myocardial iron deposits correlates well with increasing numbers of blood transfusions received. This is a restrictive cardiomyopathy. Males predominate heavily (10 to 1) in idiopathic hemochromatosis. The clinical picture is dominated by signs and symptoms of biventricular congestive heart failure. Conventional treatment is often disappointing, but removal of excess iron stores has resulted in improvement of cardiac function.

Sarcoidosis

Cardiac involvement in sarcoidosis is common but generally mild. The usual manifestations of cardiac sarcoidosis are various degrees of atrioventricular block or echocardiographic evidence of ventricular dysfunction.

Amyloidosis

Primary amyloidosis frequently involves the heart with a restrictive type of cardiomyopathy. The disease presents most commonly as an insidious and intractable form of congestive heart failure.

Beriberi Heart Disease

Severe thiamine deficiency leading to beriberi heart disease is extremely rare in the developed countries and seen almost exclusively in chronic alcoholics.

Classically, beriberi produces a reduction in systemic vascular resistance which in turn increases cardiac output and cardiac work, eventually leading to congestive heart failure. Beriberi heart disease along with thyrotoxicosis, Paget's disease of the bone and severe chronic anemia are the main causes of *high output congestive heart failure*. Clinically there is widening of the arterial pulse pressure and bounding peripheral arterial pulses are present. The heart is usually dilated and a ventricular diastolic gallop is frequently present, along with the usual signs and symptoms of biventricular congestive heart failure. Syncope and sudden death have been reported, and early treatment is therefore important. Therapy consists of parenteral thiamine in doses of 50 to 100 mg daily along with the administration of the remainder of the vitamin B complex. Bed rest and diuretics are of some help, but digitalis is said to be of little use.

PERICARDIAL DISEASE

The pericardium is affected by a large number of diseases and a variety of biological and physical agents. An abbreviated etiologic classification of pericardial disease is listed in Table 16.9.

Clinically and pathophysiologically, it is useful to consider the manifestations of pericardial disease in three separate categories: acute pericarditis, pericardial effusion, and chronic constrictive pericarditis. The reader should keep in mind, however, that these three categories most often represent different stages of the same pathologic process and frequently overlap. Thus a patient with initial signs and symptoms of acute pericarditis may later develop clinical manifestations of pericardial effusion and still later may evolve into a phase of pericardial constriction.

Acute Pericarditis

The cardinal clinical manifestation of acute inflammatory pericarditis of whatever etiology, is pain. Pericardial pain is usually retrosternal, steady, and may be difficult to differentiate from pain of myocardial ischemia. If there is associated involvement of the pleura, the character of the pain changes and becomes related to respiratory movements, is aggravated by cough or deep breathing and occasionally by swallowing. It is worse in the supine position and may be partially relieved when the patient sits up or leans forward. It is often referred to the left shoulder and the left side of the neck and occasionally may involve the upper abdomen and the back in which case it may simulate the pain of acute cholecystitis or acute pancreatitis. Since acute pericarditis may develop in a patient with a recent acute myocardial infarction, differentiation of pericardial pain from that of myocardial ischemia may be quite difficult. Pain may be a minor symptom or actually absent in some forms of acute pericarditis. In general, the less the inflammatory reaction in the pericardium the less intense the pain. Patients with uremic pericarditis rarely have severe chest pain because of their obtunded mental state as well as the blunted inflammatory response that patients with uremia exhibit. Similarly, chest pain may improve or subside in some cases of acute pericarditis if fluid separates the inflamed parietal and visceral pericardial surfaces. It is particularly important to recognize this mechanism of pain improvement, and not rely on symptomatic improvement alone in following the clinical course of a patient with acute pericarditis.

The pathognomonic physical finding in acute pericarditis is the pericardial friction rub. This is a leathery sound usually appreciated best with the diaphragm of the stethoscope applied firmly to the patient's chest wall along the lower left sternal border or between the left sternal border and the apex. Having the patient sit up and lean forward is most useful in bringing out faint pericardial friction rubs. Classically, a three component friction rub may be heard, produced by atrial systole, ventricular systole, and ventricular diastole. However, a three component friction rub is the exception rather than the rule, and frequently a two or even a single component friction rub may be all that is appreciated. The pericardial friction rub may be transitory and will only be appreciated if diligent and repeated auscultation is carried out on patients suspected of acute pericarditis.

Table 16.9 **Causes of Acute Pericarditis**

I. Infectious
   1. Viral (idiopathic or acute benign)
   2. Bacterial (tuberculosis)
   3. Fungal
   4. Parasitic
II. Metabolic
   1. Uremia
   2. Myxedema
III. Immunologic
   1. Rheumatic fever
   2. Collagen-vascular disorders (SLE, polyarteritis, scleroderma, rheumatoid arthritis)
   3. Post-myocardial trauma (post myocardial infarction, post-cardiotomy, post-traumatic)
IV. Drug-Induced
   1. Hydralazine
   2. Procainamide
V. Miscellaneous
   1. Post-radiation
   2. Neoplasm (primary or metastatic)
   3. Myocardial infarction, chest trauma

Often, the pericardial friction rub is strikingly affected by breathing, and such alterations do not necessarily imply pleural involvement.

Pericardial Effusion

Normally the pericardial space contains a few milliliters of clear fluid. When the pericardial fluid exceeds approximately 150ml, a pericardial effusion is said to be present. When pericardial effusions develop as a result of acute inflammatory pericarditis, the initial clinical manifestations are those outlined above. However, in noninflammatory cases, large pericardial effusions may develop gradually with very few if any symptoms. The hemodynamic effects of pericardial effusion depend almost entirely on the rate of fluid accumulation. If pericardial fluid accumulates rapidly only a few hundred milliliters may cause cardiac compression (cardiac tamponade) and severe hemodynamic embarrassment. On the other hand, slowly developing pericardial effusions may often fail to produce symptoms and signs even when they exceed 1,000 ml in volume.

In general, the cardinal clinical manifestation of a slowly developing large pericardial effusion is asymptomatic cardiomegaly. Percussing the left border of cardiac dullness beyond a normally located apical impulse in the 5th interspace and left midclavicular line should cause one to suspect the presence of a pericardial effusion. This sign, in general, is difficult to elicit. A number of other signs have been described, such as Auenbrugger's sign—epigastric bulging due to a large pericardial effusion, Banti's sign—dullness in the second and third interspaces at the left sternal border, and Ewart's sign—dullness and bronchial breath sounds posteriorly over the compressed left lung base between the spine and the midscapular line.

Cardiac Tamponade

Cardiac tamponade develops when sufficient fluid accumulates in the pericardial space to cause inflow obstruction of blood into the ventricles. The amount of fluid required to produce tamponade may be as little as 200 to 250 ml in rapidly accumulating effusions or may exceed 1,000 ml in slowly developing effusions, in which case the pericardium stretches gradually and adapts to the increasing size of the effusion.

The clinical manifestations of cardiac tamponade include ´yspnea and orthopnea (in the presence of clear lungs by auscultation). The mechanism of or-thopnea in cardiac tamponade is not clearly understood. Elevation of the jugular venous pressure is a constant finding. In some cases there may be a paradoxical increase in the jugular venous pressure during inspiration (Kussmaul's sign). This sign is actually much more common in constrictive pericarditis than in cardiac tamponade. A positive hepatojugular reflux may be elicited in most cases of cardiac tamponade by exerting mild to moderate pressure over the epigastrium of the patient. This finding is also not pathognomonic, as it may be seen in most cases of right heart failure. Tachycardia, hypotension, and diminution of arterial pulse pressure are commonly seen.

A most important sign in cardiac tamponade is *pulsus paradoxus*. Far from being a paradox, this manifestation is actually an exaggeration of the normal inspiratory decline in systolic arterial pressure. In severe cases the inspiratory pressure decline may be appreciated by palpation of a radial or femoral pulse. However, in the majority of cases it is necessary to listen to the Korotkoff sounds while taking the patient's blood pressure to establish the presence of pulsus paradoxus. A decline in systolic arterial pressure during inspiration of more than 10 mmHg is required to make this diagnosis. Although pulsus paradoxus is a cardinal sign and should always be sought in cases of suspected cardiac tamponade, it is important to recognize that it is not pathognomonic for this condition. Pulsus paradoxus may occur in patients with severe respiratory distress, particularly in patients with asthma, chronic obstructive lung disease, in patients with other forms of constrictive heart disease, and in some cases of severe biventricular failure.

Chronic Constrictive Pericarditis

Chronic constrictive pericarditis may rarely develop as a result of a variety of conditions, including idiopathic or acute benign pericarditis a variety of infections, hemopericardium, and mediastinal radiation. In the recent past, tuberculous infections accounted for the majority of cases of chronic constrictive pericarditis, but this is no longer true.

The cardinal clinical manifestations are produced by obstruction to the inflow of blood into the ventricles because of limited ventricular diastolic distensibility imposed by the rigid and thickened pericardium. Exertional dyspnea is frequently present and mild orthopnea is also a common symptom, although other signs of left ventricular failure are absent. The jugular venous pressure is elevated and increases further on inspiration in over 50 percent of the cases. The jugular venous pulse has an M-shaped contour with sharp and rapid X and Y descents. The liver is enlarged and abdominal ascites is a common finding, as is peripheral edema. The heart is enlarged in only one-half of patients with constrictive pericarditis and usually only to a mild degree. Heart sounds are distant except for the pericardial knock, which is an early third heart sound occurring approximately 0.08 to 0.12 sec. after aortic valve closure. The pericardial knock is usually heard widely over the entire precordium. As the disease progresses, the pericardial fibrosis and scarring process may extend into the myocardium with the result that myocardial dysfunction develops. This may account in part for some of the poor results of operative treatment of constrictive pericarditis.

Laboratory Findings

The electrocardiogram may be quite helpful in making the diagnosis of pericarditis. It usually demonstrates generalized ST segment elevation and/or PR segment depression. In contrast to the changes of acute myocardial infarction, the ST segment elevation in acute pericarditis is commonly generalized and seen in leads reflecting changes of the anterior, lateral, and inferior aspects of the heart. Furthermore, although elevated the ST segments maintain a more normal-appearing configuration (i.e., they remain concave instead of demonstrating the convex characteristic of acute myocardial infarction ST segments). As acute pericarditis evolves, the ST segments return to baseline, and days later shallow T wave inversions develop. Again, this is in contrast to the rapid T wave inversion that develops after acute myocardial infarction. In pericarditis not due to ischemic heart disease, abnormal Q waves do not appear. In large pericardial effusions, generalized low voltage of the electrocardiographic signal may be present. *Electrical alternans* (variation in QRS–T amplitude in alternating complexes) is also frequently seen in cases of large pericardial effusion and cardiac tamponade.

The chest radiograph is of some help in cases of pericardial effusion as it demonstrates cardiomegaly. The loss of the normal "waist" as the cardiac silhouette narrows above the main pulmonary artery, and development of a "flask-like" appearance of the cardiac outline are helpful but not pathognomonic and may be seen in cases of severe cardiomegaly with no pericardial effusion. Occasionally an epicardial fat pad will be seen as a semilunar line along the visceral pericardium within the cardiac silhouette. Pericardial calcification, if present, should strongly suggest the possibility of constrictive pericarditis.

The *echocardiogram* is probably the most useful laboratory study employed in the clinical assessment of pericardial effusion. It is a sensitive tool which detects even small effusions by demonstrating separation of visceral from parietal pericardium. In constrictive pericarditis, thickening of the pericardium may be detected, and in cardiac tamponade the heart may be seen to swing at a rate double the cardiac rate within the large pericardial effusion. The echocardiogram is also useful in following patients serially or in gauging the efficacy of therapy.

Treatment of Pericardial Disease

In general, treatment of pericarditis should be directed toward treatment of the primary disease. Acute idiopathic pericarditis is treated conservatively with bed rest as long as the fever persists and with salicylates for relief of pain. Corticosteroids are highly effective in relieving the pain of acute idiopathic pericarditis, but should be used with caution if the possibility of tuberculous or other forms of infectious pericarditis has not been totally excluded. Purulent pericarditis should be considered as a major medical emergency. Not only is prompt and aggressive antibiotic therapy necessary, but immediate drainage of the pericardium by a limited thoracotomy is indicated. In general, pericardiocentesis is both difficult and an inadequate form of drainage in purulent pericarditis. Tuberculous pericarditis is treated with antituberculous drug chemotherapy, and according to many investigators corticosteroids should be added to reduce the risk of subsequent constriction. Recurrences are a common problem in both acute idiopathic pericarditis and in the postcardiotomy syndrome.

The indications for pericardiocentesis in cases of pericardial effusion are: (1) therapeutic, if tamponade is present, and (2) diagnostic, if the underlying cause of the pericardial effusion is not definitely known. In general, for diagnostic purposes, a limited subxiphoid thoracotomy is preferred to simple pericardiocentesis both because it is safer and especially because it yields pericardial tissue for histologic and cultural studies in addition to the pericardial fluid. In acute cardiac tamponade, prompt pericardiocentesis may be lifesaving. In our experience it is best performed from the subxiphoid area with the needle inserted through the left xiphicostal angle and directed toward the right sternoclavicular joint. Continuous electrocardiographic monitoring with the exploring needle is necessary to prevent myocardial lacerations. At times it may be preferable to perform the procedure under fluoroscopic monitoring. In neoplastic pericardial effusions, frequently simple pericardiocentesis and aspiration of the effusion will prevent its reaccumulation. Alternatively, an antineoplastic agent or tetracycline may be instilled in the pericardial space to produce scarring and fibrosis to prevent reaccumulation of the effusion.

The treatment of chronic constrictive pericarditis is surgical pericardiectomy. Surgery is recommended when patients become symptomatically disabled. As there continues to be an appreciable operative mortality for pericardiectomy, surgery is not generally recommended when patients are only mildly limited by their disease. On the other hand, it appears that the longer pericardial constriction exists, the less the chance of optimal surgical results.

PULMONARY HEART DISEASE (COR PULMONALE)

Pulmonary heart disease (cor pulmonale) is defined as alteration of the structure and/or function of the right heart resulting from pulmonary hypertension. Left heart and congenital heart disease must be specifically excluded. It must be noted that neither right heart failure nor right ventricular hypertrophy is essential to this definition. Simple enlargement of the right ventricle or right atrium in the presence of pulmonary hypertension suffices to make the diagnosis of cor pulmonale.

PATHOGENESIS

Pulmonary arterial hypertension is an absolute requirement for the development of pulmonary heart disease. Mechanisms of pulmonary hypertension include primary pulmonary hypertension and secondary causes (see Chapter 15). In patients with chronic parenchymal lung disease (emphysema or bronchitis) the pulmonary hypertension stems mainly from the vasoconstrictive effects of aveolar hypoxia and hypoxemia. In the early stages of the disease process, pulmonary artery pressure may be normal, becoming elevated only during exercise or at times of respiratory decompensation when hypoxia, acidosis, and hypercapnia develop. How hypoxia causes pulmonary arterial smooth muscle to constrict is unclear. Two major mechanisms have been advanced: first, the release of vasoactive substances from pulmonary parenchymal cells in response to alveolar hypoxia; second, a direct stimulatory and therefore vasoconstrictive effect of hypoxia on pulmonary arterial smooth muscle. As the lung disease progresses, structural changes take place in the pulmonary arterioles and pulmonary hypertension becomes fixed.

Another large group of diseases may produce pulmonary hypertension and therefore pulmonary heart disease by causing an anatomic restriction of the pulmonary vascular bed. The pulmonary vascular bed is a capacious, low-pressure system which may accommodate three- or fourfold rises in cardiac output during exercise with only slight increases in pulmonary artery pressure. Therefore, it is estimated that the disease process must cause restriction or obliteration of more than half the pulmonary vascular bed before resting pulmonary arterial hypertension develops. Frequently, vasoconstrictive mechanisms are superimposed on the basic disease process (e.g., due to hypoxia or in acute pulmonary embolism, reflex vasoconstriction or the release of vasoactive substances from platelets may contribute).

The current consensus is that cor pulmonale is not etiologically related to left ventricular dysfunction. In elderly patients with chronic parenchymal lung disease, independent disease of the left ventricle frequently coexists. If pulmonary heart disease is responsible for abnormal left ventricular function, it may be a result of displacement of the septum into the left ventricle, the acute effects of a dilated right ventricle on intrapericardial pressure, or reduced filling of the left ventricle because of high pulmonary vascular resistance.

CLINICAL MANIFESTATIONS

Because the signs of right ventricular enlargement are subtle, all too frequently the clinical diagnosis of pulmonary heart disease is first entertained only after the right ventricle has failed and has produced systemic venous hypertension, hepatomegaly, and peripheral edema. Indeed, many clinicians continue to make the mistake of reserving the diagnosis of pulmonary heart disease until the stage of right ventricular failure has been reached.

The physical findings of right ventricular enlargement include a left parasternal lift as well as a subxiphoid systolic impulse. If pulmonary hypertension is severe and the main pulmonary artery is dilated, a systolic impulse may be visible and palpable along the upper left sternal border; however, when the lungs are hyperinflated and the anteroposterior chest diameter is increased, significant degrees of right ventricular enlargement and pulmonary arterial dilatation may be hidden from the examiner. On auscultation, the second heart sound will usually be widely split and remains split on expiration due to prolongation of right ventricular ejection. The pulmonic component of the second sound is accentuated and may be palpable in patients with a thin chest wall. A right ventricular fourth heart sound may be appreciated (frequently only on inspiration) by listening carefully along the lower left sternal border or over the xiphoid process. With severe elevations of pulmonary artery pressure, pulmonic regurgitation may develop. With progressive right ventricular dilatation, tricuspid regurgitation frequently develops. Frequently the tricuspid regurgitation murmur is only heard during a Mueller maneuver or toward the end of a long, deep inspiratory effort.

In the face of right ventricular and pulmonary arterial hypertension, the force of right atrial contraction increases. This is manifested by the development of tall dominant A waves in the jugular venous pulse. If tricuspid regurgitation is present, the V wave may become dominant on inspection of the jugular venous pulse. When right heart failure develops, the jugular venous pressure is elevated above 10 cm and the A and V waves usually become equal. In the setting of right ventricular failure, hepatomegaly and peripheral edema are also commonly seen.

ARRHYTHMIAS IN PULMONARY HEART DISEASE

Transient arrhythmias are common in pulmonary heart disease. On the other hand, persistent arrhythmias should suggest causes other than cor pulmonale. Arterial hypoxemia and acid-base disturbances predispose to arrhythmias. The usual arrhythmias encountered during an episode of acute respiratory failure are primarily supraventricular, including atrial or junctional tachycardia, wandering atrial pacemaker, and chaotic or multifocal atrial tachycardia. Less common are atrial flutter, atrial fibrillation and ventricular arrhythmias. It is important to recognize that a bout of arrhythmia may signal the onset of severe respiratory insufficiency.

LABORATORY STUDIES

Typically the *electrocardiogram* in advanced pulmonary heart disease will show right axis deviation in the frontal plane beyond 110 degrees, a rightward shift of the P wave axis in the frontal plane to beyond 60 degrees and signs of right atrial enlargement. P pulmonale is said to be present if peaked P waves exceeding 2.5 mm in amplitude are seen in leads II, III and AVF. Frank right ventricular hypertrophy pattern with a dominant R wave in V1 (Fig. 16.15) is frequently seen in cases of primary pulmonary hypertension, pulmonary arteritis, or chronic pulmonary thromboembolism but is unusual in patients with chronic parenchymal lung disease. In this setting a pattern of incomplete right bundle branch block with an RSR′ complex in V1 is more likely to be present. In earlier stages of the disease process when right ventricular enlargement rather than hypertrophy is the main pathologic change, the electrocardiogram may be less specific and show borderline evidence of right atrial enlargement, mild right axis deviation, and delayed precordial R wave progression. In this setting an R/S ratio in V6 of less than one may be the only evidence of right ventricular enlargement. The *chest radiograph* in chronic pulmonary heart disease is of help primarily in delineating the pulmonary parenchymal changes and demonstrating dilated central pulmonary arteries. Right ventricular enlargement may be detected by abnormal filling of the retrosternal clear space on the lateral radiograph. However, even this sign may be absent in the patient with chronic obstructive lung disease and increased anteroposterior chest diameter.

The *echocardiogram* is a helpful noninvasive technique in diagnosing chronic pulmonary heart disease, despite the technical difficulties imposed by hyperinflated lungs. The first clue is right ventricular enlargement, which can be best estimated from the two-dimensional echocardiogram and especially from the apical four-chamber view. A second useful feature is the echocardiographic diagnosis of pulmonary hypertension from the abnormal pattern of pulmonic valve motion on M-mode echocardiography.

HEMODYNAMIC FEATURES

The hemodynamic features of chronic cor pulmonale depend somewhat on the cause and duration of the lung disease. In patients with multiple pulmonary emboli or primary pulmonary hypertension, pulmonary arterial pressures are commonly much higher than in patients with chronic bronchitis and emphysema, even during an episode of acute respiratory failure. Patients with diffuse interstitial parenchymal disease tend to have moderate levels of pulmonary arterial hypertension until late in the disease when ventilation–perfusion abnormalities become sufficiently deranged to cause severe hypoxemia and respiratory acidosis. Mean pulmonary arterial pressures then may well reach the 60 to 80 mmHg level.

The left atrial pressure is consistently normal in cor pulmonale. Exceptions occur when cor pulmonale is complicated by left ventricular failure produced by independent coexisting left heart disease. Usually,

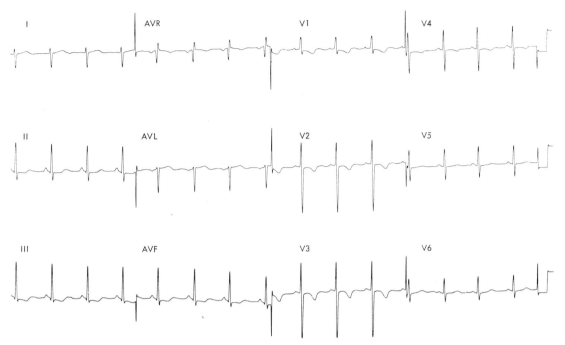

Fig. 16.15 Electrocardiogram of a 27-year-old female with severe pulmonary hypertension due to systemic lupus erythematosus. The frontal plane QRS axis is 110° (right axis deviation). Dominant R waves in V1 and prominent S waves in V6 are diagnostic of right ventricular hypertrophy. The ST–T changes in V1–V4 are consistent with the systolic overload pattern of right ventricular hypertrophy.

left atrial pressure is assessed by means of measurement of the pulmonary artery "wedge" pressure. In the face of severe pulmonary hypertension and pulmonary vascular disease, a reliable pulmonary artery wedge pressure measurement may be difficult to obtain in as many as 20 percent of patients.

THERAPY

Once the diagnosis of cor pulmonale is established and evidence of pulmonary hypertension is documented, reduction in pulmonary arterial pressure levels is of paramount importance. Specific modes of therapy will depend upon the cause of pulmonary hypertension.

In patients with parenchymal lung disease or airway disease, correction of hypoxemia and acidosis is most important (see Chapter 15). Patients with thromboembolic disease should be treated with anticoagulants as outlined in Chapter 4. Primary pulmonary hypertension and vasculitis occasionally respond to pulmonary vasodilators.

The use of digitalis in right ventricular failure in pulmonary heart disease has been debated for many years. There is no question that digitalis glycosides will strengthen the failing right ventricle and im-

prove its performance with measurable increments in cardiac output. Clinical estimation of proper digitalis dosage may be difficult if the heart rate is used as a guide, because hypoxemia as well as heart failure will evoke tachycardia. The presence of hypoxemia, hypokalemia, hypercapnia, as well as the concomitant administration of bronchodilators such as theophylline often contribute to the development of digitoxic rhythms. Taking all of the above into account, digitalis should be used only when other measures are ineffective, and then at reduced dose levels.

CONGENITAL HEART DISEASE IN THE ADULT

INCIDENCE AND NATURAL HISTORY

The incidence of congenital heart disease at birth is estimated at 6 to 8 per thousand. During the first year of life the mortality rate of patients with some of these anomalies is high. Thereafter the mortality rate declines rapidly. The exact incidence of congenital heart disease in adults is not precisely known. Freshmen evaluated during college entrance examinations had an incidence of approximately 0.7 per 1,000 students examined. This represents a reduction by a factor of 10 in the incidence of congenital cardiac anomalies from birth to age 18. Similarly the incidence of specific types of congenital anomalies changes considerably from birth to early adult life (Table 16.10). Perhaps the most striking change is in the incidence of transposition of the great arteries which decreases from a high of 8 percent at birth to less than 1 percent of congenital cardiac anomalies seen in adult life. This reduction is the result of the high mortality rate of this lesion in early life.

Of all congenital cardiac defects, patent ductus arteriosus carries the best prognosis. The mean age at death of patients with a patent ductus arteriosus has been estimated at 43 years. If patients whose ductus closes spontaneously are included in the calculations, the mean age at death is raised to 48 years. Surgical closure of a patent ductus restores the patient to near normal life expectancy.

Atrial septal defects carry the second best prognosis, although many patients become severely symptomatic during the third or fourth decade of life. The mean age at death of all patients with an atrial septal defect has been estimated at 37.5 years. This figure does not include patients with an atrial septal defect associated with an endocardial cushion abnormality which carries a much worse prognosis.

The prognosis in ventricular septal defect will depend upon its size. Patients with small ventricular septal defects and pulmonic to systemic blood flow ratios of 1.5 to 1 or less have a rather good prognosis and their survival expectancy approximates that of patent ductus arteriosus. Conversely, patients with large ventricular septal defects have a much higher mortality in early life. The mean age at death of all patients with "larger" ventricular septal defects has been estimated at 31 years.

The worst prognosis is carried by complex lesions such as transposition of the great arteries, tricuspid atresia, pulmonary atresia, and truncus arteriosus. Tetralogy of Fallot carries a slightly better but still serious prognosis, with 80 percent of patients with this lesion dying by the age of 20. Intermediate survival rates are seen in patients with coarctation of the aorta, bicuspid aortic valve, and valvular pulmonic stenosis.

MODES OF PRESENTATION

Adult patients with congenital cardiac defects usually present to a physician in one of several ways:

1. The patient may be clinically stable with a previously undiagnosed congenital cardiac defect. Such a presentation is common in patients with moderate-sized atrial septal defects who may be asymptomatic early in life but may come to a physician's attention because of an abnormal chest radiograph, or the detection of a systolic ejection murmur during a routine physical examination. Patients with small patent ductus arteriosus and a congenitally bicuspid aortic valve also fall in this category.

2. A patient may present with progressive cardiovascular symptoms and a previously undiagnosed congenital cardiac defect. A larger atrial septal defect with left to right shunting may remain undetected until the fourth or fifth decade, at which time the patient may present with supraventricular arrhythmias or signs and symptoms of congestive heart failure. Or a patient with a small ductus arteriosus may develop infective endarteritis and consult a physician because of symptoms from this complication. Patients with progressive stenosis of a congenitally bicuspid aortic valve may also fall in this category.

3. Patients may be clinically stable with a previously diagnosed congenital cardiac defect. Patients with moderate valvular pulmonic stenosis fall in this group, since this is a lesion that tends to be diagnosed early because of the intensity of the systolic ejection murmur but remains stable over many years. Similarly, patients with small ventricular septal defects and very loud systolic murmurs are usually diagnosed early in life and may remain stable for many years as a small left to right shunt causes very little hemodynamic embarrassment.

4. Another group of patients complain of progressive symptoms superimposed on a previously diagnosed congenital cardiac defect. This group includes patients with congenital aortic stenosis, commonly a progressive lesion. Patients with Ebstein's disease also tend to have progressive symptoms, and all patients with shunt lesions and Eisenmenger physiology will present with inexorably progressive symptomatology.

5. The last group of patients includes those with previous corrective surgery of a congenital cardiac defect. Such patients may be totally asymptomatic following a complete anatomic and physiologic re-

Table 16.10 **Incidence of Various Congenital Cardiac Anomalies**

Anomaly	At Birth (%)	In Adults (%)
Ventricular septal defect	28	20
Patent ductus arteriosus	11	15
Atrial septal defect	10	15
Coarctation of the aorta	9	7
Transposition of the great arteries	8	<1
Tetralogy of Fallot	7	14
Pulmonic stenosis	6	13
Miscellaneous others	21	15

pair or they may be continuously symptomatic following an incomplete anatomic or physiologic repair or palliative surgery.

CLINICAL MANIFESTATIONS

Interatrial Septal Defect

Patients with atrial septal defects and relatively large left to right shunts may remain asymptomatic until the third or fourth decade, at which time symptoms of right heart failure and recurring episodes of supraventricular arrhythmia (atrial tachycardia or atrial flutter) may develop. On examination such a patient will usually show signs of right ventricular enlargement and hyperactivity at the lower left sternal border. A systolic ejection murmur with superficial or "scratchy" characteristics is usually present along the upper left sternal border. The second heart sound is widely and persistently split in most cases with minimal if any respiratory variation. A soft, early diastolic flow rumble generated by increased blood flow across the tricuspid valve is heard at the lower left sternal border or over the xiphoid process. Occasionally patients with atrial septal defects are misdiagnosed as having mitral stenosis, since there is a superficial resemblance between the physical findings of the two lesions. The chest radiograph in atrial septal defect usually demonstrates right ventricular enlargement and large central pulmonary arteries but with increased pulmonary vascular markings of the peripheral lung fields as well (Fig. 16.16). The electrocardiogram commonly shows an incomplete right bundle branch block with an RSR' pattern in V1—the so-called diastolic overload pattern of the right ventricle. The frontal plane QRS axis is usually between +60 and +90 degrees. Patients with an ostium primum type of atrial septal defect (associated with an endocardial cushion abnormality) usually demonstrate left axis deviation in the frontal plane in association with complete or incomplete right bundle branch block patterns in the precordial leads. The echocardiogram in atrial septal defect with a left to right shunt shows an enlarged right ventricle and right atrium and in many cases paradoxic motion of the interventricular septum.

Ventricular Septal Defect

Patients with ventricular septal defects and moderate to large left to right shunts have evidence on physical examination of both right and left ventricular overactivity manifested by both apical and left

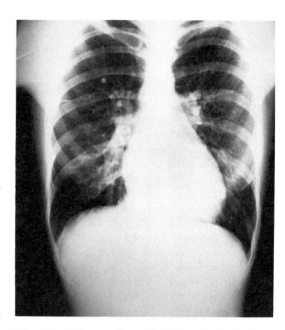

Fig. 16.16 Chest radiograph (PA projection) of a 23-year-old female with a large interatrial septal defect and left to right shunt. The overall cardiac silhouette is normal in size. The apex is rounded and lifted up from the diaphragm suggesting right ventricular enlargement. The central pulmonary arteries are enlarged and pulmonary vascular markings are increased throughout both lung fields.

parasternal lifts. Depending upon the size of the left to right shunt and the level of pulmonary artery pressure, the second heart sound may vary from physiologic splitting to single or persistently split. The murmur of ventricular septal defect is usually loud, harsh and, holosystolic. It is maximal in the third or fourth interspaces at the left sternal border and often radiates well to the right of the sternum. Because of the increased pulmonary blood flow and increased pulmonary venous return across the mitral valve, a short, early mitral flow rumble is often appreciated at the apex. The chest radiograph and electrocardiogram may vary from normal, in cases of very small ventricular septal defects with a pulmonic/systemic blood flow ratio of less than 1.5 to 1, to signs of biventricular enlargement. With large left to right shunts there is enlargement of the central pulmonary arteries and increased pulmonary vascularity on the radiograph, but these findings are not as prominent as in patients with atrial septal defects. Since the left atrium is involved in the shunt circulation, it is usually enlarged and the enlargement may be detected on the chest radiograph, the electrocardiogram and the echocardiogram.

Patent Ductus Arteriosus

Patients with a small left to right shunt through a small patent ductus arteriosus are usually asymptomatic. A high-pitched continuous murmur is present and is usually maximal at the left infraclavicular area or at the first and second interspaces and left sternal border. Faint murmurs may be accentuated by having the patient squat or perform a sustained handgrip maneuver. If a continuous murmur is heard in an atypical location—for example, the third or fourth interspace at the left sternal border—other causes for the murmur should be entertained, such as a coronary to pulmonary artery fistula or chest wall arteriovenous malformation. Patients with a large left to right shunt through a patent ductus will, in addition to the continuous murmur, exhibit signs of left ventricular enlargement with a hyperdynamic and diffuse apical impulse as well as an early diastolic mitral flow rumble due to increased diastolic blood flow across the mitral valve. The chest radiograph usually shows signs of left ventricular and left atrial enlargement and increased pulmonary vascular markings. In contrast to patients with atrial or ventricular septal defects, the aortic knob characteristically is enlarged and prominent on the chest radiograph, since the proximal aorta participates in the abnormal shunt circulation. The electrocardiogram generally shows signs of left ventricular hypertrophy and left atrial enlargement.

Valvular Pulmonic Stenosis with Intact Ventricular Septum

Patients with moderate valvular pulmonic stenosis tolerate this lesion well for many years and may remain asymptomatic to middle age or beyond. On physical examination there are signs of right ventricular hypertrophy with a left parasternal lift. A systolic thrill is commonly present along the upper left sternal border. The second sound is persistently split, and the pulmonic component is attenuated or occasionally inaudible. A long, harsh systolic ejection murmur is present along the upper left sternal border. The shape and length of this murmur correlate well with the severity of the stenotic lesion. Thus, the more severe the stenosis the longer the murmur and the later in systole its peak. In very severe cases the systolic murmur may actually extend beyond the aortic component of the second sound, since right ventricular ejection time is markedly prolonged. The electrocardiogram usually shows right axis deviation to beyond 110 degrees in the frontal plane and evidence of right ventricular hypertrophy

with a dominant R wave in V1 and a dominant S wave in V6. The chest radiograph shows signs of right ventricular enlargement with filling of the retrosternal clear space, poststenotic dilatation of the main pulmonary artery, and normal peripheral vascular markings.

Pulmonic Stenosis with Associated Ventricular Septal Defect (Tetralogy of Fallot)

Tetralogy of Fallot is the most common type of *cyanotic* congenital heart disease in adults. Anatomically this complex requires the presence of a large ventricular septal defect and right ventricular outflow obstruction either at the valvular or the infundibular level. In most cases of tetralogy of Fallot the pulmonary stenosis is severe and only right to left shunting occurs through the ventricular septal defect. This results in cyanosis, clubbing of the fingers and toes, and polycythemia. In a few cases of mild pulmonic stenosis, shunting across the ventricular septal defect may be bidirectional or predominantly left to right, and these cases are classified as "acyanotic tetralogy" or "pink tetralogy." On physical examination, signs of right ventricular hypertrophy are usually present along the lower left sternal border. In approximately 30 percent of cases, a systolic impulse may be palpated along the right upper sternal border as a result of a dilated ascending aorta. On auscultation, a harsh systolic ejection murmur is heard along the mid and upper left sternal border. It may be accompanied by a systolic thrill. The systolic murmur ends well before a single second sound. The more severe the right ventricular outflow tract obstruction, the shorter the systolic murmur, since in tetralogy of Fallot the right ventricle tends to eject predominantly across the ventricular septal defect. In severe cases a continuous murmur of patent ductus arteriosus or of bronchial collaterals may be appreciated. The electrocardiogram shows signs of right axis deviation and right ventricular hypertrophy. The chest radiograph shows a normal heart size overall with signs of right ventricular enlargement. In this lesion the apex of the cardiac silhouette is usually rounded and tilted upward above the left hemidiaphragm. This sign along with concavity in the region of the main pulmonary artery segment gives the "coeur en sabot" (boot-shaped heart) appearance. The aortic arch descends on the right in approximately 25 percent of cases of tetralogy. Pulmonary blood flow is decreased and pulmonary vascular markings are consequently diminished. The echocardiogram may show a dilated aortic root overriding the ventricular septum, but these findings are not diagnostic.

Coarctation of the Aorta

The commonest form of coarctation of the aorta seen in adults is *juxta ductal* (i.e., the stenosis occurs in the early part of the descending thoracic aorta at the approximate level of insertion of the ligamentum arteriosum either before or just after the takeoff of the left subclavian artery). The main pathophysiologic derrangement in coarctation of the aorta in adults is upper compartment hypertension. The blood pressure is elevated in the arms and distinctly decreased in the lower extremities. Coarctation of the aorta is three times more common in males. It occurs in 45 percent of children with XO Turner's syndrome (see Chapter 8).

The clinical manifestations of coarctation of the aorta include prominent arterial pulsations in the suprasternal notch, supraclavicular areas, and neck, and signs of left ventricular hypertrophy. The aortic component of the second sound is usually accentuated, and both systolic and diastolic murmurs may be present. A systolic ejection murmur initiated by an ejection sound is often heard maximally along the upper right sternal border and is due to an associated bicuspid aortic valve which occurs in 40 to 80 percent of all cases of coarctation. A mid to late systolic murmur that continues into diastole may be heard posteriorly over the spine and is thought to originate from the coarctation. Another continuous low frequency murmur may be appreciated over both lateral aspects of the thorax and is thought to result from collateral intercostal vessels. When these collaterals are well developed, their pulsations may be palpated in the intercostal spaces along the lateral aspects of the thorax. The diagnosis is confirmed by measuring at least a 30 mmHg systolic pressure gradient between the right upper arm and the lower extremity. Frequently lower extremity pulses are difficult to palpate, and in children one may have to resort to the "flush" method of measuring the blood pressure. Simultaneous palpation of the right radial and femoral pulses normally shows a simultaneous arrival of the pulse. In patients with coarctation of the aorta there is a distinct delay in the arrival of the femoral pulse; this has been called "radio-femoral pulse lag." This sign is almost as good as the blood pressure discrepancy in making the diagnosis of coarctation of the aorta.

The electrocardiogram in adolescents and adults with coarctation of the aorta reveals left ventricular hypertrophy with systolic overload (ST segment depression) and frequently left atrial abnormality. The chest radiograph may show subtle but characteristic features: left ventricular enlargement may be appreciated on the lateral projection. On the posteroanterior projection irregularities or notching of the inferior margins of the posterior ribs by tortuous collaterals is seen commonly in patients with hemodynamically significant coarctation. This sign, however, may be absent in early childhood and develops only after ten years of age. The proximal descending thoracic aorta and the aortic knob may show a "3" configuration, representing the coarctation site with proximal and distal dilatations. The echocardiogram may be useful by confirming the presence of left ventricular hypertrophy. In young children the coarctation may be visualized by two-dimensional echocardiography through the suprasternal notch. Coarctation of the aorta is usually well tolerated in later childhood and early adolescence by children who have survived infancy. Nevertheless, there is a small but finite annual mortality rate of 2 percent to age 20, and the mortality rate increases over the ensuing decades. The common complications of coarctation of the aorta are left ventricular failure, aortic rupture, infective endocarditis, and intracranial hemorrhage due to rupture of a frequently associated berry aneurysm.

The Eisenmenger Syndrome

Patients are said to have Eisenmenger's syndrome or Eisenmenger physiology or reaction if they have a shunt lesion in association with increased pulmonary vascular resistance which in turn causes reversal of the shunt. The Eisenmenger reaction develops in patients with atrial or ventricular septal defects, patent ductus arteriosus, and other more complex shunt lesions. It is caused by the development of pulmonary vascular obstructive disease which results in elevation of pulmonary arterial pressure and right ventricular hypertension. The stimulus for the development of pulmonary vascular obstructive disease is thought to be a combination of high flow and high pressure in the normally low pressure pulmonary circuit. In some patients with large left to right shunts, the initially high neonatal pulmonary vascular resistance may persist with early development of pulmonary vascular obstructive disease. The clinical manifestations of patients with the Eisenmenger syndrome are those of severe pulmonary hypertension with associated cyanosis, polycythemia, and clubbing. The clinical findings will vary somewhat according to what type of defect is present. Thus in patients with ventricular septal defect or patent ductus arteriosus and Eisenmenger physiology, the second sound tends to be single or narrowly split, whereas in Eisenmenger ASD patients persistence of the wide splitting of the second sound is often appreciated. The pulmonic component of the second sound is accentuated and frequently palpable along the upper left sternal border. In general, when pulmonary hypertension develops in this syndrome and reversal of the shunt takes place, the amount of blood shunted right to left is relatively small and murmurs may not be generated. Patients with patent ductus arteriosus with reversed shunting (right to left) will demonstrate differential cyanosis of the toes while the fingers retain normal color. The electrocardiogram usually shows signs of right ventricular hypertrophy as well as right atrial enlargement. The chest radiograph also shows signs of right ventricular enlargement in association with large central pulmonary arteries and sparse peripheral vascular markings. The hematocrit and hemoglobin values may reach remarkable levels especially in young adults; values between 65 and 75 percent are not uncommon.

THERAPY AND SEQUELAE

In general, treatment of congenital cardiac anomalies in early adult life is not particularly different from treatment of the same anomalies in childhood. Shunt lesions with left to right shunts of greater than two to one magnitude should be repaired surgically. A patent ductus arteriosus should be closed under almost all circumstances even if it is small, since the risk of surgery in this lesion is minimal and the risk of infective endarteritis considerable. Ventricular and atrial septal defects with small left to right shunts (pulmonic to systemic blood flow ratio of less than 1.5 to 1) if they are first discovered in adult life are probably best left alone with medical treatment of their complications. Considerable controversy exists as to the optimal management of shunt lesions of moderate magnitude.

Coarctation of the aorta should be repaired as early as possible, as it is now well recognized that the late incidence of cardiovascular complications in patients with coarctation is directly related to the age of repair. Thus in one study 20 percent of patients with coarctation operated after the age of 25 showed clinical evidence of cardiovascular disease as opposed to only 6 percent of patients who were operated before the age of 25.

Overall, approximately 80 percent of patients with congenital cardiac defects will benefit from currently available methods of surgery when these are properly applied. Cardiac dysfunction often persists in pa-

tients following surgery even among those with the best operative results. The undisputed value of palliative surgical treatment makes it all the more necessary for the clinician to be aware of its limitations. Table 16.11 lists a series of common congenital cardiac defects with residua, sequelae, and complications of surgical therapy.

When right or left ventricular failure develops as a result of a congenital cardiac abnormality, initial treatment is fairly standard. The use of digitalis glycosides, diuretics, and vasodilator agents usually affords modest relief of symptoms. Treatment of postoperative arrhythmias in patients with atrial septal defects may be difficult, but usually the arrhythmias subside over a period of time.

Patients with the Eisenmenger reaction are not surgical candidates. As a matter of fact, closure of the shunt in the face of pulmonary vascular obstructive disease may be deleterious and hasten the development of right heart failure. In general, patients who are markedly polycythemic should undergo phlebotomy. A reduction in the hematocrit improves blood flow through the capillaries and probably retards the development of in situ thromboses. Phlebotomies should be carried out to the individual's level of tolerance replacing the volume removed with saline. Generally the hematocrit should be maintained below 60 percent. Recurrent phlebotomies may induce an iron deficiency, in which case the judicious administration of supplemental iron is indicated.

Patients with severe pulmonary hypertension secondary to Eisenmenger physiology often develop hemoptysis and may die suddenly as a result. The mechanism of hemoptysis is variable, but pulmonary infarction is a common cause. In these patients, chronic anticoagulation may be of value in preventing future episodes of this complication.

CARDIAC ARRHYTHMIAS

A practical classification of arrhythmias follows and is summarized in Table 16.12.

DISTURBANCES OF IMPULSE FORMATION

Automaticity

Physiologic Alterations

Normal sinus rhythm. Under most physiologic circumstances, sinus nodal cells achieve threshold earliest during spontaneous diastolic depolarization and thereby retain control of the heart. The

Table 16.11   **Surgery for Congenital Heart Disease**

Defect	Residua	Sequelae	Complications

PDA	Persistent patency
	Recannalization
	Persistent endocarditis
	  susceptibility
	Pulmonary vascular
	  obstructive disease
		None	Recurrent laryngeal or
			  phrenic n. injury
			False aneurysm formation

ASD	Persistent atrial
	  communication
	Cardiomegaly. Mitral valve
	  abnormalities
		Post pericardiotomy
		  syndrome
		Arrhythmias
			None

VSD (normal PVR)	Persistent L–R shunt and
	  endocarditis susceptibility
		R. ventriculotomy. RBBB	Complete A–V block. AR.
			  TR

VSD (High PVR)	Persistent elevation of PVR	Polycythemia, cyanosis	Same

Coarctation	Persistent gradient
	Persistent hypertension despite
	  good anatomic repair (9%).
	Bicuspid Ao. valve (40–80%).
	  SBE susceptibility.
	Persistent LVH
		Stenosis L. subclavian
		  artery. Restenosis of
		  coarctation
			Spinal cord injury and
			  paraplegia

AS	Persistent gradient and SBE susceptibility Valvular calcification	Aortic insufficiency. Aneurysm at aortotomy site	None

TOF	Persistent VSD
	Persistent RV–PA gradient
	Obstruction of small
	  pulmonary arteries
		RBBB. PR. Ventriculotomy
		  scar. Outflow patch
		  aneurysm
			Complete A–V block.
			Sudden death

VPS	Persistent gradient Persistent RV hypertension and elevated RVEDP Persistent ASD	PR	None

TGA (Mustard procedure)	Dysfunction of systemic
	  ventricle (right)
		Arrhythmias. Obstruction of
		  SVC, IVC, or pulmonary
		  veins. TR
			None

Residua = remaining anatomic or hemodynamic abnormalities which existed as part of the congenital malformation.
Sequelae = anatomic or hemodynamic consequences of the operative procedure which are unavoidable at our current state of knowledge.
Complications = unexpected anatomic or hemodynamic events related to surgery.
PDA = patent ductus arteriosus. ASD = Atrial septal defect. VSD = ventricular septal defect. PVR = Pulmonary vascular resistance. AS = Aortic Stenosis. TOF = tetralogy of Fallot. VPS = Valvular pulmonic stenosis. TGA = transposition of great arteries. A–V = atrioventricular. RBBB = right bundle branch block. AR = aortic regurgitation. TR = tricuspid regurgitation. LVH = left ventricular hypertrophy. SBE = subacute bacterial endocarditis. RV = right ventricle. PA = pulmonary artery. PR = pulmonic regurgitation. RVEDP = right ventricular end-diastolic pressure. SVC = superior vena cava. IVC = inferior vena cava.

propagated impulse effectively "prematurely" depolarizes all other autorhythmic cells. The intrinsic rate of sinus autorhythmicity in the denervated human heart is approximately 100 impulses/minute. This intrinsic automatic rate is modulated by cholingergic and adrenergic influences.

Sinus bradycardia.   At rest, particularly in the physically fit individual, intrinsic vagal tone is high; the automatic discharge rate of sinus nodal cells is reduced; a rate of less than 50 impulses/minute called sinus bradycardia may occur. Beta-adrenergic blockade and administration of cardiac glycosides may also produce sinus bradycardia.

Sinus arrhythmia.   Many normal individuals, particularly at rest, have a fluctuating sinus rate, partially mediated through pulmonary stretch receptors to the sinus node producing a respirophasic waxing and waning of sinus rate (Fig. 16.17).

Sinus tachycardia   is a physiologic response to bodily stress (e.g., exercise, fright, and fever) that is mediated by vagal inhibition and sympathetic stimulation. These control mechanisms permit physiologic sinus tachycardia at times of stress to rates of approximately 190 beats/minute in adult man. The maximum heart rate decreases about 1 percent per year with age beyond 25 years.

Enhanced Automaticity

If the slope of diastolic depolarization in automatic fibers outside the S–A node becomes abnormally steep, these fibers may eventually take over the con-

Table 16.12   **Classification of Arrhythmias**

Classification	Clinical Examples
Disturbances of Impulse Information	
1. Automaticity	
a. Physiologic alterations	Sinus bradycardia, sinus tachycardia
b. Enhanced automaticity	Junctional tachycardia ventricular tachycardia
c. Depressed automaticity	Loss of one or more pacemakers
d. Normal automaticity as reserve mechanism	Escape beats
Disturbances of Impulse Conduction	
1. Simple conduction block	
a. Refractory tissue	Heart block; bundle branch block
b. Decremental conduction	Atrial fibrillation
2. Undirectional block and reentry	
a. In the A-V junction (functional longitudinal dissociation)	Supraventricular tachycardia
b. Local block and microreentry	Ventricular premature beats; ventricular tachycardia
Combined Disturbances of Impulse Formation and Conduction	
1. Ectopic rhythm with exit block	Supraventricular tachycardia with block
2. Fibrillation	Atrial fibrillation; ventricular fibrillation

trol of the atrial or ventricular excitation or both. Examples are junctional tachycardia and ventricular tachycardia. Factors that may lead to enhanced automaticity include decreased extracellular potassium, excess cardiac digitalis levels, and increased levels of circulating catecholamines.

Depressed Automaticity

This can occur either by itself or in association with disturbances of impulse conduction, especially bundle branch block.

Normal Automaticity as a Reserve Mechanism

Under normal circumstances automatic rates for areas other than the sinus node are approximately:

Zone	Rate
Atrial conduction tissue	55/min
Atrioventricular node	50/min
His-Purkinje system	35/min

With unusual degrees of sinus bradycardia, normally subservient autorhythmic cells may spontaneously depolarize first and become the dominant

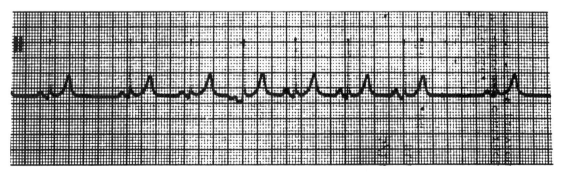

Fig. 16.17 The variation in the RR interval exceeds 0.16 sec. Increases and decreases in heart rate were recorded during inspiration and expiration, respectively. (In Laiken, N., Laiken, S.L., Karliner, J.S.: Interpretation of Electrocardiograms. A self-instructional approach. Appleton-Century-Crofts, New York, 1978, with permission.)

pacemaker zone. Similarly, a normally subservient automatic locus may become dominant if impulse propagation to this locus from a more rapid focus is impeded. These phenomena are termed "escape" mechanisms.

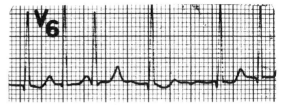

Fig. 16.18 Atrial fibrillation. Note normal QRS complexes at an irregularly irregular rate; no atrial activity is present. Coarse fibrillatory waves in leads 2,3 and aVF and in leads V1 and V2. (In Laiken, N., Laiken, S.L., Karliner, J.S.: Interpretation of electrocardiograms. A self-instructional approach. Appleton-Century Crofts, New York, 1978, with permission.)

DISTURBANCES OF IMPULSE
CONDUCTION

Simple Conduction Block

Refractory Tissue

Refractory tissue ahead of the advancing wave of excitation may occur at the junction of two fiber groups with dissimilar excitability or duration of refractoriness. The action potential becomes progressively prolonged from the atrial fibers through the atrioventricular (AV) node, His bundle and bundle branches, and to the more peripheral Purkinje fibers. Thus, at the junction of any two specialized conduction tissues, the distal fibers usually have a longer refractory period and may fail to respond to a higher frequency discharge of proximal fibers. Refractory tissue causing conduction may result from physiologic changes (increased vagal tone), drugs, (e.g., digitalis), or pathological abnormalities such as scar tissue.

Decremental Conduction

Normally, successful conduction through the AV node occurs with synchronous activation of fibers in the upper regions of the node such that a smooth excitation front invades the region. When the rate of depolarization (rate of rise of the initial phase of the action potential) is decreased and conduction is further slowed, particularly in the critical midregion of the AV node, the spread of excitation in this region becomes inhomogeneous. Such inhomogeneity of conduction could manifest itself as two or more functionally separate portions of tissue, some of which show relatively rapid conduction. Increasing decrement in all portions or in the slower conducting portions alone can cause further fractionation of the wave front, leading to failure of propagation. A common arrhythmia in which the phenomenon of decremental conduction helps to control the ventricular response is atrial fibrillation (Figs. 16.12, 16.18). The concept of decremental conduction is not confined to the AV node, and can occur in all portions of the conducting system.

Unidirectional Block and Reentry

In the A–V Junction

Functional longitudinal dissociation may occur within the A–V junction (Fig. 16.19) and is responsible for the production of reciprocal beating (repetitive supraventricular arrhythmias) (Fig. 16.20). Such inhomogeneous conduction is thought to occur as follows: There is slow but successful transmission of an impulse through one side of the A–V junction with a short refractory period (alpha pathway). The impulse then turns and reenters the opposite side of the A–V junction which had shown marked decrement or block to forward conduction but allows conduction of a retrograde impulse (beta pathway). This leads to a "circus" movement. With preexcitation (Wolff-Parkinson-White Syndrome Fig. 16.21), anatomic rather than functional separation occurs. Thus, impulses may be conducted antegrade through the accessory pathway and retrograde through the A–V junction or vice versa.

Local Block and Microreentry

The term *microreentry* implies a small geometric arrangement of the reentry pathway. Thus, local block and microreentry differ from functional longitudinal dissociation in the A–V node only by virtue of the anatomical, instead of functional, separation of two pathways conducting impulses in a forward and a retrograde fashion, respectively. Thus, in Figure 16.22, it can be seen that when an impulse spreads from point A, excitation proceeds normally in pathway AB, while propagation becomes slower and may finally be blocked in the depressed tissue X. The excitation invading X from the opposite direction

Functional Longitudinal
Dissociation

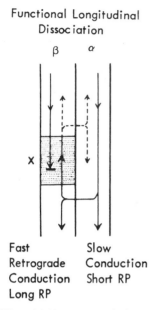

Fast
Retrograde
Conduction
Long RP

Slow
Conduction
Short RP

Fig. 16.19 Functional longitudinal dissociation in the atrio-ventricular junction. For details see text. (In Laiken, H., Laiken, S.L., Karliner, J.S.: Interpretation of electrocardiograms. A self-instructional approach. Appleton-Century-Crofts, New York, 1978, with permission.)

(C) may, however, be successful in traversing this depressed area and reexcite the originally depolarized fibers in pathway AB. A reentry circuit is thus formed.

The mechanism that prevents forward transmission of an impulse but permits subsequent retrograde

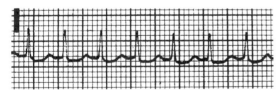

Fig. 16.20 Supraventricular tachycardia. The rate is regular and approximately 200/min. No atrial activity can be seen, but the QRS complexes are normal. Since this pattern could be produced by either atrial or junctional tachycardia, the arrhythmia can only be termed a supraventricular tachycardia. (In Laiken, N., Laiken, S.L., Karliner, J.S.: Interpretation of electrocardiograms. A self-instructional approach. Appleton-Century Crofts, New York, 1978, with permission.)

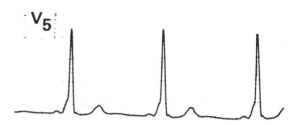

Fig. 16.21 Pre-excitation (Wolff-Parkinson-White syndrome). The PR interval is less than 0.12 sec. The QRS complex has an initial shoulder or delta wave, which causes the QRS interval to exceed 0.09 sec: (In Laiken, N., Laiken, S.L., Karliner, J.S. Interpretation of electrocardiograms. A self-instructional approach. Appleton-Century Crofts, New York, 1978, with permission.)

conduction through region X is most likely dissimilar degrees of decrement, resulting in unidirectional block. However, a longer duration of refractoriness in region X is an alternative mechanism. Local block and microreentry are important in the pathogenesis of many ventricular arrhythmias, such as ventricular

Local Block with Microreentry

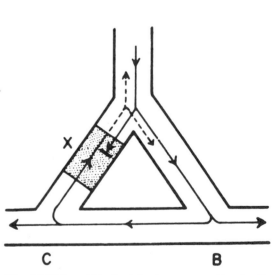

Fig. 16.22 Local block and microreentry. For details see text. (In Laiken, N., Laiken, S.L., Karliner, J.S.: Interpretation of electrocardiograms. A self-instructional approach. Appleton-Century Crofts, New York, 1978, with permission.)

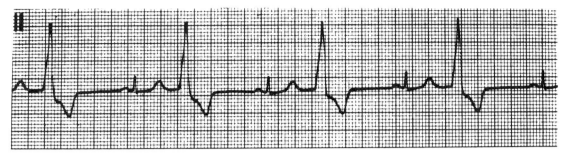

Fig. 16.23 Ventricular bigeminy. Fixed-coupled unifocal ventricular premature beats alternate with sinus beats. (In Laiken, N., Laiken, S.L., Karliner, J.S.: Interpretation of electrocardiograms. A self-instructional approach. Appleton-Century Crofts, New York, 1978, with permission.)

premature beats (Fig. 16.23) and ventricular tachycardia (Fig. 16.24).

COMBINED DISTURBANCES OF IMPULSE FORMATION AND CONDUCTION

Ectopic Rhythm with Exit Block

It is possible to have a dominant pacemaker focus exhibiting increased automaticity, in association with more distal conduction block. A classical example is supraventricular tachycardia with block that can result from excess levels of digitalis glycosides. In this instance, the digitalis both enhances automaticity in the atria (or internodal tracts) while causing increased refractoriness at the A–V junction.

Fibrillation

Fibrillation may affect both the atria and the ventricles. Fibrillation may not represent an isolated electrophysiologic entity, but may result from combinations of various mechanisms discussed above. It also appears reasonable to assume that the mechanisms that initiate the fibrillatory state and those sustaining this arrhythmia are not necessarily identical. Regarding the initiating mechanisms, three theories have classically been developed: (1) unifocal impulse formation, (2) multifocal impulse formation, and (3) reentry. Combinations are also possible.

In both clinical and experimental fibrillation, two modes of initiation have been identified. The first (Type A) is characterized by rapid onset of fibrillation with one or two premature systoles early in the repolarization phase of a previous excitation, while Type B shows a gradual development of disorganized excitation after a sustained period of tachycardia. Examples of ventricular fibrillation are shown in Figure 16.25.

ANTIARRHYTHMIC AGENTS

A convenient way to group antiarrhythmic drugs is into classes based on their electrophysiologic action:

Class I Local anesthetics. These drugs are quinidine, procainamide, lidocaine, diphenylhydantoin, and disopyramide.

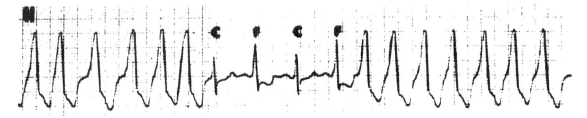

Fig. 16.24 Ventricular tachycardia with capture and fusion beats. The rate is slightly irregular but averages 135/min. While the wide and bizarre QRS complexes obscure the sinus P waves, evidence for independent atrial activity is provided by two capture beats (c) and two fusion beats (F). The fusion beat QRS complexes have a morphology that is intermediate between the normal QRS complex and the capture beats and the wide and bizarre QRS complex of the ventricular ectopic beats. (In Laiken, N., Laiken, S.L., Karliner, J.S.: Interpretation of electrocardiograms. A self-instructional approach. Appleton-Century Crofts, New York, 1978, with permission.)

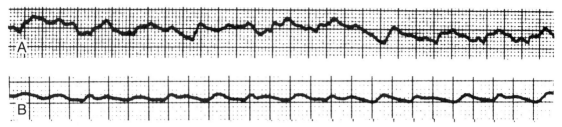

Fig. 16.25 Ventricular fibrillation. (A) The spread of impulses through the ventricles is represented by a series of rapid and irregular undulations. (B) In this rhythm strip the undulations have a somewhat finer appearance. (In Laiken, N., Laiken, S.L., Karliner, J.S.: Interpretation of electrocardiograms. A self-instructional approach. Appleton-Century Crofts, New York, 1978, with permission.)

Class II drugs produce arryhthmia suppression by blocking the effects of catecholamine stimulation of the myocardial cell, and this class encompasses all the beta-adrenergic blocking drugs.

Class III drugs share the common property of prolonging both the action potential duration and the effective refractory period of the myocardial cell, but unlike Class I drugs, they do not seem to affect resting membrane potential, rate of rise of Phase 0 of the action potential, conduction velocity, or membrane responsiveness. The drugs in this class are bretylium and amiodarone.

Class IV drugs are the so-called slow channel blocking drugs, which are selective calcium antagonists. Verapamil is the prototype drug in this class. Agents in this group produce their most profound effect in tissue in which slowly rising action potentials normally exist, such as the A–V node. Clinical use of these drugs has shown them to be effective in controlling ventricular response rates to supraventricular arrhythmias, presumably by the depressant effects on slow response potentials involved in A–V nodal conduction.

The most practical use of the classification system for the clinician occurs when therapy with two antiarrhythmic agents is required. Unpleasant side effects accompanying large doses of a single drug can sometimes be avoided by utilizing lower doses of two agents with the same electrophysiologic properties but with different side effects. A satisfactory electrophysiologic result can sometimes be achieved with two or more drugs acting in concert while the drug dose of the individual agent is low enough so that side effects are minimized. Combination therapy for arrhythmia suppression is more likely to be successful if drugs with different electrophysiologic properties are employed. However, the fact that two drugs are in the same class does not mean that they have identical electrophysiologic properties or side effects. It means only that the spectrum of major electrophysiologic effects is the same. Different subsidiary actions are possible and some drugs may possess extracardiac effects which alter the observed direct myocardial electrophysiologic effects.

The clinical pharmacology of commonly employed antiarrhythmic agents is summarized below. A number of aspects of adverse reactions associated with these agents require emphasis.

Quinidine

Fifteen to 20 percent of patients given oral quinidine in either the sulfate or gluconate dosage form develop gastrointestinal intolerance (nausea, vomiting, diarrhea) requiring discontinuation of this agent. The recently described elevation of serum digoxin among patients in whom quinidine therapy is initiated requires careful monitoring of serum digoxin levels in such individuals. Hypersensitivity reactions to quinidine manifest as fever, urticara, rash, and hematologic abnormalities, with thrombocytopenia being the most frequently reported. Prolongation of the QT_c interval may increase the possibility of reentrant ventricular arrhythmias and, in rare instances, lead to the development of "quinidine syncope" (i.e., ventricular tachycardia and fibrillation associated with quinidine therapy). Although quinidine is classified as a myocardial depressant, producing impaired left ventricular performance when the drug is used intravenously, under ordinary circumstances, oral administration of quinidine, even to patients with congestive cardiac failure, carries little if any risk of inducing clinically important left ventricular dysfunction.

Procainamide

Procainamide has the disadvantage that it must be given every four hours in order to obtain adequate drug levels and few patients can comply with such a regimen. However, a recently released sustained action preparation may obviate this difficulty. Effective therapy with procainamide is limited by the drug's ability to induce serologic abnormalities with chronic use and induction of a syndrome that resembles systemic lupus erythematosis. Most patients receiving more than 2 g of procainamide per day develop a positive antinuclear antibody test. Polyarthralgia, fever, and skin rashes may appear in up to one-third of patients maintained on chronic procainamide therapy in association with an abnormal serology. Under some circumstances, serum levels of procainamide may be lower than those of its active metabolite, N-acetylprocainamide. Patients receiving chronic therapy should be followed closely for evidence of drug-induced lupus and for agranulocytosis, which has also been reported.

Disopyramide

The major adverse reactions to dispyramide result from its anticholinergic properties. In men symptoms of prostatic obstruction may be exacerbated, and many patients complain of dry mouth and mild visual blurring. Patients with glaucoma are also at risk for the development of further increases in intraocular pressure when given this agent. Disopyramide therapy may be associated with worsening of congestive cardiac failure in up to 50 percent of patients with a history of cardiac decompensation. Unlike oral quinidine, this constitutes a relative contraindication to the use of this drug.

Lidocaine

Considerable experience with lidocaine suggests that this agent lacks significant cardiac toxicity. However, in patients with intraventricular conduction block and other conduction system disease, lidocaine may transiently increase conduction system disturbances and atrioventricular block has been reported. The major side effects of this agent involve the central nervous system: dizziness, drowziness, paresthesias, and euphoria are most frequently encountered at therapeutic lidocaine concentrations. Speech disturbances, confusion, excitement, and frank psychosis also occur, particularly in patients with previous central nervous system disease or in elderly individuals. Both petit mal and grand mal seizures with respiratory arrest and coma can accompany toxic drug levels.

Propranolol

The most commonly observed adverse reactions to beta-adrenergic blocking agents involve the central nervous system. These include generalized fatigue not due to worsening of congestive cardiac failure or to myocardial depression, emotional depression, and nightmares. Other reported adverse reactions include nausea, diarrhea, alopecia, impotence, increased peripheral vascular insufficiency, and alterations in glucose tolerance. Asthma and chronic pulmonary disease can be exacerbated by propranolol, and this drug is relatively contraindicated in such patients. However, "selective" $beta_1$ antagonists, if used cautiously, can on occasion be employed in such patients with relative safety. The cardiac actions of propranolol can result in worsening of congestive cardiac failure in patients dependent upon sympathetic nervous system tone for adequate cardiac function. Sudden propranolol withdrawal in some patients with angina pectoris has been associated with serious rebound phenomena including marked increase in the frequency of chest pain and, on occasion, myocardial infarction.

Verapamil

This agent is usually well tolerated if conditions that will amplify its pharmacologic effects are avoided, such as a high degree of unstable atrioventricular block, sick sinus syndrome, overt congestive cardiac failure, or marked hypotension. Caution should be observed in patients receiving propranolol and quinidine-like agents, as shock and asystole have been reported when these agents are used in combination with verapamil. After oral administration, approximately two percent of patients will complain of gastrointestinal disturbances; central nervous system symptoms, such as headache and dizziness, also occur.

Other Agents, Including Amiodarone

In patients refractory to one or a combination of the antiarrhythmic agents described above, a variety of other agents may be obtained by individuals at specialized centers, but these drugs are not yet available for general use. Among these agents are aprindine, tocainide, mexiletine, and amiodarone. Mexiletine and tocainide are particularly effective against ventricular arrhythmias, while aprindine may be used to treat both ventricular and supraventricular arrhythmias.

Amiodarone, a benzofurane derivative, may be effective therapy for the treatment of refractory supraventricular and ventricular arrhythmias. When given orally, its onset of action is several days and its half-life is prolonged (? several weeks). After a loading dose, usual maintenance regimens are 400–

800 mg daily for ventricular arrhythmias and 200 mg daily for supraventricular arrhythmias. The incidence of side effects increases with increasing dosage. Adverse reactions in decreasing order of incidence include corneal deposits, tremor, ataxia, bluish skin discoloration, hyper- and hypothyroidism, photosensitivity, elevation of hepatic enzymes and pulmonary fibrosis. The latter complication is sometimes fatal. Drug interactions include raised serum digoxin and chloroquine levels and an increased prothrombin time in patients receiving oral anticoagulants.

CHOICE OF AGENTS IN THE TREATMENT OF CARDIAC ARRHYTHMIAS

Supraventricular Arrhythmias

Reentrant Paroxysmal (AV Nodal) Tachycardia

Isolated premature contractions rarely require specific therapy. If they are bothersome, quinidine, procainamide, or disopyramide may be used. Patients with AV nodal reentrant paroxysmal tachycardia may often treat themselves using vagal maneuvers and can be taught to perform the Valsalva maneuver to abort the tachycardia. Other individuals have learned to employ carotid sinus massage. When attacks are infrequent, it is difficult to prescribe drug therapy and to be certain it is effective; however, when attacks are frequent and troublesome, propranolol or digoxin may be tried as initial therapy with the addition of one of the oral Class I antiarrhythmic agents if the initial approach is unsatisfactory. Generally, in patients with paroxysmal supraventricular tachycardia associated with preexcitation, one of the Class I agents or propranolol may be tried; if atrial fibrillation is not present, digoxin may also be attempted. For both AV nodal reentrant paroxysmal tachycardia and for paroxysmal supraventricular tachycardia associated with preexcitation, oral verapamil may also constitute effective therapy; in both these arrhythmias, intravenous verapamil is exceedingly effective. If either of these arrhythmias cause hemodynamic embarrassment, such as hypotension or pulmonary edema, immediate treatment with electrical cardioversion is indicated.

In some patients, a combination of bradyarrhythmia ("sick sinus syndrome") with a supraventricular tachyarrhythmia ("bradytachy syndrome") may occur. Under these circumstances, permanent pacemaker therapy along with oral antiarrhythmic treatment as described above is indicated.

Atrial Flutter

This arrhythmia often responds to small doses of DC synchronized countershock, such as 25 to 50 joules. Initially digoxin may be used to control the ventricular rate, after which quinidine administration is begun in order to convert the arrhythmia chemically; should this approach not work, cardioversion can then be used.

Atrial Fibrillation

Patients with atrial fibrillation of recent onset and those with small left atrial size can usually be converted to sinus rhythm with the use of DC synchronized electrical cardioversion. The dose required is generally 100 to 200 joules. Depending on the clinical circumstances, it is often necessary to maintain such patients on digoxin and quinidine, and these agents should be started before electrical cardioversion is attempted. In some patients, "chemical cardioversion" will occur; the usual sequence is to begin digoxin to control the ventricular response and then to add quinidine. The classical sequence of chemical cardioversion is for atrial fibrillation to be converted to atrial flutter and then to sinus rhythm. In the past it has been recommended that digoxin be withheld for one or more days prior to electrical cardioversion, but recent experience has indicated that if serum digoxin levels are below 3 ng/ml and the serum potassium is within normal limits, ventricular arrhythmias are unlikely to occur following elective cardioversion. Procainamide and disopyramide may be used instead of quinidine to maintain sinus rhythm. If digoxin alone is ineffective in controlling the ventricular response to the atrial fibrillation, propranolol may be added.

Patients with longstanding atrial fibrillation (> one year) and those with grossly enlarged left atria (left atrial dimension >50 mm by echocardiogram) tend not to remain in sinus rhythm, even if initial cardioversion is successful. In these individuals, chronic anticoagulation is indicated. Should the patient revert to atrial fibrillation, antiarrhythmic therapy, save for digoxin, should be discontinued, unless the treatment is being given for the control of ventricular ectopic beats.

Bradycardia and Heart Block

When profound sinus or junctional bradycardia or high-grade atrioventricular block is documented in patients with frank syncope or transient central nerv-

Table 16.13 Antiarrhythmic Therapy: Choice of Agents (USA)*

Arrhythmia	Therapy (In Order of Preference)
Supraventricular	
Atrial premature contractions	Quinidine, procainamide, disopyramide
Reentrant paroxysmal AV nodal tachycardia	Verapamil, propranolol, digoxin, Type I agent
Paroxysmal supraventricular tachycardia involving a bypass tract	Quinidine, procainamide, propranolol; avoid digoxin and verapamil in presence of atrial fibrillation or flutter
Atrial flutter	Cardioversion, digoxin, verapamil
Atrial fibrillation	Cardioversion, quinidine, procainamide, disopyramide (to maintain sinus rhythm) Digoxin, propranolol (to control ventricular response)
Ventricular	
Ventricular premature contractions	
Emergency	Lidocaine, procainamide, bretylium
Chronic	Quinidine, procainamide, disopyramide, combinations (see below); amiodarone
Tachycardia	Lidocaine, procainamide, bretylium, cardioversion
Digitalis-Induced	
Supraventricular or ventricular	Lidocaine (ventricular), diphenylhydantoin, propranolol

Combination Therapy for Suppression of Ventricular Ectopy
1. Quinidine—procainamide (for maximal quinidine-like effect at a lower dose for each agent)
2. Quinidine or procainamide with propranolol in patients without congestive heart failure
3. #1 above with lidocaine or diphenylhydantoin.

* As new drugs become available the order of preference may change.
(Adapted from Karliner, J. S., Gregoratos, G. (eds.): Coronary Care. Churchill Livingstone, New York, 1981.)

ous system symptoms (or even in the absence of symptoms), pacemaker implantation is indicated. Careful long-term follow-up should be undertaken, preferably at a pacemaker clinic. Recent advances in transtelephone monitoring make it feasible for patients to be followed even in rural or more remote areas. Pacemaker technology has progressed to the point where pulse generators may last as long as 10 years. In addition, versatility as to rate, pulse width, refractory period, and sensitivity settings has been enhanced with the advent of externally-programmable units.

Ventricular Arrhythmias

Ventricular Premature Beats and Ventricular Tachycardia

For emergency treatment of ventricular premature beats, intravenous lidocaine, procainamide, or bretylium may be used. These agents should also be employed in the treatment of ventricular tachycardia, and, if the tachycardia is refractory, cardioversion should be used. Electrical cardioversion is the treatment of choice for the treatment of ventricular fibrillation, but the use of bretylium is an alternative approach. For the chronic treatment of ventricular arrhythmias, quinidine, procainamide, disopyramide, and combinations of these agents may be used.

For example, for a maximal quinidine-like effect at a lower dose for each agent, a combination of quinidine and procainamide may be employed. These agents may also be employed along with propranolol in patients without congestive cardiac failure. In many instances of ventricular arrhythmias refractory to the above agents, amiodarone has been of benefit. It should be noted that the indications for the treatment of ventricular ectopic beats in outpatients are not well defined. It seems clear that in patients with chronic ischemic heart disease increasing complexity of ventricular arrhythmias is associated with a higher incidence of sudden death, but there is yet no proof that prophylactic antiarrhythmic therapy will prevent such occurrences.

The choice of antiarrhythmic agents is summarized in Table 16.13.

REFERENCES

1. Hurst, J.W., (ed): The Heart. McGraw Hill Book Co., New York, 5th ed. 1982.
2. Karliner, J.S., Gregoratos, G.: Coronary Care. Churchill Livingstone, New York, 1981.
3. Zelis, R.: Calcium-blocker therapy for unstable angina pectoris. N. Eng. J. Med. 306:926, 1982.
4. Doherty, James, E.: The digoxin-quinidine interaction. Ann. Rev. Med. 33:163, 1982.

5. Stollerman, G.H.: Global strategies in group A streptococcol diseases and strategies for their prevention. Adv. Int. Med. 27:373, 1982.

6. Swan, H.J.C., Ganz, W.: Measurement of right atrial and pulmonary arterial pressures and cardiac output: Clinical application of hemodynamic monitoring. Adv. Int. Med. 27:953, 1982.

7. Cohn, Jay, N.: Vasodilator therapy of congestive heart failure. Adv. Int. Med. 26:293, 1981.

8. Hunt, S.A., Stinson, E.B.: Cardiac transplantation. Ann. Rev. Med. 32:213, 1981.

9. Weisfeldt, M.L., Chandra, W.: Physiology of cardiopulmonary resuscitation. Ann. Rev. Med. 32: 435, 1981.

17

DISORDERS OF THE BLOOD AND RETICULOENDOTHELIAL SYSTEM

Scott N. Swisher, M.D.

The practice of hematology is commonly but erroneously regarded as primarily a laboratory-based discipline. Patients with disorders of the hematopoietic system require exactly the same clinical approach as do patients with illnesses involving any other organ system. A carefully obtained and analyzed base of information derived from skilled use of the technics of interviewing and physical examination is essential in guiding the further study of all patients. Although the role of the laboratory is important in hematology, it does not substitute for the classical clinical information about the patient.

HEMATOLOGICAL LABORATORY TESTS

Sometimes blood disorders are first discovered through routine hematological studies. These studies usually include enumeration of white blood cells (WBC), red cells (RBC), measurement of the packed volume of red cells (hematocrit, Hct or PCV), hemoglobin (Hgb) concentration, enumeration of the proportion (percentage) of the leukocytes in the various categories of cell types from examination of a Wright's stained blood film. The latter is the differential leukocyte count. The cell types normally present among the neutrophils include the polymorphonuclear neutrophil (pmn), eosinophil (eos.), basophil (baso), monocyte (mono), and lymphocyte (lymph). Because only one or two hundred cells are routinely identified in the differential leukocyte count, there is a substantial variability in these percentages (Table 17.1).

Frequently, these data are supplemented by calculation of the red cell indices mean corpuscular volume (MCV), mean corpuscular hemoglobin (MCH), and mean corpuscular hemoglobin concentration (MCHC). These data are usually provided by automated blood cell counting equipment. In some laboratories, a count of the blood platelets is routinely done, again usually by electronic means.

The usually available data of a routine blood examination ("CBC" or Complete Blood Count) are summarized in Table 17.1 along with generally accepted normal limits for these measurements. Figure 17.1 shows an example of a laboratory report form for these data which has been generated by an automated blood cell counter. The differential leukocyte count reported on this form and the comments on platelet numbers and red cell morphology are done by a technician employing a stained blood film examined microscopically. Automated systems for performance of differential leukocyte counts are being introduced into clinical laboratory practice.

For many purposes, a skilled clinical hematologist could rely on a measure of Hct or Hgb and a *personal* examination of a well-stained blood smear. Most of the other information provided in numerical form can be routinely estimated with clinically useful precision by careful examination of the blood smear. Unfortunately, this skill is being lost by modern clinicians who rely increasingly on laboratories to provide these services. It is strongly recommended that medical students, house officers and fellows make a practice of going to the laboratory, examining the blood films of all their patients and learning these important skills with the help of people available in most laboratories. The information available from the blood smear is always much enhanced by knowledge of the patient's illness obtained previously from the history and physical examination.

Table 17.1   Normal Values of the Peripheral Blood of Adults

		Range
White Blood Cells		$4.8-10.8 \times 10^3$/cu. mm.
Red Blood Cells		
Male		$4.7-6.1 \times 10^3$/cu. mm.
Female		$4.2-5.4 \times 10^3$/cu. mm.
Hemoglobin Concentration		
Male		14–18 gm./dl.
Female		12–16 gm./dl.
Red Cell Indices		
Mean Corpuscular Volume		
Male		$80-94\mu^3$
Female		$81-99\mu^3$
Mean Corpuscular Hemoglobin		
Both Sexes		$27-31\mu\mu$ gm./cell
Mean Corpuscular Hemoglobulin Concentration		
Both Sexes		32–36%
Reticulocyte Count		0.5–1.5%
Platelet Count		$150-400 \times 10^3$/cu. mm.
Differential Leukocyte Count	%	Absolute Numbers/cu. mm.
Neutrophils		
Segmented Cells	50–75	2500–7500
Band Forms	2–6	100–600
Lymphocytes	20–44	1000–4400
Monocytes	2–9	100–900
Eosinophils	1–5	50–400
Basophils	0–2	0–200

Data given for WBC, RBC, hemoglobin, hematocrit and red cell indices are based upon normals determined by an automated blood cell counter (Coulter Electronics). Data given for leukocyte differential counts are after Hyun, et. al.

INTERPRETATION OF HEMATOLOGICAL TESTS

It is important to have a clear conception of normalcy as applied to clinical laboratory results, that is the statistical interval which will contain 95 percent of the individuals from a population defined as normal. In general, the 5 percent of values which lie outside the statistical normal range but which are nevertheless normal lie quite close to the upper or lower interval value. Values which are substantially higher or lower than normal can be assumed to be abnormal in most instances.

Blood values related to the red cells are also affected by sex. At the time of puberty hemoglobin, hematocrit, and red cell count rise to levels significantly higher in males than in females. These systematic differences persist at least until very late life. Furthermore, prior to the onset of maturity all blood cell values are influenced by age. Infants and very young children have normal values for both the red cells and white cells which differ markedly from those which are normal in later life.

White blood cell counts, hemoglobin or hematocrit values and platelet counts that lie just above or just below the range defined as normal may be interpreted better if previous values are known. If they were closer to the middle of the normal range,

slightly high or slightly low values could then be interpreted as a change from a presumed normal prior state, and the value under consideration could be regarded as abnormal. Known prior blood values, preferably obtained during a period of apparent good health, are thus of great value in interpreting values encountered during the study of a patient for an apparent disease process.

Blood values may vary slightly in differing geographic areas and between various ethnic groups. In areas where the altitude is significantly above sea level, usually above 5,000 feet, values for red cells may be higher than those encountered in lower altitudes. Similarly, somewhat lower normal values than those found in Caucasian populations are found in black populations in the United States. In parts of the world with common disorders, such as hookworm infestation, malaria, and dietary iron deficiency, it may be difficult to establish truly normal values and to identify a truly "healthy" normal population. In these instances, values extrapolated from areas where similar healthy populations do exist may be the most appropriate reference.

Normal values also depend to some extent upon the measuring methods used in a laboratory. Although it is beyond the scope of this chapter to discuss these methods in any detail, they are well described in a number of current textbooks of clinical

| TECH: |
| CHARGE: |
| DATE: |

□ REPEAT □ EMERGENCY □ PRE-OP □ ROUTINE

DATE REQUIRED | NURSE

□ ALL □ RBC □ WBC □ CBC

□ HCT □ HGB □ DIFF

	TEST	NORMAL VALUES COULTER COUNTER*
•	WBC × 10³	M 4.8–10.8 F 4.8–10.8
•	RBC × 10⁶	M 4.7–6.1 F 4.2–5.4
•	HGB g/dl	M 14–18 F 12–16
•	HCT %	M 42–52 F 37–47
•	MCV μ³	M 80–94 F 81–99
•	MCH μμg	M 27–31 F 27–31
•	MCHC %	M 32–36 F 32–36

DIFFERENTIAL		MORPH	1	2	3	4
SEG		POLYCHROM				
BAND		HYPOCHROM				
LYMPH		POIK				
MONO		TARGET				
EOSIN		SPHERO				
BASO		ANISO				
ATYP LYMPH		MICRO				
META		MACRO				
MYELO		SICKLE CELLS				
PROS		BASO STIP				
OTHER		VACUOLES				
TOTAL CELL COUNT		TOXIC GRAN				
NRBC/100 WBC						
NORMAL RBC						
PLATELET EST.	NORM	INC.	DEC.			

1 - SLIGHT BUT SIGNIFICANT
2 - MODERATE
3 - MOD TO MARKED
4 - MARKED

COMMENTS (OTHER):

Fig. 17.1 Report form, automated blood analyzer

pathology. Many laboratories now employ automated methods for determining white blood cell count, the red cell related measurements, and platelet counts. In some laboratories, automated methods for performing the differential leukocyte count are also employed. Ideally, every laboratory would define its own normal reference values. This is infrequently done. At the very least, laboratories must carry out quality control procedures to ensure that whatever procedure is being used is, in fact, giving accurate reproducible results.

RELATIVE AND ABSOLUTE BLOOD CELL COUNTS

Although the reticulocyte count and the differential leukocyte count are commonly reported in percentages, it is very useful to convert these to absolute counts. Normally, reticulocytes make up approximately 1 percent of the red cells based upon the life span of red cells of about 120 days in the circulation. If the red cell count is 5×10^6/cu mm, this is equivalent to approximately 50,000 reticulocytes/cu mm. On the average, there are about 60,000 reticulocytes per cu mm normally. On the other hand, in a case of moderately severe anemia where the red blood cell count is 2.5×10^6/cu mm, 1 percent is equivalent only to 25,000/cu mm, an abnormally low value. This calculation should be made in all cases where any degree of anemia is encountered. A more elaborate calculation can be employed, the red cell production index, but this refinement provides little additional useful information.

In the case of the differential leukocyte count, it is important to know the absolute number of neutrophil leukocytes/cu mm, particularly in patients who are leukopenic. If the white blood cell count is 7,500/cu mm and there are 60 percent neutrophil leukocytes, including the few relatively immature forms normally present, the absolute neutrophil count is approximately 4,500/cu mm, a normal value. In situations where the total granulocyte count is low, there is an increasing hazard of infection when the absolute neutrophil count falls below about 1,000/cu mm. The lower limit of normal total granulocytes is about 1,500/cu mm. This simple calculation of absolute neutrophil count should be made in every instance where the total white cell count or the proportion of neutrophils is found to be below the lower limit of normal.

INTERPRETATION OF THE BLOOD SMEAR

In addition to the differential leukocyte count, much more information is available from a careful examination of the blood smear. The erythrocytes are evaluated for hemoglobin content (hypochromia or normochromia), variability in size (anisocytosis or aniso), shape (poikiloytosis or poik), abnormal pigmentation (punctate basophilia, Howell-Jolly bodies), and the proportion of erythrocytes showing diffuse basophilia (polychromasia). The degree of red cell polychromasia reflects the number of new red cells in the circulation; this is more directly measured by the reticulocyte count (retic) in which the diffuse basophilic material is precipitated and stained by a supravital dye, such as New Methylene Blue. Although these observations will be correlated to some degree with the calculated red cell indices, it is important to know if the red cell size varies widely from very large macrocytic cells to very small microcytic forms; if this were the case, the mean value for red cell size might be nearly normal. Similarly, marked variation in the shape and an estimate of the average hemoglobin per cell as well as variations in hemoglobin per red cell are of importance. These data may reflect abnormalities of red cell production or destruction.

The leukocyte population, particularly the neutrophils, should be examined for size, shape, and nuclear configuration. In normal blood smears, between two and three lobes of the nucleus are found in the average neutrophil. In inflammatory conditions, not only does the total number and thus the proportion of neutrophils commonly rise, but the cells become less mature as new leukocytes are delivered to the circulation from the bone marrow. The latter is referred to as "shift to the left" and is manifest by a decrease in the number of nuclear lobes per cell. So-called "band-form" neutrophils are found which have a single ribbon like nucleus. Even less mature forms, the neutrophil metamyelocytes with bean-shaped nuclei may appear. In addition, the cytoplasm of neutrophils in severe bacterial infections may show the appearance of tiny black to purple flecks of granulation, the "toxic" granulations. In some instances, areas of residual blue staining cytoplasm, the so-called Doehle bodies are seen. The latter finding is associated with relatively severe infection. Because problems of infection are very common in medical practice, these abnormalities of the leukocytes are frequently encountered.

The lymphocytes are ordinarily relatively uniform in size, shape, nuclear configuration and nucleus to cytoplasm ratio. The predominant lymphoid cells are small lymphocytes with scanty cytoplasm. However, in response to a number of viral infections, the lymphocytes may become more variable in size and shape with notching and indentation of the nucleus, the appearance of purple granules in the cytoplasm, and an increase in large lymphoid cells with more open nuclear structure. These findings, termed a lymphatic reaction, are most pronounced in the disorder infectious mononucleosis.

An increase in blood eosinophils is not infrequent due to the prevalence of allergic disorders in North American populations. An increase in basophil leukocytes is rare in other than the myeloproliferative disorders, and its presence should always be regarded as abnormal. The number of blood monocytes/cu mm varies quite widely in normal individuals and when elevated commonly implies recovery from a recent bacterial infection if the monocytes present are all mature.

Disorders of hemostasis are considered in Chapter 4; however, assessment of platelets will be discussed here. With only moderate experience, the number of platelets present can be usefully estimated if the smear is examined over a large part of its area under relatively low power. Very low platelet counts, those below 20,000/cu mm, can be quite easily recognized, as can significant increases in the platelet count, those over 1 million/cu mm. Somewhat more experience is required to distinguish between normal values of platelet count and decreased numbers in the neighborhood of 100,000/cu mm to 50,000/cu mm.

The platelets should also be examined for their morphology with attention to their size, granulation, and degree of aggregation. Newly produced platelets tend to be larger than average. These have been referred to as "shift" platelets; an increased number of such platelets may indicate an increased rate of platelet destruction and production. Similarly, platelets nearing the end of their life span in the circulation tend to be small with the granules remaining tightly clumped in the center. Since the hemostatic function of newly released platelets is greater than that of aged platelets, it is important to evaluate this finding on the blood smear in situations where the platelet count is low. Significant clinical bleeding is not common when the platelet count is reduced (but still above 20,000/cu mm) particularly if a substantial proportion of the platelets that remain are young, newly released forms.

EXAMINATION OF THE BONE MARROW

The bone marrow can be safely and conveniently examined. Prior to the development of small trephines which permit the removal of a core of bone and bone marrow, this examination was limited to cells which could be aspirated freely from a puncture of the bone marrow cavity. At present, both techniques are employed in virtually every examination. Stained smears of bone marrow cells permit evaluation of the proportion of several marrow cell groups and their morphology. Core biopsy specimens, which are sectioned and stained like other tissue biopsy materials, permit evaluation of the cellularity of the bone marrow, the uniformity of the marrow cell population from area to area, and detection of abnormal focal collections of hematopoietic cells or cells foreign to the marrow such as metastatic tumor. Special examinations such as electron microscopy, histochemical staining, and immunological reactions may also be performed upon specific indication from samples obtained from the marrow. A variety of microbiological cultures of the bone marrow may also be carried out; this procedure, however, appears to be of less value than previously thought if carefully obtained repeated blood cultures have been done.

In most instances, the findings of the bone marrow examination are predictable after careful evaluation of the peripheral blood, except in an early leukemic disorder which has not yet appeared in the peripheral blood, a granulomatous disease involving the bone marrow, a storage disease or a lymphoma or metastatic tumor. The examination of the bone marrow is therefore not a routine procedure necessary to evaluate or manage every patient with a hematological disorder. Its simplicity and safety have probably lead to its overuse.

Commonly a differential count of two to five hundred bone marrow cells is carried out as part of a bone marrow examination. This is done by examining and identifying sequentially encountered cells of the bone marrow in a well-stained and representative area of a bone marrow aspiration smear. Statistical variability is reduced by counting more cells. A representative set of normal values for this type of examination is given in Table 17.2. As in the case of the differential peripheral blood leukocyte count, only a part of the significant information obtained from the bone marrow examination is conveyed by a differential cell count. Of greater importance is careful evaluation of the stained marrow slides of the aspiration and histologically sectioned material by an experienced observer. The normality of the several cell types involved, the orderly progression of the maturation of both the myeloid and the erythroid series, the presence of abnormal cells such as those characteristic of the lipid storage diseases, metastatic tumor and elements of granulomas, and the quantative and qualitative characteristics of the lymphoreticular cells also found in the normal bone marrow should be evaluated.

An important observation in the bone marrow examination is the ratio of developing myeloid cells to erythroid cells of the normoblast series. Normally this ratio ranges from two to four myeloid cells to one cell of the erythroid series. This reflects the more rapid formation and delivery of myeloid cells, particularly the granulocytes, which have relatively short life spans in the circulation compared to the 120 day life span of a newly released red cell. If either the erythroid or the myeloid series of cells is hy-

Table 17.2 **Normal Values for Bone Marrow Differential Cell Count of Adults**

Cell Type	Range in Percent
Undifferentiated cells	0.0
Myeloblasts	0.0–3.5
Promyelocytes	0.5–8.0
Myelocytes	
Neutrophil	7.0–34.6
Eosinophil	0.3–3.0
Basophil	0.0–0.5
Metamyelocytes and band cells	
Neutrophil	20.0–45.0
Eosinophil	0.3–3.7
Basophil	0.0–0.3
Segmented cells	
Neutrophil	7.0–25.0
Eosinophil	0.1–3.0
Basophil	0.0–1.0
Pronormoblasts	0.1–3.5
Basophilic normoblasts	1.7–5.5
Polychromatic normoblasts	5.0–20.0
Orthochromic normoblasts	5.0–23.8
Megakaryocyte series	0.05–1.2
Histiocytes	0.3–2.6
Monocytic series	0.1–3.2
Lymphocyte series	2.5–25.0
Plasmacyte series	0.1–1.2

Modified from R. P. Custer: An Atlas of the Blood and Bone Marrow. 2nd edition. Philadephia, W. B. Saunders Company, 1974.

poplastic or hyperplastic relative to the other, it will generally be found that this is correlated with relative hypo or hyper activity of marrow cell formation. In general, pancytopenic states are associated with hypoplastic bone marrow samples in which less than 10 percent of a core biopsy sample of bone marrow is found to be cellular, in the absence of infiltration with abnormal cells. Hypocellularity of the normoblastic series of cells is usually accompanied by a low absolute reticulocyte count. Conversely, in all but a very few instances, a hyperplastic normoblastic series in the marrow will be associated with a high reticulocyte count both absolutely and proportionately. Since there is effectively no technique equivalent to the reticulocyte count for the identification and counting of newly delivered granulocytes, it is difficult to establish a useful correlation of the degree of marrow cellularity of these precursors with the granulocyte count. A hyperplastic myeloid series of cells is generally associated with neutrophilia, some degree of shift to the left and the presence of neutrophil band forms and metamyelocytes in the peripheral blood.

Aspiration and core biopsies of the bone marrow are usually obtained from the posterior superior region of the iliac bone. This site has the advantage of easy accessibility, a relatively large marrow cavity, little possibility of injury to adjacent organs and greater patient acceptance. Many other anatomical sites have been employed and can be used under special circumstances. These include the upper one centimeter of the sternum below the sternal angle, the anterior superior spine of the ilium, sites along the anterior iliac crest, and the lumbar vertebral processes. Since most disorders of the bone marrow are diffuse in nature, a biopsy from any site is very likely to be representative of the marrow in general. However, in certain disorders, multiple biopsies from different sites may be useful. If the bone marrow as a whole is severely hypoplastic, several biopsies may be necessary to demonstrate this. Carcinomas metastatic to bone marrow, lymphomas and occasionally granulomas and the neoplastic plasma cells of multiple myeloma may not be uniformly distributed within the marrow. Equivocal diagnostic findings may then be encountered. Normal marrow occasionally may be aspirated from one site with the disease process demonstrable in other aspirates. Multiple aspirations are not commonly needed for diagnostic purposes, but if the clinical situation strongly suggests involvement of the marrow and a normal examination is found from one site, a second aspiration from another site is well justified.

LYMPH NODE BIOPSIES

The diagnosis of a number of disorders of the hematopoietic system, particulary the neoplastic diseases of the lymphoreticular system, depends upon lymph node biopsies. Persistent lymphadenopathy confined to one group of lymph nodes or generalized adenopathy may justify a lymph node biopsy if diagnostic findings are not present in the peripheral blood or bone marrow. A lymph node biopsy is of great value in establishing the appropriate classification of lymphomas according to the several modern classification systems; this classification frequently provides both diagnostic and prognostic information and guidance in the selection of treatment. In most cases in which there is diffuse lymphadenopathy, there is little urgency about early biopsy. However, in cases where only a single enlarged and clearly abnormal lymph node is present, an early biopsy may be of clinical importance, especially if Hodgkin's disease is discovered. This is particularly true of a single enlarged lymph node or a group of enlarged lymph nodes in the lower cervical region, which may be a manifestation of stage I Hodgkin's disease (where there is a high probability of curability). In general, lymph nodes which enlarge rapidly

are tender, have overlying redness and edema and are associated with inflammatory diseases; a localized regional source of infection should be sought. Diffuse lymphadenopathy associated with a febrile illness may reflect a systemic viral infection and does not require biopsy if other clinical evidence also favors this diagnosis. However, a group of enlarged lymph nodes in one anatomical region, which is not explainable on the basis of local infection and which remains enlarged or slowly increases in size over several weeks, justifies biopsy in most instances. It should be pointed out that occasionally lymph nodes involved with lymphoma or metastatic cancer will be tender and exhibit some inflammatory phenomena in the overlying tissue. Thus the presence of these signs should not defer biopsy if other evidence points to the presence of neoplastic disease.

In virtually all instances, a lymph node biopsy should be carried out by surgical removal. Biopsy of inguinal nodes should be avoided if other nodes are available; chronic and recurrent infections of the feet commonly result in changes in the histology of these nodes making their interpretation difficult. In the laboratory, material should be set aside for culture and possible immunological, immunochemical and histochemical studies.

The pathological examination and interpretation of lymph nodes is among the most difficult of all problems in surgical pathology. An accurate diagnosis and classification can be made only with the very best preparation of properly fixed tissue, sectioned as thin as possible and carefully stained. Inadequately prepared material is, in most instances, better ignored than interpreted. It is frequently better judgment to rebiopsy nodes, if available, than to risk interpretation of inadequately prepared material.

Lymph Node Aspiration Biopsies

It is possible to remove small numbers of cells for cytological examination from enlarged lymph nodes by obtaining core biopsies with a needle. Whereas these procedures avoid a surgical biopsy, they are very much inferior for diagnostic purposes and there is little to recommend them. Aspiration biopsies of a node to obtain material for microbiological cultures may be justified in certain circumstances. Similarly, in the presence of known malignant disorders such as breast, lung, or gastric cancer, an aspiration biopsy of a regional lymph node may be adequate to demonstrate the presence of metastatic tumor. This procedure, however, should be employed only when there are quite specific contraindications for an open surgical biopsy of the node.

OTHER DIAGNOSTIC PROCEDURES EMPLOYED IN HEMATOLOGY

It is possible to biopsy the enlarged spleen by an aspiration technique. This procedure is now rarely used because the diagnostic findings may not be sufficiently specific and there is a significant risk of subcapsular hemorrhage, particularly in patients who are thrombocytopenic or have other hemostatic abnormalities.

Liver biopsy, employing a needle which removes a core of liver tissue, is also of use in the study of some patients with hematological disorders. It may be useful in demonstrating metaplastic foci of hematopoiesis in myeloid metaplasia. Liver biopsies also may be useful in demonstrating the presence or absence of hepatic involvement in patients with malignant lymphomas.

A wide range of specific biochemical, immunochemical and physiological procedures of use in evaluating patients with hematological disorders will be discussed in relation to the specific disease entities where they are useful.

ANEMIA

Although anemia is commonly defined in terms of one of the concentration measurements of red cells (the hemoglobin, hematocrit, or red blood cell count), a more physiologically significant definition is based upon the patient's total body red cell mass. Total body red blood cell mass can be measured directly by the infusion of a known volume of red blood cells carrying a measurable radioactive tag such as ^{51}Cr. This measurement is cumbersome, time consuming,

and cannot be repeated more than a few times within a matter of weeks or months because of the rise in radioactive background count caused by the earlier measurements. Therefore, normal values for red blood cell mass are usually estimated based upon body weight, with 26–33 ml/kg and 22–29 ml/kg being considered normal for men and women respectively. The plasma volume, normally 35–45 ml/kg is the other variable in determining the total blood volume. It also can be measured directly but with somewhat less accuracy. Most labelled materials used to measure the plasma volume redistribute relatively rapidly to the extravascular volume resulting in imprecision of the measurement. Plasma volumes can be estimated reasonably accurately in normal circumstances by the following equation: body weight in kg × 39 = plasma volume in ml. The whole body hematocrit is lower than the venous hematocrit; it averages about .91 × venous hematocrit in percent.

Figure 17.2 illustrates the relationship between total blood volume, red cell mass and plasma volume under a number of normal and abnormal circumstances. The area of the rectangle enclosed by the heavy line indicates the blood volume; the red cell mass is shown in the shaded section of the rectangle. The hematocrit is indicated by the height of the shaded section of the rectangle. Assuming a normal hematocrit of approximately 45 percent, it can be seen in A that a sudden contraction of total blood volume as in acute hemorrhage may leave the hematocrit essentially unchanged for a period of time until additional plasma volume can be developed from extravascular water, electrolytes and proteins. When the blood volume has returned to normal by this physiological process of hemodilution or as a result of infusion of water and electrolyte, the hematocrit will have fallen, although the remaining red cell mass will be unchanged. By contrast, if the plasma volume is contracted as in B with the red cell

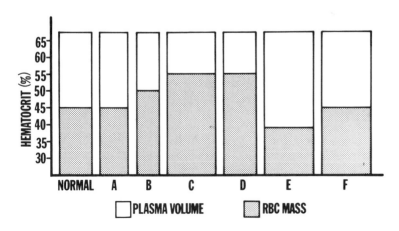

Fig. *17.2* Relationship between blood volume, red cell mass, plasma volume and hematocrit. Changes in the width of the bars reflect changes in blood volume. See text for interpretation of the several bars.

mass remaining normal, the hematocrit will rise sometimes to abnormal values. This is a situation referred to as spurious polycythemia. Expansion of red blood cell mass, even with some expansion of total blood volume as in C, generally results in elevation of the hematocrit as in polycythemia rubra vera. In a variety of disorders leading to chronic hypoxemia, such as residence at high altitude, the red cell mass may rise without appreciable expansion of the total blood volume and a very high hematocrit may be achieved as in D. When the plasma volume increases, as in the third trimester of pregnancy, the blood volume increases, the red cell mass remains approximately the same, there is a decrease in the hematocrit and the appearance of spurious anemia if evaluated only by measures of red cell concentration as in E. Finally, it is theoretically possible, as illustrated in F, that both the plasma volume and the red cell mass may expand proportionately with a rise in total blood volume and an unchanged hematocrit, a situation uncommonly encountered in clinical medicine.

From Figure 17.2, one can appreciate that concentration measurements of red blood cells do not always directly reflect the measurement of greatest physiological importance, red blood cell mass. This is particularly true in cases of acute blood loss which tend to be occult or underestimated, when there has been significant loss of plasma volume due to dehydration or exudative loss, or where the plasma volume is increased. It is only by a comprehensive evaluation of the patient that a reasonable estimate of the red blood cell mass can be made from concentration measurements.

INCIDENCE OF ANEMIA

Anemia, usually of relatively mild degree, is a common finding in clinical practice. This reflects the coincidence of anemia with a wide variety of other disorders. Disorders such as chronic renal insufficiency, chronic infections, chronic inflammatory disorders such as rheumatoid arthritis, and metastatic malignancies fall in this category of anemia secondary to another disease. Anemias due primarily to disorders of the hematopoietic system itself are much less common. One of the first tasks in the evaluation of the anemic patient is to decide whether the anemia is most probably a manifestation of a known or unknown primary illness, or whether it is a manifestation of an abnormality of the hematopoietic system or due to red cell loss or hemolysis. The rational management of the patient with anemia depends upon a precise diagnosis of the cause and mechanism of the anemic state. There is no place in the modern practice of medicine for empirical treatment of the anemic patient. Indeed, in many instances, empirical treatment can be shown to influence adversely the patient's long-term welfare by concealing an important primary diagnosis at a time when it might be treated definitively. For example, empirical administration of iron therapy to a patient with unrecognized slow gastrointestinal bleeding due to a carcinoma of the right side of the colon may well delay the diagnosis and surgical treatment of this potentially curable disease. Similarly, the simultaneous administration of large doses of vitamin B-12 and folic acid may make it difficult or impossible to establish the specific deficiency state which the patient presents and prevent a more rational program of treatment which may be necessary for the patient's remaining life.

The exact incidence of anemia is difficult to determine in the American population as a whole or among so-called "average" patients presenting themselves for health care. It is clear that the incidence of true anemia varies substantially from area to area in the country, depending upon the socioecomonic and demographic factors of a given patient population.

An aphorism which has withstood the test of time directs the physician to search for more than a single cause of anemia in the individual patient. Even though another reasonable explanation for a patient's anemia may be present, occult gastrointestinal bleeding should be searched for in every such patient. This is true even in patients who have obvious blood loss from one source, such as excessive uterine bleeding. At times a disorder of hemostasis results in significant bleeding from preexisting gastrointestinal lesions which might not otherwise result in significant blood loss. Patients with primary disorders of the bone marrow, such as hypoplastic states, may become severely anemic with even minor simultaneous gastrointestinal blood loss, since the bone marrow may be unable to compensate for the lost erythrocytes. If the gastrointestinal blood loss can be readily controlled, this may make a great difference in the management of such a patient by reducing the requirement for blood transfusion. The search for occult gastrointestinal blood loss and the evaluation of uterine and other possible sources of blood loss is part of the evaluation of every anemic patient.

THE ERYTHRON

The red cell mass in the circulation and the erythropoietic cells of the bone marrow can be considered functionally as a single organ termed the erythron.

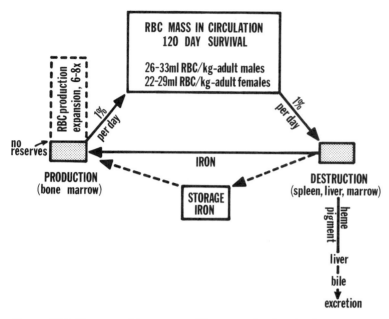

Fig. 17.3 The Erythron. The red cells and marrow precursors viewed as an organ system.

Figure 17.3 illustrates this concept. The normal red cell survives in the circulation for approximately 120 days. The dynamic steady state of the red cell mass implies that approximately 1 percent or slightly less of the red cells are destroyed and replaced daily. Normal and abnormal rates of red cell production and destruction have been measured by a wide variety of techniques and have validated this model. Measurements of the red cell production rate by the incorporation of a radioisotope of iron and the survival of red cells in the peripheral blood as a measure of rate of red cell destruction are of clinical value in a number of circumstances. However, in most instances, careful evaluation of the absolute reticulocyte count gives a clinically useful measure of red cell production; from this the approximate rate of red cell destruction can be inferred if the hematocrit is stable.

Normally, reticulocytes undergo maturation in the peripheral blood with loss of the diffusely basophilic staining material over about two days. When increased red cell production is called for, the new red cells delivered to the circulation may be somewhat less mature with a slightly prolonged period of maturation in the peripheral blood. Thus, the reticulocyte count is not a direct measure of the rate of red cell production, even though it provides clinically useful information.

The normal bone marrow provided with an adequate supply of iron and other essential nutrients for hematopoiesis is capable of increasing red cell production six- to eight-fold. In the presence of a hemolytic disorder in which iron derived from the destroyed red cells is immediately available for the production of new cells, the capacity to expand production may increase substantially. The ability of the marrow to replace red cells lost for any reason will vary substantially from patient to patient, depending upon the presence or absence of factors which may suppress red cell production. Chronic infection or inflammation, renal insufficiency, the presence of a tumor, particularly one that is metastatic, or recent chemotherapy with a cytotoxic agent are examples of factors which will limit the capacity of the bone marrow to respond to the need for new red cell production.

Requirements For Normal Erythropoiesis

Normal red cell production is a process whereby red cell precursors proliferate with progressive differentiation from a primitive stem cell to the definitive red cell which has lost its nucleus. Morphologically, the sequential changes of maturation are called the normoblastic series of cells of the bone marrow; the term erythroblastic is also used in the same sense. This series of red cell precursors is shown in Figure 17.4 along with the approximate normal proportions of these cells at the several levels of maturation. More mature forms are more common than immature cells. The ability to undergo mitotic division and thus to increase the number of red cells is normally lost during the stage defined as the orthochromatic normoblast. The bulk of red cell proliferation appears to occur during the polychromatic stage of red cell differentiation. This stage is characterized by the synthesis of an increasing amount of hemoglobin in the individual cell.

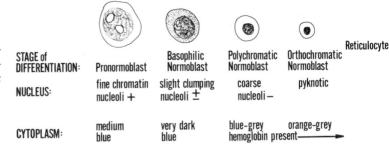

Fig. 17.4 Diagrammatic representation of stages of differentiation in normoblastic erythropoiesis.

STAGE of DIFFERENTIATION:	Pronormoblast	Basophilic Normoblast	Polychromatic Normoblast	Orthochromatic Normoblast	Reticulocyte
NUCLEUS:	fine chromatin nucleoli +	slight clumping nucleoli ±	coarse nucleoli −	pyknotic	
CYTOPLASM:	medium blue	very dark blue	blue-grey hemoglobin present———	orange-grey	

A more physiologically significant description of the pattern of red cell proliferation and differentiation can be shown by in vitro bone marrow culture techniques. These methods which are still largely restricted to research applications recognize a basic stem cell, which when properly stimulated and provided with hormonal support in the form of erythropoietin and probably other factors produced by lymphoid cells, forms an erythroid colony forming unit (CFU-E). This is followed by formation of a so-called "burst forming unit" (BFU-E), a red cell precursor with major proliferative potential. This schema is shown in Figure 17.5. At the present time, there is uncertainty as to the morphology of these two major red cell procursors recognized by in vitro culture. Nevertheless, studies of this type have revealed clinically important information about erythrokinetics, particularly in those disorders characterized by inadequate numbers of stem cells and failure of appropriate erythroid differentiation to occur in the early stages of red cell production.

Although erythropoietin has been identified as a

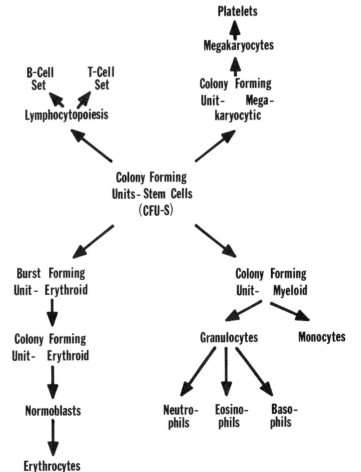

Fig. 17.5 Relationships of stem cells to proliferation of the blood cells.

Table 17.3 **Classification of Anemia Based Upon Red Cell Size and Hemoglobin Content**

RBC Size	HGB Concentration/ Cell	Examples
Normocytic	Normochromic	Acute hemorrhage, hemolytic and hyporegenerative anemia, anemia of chronic disease
Macrocytic	Normochromic	Megaloblastic anemia, anemia of chronic liver disease
Microcytic	Hypochromic	Iron deficiency, Thalassemia, abnormalities of iron metabolism and hemoglobin synthesis.

major hormone required for normal erythropoiesis, the hormonal support of red cell production is clearly more complex. The erythropoietin mechanism itself may involve more than a single substance. Although erythropoietin is derived principally from the kidney, total nephrectomy does not abolish all erythropoiesis. This may reflect the secretion of small amounts of erythropoitein from other organs or the existence of other stimulatory materials which support a basal level of red cell production. Additionally, erythropoietin can be stimulated in vivo by androgenic steroids. Marked hypothyroidism also results in decreased red cell production, although in part this may reflect a requirement for fewer red cells in severe states of hypometabolism. Neither androgens nor thyroid hormone appear to be required for erythropoiesis at the cellular level in vitro, although they may play some indirect regulatory role in control of the red cell mass in vitro.

Another view of the processes of red cell production and destruction is provided by tracking the metabolism of iron as it moves into and out of the red cell mass. The iron present in hemoglobin represents the principle pool of the body iron; its turnover within the red cell mass reflects the processes of red cell production and destruction. This topic will be discussed in more detail in connection with iron deficiency anemia. Iron, vitamin B-12 and folic acid are three known substances of dietary origin which are essential for normal red cell production. The role of other nutrients which may be important for hematopoietically Active Substances. Since the average diet in developed countries is rich in critical nutrients, it requires a radically abnormal diet to induce anemia in otherwise normal people. The American public has a strong belief in the direct connection between diet and anemia, a belief which probably dates to the discovery that eating large amounts of liver would correct pernicious anemia associated with lack of vitamin B-12. Many anemic patients are concerned about their diet as a possible cause of anemia or as a way of treating a known anemic state. Adequate nutrition is undoubtedly important for good health and patients should be educated in this regard. However,

unrealistic expectations about the influence of an otherwise reasonable diet on anemia should also be part of patient education to assist the patient in focusing on the real problem which may underlie the anemia.

BASIC MECHANISMS OF ANEMIA

There are only three basic mechanisms by which the red cell mass can be reduced in size and a state of anemia produced. These are:

1. Blood loss
2. Inadequate red cell production
3. Excessive red cell destruction

In any given anemic state, more than one of these mechanisms may operate. Blood loss may be acute resulting in hypovolemia, and, if severe, shock may be induced and acute anemic anoxia may occur. Chronic blood loss generally induces anemia by depleting the body iron stores resulting in inadequate hemoglobin regeneration. The mechanisms of inadequate red cell production include those conditions termed hyporegenerative in which the marrow responds inadequately to the requirement for increased red blood cell production. Processes which destroy the bone marrow by toxic chemicals or invasion of the marrow with metastatic tumor are examples of this mechanism. In severe states of marrow hypoplasia, termed aplastic anemia, pancytopenia is produced, and the clinical picture may be complicated by problems of infection or bleeding. Excessive red cell destruction refers to the hemolytic anemias due either to an inherently abnormal red cell with a limited ability to survive in the circulation or normal red cells which are destroyed by an abnormal milieu into which they are delivered.

Anemic disorders have also been classified for clinical purposes on the basis of the size and hemoglobin content of the patient's red cells. Table 17.3 illustrates this approach to the classification of anemia and some of the major diagnostic categories. Red cell size can be measured directly by the red cell indices, or it can be estimated by careful examination of the peripheral blood smear. Classification by red cell size and hemoglobin content results in grouping the causes of anemia with some overlap. For example, disorders characterized by dysplastic erythropoiesis in the bone marrow may result in the production of red cells of normal size, larger or smaller than normal size, or a very wide range of red cell sizes in which the mean cell size may be within the normal range.

The study of anemia should be carried out in a logical, step-by-step fashion rather than by indiscriminately collecting all possible kinds of laboratory information in a random search.

ANEMIA DUE TO BLOOD LOSS

Acute Blood Loss

The acute loss of blood induces a state of acute anemia through reduction of the red cell mass. If the acute blood loss is less than 10 percent of the total blood volume in an otherwise normal individual, it is unlikely to be of major physiological significance. The normal cardiovascular system quickly accommodates to this degree of blood loss by increasing cardiac rate and output; relatively rapid mobilization of extravascular fluid into the plasma compartment soon restores the blood volume, albeit at a somewhat lower hematocrit than prior to bleeding. An essentially normal state of cardiovascular function returns. Blood donors regularly experience hemorrhage of about this extent with no adverse effects. Limitations on the cardiovascular system's ability to compensate for acute blood loss or preexisting contraction of the blood volume or red cell mass may make hemorrhages of this size physiologically significant. Thus, the preexisting state of the patient, the size of an acute blood loss and the rate at which it is lost are the primary determinants of the effects of acute bleeding.

As the size of an acute hemorrhage increases to approximately 20 percent of blood volume the capacity of the cardiovascular system to adjust is progressively exceeded and the complex abnormal physiological state known as shock begins to develop. Failure of perfusion of the capillary bed due to inadequate intravascular volume appears to be of much greater importance in the pathogenesis of shock than does decreased oxygen carrying capacity of the blood. Restoration of blood volume thus is usually more important in the treatment of such patients than is immediate replacement of the red cell mass. If the intravascular volume is restored with crystalloid solutions patients can survive massive blood loss even when it results in a very low hematocrit. This is not to say, however, that it is unimportant to restore the red cell mass in the treatment of massive blood loss.

As acute blood loss approaches approximately 50 percent of the blood volume, without replacement, the severity of the shock syndrome increases to an irreversible point, even with intensive treatment designed to restore both the plasma volume and the red cell mass. The number of patients with severe acute blood loss who survive has increased due to improved techniques of resuscitation. Unfortunately, many such patients also suffer from severe accidental or surgical trauma, a factor which further limits their chances of recovery from shock. Deaths from shock will continue to occur in spite of the most vigorous management possible. Further discussion of the management of shock is included in Chapters 7, 15 and 16. This is an important topic about which every physician should be knowledgeable. Additional discussion regarding replacement fluids is in the section dealing with blood transfusion.

The peripheral blood picture, including measurements of red cell concentration, may be unchanged for a period of several hours following an acute loss of blood. Significant hemodilution may be seen within 4 hours, and this continues progressively up to about 24 hours. The severity of hemorrhage should be assessed by estimation of the apparent loss of blood if this can be determined. Overt blood loss such as that from even relatively severe nose bleed, uterine bleeding, or a major laceration tend to be overestimated both by the patient and by the medical personnel in attendance. Acute blood loss which is concealed, such as bleeding into the tissues surrounding a major fracture of the femur or bleeding into the gastrointestinal tract which has not been ejected by vomiting or diarrhea, may be seriously underestimated. In these instances, evaluation of the patient's physiological response to blood loss, including heart rate, blood pressure, peripheral skin vasoconstriction, urinary output, and level of consciousness become much more important in assessing the degree of blood loss. In all such instances, particularly if blood loss is continuing and occult, meticulous and frequent evaluation of the patient as well as early treatment may be life saving. Overestimation of blood loss may lead to rapid overreplacement, which in the patient with limited cardiovascular reserves may result in congestive heart failure. Underestimates of the severity of blood loss can lead to underreplacement, seriously jeopardizing the patient who may be at risk of further unpredictable bleeding. In the management of the patient who is experiencing acute blood loss, it is always important to make the best possible estimate of the amount of blood lost and, if this is uncertain, to recognize that uncertainty in planning the patient's management.

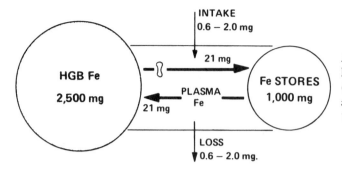

Fig. 17.6 Diagram of whole body ferrokinetics and principal body iron pools. (From Rapaport SI, Introduction to Hematology. Harper and Row, New York, 1971, with permission.)

Chronic Bleeding

In some patients, bleeding is intermittent and occult. Multiple stool samples tested for occult blood over a period of many weeks may be required to document gastrointestinal bleeding. If blood loss is not detected, the gastrointestinal tract may be examined by radiological procedures and direct visualization. If, however, a lesion is not encountered which might produce gastrointestinal bleeding, the search for the source of occult blood loss should not stop (see Chapter 12), but other possible mechanisms of iron depletion should then be investigated.

IRON DEFICIENCY ANEMIA

The Metabolism of Iron

Most of the details of the overall body metabolism of iron have been clarified in the last 25 years; much is also known about the role of iron in intracellular metabolism, its function in a wide variety of enzyme systems, and its role in oxygen transport as part of the hemoglobin molecule.

The term ferrokinetics is commonly used to describe the overall movement of iron into, out of, and through the various iron compartments of the body. This concept is particularly useful because it provides a number of specific measurements that can be made as iron is absorbed, transported, stored and utilized. A simplified diagram of over-all ferrokinetics is given in Figure 17.6. The most important aspect of iron metabolism involves the equilibrium between iron absorption and iron loss. Once absorbed, iron is highly conserved. In normal males, a steady state absorption of approximately 1 mg of iron per day is balanced by a loss of approximately 1 mg, largely in exfoliated cells. Normal women in the child-bearing years require an increased amount of iron absorption to balance the additional iron lost by menstruation and transferred to developing fetuses. This more than doubles the iron absorption requirement for women

until the time of menopause when the requirement for additional iron declines to levels comparable to males. Although anemia appears to increase the absorption of iron to some degree, limitations in dietary iron may prevent compensation for even minor amounts of chronic blood loss over a long period of time.

The other clinically important feature of iron metabolism is the amount of iron in storage, approximately 40 percent of the total body iron under normal circumstances. This iron, stored in the bone marrow, liver and spleen, can be mobilized to support production of hemoglobin and new erythrocytes when iron absorption is exceeded by iron loss. Storage iron exists in two chemical forms: *ferritin*, a labile and rapidly mobilizable form which is a highly structured iron protein compound, and a more amorphous and chemically less well defined iron protein complex termed *hemosiderin* from which iron is mobilized more slowly. Iron in storage as hemosiderin can be stained permitting the amount of iron in storage in the bone marrow or liver to be roughly estimated.

When iron loss exceeds iron absorption for a prolonged period, iron stores will be mobilized and progressively transferred to the circulating red cell mass until reserves are nearly exhausted. Thus, there is a point in the progressive depletion of body iron where the hemoglobin or hematocrit may be only minimally decreased, but the normal amount of iron in storage has largely disappeared. Further depletion of the body iron then results in progressive failure of hemoglobin synthesis, the onset of hypochromia and microcytosis of the red cells, and the appearance of anemia of variable severity. These progressive changes indicate that examination of the bone marrow for iron in storage may be clinically useful, even though the classic findings of iron deficiency anemia have not yet fully developed in the peripheral blood.

Iron in the plasma is transported bound to a protein, *transferrin*. This protein with its attached iron has a marked affinity for developing normoblasts of the bone marrow in which new hemoglobin is being synthesized. Transferrin carrying iron is bound to a specific binding site on the normoblast cell surface where the iron is released and taken into the cell. Following this, the binding site affinity for the iron-free transferrin is much reduced and the transport protein is released into the plasma. Not all of the transferrin in plasma is normally bound to iron. Measuring the amounts of serum iron and the total capacity of the plasma to bind added iron permits calculation of the unsaturated portion of the trans-ferrin of the plasma. In clinical situations where there has been simple iron depletion, serum iron will be low, but the total binding capacity of the plasma for iron will be high. Certain chronic diseases, particularly those associated with chronic infection or inflammation, depress the serum iron and decrease the iron binding capacity. This provides an important diagnostic test to differentiate iron deficiency states from the so-called anemia of chronic disease. Abnormal red cell development may result in hypochromic and microcytic red cells not due to iron deficiency, with elevated or normal levels of serum iron. Similarly, when body stores of iron are increased, as in the disorder hemochromatosis, the serum iron will be elevated and the transferrin will be more nearly saturated with bound iron. Table 17.4 summarizes these aspects of serum iron measurements.

The ferritin present in serum can now be measured by radioimmunoassay. Serum ferritin falls as iron stores are depleted. Values below about 20 ng/ml may be found before iron deficiency anemia appears. Serum ferritin measurements appear to reflect storage iron depletion in this situation.

Dietary Intake of Iron

The average American and Western European diet contains approximately 10 to 25 mg of iron per day. Dietary sources of iron vary widely in their availability for absorption. Table 17.5 lists the iron content of a number of common foods along with estimates of their availability for absorption.

Although the average diet in the developed countries appears to contain adequate amounts of iron for

Table 17.4 Normal Values for Serum Iron, Iron Binding Capacity and Ferritin

Serum Iron	50–150μg/100 ml.
Total Iron Binding Capacity	200–400μg/100 ml.
Iron Binding Capacity Saturation	25–30%
Serum Ferritin	12–250μg/l.

Normal values for adult females and very elderly people are slightly lower than adult males.

Table 17.5 Food Iron Content and Availability for Absorption

Food	Iron Content (mg./100 gm.)	Availability
Foods Containing High Iron		High
(Muscle meats, liver, etc.)	1.5–2.5	
Grains		Low
Wheat	1.0–4.0	
Corn	1.8–2.3	
Rice	0.9–1.4	
Vegetables		Very low
Green leafy	1.1–2.9	
Potatoes	0.7–1.1	
Fruits	0.4–0.8	Very low
Eggs	2.5	Low
Milk	0.1	Low

Iron content of grains and vegetables variable depending upon cultivation conditions. Significant inhibition of iron absorption may be produced by other dietary items—e.g., those containing phytates or phosphates. Ascorbate increases absorption. Average American diet contains 10–15 mg. iron/day with absorption of about 10%.

the majority of people, there is a substantial population with poor socioeconomic status, particularly children during rapid growth, whose intake of iron is marginal or inadequate. A number of proposals have been made to require that bread be supplemented with iron in an attempt to improve the dietary availability of iron for these people. This proposal has been highly controversial. The question hinges around whether the increased intake of iron by people who do not require it would in any way be harmful. For example, the exact incidence of the genetic predisposition for the iron storage disease hemochromatosis is unknown. Potentially people with enhanced iron absorbing capability might more rapidly accumulate injurious stores of iron. A carefully obtained history of the iron deficient patient's dietary habits will usually reveal any dietary deficiencies.

Although iron is one of the most common metals in the earth's crust, iron deficiency is a common phenomenon world-wide. This reflects not only diets inadequate in iron, such as those which are based primarily on grains, but also the high incidence of hookworm infestation among tropical populations which result in chronic gastrointestinal blood loss to the parasite.

Clinical Picture of Iron Deficiency Anemia

Relatively mild iron deficiency anemia, with hemoglobin levels of 8 gm/dl and above, may be both clinically asymptomatic and without significant clinical findings. Since chronic iron deficiency commonly develops rather slowly, patients usually compensate for the slowly declining hemoglobin and may be unaware of these compensations. It is commonly assumed by patients and physicians alike that iron deficiency of approximately this degree of severity results in symptoms of lassitude, weakness, and a sense of malaise. This is probably incorrect. Several studies have shown that patients are unable to detect improvement in their hemoglobin levels when treated. These studies strongly suggest that most symptoms attributed to iron deficiency anemia of this degree are of psychological origin. The same is probably true of most types of chronic anemia not due to lack of vitamin B-12 or folic acid.

As iron depletion becomes more severe and the accompaning anemia increases, the patients very commonly become symptomatic when the hemoglobin reaches levels of 5 or 6 gm/dl. Shortness of breath, exercise limitation, awareness of tachycardia and pounding pulse on exertion are the principal symptoms of note (i.e., findings which reflect cardiovascular compensations for anemia). In addition, the patient may note cheilosis, glossitis, and perhaps even dysphagia. The nails may become soft and split easily. The latter are probably manifestations of the depletion of iron in skin and mucosal cells. The patient is frequently aware of pallor. Many patients have voluntarily limited their activity.

Physical findings are mainly those associated with cardiorespiratory compensation for anemia. Other findings are those referred to in the mouth, lips, skin and nails. Pallor may be striking if the hemoglobin level is below 5 gm/dl. It is of great importance to search for possible lesions which may have resulted in bleeding. The lips, nose, anus, rectum and skin should be examined carefully for the lesions of hereditary hemorrhagic telangectasia (Weber Osler Rendu syndrome, see Chapter 19). The abdomen should be palpated carefully for abnormal masses and hepatic enlargement. Evidence of portal hypertension including abdominal venous distention, ascites, and splenomegaly should be sought. A pelvic examination and cervical cytology should be carried out as well as a digital rectal examination and proctosigmoidoscopy.

Blood Picture

The blood film will show striking microcytosis and hypochromia in the presence of even moderately severe iron deficiency anemia. Red cells vary in size, shape and hemoglobin content when severe iron deficiency is present; some cells may be essentially achromic. If red cell polychromasia is increased and the reticulocyte count is elevated, the patient may have recently received some additional iron either in therapy or in the diet. The red cell indices will confirm the presence of hypochromia and microcytosis by reduced MCV, MCH and MCHC. The white blood cell picture is commonly within normal limits, but frequently there is a mild to moderate increase in blood platelets.

During the period when the patient with chronic blood loss is mobilizing body iron stores, but has not yet become significantly anemic, the red cells may be somewhat decreased in size and mildly hypochromic. These patients usually have an increase in reticulocyte count as long as some iron is avilable from body stores. The reticulocyte count and red cell polychromasia then decreases as body stores are totally depleted.

Differential Diagnosis

Iron deficiency anemia should be carefully distinguished from thalassemia minor which also results in a microcytic but not hypochromic blood picture. The thin leptocytic ("target") cells of this genetic trait may appear somewhat hypochromic on superficial examination. The poikilocytosis and punctate basophilia of the erythrocytes as well as the stability of the blood values and the genetic characteristics of thalassemia trait should serve to establish this diagnosis. Acquired dysplastic states of erythropoiesis associated with sideroblastic anemia and preleukemic states may produce both microcytosis and some degree of hypochromia of at least part of the red cell population. Under these circumstances, measurements of serum iron as well as determinations of iron stores may be particularly valuable; both will usually be normal or even slightly increased.

Treatment of Iron Deficiency

The treatment of iron deficiency is both simple and effective: oral administration of an absorbable ferrous iron salt in doses equivalent to approximately 60 mg of elemental iron two or three times per day with meals for a prolonged period is usually well-tolerated and effective. Ferrous sulfate is both cheap and effective if the tablets are fresh. Rarely is a more complex preparation justified. The patient should be informed that stools will turn black, one of the few disadvantages of oral iron therapy since it makes the detection of recurrent melena more difficult. However, if the patient has had occult gastrointestinal bleeding the stools should be tested periodically for recurrent blood loss. Serious iron intolerance with gastric distress, diarrhea or constipation is not common. If iron is poorly tolerated, the dose can be reduced and the timing (in relation to meals) changed to reduce the gastrointestinal symptoms. If the dose of iron must be reduced, the period of treatment can be extended. The anemic patient without significant iron stores may require treatment for a year or more to rebuild at least some storage iron.

If possible, iron treatment should be carried out as a therapeutic trial. Treatment should be instituted after base-line reticulocyte counts have been obtained. Reticulocyte counts should then be obtained 5, 10 and 15 days following treatment. A prolonged rise in reticulocyte count with a prompt rise in hemoglobin level both confirms the diagnosis and indicates that the patient probably has no other significant limitation on erythropoiesis and synthesis of hemoglobin.

The patient under treatment should have repeated peripheral blood examinations until the blood picture including the reticulocyte count has become normal. Treatment should be extended beyond this time, although it may not be fully effective in reestablishing normal iron stores. Patients who have been significantly iron depleted should be re-treated with iron periodically if they experience recurrent bleeding, including menstruating women, and women who are bearing children.

The routine administration of parenteral iron as a treatment for iron deficiency is not justified. In rare circumstances when true malabsorption of iron has been demonstrated or under circumstances where a patient continues to experience blood loss at a more rapid rate than can be compensated for by oral iron treatment, parenteral iron therapy is useful. It is rarely justified by iron intolerance or the need for rapid response. Relatively severe iron deficiency in the third trimester of pregnancy may be an indication for parenteral therapy. The most serious risk of parenteral iron therapy is the risk of an anaphylactic response, for which treatment should be available whenever it is administered. Local inflammation and discomfort may occur at the injection site, and if the "Z" technique of injection is not employed, tattoo marks may be produced in the skin.

Unless the source of abnormal blood loss can be identified and controlled, iron therapy in any form may not successfully correct anemia. Most patients who are thought to be "resistant" to iron therapy are in fact continuing to lose blood. The patient whose hemoglobin does not rise to near normal during a 3 to 4 week period of iron therapy should be carefully reinvestigated for recurrent bleeding as a first priority. One should not assume that the patient has failed to absorb oral iron. In the rare instance of true failure of iron absorption, one or two injections of parenteral iron administered as a therapeutic test may be helpful in establishing the diagnosis. Iron absorption tests involving the use of a radioactive isotope of iron are seldom necessary for clinical purposes. An iron absorption test employing ferrous sulfate administered by mouth with pre- and one hour post-administration measurements of serum iron may be useful in identifying patients with iron malabsorption, most of whom also have evidence of a general malabsorptive state. If this test demonstrates the absorbability of oral iron, another cause of failure of erythropoiesis should be sought.

Summary

Iron deficiency anemia by itself is not a diagnosis, but a manifestation of some mechanism, usually chronic blood loss, which has resulted in depletion of body iron stores. The anemic state should not be treated without an intensive effort to discover the mechanism of iron depletion and to correct it. Dietary deficiency of iron is uncommon; chronic, frequently occult blood loss is the most common and most important cause of iron deficiency anemia.

INADEQUATE RED CELL PRODUCTION

Inadequate red cell production can be absolute or relative. When red cell production is inadequate to replace the normal daily destruction of senescent red cells, anemia will occur; this is termed a hyporegenerative state. The red cell mass will stabilize at a lower than normal level determined by the lower rate of red cell replacement. Relatively decreased red cell production is a situation which requires increased red cell production to replace erythrocytes lost by bleeding or accelerated red cell destruction, but under the circumstances the bone marrow is unable to respond with the expected level of compensation. Therefore, the number of new red cells delivered to the circulation daily is increased over normal and the reticulocyte count is elevated, but to a lesser degree than would be expected were the bone marrow to respond fully to the physiological requirement for new red cell production. This also contributes to the development of the anemia; the state is termed relative hyporegeneration of red cells.

Mechanisms of inadequate red cell production:
  1. Lack of hematopoietically active substances
     a. Nutritional (iron, vitamin B-12, folic acid, and others)

b. Endocrine (erythropoietin, thyroid hormone, and others)
2. Destruction of bone marrow
   a. Toxins
   b. Ionizing radiation
   c. Tumor invasion
   d. Infection
   e. Idiopathic marrow failure
3. Suppression of erythropoiesis
   a. Toxins
   b. Acute or chronic inflammation (infection)
   c. Presence of malignant tumor, particularly metastatic
   d. Congenital marrow failure
   e. Immunological mechanisms
   f. Idiopathic
4. Primary neoplastic disorders of the bone marrow
   a. Preleukemia and leukemia
   b. Multiple myeloma and lymphoproliferative disorders
   c. Clonal abnormalities of the bone marrow
      1) Myeloproliferative disorders
      2) Paroxysmal nocturnal hemoglobinuria

As with any classification system, specific disease entities may fall into several of these mechanistic categories.

Lack of Hematopoietically Active Substances

The Megloblastic Anemias

Deficient absorption of vitamin B-12 (cyanocobalamin) and folic acid (FA) lead to suppression of DNA synthesis in all regenerating and renewing cell systems. The hematopoietic system and the mucosal cells of the gastrointestinal tract are the main systems in which this metabolic defect expresses itself.

The cellular pattern of hematopoeisis induced by severe deficiencies of either of these substances is termed megaloblastic. It reflects a slow rate of nuclear replication, asynchronous maturation of cytoplasm and nucleus, slowed blood cell production, and production of defective blood cells which may undergo destruction in the marrow (ineffective erythropoiesis) and have shortened life span in the circulation. The megaloblastic pattern of hematopoiesis affects all cells produced by the marrow, not just the erythrocytes.

In these deficiency states, the red cells produced are on the average macrocytic with increased variability of red cell sizes and shapes (i.e., anisocytosis and poikilocytosis). Figure 17.7 illustrates the altered marrow pattern of megaloblastic hematopoiesis and the changes induced in the peripheral blood. Not all macrocytic anemias are due to megaloblastic hematopoiesis. Macronormoblastic anemias frequently accompany chronic liver disease and severe hypothyroidism. These anemias are seen with other diseases for unknown reasons.

Megaloblastic anemias, regardless of the specific deficiency involved, commonly are pancytopenias with white blood cell counts as low as 2,000/cu mm and platelet counts under 100,000/cu mm. Thrombocytopenia severe enough to result in bleeding is rare. The earliest changes in the development of a megaloblastic anemia frequently appear in the neutrophils which turn over rapidly. Hypersegmentation of the nucleus, pale staining of nuclear chromatin (which has an open, fine-stranded appearance), and an increase in cell size may be seen in peripheral blood neutrophils and in their marrow precursors before significant anemia has developed. The giant metamyelocyte of the marrow is typical of this change. Megaloblastic hematopoiesis is best shown by a bone marrow examination, although enough late developmental stages of megaloblastic erythroid cells and typical neutrophils may be found in peripheral blood films to establish this in some patients without marrow biopsy.

Megaloblastic anemias usually develop slowly and cardiovascular compensations delay the onset of symptoms. Folic acid deficiency, particularly that associated with pregnancy, may present as a rapidly developing anemia associated with a severe, even life-threatening illness. After appropriate diagnostic procedures, the ultimate clinical proof of the existence of B-12 or folate deficiency is the response to physiological replacement doses of the depleted vitamin.

Vitamin B-12 Deficiency

B-12 is a specific nutritional requirement of man. Many life forms can synthesize this substance or obtain it from gastrointestinal organisms as in the case of ruminant animals. Its chemical name, cyanocobalamin, includes a number of related compounds. Structurally, it consists of a tetrapyrrole bound to an atom of cobalt with a complex of substituent groups; the structure is shown in Figure 17.8.

B-12 deficiency can develop by a number of mechanisms. Failure of absorption may be due to disappearance of the specific absorption mechanisms, the intrinsic factor secreted by the stomach. When pri-

Maturation of the Erythrocytic Series

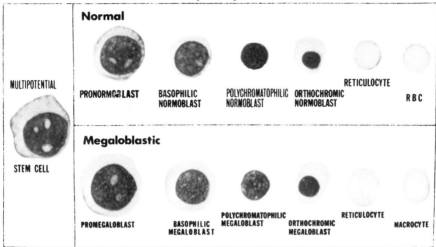

Fig. 17.7 The comparative morphological picture of normoblastic and megaloblastic erythropoiesis. (From Hyun BH, Ashton JK, Dolan K: Practical Hematology. WB Saunders, Philadelphia, 1975, with permission.)

Fig. 17.8 A. Chemical structure of vitamin B_{12} (cyanocobalamin). B. Chemical structure of pteroylglutamic acid (folic acid) (both from Chanarin J, Brozović M, Tidemarsh E, Waters DAW: Blood and its Diseases. 2nd ed. Churchill Livingstone, Edinburgh, 1980, with permission.)

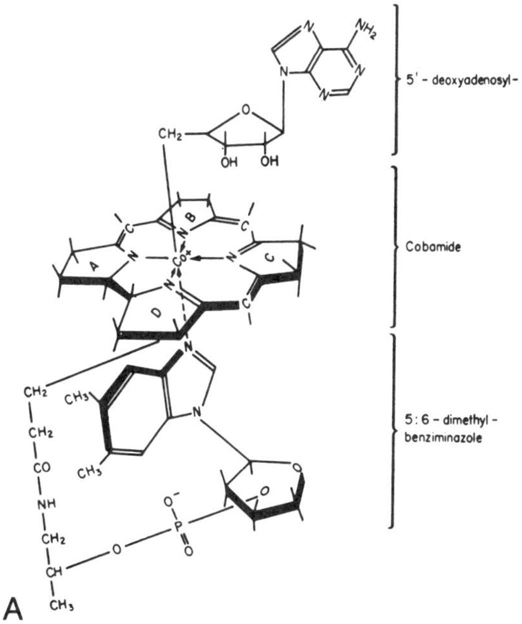

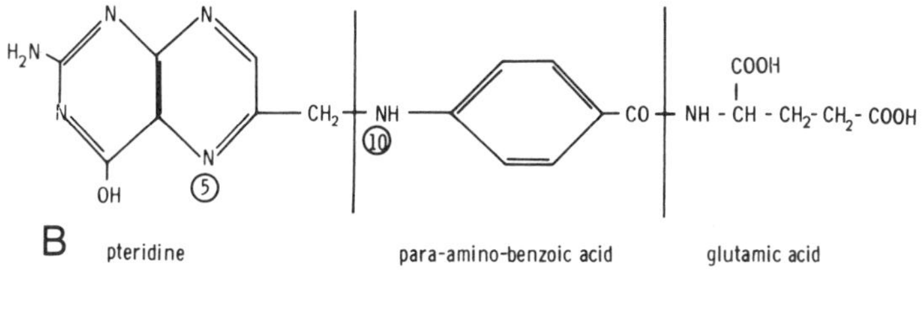

Table 17.6 **Normal Blood Levels of Vitamin B$_{12}$ and Folate, with Values in Deficiency States**

	Serum B$_{12}$ pg/ml	Serum Folate ng/ml	RBC Folate ng/l
Normal Subjects	300–900	5–21	200–700
Deficient Subjects	<200 (usually <100)	<3	<140

Values given are measured by radioisotopic methods which depend upon a binder for B$_{12}$ or folate. These methods are now widely used, but yield results somewhat higher than the more specific microbiological assays. (From Maslow WC, et al: Practical Diagnosis, Hematological Disease. New York, © John Wiley and Sons, Inc., 1980, with permission.)

mary gastric atrophy, probably of autoimmune origin, is responsible for this, the disease is referred to as pernicious anemia. Total gastrectomy produces essentially the same result. Dietary B-12 bound to intrinsic factor, a glycoprotein secreted by the chief cells of the gastric fundus, is absorbed in the last two meters of the ileum. Inflammatory or other disease in this segment may also impair B-12 absorption. Intrinsic factor bound to B-12 rather surprisingly resists peptic digestion.

Man's daily nutritional requirement for B-12 is miniscule but crucial, about 2 to 4 μg/day. The average daily diet containing some animal protein contains about 6 to 15 μg. On absorption and resecretion into the plasma, B-12 is bound to transport proteins, transcobalamin I and II, which are synthesized in the liver and by leukocytes. The liver accumulates relatively large stores of B-12, about 3,000 μg normally. In the absence of B-12 absorption, stores are slowly mobilized. If B-12 stores are normal, findings of B-12 lack may not appear in the blood for about 3 years after cessation of absorption.

The metabolic role of B-12 in man is still incompletely understood. It is clearly an enzyme cofactor which participates in the synthesis of components of DNA. It also participates in other metabolic reactions. The best known of these is the conversion of methylmalonate to succinate. In the absence of adequate amounts of B-12, methylmalonic acid is excreted in the urine. B-12 also is involved in unknown ways in the metabolism of the central nervous system. Subacute combined degeneration of the spinal cord with loss of deep sensation, including vibratory sensation and fine motor functions, occurs as a prominent manifestation of severe and prolonged B-12 deficiency. Delerium is also a common finding in severe B-12 lack; this is not due primarily to anemia, since it does respond to the administration of small amounts of B-12 before the anemia has been significantly corrected. Pernicious anemia patients treated with B-12 subjectively feel better after about 3 days; this is correlated with relief of delerium. At about

the same time, there is onset of reticulocytosis, which becomes maximal about 7 days after starting treatment. Other metabolic functions of B-12 in many cell systems remain unclear.

Clinical picture and diagnosis of B-12 deficiency. B-12 deficiency of any origin resulting in anemia is a relatively rare clinical condition. The majority of these patients will have pernicious anemia. Typical pernicious anemia patients are usually beyond 50 years of age, of northern European origin, frequently with premature grey hair. There is a slight preponderance of females. They exhibit striking pallor, at times with a faint yellow tinge to the skin. If the anemia is severe, the cardiovascular system will be hyperdynamic with sustained tachycardia, wide pulse pressure and hyperactive precordium; in spite of this many patients are still able to engage in normal activities of daily living. Delerium and neurological manifestations of subacute combined spinal cord degeneration will be detected in over half of severely anemic patients. The neurological manifestations may be severe in the presence of only mild anemia in some patients.

The blood picture has been described. If hypersegmented macroneutrophils are present or if even a rare nucleated red cell showing a megaloblastic nuclear pattern can be found, the pattern of hematopoiesis in the bone marrow is very likely to be megaloblastic. In most patients, a bone marrow examination is desirable, but it may not be essential to establish a diagnosis.

The typical clinical profile, in the presence of a normal diet and gastric achlorhydria and in the absence of generalized malabsorption or disease of the terminal ileum, makes the diagnosis of B-12 deficiency secondary to pernicious anemia virtually certain. Measurement of serum B-12 and folate levels will confirm this; typical findings in deficient patients and normal values are given in Table 17.6.

Patients have frequently been treated for B-12 deficiency before firm establishment of the diagnosis. In these patients, the ability to absorb B-12 can be assessed by use of the Schilling test employing B-12 labelled with radiocobalt. The radiolabelled material is given orally followed shortly by a large parenteral dose of non-labelled B-12. The excess B-12, including a proportion of the labelled material which may have been absorbed orally, will be excreted in the next 24 hours in the urine where the excreted radioactivity can be measured. Normal individuals excrete at least 10 percent of the oral dose; patients with B-12 absorption defects excrete little or none of the labelled material. The test can be made more specific for pernicious anemia by repeating it in those patients who do not absorb B-12 by oral administration of labelled B-12 with active intrinsic factor; this should result in nearly normal absorption of the labelled B-12 in patients who lack their own intrinsic factor.

Differential diagnosis. Pernicious anemia, or other causes of vitamin B-12 deficiency, must be distinguished from deficiency of folic acid. During the so-called "herald state" of acute myeloblastic leukemias, at times the bone marrow has a partial megaloblastic-like appearance. This is particularly true in the disorder erythroleukemia, in which the abnormally developing line of erythroid cells may resemble megaloblasts quite closely. These latter disorders are differentiated from megaloblastic states of metabolic and nutritional origin by determinations of serum B-12 and/or folic levels as well as by failure of the patient to respond to therapeutic trials with these vitamins.

Therapy of pernicious anemia. The treatment of vitamin B-12 deficiency is specific and effective: the replacement of vitamin B-12 by injection. Monthly doses of 50–100 µg is adequate both to induce and maintain hematological remission. Treatment must be carried on for the remainder of the patient's life in the case of typical pernicious anemia. In the presence of significant subacute combined degeneration of the spinal cord somewhat higher doses of vitamin B-12, 100 µg per week by injection for a period of 6 to 12 months or for as long as spinal cord function appears to be improving, may be of value. Patients so treated respond quite variably in the amount of neurological function that appears to be restored by this treatment program. Larger doses of vitamin B-12 have no proven use. There is no place for oral vitamin B-12 treatment in the management of this disease. Reliable oral absorption of vitamin B-12 in adequate amount cannot be depended upon and is significantly more costly.

Complications. Gastric atrophy associated with pernicious anemia has been regarded as a precursor of carcinoma of the stomach. However, the incidence of this complication has decreased markedly in pernicious anemia patients as the incidence of this malignancy has declined in the general population. Nevertheless, periodic examinations of the stools for occult blood and regular surveillance of the patient's state of general health is wise in these patients.

Folic Acid Deficiency

The second, and most frequent cause of megaloblastic anemia, is the deficiency of folic acid. Dietary deficiency, particularly in alcoholic patients, is most frequently encountered. There may also be a block in the metabolism of folic acid in alcoholic patients. Drugs such as methotrexate, now being employed as agents for the treatment of psoriasis, will also block the metabolism of folic acid since this is the basis of the therapeutic effect. Generalized malabsorption syndromes, particularly sprue, may also be associated with deficient absorption of folic acid. An increased metabolic demand for folic acid appears to be responsible for a particularly severe type of megaloblastic anemia, the megaloblastic anemia of pregnancy, although other factors may be involved such as dietary deficiency.

Folic acid is found in dietary sources including organ meats, green vegtables, beans and fruits. Food preparation may destroy a substantial part of the folic acid content of fresh foods. Food sources of the vitamin are in the form of polyglutamate, which is converted during the process of absorption to monoglutamic folic acid. Monoglutamate is then converted enzymatically to methyltetrahydrofolate, the metabolically active form of the vitamin. Folic acid is involved in the transfer of one carbon fragment in a variety of metabolic processes. In the case of erythropoiesis, folic acid deficiency results in a decreased rate of DNA synthesis in the rapidly turning over cells of the bone marrow. There is metabolic interaction of folic acid with vitamin B-12, although the simultaneous deficiency of both of these vitamins is clinically very rare.

The daily metabolic requirement for folic acid is in the range of 100 to 200 µg absorbed per day. Pregnancy nearly doubles the requirement for folic acid and marginal folate deficiency is found in the latter half of pregnancy in a substantial proportion of women, particularly those with inadequate diets. Because of relatively low efficiency of absorption, the dietary requirement for folic acid intake is substantially higher than the daily metabolic requirement, on the order of 1 to 2 mg per day. Tissue storage of folate, estimated at 5 to 10 mg total body stores, provides a relatively much smaller reserve of this vitamin compared to stores of vitamin B-12, because of the higher daily metabolic requirement for folate.

Clinical manifestations. The clinical picture of folic acid deficiency depends substantially upon the mechanism responsible for the disorder. The clinical picture may be that of specific or generalized malnutrition, alcoholism, sprue, late pregnancy or the early postpartum period. The development of anemia may be quite rapid, as in the case of megaloblastic anemia of pregnancy in which the patient may become acutely ill, or slowly developing in situations where the absorption of folate is only marginally inadequate. The blood and bone marrow picture is indistinguishable from that associated with megaloblastic anemia due to B-12 deficiency. The differential diagnosis is made largely on the basis of the clinical setting in which the megaloblastic anemia is encountered. A history of a mechanism which will lead to folate deficiency is critical. The presence of free gastric acid virtually rules out typical pernicious anemia, but does not necessarily rule out other forms of vitamin B-12 deficiency.

Serum folate measurements are of some value in establishing the presence of folic acid deficiency. Normal serum levels range from 6 to 16 ng/ml, but low levels may be encountered within a month of an abrupt decrease in folic acid intake at a time when body stores of folate are still adequate to maintain hematopoeisis. Decreased levels of red cell folate reflect a more long term folic acid deficiency.

Treatment. Initiation of therapy for folic acid deficiency should almost always be carried on as a therapeutic trial. If there is any question of vitamin B-12 deficiency, normal therapeutic doses of this vitamin should be administered first and a reticulocyte response looked for over a period of 5 to 7 days. Ordinarily, this will not occur if the patient is folate deficient. The patient can then be treated with 1 to 2 mg of folic acid by injection daily. Again, the patient should be observed for a reticulocyte response which should occur within 4 to 7 days if the megaloblastic state is due to folic acid deficiency. Afterwards treatment can usually be administered orally. Five milligrams of folic acid per day, unless there is marked persistent malabsorption is usually adequate. In tropical sprue a period of relatively prolonged parenteral administration of folic acid may mitigate the severity of the sprue and allow the patient to later take the folic acid supplement orally. Ordinarily, the requirement for folic acid therapy is not life-long, but will be required until the mechanism which induced the deficiency can be corrected. Patients with severe congenital hemolytic anemia of long standing probably require permanent folate supplementation. All patients with hemolytic anemia

in whom the reticulocyte response is submaximal should be treated with supplemental folic acid.

When conducting a therapeutic trial, it is important to recognize that the patient with vitamin B-12 deficiency may have a substantial reticulocyte response after administration of folic acid. However, this response will not be permanent. Folate treatment in pernicious anemia is hazardous in that it may accelerate the progression of neurological injury.

Other Nutritional Aspects of Anemia

Although nutrition is undoubtedly related in complex and multiple ways to normal hematopoiesis, no other nutritional deficiencies in addition to iron, vitamin B-12 and folic acid have been identified as specific causes of anemia. Anemia accompanies generalized protein malnutrition quite regularly. However, this may reflect deficient intake of the three essential dietary substances. Also, many patients with severe protein malnutrition have other active illnesses which may supress normal hematopoiesis. It should be emphasized that only severe malnutrition may be associated with anemia. Minor anomalies of the diet cannot be held responsible for anemia, even though this is a popular belief.

A very rare hypochromic microcytic refractory anemia has been found to be responsive in some cases to pharmcological doses of pyridoxine. This disorder is not accompanied by other findings of pyridoxine deficiency and cannot be regarded as a nutritional deficiency disease.

Suppression or Failure of Hematopoiesis

This large and diverse group of disorders is usually referred to as aplastic, hypoplastic or hyporegenerative states of the bone marrow. Usually some degree of hypocellularity of the marrow accompanies them, however, marrow cellularity may be normal or increased in the face of decreased production of blood cells.

Although single cell type cytopenias due to hyporegeneration do occur clinically, more commonly some degree of hyporegeneration of all cell types occurs, particularly when the bone marrow is hypocellular. These disorders are termed pancytopenias where anemia, granulocytopenia and thrombocytopenia in variable degrees of severity occur together. Granulocytopenia, resulting in neutropenia of less than 500 cells/cu mm, is associated with increased frequency and severity of infection. Thrombocytopenia, with fewer platelets than 20,000/cu mm, results in increasing incidence of clinically important hemorrhage as the platelet count decreases. The total clinical picture will depend upon the combination and severity of the three major blood cell deficits.

The clinical outcome of a hyporegenerative process is largely determined by the reversibility of the cause. Many hyporegenerative disorders are transient or promptly reversible when a known offending drug or chemical exposure is removed; others may not recover on cessation of exposure as is the case in some patients treated with chloramphenicol. Unfortunately, many patients in whom an etiological agent cannot be identified have marrow hypoplasia which is severe, chronic and frequently fatal.

Anemia of Chronic Disease

This term includes a very large number of causes of a hyporegenerative anemia and represents the most common causes of anemia encountered in general medical practice. Metabolic disorders, particularly hypothyroidism and uremia, chronic infections or inflammatory diseases, such as chronic osteomyelitis or rheumatoid arthritis and malignant neoplasms, constitute the primary disorders associated with the anemia of chronic disease.

The clinical picture is usually that of a minimal to moderate anemic state with the hemoglobin concentration usually above 6 to 7 gm/dl. Patients with end-stage renal insufficiency, particularly those that have been nephrectomized, usually have more severe anemia. The blood picture is a normocytic and normochromic anemia; characteristically, the reticulocyte count is low in relation to the degree of anemia present. The bone marrow shows a normoblastic pattern of red cell development; granulocytopoiesis is commonly increased in those cases associated with chronic inflammation or infection. Occasionally, the peripheral blood picture is to some degree macrocytic with similar enlargement of the erythroid precursors in the marrow but without typical megloblastic changes in nuclear structure. Serum iron concentration and iron binding capacity are usually reduced.

Treatment must be thought of in terms of management of the underlying disease. When this cannot be alleviated, the patient's symptoms secondary to anemia should be carefully evaluated and a program of chronic transfusion therapy instituted, if it is justified by significant physiological limitations imposed on the patient by anemia. Patients whose hemoglobin levels stabilize in the neighborhood of 8 gm/dl or above rarely require transfusion. Over transfusion of this group of patients is common practice and exposes the patient to significant, unnecesary risks. The prognosis for the patient and the course of the anemic state depend upon the nature and clinical course of the primary disease.

Bone Marrow Hypoplasia and Aplasia

Although infrequently encountered, a severe hypoplastic state of the bone marrow with pancytopenia is a serious and commonly lethal disorder. The clinical onset may vary from slow to very rapid, particularly when a severe infection or hemorrhage calls attention to the problem. The prognosis for the individual patient depends upon the reversibility of the aplastic or hypoplastic process and the possibility that by appropriate therapy the patient may withstand severe marrow hypofunction.

Sudden aplasia of the red cell precursors in the marrow is encountered as an "aplastic crisis" in a few patients with chronic hemolytic disorders. In this situation, marrow production of red cells stops, frequently in association with a transient, ill-defined illness (probably of viral origin). After approximately 10 to 14 days, red cell production begins again with an intense outpouring of reticulocytes and late nomoblasts into the peripheral blood. This type of transient red cell aplasia is recognized in patients with chronic hemolytic states because of the short survival of their red cells in the peripheral blood, which leads to prompt appearance of severe anemia when red cell production stops. Transfusion may be necessary during this period to allow the patient to survive until red cell production is reestablished. The mechanism of this type of transient red cell aplasia is unknown. It is possible that it also occurs in people with normal red cell survival who do not become significantly anemic because of the brief duration of surpressed red cell production.

More chronic forms of pure red cell aplasia have been described, but they are very uncommon. One such disorder is congenital. Failure of proliferation of a very early red cell precursor is thought to be responsible for acquired chronic red cell aplasia. An autoimmune process in which an autoantibody somehow interferes with red cell precursor proliferation is thought to account for at least some patients with acquired red cell aplasia. The strategy of managing such patients is appropriate chronic transfusion therapy in most instances. Some patients respond to treatment with a variety of combinations of corticosteroid and androgenic compounds. When an autoimmune process has been found to be involved, immunosuppressive therapy has been successful in some cases.

When the anemic patient is also granulocytopenic and/or thrombocytopenic, the management problem becomes much more difficult. Careful surveillance of the patient for infection with prompt treatment of infections that are identified or even suspected is crucial. Even so, many patients who are severely granulocytopenic for more than a few weeks will succumb to infection and sepsis. Granulocyte transfusions can be given to such patients with infection for periods of several weeks before the development of alloantibodies to donor granulocyte antigens renders them no longer effective.

In patients who are severely thrombocytopenic, bleeding manifestations may be minimal in spite of severely depressed platelet counts. Even small numbers of newly produced platelets may offer the patient substantial protection against hemorrhage. In other patients, more severe degrees of hemostatic impairment are seen. This may result in blood loss, such as gastrointestinal bleeding or epistaxis, which, unless massive and uncontrollable, can be dealt with by transfusion. On the other hand, relatively minor bleeding into a vital site such as the central nervous system may result in the patient's death in a short period of time.

Platelet transfusions are effective in the control of hemorrhage caused by thrombocytopenia, again for relatively short periods of time, up to about 2 weeks. Although platelet transfusions have been administered prophylactically, it is probably better strategy to administer them to control bleeding episodes. As in the case of granulocyte transfusions, platelet transfusions are useful only in supporting the patient during a relatively short period of recoverable marrow aplasia, up to about 4 to 6 weeks. It should be recognized that patients who are both thrombocytopenic and granulocytopenic are more likely to die of infection than of hemorrhage, even though hemorrhage may be an alarming and serious clinical problem.

Hyporegenerative Anemia with Normally Cellular or Hyperplastic Bone Marrow

Occasionally, patients are encountered who have marked suppression of peripheral blood cell production but in whom the bone marrow is normal in cellularity or hypercellular. This situation is commonly a precursor of a true neoplastic disorder of hematopoiesis. After a variable period of time, a more typical picture of acute leukemia frequently appears. In some instances, changes in the nuclear structure of the developing erythroid cells cause them to resemble megloblasts. These changes, referred to as "megloblastoid", are unresponsive to therapy with vitamin B-12 or folic acid, and commonly the serum levels of these two vitamins are normal.

These patients should be treated as any other patient with a hyporegenerative process until the basic leukemic process expresses itself, at which time treatment can be directed toward the neoplastic disease. Frequently such patients are relatively unresponsive to antileukemic therapy.

Sideroblastic anemia. A disorder related to this group of hyporegenerative anemias is termed sideroblastic anemia because of the presence of relatively large numbers of red cell precursors in the bone marrow which contain stainable iron. These erythroid precursors are called sideroblasts. The iron may be present in the form of large and/or small granules. Large aggregations of stainable iron in the perinuclear area may form a virtual ring around the nucleus, the "ringed sideroblast". The peripheral blood picture in these patients may show variable degrees of hypochromia, anisocytosis and poikilocytosis. The serum iron levels are generally normal or elevated, and the patient does not respond to therapeutic iron. Some patients in this group have been found to be responsive to pharmacologic doses of pyridoxine. They form a sub-group called pyridoxine responsive sideroblastic anemia. The majority of patients have a prolonged clinical course characterized by moderate to severe hyporegenerative anemia which at times requires transfusion. A substantial portion of these patients will terminate with an acute leukemic process. The relationship between the sideroblastic state and the appearance of leukemia is unknown but probably represents the occurrence of an oncogenic event in a particularly susceptible cell population in the bone marrow.

DISORDERS ASSOCIATED WITH INCREASED RED CELL DESTRUCTION

The Hemolytic Disorders

These disorders are defined by shortened red cell life-span in the peripheral circulation (i.e., less than the normal value of approximately 120 days). If the shortening of life-span is minimal (70 to 80 days) it may only be detectable by a measurement of red cell life-span. In other situations, it may be extremely short, a matter of hours to a few days as may be seen in the immunologically mediated hemolytic diseases, and cause severe anemia.

Patients with hemolytic disorders become anemic when their capacity for new red cell production exceeds the increased rate of destruction; at this point a new and lower level of the hematocrit will occur and remain stable as long as the rates of red cell destruction and production do not change. The patient who has shortened red cell life-span without anemia has a compensated hemolytic disorder; after the onset of anemia the term uncompensated is applied. Although clinically feasible methods for measuring red cell life-span are available and may help to define hemolytic disorders in which life-span is only minimally decreased, they are rarely necessary in clinical practice. The most reliable evidence of the existence of a hemolytic disorder is persistent reticulocytosis indicative of the regenerative effort of the bone marrow to replace the excessive destruction of red cells. Normal liver function can clear substantially increased heme pigment loads and prevent the patient from becoming clinically jaundiced, however, the total serum bilirubin concentration may rise slightly with an increase in the unconjugated bilirubin fraction in the face of relatively slow hemolysis. When hemolysis is more vigorous, the patient becomes jaundiced. After serum bilirubin concentration has risen to about 4.0 mg/dl, both the conjugated and unconjugated fractions will be increased in most patients.

Classification of Hemolytic Disorders

Two large groups of hemolytic disorders are recognized (Table 17.7). In the first group, a red cell defect limits the life-span of the cell. Disorders of this nature are largely congenital and of genetic origin. They reflect a wide range of biochemical defects of the metabolism and structure of the red cell. Characteristically, these abnormal red cells have a short life-span in the circulation of the patient and very nearly as short a life-span in the circulation of a normal recipient.

The second large group is the acquired hemolytic disorders in which an essentially normal red cell is delivered into the peripheral circulation but is destroyed there by a pathophysiological process operating in the circulatory milieu. The defect in these disorders is extracorpuscular in nature. Neither the patient's own red cells nor red cells of a normal donor will have a normal life-span in the patient's circulation.

Genetically Determined Defects of Red Cell Metabolism

Erythrocytes derive energy by the process of anaeorobic glycolysis. Two highly interrelated metabolic pathways are present in normal red cells, the

Table 17.7 Classification of Congenital and Acquired Hemolytic Disorders

I. Congenital disorders
  A. Genetically determined defects of red cell metabolism
    1. Abnormalities of glycolysis (see Table 8)
    2. Abnormalities of other enzyme systems that are:
      a) Associated with glutathione metabolism
        Glutathione reductase
        GSH synthetase
        GSH peroxidase
      b) Associated with nucleotide metabolism
        Adenylate kinase
        Pyrimidine-5'-nucleotidase
  B. Hemolytic anemia associated with abnormalities of hemoglobin synthesis
    1. Reduced globin synthesis
      Alpha Thalassemias
      Beta Thalassemias
    2. Abnormal Hemoglobin
      Sickle cell anemia
      Hemoglobin C disease
      Other hemoglobinopathies
  C. Associated with undefined ultrastructural abnormalities
    1. Hereditary spherocytosis
    2. Hereditary elliptocytosis
    3. Hereditary stomatocytosis
    4. Acanthocytosis
II. Acquired disorders
  A. Immunologically mediated hemolyis
    1. Autoimmune hemolytic diseases
      Warm-reacting autoantibodies
      Cryopathic hemolytic syndromes
    2. Drug-induced immunological mechanisms
      Drugs acting as haptenes
      Immune complex formation
      Induction of an autoimmune response
    3. Due to passive transfer of blood group alloantibodies
  B. Hemolysis induced by physical and chemical agents
    1. Red cell trauma
      March hemoglobinuria
      Circulatory trauma
        Aortic cardiac valves
        Blood flow at high pressures through small openings
        Microangiopathic hemolysis
        Thermal injury
    2. Strongly oxidant chemicals and poisonings
    3. Osmotic hemolysis
    4. Toxic bites
  C. Secondary to infection
    1. Malaria
    2. Bartonellosis
    3. *Clostridium welchii*
  D. Undefined membrane defects
    Paroxysmal nocturnal hemoglobinuria

Embden-Meyerhoff hexose pathway and the pentose or so-called "shunt" metabolic pathway. Both pathways have as their ultimate purpose the regeneration of adenosine triphosphate (ATP) which is coupled to

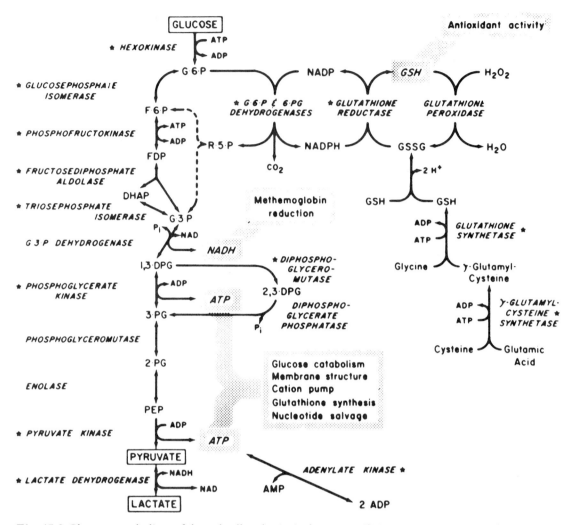

Fig. 17.9 Glucose metabolism of the red cell and principal energy utilizing reactions (From Valentine WN: Hemolytic anemia and inborn errors of metabolism. Blood, 54:549, 1979, with permission.)

energy requiring processes of the red cell. Maintenance of NADH and glutathione in the reduced state is also dependent upon glycolysis. The glycolytic processes of the red cell are shown in Figure 17.9.

Another product of red cell glycolysis is the intracellular pool of 2,3 diphosphoglycerate (2,3, DPG) which is important in maintaining the normal hemoglobin affinity for oxygen. Maintenance of the iron of hemoglobin in the reduced state is also dependent upon glycolysis. A number of energy requiring reactions of the red cell such as Na^+ and K^+ transport are known. Undoubtedly other linkages of red cell sources of energy to important functions remain to be defined.

At virtually every point in this metabolic schema, an enzymatic defect has been identified which has been associated with shortening of red cell life-span.

Table 17.8 lists the more common red cell abnormalities of glycolysis and indicates the principle clinical features of each disorder.

Glucose 6 Phosphate Dehydrogenase Deficiency

Pathophysiology. This disorder is of particular importance because it was the first metabolic disorder of red cells shown to result in hemolysis. Alving and colleagues, while studying the antimalarial drug primaquine, found that in certain subjects, primarily black males, this mildly oxidant compound resulted in hemolysis. The hemolytic process was found to stabilize usually when the hematocrit was only moderately depressed and newly formed red cells were

Table 17.8 **Defects of Glucose Metabolism Leading to Congenital Hemolytic Anemia**

Metabolic Abnormality	Genetic pattern of transmission	Clinical features
Abnormalities of Embden-Meyerhof pathway		
Hexokinase (HK)	Autosomal Recessive	All have hemolysis and anemia-variable severity
Glucose phosphate isomerase (GPI)	"	"
Phosphofructokinase (PFK)	"	Muscle glycogenosis in some cases. Also neurological disorder
Aldolase (ALD)	"	"
Triosephosphate isomerase (TPI)	"	Systemic disease including neurological and cardiac abnormalities
Diphosphoglycerate mutase (DPGM)	"	"
Phosphoglycerate kinase (PGK)	X-Linked	Also neurological disorder
Pyruvate kinase (PK)	Autosomal Recessive	Splenectomy may improve
Abnormalities of the hexose monophosphate shunt pathway		
Glucose-6-phosphate dehydrogenase (G-6-PD)	X-Linked	Hemolysis after exposure to oxidant drugs

delivered to the circulation. Subsequent biochemical investigations revealed that the enzyme, glucose 6 phosphate dehydrogenase (G6PD), in the shunt or pentose pathway of red cell glucose metabolism was low in activity. Since the shunt metabolic reactions are coupled to the biochemical reactions which maintain glutathione (GSH) in the reduced state, gradually GSH becomes oxidized thereby reducing the capacity of the red cell membrane to defend itself against oxidant attack by the drug. This hemolytic process preferentially destroys older cells in which G6PD activity is lowest. The rate of red cell destruction stabilizes as newly delivered cells with higher enzyme content are delivered to the peripheral blood in response to hemolysis. These important observations initiated the systematic investigation of a variety of unexplained congenital hemolytic anemias.

Clinical features. G6PD deficiency is found largely in people of African and Mediterranean origin. It is estimated to be present in about 10 percent of American blacks. The disorder affects largely males since the gene which determines this enzyme is present on the X chromosome for which males are hemizygous. Homozygous females are also affected. Rarely a heterozygous female will have a large enough proportion of her red cells containing only the defective enzyme to cause significant hemolysis on exposure to an oxidant drug. G6PD deficiency in the heterozygous state is thought to confer some protection against malaria, which through increased survival may contribute to its frequency in some malarious areas of the world.

The enzyme G6PD can be isolated from red cells and subjected to chromatographic analysis. Over 150 variants of this enzyme have been discovered with a wide range of decrease in activity. The type B enzyme predominates among caucasian populations and about three quarters of American blacks; about 20 percent of blacks of African origin have a variant termed A$^+$ which is also normal in enzymatic activity. The A$^-$ variant is the most frequent defective enzyme among blacks. The most severely G6PD deficient patients are frequently northern Europeans who are found to have a chronic low level of hemolysis, which becomes very much more severe on exposure to oxidant drugs or during infections. They may require urgent transfusion support during severe hemolytic episodes.

Treatment. It is important that patients with G6PD deficiency be identified so that they may be counseled to avoid exposure to oxidant drugs (Table 17.9). Also, relatively severe infections will result in onset of hemolysis in patients with more markedly decreased G6PD function. A number of tests exist for screening patients suspected of G6PD deficiency. These tests may be negative after an episode of hemolysis, when a large number of G6PD rich reticulocyte and newly formed red cells are present in the circulation. The test should be carried out 2 to 3 months after a hemolytic episode. G6PD testing may be useful as part of a screening program for genetic counseling purposes among ethnic groups at increased risk.

Other enzymes in the metabolic pathway between G6PD and glutathione have been found to be deficient in certain patients whose clinical picture very much resembles G6PD deficiency. Specifically, glutathione reductase deficiency and a number of metabolic defects which lead to a deficiency in the synthesis of glutathione itself form a related group of disorders involving this important metabolic pathway of red cell energy production.

Table 17.9 **Drugs Which May Induce Hemolysis in Patients with G-6-PD Deficiency**

Antimalarials
  Primaquine
  Pamaquine
Analgesics
  Acetanalid
  Aspirin—large doses
  Phenacetin—large doses
Antibacterial agents
  Sulfonamides and sulfones
  Furazolidone
  Nitrofurantoin
  Para-aminosalicylic acid (PAS)
Others
  Naphthalene
  Nalidixic acid
  Phenylhydrazine

Favism

This interesting disorder, found principally in southern Italy, Sicily, Sardinia, the Middle East and Greece, is characterized by a severe hemolytic process induced by exposure to fava beans in the diet (vincia faba). Severely sensitive people also hemolyze on exposure to the pollen of this bean when it is in flower. The process by which the fava bean induces hemolysis remains unclear. Patients with favism are also severely G6PD deficient; however, not all patients with severe forms of G6PD deficiency have favism. The disorder has been regarded as a hypersensitivity state, but the mechanism of the hypersensitivity has not been demonstrated. Although it is uncommonly encountered in the United States, it can present a severe and life threatening hemolytic anemia, treatable only with transfusion support. These patients should be identified and warned to refrain from exposure to the fava bean.

The Hemoglobinopathies and Thalassemia Syndromes

This diverse group of disorders have in common abnormalities of hemoglobin structure or synthesis which are genetic in origin. The hemoglobinopathies are characterized by synthesis of hemoglobins with abnormal primary aminoacid sequences secondary to mutations in the DNA code which specifies the structure of the globin moiety of hemoglobin. By contrast, the thalassemia syndromes are characterized by varying degrees of suppression of normal globin chain production. Here the abnormality residing in the DNA is either complete or partial deletion of one or more of the genes for globin production or the presence of a gene which does not permit globin production at a normal rate.

The frequency of both types of genetic abnormalities vary from extremely rare to relatively common in differing world populations. They are more frequent among African, Mediterranean (including middle eastern), and oriental populations. It is thought that certain hemoglobinopathies such as hemoglobin S, associated with the clinically benign sickling trait in the heterozygous state, have a selective survival advantage in areas with endemic malaria.

The full clinical spectrum of these disorders is not appreciated in the practice of internal medicine. Not only do a significant proportion of the most severely affected individuals die during childhood, but the problems of anemia and hemolysis are relatively more severe in the growing and developing child. The milder disorders recognized with increasing frequency among adults have significance in genetic counselling. It is also important to identify patients with these causes of anemia to separate them from those who have an important treatable cause of anemia and to establish appropriate therapy for both groups of patients based upon a firm diagnosis.

Normal structure, function and synthesis of hemoglobin. Normal human hemoglobins have four globin chains, each of which bears an iron-heme moiety responsible for reversible oxygen binding in the oxygen transport process. Two of the chains are of the α (alpha) type. The nature of the remaining two chains determine three specific normal hemoglobin types termed A, A_2 and F. These chains are termed β, δ and γ (beta, delta and gamma) respectively. Normally, four α chain genes and two each of the genes for β, δ and γ chains are present in the DNA; they direct the synthesis of these specific globin proteins. Assembly of the four protein chains into tetramers appears to depend upon balanced synthesis of the component chains and the configurations of the chains themselves. A diagramatic illustration of the tetrameric structure of the hemoglobin A molecule is shown in Figure 17.10. Note that a cavity is depicted in the center of this symmetrical structure where the four chains approach each other. The chains move one upon the other during oxygenation and deoxygenation. This is the region of the molecule in which the compound 2, 3 DPG interacts to affect oxygen association and disassociation. Abnormalities in the chain structures which affect the areas of interchain contact result in hemoglobins with altered affinity for oxygen. The heme moiety is bound to histidine in a hydrophobic

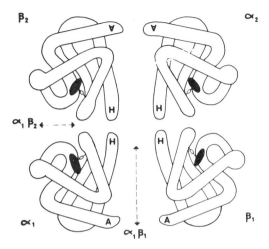

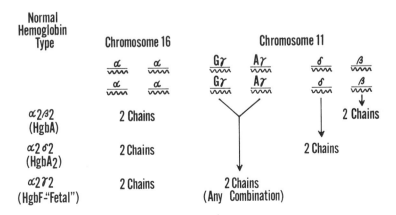

Fig. 17.10 Diagramatic structure of normal human hemoglobin. A. (after White JM, cited by Chanarin J, Brozović M, Tidemarsh E, Waters DAW: Blood and its Diseases. 2nd ed. Churchill Livingstone, Edinburgh, 1980, with permission.)

Table 17.10   Evolution of Hemoglobin Patterns in Fetal and Post-Natal Life

Hemoglobin type	Stage of Development			
	Fetal*	Birth	Age 1 yr.	Adult
HgbA($\alpha_1\beta_2$)	<10%	<1/3	>96%	>96%
HgbA2($\alpha\delta_2$)				<3.5%
HgbF($\alpha_2\gamma_2$)	90–95%	>2/3	2–3%	<1.5%

* Other hemoglobins also found only in very early embryonic life

pocket. Substitutions of amino acids in this region which result in a polar pocket cause instability of those hemoglobin variants.

The gene complex responsible for the structure of normal human hemoglobin is shown diagrammatically in Figure 17.11. The proportion of the three non α chains synthesized, which results in the formation of variable amounts of the three normal hemoglobins A, A_2 and F, is regulated by a complex and poorly understood mechanism during fetal life, early infancy and adulthood as summarized in Table 17.10.

To function as an oxygen transport protein, the iron of the heme moiety must be maintained in a reduced, ferrous state. When iron is in the ferric form, the hemoglobin is referred to as *methemoglobin*. Reduction is normally carried out enzymatically by methemoglobin reductase linked to NADH derived from the red cell glycolytic cycle. A second enzyme system linked to NADPH derived from the shunt or pentose glycolytic pathway exists but requires an artificial electron carrier such as methylene blue to function. This property of methylene blue has been used to reverse rapidly acquired types of methemoglobinemia. Rare abnormal hemoglobins in which the heme iron is unprotected from oxidation to the ferric state are termed M hemoglobins. They are commonly the result of replacement of one of the two histidines of the heme pocket of the globin chain by tyrosine.

As hemoglobin is oxygenated, there is cooperative interaction of the four chains, termed heme-heme interaction, which results in an approximately 20 fold difference in the affinity with which the oxygen molecules from the first to the fourth are bound. This differential affinity results in a sigmoid shape of the curve describing the hemoglobin-oxygen association. (see Chapter 15 and Fig. 15.3). The position of this curve of oxygen saturation of hemoglobin vs. partial pressure of O_2(pO_2) varies under a number of influences (Table 17.11).

HUMAN HEMOGLOBIN GENES

Fig. 17.11 Gene structure determining globin chain and structure of normal human hemoglobins. The two types of γ genes reflect the presence of glycine or alanine at position 136 of the chain; they appear to have equivalent properties.

Table 17.11 Factors Which Influence the Affinity of Hemoglobin for Oxygen (See also Fig. 15.3)

Factor	Change	Shift of Dissociation Curve	Change in O_2 Affinity	Change in P50
H+ conc.	Increased	Right	↓	↑
CO_2 conc. Temperature 2,3, DPG Conc.	Decreased	Left	↑	↓

The most useful measurement to define the hemoglobin affinity for oxygen is provided by determination of the partial pressure of O_2 at which 50 percent of the hemoglobin is oxygenated, P_{50} value. Normally this is 27.0 ± 1 mm Hg partial pressure of O_2 when measured at standard conditions (37°C, pH 7.4, PCO_2 40 mm Hg). The level of intracellular 2,3 DPG influences the hemoglobin affinity for oxygen and oxygen transport. Pulmonary insufficiency, right to left cardiovascular shunts, chronic anemia and other causes of chronic tissue anoxia all activate synthesis of increased 2, 3 DPG and shift the curve to the right.

Hemoglobinopathies

Human hemoglobin is one of the most structurally variable proteins known with more than 350 recognized variants. A surprising range of altered properties of this protein are either asymptomatic or only minimally disabling in affected patients, particularly in the heterozygous state. The majority of known variants are single point mutations (about 300 in all), involving a single amino acid substitution or deletion in the α and β chains in a ratio of nearly 1:2. Except for a small number of known single point mutations of the δ and γ chains, all other abnormalities are more complex and involve gene fusion, deletions, extended chains, and a small number of two point mutations. Most of these complex abnormalities are rare and also usually involve the β chain which appears to be more mutation prone than the other hemoglobin genes.

Abnormal hemoglobins produce pathophysiological changes when the structural abnormality significantly alters the function or solubility of the molecule. The severity of the clinical disease caused by the abnormality will also depend upon the relative amounts of abnormal hemoglobin and the other normal hemoglobins present. The zygosity of the patient for the abnormal gene, presence or absence of abnormalities of hemoglobin synthesis (such as thalassemia and other less well understood factors which regulate hemoglobin synthesis), and other environmental and individual factors determine the ultimate clinical expression of these genetic abnormalities. The major groups of abnormal hemoglobins are summarized in Table 17.12.

Clinical importance of these disorders is determined by the incidence of the disorder and its severity. Only those disorders which are relatively common can be discussed here. Many of even the more severe disorders are so infrequently encountered that they remain in the province of research or reference laboratories.

Sickle Cell Hemoglobinopathy

This disorder, affecting blacks, almost exclusively, is usually discussed in the group of hemolytic anemias, since shortened red cell life span is part of the

Table 17.12 Major Groups of Abnormal Hemoglobins and Pathophysiological Consequences

Major Abnormality	Example	Pathophysiological Consequences
Decreased stability	Sickle Hgb (HbS)	Decreased solubility in deoxygenated state with precipitation, rigidification of RBC, hemolysis and microvascular occlusion
Unstable Hgbs.	HB Koln	Denaturation—precipitation of Hb, Heinz body formation, Hemolysis
Hemoglobins with altered O_2 affinity		
High affinity	Hb Chesapeake	Oxygen dissociation curve shifted left, ↓ O_2 delivery erythrocytosis
Low affinity	Hb Boston	Curve shifted right, ↑ O_2 delivery, "spurious anemia" (i.e., lower than normal RBC mass adequate for normal O_2 delivery)
M Hemoglobins	HbM Boston	$Fe^{++} \rightarrow Fe^{+++}$, ↓ O_2 uptake, cyanosis, variable erythrocytosis

pathophysiological process caused by presence of an abnormal hemoglobin, Hgb S. The elongated "tactoids" of insoluble deoxyhemoglobin S are a hallmark of the disease.

Sickle trait.   This genetic trait caused by inheritance of a single β gene for Hb S exists in many black people without symptoms or abnormal physical or laboratory findings. The blood film, if produced from well-oxygenated blood, is usually normal. A variety of tests for sickling of red cells will be positive. These tests are primarily important for genetic counselling purposes. The patients are not anemic although it should be recognized that black people as a group have slightly lower normal values of hemoglobin and hematocrit. Sickle trait is frequently associated with fixed or low specific gravity of the urine without significantly abnormal renal function. Thrombotic episodes secondary to intravascular sickling must be very uncommon in true HbS trait, although it may occur with severe anoxia. In general, the concentration of HbS in the heterozygote will be about 30 percent. If the concentration of HbS approaches 50 percent or greater consideration must be given to the likelihood that the patient also has a second abnormal gene of the thalassemia group which has limited the synthesis of HbA.

Treatment is not required for this genetic trait. It is important to explain the clinical significance and genetic transmission of HbS trait and to be sure the patient understands that this disorder does not become sickle cell anemia.

Sickle cell anemia.   Homozygosity for the HbS gene results in a severe, devastating disorder often leading to demise in early adulthood. The hallmarks of the disease are a severe hemolytic anemia and recurrent vaso–occlusive crises which produce a wide range of manifestations, particularly recurrent episodes of abdominal pain. These crises do not in general involve accelerated red cell destruction; they are inappropriately referred to as hemolytic crises. They frequently resemble acute surgical problems in the abdomen. These patients, of course, may have true surgical problems unrelated to sickle cell anemia, a serious differential diagnostic dilemma requiring great experience and clinical acuity to resolve. There may be neutrophilic leukocytosis and some fever associated with crisis. Ileus may occur. In spite of the fact that the abdomen may be tender either diffusely or in a localized region, true signs of peritoneal inflammation occur uncommonly. Many such patients have been subjected to abdominal exploration unnecessarily, but there are times when the abdominal manifestations of sickle cell crisis so closely resemble a surgical condition that exploration seems necessary.

As a result of repeated small splenic infarctions secondary to aggregations of red cells within the splenic pulp which occlude circulation, many patients have effectively lost splenic function by the time they reach late childhood or early adulthood. This has been referred to as autosplenectomy, an abnormality of some importance since it increases the likelihood that the patient will have septic infections, particularly pneumonia or osteomyelitis with gram negative organisms. The white blood cell count may become chronically elevated secondary to loss of splenic function.

Chronic anemia as well as vascular occlusions at the microcirculatory level are thought to be responsible for decreased cardiac reserve, cardiac enlargement and at times the onset of overt cardiac failure. A high incidence of chronic ulcerations of the lower extremities, frequently just above the ankle, have been associated with this disorder. The pathogenesis of these lesions is unclear, but they probably also reflect some degree of vascular occlusion and ischemia. The incidence of this complication of sickle cell anemia may be declining.

The blood picture shows chronic anemia with hemoglobin levels commonly below 5 gm percent with persistent, marked reticulocytosis and normoblastemia. A careful search of the blood film usually reveals irreversibly sickled red cells. All tests for red cell sickling are strongly positive. Although these findings are adequate to establish the diagnosis of sickle cell anemia in most instances, hemoglobin electrophoresis provides strong confirmation and may also suggest the presence of other abnormal hemoglobins.

The treatment of sickle cell anemia is still a subject of some controversy. Transfusion is certainly necessary if the patient's symptoms are due primarily to chronic anemia per se. Under these circumstances, only enough transfusion need be administered to improve the patient's functional capacity to a reasonable point. Significant cardiac impairment justifies maintenance of a higher level of hemoglobin (in the neighborhood of 10 gm/dl). During aplastic crises in which red cell production virtually ceases for a period of 7 to 10 days, transfusion may be required urgently. Hemolytic crises which are uncommon also usually require transfusion therapy.

It is generally agreed after one is convinced that a surgical condition does not exist, that the painful crises can be managed by rest, correction of dehydration and electrolyte abnormalities, and control of pain by analgesics. Transfusion therapy does not significantly change the course of an attack or crisis after it has been established. However, chronic hypertransfusion with normal red cells, which is designed to supress the production of the patient's own abnormal red cells, does appear to decrease the frequency and/or severity of attacks. What is controversial is whether the risks associated with chronic transfusion, including cost and inconvenience, are adequately offset by the benefits that may be obtained. Patients with severe, frequent recurrent crises may well justify a trial of transfusion designed to reduce the concentration of hemoglobin S to a level below about 50 percent. Patients with sickle cell anemia who may become anoxic during the administration of an anesthetic and surgery or who become acutely anoxic due to any type of disturbed pulmonary function should be transfused again to reduce the level of hemoglobin S to less than 50 percent.

The administration of folic acid, 1 to 2 mg per day by mouth, is probably of value in these patients, as in any patient with a severe and chronic hemolytic disorder. This provides adequate folic acid to support the necessary regeneration of blood. In recent years, several methods have been proposed for the chemical or physico-chemical modification of hemoglobin S to prevent its sickling. The use of urea and glycerol or carbamylation of the hemoglobin, all of which in vitro limit the formation of the long tubular polymers of hemoglobin S in the deoxygenated form, have proved neither clinically valuable nor sound as preventive measures to control crises.

The outlook for the patient with sickle cell anemia remains poor. However, the life-span of those patients who have less severe disease and who have been well managed has increased over the last several decades. A substantial number of them are now surviving into middle age. At present, genetic counseling appears to offer the greatest hope for the reduction in the incidence of this serious disease. It is now possible by amniocentesis to detect the presence of a homozygous fetus during pregnancy. Since these methods are available to only a small proportion of people at risk, it is likely that sickle cell anemia will continue to be a major medical problem for the foreseeable future among people of African origin.

Hemoglobin C Disease

Hemoglobin C is also an anomaly of the β chain. In the heterozygous form, it is without clinical significance, although the blood picture is quite strikingly abnormal. On the blood film, numerous thin (leptocytic) cells are seen which also have a concentration of hemoglobin in the center of the cell giving rise to an appearance which has been called a "target cell". The mean cell diameter is increased, and there is some variation in size and shape of the erythro-cytes. Levels of hemoglobin and hematocrit are usually in the normal range unless there is another cause of anemia present.

In the homozygous state, the patient may have some shortening of red cell life span with mild anemia. The spleen may be moderately enlarged. Some patients have unexplained joint discomfort. Nevertheless, life expectancy is essentially normal in these patients. The blood smear is strikingly abnormal with large numbers of target cells, a large population of small highly distorted poikilocytes and reticulocytosis proportionate to the increased rate of blood destruction.

SC Double Heterozygote

Normally the heterozygote with S hemoglobin has more than 50 percent hemoglobin A. Similarly the heterozygote for hemoglobin C has at least 50 percent hemoglobin A. It is the predominance of hemoglobin A which appears to prevent intravascular sickling in SA patients under all but exceptional circumstances and to prevent the hemolytic process which characterizes both of these abnormal hemoglobins in the homozygous state. The patient who inherits one gene for hemoglobin S and another for hemoglobin C, however, presents a clinical picture less severe than that of the hemoglobin SS patients but, nevertheless, a picture indicative of significant disability. The degree of anemia is usually less severe than that encountered in hemoglobin SS disease, but vaso-occlusive crises occur. Bone infarcts and predisposition to infection also are seen in SC disease.

This disorder can be best diagnosed by hemoglobin electrophoresis in which roughly equal amounts of hemoglobin S and C will be found. It should be suspected in patients who otherwise resemble less severe forms of SS disease but who are less anemic than might be expected and who have prominent target cells in the blood film. Alternatively, a family study commonly reveals segregation of the S and C traits among siblings and one parent with each trait.

The treatment of SC disease patients is patterned after the management of the SS patient, although it is in general a somewhat less serious disorder. The same issues with regard to the use of transfusion therapy apply in both diseases.

Many other double heterozygotes for abnormalities of hemoglobin structure have been described but are infrequently encountered. Their identification depends on reference and research laboratories. The double heterozygotes involving the genes for thalassemia will be discussed in the next section. Hemoglobin D is notable in that it has essentially the same electrophoretic mobility as hemoglobin S. Such patients may appear to have all hemoglobin S but few, if any, clinical manifestations of SS disease. Other separation techniques are available which differentiate these two hemoglobins.

Other Abnormal Hemoglobins of Significance

Some abnormal hemoglobins are characterized by instability which leads to the formation of intraerythrocytic precipitates of denatured hemoglobin. These aggregates stain as so-called "Heinz" bodies. A hemolytic process results, probably because these hemoglobin aggregates are removed by splenic macrophages as a normal function. As a group, these patients are referred to as congenital Heinz body hemolytic anemia.

Abnormal hemoglobins may have either high or low affinity for oxygen, depending on their effects on 2-3 DPG and configuration of the hemoglobin molecule (Table 17.12).

The abnormal M hemoglobins maintain the iron in the ferric state, thus preventing normal transportation of oxygen. This is a rare cause of chronic methemoglobinemia, the principal manifestation of which is chronic cyanosis. In the heterozygous state for an M hemoglobin, the hemoglobin A present is usually able to transport adequate amounts of oxygen. The M hemoglobins are able to transport some oxygen, depending upon the efficiency with which the hemoglobin can be reduced and maintained in the ferrous state.

More common causes of methemoglobinemia are poisoning of the diaphorase responsible for reduction of iron from the ferric to ferrous state. A substantial number of chemicals and compounds have this potential. High levels of nitrates in the water drawn from shallow wells was at one time a common cause of methemoglobinemia and cyanosis in infants. This type of methemoglobinemia spontaneously reverses itself on withdrawal of the offending chemical or drug. In some instances, the methemoglobinemia may be so severe as to require prompt reversal by the administration of methylene blue to activate the NADPH linked hemoglobin reduction system.

Thalassemia Syndromes

The thalassemia syndromes, seen primarily among ethnic groups derived from the area of the Mediterranean basin, are fundamentally disorders characterized by suppressed synthesis of hemoglobin A.

Suppression of hemoglobin synthesis is now recognized to be due to decreased production of either α (alpha) or β (beta) chains of the hemoglobin molecule. These two major types of thalassemia are thus known as alpha or beta thalassemia. Multiple abnormalities exist at the genetic level in both of these groups, leading to an extraordinary complexity of the resultant clinical pictures. Actual deletion of the genetic information itself, defects in transcription which result in production of little mRNA, and other anomalies of gene transcription all appear to have a common effect: inhibition of the synthesis of normal amounts of α or β chains. Since the total amount of hemoglobin synthesized is reduced, these disorders have in common some degree of hypochromia and microcytosis. Furthermore, since the inhibition of synthesis may involve only a single type of chain, the remaining chains may be produced in relatively excessive amounts, leading to unbalanced chain synthesis. Variable amounts of hemoglobins A_2 and F are found in these patients; in some instances this appears to be compensatory in nature and in other cases under independent genetic control. The complete characterization of patients in this very complex group of disorders remains difficult, but the more common alpha and beta thalassemias can be recognized with some probability by standard hematological techniques and analysis of family pedigrees.

Alpha thalassemia   The recognition that there are normally four genes for the synthesis of alpha chains rather than two resulted in the classification of this group of disorders into four basic levels of increasing severity of suppression of A hemoglobin production. The disorder in which only a single abnormal alpha chain gene is present is effectively silent. When two genes are abnormal, alpha thalassemia trait results in which mild hypochromia, microcytosis with a relatively increased red cell count, and minimal or no anemia is present; it is also a clinically silent disorder. Its importance is based upon confusion with hypochromic microcytic anemia secondary to iron deficiency. The normal serum iron and iron binding capacity and studies of family members serve to distinguish this disorder which requires no treatment.

When three alpha genes are absent or dysfunctional, a severe disorder is created in which hemoglobin H is found. This abnormal hemoglobin consists of a tetramer of β chains and as such reflects the unbalanced increased synthesis of β as compared to α chains. Heinz bodies are present in the cells; red cell life-span is short; and moderately severe anemia is present.

When four alpha chain genes are absent, no alpha chains are synthesized thereby eliminating all hemoglobin A, F and A^2. This abnormality is lethal with hydropic infants still-born. Some hemoglobin Bart's is present, a tetramer of γ chains.

Beta thalassemia. Several abnormal β chain thalassemic genes are recognized. The β_0 gene is translated to mRNA, but this does not result in the synthesis of β chains. Heterozygotes have a variable degree of anemia with elevated A$_2$ hemoglobin and a "thalassemia trait" blood picture on the blood film. Homozygotes with this thalassemic gene have a severe anemia which commonly requires transfusion support throughout life; early death in childhood or adolescence is common.

The β + thalassemia gene results in synthesis of diminished amounts of beta chains with minimal or no anemia in the heterozygous state and a severe chronic anemia which ultimately is lethal in homozygotes. A type of combined thalassemic disorder in which both the β and δ genes are deleted is characterized by the presence of large amounts of hemoglobin F, apparently as a compensatory mechanism. Again homozygotes are severely affected with variable but less severe clinical manifestations than those seen in heterozygotes. Because of the multiple genetic abnormalities involved in this group of disorders, a large variety of mixed heterozygotes can be encountered with a variety of clinical manifestations. These patients are likely to present with moderate anemia, thalassemic findings in the blood film and variable, frequently minimal, clinical manifestations. At present they can be identified only in reference laboratories.

Interactions of thalassemia with hemoglobinopathies. When one or more genes for thalassemia are present along with a mutant gene specifying synthesis of an abnormal hemoglobin, a wide variety of possible interactions exists. This is particularly true in situations where the thalassemic gene and the gene for an abnormal hemoglobin both affect the same hemoglobin chain. Of these, the double heterozygote for beta thalassemia and hemoglobin S is the most important. In this situation, the synthesis of normal β chains may be markedly or virtually completely suppressed, with the result that all of the patient's β chain synthesis, or a very large part of it, is the abnormal beta chain of hemoglobin S. These patients have a severe disorder which closely resembles homozygous hemoglobin S disease. On electrophoresis, their hemoglobin may be virtually all hemoglobin S if the production of normal beta chains has been severely suppressed by the thalassemic gene. The true genetic situation can usually be clarified best by family studies, particularly if both parents are available. In this situation, one parent will be found to carry the S gene and the other the thalassemic

gene. In spite of the fact that this disorder is clinically more severe than that of the SC double heterozygote, the overall prognosis is still somewhat better than that of patients with homozygous hemoglobin S disease. It is important to identify these patients because of the possibly better prognosis. Also, the information obtained may be valuable for purposes of genetic counseling. The management of the patient is again comparable to that of homozygous hemoglobin S disease.

Undefined Ultrastructural Defects of the Red Blood Cell

This group if disorders has in common genetically determined abnormalities of red cell structure which involve primarily the red cell membrane and its cytoskeleton. The specific structural abnormality involved has not been identified biochemically in any of these disorders, although it is thought to primarily involve the proteins of the cytoskeleton rather than the lipid bilayer of the membrane itself. This group of disorders is also quite diverse, with variable patterns of genetic transmission, clinical expression, and in all probability substantially differing biochemically defined abnormalities. Fortunately, for clinical purposes, the disorders can be dealt with in three groups.

Hereditary spherocytosis. Hereditary spherocytosis (HS) is the best known disorder of this group. The disease is characterized by delivery from the bone marrow of red cells which are morphologically normal as they enter the circulation. Later, they assume a spherical shape, lose their normal plasticity and are ultimately fragmented in the spleen and removed by filtration. Chronic reticulocytosis, variable degrees of anemia and elevated serum bilirubin with splenomegaly are the clinical hallmarks of the disease. The spherocytic cells appear as dense, thick cells of reduced diameter on the blood film. The osmotic fragility of these spherocytes is increased over that of normal cells; they rupture in a less hypotonic medium than do normal red cells because they have less excess membrane to accomodate the increase in intracellular volume. Incubation of red cells from these patients without added glucose markedly accentuates the increase in osmotic sensitivity. The cause of the disorder is unknown, but investigation now centers around the structural protein spectrin.

HS is a relatively uncommon disorder, seen primarily among peoples of Northern European and English derivation. In the most common form of the disease, it is inherited as an autosomal dominant, although it has been noted for some time that there is a shortage of affected siblings and relatives. This has been interpreted as due to a relatively high mutation rate at this genetic locus. Also within a sibship, the disorder is commonly found to have variable severity, a situation referred to as variable expressivity. It is possible that the minimum genetic expression of this abnormality may be beyond the range of detection at present, in which case some family members may be misclassified as normal.

Because of the highly variable expression of HS, the associated clinical picture is equally variable. Patients with minimal clinical manifestations are frequently identified in family studies where a more significantly affected propositus has chronic anemia, reticulocytosis and splenomegaly. Severe anemia is uncommon and when present is associated with marked enlargement of the spleen. Many patients who have a high turnover of heme pigments will develop pigment gallstones by the second or third decade. Biliary obstruction may then occur, further complicating the clinical picture and the diagnosis.

Splenectomy is virtually curative of HS, although it does not reduce the abnormality of the red cells; indeed it may accentuate it. However, removal of the spleen, the principal site of damage and destruction of the spherocytic erythrocytes, greatly increases the survival of these cells in the circulation. It is probably wise to splenectomize virtually every patient with HS who has even mild chronic anemia with persistent reticulocytosis above 5 percent. The size of spleen tends to increase with age, and the hemolytic process may become more severe as a result. The risk of the surgical procedure itself is minimal, but there is increasing concern about susceptibility of the asplenic patient to infections, regardless of the age at which splenectomy is performed. If the patient is not anemic or is only minimally anemic with reticulocytes less than 3 to 4 percent, deferral of splenectomy may be reasonable, particularly if the patient is middle-aged or older.

Transfusion is rarely necessary except in the uncommon situation of an aplastic crisis at which time it may become urgently necessary as the patient's hematocrit falls rapidly. Following splenectomy, careful surveillance for infections with prompt treatment is necessary. Immunization against pneumococci may be of value in these patients as well. Excessive morbidity and mortality in this group of patients is minor and primarily the result of complications of surgery, infections or rarely transfusion. Genetic counseling should be provided to patient and affected family members.

Hereditary elliptocytosis. This rare disorder appears to be closely related to HS. It is again, undoubtedly, a heterogenous group of patients. In caucasians minimal or no anemia is usually present, with normal or minimally elevated reticulocyte counts. The diagnosis is most commonly made by identifying elliptical cells in a blood film prepared for another reason. No therapy is necessary.

Chronic ovalocytosis among blacks is associated with mild to moderate anemia, and blood films show more variability in size and shape of the red cells with increased reticulocytes.

Hereditary stomatocytosis. This rare disorder is characterized by the presence of red cells having a "stoma" (mouth) which can be observed both on the stained blood film and by scanning electron microscopy. The cells have a spherocytic form with the stoma appearing as a slit-like opening or cleft in the cell. Frequently this disorder is more severe than that seen in hereditary spherocytosis, but minimally affected patients and sibships have been encountered.

Acanthocytosis. The absence of beta lipoproteins in the plasma (abetalipoproteinemia), a rare congenital anomaly, results in the appearance of bizarre looking red cells termed acanthocytes. These red cells have a surface covered with nobby and spiny projections. The lipid composition of these erythrocytes is markedly deranged. In spite of their bizarre appearance, these red cells may have a nearly normal life-span with little evidence, therefore, of a hemolytic state.

Abnormalities of lipid metabolism associated with alcoholism and cirrhosis of the liver, as well as other genetically determined abnormalities of serum lipids, may result in the formation of red cells which resemble acanthocytes. Of the acquired types of acanthocytosis, that associated with alcoholism, liver disease and hypercholesterolemia, termed Zieve's syndrome, is the most frequently encountered and the most commonly associated with evidence of excessive hemolysis.

Acquired Hemolytic Disorders

Hemolytic Anemias Caused by Autoimmunity

Although the entire pathogenesis of the autoimmune response is still unknown, it is clear that abnormal immune responses against a wide variety of the body's own tissues is a major cause of disease. Autoimmunity directed against a patient's own red cells was one of the earliest recognized members of this large and expanding group of disorders. Until the immunological nature of the autoimmune acquired hemolytic anemias (AIHD) was recognized, these disorders were confused with the congenital

Table 17.13 **Comparison of Cold and Warm Reactive Autoantibodies**

Characteristic	Cold Reactive	Warm Reactive
Ig Type	Usually IgM.	IgG, rarely IgA.
Specificity	Ii, H systems	Rh related or Wr related
Thermal optimum	2°–4°C—may react up to 30°C+	22°–37°C
Complement fixation	Yes, usually C3	Usually not in vitro ? in vivo
Serological detection	Cold agglutination or hemolysis	Antiglobulin test (Coombs' test)

types of spherocytosis, since spherocytosis is a variably prominent feature of the blood picture in patients with active AIHD.

Two large groups of immunologically mediated acquired hemolytic disorders are recognized, based upon the physical and biochemical characteristics of the autoantibody. In the larger group of patients with AIHD, the autoantibody belongs to the 7S, IgG class of immunoglobulin and is serologically active at body temperature. A few autoantibodies of the IgA class also produce AIHD. This group of patients is referred to as the "warm autoantibody type" (Table 17.13). In the second major group, an IgM immunoglobulin autoantibody is involved which is serologically most active at lowered temperatures, usually less than 20°C, with optimal activity in vitro around 4°C. This group is referred to as the "cold reactive autoantibody type". The second group of disorders is also referred to as the "cryopathic hemolytic syndromes". Autoantibodies may react with many different antigenic determinant groups on the red cell surface. In general, the warm type of autoantibody reacts most frequently with a component of the Rh antigen complex. The Rh complex is found on the red cells of virtually every person except for a very small number of people in whom expression of this antigen has been completely or partially suppressed. Autoantibody components which react with other specific parts of the Rh antigen complex, for example the Rh antigens, E,C,e and c, are also found in AIHD. Other autoantibodies with specificities outside the Rh blood grouping system occur in about one-half of cases of warm autoantibody AIHD; those reactive with a complex of antigens termed Wr are the most frequently seen. Among cold reactive autoantibodies, the specificities are largely directed toward the antigens of the Ii and H complex. The specificity of the autoantibodies is important in these patients because of the complexities which autoantibodies produce in cross-matching them for transfusion.

Autoimmune acquired hemolytic anemia induced by warm autoantibodies. This disorder occurs in virtually all age groups. Two large groups are recognized: those in whom the disorder is un-associated with any apparent disease process, termed *idiopathic*, and those who have an associated disease, commonly a lymphoreticular proliferative disorder or another autoimmune disorder such as lupus erythematosus (Table 17.14). In the latter group screening with direct antiglobulin tests of the red cells may be useful, particularly if the patient is found to be anemic or to have persistent reticulocytosis.

The onset of the hemolytic process may be either insidious or explosive in nature. In the latter instance, there may be hemoglobinemia and a delay of several days before a significant reticulocyte response develops. More typically, the patient is anemic with a relatively high reticulocyte count, commonly above 10 percent, mildly icteric with an increase in unconjugated serum bilirubin and with some evidence of spherocytosis on examination of the blood film. Intense spherocytosis is seen in the presence of very rapid hemolysis. Serum haptoglobin levels will be reduced or absent, and the serum lactic dehydrogenase activity will be increased reflecting release of this enzyme from hemolyzed blood cells; it is usually not necessary, however, to make these latter two measurements to establish the presence of a hemolytic process.

Table 17.14 **Disorders Associated with Autoimmune Acquired Hemolytic Disease with Warm-Reactive Autoantibodies**

I. Neoplastic Disorders of the Lymphoreticular System
   A. Chronic lymphocytic leukemia
   B. Lymphocytic and lymphoblastic lymphomas
   C. Hodgkin's disease
   D. Infrequently with other lymphoproliferative disorders
II. Other Disease of Autoimmune Etiology
   A. Lupus erythematosus
   B. Scleroderma
   C. Rheumatoid disease
   D. Infrequently with other diseases of this group
III. Infectious and Inflammatory Diseases
   A. Sarcoidosis
   B. Viral infections
   C. Ulcerative colitis
IV. Immunodeficiency Syndromes
   A. Congenital
   B. Acquired
V. Benign and Malignant Tumors

In addition to the autoantibody of IgG type, the red cells of many patients with AIHD have components of the complement system bound to their surfaces. These are most commonly components of C3 and occasionally C4. In some instances, only complement components are detectable on the red cell surface. Therefore, be sure that the antiglobulin reagent employed for this type of red cell testing also reacts with at least C3.

Although when hemolysis is overt red cell antiglobulin tests are often strongly positive, a small number of patients with less severe hemolysis have been found in which the total burden of either IgG or C3 components on the red cell surface was too low to be detectable by the standard antiglobulin testing methods. These patients have all of the other clinical characteristics of AIHD, including typical patterns of response to therapy, but the diagnosis depends on techniques that are available only in serological reference laboratories.

One of the most poorly understood features of patients with AIHD is the relationship of hemolysis to serological examinations of the red cells. Many patients who have an attack of hemolysis, commonly precipitated by a stressful circumstance (e.g., infection, surgery, pregnancy), have a strongly positive direct antiglobulin test. As the attack of hemolysis subsides, spontaneously or under treatment, the apparent strength of the antiglobulin test of the red cells may remain virtually unchanged. Routine antiglobulin testing of people who have no history or evidence of hemolysis reveals a small proportion of patients with positive antiglobulin tests. Thus, the presence of a positive red cell antiglobulin test does not predict whether or not the patient will have hemolysis. Nevertheless, patients who have positive antiglobulin tests of their red cells, particularly of IgG type, should be kept under some degree of surveillance for the onset of hemolysis, particularly if intercurrent illnesses or injuries occur.

The physical findings in this group of patients depend primarily upon whether or not there is an associated disorder. When an associated disorder is present the physical findings will be primarily those of the associated disease. In idiopathic patients splenic enlargement slowly increases with increasing duration or severity of hemolysis, although massive splenomegaly secondary to AIHD alone is rare. Icterus of variable degree and other physical findings proportionate to the severity of the anemia are also found.

Patients with a rapid onset of hemolysis and hematocrits in the range of 10 percent may have dyspnea, fluctuating level of consciousness, and, occasionally, congestive heart failure. These patients present a major medical emergency.

Corticosteroid therapy, by mechanisms still imperfectly understood, is able to reduce the rate of red cell destruction in most patients. Initial treatment with 60 mg/day in divided doses of a synthetic corticosteroid such as prednisone should be maintained until the patient demonstrates a rising hematocrit and falling reticulocyte count; this should then be followed by a slow reduction in the dosage of the drug to approximately one-half the initial level. This dosage should be maintained until the hematocrit and reticulocyte count approach normal values. Usually the drug can then be slowly withdrawn (over a period of several months) with maintenance of the majority of patients in some state of remission. In other patients, the slow withdrawal of corticosteroid therapy is accompanied by a relapse of hemolysis. Doses between 20 and 30 mg of prednisone per day may be necessary to maintain an adequate hematocrit. Abrupt discontinuance of prednisone therapy, even after a full remission of the hemolytic process, is commonly associated with recurrent hemolysis. In some patients, corticosteroid appears to have little effect. Occasionally remissions of hemolysis are spontaneous.

When the patient requires intolerably large doses of corticosteroid over a long period or when this therapy is otherwise ineffective, splenectomy can be of some value. Splenectomy and corticosteroid therapy together may terminate an attack of hemolysis for a variable period of time, sometimes permanently. Alternatively, it may allow the patient to remain in a relatively stable state with a tolerable daily dose of corticosteroid. Patients who have serious relapses following splenectomy or who are not surgical candidates may be effectively treated with immunosuppressive agents.

Transfusion therapy is very difficult in these patients. Due to the presence of free autoantibody in the serum, the patient's serum reacts with red cells of virtually every proposed donor. In addition, the patient may have a true alloantibody as a result of previous transfusion or pregnancy. This may be difficult to detect in the presence of an autoantibody and may present a problem beyond the capabilities of many hospital blood banks to resolve. In this case, the services of a reference laboratory are crucial.

Even though the patient cannot be cross-matched in a serologically compatible sense, donor red cells can be administered to many such patients, when necessary, as a life-saving procedure. The transfusion should be administered slowly under constant medical supervision with prompt discontinuation if untoward results occur. The object of transfusion is to give the minimum amount of donor blood necessary to support the patient until other efforts to control the hemolytic process have had sufficient time to be effective. Thus, the amount of transfusion should be guided by the patient's status rather than by the hemoglobin or hematocrit value achieved at any one time. At times, a half unit of sedimented red cells administered every 6 to 8 hours may accomplish this more effectively than a single unit or two given at one time.

Although the majority of patients with even severe attacks of hemolysis can now be stabilized by therapy, the disorder is still fatal in 5 to 10 percent of such cases. A variant of the more typical AIHD also has simultaneous autoimmune thrombocytopenia which results in hemorrhage in addition to hemolysis. This situation, referred to as the Evans syndrome, is particularly hazardous and may justify early splenectomy.

Cryopathic hemolytic syndromes. Low levels of cold reactive autoantibodies with titers less than 1:16 are not uncommon in patient populations. They are not in general associated with hemolytic disorders. This type of autoantibody may be elicited by infection and is commonly associated with mycoplasmal pneumonias. These patients may have mild to moderate attacks of hemolytic anemia when the titer of cold reactive autoantibody either rises to high levels or demonstrates activity at temperatures above 20°C. More commonly, hemolytic anemia is associated with the presence of a spontaneously occuring very high titered cold agglutinin, which may reflect monoclonal proliferation of an antibody producing lymphoid cell. In these patients, a mixed clinical picture is produced. They may have hemolysis of variable severity, but more significant are vaso-occlusive phenomena in the extremities due to autoaggregation of red cells in these cooler parts of the body. It is the latter group of symptoms, rather than the hemolytic process, which dominates the clinical picture of this relatively rare disorder, termed the cold agglutinin syndrome.

All types of cold agglutinin related hemolytic processes are much less common than those due to warm reactive autoantibodies. In general, severe hemolysis is less frequent. The cold agglutinin is easily demonstrated in the laboratory.

The principal aim of therapy in this group of patients is to minimize the vaso-occlusive manifestations by keeping the patient warm. Many patients are more comfortable on moving to a warm climate. The hands, feet, face and ears should be carefully protected before exposure to the cold. If a lympho-proliferative disorder is associated with cold agglutinin syndrome, its treatment with cytostatic drugs may improve the manifestations of the cold agglutinin disease. Corticosteroid therapy and splenectomy are much less effective in this disorder than in the warm reactive autoantibody counterpart disease. Removal of the autoantibody from the plasma by plasma exchange may be of temporary benefit in these patients.

Paroxysmal cold hemoglobinuria. This rare disorder is associated with presence of an autoantibody which is able to fix the early reacting components of complement to the red cells during a cold phase, followed by completion of the complement sequence and hemolysis on rewarming. Since complement dependent hemolysis is rapid, it results in free plasma hemoglobin, which then appears in the urine. There may be no associated disorder or the patient may have a chronic granulomatous disease or other evidence of a chronic stabilized infectious process.

Immunologically Mediated Drug Induced Hemolysis

Immunologically mediated drug reactions resulting in hemolysis must be separated from those drugs which attack the structure of the red cell directly. Certain chemicals, such as phenylhydrazine, are able to induce hemolysis of normal red cells in vivo. Erythrocytes which are biochemically abnormal, such as those with G6PD deficiency, may be hemolyzed by agents which are well-tolerated by normal people. These reactions do not involve immunological processes.

Three major types of immunologically mediated hemolytic processes are summarized in Table 17.15.

Haptene type. Hemolysis associated with penicillin therapy is the best example of the haptene type of drug hypersensitivity. When administered in high doses as the treatment of subacute bacterial endocarditis, penicillin may become covalently bonded to the red cell membrane. When penicillin also evokes the formation of an antipenicillin antibody of IgG type, a reaction between this antibody and the bound penicillin haptene will occur which may result in the destruction of the penicillinized red cells. IgM antibodies to penicillin which do not cause hemolysis are common among the North American general population, probably as a result of the widespread use of this antibiotic and environmental exposure to it. Hemolytic anemia secondary to penicillin therapy is uncommon, probably because high doses of drug are required and the formation of an antibody to peni-

Table 17.15 Immunological Mechanisms of Hemolysis Induced by Drugs

Mechanism	Example	In Vitro Demonstration
Haptenic	Penicillin	Patient's serum + haptene coated normal cells, then antiglobulin test
Immune Complex ("innocent bystander")	Stibophen	Patient's fresh serum, drug, normal red cells. Hemolysis or sensitization for anticomplement antiglobulin test
Induction of Autoimmunity	alpha methyldopa	Patient's red cells are positive in direct anti Ig antiglobulin test

cillin capable of inducing hemolysis is also infrequent.

In vitro demonstration of this mechanism of hemolysis requires the presence of the haptene drug attached to the test red cells. Normal red cells are not hemolyzed by the antibodies of these patients since presence of the significant antigenic determinant depends upon drug exposure.

Treatment is based upon withdrawal of the involved drug and transfusion, if necessary, to support the patient until the population of haptene bearing cells has been significantly reduced and the hemolytic process has subsided.

Immune complex type. In this circumstance, a drug-anti-drug immune complex forms in the plasma which is capable of attaching complement to red cells without becoming firmly bound to the red cell membrane itself. This mechanism is also responsible for thrombocytopenia in some cases, and both manifestations may be found in a few patients. Again, the responsible drug must be present in in vitro tests designed to demonstrate the presence of this mechanism of hemolysis.

Drug induced autoantibodies. The prototype disorder in this group is that induced by the administration of alpha methyldopa for the treatment of hypertension. Up to ten percent of patients so treated develop a positive direct red cell antiglobulin test, although only a small proportion of those who become antiglobulin positive develop hemolysis. The autoantibody produced has many of the characteristics and specificity of an IgG warm reactive autoantibody encountered in spontaneously occurring AIHD. The mechanism responsible for autoantibody formation is unknown.

Treatment, other than withdrawal of the offending drug, is rarely necessary. The hemolysis usually subsides promptly although the Coombs test may remain positive for a number of months. It may be possible to retreat the patient with the same agent later without again evoking a hemolytic response. A number of other drugs induce a similar response and more, undoubtedly, will be added to the list in the future.

Hemolytic Processes Due to Passively Acquired Alloantibodies

Hemolytic disease of the newborn (secondary to transplacental transfer of an IgG type of alloantibody commonly of Rh blood group specificity from an alloimmunized mother to an infant having that blood group antigen) is the prototype of hemolytic processes secondary to passive transfer of alloantibodies. This disorder has largely disappeared with the suppression of Rh immunization during pregnancy by the passive administration of Rh antibody to the mother at risk during the pregnancy and at the time of delivery.

Transfusion of donor plasma containing high titers of anti-A to patients having the A antigen rarely results in a hemolytic transfusion reaction. This is uncommon also because current blood transfusion practice selects donors that are ABO group matched to recipients. Very rarely, passive transfusion of plasma containing an alloantibody of another blood group specificity will result in increased destruction of red cells.

Hemolytic Processes Due to Physical and Chemical Agents

A substantial number of physical and chemical effects can induce hemolysis. Extensive burns result in thermally induced hemolysis; red cell fragmentation and the induction of spherocytosis appears to be the mechanism of thermal hemolysis.

The accidental infusion of very hypotonic solutions into the circulation may also result in hemolysis. This has been seen in the past when distilled water was used to irrigate the surgical field in transurethral prostatectomy. Iso-osmotic, nonconducting solutions are now employed.

Physical trauma to the red cells causes a disorder known as march hemoglobinuria. This is seen in a small proportion of persons who run or march long distances. It is thought to be secondary to direct physical disruption of red cells in the feet and possibly other joints. Some evidence of hemolysis without hemoglobinuria may be much more common than is generally appreciated among people who run or jog regularly.

Certain types of artificial cardiac valves induce hemolysis by direct trauma to the red cells as the valve closes. Blood forced at high pressure through small orifices in the circulation also may cause traumatic hemolysis, as may be seen with leaks next to artificial valves and high grade calcific aortic stenosis. Red cell fragmentation can be identified on the blood film where crescentic forms, irregular small poikilocytes, and tiny red cell fragments of variable small size can be found.

Microangiopathic hemolytic anemia. This group of disorders is due to diffuse obstruction of the microcirculation which results in fragmentation as red cells are forced past the obstructions. Diffuse arteritis involving multiple small vessels, widespread vascular obstruction due to micrometastatic tumor deposits, and a disorder termed *thrombotic thrombocytopenic purpura* with hemolytic anemia (TTP) are examples of microangiopathic states which produce red cell fragmentation (see Chapter 4, Thrombocytopenia).

Hemolysis secondary to infectious agents. Intraerythrocytic parasites, of which *malaria* is the most common, may result in overt hemolytic anemia when heavy levels of parasitism are present. Other hemoparasites occur in other parts of the world, but these are uncommon causes of hemolysis in North America. Some degree of hemolysis may be encountered in patients with a wide variety of septic infections, but this seldom presents a major problem. Patients with G6PD deficiency and allied conditions may hemolyze quite severely in the face of severe bacterial infection.

Paroxysmal nocturnal hemoglobinuria (PNH). PNH is a rare, acquired hemolytic process characterized by episodes of hemolysis while the patient is asleep. On awakening, the patient may pass dark urine due to the presence of free hemoglobin. The disorder is of importance because it is now thought to represent an acquired abnormality in which an abnormal clone of marrow cells displaces the normal marrow hematopoietic cells. Because the disorder may spontaneously remit, it is thought that normal precursor cells may ultimately be able to reestablish themselves in the marrow and recover their function. The onset of the disease is usually slow, with variable anemia appearing before frank hemoglobinuria. Because of renal loss of iron, the patient may become iron deficient. In some instances, the disorder is ushered in by a period of marked marrow hypofunction with hypocellularity resembling other hypoplastic or aplastic states. The relationship between PNH and aplastic anemia of other types is unclear. Some patients with aplastic anemia who do not develop PNH may have some red cells which resemble those present in PNH.

The primary abnormality in PNH is in the heightened ability of these red cells to fix complement in vivo particularly C_3. They are markedly sensitive to complement induced hemolysis in vitro as well. Several diagnostic tests are based on this abnormality. It is possible to demonstrate several populations of PNH red cells, one with nearly normal complement sensitivity (although this population may fix increased amounts of C_3), a population with an intermediate sensitivity, and a third highly sensitive population. The three red cell populations are found in various combinations and proportions in PNH patients.

The platelets and leukocytes of PNH patients also are abnormal. Thrombocytopenia and neutropenia are seen in the majority of cases. Infection occurs commonly and accentuates the hemolytic process.

PNH patients also have a tendency to develop spontaneous thrombosis which may be life threatening. Central nervous system thrombosis and thrombosis in the hepatoportal system are particularly hazardous. Unexplained chest, abdominal, and back pain, suggestive of the vaso-occlusive crises in sickle cell anemia, also occurs.

Transfusions with plasma free red cells can be given when absolutely necessary for the treatment of acute anemia. Corticosteroid therapy, as in the case of autoimmune acquired hemolytic anemia, may decrease the rate of red cell destruction. Correction of iron deficiency will increase the number of new red cells, but if the new population of red cells are very sensitive to complement, iron therapy may paradoxically increase the rate of hemolysis and the hemoglobinuria. Therapy with androgens may be useful in patients with hypoplastic bone marrows. Recently, some patients with severe marrow aplasia associated with PNH have received bone marrow transplants. Many other treatment modalities have been suggested, including the administration of dextran and anti-coagulation, all with little evidence of effectiveness. The basic mechanism by which sleep activates the complement system remains unknown.

ERYTHROCYTOSIS

Erythrocytosis is an increase in red cell mass without a proportionate increase in other cellular elements of the blood. When all cellular elements increase simultaneously, the disorder is called polycythemia vera (discussed in the section dealing with the myeloproliferative syndromes). Any disorder characterized by chronic anoxia and inadequate oxygen transport will, in most instances, increase the red cell mass. The hematocrit rises and, in some instances, reaches very high levels, in the range of 70-75 percent. Renal lesions, particularly renal cysts and carcinomas, are occasionally associated with erythrocytosis, presumably due to abnormal production of erythropoietin and other erythrostimulatory substances. These latter patients can be distinguished from those with the erythrocytosis secondary to hypoxemia by the presence of normal oxygen saturation of arterial blood.

In those circumstances in which erythrocytosis is a compensatory mechanism for chronic hypoxemia, the patient may not require therapy. However, when the hematocrit rises markedly a sharp increase in whole blood viscosity may decrease capillary perfusion and oxygen transport. In these circumstances, a trial of phlebotomy, designed to reduce the hematocrit to about 55 percent, may be of value. It is important to assess carefully the patient's functional capabilities as the hematocrit reduces in order to find the optimal point for the individual. Removal of renal or other lesions responsible for abnormal erythropoietin production usually cures erythrocytosis due to that cause.

True erythrocytosis must be differentiated from a situation referred to as spurious erythrocytosis. As shown in Figure 17.2, if the plasma volume becomes contracted, the hematocrit rises suggesting an increase in red cell mass. Patients in this situation, also termed stress polycythemia, present with stable, moderately elevated hematocrits, usually in the range of 55 percent, without hypoxemia. They are usually under relatively severe, chronic psychological stress which is easily detected. These patients do not require treatment designed to reduce the hematocrit. The stability of the elevated hematocrit coupled with the remainder of the clinical picture usually leads to the proper diagnosis. Occasionally, a measurement of red cell mass may be useful to demonstrate that it is within the normal range.

DISORDERS OF LEUKOCYTES

The wide range of disorders which affect this diverse group of blood cells are classified first by the cell's tissue of origin: myeloid (bone marrow) and lymphoid (the lymphoreticular apparatus). A secondary classification depends upon the class or specific cell type involved: *granulocytic* including neutrophils, eosinophils and basophils, *monocytic*, and *lymphoreticular*, including lymphocytes, their precursors, histiocytes and plasma cells. All leukocytes are primarily tissue cells whose presence in the blood reflects the need to transport them from site to site where they are produced, modified or utilized.

CLINICAL SIGNIFICANCE OF MYELOID CELL PHYSIOLOGY

Granulocytes and monocytes are both produced in the marrow, probably from a common precursor which very early differentiates definitively into the three varieties of granulocyte and the monocyte. Proliferation, increasing cell numbers, proceeds simultaneously with maturation during which the definitive functional biochemical apparatus of the cell is formed. Neutrophils and monocytes are the most important cells of acute body defense reactions. They are motile and actively phagocytic. After phagocytosis, granulocytes form lysosomal vacuoles into which the granules discharge enzymes that destroy and digest the ingested material. Phagocytosis induces a burst of oxidative metabolism during which peroxides and other active forms of oxygen are formed; these compounds are important in killing ingested bacteria and may play a role in tissue injury associated with inflammation. Ability of the leukocytes to reduce the dye, nitroblue tetrazolium, tests this important function.

Eosinophils contain a number of cationic proteins. Their phagocytic functions are similar to neutrophils. They respond to sites of allergic reactions, although their function there is unknown. Eosinophils are also present in increased numbers in the peripheral blood of patients with a wide variety of parasitic diseases in which the parasite invades tissue. Basophil granules contain both histamine and heparin. Their physiological role remains obscure but they are probably involved in histamine release at sites of allergic reactions. Increased numbers of basophils in the peripheral blood are rarely encountered outside myeloproliferative disorders, such as myeloid metaplasia and chronic myelocytic leukemia.

Monocytes, though actively motile and phagocytic, do not have the enzymatic apparatus of the granulocytes. They respond later in the course of inflammation and are involved in removal of debris and early tissue repair, as well as in development of chronic (round cell) inflammatory reactions. They appear to be of critical importance in the immune response where they are involved in antigen uptake, processing and transport. Marked increases in peripheral blood monocytes are uncommon in other than monocytic leukemia, although transient in-

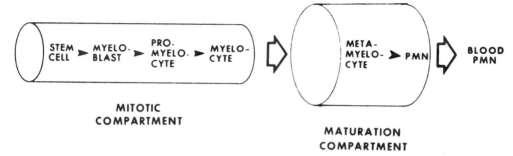

MITOTIC COMPARTMENT

MATURATION COMPARTMENT

Fig. 17.12 Granulocyte compartments; production, storage and utilization times (Reprinted by permission of the publisher from The White Cell, by Martin J. Cline, M.D., Cambridge, Mass.: The Commonwealth Fund, Harvard University Press, © 1975 by The President and Fellows of Harvard College. (Conflicting data re: cell production times exist; overall, probably 6–8 days; about equal times in proliferation and maturation and storage compartments; T ½ in peripheral blood 6–8 hours.)

creases accompany a variety of infections and inflammatory disorders.

Leukocyte Kinetics

Granulocyte production requires 4 to 6 days. The several compartments of granulocytes are shown in Figure 17.12. Within the peripheral blood transport compartment, they are in a well-mixed central pool and a slowly exchanging less well-mixed pool (the marginal pool) near the walls of blood vessels. These pools are roughly the same size. Acute inflammatory stimuli and drugs, such as adrenalin and corticosteroids, mobilize the marginal pool and increase the peripheral blood leukocyte count with little modification of the granulocytes' immaturity. A continuing inflammatory stimulus evokes release of granulocytes stored in the marrow which, on the average, are less mature. This leads to a "shift to the left". Severe continuing inflammation causes even more immature cells to be released, including metamyelocytes and occasionally myelocytes. A very high white cell count, which may range from 30,000 to 100,000/cu mm, may result from continued severe stimulation and is termed a *leukemoid* response. This can usually be differentiated from a leukemic disorder by the virtual absence of very immature myeloid cells, myeloblasts, and promyelocytes, and by the marked elevation of the enzyme leukocyte alkaline phosphatase. Severe leukemoid reactions are occasionally encountered in which the peripheral blood contains a few myeloblasts, promyelocytes, megakaryocyte fragments and erythroid cell precursors.

Neutrophils leave the capillary bed at a site of inflammation in response to humoral chemotactic stimuli such as those derived from the complement system. They do not return to the circulation but rather are consumed in situ after performing their physiological functions. Methods to evaluate these essential functions for clinical purposes are unavailable in most laboratories.

ABNORMALITIES OF GRANULOCYTE STRUCTURE AND/OR FUNCTION

A number of genetically determined abnormalities of granulocytes have been recognized. These are rare and widely variable in clinical severity. Those associated with severe impairment of function lead to chronic and recurrent infections and frequently early death from sepsis (Table 17.16).

Granulocytopenia

The absolute granulocyte count of normal Caucasian populations varies considerably with 1,500/cu mm widely accepted as the lower limit of normal. Normal blacks appear to have a slightly lower average value. Values as low as 1,200/cu mm are seen in individuals who have no recognizable propensity for infection. Values below 1,000/cu mm can be assumed to be abnormal, with increasing risk of infection, particularly sepsis, as the count decreases; below 500/cu mm the risk increases greatly, and at counts of 200-300/cu mm virtually all patients become bacterially infected after a few days. An increase in monocytes may offset the risk of infection to some degree. Granulocyte counts less than 100/cu mm are referred to as agranulocytosis.

The manifestations of acute agranulocytosis are those of infection. Sudden onset of a severe pharyngitis, fever, or septic shock may be the presenting

Table 17.16   Inherited Anomalies of Granulocyte Structure

Anomalies with No Associated Illness	Description	Clinical Significance
I. Pelger-Huet	Round or bilobed nuclei	Normal function; may be confused with "left-shift". Autosomal dominant.
II. Hereditary Hypersegmentation	Nucleus with more than 4 lobes/cell. Cells may also be macrocytic	Autosomal dominant. No associated abnormalities
III. May-Hegglin	Leukopenia, Döhle bodies and giant platelets	No associated illness
Anomalies Associated With Illness		
I. Alder's Anomaly	Giant cytoplasmic granulation	Associated with abnormalities of polysaccharide metabolism, gargoylism.
II. Chediak-Higashi	Giant cytoplasmic granules (also in monocytes and lymphocytes)	Autosomal recessive; albinism, accelerated phase leads to death
III. Chronic Granulomatous Disease (CGD)	No morphological abnormality. Failure to generate peroxide after phagocytosis	X linked usually. Recurrent infection; related to McLeod phenotype of Kell blood group system

picture. In most instances, acute severe granulocytopenia is due to an idiosyncratic drug toxicity or to intensive chemotherapy with myelosuppressive drugs. In some instances a known toxic agent is not present; nevertheless, an occult environmental toxic exposure still may be responsible. Other unknown mechanisms, including autoimmunity, may be involved in some cases. Treatment depends upon removal of all suspect toxic exposures and control of infection while awaiting return of granulocyte production. Leukocyte transfusions, discussed in the last section of this chapter, may be of value, but are not widely available. Unfortunately, the mortality of acute agranulocytosis remains high. Risk may be decreased by periodic monitoring of the WBC of patients receiving long-term treatment with drugs known to cause leukopenia, but not all such cases can be prevented in this way. Recovery of granulocyte production, if it is to occur, usually is seen after 2 or 3 weeks. A rise in monocyte count frequently heralds recovery from acute agranulocytosis.

Chronic granulocytopenia usually involves less severe depression of the granulocyte count with recurrent infections in various sites, particularly pneumonia, skin infections, otitis and sinusitis. The clinical picture may resemble that of an immunodeficiency disease. Toxic drug or chemical reactions, autoimmune processes, congestive splenomegaly and unknown causes are all encountered in this group of patients. It is important to recognize that sepsis in its early stages frequently results in transient granulocytopenia; such patients may not be infected as a result of granulocytopenia. Moderate granulocytopenia may persist for several weeks or more after a variety of acute viral illnesses. At times, residual findings of a lymphatic reaction in the blood smear may be found. Granulocytopenia persisting more than 2 months is probably not secondary to a viral illness.

Felty's syndrome is the combination of granulocytopenia, splenomegaly and rheumatoid arthritis. The mechanism of granulocytopenia probably involves excess destruction by both an autoimmune mechanism and by a hyperfunctional enlarged spleen. Splenectomy for hypersplenic states should be carried out only if the patient is experiencing repeated significant infections.

Cyclic neutropenia is a rare disorder of unknown cause in which neutrophil production stops for a period of several days every 2 or 3 weeks. At the time of the lowest granulocyte count, the marrow may be devoid of granulocyte precursors. Infections frequently occur at this time. An animal model of this disorder exists in the grey collie dog in which it has been investigated extensively. No effective treatment is known, but prompt treatment of infections may be life saving.

THE MYELOPROLIFERATIVE SYNDROMES

This group of disorders, listed in Table 17.17, has come to be considered as a whole not because of known common etiological factors but rather because the term recognizes that some type of disturbed and/or increased proliferation of one or more cellular elements of the marrow is common to all disorders of the group. In some instances, the clinical pictures merge or appear to convert from one diagnostic category to another. All of these disorders are thought to reflect clonal proliferation of an abnormal myeloid precursor cell which has a proliferative advantage over the normal cells of the marrow. This leads to replacement of the normal cells by the clonal cells. Clones are probably established as a result of a cel-

Eosinophilic and basophilic leukemia, monocytic leukemias and the acute leukemias of myeloblastic origin are sometimes included in this group of disorders.

lular mutation, although the mechanism of such an event is unknown.

The first three disorders listed in Table 17.17 are generally regarded as non-malignant, whereas those designated as leukemia are thought to be neoplastic. All these disorders share a greatly increased risk for the development of an acute leukemia. The clones may be regarded as unstable or metastable, thus increasing the probability that an oncogenic event will result in emergence of a fully autonomous leukemic cell line.

Polycythemia Vera (P. Vera)

This is a disorder, usually seen in people of middle age and beyond characterized by an increase in red cell mass, blood volume and hematocrit as well as by leukocytosis, thrombocytosis and splenomegaly. The bone marrow is moderately hypercellular with normal orderly appearing myeloid and erythroid precursors. Absence of hypoxemia, best measured after the hematocrit and red cell mass have been reduced to near normal by phlebotomy, virtually excludes secondary types of polycythemia. Rubor of the face, vee area of the chest, hands and feet are frequently physical findings. Splenomegaly and slight hepatomegaly are usually easily palpable, but the spleen and liver are not massively enlarged in uncomplicated P. vera. The hematocrit may be between 55 and 70 percent; the WBC is usually between 15,000 and 30,000/cu mm and the platelet count between 400,000 and 800,000/cu mm, with substantial variation from case to case. The leukocyte alkaline phosphatase activity is high, with scores usually above 200. These patients are prone to increased venous and arterial thrombosis, related to the high platelet counts, and increased viscosity due to red cells.

Initial treatment of P. vera is designed to reduce the hematocrit and blood volume promptly by repeated phlebotomies, daily or every other day, until it is in the range of 50 percent or less. This usually relieves the sense of head congestion and mental dysfunction which may be associated with hypervolemia or increased blood viscosity. The patient should then be observed for a period of weeks to see how rapidly the hematocrit rises. If the hematocrit does not rise above 55 percent within 4 to 6 months, it may be possible to control the disorder by phlebotomy alone. Ultimately, however, repeated phlebotomy leads to iron deficiency. Administration of therapeutic iron frequently accelerates the rise in hematocrit. Blood cell production may be suppressed by administration of an alkylating drug such as chlorambucil or by giving a calculated dose of ^{32}P. A recent study indicates that the latter program of treatment is best in establishing good control of hematocrit and minimizing thrombotic and hemostatic complications.

After a variable period of a few to many years, the proliferative process slowly subsides in most patients and at times is replaced by a chronic hyporegenerative state with variable anemia, leukopenia and thrombocytopenia. The spleen and liver may continue to enlarge, sometimes massively, and the clinical and blood picture of myeloid metaplasia emerges. This occurs in about one-third of P. vera patients. The marrow is then usually fibrotic, with extensive hematopoietic activity in spleen and liver. These states are termed "burned out" P. vera; they may in part be due to therapy and/or reflect the natural evolution of the disease. About 10 percent of the patients with P. vera terminate in an acute leukemic state which is usually refractory to treatment.

Myeloid Metaplasia (M.M.)

This disorder, once thought to be rare, is now recognized with increasing frequency. Its incidence has been estimated in several clinics to be about twice that of chronic myelocytic leukemia. Its cause is unknown. Both sexes are affected about equally. Although it has been encountered throughout the entire adult age spectrum, it is most common in middle life and beyond. About 20 percent of patients with M.M. have had polycythemia vera previously; these patients seem to behave during the metaplastic phase in the same way as patients without preexistent polycythemia.

Myeloid metaplasia presents an extremely variable clinical picture and course. In some patients, the disorder is stable over many years. Most patients however have a progressive disorder with ultimate development of massive hepatosplenomegaly, anemia and frequently leukopenia and thrombocytopenia as well. Perisplenitis and splenic infarctions are common at this stage. Hypermetabolism, heat intolerance, pruritis and weight loss are common. Gastric crowding may reduce food intake. Hemorrhagic or thrombotic episodes may occur, as may infections. Active portal hypertension with esophageal varices occurs in some patients with massive splenomegaly. Ultimately, a substantial proportion of M.M. patients succumb to some combination of these complications.

The blood picture is quite characteristic. Intense poikilocytosis with target cells, teardrop shaped cells, some spherocytes and elongated forms are present, as is normoblastemia. The platelets are usually increased in numbers at the time of diagnosis with large and giant forms; frequently megakaryocyte fragments are present. The granulocytes show immaturity with large numbers of the more mature forms and progressively fewer cells of increasing immaturity. A few myeloblasts can usually be found. Eosinophils and basophils are increased in most cases.

The bone marrow examination commonly does not yield an aspirated sample due to fibrosis. A core biopsy will show large areas of fibrosis with many megakaryocytes still present in these areas. Small scattered islands of hematopoiesis remain. Extramedullary hematopoiesis will be found in liver, spleen, lymphatic structures and, at times, in other areas which reflect sites of embryological hematopoiesis. Liver and splenic biopsy are not needed to establish the diagnosis and are hazardous because of the risk of hemorrhage.

The leucocyte alkaline phosphatase (LAP) score will be normal or elevated in about 80 percent of MM patients. In the remaining patients it will be low or near zero; these two groups of patients are not distinguishable on other grounds. When the MM patient presents with a high WBC, elevated LAP activity may be of value in differentiating myeloid metaplasia from chronic myelocytic leukemia where it is uniformly low. Cytogenetic studies of the marrow and blood in MM are difficult for technical reasons, but it is generally agreed that the Ph[1] chromosome is not found in this disorder.

Other diseases which cause widespread marrow destruction by replacement may present with compensatory extramedullary hematopoiesis. Tuberculosis of the bone marrow and disseminated cancer, especially of breast and prostate, are examples of this. A well-developed leukoerythroblastic blood picture may be present. True diagnostic confusion rarely occurs if an adequate core biopsy of the marrow has been obtained and evaluated in light of the rest of the clinical picture.

Early in the course of myeloid metaplasia treatment with the myelosuppressive drug busulfan may dramatically reduce the size of an oppressively enlarged spleen; WBC and platelet count usually fall, and anemia, if present, improves. The beneficial effect sometimes persists for many months, but usually splenomegaly recurs and repeated courses of treatment are required, with decreasing effectiveness. Ultimately massive splenomegaly develops, usually with pancytopenia. Transfusions may be required to maintain even a low hematocrit. Hemolysis can be assumed to be present when an adult patient's transfusion requirements exceed 2 to 3 units of red cells every 2 weeks in the absence of bleeding. Even though the spleen may be a major site of hematopoiesis, it may be destroying more blood cells than it produces. Under these circumstances, splenectomy is frequently carried out with favorable, if temporary, results in many patients. Leukemic transformation occurs as a terminal event in about a third of MM patients. The disorder has a high fatality rate ultimately in those patients who exhibit an aggressive course at the onset.

Thrombocythemia

The principal clinical feature of the disease is a persistently high platelet count. Platelet counts of well over 1×10^6/cu mm are common. On the blood smear, platelets are greatly variable in size with many giant forms. Megakaryocyte fragments, including nuclear material, are easily identified. There may be splenomegaly and features suggesting myeloid metaplasia in the blood and marrow. Hemorrhagic and thrombotic complications are common. In a few patients who survive for a long period, acute leukemia may emerge. The disorder is further discussed in the chapter on hemostasis (see Chapter 4).

Erythroleukemia

Classification of disorders in this group remains imprecise. In a few patients with what is basically an acute myeloblastic leukemia, some evidence of partial differentiation of the leukemic cell line into erythroid precursors of abnormal type may be found early in the course of the disease. These cells commonly resemble megaloblasts and are referred to as megaloblastoid. As the disorder progresses, evidence of erythroid differentiation usually disappears, leaving the picture of an acute myeloblastic leukemia usually rapidly progressive and resistant to treatment. This is a neoplastic disorder which may be better termed erythroblastic leukemia.

A disorder more typically akin to the myeloproliferative disorders is frequently referred to as the di

Guglielimo syndrome. In this state, proliferation of later erythroid precursors is common, there is intense normoblastemia, and many multinucleated erythroid cells are found in the bone marrow. The disorder may pursue a relatively indolent course for a while, with moderate anemia as the principal clinical manifestation. Most often it terminates in acute myeloid leukemia. Prior to this phase, treatment is directed towards controlling the symptoms. Chronic transfusion may be required.

Chronic Leukemias of Granulocytes and Monocytes

Chronic Myelocytic Leukemia (CML)

At least two quite different disorders are included under this designation. The more common disease is characterized by presence of the Ph[1] chromosome (Philadelphia 1 chromosome). This is a small variant chromosome 21 in which the short arms have been translocated, usually to the long arms of chromosome 9. This marker defines a relatively homogeneous group of patients, about 90 percent of all patients who present with the clinical, blood and marrow picture of chronic granulocytic leukemia. The remaining 10 percent, as a rule, lack this or other cytogenetic markers, have a much more aggressive disease, and are relatively resistant to therapy. Thus the distinction provided by the Ph[1] chromosome is of major clinical importance.

Ph[1] Positive CML. Although more common in the middle years of life, this disease occurs throughout the entire adult age range. It is a panmyelopathy; all of the cells of myeloid origin are involved in physiologically unregulated proliferation. The clinical onset is almost always subtle with weight loss, mild fever or heat intolerance, fatigue, vague feelings of illness and, at times, a sense of upper abdominal fullness due to splenomegaly. Later, pallor may appear and the patient may find the enlarged spleen before seeking medical care. Occasionally, bleeding is the presenting complaint. The diagnosis is sometimes made while the disease is still asymptomatic; a blood study obtained for an unrelated purpose often first indicates the presence of the disorder.

The blood picture shows all three types of granulocytes in large numbers, with neutrophils and their precursors (including some myeloblasts) predominating. Usually less than 5 percent blast cells are present. Larger numbers of myeloblasts suggest that the disease will run a more acute course. The platelet count is usually increased with large, bizarre forms present. Normoblastemia of variable degree is also usually seen. The red cells may show moderately increased anisocytosis and poikilocytosis, but frequently they appear normal. Sometimes moderate numbers of agranular neutrophils will resemble monocytes. This can lead to an erroneous diagnosis of myelomonocytic leukemia.

The bone marrow is densely hypercellular and usually aspirates freely. Specimens should be submitted for cytogenic analysis by direct culture of the marrow cells. The myeloid:erythroid ratio, normally from 2 to 4:1, is always increased and may exceed 20:1. Erythropoiesis, although relatively reduced, is usually normal in appearance. The proportion of myeloblasts is usually below 5 percent.

Leukocyte alkaline phosphatase activity is nearly zero. Serum B_{12} level is usually elevated due to an increase in the transport protein transcobalamin I. Lactic dehydrogenase and uric acid levels are also increased, reflecting increased cell turnover. The WBC at time of diagnosis is frequently about 50,000/cu mm, but it may exceed 200,000/cu mm. The clinical manifestations of the disease are correlated to some degree with the level of the WBC, but a general evaluation of the patient must be employed in making decisions about treatment. Mild anemia, with the hematocrit decreased to the range of 30 percent, is common, Centrifuged hematocrit tubes show the markedly increased "buffy coat" containing the nucleated cells and platelets, which may be in the range of 3 to 6 percent of the cellular sediment.

Most patients require treatment at the time of diagnosis. Many therapeutic agents are effective. Currently, treatment with busulfan is most generally employed. If the WBC is markedly elevated and the spleen enlarged with elevated blood uric acid, blocking of uric acid synthesis with allopurinol for several days prior to administration of this cytotoxic agent prevents renal damage due to tubular deposition of uric acid crystals. Fluid intake and urine volume should be kept high during treatment. Therapy is stopped when the WBC decreases to about 25,000/cu mm; it will continue to decline into the normal range in most patients. This therapy usually induces a nearly complete remission of all symptoms and findings after 1 or 2 months. The duration of remission is variable. The WBC may start to climb again within a month or two, and early symptoms will return in another several months. Symptomatic relapse commonly occurs soon after the WBC reaches 50,000/cu mm. At times, long remissions, a year or more, are induced. Retreatment often succeeds. There appears to be no advantage to maintenance therapy. Busulfan induces a dusky bronze skin pigmentation and some features of Addison's disease in a few patients. Suppression of ovarian function and reduction in spermatogenesis are also frequent complications. Pulmonary fibrosis, a less common but more serious complication, requires changing to another drug for further therapy. Periodic pulmonary function studies should be carried out in patients who receive frequent courses of therapy.

Early splenectomy has been carried out in this disorder in an effort to prevent the late complications associated with refractory splenomegaly, gastric crowding, splenic infarction and perisplenitis. It has no influence on survival and is of doubtful value.

Although busulfan therapy has improved the quality of life for CML patients, their survival rate remains largely unchanged, with median survival of less than 3 years following diagnosis. Annually, about 10 percent of CML patients develop acute leukemia, usually myeloblastic in type, termed blastic crisis, with short survival thereafter, even if remission can be induced with intensive chemotherapy. In 10 to 15 percent of these patients, the blastic cells have characteristics of lymphoblasts, as judged by the presence of surface immunological markers and the enzyme TdT (terminal deoxynucleotidyl transferase). These patients also respond to the remission induction regimen used for acute lymphocytic leukemia with vincristine and prednisone. They have a better but still poor prognosis. This important observation suggests that the cell of origin of the CML clone is capable of differentiation in a lymphoid as well as myeloid direction (i.e., it is essentially a totipotent stem cell).

The onset of blastic crisis is usually signalled by a rising number of blastic cells in blood and bone marrow, marrow failure with anemia and thrombocytopenia, and poor to no response to busulfan therapy. Additional cytogenetic abnormalities may appear in the marrow, including reduplication of the Ph^1 chromosome, other chromosomal markers, random chromosomal changes and aneuploidy. Unfortunately, this information is currently of little practical value. Bone marrow transplantation may be of value in some patients, but tested criteria for deciding when, in the course of the illness, to undertake this difficult, hazardous and still investigational procedure are not agreed upon.

Patients who do not experience a blastic crisis may survive in relatively good health for years. Others gradually lose responsiveness to busulfan treatment, develop marrow failure, inanition, severe weight loss and massive hepatosplenomegaly as well as a wide range of complications due to leukemic infiltrations in bony, cutaneous and other organ sites. Infection,

hemorrhage and combinations of these complications result in death.

Ph^1 negative CML.   The onset of this disorder resembles that of its Ph^1 positive counterpart, although in some patients it is somewhat more abrupt. The blood and bone marrow findings, as well as the physical findings, are also similar. If the Ph^1 chromsome is not found initially the study should be repeated to reduce the possibility of a technical error. Other variable cytogenetic abnormalities have been reported in some of these patients.

Response to busulfan therapy is poor. The WBC may diminish only slightly, splenomegaly persists and the patient's symptoms mildly improve. After stopping therapy there is rapid recurrence and early onset of marrow failure with persistent anemia and frequently thrombocytopenia. Patients usually survive less than 18 months, with death due to infection, bleeding, or tumor associated cachexia. Acute leukemia which is usually refractory to treatment emerges in some patients. No satisfactory treatment is available for this probably heterogeneous group of patients.

Chronic myelomonocytic leukemia (Naegeli type).   Myelomonocytic leukemia usually pursues an acute or subacute course. A relatively chronic form of this disorder is now recognized in which a few patients may survive for more than 5 years. The proliferative process appears to arise in a precursor cell which is capable of differentiating into both monocytic and granulocytic cells in widely variable and fluctuating proportions. The diagnosis is based upon recognizing both cell types and their precursors in the blood and marrow films. The Ph^1 chromosome is not found.

The clinical features and course of this disorder may resemble those of Ph^1 negative CML. Response to therapy is limited in most instances, but in those patients who have a chronic course, the clinical picture and laboratory findings may remain relatively stable for long periods without treatment. Monocytic leukemia is prone to produce infiltrations of gums, rectum and skin. The characteristic lesions are red-purple macules which in the skin tend to form clusters over the trunk and extremities. They may be mistaken for petechiae. Acute leukemia develops as a terminal event in some patients. The remainder succumb mainly to complications of bone marrow failure.

Other granulocytic leukemia.   A rare variant of CML is neutrophilic leukemia in which the proliferation is restricted to the neutrophil series. Eosinophilic leukemia is also rare; its status remains controversial because of the difficulty of separating it from several poorly understood hypereosinophilic syndromes which appear to be non-neoplastic. Many authors regard it as a variant of CML. The disorder has a variable course and is frequently associated with a variety of pulmonary abnormalities which remain poorly defined. The Ph^1 chromosome is absent. Basophilic leukemia is even rarer with only a few well-defined cases reported. It appears to have a more rapid clinical course than other myeloid leukemias.

Promyelocytic leukemia is a recently recognized entity of interest even though it is uncommon. The proliferating myeloid cells do not differentiate appreciably beyond the promyelocyte stage. There is frequent association with bleeding and deficiencies of a number of coagulation factors, including Factor V and fibrinogen. These deficiencies may reflect a consumption coagulopathy. Bleeding due to this complex coagulation deficiency is sometimes fatal. The clinical course is usually subacute or acute, and treatment appropriate for acute myelocytic leukemia is usually administered. Administration of Factor IX concentrates, fresh frozen plasma, or cryoprecipiate may temporarily control hemorrhage associated with impaired blood coagulation.

Acute Leukemia, Non-lymphocytic

In practice, leukemias are most often classified on the basis of morphological characteristics of the cells involved. This is quite straightforward in the chronic leukemias where the cells are recognizably differentiated; it becomes much more difficult and unreliable in the acute leukemias. Many efforts are underway to reclassify the acute leukemias based upon cytochemical, immunological, and cell culture characteristics. This work has great promise for improved clinical management of the acute leukemias by recognizing subgroups which respond more effectively to different specific treatment programs. A number of nomenclature systems based upon these characteristics already exist, but they have not come into common use. For the purpose of this discussion, the large groups of acute leukemias, as defined by morphological criteria, will be employed.

Although acute leukemia is clearly a neoplastic disorder involving unregulated proliferation of hematopoietic precursor cells, it can also be viewed as a disorder in which there is failure of normal blood elements to differentiate and produce. The clinical picture presented reflects in varying proportion the pathophysiological consequences of this failure.

Acute leukemia of all morphological types occurs throughout the entire age spectrum. Acute lymphoblastic leukemias are much more common

among children. At adolescence, the incidence of the non-lymphoblastic leukemias rises and becomes the predominant group of acute leukemias affecting adults. Three large groups of acute leukemias arising from myeloblastic cell are (1) acute myeloblastic leukemia, (2) acute myelomonocytic leukemia and (3) acute monoblastic leukemia.

Acute leukemias are characterized by large numbers of highly immature precursor cells which show little or no evidence of differentiation into the definitive cell types of blood, bone marrow and tissues. These disorders run an accelerated clinical course, largely because bone marrow failure occurs very early and results in anemia, granulocytopenia and thrombocytopenia. In many instances, the patient presents for medical care because of symptoms associated with one or more of these types of marrow failure. Pallor, other manifestations of anemia, spontaneous bleeding from the nose or gums, petechiae and bruising, and fever are thus common presenting symptoms. The physical findings vary. In addition to those related to bone marrow failure, there may be hepatosplenomegaly and leukemic infiltrations of the gums and skin. The latter is seen particularly in disorders involving myelomonocytic proliferation.

The diagnosis of acute leukemia is usually easily established by examination of the peripheral blood. The WBC is usually elevated, sometimes markedly so, with counts over 100,000/cu mm. Some patients, however, present with a very low white count, and it may be difficult to identify the distinctive blast cells in ordinary films of the peripheral blood. Concentration by gentle centrifugation of the leukocytes in a specimen of anticoagulated blood will usually demonstrate the presence of blastic cells. The bone marrow examination is particularly useful in patients with a leukopenic onset where intense proliferation of blast forms will be found. Normal erythroid and myeloid cells as well as megakaryocytes are few or virtually absent.

Prior to the advent of modern aggressive chemotherapy, these disorders usually resulted in death within 6 to 9 months and, frequently, within a few weeks. Survival has been markedly improved through intensive chemotherapy which induces remissions, of variable duration, in the majority of these patients. In many clinics more than 75 percent of patients with acute myeloblastic leukemia achieve a first remission and frequently a second and third. Remission may be as long as several years. Those patients with monocytic elements in the leukemic process respond somewhat less frequently and with shorter duration of remission. Death in acute leukemia is usually the result of a complication of bone marrow failure: infection or bleeding. Occasionally infiltrations of the meninges with leukemic cells or infiltration of other organs contribute to the cause of death. Inanition, cachexia, and the adverse effects of intensive chemotherapy also contribute to the morbidity and mortality of these patients.

The treatment of patients with acute leukemia is based upon administration of an intensive course of chemotherapy called an induction regime. In myelocytic leukemias three different drugs are usually employed, including an anthracycline antibiotic anti-tumor agent such as doxorubicin, cytosine arabinoside, and a pseudopurine such as 6-mercaptopurine or 6-thioguanine. These drugs are administered over a course of about seven days. The three agents kill cells by differing biochemical mechanisms. This treatment commonly produces bone marrow aplasia and, if effective, destroys the large mass of leukemic cells. Recovery of normal bone marrow function then usually occurs in the following 2 to 3 weeks. During the period of marrow aplasia, infection and bleeding are common. Supportive treatment with antibiotic therapy, transfusions of red cells, platelets and occasionally granulocytes usually tide the patient over this critical period until normal hematopoeisis begins to reappear. Transfusion support of acute leukemia patients is discussed in more detail in the section on transfusions.

The induction regimen for patients with acute lymphoblastic leukemia is simpler and safer. Vincristine and prednisone treatment alone commonly induce remission without induction of marrow aplasia and its serious attendant difficulties.

After induction of remission, some form of recurrent maintenance treatment is usually administered, although optimal maintenance programs have not yet been defined. About 20-25 percent of patients with myeloblastic leukemias so treated can survive for 5 years. Adult patients with lymphoblastic leukemia frequently have somewhat better survival, and some may achieve the same type of cure that is seen in the childhood disease. Relapse is heralded by the reappearance of blasts in the peripheral blood or bone marrow and ultimately by recurrence of the symptom complex of acute leukemia. Thus, careful monitoring of the patient in remission is needed to detect early relapse when retreatment may be most effective.

A wide variety of new agents as well as new combinations and schedules of dosage with existing drugs is being evaluated for the treatment of acute leukemia. The current literature should thus be consulted for details of the most effective treatment protocol available.

Pre-Leukemic Syndromes

At times, acute leukemia is preceded by a variable period of abnormal bone marrow function usually characterized by anemia of a hyporegenerative type. This has been referred to as a "herald state". The bone marrow picture is nondiagnostic, but commonly the marrow is normal in cellularity, at times with a variety of non-specific changes in the appearance of the erythrocyte precursors. Red cell precursors resembling megaloblasts are seen in some cases, as are sideroblastic forms. The picture of sideroblastic anemia may precede the development of acute leukemia by many years.

All of the myeloproliferative disorders must be regarded as possible precursors of acute leukemia. Patients exposed to radiation and to certain alkalating agents employed in chemotherapy of other malignant disorders have an increased likelihood of developing acute leukemia, with widely variable relative risk. In these latter instances, however, there is infrequently a recognizable clinical or laboratory connecting link on which to base a prediction that acute leukemia will develop.

Hypoplastic Marrow with Excess Blasts

This is a relatively recently recognized diagnostic entity. Its relationship to acute leukemia is unclear, although some patients apparently develop more typical acute leukemia after a variable period of time. Pancytopenia due to hyporegeneration of all of the cells of the peripheral blood is typical. A markedly hypoplastic bone marrow in which a large proportion of the remaining cells are blastic characterizes this disorder. Its management is that of a severe hypoplastic state. If acute leukemia develops, it is treated as are other acute leukemias. A large proportion of these patients succumb to the complications of the severe marrow hyporegenerative state. Others have survived for a prolonged period without development of acute leukemia.

DISORDERS OF THE LYMPHORETICULAR SYSTEM

LYMPHORETICULAR CELL FUNCTIONS AND THEIR CLINICAL SIGNIFICANCE

Understanding of the biological functions of this complex cell system has increased dramatically in the last 20 years with the rapid development of the field of cellular immunology. Indeed, the lymphoreticular cell system has moved largely into the domain of the immunologist-investigator in recent years, with the exception of certain aspects of the proliferative and neoplastic disorders of lymphoreticular cells.

Structure and Function of the Lymphoreticular Cell System

The reticuloendothelial system is still conceptualized as a network of fixed and free totipotential cells of mesenchymal origin distributed throughout the body. Certain of these cells, described as "littoral", form the lining of blood vessels, lymphatics, and sinusoidal structures within the lymphatic organs. In some sites, such as in the liver and lymphatic organs, they are intimately associated with the function of phagocytosis. The fixed cells are invested in the network of reticulin fibers, which form a kind of structural skeleton within which the free cells of the hematopoietic and lymphoid organs are formed, moved, or stored. Free cells, close derivatives of those of the fixed reticulum, appear to provide the precursor cells for hematopoeisis of all types. Some also differentiate into phagocytic macrophages. The exact morphological characteristics of the hematopoietic precursors or stem cells remains unclear, but there is evidence that at least in their resting form they resemble small lymphoid cells.

In man, the lymphatic apparatus has three major functional components. These are:

1. the bone marrow, where some lymphoid cells are produced and from which other lymphatic organs have been populated during embryological and early postpartum life;
2. The thymus, which is a specialized organ that processes uncommitted lyphoid cells to perform the functions of cellular immunity, termed the T-cells;
3. The peripheral lymphatic system, consisting of the widespread depositions of lymphoid tissues in many organs, the lymph nodes, and the spleen.

Antibody synthesis is carried out by a subset of lymphoid cells, the B-cells, which are recognizable because they have immunoglobulins bound to the surface of the cell membrane. Antigens, appropriately processed by phagocytic cells, stimulate B-cells selected because they have been able to interact with the antigen to form antibodies; this is the humoral immune system. Plasma cells represent a matured, stable population of lymphoid cells which produce immunoglobulins.

T-cells, recognizable by their ability to form a ring or rosette with sheep red blood cells, are divided into a number of subsets capable of modulating the immune response. These are the helper and suppressor subsets of T-cells. Other T-cells exert cytotoxic effects upon cells which they have immunologically recognized, sometimes called killer or K-cells.

The kinetics of the several types of lymphoid cells are discussed in detail in Chapter 6.

Lymphoid cells recirculate between the blood and lymphatic organs with many cells leaving the blood circulation, traversing the lymphatic system and returning to the blood by way of the thoracic duct. They may remain within the lymphatic organs for variable periods. The two major types of lymphoid cells have different locations within the lymph nodes, an important point in understanding the histology of the lymphoproliferative disorders. The cortical lymphoid follicles contain primarily B-cells, whereas the T-cells are found deeper within the lymph node, in the subcortical and hilar areas. Within the lymphoid follicles, the actively proliferating, stimulated cells are found in the centers of the follicles, and the more completely differentiated plasma cells and plasmacytoid lymphocytes are found toward the periphery. Normally, 60-70 percent of the peripheral blood lymphocytes are T-cells, and 15-20 percent are B-cells. The remainder are classified as "null cells".

Participation of Lymphoid Cells in Inflammation

Lymphoid cells participate in the late stages of many inflammatory processes. They are an important element in the granulomatous inflammatory reactions evoked by certain classes of bacterial and fungal pathogens. They also respond primarily to infections whose viral agents activate both cellular and humoral immune responses. Many viral infections result in a lymphatic reaction which is identifiable in the peripheral blood. The normal population of lymphoid cells, cells predominantly small in size with a few medium-sized forms and rare large forms, is shifted to include increased numbers of medium-sized and large-sized lymphocytes. The larger cells may show open reticular nuclei which have a blast-like appearance. These are probably cells stimulated to proliferate by contact with antigens. Some lymphocytes have increased amounts of cytoplasm, sometimes with irregular blue staining properties or with small amounts of purple or dark blue granulation. Other cells show increased blue staining of the cytoplasm, contraction of the nuclear chromatin, and what appears to be early differentiation into the plasma cell form (i.e., the plasmacytoid lymphocyte). Still other changes may be observed in the small lymphoid cells where the nucleus may become contorted and irregular with a very thin rim of cytoplasm which at times shows dark staining granulation. Combinations of these changes result in lymphoid cells which somewhat resemble monocytes. When all of these features are present, along with an absolute lymphocytosis, the picture is that of a fully developed lymphatic reaction.

A fully developed lymphatic reaction is most commonly seen in infectious mononucleosis cuased by the Epstein-Barr virus. However, a wide variety of viral infections, particularly infections with cytomegalovirus, hepatitis, and measles, may also be associated with a lymphatic reaction in the peripheral blood. Lymphatic reactions are frequently accompanied by enlargement of lymph nodes and splenomegaly, which may also be tender and painful. The findings of a lymphatic reaction may remain in the peripheral blood for a long period of time following some infections such as infectious mononucleosis. Some changes may be identifiable for 2 to 3 months after clinical recovery from the acute infection.

An unusual rare disorder of childhood is infectious lymphocytosis, which produces quite a different peripheral blood picture. Here large numbers of small mature appearing lymphocytes appear in the peripheral blood. This resembles the blood picture of chronic lymphocytic leukemia, but since it occurs at an age where chronic lymphocytic leukemia is not seen, the differential diagnosis is easily established. The nature of the infectious agent is unknown.

PROLIFERATIVE DISORDERS OF LYMPHORETICULAR CELLS

Lymphoma

The classification of lymphoreticular neoplastic disorders has been revolutionized in recent years by the large body of new information about the structure and function of the diverse members of this cell system. New information derived from fine scale morphological methods, from biochemistry, cell physiology and immunology have been of particular importance. The use of cell surface markers which relate subsets of lymphatic cells to specific functions has resulted in the definition of new categories of lymphoreticular proliferative disease. As yet, the clinical significance of these new classification systems, particularly as they define optimal therapy, remains incompletely understood.

A revised histopathological classification in wide clinical use, based upon morphological cell charac-

teristics and immunological methods, will be used here for the non-Hodgkins lymphomas. Classification of lymphatic leukemias based upon both morphological and immunological determinations of cell surface characteristics will be used in this discussion. This field is rapidly changing and it is difficult to interpret much of the current medical literature because there are still unresolved questions of nomenclature. At present, no easy specific translation from one system to another exists, although there are large areas of correspondence.

Neoplastic disorders of lymphoreticular cells present as lymphomas (diseases in which the proliferative process arises in a peripheral lymphatic organ) and as leukemias in which the disorder seems to first involve the bone marrow and peripheral blood. This is a clinically useful distinction, but a great deal of overlap between these two processes must be recognized. Many patients with lymphoma, with the exception of Hodgkin's disease, will from time to time have variable numbers of lymphoma cells identifiable in the peripheral blood. Invasion of the bone marrow by patchy deposits of non-Hodgkin's lymphoma is common even early in the course of the disease and widespread later on. Similarly, leukemic disorders which involve the bone marrow diffusely at the onset soon infiltrate a variety of other lymphatic structures where they produce a histological picture which resembles lymphoma. The morphological type of cell involved in all lymphatic leukemias has a counter-part among the lymphomas, although this does not imply that the cells are identical. The determinants of these two different expressions of malignant lymphoproliferation are still unknown.

Hodgkin's Disease (HD)

About a third of all patients with lymphoma suffer from this disorder. Both biologically and clinically distinctive, it is characterized by the presence of the Reed-Sternberg cell, a large binucleated cell with prominent nucleoli which may be present in variable numbers; at times it is difficult to unequivocally find and identify this cell. Many large mononuclear cells which appear to be of reticular origin are also found, as are variable numbers of lymphoid cells, eosinophils and areas of fibrosis. There is now good evidence that HD starts at a single anatomical site, usually within a lymph node, and spreads through the lymphatic system by way of contiguous nodes. Hematogenous spread may also occur.

HD is classified both histopathologically and anatomically (Table 17.18). Classification by the anatomical site of involvement is called staging. Both

Table 17.18 **Histological Classification and Clinical (Anatomical) Staging of Hodgkin's Disease**

Histological Classification (Lukes-Butler)	Prognosis
I. Lymphocytic and/or histiocytic	Generally good for cure
A. nodular	Best outlook
B. diffuse	Not as good as nodular
II. Nodular sclerosis	Good for cure
III. Mixed	Guarded
IV. Diffuse fibrosis (Lymphocyte depleted)	Poor
V. Reticular (Lymphocyte depleted)	Very poor
Clinical/Anatomical Stage	
Stage I: Single lymph node region or extra nodal site	Good for cure with favorable histology
Stage II: Two or more node regions, or extra nodal site and lymph node region on same side of diaphragm	Fair for cure; Recurrence common
Stage III: Two or more node regions and/or extra nodal sites involving both sides of diaphragm	Poor for cure; may have long-term remission
Stage IV: Diffuse involvement	Poor
Symptoms present, any subtype	
A. None	
B. Fever, weight loss and night sweats	Prognosis somewhat poorer when present

methods are valuable in planning therapy. The mode of spread of the disease makes staging of particular clinical value in this regard.

A more aggressive clinical course is associated with diffuse histology and with depletion of normal lymphocytes. Nodular histology, particularly with sclerosis of the node, usually runs a more benign course and responds better to therapy. Stages I and II of the disease, which reflect early evolution of the disease process, are associated with a high probability of cure after modern radiotherapy and chemotherapy programs. More advanced stages of the disease, particularly when systemic symptoms of fever and hypermetabolism are present, are unfavorable for curative therapy, but they may still respond to treatment, resulting in long disease free periods.

Histopathological classification of all lymphomas is a specialized discipline of pathology. Clinical (anatomical) staging is based upon a careful physical assessment of the areas of lymph node involvement as indicated by presence of firm frequently matted nodes. Presence of palpable splenomegaly and/or hepatomegaly is also an important indicator of disease within the abdomen. The chest roentgenogram will usually indicate significant involvement of mediastinum and hilar lymph nodes. Lymphangiography may define nodal involvement in the iliac and periaortic lymph node chains which are too small to be palpable. Lymphangiograms, however, may be negative in the presence of minimal or moderate nodal involvement. An exploratory ("staging") laparotomy with splenectomy and liver biopsy may be necessary to determine the extent, if any, of abdominal involvement; available lymph nodes should be obtained from throughout the abdomen for histological investigation even when not apparently enlarged or involved. At present, most patients with clinically anatomical Stage II disease are subjected to staging laparotomy. A significant number are found to be in Stage III.

Clinical picture of HD. HD occurs throughout the age spectrum but most frequently among post-adolescents, young adults, and people beyond age 50. Among adults, males predominate by about 3:2. Painless, progressive enlargement of one or more closely related peripheral lymph nodes, most frequently in the neck, is a common pattern of presentation. Recognition of the disease is usually delayed when it arises in the retroperitoneal or mediastinal nodes and when fever, hypermetabolism and weight loss, persistent cough and other chest symptoms form the presenting picture. Atypical onsets are associated with lesions which involve organs such as the gastrointestinal or urinary tract, or bones. Although extranodal disease and systemic symptoms are associated in general with a poorer prognosis, aggressive therapy still can result in very prolonged stabilization or even cure.

Patients with HD of more than minimal extent have associated abnormalities of immune responsiveness. Decreased cellular immunity is manifest by failure to respond to common skin test antigens, such as mumps or tuberculin, or to sensitization with dinitrochlorobenzene. Later in the course of the disease, if it becomes widely disseminated, humoral antibody synthesis may be impaired. As a result, these patients have a propensity to become infected by viruses, fungi and tuberculosis. When splenectomy has been carried out as part of a staging procedure an additional hazard of sepsis is present.

Therapy of HD. There remains a great deal of controversy and uncertainty about optimal treatment programs. Recent advances, however, make it reasonable to aim for cure in all patients with limited disease of the more favorable histological types. Radiotherapy (RT) delivered in high doses to areas of involvement and contiguous node fields is the present cornerstone; effective cures will result in up to 85 percent of favorable patients. With more widespread involvement and less favorable histology, various combinations of radiotherapy and multiagent chemotherapy are available which result in some long term remissions which may be equivalent to a cure. The MOPP program of chemotherapy (nitrogen mustard, oncovin, procarbazine and predisone) administered in monthly cycles until objective evidence of disease control has occurred has proven most effective in Stage III HD, but how it is best combined with RT is still controversial. MOPP treatment without RT is now regarded as optimal for Stage IV disease, where the expectation is for control of the disease for a variable, sometimes disappointingly short time, usually less than 5 years.

Uncontrolled disease is characterized by relapses of symptoms with evidence of recurrent disease in nodes, organs and, at times, bone. Cord compression may occur secondary to vertebral or epidural involvement. Intolerance to further intensive therapy due to bone marrow suppression reduces the effectiveness of treatment. Marrow failure, infection, inanition and progressive debilitation ultimately lead to death. Because HD must now be considered a curable neoplastic disease, it is important that these patients be managed by physicians in centers fully familiar with the disorder and its most current management.

Non-Hodgkin's Lymphomas

The clinical features of this large group of disorders (Table 17.19) are somewhat more diverse than those encountered in HD. As in HD, more benign clinical courses are associated with nodular patterns of histology as well as with diffuse, well-differentiated, lymphocytic tumors. The variability noted in incidence may reflect in part the use of somewhat variable diagnostic criteria. Histological classification of non-Hodgkin's lymphomas is even more difficult and controversial than classification of HD.

Anatomical staging of the non-Hodgkin's lymphomas is of less value than in HD. In general, prognosis also correlates inversely with extent of disease at diagnosis. It is uncertain if these neoplasms arise unicentrically or in multiple sites. Very frequently staging procedures, including bone marrow sections, show relatively widespread disease at the time of presentation, even when only a single group of nodes is clinically involved. The results of complete staging, including laparotomy, have much less influence on decisions about treatment; most initial treatment programs are based on the high probability that the disease is widespread at time of diagnosis. Chemotherapy (CT) is thus more frequently employed initially, with RT used to control specific lesions that are critically situated anatomically or which do not respond to CT. Cure is less often a feasible goal of therapy, although long-term disease control can frequently be accomplished with optimal management.

Clinical presentations vary from slowly developing, isolated asymptomatic node enlargement, to rapid onset with anemia, fever, inanition, malaise, weight loss and diffuse lymphadenopathy. Unexplained anemia may be due to early onset of marrow failure because of tumor infiltration. Occasionally, patients present with acquired autoimmune hemolytic anemia.

The physical findings reflect the extent of the disease at presentation and are quite variable. The blood picture will reflect the degree of marrow failure with anemia most prominent. Leukemic lymphosarcoma cells may be present in variable numbers in the blood smears, with at times substantially elevated total WBC and 80 percent or more lymphoid cells. Bone marrow sections may show such extensive infiltration that the involvement appears to be diffuse. More usually, areas of residual normal hematopoiesis remain between intervening deposits of lymphosar-

Table 17.19 **Revised Rappaport Classification for Non-Hodgkin's Lymphoma**

Histological Subgroups	Relative Incidence (%)	Five Year Survival (%)
Nodular pattern		
Lymphocytic, well differentiated	1–2	75
Lymphocytic, poorly differentiated	15–20	70
Mixed lymphocytic-histiocytic	15–20	50
Histiocytic	4–7	70
Diffuse pattern		
Lymphocytic, well differentiated (with or without plasmacytoid features)	2–3	65
Lymphocytic, poorly differentiated (with or without plasmacytoid features)	8–15	40
Mixed lymphocytic-histiocytic	8–12	35
Histiocytic (with and without sclerosis)	28–35	40
Undifferentiated	1–2	<10
Burkitt's tumor	1–2	<5
Lymphoblastic (with or without convoluted cells)	2–3	30
Unclassified		

(Modified from Golomb H, Gams R, Hoppe R: Educational Program Abstracts. American Society of Hematology, December 1981.)

coma cells. Splenic and hepatic enlargement are variably present at the time of diagnosis, but they almost always occur sometime during the evolution of the disease. Skin infiltration, typically rose colored lesions particularly in the scalp, are frequently seen in cases with aggressive clinical course.

Treatment employs primarily CT with multiple agents. The COP program (cytoxan, Oncovin, prednisone), at times with addition of an anthracycline antibiotic, is presently the most commonly employed initial treatment. In those disorders which are probably less aggressive and where cure is unlikely, initial treatment with a single agent may be appropriate. It is important that initial treatment be given to the point of objective control of disease, within the limits of tolerance of the patient's bone marrow function. Optimum programs of continued management, including the possible role of maintenance CT as well as criteria for treatment of relapses, have not been defined for most of the disorders in this large and diverse group of neoplastic diseases.

Burkitt's lymphoma deserves a brief comment. This highly malignant neoplasm was first recognized in a restricted geographic distribution largely among children in East Africa. It has a distinctive histology in which many large irregular phagocytic reticular cells with abundant cytoplasm are scattered about in a more uniform closely packed population of large round blastic cells, the so-called "starry sky" histology. The disease has a predeliction for tumor formation particularly in the jaws and ovaries or testes. It is uncommon in America. Its importance is due to the close relation this tumor has to the Epstein-Barr virus which is also the causative agent of infectious mononucleosis. Although definitive evidence that this virus is the responsible oncogenic agent is still lacking, it suggests that the outcome of this infection may vary greatly depending upon both host and environmental factors.

Chronic Lymphocytic Leukemia (CLL)

This is also a heterogeneous group of diseases which was previously regarded as quite homogeneous. Recent studies, including cell surface markers and refined morphological examinations, have lead to the development of useful correlations of identifiable sub-types of CLL with clinical features of the disease. Both B and T cell types produce a hematological picture of chronic lymphocytic leukemia, although B cell types predominate substantially. Table 17.20 lists the currently recognized variants of this disease group.

These disorders occur primarily in late life with median onset at about age 60. In general, males pre-

Table 17.20   Classification of Chronic Lymphocytic Leukemias

A. Chronic B-lymphoid leukemias:
  1. Small B-lymphocyte (B-CLL)
  2. Prolymphocyte
  3. Plasmacytoid lymphocyte
  4. Small cleaved follicular center cell
  5. Hairy cell
B. Chronic T-lymphoid leukemias
  1. T-lymphocyte CLL:
    a. Japanese T-cell leukemia (Knobby variant)
    b. Cytoplasmic variant (T-CLL)
    c. Prolymphocyte
  2. Sezary cell
  3. Hairy cell

(Modified from Gale RP, Levine A, Golde DW: Educational Program Abstracts. American Society of Hematology, December, 1981.)

dominate in a ratio of about 2:1 in most disease categories, particularly in the most common small B cell type. True clinical chronicity, with median survivals of between 4 and 5 years, is the hallmark of CLL. Many patients survive for much longer periods. Some patients have a more accelerated course with aggressive disease at the onset; the patients with prolymphocytic B cells and most of the T cell types of CLL are in this category.

The blood picture early in the course of CLL frequently shows only an absolute and relative lymphocytosis, most commonly with small, densely stained, mature-appearing lymphocytes having little cytoplasm. These cells are mechanically fragile and many distorted "basket" cells may be seen in blood films. The WBC may range from $15–20 \times 10^3$/cu mm to over 100×10^3/cu mm at diagnosis. The diagnosis is frequently made when a routine blood study is done for another purpose. Later in the developing course of CLL, patients seek medical care for recurrent infections, diffuse lymphadenopathy or symptoms associated with spenomegaly. Still later, symptoms secondary to marrow failure, anemia, and thrombocytopenic bleeding may be presenting complaints. Autoimmune acquired hemolytic anemia (AIHD), with abrupt onset of severe anemia, may occur at any point in the clinical course. Positive red cell antiglobulin tests and/or AIHD has been estimated to occur in about 10 percent of patients with CLL at some time in their clinical course.

The bone marrow shows diffuse infiltration with the same type of small lymphoid cell that is found in the peripheral blood; early in the course of CLL, 30 to 40 percent of the marrow cells will be of this type. As the disease progresses, the degree of marrow infiltration increases until marrow failure results. Recently, several clinical staging systems have been proposed; their clinical usefulness is still being evaluated.

Cytogenetic studies utilizing methods for stimulating B cells show that non-random abnormalities, particularly involving chromosomes 12 and 14, occur in nearly half of patients with B cell CLL. This contrasts with previous results which yielded normal cytogenetic findings when primarily stimulated T cells were studied. Failure of full functional differentiation in CLL apparently results in the inability to (1) respond to antigenic challenge, (2) produce immunoglobulin and (3) differentiate into plasma cell forms. This is at least part of the pathogenetic mechanism which leads to progressive accumulation of nonfunctional lymphoid cells in the blood, marrow and lymphoreticular organs.

To know when treatment of CLL will be beneficial requires experience and sound judgement. Alkylating drugs (such as chlorambucil and cytoxan) and prednisone are most commonly employed. The degree of elevation of the WBC is by itself of little value in making treatment decisions. Evidence of marrow failure, the bulk of lymphatic infiltration, and presence of hypermetabolism with weight loss are more important indicators of the need for treatment. Unfortunately, many patients are over-treated which adds the marrow suppressive effects of the therapy to the results of infiltration; this results in progressive early onset of marrow failure. Death results from infection or from development of a refractory state in which the patient no longer responds to therapy. Only very rarely does an acute leukemia develop. Many patients with CLL die of unrelated causes.

Hairy Cell Leukemia

This sub-group of CLL has been frequently diagnosed in recent years. Although some of the morphological features of the disease which classified it as a reticuloendotheliosis have been recognized for some time, the advent of the scanning electron microscope revealed the prominent surface projections which characterize these cells. Tartrate resistant acid phosphatase can be demonstrated cytochemically in hairy cells. Both B and T cell types exist. The clinical course is indolent as a rule, and splenectomy alone may induce a prolonged remission. Optimal chemotherapy for patients unresponsive to splenectomy has not been defined.

Sezary Syndrome

The T cell variant of CLL clinically resembles and is closely related to mycosis fungoides in that widespread plaque-like skin infiltration with T lymphoid cells occurs in both. In the Sezary syndrome, a leu-

kemic process develops. Relatively large cells with contorted cerebriform clumped nuclei and PAS postive cytoplasmic granules are typical. After onset of leukemia, the disease is relatively rapidly progressive and poorly responsive to therapy with survival of about a year.

Acute Lymphocytic Leukemia

Although primarily a children's disease, occasional cases are encountered among adolescents and young adults. It also may follow typical CML as a blastic crisis. The clinical features of this acute leukemia greatly resemble those of acute non-lymphocytic leukemia (q.v.). The major clinical difference is the relative ease and safety with which remissions can be induced with prednisone and vincristine (Oncovin). These agents, coupled with more intensive and repeated courses of chemotherapy and prophylactic treatment of the CNS with radiation, have resulted in a high proportion of apparent cures or at least very long remissions among childhood cases. Among older children and adults the results are less satisfactory, but long periods of useful life interrupted by the need for periodic treatment are not uncommon.

Because of the very different clinical course and treatment of the lymphocytic type of acute leukemia, it is important to establish or exclude this diagnosis quickly in every patient with acute leukemia. The characteristics of acute lymphocytic leukemia cells which are of differential diagnostic value are listed in Table 17.21 along with a classification of recognized

Table 17.21   Cell Characteristics in Acute Leukemia

Acute Lymphoblastic Leukemia (ALL)	Surface Immuno-globin	Anti[1] T	Anti[2] CALLA	TdT[3]
Subtypes				
Common	–	–	+	+ +
Null Cell	–	–	–	+
T Cell	–	+	–	+ +
B Cell	+	–	–	–

Acute Myeloid Leukemias:
  a. Lack ALL markers (above)
  b. Stain for peroxidase of Sudan black; negative in ALL.
  c. Have Auer bodies in cytoplasm in some cases; not seen in ALL. Other cytochemical staining procedures have less specificity for AML or ALL.

[1] Anti-T Antibody against T cell determinants
[2] CALLA Common acute lymphocytic leukemia antigen
[3] TdT   Terminal deoxynucleotidyl transferase

(Modified from Bennett JM, Brennan JK, Catovsky D: Educational Program Abstracts. American Society of Hematology, 1981.)

subtypes. No single characteristic should be regarded as specific. When a group of cytochemical and immunochemical characteristics have been evaluated, a specific diagnosis can usually be established. This field is also rapidly changing and better clinical correlations with related recommendations for therapy will no doubt be developed.

Stem Cell Leukemia

This relatively rare disorder reflects neoplastic proliferation of essentially totally undifferentiated reticuloendothelial cells. Its counterpart among the lymphomas is diffuse histiocytic lymphoma. Acute leukemic undifferentiated reticuloendotheliosis may be a more appropriate name. It is usually a highly aggressive and unresponsive disease in which fever and rapid deterioration of the patient frequently occur. Some patients may run a more subacute course.

Plasma Cell Disorders

The benign disorders of plasma cells are primarily those associated with humoral immunodeficiency disorders in which failure of lymphoid cells to mature and differentiate into this functional form is a prominent feature. These will not be discussed here.

Plasma cells are rarely seen in the peripheral blood. They may be found following acute viral infections such as measles. Plasmacytoid lymphocytes are seen more commonly. In the bone marrow, the number of mature plasma cells is usually less than 1 percent. In some situations involving chronic infections or chronic liver disease, benign marrow plasmacytosis may be quite striking with about 5 percent of cells of this nature.

Plasma cells and lymphocytes present in many stimulated lymphoid clones produce a large variety of immunoglobulins reflected by broad-based groups of γ globulins on electrophoretic analysis of the plasma proteins. Presence of large amounts of a sharply defined single-species of immunoglobulin, termed a monoclonal Ig, frequently is a finding indicative of neoplastic plasma cell or lymphoid proliferation. When this is the case, the monoclonal Ig is referred to as an M (for *m*yeloma) protein.

Monoclonal proteins may be found in patients who do not have other morphological, clinical or radiological evidences of multiple myeloma or other malignant proliferation of plasma cells or lymphocytes. The etiology and clinical course of this situation, termed benign monoclonal gammopathy, is still poorly understood. No treatment is required, but periodic observation is usually recommended. Depending upon the criteria employed for diagnosis and the period of observation prior to acceptance of this diagnosis, a variable small proportion of patients with what appears to be benign monoclonal gammopathy go on to develop true multiple myeloma or are later found to have an isolated malignant plasmacytoma. The latter are usually associated with the gastrointestinal or respiratory tracts, including the upper airway.

Neoplastic Disorders of Plasma Cells

Multiple myeloma. Multiple myeloma (MM) is the most common of this group of malignant plasma cell proliferations. It is a disease of older people characterized by infiltration of plasma cells throughout the bone marrow. At times, the infiltrates form tumorous collections. Early in the disease, the bone marrow may not be uniformly involved and several biopsies may be needed to identify the immature neoplastic plasma cell infiltrate.

Multiple myeloma results in bone mineral mobilization which leads to diffuse osteoporosis and/or lytic bone lesions. Typical lytic lesions are more easily identified radiographically. Vertebral involvement leads to collapse and nerve root compression with back pain. Acute cord compression which may require emergency laminectomy may occur. Anemia secondary to suppression of erythropoiesis is also a consistent early clinical manifestation. Propensity to develop serious bacterial infections is also an important clinical problem.

The diagnosis is usually established by demonstrating presence of an M protein and marrow infiltration with neoplastic plasma cells. In about half of MM patients, the M protein is IgG; it is an IgA in another quarter. Some patients do not have a demonstrable M protein. Many MM patients excrete variable, sometimes large, amounts of light chains of the immunoglobulin molecule in the urine, the so-called Bence-Jones protein. These are best characterized immunochemically, although classically they have been demonstrated by heat precipitation at temperatures from 50–60°C with redissolving near the boiling point. This protein is present in the urine of about three-fourths of patients with MM, including those that do not have a demonstrable serum M protein. Renal damage leading to renal failure is common in MM and is thought to be associated with filtration of large amounts of free light chains.

Treatment is based upon destroying the myeloma cells with alkylating drugs. L-plenylalanine mustard

(L-PAM) and cytoxan are most commonly employed, frequently with prednisone. Because of the production of an identifiable and measurable tumor product, the M protein, the synthesis of which can be measured in in vitro cultures, it has been possible to estimate tumor burden, tumor kill after treatment and rate of tumor recurrence in this disease. This has shed important light on tumor kinetics; prognosis is dependent upon tumor burden and tumor destruction accomplished by therapy.

Radiotherapy is useful in treatment of painful or collapsing bone lesions. Orthopedic support of the spine and pain control with drugs are also of great symptomatic importance. Hypercalcemia may occur acutely requiring emergency therapy. Death is due in most cases to some combination of resistance to treatment, marrow failure, renal insufficiency and infection. Survival is quite variable, but averages about 2 years from diagnosis.

Macroglobulinemia. This disorder is less frequently seen than MM, but it is not as rare as once thought. Better techniques now available to measure and characterize the immunoglobulins have disclosed a substantial group of patients with high levels of IgM immunoglobulin. The associated clinical picture is quite variable but usually much less aggressive than that seen with MM. Rarely a patient with otherwise typical MM will be found to have a monoclonal IgM in the serum. More commonly, the marrow and blood picture reflects a lymphoid and plasmacytic proliferative process with increased numbers of tissue mast cells in the marrow. The disease is usually slowly progressive, sometimes over many years. The concentration of IgM protein in the serum may be in the range of 1–2 gm percent. This may lead to elevated viscosity, poor perfusion and manifestations in the central nervous system of confusion, slowed thinking and responsiveness, the so-called *hyperviscosity syndrome*. Because the IgM protein remains intravascularly where it exerts an oncotic effect, the plasma volume may be expanded with spurious anemia. The high concentration of IgM may interfere with platelet function and induce abnormal bleeding from wounds. Susceptibility to infection is also frequently increased. Cryoglobulins and pyroglobulins may be demonstrable.

Treatment is usually initiated with alkylating drugs, which, if effective, slowly reduce the serum IgM level. Plasma exchange may be needed to control abnormal bleeding or hyperviscosity. Late in the course of the illness, these patients increasingly resemble patients with MM with a terminal picture that is much the same.

Plasma cell leukemia. This is a rare disorder in which large numbers of malignant plasma cells are consistently present in the peripheral blood. Occasional plasma cells may be found in the blood of patients with typical MM. The leukemic form of plasma cell neoplasia usually follows an acute or subacute course. Some clinical features of MM may also be present. Several reported cases have been associated with rarely encountered IgE or IgD M proteins.

Other Dysproteinemic Disorders

Neoplastic proliferation of immunocytes, usually presenting with a clinical picture of lymphoma or chronic lymphocytic leukemia, has been associated with the production of abnormal amounts of immunoglobulin heavy chains (H Chains) of several types. Gamma H chain disease overproduces a peptide related to the FC fragment of IgG. Alpha H chain disease is associated with overproduction of an IgA related peptide. Mu H chain disease has also been identified in patients with a benign CLL like picture.

TRANSFUSION OF BLOOD AND BLOOD PRODUCTS

Transfusion of donor blood and its components is a type of transplantation procedure in which, fortunately, the immunobiological rules governing donor-recipient compatibility are relatively simple, well-understood and useable in a practical sense. Discovery by Landsteiner in the early years of this century of the major ABO blood grouping system and its significance and the elucidation in the 1940s and 1950s of the Rh blood group system provided the basic understanding of the immunology involved in donor-recipient compatibility.

Much of modern medical and surgical therapy depends upon availability of blood or blood components. Treatment of military casualties has provided great impetus to development of this science and its supporting technology. Research in blood preservation has also lead to true blood banking. Simple anticoagulants preserve red cell viability only for a few hours. Refrigeration at 2 to 4°C extends this period only a little. Development of acid-citrate-dextrose solution (ACD) resulted in a 21-day period of useful viability. Adding small amounts of adenine (citrate-phosphate-dextrose-adenine, CPD-A) to supplement ATP regeneration has now extended this period to 35 days, with substantial improvements in the quality of transfused blood.

The development and maintenance of a reliable, adequate and safe blood supply has been an area of great medical and social progress in America and much of the world in the last two decades. Almost all of the United States blood supply, estimated at 10 to 11 million donations annually, comes from volunteer donors. Large regional blood banks operated by the American Red Cross or by voluntary community agencies supply the bulk of the transfusion materials required. In Canada, a government sponsored national blood service program operated by the Canadian Red Cross provides comprehensive services. Some hospitals in the United States also operate their own donor recruitment and blood banking programs. National and regional programs now exist which exchange blood products to deal with shortages which may develop in an area where adequate numbers of donors are not available or where a major disaster has occurred. It is the responsibility of every physician to support donor recruitment in the area of his or her practice and to become familiar with the way in which the local blood supply is managed. Over all in North America, the supply of blood is probably adequate to meet real needs. Localities may have an inadequate supply temporarily, or longterm. In the latter case, blood imports may supplement the local supply, but improved blood program organization and operation will be needed in these areas to secure an adequate stable supply in the future. Unfortunately, a significant part of the blood supply is still inappropriately administered to patients who could be equally well-managed without transfusion or with smaller amounts of blood. Practice is improving in this regard, but continued surveillance of blood usage in each hospital administering transfusions remains an important professional responsibility.

THE IMMUNOBIOLOGICAL BASIS OF BLOOD TRANSFUSION

The ABO and Rh Blood Group Systems.

Discovery of the ABO blood grouping system permitted classification of donors and recipients into four major categories as shown in Table 17.22. The groups are named for the red cell antigens present. The ABO system is unique in that an antibody against the antigens not present is almost always found in the individual's serum. Good practice involves administering donor blood of the same ABO group as that of the recipient, although donor red cells which lack the antigen(s) which would react with antibodies in the donor's serum can be administered safely. Blood lacking both the A and B antigens, Group O, is most commonly employed for this purpose.

The A and B antigens are determined by autosomal dominant genes. These genes produce a sugar transferase responsible for assembly of the carbohydrate moiety which forms the antigenic determinant group on the red cell membrane. A related precursor antigen, termed H, is also part of this system and is found on virtually all human red cells. A and B antigens have a number of genetically determined variants, the most important of which is a weaker reacting form of A, called A_2. The Lewis blood grouping antigens are also related immunochemically to the ABO antigens.

Occurrence of hemolytic transfusion reactions in ABO compatible transfusions among recipients previously transfused with ABO group compatible blood as well as investigation of hemolytic disease of the newborn lead to discovery of the Rh blood grouping system. Antibodies to the Rh complex of antigens are evoked by an immunizing exposure of a patient who lacks the antigen to red cells which carry it. Transfusion and feto-maternal bleeding at the time of delivery are the main routes of blood group antigen alloimmunization. Although earlier serological studies demonstrated the existence of the important Rh blood group system, it was not until development of the antiglobulin technic by Coombs and associates that the system could be fully investigated. The majority of alloantibodies induced by immunization are non-agglutinating in simple serological tests. They are mainly 7S IgG immunoglobulins. Modification of the test cell surface by enzyme treatment which reduces its net negative charge, or carrying out agglutination tests in a high dielectric colloid medium which effectively reduces the electrostatic effect of the surface charge are other methods which have been employed to enhance the agglutinating activity of antibodies of this class.

The Rh antigen system is a complex consisting of a large number of recognizable, inherited, antigenic determinants. The principal antigens of clinical importance are listed in Table 17.22. Because all other antigens of this complex are less antigenic than the principal antigen, D, donors and recipients are routinely matched for only this antigen in the United States and Canada. Bloods containing the D antigen are termed Rh positive, all lacking it, Rh negative.

When Rh positive blood has been administered accidentally to an Rh negative recipient, immunization may still not occur; 15 to 20 percent of North American Caucasians resist this alloimmunization for reasons not understood. Immunization can also usually be prevented following this transfusion error by administering appropriate amounts of Rh antibody in the form of an anti-Rh immune human globulin preparation, as is done when an Rh negative mother delivers an Rh positive child. The passively acquired Rh antibody accelerates removal of the potentially

Table 17.22   **ABO and Rh Blood Groups**

		Group	Antigens Present	Incidence (%) North American Caucasians
I.	ABO Systems	O	None	45
		A	A	41
		B	B	10
		AB	A and B	4
	Related Antigens		A$_2$	20% of A & AB
			H	Virtually 100% (variable amount)
II.	Rh System	Rh positive	D★	85
		Rh negative	D not present	15
	Related Antigens		C	70
			E	30
			c	80
			e	98
			f	64
			G	85

★ A weaker reacting group of variant D antigens, Termed D^u exist. These indivduals are classified as Rh positive as donors and Rh negative as recipients. Weaker reacting variants of the C and E antigens are also known.

antigenic donor erythrocytes from the circulation and interferes with the immune response to them by other mechanisms as well. With these several measures, recipients are now rarely alloimmunized to the D antigen.

Other Blood Grouping Systems

In addition to the ABO and Rh systems, there are at least nine other known and well-studied human blood grouping systems. All are inherited as autosomal dominant traits except the Xg system, which is sex linked and found on the X chromosome (Table 17.23). Altogether, over 350 blood group antigens are known. Combinations of these characteristics

Table 17.23   **Other Human Red Cell Antigen Systems**

Recognized Antigen Systems★	Symbol
Lewis	Le
MNSs	(same)
Lutheran	Lu
Kell	Kk
Duffy	Fy
Kidd	Jk
Ii	(same)
Xg	(same)
Less Well Established Systems★★	
Ena	(same)
SID	Sd

★ A system is defined as a group of genetically related antigens dependent upon an independent genetic locus, not part of any other system.
★★ At least eight other well characterized antigens are known which may be part of a known or unknown blood group system.

alone indicate that, except for identical twins, all donors and recipients differ in the antigenic structure of their red cells. Yet the frequency of alloimmunization following administration of ABO and Rh compatible blood is low. This is due to the relatively much lower antigenicity of all other red cell antigens. Occasionally, antigens of the Kell and Duffy systems evoke an immune response, as do the Cc, E and e antigens of the Rh complex. Incompatibilities involving these antigens must be detected and avoided when subsequent transfusions are administered to a patient alloimmunized to one or more of them.

The Cross-Match and Recipient Antibody Screening

Two alternative strategies are employed to detect and avoid donor-recipient incompatibility when a recipient has been previously alloimmunized. In the cross match, the recipient's serum is tested in an agglutination reaction with the red cells of a proposed donor. If agglutination is not observed, the test red cells are subjected to an antiglobulin test to detect non-agglutinating IgG antibody molecules bound to their surfaces from the recipient's serum. If this test is also negative, there is a very high probability but not certainty, that the donor red cells will survive normally, at least initially, in the recipient's circulation. Other serological methods to demonstrate antibodies in the recipient's serum are also employed, but the antiglobulin test remains the accepted standard.

Alternatively, the recipient's serum may be screened for the presence of alloantibodies of a wide range of specificities by testing it with erythrocytes of 10 to 20 individuals (called a panel) chosen for their representation of a wide range of antigens, including all those of major clinical importance. If an antibody is detected, its specificity is determined by retesting with red cells of known antigenic content, and donors lacking the identified antigen(s) are chosen. This approach, called "type and screen", is now being employed in some large medical centers in place of the antiglobulin cross-match test, since it has been found to provide essentially the same safety for recipients as the cross match. A "quick cross-match" prior to release of the blood for transfusion is still carried out to detect clerical errors which might lead to serious incompatibility within the ABO system.

Not all serologically detectable red cell alloantibodies lead to rapid in vivo destruction of incompatible erythrocytes. Some induce slowly accelerated destruction over 10 to 30 or more days leading to inefficient transfusions. Alloimmune responses may occur while donor red cells are still present in the circulation, leading to delayed hemolytic transfusion reactions sometimes sufficiently rapid to cause symptoms of back pain, chest discomfort and hemoglobinuria. It is important to recognize these situations clinically and to investigate them in the laboratory so that future transfusions may be administered safely.

Administration of Blood Transfusions

The final test of donor-recipient compatibility is the administration of the blood itself. In elective transfusions, the first 25 to 30 ml of sedimented red cells (or 50 ml of whole blood) should be administered slowly over 20 to 30 minutes with careful observation of the patient. Appearance of virtually any new symptoms, but particularly back pain, chest discomfort, a feeling of suffocation, restlessness and alarm, requires prompt stopping of the transfusion. Venous access should be maintained and existing dehydration promptly corrected. The remainder of the blood which was being transfused and a fresh sample of the recipient's blood (drawn at a different location into a dry tube) should be sent immediately to the blood bank laboratory for investigation. Further management of overt hemolytic reactions is designed to minimize renal injury by correction of hypovolemia, maintenance of blood pressure and transfusion with compatible blood if necessary. Alkalinization of the urine with sodium bicarbonate is not of value; it may provide a hazardous sodium load if the patient develops acute renal tubular failure and anuria.

If no symptoms are encountered after slow administration of the small amount of blood, the re-

maining transfusion can be administered more rapidly over the course of 60 to 90 minutes. Intermittent observation of the patient should continue. It is an unfortunate practice that many transfusions are administered with inadequate observation. Late in the course of blood administration, particularly in patients who have received many transfusions, some recipients will develop chilly sensations and fever, called a febrile reaction. These symptoms rarely are of serious importance, but occasionally in elderly or debilitated people they may induce hypotension and, even more rarely, result in death. Thus, most transfusions which cause febrile reactions, are stopped and investigated. The reactions are in the main due to immunization to platelets and leukocytes or their debris remaining with the red cells; the term "buffy coat" reaction is also employed to describe them. Removal of leukocytes and platelets from red cells for transfusion may eliminate or ameliorate the reaction. Pretransfusion treatment of patients who exhibit recurrent mild febrile reactions with aspirin and/or an antihistamine compound also frequently reduces the severity of the reaction.

PRINCIPLES OF COMPONENT AND REPLACEMENT TRANSFUSION THERAPY

In the past, only whole blood anticoagulated and preserved in bottles at 4°C in Acid Citrate Dextrose solution (ACD) was available for transfusion. Development of plastic blood transfusion equipment and related technology resulted in a major advance: component therapy. Red cells separated by gentle centrifugation can be provided for correction of anemia. Platelets can be centrifugally concentrated from the separated plasma, pooled from multiple donors (usually seven or eight), and administered to patients with bleeding due to certain types of transient thrombocytopenia. Although the leukocytes of individual blood donors can also be concentrated and pooled, this is not an efficient way to provide granulocytes for transfusion. Rather, granulocytes are collected selectively in large numbers from single donors by the process of leukapheresis in which the red cells and plasma are returned to the donor. Platelets, platelets plus granulocytes, or plasma only can also be collected by this method. It has the great advantage of exposing the recipient to the leukocyte and platelet antigens (as well as the hepatitis risk) of only one donor and delays appearance of broad immunity against this class of cellular antigens which reduces the effectiveness of the cell replacement process.

If the blood has been processed within 4 to 6 hours of drawing and carefully refrigerated in that interval, the recovered plasma can be frozen, thawed at 0°C

Table 17.24   **Characteristics of Blood Components for Transfusion**

Red Cell Preparations	
Concentrated red cells	300 ± 20 ml., Hematocrit 70–80%
Leukocyte and platelet poor red cells	Prepared by washing or filtration
Platelet Concentrates (pools of 6–8 donors)	
Each donor	About 50 ml. 5–10 × 10^{10} platelets
Plasma Products	
Fresh frozen plasma	About 200 ml./unit. Frozen shortly after drawing to preserve humoral coagulation factors
Cryoprecipitate	10–15 ml. 80–120 units Factor VIII 300–400 mg. fibrinogen

White blood cells for transfusion prepared only by leukopheresis. Platelets for transfusion prepared by plateletpheresis are preferred to pooled donor platelets when available.

and a precipitate rich in coagulation Factor VIII can be obtained for treatment of patients with hemophilia A. This product, termed cryoprecipitate, is also the starting material for manufacturing concentrated, lyophilized Factor VIII preparations. Most of the plasma employed for fractionation is obtained commercially by plasmapheresis. The remaining plasma from a unit of whole blood can be used as a volume expander in patients requiring expansion of plasma volume; it should not be employed to replace hemostatic system components since it lacks Factor VIII and has reduced fibrinogen content. Cryoprecipitate is also useful as a source of therapeutic fibrinogen, although there are very few indications for this use. The principal blood bank products and some of their characteristics are listed in Table 17.24.

Residual plasma lacking Factor VIII and plasma salvaged from the preparation of concentrated red cells can be employed in the manufacture of either human serum albumin or a partially fractionated albumin preparation called PPF as well as in an immunoglobulin fraction containing the antibodies generally present in blood donors. If plasma is collected from deliberately immunized donors who have received specific antigens, such as tetanus or rabies vaccine or the Rh antigen, immunoglobulins of high specific antibody content can be prepared. Serum of patients convalescent from an infection such as Herpes zoster also contain higher amounts of specific immunoglobulin. These products collectively are known as *hyperimmune serum globulins*. They are important therapeutic and prophylactic materials and are discussed elsewhere in relation to specific conditions.

Transfusion of Red Blood Cells, Whole Blood and Plasma Volume Expanders

Red blood cells are tranfused primarily to increase the oxygen carrying capacity of the blood; acute and severe chronic anemic states are thus the primary in-

dication for their administration. Red cells also increase the blood volume, a physiological fact that must be considered when red blood cells are administered to hypovolemic patients or to patients whose circulation is overloaded in relation to the pumping capacity of the heart. Although stored red cells have decreased amounts of 2, 3, DPG and a higher affinity for oxygen than normal red cells, they still will transport oxygen to tissues. Returned to the circulation, they metabolically regenerate the normal pool of intracellular 2, 3, DPG in about 6 to 12 hours, and thereafter function more efficiently in oxygen transport. Not all losses of oxygen carrying capacity, acute or chronic, need to be replaced. Circulatory adjustments compensate to a great degree for reduced red cell mass, as discussed in the section on anemia.

Acute blood loss reduces not only oxygen carrying capacity but also intravascular volume. In many instances, the latter factor is of greater clinical importance. If severe enough, it leads ultimately to failure of tissue perfusion and the complex pathophysiological state called shock. It is clear that prevention of shock by intravenous administration of fluids designed to increase the intravascular volume is of paramount clinical importance in preventing a fatal outcome. Control of blood loss, replacement of lost red cells and sufficient other colloid and/or crystalloid solutions to restore perfusion are the main aims of shock prevention and therapy. Controversy exists about the use of colloids such as serum albumin products versus crystalloids: normal saline, Ringer's solution or lactate Ringer's solution. Larger volumes of crystalloid solutions than of colloids must be given for equivalent expansion of the intravascular volume, but clinical experience indicates that the outcome of these two approaches is essentially equivalent. Albumium is rapidly synthesized by the normal liver, but synthesis virtually stops in the face of acute undernutrition, widespread trauma, or a severe inflammatory process. The assessment of individual patient's needs for albumium administration is complex and not agreed upon. It is inappropriately used for nutritional purposes.

The amount of acute blood loss tends to be over estimated when bleeding is overt and external as from an epistaxis, vaginal bleeding or a laceration. There is a tendency to over-replace this type of blood loss. In many instances no replacement is physiologically necessary. Occult blood loss, as into a body cavity, the GI tract or the site of a severe fracture, tends to be underestimated and thus underreplaced. Changes in hemoglobin concentration of hematocrit are of little or no value in estimating the amount of blood lost acutely. Rather, attention should be focused on presence or absence of continued or recurrent bleeding, the state of the circulation with careful frequent measurements of blood pressure, pulse rate, urine flow, and state of consciousness, and, above all, trends in these observations. Blood replacement should be guided by these data.

If only a few units of red cells need to be replaced, up to four or five, concentrated red blood cells can be given, along with adequate crystalloid solutions. If a larger volume of blood replacement is required, whole blood is frequently employed, although continued use of red cells, crystalloid solutions and possibly albumiun solutions can be employed.

Massive transfusion, in which the total blood volume may be replaced several times, presents a number of additional unresolved problems. Blood platelets do not survive for more than a few hours in a functionally effective form in refrigerated anticoagulated blood. Similarly, the activities of many of the protein components of the coagulation system decline on storage. Serum albumin and, of course, crystalloid solutions contain none of these proteins. After massive transfusion, the concentration of platelets and coagulant factors is reduced. Thus, the question frequently arises, should efforts be made to replace these hemostatically important materials by administration of concentrated donor platelets, Factor VIII concentrates, or fresh frozen plasma in which the other coagulant components are preserved? Although these questions remain incompletely resolved, a number of recent clinical investigations indicate that replacement is not necessary, and, when done, does not significantly improve the outcome.

Chronic anemia and its management by transfusion have been discussed in the section dealing with hyporegenerative anemias. Two points should be reemphasized. The patient who depends upon chronic transfusion for survival is usually best managed by regularly scheduled transfusions rather than "chasing the hemoglobin level". Over-transfusion of these patients with more than the amount needed to maintain a reasonably functional status should be avoided to delay onset of complications induced by transfusion itself: alloimmunization, febrile reactions, iron overload and the probability of transmission of hepatitis.

Platelet Transfusion

Platelet transfusions are currently widely used in virtually all thrombocytopenic states. They are usually ineffective and possibly contraindicated in those disorders characterized by rapid platelet destruction or platelet consumption. Platelets are highly antigenic and readily evoke antibody responses to HLA antigens as well as other intrinsic alloantigens which they bear. Thus, platelet transfusions are most effective for about 2 to 3 weeks, after which their effectiveness may be seriously limited by short life span in the recipient's circulation. This is termed refractoriness and is due, at least in part, to alloimmunization. Platelet transfusions are most effective in patients with severe but short-term suppression of platelet production and in patients in whom recovery of platelet formation can be reasonably expected. Severe marrow hypoplasia secondary to drug toxicity, or deliberately induced by chemotherapy (as is done in the treatment of acute leukemia) are examples of situations in which platelet transfusions are most effective.

Platelet transfusions should be administered to control bleeding due to thrombocytopenia, not on the indication of even a very low platelet count. Many patients with platelet counts less than 10,000/ cu mm do not bleed. Administration of platelets in the absence of bleeding hastens the onset of refractoriness and decreases the effectiveness of later platelet transfusions that may be needed to control serious hemorrhage.

Transfused platelets survive long enough in the circulation in the absence of alloimmunization to permit transfusions to be given every 24 to 48 hours (7 to 8 donors, or about 4 to 4×10^{11} platelets per transfusion), unless there is severe continuing bleeding when more frequent transfusions may be required. Platelet administration, frequency and amount should be gauged by hemostatic effect rather than by the platelet count; platelet numbers greater than 20,000/cu mm are rarely needed to achieve hemostasis if bleeding is due primarily to thrombocytopenia.

Complete or partial matching of recipient for antigens of the HLA system with use of one or a small number of donors of platelets collected by plateletpheresis can most easily be done employing siblings of the recipient as donors. Although alloimmunization may be delayed or avoided, a single donor can usually be employed for platelet procurement for only a limited time, usually less than a week of daily transfusions. Matching donor and recipient for certain antigens of the HLA system has been reported to delay or prevent alloimmunization in a significant proportion of recipients. Panels of platelet and leukocyte donors who have been typed for ABO, Rh and HLA antigens are being developed in many areas from which "best matched" donors may be selected. In spite of these strategies, the high probability of ultimate alloimmunization and refractoriness of the recipient must be considered in planning treatment programs.

Leukocyte Transfusions

At present, leukocyte transfusions, although relatively widely employed on empirical grounds, are still under clinical investigation in efforts to define their effectiveness, indications for use, limitations and risks. There is little doubt that they are of value in some septic or seriously infected severely leukopenic patients. Whether they should be administered to febrile severely leukopenic patients without obvious sites of infection is controversial. It is difficult or impossible to assess their contribution to an apparently favorable outcome since such patients are always treated with multiple antibiotics and frequently with other active pharmacological agents such as corticosteroid. There is certainly no established standard of practice in this regard. It is widely agreed, however, that present technology does not allow collection of enough granulocytes for fully effective treatment regimens. Because of the difficulty of carrying out a critically controlled study of this problem, further refinements in the use of transfused granulocytes may not develop for some time.

Most of the same problems of procurement, preparation and immunological incompatibility of donor and recipient encountered in platelet transfusions also apply to granulocyte transfusions. Practically, these transfusions can be prepared only by leukapheresis. Most are employed in the treatment of acute leukemia or other neoplastic diseases where severe marrow depression has been induced by intensive chemotherapy. Most such patients have total granulocyte counts well under 500/cu mm and are overtly infected. Transient, severe agranulocytosis due to a drug reaction with sepsis is another circumstance where granulocyte transfusion may be useful.

HAZARDS OF TRANSFUSIONS

Hemolytic Reactions

Severe hemolytic reactions occur rarely in a well-managed transfusion service. Those that do occur are most frequently due to clerical errors such as mislabelling or misrecording of ABO blood types or cross-match results or misidentification of the recipient or of the unit of blood prepared for a specific patient. Technical errors or failure of serological test systems to detect donor-recipient incompatibility account for a small proportion of identified hemolytic reactions, usually well below 10 percent. Administration of a transfusion is a disarmingly simple procedure. Great care must be taken at all points in the chain to assure that a recipient receives blood which has been correctly prepared. The recognition and principles of management of hemolytic reactions have been discussed in the section on donor-recipient compatibility.

Hepatitis and Other Infections Transmitted by Transfusion

Any blood product which cannot be subjected to heat inactivation must be regarded as potentially able to transmit the infective agents of hepatitis. At present in North America and much of the rest of the world, all such products must be tested for the presence of the hepatitis B surface antigen (HbSAg). Elimination of most commercially donated blood, in which there is a high incidence of this infection, plus development of highly sensitive tests for presence of this agent have reduced the incidence of hepatitis B infection in blood recipients to the same level in untransfused control patients. Increased sensitivity of a test for hepatitis B would not be expected to lower this incidence much further. The infective agent of hepatitis B has multiple modes of transmission in addition to transfusion.

Transmission of hepatitis A is not a significant problem among transfusion recipients. This disorder, fundamentally an enteric disease, appears to have only a brief viremic phase. However, hepatitis due to other currently undetectable infectious agents that remain in the donor's blood for long periods remains a significant problem among blood recipients. At present, about 10 percent of recipients who receive 4 to 10 units of blood develop at least biochemical evidence of hepatitis. Probably at least two agents, collectively termed non A-non B (NANB) hepatitis, are responsible for these infections. No specific test for their detection exists and nonspecific tests are not of proven effectiveness as yet. This problem strongly supports the recommended policy of administering only necessary transfusions in the smallest effective amount. Treatment of transfusion acquired hepatitis and its long-term sequelae is discussed in Chapter 12.

Transmission of cytomegalovirus by transfusion is becoming of increasing concern. It induces an acute disease resembling infectious mononucleosis. This infection may be more serious in immunocompromised patients and in renal grafted patients. No adequate test of the infectivity of blood products is available for screening use.

Other infectious agents may be transmitted by transfusion. Of these, malaria is the most important. Donors who have been in malarious areas are screened out for variable periods. However, donors who have had quartan malaria even many years before may still be infectious. Other hemoparasites are hazards of transfusion in tropical areas.

Other Adverse Effects

In addition to those adverse effects already discussed, transfusion may produce other undesirable or dangerous complications. Air embolism is a rare complication, encountered mainly when blood is administered under pressure from a container into which air had inadvertently been introduced. Cardiovascular overload with precipitation of acute heart failure and pulmonary edema may occur in patients with low cardiac functional reserve who have been given blood too rapidly. Prompt cessation of the transfusion, and measures to control heart failure should be initiated at the first sign of this complication. A small phlebotomy into a sterile donor blood bag may be necessary to control a severe failure episode. This blood with plasma removed can be readministered to the patient later when congestive failure has subsided.

Chronic transfusion, in the absence of chronic blood loss, results in accumulation of large stores of iron in all the physiological and some pathological storage sites. This situation, termed transfusion siderosis, sometimes is associated with abnormalities of heart, liver and pancreatic function which resemble those of the primary iron storage disease hemochromatosis. The relationship between these two disorders is unclear at present. Removal of iron accumulated by transfusion is difficult, since phlebotomy cannot be employed. Newer programs of administration of iron chelating compounds by slow continuous infusion may prove to be effective preventive or therapeutic measures.

REFERENCES

Clinical Laboratory Methods in Hematology

1. Hyun, B.H., Ashton, J.K., and Dolan, K.: Practical Hematology. W.B. Saunders, Philadelphia, 1975.
2. Chanarin, I., Brozović, M., Tidmarsh, E., Waters, D.A.W.: Blood and its Diseases. 2nd ed., Churchill Livingstone, Edinburgh, 1980.
3. Maslow, W.C., Beutler, E., Bell, C.H., Hougie, C., and Kjeldsberg, C.R.: Practical Diagnosis, Hematological Disease. Houghton Mifflin, Boston, 1980.
4. Custer, R.P.: An Atlas of the Blood and Bone Marrow. 2nd. ed., W.B. Saunders, Philadelphia, 1974.
5. Zucker-Franklin, D., Greaves, M.F., Grossi, C.E., and Marmont, A.M.: Atlas of Blood Cells, Function and Pathology. Lea and Febiger, Philadelphia, 1981.

Nutritional Requirements for Hematopoiesis

6. Chanarin, I.: The Megaloblastic Anemias. 2nd. ed., Blackwell, Oxford, 1979.
7. Bothwell, T.H., Charlton, R.W., Cook, J.D., and Finch, C.A.: Iron Metabolism in Man. Blackwell, Oxford, 1979.
8. Finch, C.A., and Huebers, M.D.: Perspectives in iron metabolism, NEJM, 306, 1520, 1982.
9. Valentine, W.N.: Hemolytic anemia and inborn errors of metabolism. Blood, 54:549, 1979.
10. Harris, J.W., and Kellermeyer, R.W.: The Red Cell. Harvard University Press, Cambridge, 1970.
11. Petz, L.W. and Garatty, A.: Acquired Immune Hemolytic Anemias. Churchill Livingstone, New York, 1980.

Abnormal Hemoglobins

12. Bunn, H.F., Forget, B.G., and Ranney, H.M.: Human Hemoglobins. W.B. Saunders, Philadelphia, 1977.
13. Harkness, D.R.: Hematological and clinical manifestations of sickle cell disease: a review. Hemoglobin, 4, 313, 1980.
14. Weatherall, D.J., and Clegg, J.B.: The Thalassemia Syndromes. 2nd ed., Blackwell, Oxford, 1972.

White Cells, Myeloproliferative Syndromes and Acute Leukemia

15. Beard, M.E.J., and Fairly, G.H.: Acute leukemias in adults. Sem. Hematol. 11, 5, 1974.
16. Cline, M.J.: The White Cell. Harvard University Press, Cambridge, Mass., 1975.
17. Cline, M.J., ed:, Leukocyte Function. Churchvill Livingstone, New York, 1981.
18. Dameshek, W., and Gunz, F.: Leukemia. 2nd ed., Grune and Stratton, New York, 1964.
19. Miller, D.: Acute lymphoblastic leukemia. Pediatr. Clinic., North America, 27, 269, 1980.
20. Kaplan, H.S.: Hodgkin's Disease. Harvard University Press, Cambridge, 1972.

21. Lichtman, M.A., ed: Hematology for Practitioners. Little, Brown, Boston, 1978.
22. Mollison, P.A.: Blood Transfusion in Clinical Medicine. 7th ed., Blackwell, Oxford (in press), 6th ed., 1979.
23. Petz, L.D., and Swisher, S.N.: Blood Transfusion in Clinical Practice. Churchill Livingstone, New York, 1981.

General Hematology

24. Williams, W.J., Beutler, E., Erslev, A.J., and Rundles, R.W.: Hematology. McGraw-Hill, New York, 1977.
25. Wintrobe, M.M., Lee, G.R., Boggs, D.R., Bithell, T.C., et al: Clinical Hematology. Lea and Febiger, Philadelphia, 1974.

18

Disorders of Joints and Connective Tissues

Raymond M. Lewkonia and T. Douglas Kinsella

PRINCIPLES OF RHEUMATOLOGY

NOMENCLATURE

The causes of most rheumatic diseases are not immediately apparent, and, at first sight, many of the diseases appear to have similar symptoms and signs. The number of words used by physicians to describe these disorders was, therefore, quite restricted for many centuries, and conceptual recognition of distinct entities was hindered by the application of a limited vocabulary based on ancient and often inappropriate ideas. *Gout* was well known by the time of Hippocrates, when it was believed that the disorder was caused by invisible evil humors dropping incessantly onto the affected joint (Latin, *gutta*—a drop). Gout slowly became the generic name for many types of acute and chronic rheumatic disease, because of the mistaken belief that all had a shared basis. *Rheumatism* is from a Greek word meaning a flow of mucus or catarrh, and in the 16th century rheumatism was described as "a defluxion of pernicious humors." Rheumatic fever was probably so named to reflect the flowing, or migratory, pattern of the acute polyarthritis of the disease. A similar derivation provides the modern usage of rheumatism to describe poorly localized nonarticular musculoskeletal pain. At the dawn of the application of biochemistry to medicine, Garrod discovered in 1848 that typical gout is associated with hyperuricemia. It was soon realized that a form of chronic arthritis that had been called "rheumatic gout" was not associated with hyperuricemia, and in 1859 Garrod suggested the name *rheumatoid arthritis* for a disease not hitherto defined as a separate entity. Having recognized that common disease, he was later able to separate rheumatoid arthritis and osteoarthritis by further clinical observation.

Joints become symptomatically involved in several chronic multisystem diseases that have protean manifestations. The best known example is systemic lupus erythematosus. Facial lupus erythematosus was considered to be a variant of cutaneous tuberculosis, lupus vulgaris, (Latin, *lupus*—wolf) in the late 19th century. It was then found that lupus erythematosus is sometimes associated with diseases of joints and internal organs, hence the modern name systemic lupus erythematosus. The variability of clinical presentations of this disease and of other apparently related disease processes such as scleroderma prompted much speculation regarding possible pathogenesis. In 1942 a hypothesis was advanced that the central feature in the group of disorders was a pathological abnormality of collagen, and the term *collagen disease* was introduced. The group was enlarged to embrace other diseases involving joints, connective tissues, and skin, including polyarteritis nodosa and dermatomyositis. These disorders are now known to have an autoimmune basis, and, although autoimmunity directed against collagen has been demonstrated, it appears to be of secondary importance in most of the diseases. Vasculitis appears to be a more important unifying pathological process, so the group is, therefore, often now referred to as *collagen-vascular diseases*. It is important that these be distinguished from the nonimmunological heritable disorders of collagen structure and metabolism.

BIOLOGY OF JOINTS AND CONNECTIVE TISSUE

Joint Morphology

Diarthrodial joints show much variation in structure and function but share characteristic features (Fig. 18.1). The joint cavity is only a potential space in the normal healthy state. Synovial membrane lines the whole of the joint interior except for the cartilage-covered ends of articulating bones. Stability and constraint from excessive movement are achieved by the complementary shapes of articulating surfaces, by a resilient fibrous external capsule, and in some joints by internal ligaments or fibrocartilagenous spacers. It is necessary to consider the structure, biochemistry, and physiology of the cellular and fibrillar elements of articular cartilage and of synovium to understand the mechanisms and effects of disease in joints and other connective tissues.

Articular Cartilage

Articular cartilage covers the bone ends in synovial joints, and its highly specialized structure serves the functions of low friction movement, distribution of weight-bearing forces, and shock absorption. During a normal lifetime, articular cartilage is subjected to repeated compressive and impact forces. It is estimated that every year each of the weight-bearing joints in the lower limb receives approximately 2,000,000 impact strains during normal walking activities, and these mechanical forces are transmitted across a limited area of contact rather than the whole articular surface. During movement of limb joints, the shear forces are greatly minimized by the extraordinarily efficient lubrication apparatus of arti-

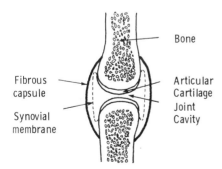

Fig. 18.1 Anatomy of a typical diarthrodial (synovial) joint.

cular cartilage and synovial fluid. The coefficient of friction of synovial joints is in the range of 0.02 to 0.002, which compares very favorably with the coefficient of friction between steel surfaces in oil lubricated machine joints, which is usually in the range of 0.1 to 0.5. Not only are the large weight-bearing joints of the lower limbs subject to great mechanical stress, but also the small peripheral joints of the limbs. The stresses generated in repetitive movement of finger joints in grasping actions have been estimated to be in the same range of magnitude as the forces exerted across the knee joint in walking.

Articular cartilage has a fibrillar scaffold containing a relatively small mass of cells. Water constitutes 70 to 80 percent of the wet tissue weight and it serves a vital role in the nutrition and mechanical function of articular cartilage. It facilitates the flow of nutrients and waste materials from cartilage to synovial fluid and also has an important role in the "weeping lubrication" of cartilage, in which water flows from the cartilage surface as load increases and re-enters the surface as load decreases.

The cells, or chondrocytes, of hyaline articular cartilage constitute less than 10 percent of the volume of the tissue. They lie embedded in a matrix which has a Type II collagen fiber scaffold enclosed in a ground substance of proteoglycans and water. Several discrete layers can be recognized in sections of articular cartilage and these correspond with varying alignment of the collagen fiber network (Fig. 18.2). The tensile properties of Type II collagen fibers and the arrangement of the collagen network confer resistance to shearing forces. In addition, the architectural arrangement of the collagen fibers is thought to restrain proteoglycans from excessive expansion when fully hydrated.

Chondrocytes in normal adult cartilage do not show mitotic activity or even evidence of DNA synthesis. However, they should not be regarded as effete cells; they play an essential role in the production of cartilage collagen, glycosaminoglycans, and the degradative enzymes concerned with turnover of matrix components. The turnover of collagen in adult articular cartilage is very slow, but the proteoglycan protein core and glycosaminoglycans undergo more rapid metabolic breakdown and renewal. Not possessing a direct blood supply, chondrocytes use an anaerobic system for energy production and for their metabolic activities. These activities and consequently the vitality of articular cartilage are influenced by local concentrations of prostaglandins, corticosteroids, and somatomedins. In diseases such as osteoarthritis, or following direct injury to arti-

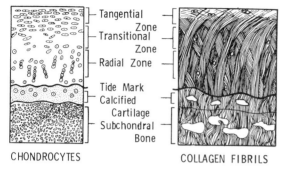

Fig. 18.2 Alignment of chondrocytes and collagen bundles in mature articular cartilage.

cular cartilage, chondrocytes are capable of increased metabolic activity, reactivation of DNA synthesis, and replication.

Aging of Articular Cartilage

Articular cartilage shows a number of important changes with aging, which are clearly significant to the etiology of degenerative joint disease. Aging is accompanied by a color change in the macroscopic appearance from white to a slightly yellow tinge, and the smooth glistening surface tends to become slightly roughened. On microscopic examination the loss of surface continuity appears as "fibrillation." Fibrillation commences at the periphery of joint surfaces before it is seen in the central weight-bearing areas and may progress to the formation of deeper clefts penetrating beyond the superficial cartilage layers.

Severe biochemical changes of aging have been demonstrated in the femoral head and other articular cartilages. The overall collagen content of articular cartilages decreases slightly and shows even less water solubility than does young cartilage, probably as a consequence of increased cross-linkage of collagen fibers. The mechanical properties of articular cartilage are also altered, and histological examination suggests that the collagen network becomes more prone to fatigue and stress failure. Articular cartilage from the elderly shows a relative total depletion of proteoglycans with an overall decreased polysaccharide content, decreased chondroitin-4-sulfate, and increased keratan sulfate content. The total water content decreases slightly with aging. The total number of cartilage chondrocytes also decreases, but local increase of chondrocyte numbers is seen around areas of fibrillation and clefts in the cartilage surface.

Synovium

The synovial membrane which secretes joint fluid is just a few cells thick in normal diarthrodial joint but is capable of very considerable hypertrophy in disease. In health it has a smooth velvety appearance and is thrown into redundant folds and villi, giving flexibility for movement and a large surface area for metabolic activity. The highly specialized inner lining cells do not rest on a basement membrane but rather on a loose weave of areolar, adipose, and fibrous connective tissue that is permeated by vascular capillaries and lymphatics. The subsynovial capillary plexuses have a specialized intimal lining comparable with that of other vascular plexuses such as the renal glomerulus and choroid plexus. The intimal structure is believed to facilitate rapid exchange of water and solutes and thus play an important part in intra-articular metabolism. There are two predominant varieties of synovial lining cells: Type A cells being macrophage derived and Type B cells probably related to fibroblasts. The majority of Type A cells have prominent Golgi apparatus, and more numerous vacuoles, mitochondria, and intracellular fibrils than the Type B cells, which have abundant rough endoplasmic reticulum. Type A cells are more active in phagocytosis and are presumed to have an important immunological function. Receptors for C3 of the complement system and the Fc fragment of immunoglobulin molecules have been demonstrated on synovial membrane; this finding is almost certainly pertinent to the occurence of synovitis as a complication of many diseases in which immune complexes are present in the circulation. Type B cells have a secretory function and synthesize proteins that are added to the plasma-derived proteins in the joint cavity. In addition to the differentiated Type A and Type B cells, normal synovial membrane contains cells with intermediate morphology, fibroblasts, and some mast cells. Tendon sheaths and bursae are lined by a synovial membrane with similar structure to that of the synovium of joints, and these structures are susceptible to many of the disease processes seen in joints.

Synovial Physiology

Alteration of the rate of blood flow through the subsynovial capillary plexus and of capillary permeability has profound effects on the composition of synovial fluid. The rate of blood flow is subject to control by a number of factors, including autonomic nerve stimulation and chemical agents such as the prostaglandins E1 and E2, and histamine. Attenuation of blood flow by these agents is important in inflammatory joint disease and in pharmacological attempts to manipulate inflammatory processes. Aging is accompanied by fibrosis in the subsynovial tissues and by decreased blood flow, changes which may impede the flow of nutrients to articular cartilage and perhaps contribute to the changes in degenerative joint disease.

Synovial lining cells have a number of important metabolic products. Hyaluronic acid is assembled from uridine disphosphate sugars in the Golgi apparatus of Type B cells and secreted as a high molecular weight polymer containing equimolar concentrations of glucosamine and glucuronic acid. The rate of hyaluronic acid synthesis is influenced by local concentrations of mediators including prostaglandin E1, but sustained high concentrations of this prostaglandin as may occur in inflammatory joint disease may actually inhibit hyaluronic acid synthesis.

Synovial tissue secretes several proteinases, including a plasminogen activator that helps to impede fibrin clot formation within joints, collagenases, and proteoglycan proteinases, which are thought to participate in synovial fluid protein catabolism. Proteins and other large macromolecules are cleared from the joint cavity by lymphatics in the subsynovial tissues. Small molecular weight joint nutrients and electrolytes leave the joint cavity by diffusion into the intravascular compartment of the subsynovial capillary plexus.

Synovial Fluid

Normal synovial fluid is clear, slightly yellow, and highly viscous. It may be regarded as an ultrafiltrate of plasma that is modified in composition by products of the synovium. In health the volume of synovial fluid within most joints is very small and even in a large synovial joint such as the knee the normal volume of fluid is less than 4 ml. The permeability of synovium to proteins depends on their molecular weight and shape. High molecular weight molecules, such as IgM and Clq and other proteins of the complement system, or highly asymmetrical molecules, such as fibrinogen, are mostly excluded from the joint cavity. Some of the antiproteinases of high molecular weight, for example alpha-2-macroglobulin, which inhibit the actions of lytic enzymes released during acute inflammatory responses, do not gain access to the joint cavity in more than trace amounts

until synovial vascular permeability has been increased by disease. Molecular size is unlikely to be the only factor which restricts protein entry into joints, because albumin with a molecular weight of 70,000 is present at almost the same concentration as in plasma, whereas prothrombin is absent and yet has a molecular weight of 63,000. The absence of the latter protein is one of the several important factors which explains the lack of clotting of normal synovial fluid. The total protein content of normal synovial fluid is in the range of 1.8 to 2.0 g/dl of which 60 percent is albumin and 40 percent is globulin. Hyaluronic acid comprises less than 1 percent of the total solutes, yet it determines the viscosity and remarkable hydrodynamic properties of the fluid. The flow characteristics of normal synovial fluid are such that its viscosity is high at low shear rates and falls with increased shear rate during movement. The rheological properties of synovial fluid confer resistance to impact pressure and yet tend to facilitate the acceleration of gliding movements of joints. In normal synovial fluid the hyaluronic acid molecular weight is of the order of 10×10^6. In inflammatory diseases, such as rheumatoid arthritis, the hyaluronic acid molecular weight is reduced by the effects of proteolytic enzymes, and alterations in synovial synthesis. The low viscosity synovial fluid of inflammatory and purulent arthritides has a hyaluronic acid molecular weight in the range of 1×10^6 to 2×10^6. Synovial fluid constituent concentration changes found in disease must be assessed in the context of overall dilution resulting from altered capillary permeability.

Normal synovial fluid has a low cell concentration of less than $200/mm^3$. Almost all of the cells present are white blood cells, but a few synovial lining cells may be seen. In health 80 percent or more of the white cells are monocytes or lymphocytes and only a small number of granulocytes is present. Synovial fluid analysis is an important diagnostic tool, and the changes found in disease are described in subsequent sections of this chapter (Table 18.3).

FIBRILLAR ELEMENTS OF JOINT TISSUES AND OTHER CONNECTIVE TISSUES

The fibrillar elements of connective tissues are responsible for the tensile strength and resilience necessary to hold the body together under mechanical stress. The functional importance of these macromolecules is especially evident in joints, but the widespread importance of collagen, proteoglycans, and elastin throughout the body has become evident as the consequences of biochemical abnormalities of these substances has been recognized.

Collagen

Collagen is the major structural molecule of the musculoskeletal system and accounts for 40 to 50 percent of all body proteins. It occurs in slightly different molecular forms (Types I to V) in bone, ligaments, fasciae, cartilage, large blood vessels, basement membranes, and other specialized tissues and organs. The typical collagen molecule has an average length of 3,000 Å but is only 15Å wide. Each molecule is made of three intertwined alpha chains of approximately 1,000 aminoacids in a repeating sequence of glycine, proline, and hydroxyproline. The long rope-like molecule forms a triple-stranded super-helix bound together by cross-links. The helical structure depends on the presence of glycine, which holds the chains together by hydrogen bonding. Cross-linking of molecules results from covalent reactions between lysyl and hydroxylysyl side chains. The distribution of cross links is probably the major determinant of collagen strength and is also an important determinant in resistance to collagenases.

Collagen is synthesized first as a precursor molecule, procollagen, which is about 40 percent larger than the final molecule. Molecular extensions at the carboxy-terminal and amino-terminal ends appear to facilitate solubility and intracellular transport of the molecule. It is necessary to briefly consider the biosynthesis of collagen in order to understand the heritable collagen diseases. Translation of procollagen messenger-RNA determines the primary structure of alpha chains. These are subject to three important post-translational modifications, namely hydroxylation, glycosylation, and disulphide bond formation. Ascorbate is one of the cofactors necessary for hydroxylation of prolyl and lysyl residues. The connective tissue abnormalities of scurvy can thus be explained by defective hydroxylation of alpha chains, which proceed to disulphide linkage without a stable triple helix conformation. Following post-translational modifications the procollagen molecule passes from the smooth endoplasmic reticulum to the Golgi apparatus prior to secretion from the cell. Specific procollagen peptidases remove the propeptides from each end of the molecule, converting it to the less soluble collagen fibril which then becomes reinforced by covalent cross link formation through aldehydes derived from hydroxylysine and lysine residues. This last step requires the enzyme lysyl oxidase.

Investigation of collagen metabolism has shed light on the nature of several of the heritable disorders of connective tissue, especially the *Ehlers-Danlos syndromes* (EDS) and osteogenesis imperfecta (OI). EDS are characterized by extensive connective tissue abnormalities, including hypermobile joints subject to recurrent dislocation and effusion, fragile and bruisable skin with poor healing characteristics, rupture of large arteries or of the bowel, retinal detachment, varicose veins, and even fragile fetal membranes giving rise to premature birth. Careful observation of patients with EDS and of the patterns of inheritance has divided the syndromes into several distinct entities, and the biochemical basis of several of the varieties of EDS has been discovered. For example, death due to aortic rupture in Ehlers-Danlos syndrome Type IV has been attributed to absent or highly defective Type III collagen synthesis (aortic and large artery collagen is predominantly of the Type III variety). See Chapter 8, Table 8.7.

The *osteogenesis imperfecta syndrome* also represents a heterogeneous group of heritable connective tissue diseases in which the major feature is fragility of bone. Other features in addition to frequent fractures are joint hypermobility, blue sclerae, dental abnormalities, and progressive deafness. Several abnormalities of collagen have been identified in patients with OI.

The *Marfan syndrome* includes skeletal abnormalities as well as connective tissue abnormality. It is usually inherited in a dominant pattern and has some resemblance to EDS. Affected individuals are very tall and have long thin limb bones with spidery digits (arachnodactyly), ectopia lentis, susceptibility to dissecting aneurysm of the aorta, valvular abnormalities including aortic regurgitation and prolapsed mitral valve. Many patients have hypermobile joints and hyperextensibility of the skin comparable with the findings in EDS. The biochemical abnormality in the Marfan syndrome has not been fully defined, but abnormalities in collagen cross linkage have been reported.

Most of the phenotypic features of the Marfan syndrome are seen in homocystinuria, with generalized osteoporosis as an additional skeletal feature. This has a recessive pattern of inheritance and the underlying defect concerns cystathionine synthetase activity.

Collagen in articular cartilage and other connective tissue is slowly degraded subject to enzymatic action. Several proteinases have collagenase activity. Elastase and other enzymes cleave cross links between collagen fibrils outside cells, cathepsin B and other enzymes degrade fragments of collagen fibril within cells at acid pH, and other enzymes have collagenase activity at neutral pH in extracellular fluid. The activation and inhibition of collagenolytic enzymes is of major importance in the destruction of articular cartilage in disease.

Proteoglycans

The amorphous matrix, or ground substance, of articular cartilage and other connective tissues such as heart values, cornea, and tendons, is largely composed of hydrated proteoglycans. These macromolecules have a filamentous backbone of hyaluronate to which is attached carbohydrate side chains called glycosaminoglycans (formerly called acid mucopolysaccharides) through a link-protein region. The structure of proteoglycan molecules resembles a very long bottle brush (Fig. 18.3). In the biosynthesis of proteoglycans, the protein core is assembled on a ribosomal template and then the carbohydrate chains are added. The sugars are sulfated on the endoplasmic reticulum before passing through the Golgi apparatus. The carbohydrate chains comprise a hexosamine, which is either glucosamine or galactosamine, alternating with a monosaccharide, which is either glucuronic acid or iduronic acid.

The physical chemistry of proteoglycans has functional significance in articular cartilage physiology. The large number of sulfate and carboxyl anion groups gives a high net negative charge, which contributes to electrostatic binding to adjacent collagen molecules. Proteoglycans in cartilage are associated with hyaluronate, and, in normal articular cartilage, about 75 percent of the proteoglycans are bound in aggregates in the form of gel. The proteoglycan gel is very successful in holding water, to the extent that the volume of hydrated cartilage proteoglycan is approximately 100 times larger than that of the dry molecule. Water held in the gel gives articular cartilage its weight-bearing and shock-absorbing properties, and yet the gel allows water molecules and nutrient solutes to diffuse through its substance. Proteoglycans swell further if the restraining collagen network in articular cartilage is damaged by mechanical or enzymatic agents.

In normal adult articular cartilage, proteoglycans are believed to have a turnover half-life of approximately 900 days, but in joint disease degradation may become rapid. Catabolism of proteoglycans involves breaking the glycosaminoglycan chain, desulfation of the sugars, and proteolysis of the backbone. Proteinases present in synovial fluid are unlikely to diffuse readily into healthy articular cartilage, and it is likely that most proteoglycan degradation is brought about by lysosomal enzymes. The most important enzyme seems to be cathepsin D, which is not active at the pH of the extracellular ground substance and is believed to have its effects close to the chondrocyte cell wall.

Abnormalities of degradation of glycosaminoglycans occur in a group of rare heritable disorders (the mucopolysaccharidoses) in which undegraded glycosaminoglycans accumulate in lysosomes throughout tissues and organs, resulting in widespread cellular damage. The clinical features vary with the type of glycosaminoglycans that accumulate. An abbreviated classification of some of the more common mucopolysaccharidoses (MPS) is shown in Table 18.1.

Elastin

Elastin is the third major fibrillar element found in most connective tissues throughout the body. It is present in high concentration in the vertebral ligamenta flava, the great vessels, and in elastic cartilages such as those in the pinna of the ear. It is a highly insoluble long molecule rich in glycine and proline, but, in contradistinction to collagen, there is little hydroxyproline or hydroxylysine. Elastin chains contain a greater number of cross links than found in collagen. It has a soluble precursor, tropoelastin, which is degraded during the latter stages of elastin biosynthesis in fibroblasts. Formed elastin is degraded by granulocyte elastase. The important disorders of elastin metabolism are nonrheumatic and may include varieties of emphysema and atherosclerosis, due to abnormal elastin in the lungs and large arteries. Elastase is inhibited by alpha-1-antitrypsin and the association of emphysema with deficiency of

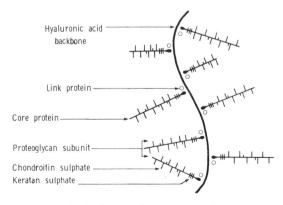

Hyaluronic acid backbone

Link protein

Core protein

Proteoglycan subunit

Chondroitin sulphate

Keratan sulphate

Fig. 18.3 Articular cartilage, proteoglycan aggregate.

Table 18.1   Mucopolysaccharidoses

Disease	Inheritance	Enzyme Defect	Clinical Features
Hurler's syndrome (MPS IH)	Recessive	Alpha-L-iduronidase	Death in childhood, mental retardation, corneal clouding, kyphosis
Scheie's syndrome (MPS IS)	Recessive	Alpha-L-iduronidase	Stiff joints, corneal clouding, normal life span, aortic valve disease
Hunter's syndrome (MPS II)	X-linked	Iduronase and sulfatase	Death in teens, mental retardation
Sanfillipo's syndrome Syndrome (MPS III)	Recessive	Heparin-N-sulfatase	Mental retardation, mild growth disturbance
Morquio's syndrome	Recessive	Hexosamine-6-sulfatase	Dwarfism, corneal clouding, osteoporosis, absence of the odontoid process
Maroteau-Lamy syndrome (MPS VI)	Recessive	Aryl sulfatase B	Corneal clouding, severe skeletal abnormality

this inactivator has been attributed to excessive elastin degradation. Two rare heritable disorders of connective tissues have been described with elastin abnormalities. In the autosomal dominant form of pseudoxanthoma elasticum, hypermobility of joints is associated with hyperextensile skin and atherosclerosis as well as myopia. Ehlers-Danlos syndrome Type V is also associated with joint hypermobility, and defective cross link formation has been found in elastin as well as collagen.

INFLAMMATORY JOINT DISEASE

The mechanisms of acute and chronic inflammation within joints are complex. They culminate in the classical signs of inflammation, namely hyperemia (rubor), warmth (calor), edema (turgor), pain (dolor), to which may be added in joint disease damage to articular cartilage and joint capsules, and bone reabsorption. A general scheme of some of the pathways of the inflammatory response is shown in Figure 18.4. The initial stimulus and early steps in the inflammatory response vary among diseases, but the products of inflammation and the final common pathway of damage are similar for most of the rheumatic diseases. The central process in the early stages of the acute inflammatory response is the activation and recruitment of phagocytic cells, granulocytes and macrophages. Within joints, the Type A cells of synovial tissue have a macrophage-like function and the major initial step in several arthropathies is probably the phagocytosis of insoluble material such as immune complexes, crystals, or fragments of infective agents. Normal synovial fluid contains relatively few granulocytes, but when an inflammatory response has been established, a great number of cells enter the joint cavity.

The early inflammatory response is amplified by the attraction of increased numbers of phagocytic cells. Factors that are chemotactic for granulocytes and monocytes include C5a of the complement system, fibrin fragments, collagen fragments, histamine, kallikrein, prostaglandins, lymphokines produced by stimulated lymphocytes, and some bacterial wall components such as N-formylmethionyl peptides. Activation of phagocytosis depends on the recognition of an insoluble particle as being "foreign." This process is facilitated by immunoglobulin acting as specific antibody to either foreign antigens or altered native antigens. In other circumstances there may be nonspecific binding of immunoglobulin to particles such as crystals; or components of the complement system such as C3b may bind in a nonspecific manner to extraneous material. Immunoglobulin or complement components act as opsonins and combine with Fc or C3b receptors on the surfaces of phagocytic cells. Ingestion of particulate material by phagocytic cells is rapidly followed by discharge of potent lysosomal enzymes into the phagocytic vacuole. Permeation of these enzymes beyond the cell can then activate a remarkable array of chemical mediators of inflammation. The lysosomal enzymes possess potent capability of lysis of ingested material, but if released in excessive quantities the potential for damage to surrounding tissues is great. This is especially so if the ingesting cell is itself damaged to the point of cell death and release of all of its lysosomal enzymes. This occurs, for example, following ingestion of monsodium urate crystals in acute gout, a situation in which it is believed that the crystal surface directly causes lysosomal enzyme discharge. Some bacterial toxins are also capable of disruption of neutrophil cell membranes with consequent release of intracellular enzymes. This is of significance in pyogenic arthritis where massive lysosomal enzyme release leads to particularly rapid destruction of articular cartilage and other tissues. The chemical mediators of the inflammatory response have many complex actions and interactions, which

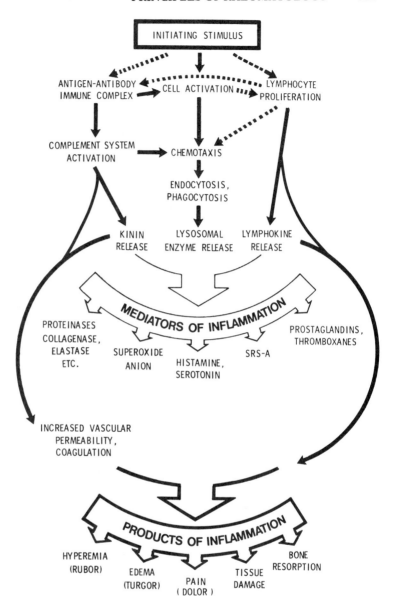

Fig. 18.4 Pathways of the inflammatory response.

will be reviewed briefly as they pertain to inflammatory arthritis and the destructive mechanisms of joint disease.

Complement

The classical complement pathway is activated through the Fc portion of immunoglobin molecules following antigen-antibody interaction (see Chapter 6). This occurs in the joint space in established rheumatoid arthritis as the major inflammatory consequence of immunoglobulin combining with anti-immunoglobulin (rheumatoid) factors. The major pathway may also be activated by other substances, including DNA released from damaged intra-articular cells. The alternative pathway of complement activation can be activated by lysosomal enzymes and by bacterial products such as may be present in the joint cavity in pyogenic arthritis. Plasmin is another alternative pathway activator, and this in turn may be generated from plasminogen precursors via lysosomal enzymes. Complement components can be demonstrated within immune complexes inside synovial phagocytic cells, and this indicates participation of the complement system in intra-articular inflammatory responses. However, the extent to which complement activation is a direct cause of articular damage is uncertain. The complement fragments C3a, C5a and the C567 complex released in activation of the complement cascade have important actions in phagocyte chemotaxis and in altering vascular permeability, but it is uncertain whether complete activation of the complement system through to C9 is an important cause of cell membrane damage within joints. Release of low molecular weight fragments of C3 and C5, namely C3a and C5a, stimulates the release of histamine from mast cells, increasing local vascular permeability. It is also increased by kinin-like activity possessed by C3a and a fragment of C2. Complement components, especially C3, bind in a nonspecific manner to some bacteria and also to crystals. This opsonic property is an important prelude to phagocytosis and has the consequences already discussed.

Lymphokines

Lymphocyte activation and proliferation lead to the production of a variety of hormone-like chemicals termed lymphokines (see Chapter 6). Among the lymphokines important in inflammatory responses in joints are macrophage activating factor, factors which affect the migration of macrophages, mediators that are chemotactic for neutrophils and other granulocytes, and lymphotoxin, which may be directly toxic to synovial and other cells. Lymphokines which recruit and activate other lymphocytes are probably important in accumulating the synovial lymphocyte infiltration found in rheumatoid arthritis and other inflammatory joint diseases. A lymphokine of particular interest in joint disease is osteoclast activating factor, which may be involved in the periarticular demineralization and bone erosion of chronic inflammatory joint disease.

Superoxide

Superoxide anion ($O\bar{2}$) is a particularly destructive product of the early stages of phagocytosis. It is formed by a membrane surface oxidase and most is converted to hydrogen peroxide (H_2O_2), which, like superoxide itself, is locally destructive. Free superoxide anions are scavenged and inactivated by the enzyme superoxide dismutase. In addition to direct damage to surrounding materials, superoxide indirectly contributes to the inflammatory response. Its oxygenation of membrane arachidonic acid contrib-

utes to the formation of members of the prostaglandin and thromboxane family of inflammatory mediators. Superoxide can depolymerize hyaluronic acid and also probably damages collagen molecules. The antiproteinases that inhibit the action of lysosomal enzymes are themselves inhibited by superoxide.

Lysosomal Enzymes

Degranulation of neutrophil granulocytes has been found in studies of synovial histology in several types of rheumatic disease. The enzymes released from lysosomes have protein degrading actions at neutral or acid pH. The major neutrophil enzymes of importance are collagenase, elastase, cathepsin G, and cathepsin D. Type I collagen present in bone and ligaments is especially susceptible to neutrophil collagenase, whereas Type II collagen in articular cartilage is relatively resistant. Granulocyte elastase is capable of degrading proteoglycans and elastin in ligaments and blood vessels. Cathepsins G and D are both capable of degrading proteoglycans, cathespsin D being the more important enzyme in joint disease. Cathepsin G is able to cleave C5 and thus may interreact with the complement system. Cathepsin D has been demonstrated in tissue cultures of articular cartilage and also in rheumatoid synovium.

Plasmin is a trypsin-like enzyme which degrades fibrin, but it also has lytic activity. It is able to degrade proteoglycans and can also activate collagenase. Production of plasmin from its precursor plasminogen can be brought about by a number of other proteolytic agents, including products of activated monocytes and the products of complement activation. Specific hyaluronidase has not been demonstrated in human granulocytes or synovial cells, the leading candidates for this activity being superoxide anion, with proteolytic enzymes probably taking a secondary role. Most of the lysosomal and other enzymes discussed here are inactivated by alpha-2-macroglobulin, alpha-1-antitrypsin and other high molecular weight proteins. These inactivators of the products of inflammation reach normal joints in low concentrations because of their large molecular size, and, even in active inflammatory joint disease, their level of activity is likely to be lower than in plasma.

Histamine

The synovial membrane cells include a small number of mast cells. These cells and basophils drawn into joints by chemotactic stimuli are the source of histamine released in inflammatory joint disease. The histamine is released under the influence of activated complement component fragments and some of the other products of inflammation. The reactions of importance in inflammatory joint disease are mediated through the H-2 class of histamine receptors and the most obvious result is increased vascular permeability. Histamine also appears to have anti-inflammatory activity, including inhibition of neutrophil chemotaxis and lysosomal enzyme release, as well as possible inhibition of some T-lymphocyte functions.

Serotonin

Serotonin is released from platelets, and its role in joint inflammation is probably of minor importance when the inflammatory process is well established. Serotonin is able to induce mononuclear cells to produce a factor chemotatic for granulocytes. Serotonin has been shown to aid collagen formation by promoting cross linkage of collagen molecules.

Prostaglandins, Thromboxanes and SRS-A

The prostaglandins and thromboxanes are a family of mediators of inflammation derived from phospholipids in cell membranes from the parent compound arachidonic acid. The primary step in arachidonic acid metabolism takes place under the influence of the enzyme cyclo-oxygenase. Inhibition of this enzyme is one of the most important effects of anti-inflammatory drugs. Some of the important effects of prostaglandins are shown in Table 18.2.

The effects of prostaglandins on cyclic AMP are of some importance in the modulation of inflammatory responses. Elevated tissue cAMP levels tend to inhibit histamine release and also inhibit the release of lymphokines. Prostaglandin E stimulates osteoclastic bone reabsorption in experimental models, and it has been shown that the synovium in rheumatoid arthritis contains large amounts of PGE2. This is likely to be of importance in the production of juxta-articular osteopenia and erosions in rheumatoid arthritis.

Slow-reacting substance of anaphylaxis has an uncertain role in joint inflammation. This group of lipids known collectively as the leukotrienes is derived from arachidonic acid by the action of the enzyme lipoxygenase. The leukotrienes are known to be liberated by granulocytes in inflammatory reactions,

Table 18.2 Effects of Prostaglandins

Prostaglandins	Activity
PGE$_2$	Vasodilatation
	Stimulates bone reabsorption
	Hyperalgesia
	Increases cAMP
PGF$_2$ alpha	Vasoconstriction
	Neutrophil chemotaxis
	Decreases cAMP
	Stimulates platelet aggregation
Prostacyclin (PG$_I$)	Vasodilatation
	Hyperalgesia
	Inhibits neutrophil chemotaxis
	Increased cAMP
	Inhibits platelet aggregation
Thromboxane A$_2$	Vasoconstriction
	Inhibits platelet aggregation
	Decreases cAMP

the release of some being mediated by prostaglandins and thromboxanes.

It is likely that the thromboxanes and leukotrienes have important roles in altering the caliber and permeability of blood vessels and in affecting chemotaxis in acute inflammatory responses comparable with the effects of prostaglandins.

PHARMACOLOGY OF JOINT INFLAMMATION

The mechanisms of inflammation in joint disease are important when considering the pharmacological means available to treat the consequences of disease. The exact mechanisms of action of most of the drugs used in treating rheumatic disease are not fully known, and the therapeutic value of many, like aspirin and colchicine, were discovered accidentally.

Aspirin

Aspirin has analgesic, antipyretic, and anti-inflammatory effects. All three seem to be mediated by inhibition of the cyclo-oxygenase concerned in the synthesis of prostaglandins. Prostaglandin E2 and prostacyclin reduce the threshold of sensory nerve endings to stimulation by histamine and kinins. Prostaglandin E1 produces fever when its concentration rises in the region of the third ventricle, and the beneficial effect of treating the pyrexia of rheumatic fever may be mediated by blocking this reaction.

In recent years many aspirin-related compounds have been synthesized and are collectively referred to as "non-steroidal anti-inflammatory drugs." The most consistently demonstrated mode of action of these drugs is inhibition of cyclo-oxygenase, but many other possible modes of actions have been suggested based on in-vitro actions. The other postulated modes of action include inhibition of lysosomal enzyme release, antagonism of proteolytic enzymes, stimulation of anti-proteinases, uncoupling of oxidative phosphorylation in cells in the inflammatory response, and immunosuppressive activity. The various drugs differ in their pharmokinetics, therapeutic half-life, protein-binding, and interaction with other drugs. Indomethacin is the most potent of these drugs in causing cyclo-oxygenase inhibition, but other members of the group also have potent effects in disease, suggesting that mechanisms other than cyclooxygenase inhibition are also important. There is considerable variation among individuals in responsiveness to different non-steroidal anti-inflammatory drugs. In addition to aspirin, commonly used non-steroidal anti-inflammatory drugs include (1) indole derivatives, e.g., indomethacin, sulindac, tolmetin; (2) proprionic acids, e.g., ibuprofen, naproxen, fenoprofen, ketoprofen; (3) fenamates, e.g., mefenamic acid, sulfenamic acid (4) pyrazolones, e.g., phenylbutazone, azaproprazone; and (5) phenylacetic acids, e.g., alclofenac, diclofenac.

Colchicine

Colchicine is a traditional treatment for acute gout which still has a place in modern therapy. It stimulates the secretion of elastase and collagenase; this has led to its use in treating scleroderma. Its more important effects inhibit the earlier stages of inflammation. Cellular microtubule formation is inhibited, which decreases phagocytosis of particles such as crystals by neutrophils, and it also inhibits mitosis.

Corticosteroids

Steroid drugs have a profound anti-inflammatory effect which is of value in treating inflammatory diseases. However, the chronic nature of many rheumatic diseases and consequent requirement for long-term treatment necessitates care and selectivity in the use of these potent drugs. Among the many effects of steroids on the inflammatory response are suppression of the synthesis and secretion of collagenase, elastase, and other proteinases, and suppression of the release of superoxide anion. The generation of arachidonic acid from membrane phospholipids is inhibited. Antigen-induced lymphocyte proliferation is suppressed, as are several other aspects of cell-mediated immunity. There is an overall depletion of lymphocytes in the peripheral circulation, which affects T-lymphocytes more than B-lymphocytes.

Gold Salts

Gold salts have a remittive action in rheumatoid arthritis, but the mechanism of action remains obscure. Its success in treating rheumatoid arthritis appears to be due to a specialized form of immunosuppression. Gold accumulates in macrophages, including synovial Type A cells, and experimental studies have shown that macrophage and neutrophil phagocytic activity is inhibited by gold. It also inhibits in-vitro proliferative lymphocyte responses.

D-Penicillamine

This drug is used as a remittive agent in rheumatoid arthritis. Immune complexes are dissociated in vitro by D-penicillamine and prolonged administration of the drug is associated with reduction or disappearance of immune complexes from serum and synovial fluid in some treated patients. The chelate of penicillamine and copper has been shown to have a superoxide dismutase-like effect and may therefore be important in scavenging superoxide anions in inflammatory disease. Penicillamine may also affect lymphocyte proliferation and other aspects of the cellular immune response. Penicillamine interferes with the formation of aldehyde cross links in Type I collagen and this property has been used therapeutically in scleroderma.

Cytotoxic Drugs

Cytotoxic and immunosuppressive drugs are of limited value in the treatment of the more serious complications of collagen-vascular diseases and extensive psoriatic arthritis. Most of the drugs interfere with DNA replication in the rapidly proliferating cells concerned in the immune response.

ORIGINS OF PAIN IN ARTHRITIS AND RHEUMATIC DISEASE

Pain is the predominant symptom of most rheumatic disorders. Rational symptomatic treatment would be based on understanding the origins of pain, but in many instances this is uncertain. Articular cartilage is aneural, but sensory receptors for pain are widely distributed in other articular tissues, including the walls of arteries, joint capsule, periosteum, subchondral bone, juxtaarticular muscles and in the skin overlying joints. Kinins, histamine, complement components, and prostaglandins are all believed to give rise to direct stimulation of pain fibers, and some of the prostaglandins may sensitize nerve endings, thereby reducing the threshold for stimulation of pain. Pain is also caused in inflammatory joint diseases by pressure effects on blood vessels containing sensory nerve endings, e.g. by increased vascular permeability causing edema and synovial effusion causing stretching of the joint capsule, and by extension of the inflammatory process to skin. Joint deformity resulting from chronic inflammatory disease is not of itself painful except when the joint capsule and periarticular ligaments become distorted in use.

The pain of degenerative joint disease is poorly understood. Among the possible origins of pain are subchondral microfractures, products of secondary inflammation, muscle spasm and increased bone intra-medullary venous pressure. The basis for increased joint pain during periods of climatic change is unclear, but it seems that the synovium and its contents react in the manner of an aneroid barometer, reflecting atmospheric pressure and humidity changes.

Pain originating in joints gives rise to a reflex type of spasm in the neighboring musculature. If prolonged, this spasm of itself becomes painful, thereby inducing yet further muscle spasm. This cycle of pain and spasm is important in the pain of degenerative joint disease especially involving large joints such as the hip, and in forms of non-articular rheumatism such as the fibrositis syndrome.

The word "pain" indicates both physical discomfort and mental anguish. Both of these facets become important in chronic rheumatic disease when pain is a constant accompaniment of every type of daily activity. Observation of a group of patients with a chronic disease such as rheumatoid arthritis demonstrates the extent to which "illness" is a function of both the individual's psychological adjustment to disease as well as the actual physical pathology present. Individuals vary in their threshold for pain appreciation, and the threshold itself appears to depend on many factors, including the premorbid personality of the individual, concomitant psychological stress, anxiety about the illness and its prognosis, and associated psychological events such as mental depression. Factors which may attenuate the pain of chronic arthritis include the occupational activities of the patient, systemic illness associated with the disease, and pharmacological intervention.

Symptomatic treatment of pain is accomplished by the analgesic and anti-inflammatory drugs described in the previous section, which reduce the rate of synthesis or antagonize the effects of chemical mediators. In most rheumatic diseases effective pharmacological means are available to control pain, but the psychological elements of chronic pain must also be treated. The anguish element of pain requires non-pharmacological management by the careful choice of reassuring explanation. Many patients at the outset of a rheumatic disease have fears of chronic crippling disability and loss of their livelihood or family structure. Explanation of the disease process, its likely course and the rationale for treatment must be regarded as part of the overall problem of pain amelioration in rheumatic disease.

INVESTIGATION OF RHEUMATIC DISEASE

Synovial Fluid

Aspirated synovial fluid should be examined at the bedside for its colour, clarity or opacity, viscosity, and the volume of fluid aspirated should be noted (Table 18.3). Normal synovial fluid is almost clear, slightly yellow in colour and is highly viscous. The clarity of synovial fluid is reduced by the presence of leukocyte or erythrocyte pleocytosis, crystals or bacteria. Very high white cell counts in acute crystal arthropathy or in pyogenic arthritis may render the

Table 18.3 **Synovial Fluid Characteristics in Disease**

Fluid Characteristic	Normal	Non-Inflammatory	Inflammatory	Pyogenic
Clarity	Transparent	Transparent	Translucent or opaque	Opaque
Colour	Yellow	Yellow	Yellow or cream	Yellow or green
Viscosity	High	High	Low	Low
White cell count (per mm^3)	<200	200–2,000	2,000–60,000	20,000–100,000 or more
Polymorphs (%)	<25%	<25%	50% or more	75% or more

fluid totally opaque. In cases of suspected gonococcal arthritis, synovial fluid should be inoculated onto chocolate agar or Thayer–Martin culture media at the bedside.

A total and differential white blood cell count should be done on all synovial fluids. The total white cell count in acute crystal arthritis may reach or exceed 50,000/mm³ and may reach or exceed 1000,000/mm³ in a pyogenic arthritis. In rheumatoid arthritis mononuclear and polymorph leukocytes may be noted to contain vacuoles (ragocytes) which can be shown to contain immunoglobulin on fluorescent microscopy. Crystals may be seen in wet mount preparations under regular light microscopy but positive identification requires examination under polarised light. A Gram stain should be done in any case of suspected pyogenic arthritis. Biochemical and immunochemical analysis of synovial fluid is often useful, but it must be recognized that variable dilution occurs according to the magnitude of the synovial effusion and, therefore, synovial fluid concentrations of proteins must be interpreted with some caution. The synovial fluid glucose concentration usually approximates that of plasma, but in pyogenic arthritis the synovial fluid glucose concentration may be appreciably lower than that of plasma.

Erythrocyte Sedimentation Rate

The rate of sedimentation of erythrocytes is determined by the size of cellular aggregates and by plasma viscosity. Changes in plasma concentration of several proteins markedly alters the sedimentation rate. In inflammatory disease, the plasma concentrations of several so-called acute-phase reactant proteins may rise considerably and influence the erythrocyte sedimentation rate. These proteins include fibrinogen, alpha-2-macroglobulin, C-reactive protein, and immunoglobulins, especially IgG and IgM. The Westergren method tends to give better discrimination and more marked elevation in rheumatic disease than the Wintrobe method.

Anti-globulin Rheumatoid Factor Tests

The tests routinely used to detect anti-globulin rheumatoid factors use either latex particles coated with human IgG or sheep red blood cells coated with sublytic doses of rabbit anti-sheep red blood cell antibody. The antiglobulins present in patients with rheumatoid arthritis typically react to a greater extent with non-human IgG, or altered human IgG, than

they do with native human IgG. Antibodies to human IgG are present in many of the rheumatic diseases and may be present in a small proportion of healthy subjects, particularly the elderly.

The latex agglutination tests show less specificity but greater sensitivity than the sheep cell agglutination tests in the diagnosis of rheumatoid arthritis. The latex test is more convenient to perform routinely in laboratories and is used far more widely than the sheep cell agglutination test.

Because low-titre positive results occur in many diseases and in healthy individuals, it is necessary that positive results be expressed as a titre. In the latex test a titre greater than 1 in 160 is unusual in healthy individuals, and the titre may rise to greater than 1 in 10,000 in patients with active rheumatoid arthritis.

The routine agglutination tests demonstrate the presence of IgM antiglobulins capable of agglutinating the substrate-coated particles. Other types of nonagglutinating antiglobulins such as IgG-anti-IgG can be detected by research methods, but their value in clinical diagnosis is uncertain.

Table 18.4 indicates the approximate frequency of positive latex agglutination tests in rheumatoid arthritis and other conditions.

Antinuclear Antibodies

Antibodies to nuclear and cytoplasmic antigens are typically found in systemic lupus erythematosus, but also appear in other rheumatic diseases. Profiles of

Table 18.4 **Frequency of Positive Latex Agglutination Tests in Rheumatic and Other Diseases**

Positive Latex Agglutination Test	Approximate Frequency (%)
Normal individuals over 60 years	8
Rheumatoid arthritis	80
Rheumatoid arthritis with nodules and erosions	95
Sjögren's syndrome	98
Felty's syndrome	98
Healthy relatives of patients with rheumatoid arthritis	10
Systemic lupus erythematosus	15
Scleroderma	15
Waldenstrom's macroglobulinemia	30
Cirrhosis	25
Chronic interstitial pulmonary fibrosis	40
Pulmonary silicosis	40
Infective endocarditis	40
Leprosy	25
Chronic parasitic diseases	50

antinuclear antibodies of differing specificities have been described, which help to differentiate systemic lupus erythematosus and other diseases.

The LE-cell phenomenon is dependent on an IgG antihistone antibody and demonstrates phagocytosis of nuclei by polymorph neutrophils. It was initially observed in bone marrow cells, but the phenomenon can be demonstrated in defibrinated blood and is sometimes observed in synovial fluid or other body fluids in patients with SLE. The LE cell test is now rarely used in clinical diagnosis because of its low sensitivity for disease.

Immunofluorescent demonstration of antinuclear antibodies is the most frequently used screening test for SLE. The substrate is usually a section of frozen rat liver or kidney. Diluted sera are added to the tissue and subsequently stained with fluorescein tagged anti-immunoglobulin antibodies. Positive staining at a serum dilution of less than 1 in 20 is usually regarded as being insignificant. This technique detects antibodies to many different nuclear and cytoplasmic constituents and therefore has great sensitivity but relatively low specificity for SLE.

Anti-DNA antibodies are usually measured by radioimmunoassay. Low titres of antibodies to native double-stranded DNA are present in many normal individuals but high titres of antibodies are almost specific for SLE. Radioimmunoassay for DNA antibodies is indicated in a patient who has symptoms and signs suggestive of SLE if the routine fluorescent staining test for antinuclear antibodies is positive.

Antibodies to specific nuclear components may be isolated and identified by special methods, including counterimmunoelectrophoresis and gel precipitation, and comparison with standardized antisera. Simple extracts of calf thymus are used as substrates to define specific antibodies to antigens such as Sm and ribonucleoprotein. Table 18.5 illustrates the frequency of antibodies to various nuclear antigens and their associations with disease.

Histocompatibility (HLA) Phenotyping

HLA phenotyping determines a characteristic of the individual rather than a feature or consequence of any disease. It can, therefore, not be taken to represent a diagnostic test, but in many rheumatic diseases the presence of particular HLA phenotypes may provide circumstantial support for a diagnosis made on other grounds. HLA phenotyping cannot exclude a particular disease. Testing is performed on viable peripheral lymphocytes. Table 18.6 indicates the approximate frequencies of HLA phenotypes in various rheumatic diseases.

Radiographic Investigation

Radiographic evaluation of joints and supporting structures remains a major asset in determining type and extent of severe disease. The characteristic changes are dealt with in relation to each condition. Radioisotope studies in inflammatory joint disease show some promise, and are commented on in relation to the appropriate diseases.

Table 18.5 **Frequency of Antinuclear Antibodies in Rheumatic Diseases**

Test or Antigen	Disease Association	Frequency in Patients (%)
LE cell test	SLE	70
Fluorescent antinuclear antibody test (ANF or ANA)	SLE	99
	Mixed Connective Tissue Disease	95 (speckled staining pattern)
	Rheumatoid Arthritis	15–25
	Sjögren's syndrome	40–60
	Felty's syndrome	60–80
	Scleroderma	70–90 (speckled or nucleolar staining pattern)
	Normal individuals over 60 years	10
Double-stranded DNA	SLE	60–90
	Mixed connective tissue disease	15
Extractable nuclear antigen (RNase sensitive)	Mixed connective tissue disease	100
Extractable nuclear antigen (RNase insensitive) Sm	SLE	40

Table 18.6   **Frequencies of HLA Phenotypes in Various Rheumatic Diseases**

Disease	HLA Antigen Association	Disease (%)	Frequency in Normal Population (%)
Ankylosing spondylitis	B27	90	8
Reiter's syndrome	B27	80	8
Reactive arthritis	B27	75	8
Rheumatoid arthritis	DR4	65	23
Sjögren's syndrome	DR3	52	21
Systemic lupus erythematosus	B8	30	20
Systemic lupus erythematosus	DR2	55	25
Psoriatic arthritis (spondylitis)	B27	40	8
Psoriatic arthritis (peripheral)	B17	25	8
Psoriatic arthritis (peripheral)	B27	15	8
Behcet's syndrome	B5	35	11
Scleroderma	DR5	50	18

JOINT DISEASES

GENERAL CLASSIFICATION

A diverse range of pathological processes may occur within the tissues enclosed by the capsule of a diarthrodial joint. The simplified classification shown in Table 18.7 lists the major varieties of joint disease according to the principal type of pathological process.

DEGENERATIVE JOINT DISEASE

Degenerative joint disease is responsible for a greater amount of morbidity than any other disease process of mankind. As many as 85 percent of individuals aged over 70 years have symptoms attributable to this process. Radiographic evidence of degenerative joint disease, which may not be symptomatic, can be found in 80 percent of individuals aged over 55 years, and may be evident in some

Table 18.7   **Classification of Joint Diseases**

1. Degenerative joint disease
   a. Primary generalized osteoarthritis
   b. Localized osteoarthrosis:
      (i) Secondary to abnormal mechanical stresses
      (ii) Secondary to chronic joint disease, e.g., rheumatoid arthritis
2. Crystal arthropathies
   a. Uric acid—gout
   b. Calcium pyrophosphate—pseudogout
   c. Hydroxyapatite
3. Immune complex arthropathies
   a. Intra-articular source—rheumatoid arthritis
   b. Articular deposition of circulating immune complexes, e.g., systemic lupus erythematosus
4. Sero-negative arthropathies
   a. Ankylosing spondylitis
   b. Reiter's disease and other HLA-B27 related arthropathies
   c. Psoriatic arthropathies
   d. Enteropathic arthropathies
5. Arthropathy due to infective agents
   a. Specific bacteria—pyogenic arthritis
   b. Viral and other nonbacterial types of infection
   c. Reactive arthritis, e.g., rheumatic fever
6. Arthropathies associated with systemic disease
   a. Neuropathic arthropathies
   b. Arthropathy associated with hemorrhagic disease
   c. Metabolic and endocrine arthropathies, e.g., hemochromatosis, ochronosis, acromegaly
   d. Miscellaneous, e.g., hypertrophic pulmonary osteoarthropathy, erythema nodosum

persons as early as the third decade. Because of its association with aging, the name degenerative joint disease is appropriate. This tends to obscure the fact that related processes may be observed in relatively young persons and also that many different pathological processes may culminate in the same clinical picture. Osteoarthritis is generally regarded as being synonymous with degenerative joint disease; the "itis" in this word suggests that there is an inflammatory component to the disease, and clinical observation of some patients suggests that this is indeed so. Exacerbation and remission of symptoms may occur with clinical features of inflammation in affected joints. In addition, these symptoms may respond to anti-inflammatory drugs in a manner beyond the expected analgesic effect of the drugs. However, inflammatory features are not prominent in the majority of patients and some authors prefer the term *osteoarthrosis*. There is an assumption in both osteoarthritis and osteoarthrosis that an abnormality is present in the subjacent bone; although there are bone changes, it is uncertain whether these precede or follow the major changes seen in articular cartilage.

Degenerative joint disease observed to follow some other pathological process is called secondary degenerative joint disease or secondary osteoarthritis. Primary osteoarthritis indicates disease occurring without obvious cause, but is also sometimes used to describe a characteristic pattern of disease seen most commonly in middle-aged women and affecting small peripheral joints rather than large joints.

Pathology

The cardinal feature of degenerative joint disease is loss of structural integrity of articular cartilage.

Aging is undoubtedly the most important single factor (see Aging of Articular Cartilage above). As damage to articular cartilage progresses, evidence of attempted repair may be seen in both cartilage and underlying bone. Although the overall number of chondrocytes per unit volume in articular cartilage decreases, clusters of chondrocytes are seen around the base of cartilage fissures. Proliferation and hypertrophy of subchondral bone is most evident in areas which have been denuded of cartilage. In advanced disease with extensive loss of cartilage, the underlying cortical bone becomes thickened and polished like ebony, hence the term *eburnation*. At the margins of articular cartilage small bony outgrowths termed *osteophytes* appear, and often these outgrowths are capped by a layer of hyaline or fibrocartilage. In advanced disease, especially when there is eburnation, cystic areas of rarefaction are seen in the subchondral bone. It is suggested that these start as microfractures which become enlarged through the entry of synovial fluid forced in under the pressures generated in normal joint movement.

Etiology

Many clinical concomitants of degenerative joint disease are observed which in their diversity demonstrate different pathogenetic mechanisms (Fig. 18.5).

1. Aging. Degenerative joint disease shows a rising prevalence with age in all populations which have been studied.

2. Usage or "wear-and-tear" of joints. Cumulative mechanical use of joints would be expected to increase the rate of surface attrition of articular cartilage, and prolonged overusage does indeed predipose to premature joint wear. Disease is seen in the

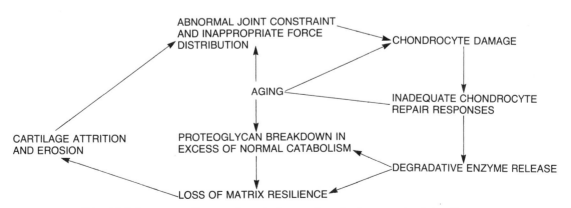

Fig. 18.5 Sequence of events in articular cartilage in degenerative joint disease.

limb joints of workers subject to physical stress, for example in the knees of carpet layers. In individuals with hemiplegia and generalized degenerative joint disease, the disease progresses more rapidly in the normal limb than in the weak limb. This may be interpreted to indicate greater wear and tear in the sound limbs or less wear and tear in the weak limbs.

3. Inappropriate mechanical stress. Prolonged application of forces inappropriate to the customary use or function of a joint is often seen to result in degenerative joint disease. For example, unilateral disease of a hip joint may be seen following injury to the ipsilateral knee some years previously, or may occur with the pelvic tilt of an uncorrected lumbar scoliosis.

4. Abnormal joint constraint. Alteration of congruity of complementary articular surfaces or excessive movement at these surfaces is frequently followed by disease. The hip provides the best example. It is estimated that as many as 60 percent of cases of unilateral degenerative disease of the hip occur as a consequence of structural defects, including congenital dysplasia and slipped capital epiphysis in childhood. It is of interest that this type of hip disease is rare in African and Oriental populations in whom congenital hip dysplasia is rare. Amongst patient groups with generalized degenerative joint disease, hypermobility of joints is more frequent than in matched controls. Joint hypermobility occurs in the rare heritable disorders of connective tissue, but minor degrees of hypermobility are of relatively common occurrence.

5. Previous inflammatory joint disease. Articular cartilage damage from chronic inflammatory disease such as rheumatoid arthritis, the seronegative arthropathies or previous pyogenic arthritis. Symptoms arising in extensively damaged joints are sometimes mistakenly attributed to continuing inflammatory disease activity.

6. Metabolic and endocrine disease. The biosynthetic pathways of collagen and proteoglycans may be extensively deranged by heritable metabolic defects. These uncommon diseases illustrate the susceptibility of articular cartilage to generalized disease. Chondrocalcinosis (see below) is a frequent accompaniment of degenerative joint disease, but it is not clear whether cartilage matrix degradation precedes or follows the deposition of calcium pyrophosphate dihydrate.

Hemorrhagic diatheses such as hemophilia complicated by recurrent hemarthroses often give rise to premature degenerative joint disease (Ch. 4). Hemosiderin deposits within chondrocytes have been observed, and articular cartilage damage is probably a consequence of chondrocyte incapacitation.

7. Avascular osteonecrosis. This curious process has clinical associations that suggest microvascular damage to subchondral bone as its pathological basis. Avascular osteonecrosis occurs in the head of the femur, the tibial plateau, the head of the humerus, and occasionally in the ends of other long bones. It is seen in sickle cell disease and other hemoglobinopathies, caisson disease, some collagen-vascular diseases, especially systemic lupus erythematosus, and in patients who have received high doses of immunosuppressive drugs. Loss of subchondral bone is followed by rapid collapse of weight-bearing surfaces and the resultant intra-articular distortion leads to rapidly progressive degenerative joint disease.

8. Familial degenerative joint disease. Pedigrees have been described with familial disease of hips and other joints, perhaps indicating a familial morphological abnormality. A more common familial pattern is the primary osteoarthritis of the finger joints sometimes known as Kellgren's disease. This is more common in women than men and an autosomal dominant mode of inheritance with incomplete penetrance in males has been claimed. An alternative theory to incomplete penetrance is that there is some endocrine influence on the process, because it often appears around the time of the menopause.

Clinical Features

The major symptom of degenerative joint disease is pain on use of affected joints. In population surveys symptomatic disease is less common than radiographic disease. It is not clear why some individuals experience symptoms of the disease earlier in its course than do others. Symptoms due to osteophyte formation are uncommon except in the fingers.

Osteophyte formation at the distal interphalangeal joints produces characteristic knob-like swelling (Heberden's nodes), and similar lesions are slightly less common at the proximal interphalangeal joints (Bouchard's nodes). Progression of the disease in the hip causes attrition of the joint surfaces with leg "shortening" due to protrusion of the femoral head into the iliac bone. In very advanced disease the patient may complain of grating of weight-bearing joints. Variability in the severity of symptoms with changes in climatic conditions is common and has given rise to the mistaken lay belief that damp weather is a cause of arthritis. Periodic exacerbations lasting a few days or a few weeks occur in patients with primary generalized osteoarthritis. There may be increased swelling, warmth, and tenderness of affected joints and this is most usually evident in the fingers and knees. Severe periodic exacerbations of symptoms should raise suspicion of associated pseudogout.

Physical Findings

Bony swelling around interphalangeal joints is a frequent finding, and Heberden's nodes when small may be more easily palpated than seen. Involvement of the metacarpophalangeal joints is very unusual. Progressive limitation of the range of motion of larger joints is accompanied by crepitus on movement. In the knee it is helpful to try to distinguish between patellofemoral crepitus and femorotibial crepitus by putting the knee through its range of motion and by moving the patella against the femoral condyles. Muscle spasm may be evident in degenerative disease affecting the vertebral joints and is probably a significant cause of pain.

Since degenerative joint disease is almost universal in the elderly, it is not infrequent to find signs of this process as well as signs of other joint disease. The presence of synovial thickening or of inflammatory synovitis, especially in elderly patients, should suggest the possibility of two joint diseases being present.

There are no systemic symptoms of untreated degenerative joint disease. Local complications of disease are uncommon except where there is extensive involvement of vertebral joints. Disease in the cervical and lumbar spinal joints, especially when there is exuberant osteophyte formation, may partly occlude neural foramina with resulting radiculopathy. This process is sometimes referred to as cervical, or lumbar, spondylosis.

Erosive osteoarthritis is an uncommon variant of primary osteoarthritis affecting the finger joints in women. There is a marked inflammatory reaction and often deformity of the fingers. Radiographic examination demonstrates erosive changes partly resembling rheumatoid arthritis but without involvement of the metacarpophalangeal joints.

Laboratory Findings

All blood tests are normal in uncomplicated degenerative joint disease. Radiographic examination will show narrowing of the joint space due to loss of cartilage (cartilage is radiolucent). Later in the course of disease marginal osteophytes become visible and subchondral sclerotic changes are seen. Subchondral cysts generally represent advanced disease and are unusual in joints other than the hips. Chondrocalcinosis is a feature of advanced disease and also may be a pertinent finding in patients subject to episodes suggesting pseudogout.

If synovial effusion is present, aspiration of the joint will usually give a high viscosity fluid with a normal cell count (less than 600 cells/mm^3) approximating to the composition of normal fluid. Inflammatory changes in the synovial fluid should stimulate a search for calcium pyrophosphate dihydrate crystals or consideration of two diseases being present.

Treatment

Many middle-aged patients with mild osteoarthritis affecting the finger joints or knees are often worried that they may have potentially crippling disease. It is important to explore that anxiety and reassure the patient. Obese patients should be encouraged to attempt weight reduction. Simple physical forms of therapy including gentle exercise are to be encouraged.

Anti-inflammatory drugs are usually more effective than simple analgesics, reinforcing the notion that low-grade inflammatory mechanisms are probably important in this group of diseases. Aspirin is the preferred agent and is effective in lower dosage than is necessary for treating rheumatoid arthritis. Non-steroidal anti-inflammatory agents are indicated in patients with gastric intolerance to aspirin and also in elderly patients who often have to take other medications for concomitant illness. Proprionic acid derivatives are helpful in mildly symptomatic disease and indole derivatives are indicated in more painful disease. It is usually unnecessary to require the patient to take these drugs continuously, but courses of treatment lasting one to two months are often helpful at times when symptoms become more obtrusive. There is great individual variation in responsiveness to these drugs, and trials of different agents for two or three weeks may be necessary to find the most effective drug for the individual patient. Systemic steroid treatment has no place in the treatment of degenerative joint disease, but intra-articular administration of depot steroid preparations may be useful at selected sites such as the knee or carpometacarpal joints. If effective, these injections should not be repeated more than once every six months because of the risk of iatrogenic crystal arthritis and consequent articular cartilage damage.

Disease in the hips and knees is especially amenable to physical forms of treatment. Physiotherapy to strengthen the hip abductor muscles for hip disease, or the quadriceps for knee disease is often useful. Relief of weight-bearing by the simple expedient of a cane, crutches, or a walking frame will greatly lessen symptoms by reducing weight-bearing forces. Patients who have leg length discrepancies may gain some pain relief by corrective elevation of their shoes. In unilateral hip disease the cane should be held in the hand of the contralateral side. By applying 45 kg to a cane held with the left hand, an involved right hip can be relieved of more than 330 kg of force.

Joint replacement surgery has transformed the prognosis in severe disease of the hips and knees. The major indication for these steel and high density plastic prostheses is pain not relieved by simple measures. Joint replacement surgery should not be considered until the other therapeutic measures mentioned have been adequately explored. Nor should replacement surgery be contemplated when radiographic examination shows adequate remaining articular cartilage as indicated by the joint space. Advanced disease shown on radiographic examination, with decreasing functional ability due to pain, indicates the need to consider joint replacement surgery. The major complication and risk of joint replacement surgery is infection; the only effective means of treatment for prosthetic joint sepsis is removal of the prosthesis. The longevity of prosthetic joints is such that the average rate of wear in the plastic component of hip prostheses is estimated to be 0.15 mm/year. Therefore, unless a prosthetic joint is abused by excessive physical strain, the average patient may expect up to 30 years of service from the acetabular component of a prosthetic hip joint.

CRYSTAL ARTHROPATHIES

Gout results from intermittent crystal formation in synovial fluid or other body tissues when they become super-saturated with monosodium urate. The crystals are intensely phlogistic and induce a very active and painful inflammatory response. The syndrome and its name have been familiar to physicians for many centuries. In addition to its medical antiquity, the historical interest extends to the belief that many important characters in history suffered from "the gout" and that on occasion acute attacks of gout may even have altered the course of the history of nations. This has given rise to an erroneous belief that gout is a disease which only affects ambitious or successful individuals. Before 1850, when the association of hyperuricemia and gout was discovered, many forms of arthritis were referred to as "the gout." It is probable that some of the famous historical figures said to have suffered from gout in fact suffered other forms of acute episodic arthritis such as Reiter's syndrome.

Understanding of the mechanisms of inflammatory arthritis has been followed by the recognition of comparable disorders caused by crystal formation within joints. The other types of crystal arthropathy are caused by precipitation of various molecular forms of calcium phosphate, the most important being calcium pyrophosphate dihydrate (CPPD) which is associated with the clinical syndrome of pseudogout. Uric acid crystals and CPPD crystals can be identified by light microscopy of synovial fluid, but it was not until the application of specialized methods of identification of very small crystals that other types of crystal arthropathy were delineated. Table 18.8 classifies the varieties of crystal deposition diseases and crystal arthropathies.

Gout

Uric Acid Metabolism

It is necessary to consider the pathways of uric acid metabolism to understand the pathogenesis and treatment of gout. Uric acid is the end-product of purine metabolism in man (in most other species a

Table 18.8 Crystal Types and Rheumatic Diseases

Crystal	Disease	Identification
Monosodium urate monohydrate	Gout	Polarizing microscopy
Calcium pyrophosphate dihydrate	Pseudogout	Polarizing microscopy
Hydroxyapatite	Osteoarthritis, calcific tendonitis	Electron microscopy
Mixed calcium phosphate crystals	Osteoarthritis	Light microscopy
	None	Light microscopy
Synthetic steroids	Iatrogenic crystal arthritis	Light microscopy

uricase enzyme is able to further degrade urate to more soluble derivatives). It is formed from the purines, adenine and guanine. Purines are formed in the biosynthesis of nucleic acids and, to a lesser extent, from dietary sources of preformed purines. The latter appear to be relatively unimportant sources, because a completely purine-free diet reduces the serum uric acid concentration by only 1 mg/dl, and large amounts of uric acid continue to be excreted in urine. Two-thirds of all the uric acid produced in the body is excreted in urine. At the pH of body fluids uric acid is present in the ionized form as a monovalent ion, and because sodium is the principal extracellular cation, the solubility of monosodium urate is of major importance in the pathogenesis of gout. The solubility of monosodium urate in plasma is close to saturation, which occurs at about 7 mg/dl.

Urate binds to albumin and other proteins, thus increasing the quantity necessary to saturate plasma. The total body pool of uric acid in an average-sized male is approximately 1.2 grams, and 60 percent of this amount is replaced daily by newly synthesized uric acid. Since two-thirds of the amount formed is eliminated by the kidney, the average renal excretion amounts to approximately 450 mg in 24 hours. The remainder is eliminated via the gastrointestinal tract and most of this is degraded by intestinal bacteria.

In the kidney, uric acid passes freely into glomerular filtrate. At least 90 percent of the filtered load is absorbed in the proximal renal tubule and is then subject to secretion into the distal tubule. The renal handling of uric acid is affected by drugs and alteration in acid-base balance. Proximal reabsorption is inhibited by several drugs, including phenylbutazone, several types of diuretic, high-dose salicylate, and probenecid. The uricosuric property of probenecid can be utilized to reduce serum uric acid levels in the treatment of gout. The distal secretion of uric acid is inhibited by some diuretics and by low-dose salicylate. Acidosis inhibits distal secretion and this probably explains the hyperuricemia observed in diabetic ketosis, starvation, and glucose-6-phosphatase deficiency. This phenomenon may contribute to the occurrence of attacks of acute gout in susceptible individuals following surgery or alcoholic overindulgence. The effects of diuretics and low-dose salicylate are important as potential precipitants of hyperuricemia and thereby lead to acute attacks of gout in susceptible individuals. Gouty patients who take one or two aspirin tablets (rather than a high dose of aspirin) for pain relief early in the course of an attack may exacerbate their metabolic situation by inhibiting urate excretion. Contrariwise, an erroneous diagnosis of gout may be made in patients with other types of acute arthritis who have taken low-dose aspirin and thereby caused a temporary and spurious rise in their serum acid concentrations.

The pH of urine falls as it flows along the renal tubule and as urinary urate is converted to uric acid. The solubility of uric acid is substantially less than that of urate; this is of importance in patients with hyperuricemia and in patients with gout because of their tendency towards impaired ability to excrete alkaline urine. Uric acid urinary calculi occur in up to 25 percent of patients with gout, a figure vastly in excess of the incidence in whole population surveys. Uric acid precipitated in and around renal tubules also favors the development of diffuse hyperuricemic nephropathy. This occurs as a complication of treatment of acute leukemias and has occasionally been caused by infusion of radiocontrast media, some of which have potent uricosuric acitvity. The major pathways of uric acid synthesis are shown in Figure 18.6. The conversion of inosinic acid to hypoxanthine is subject to rate-limiting control by feedback of PRPP, and this interaction is catalyzed by hypoxanthine guanine phosphoribosyl transferase (HG-PRTase). Deficiency of HG-PRTase occurs in the X-linked Lesch-Nyhan syndrome. Boys who have this rare disease have severe hyperuricemia, gout, neurological complications such as choreoathetosis, and extraordinary tendencies to aggression and self-mutilation. Incomplete forms of the Lesch-Nyhan syndrome with partial HG-PRTase deficiency have been described, and the importance of this rare syndrome is that it may provide clues to the pathogenesis of hyperuricemia in the more common clinical problem of idiopathic gout. Knowledge of the terminal steps in the biosynthesis of uric acid has permitted the development of a successful means of reducing serum uric acid production and of gout prophylaxis. Allopurinol is a structural analogue of hypoxanthine and inhibits the enzyme xanthine oxidase by substrate competition (Fig. 18.7). Prolonged administration of allopurinol is an effective means to reduce the propensity to acute attacks of gout. The increased quantities of xanthine produced are excreted or stored in skeletal muscle, where it is innocuous.

Frequency-distribution curves plotted to show serum uric acid levels in large population surveys generally show a Gaussian distribution with mean serum levels of 5.0 mg/dl in adult men and postmenopausal women and 4.0 mg/dl in adult premenopausal women. In addition to sex differences, racial differences in serum uric acid concentrations have been observed. Polynesian races have a tendency to relative hyperuricemia and also have a greater inci-

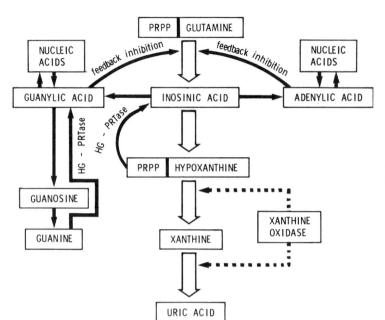

Fig. 18.6 Metabolism of uric acid precursors.

dence of gout than is found in most other populations.

The risk of gout increases with serum uric acid concentrations, but the exact risk is unknown. Less than 20 percent of males with serum uric acid values about 7 mg/dl have a history of symptoms suggestive of gout. Between 10 and 15 percent of adult males admitted to hospital are found to have serum uric acid concentrations greater than 7.0 mg/dl on autoanalyzer screening. However, study of such patients reveals a history of gout in 10 per cent, and more commonly the hyperuricemia is associated with chronic renal failure, acidosis, or prior ingestion of drugs such as diuretics and salicylates. Causes of hyperuricemia and hypouricemia are listed in Table 18.9.

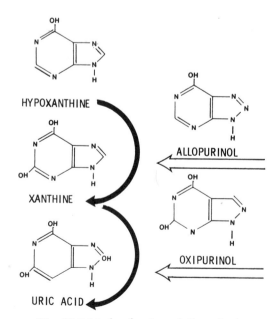

Fig. 18.7 Mode of action of allopurinol.

Clinical Features

Gout is now an uncommon cause of major disability. It occurs more commonly in males than in females, although after the menopause the incidence in females rises. In males the peak age for onset of symptoms is in the fifth decade, but attacks may occur at almost any age after puberty. Ninety percent of patients experience acute episodes in the first metatarsophalangeal joint some time during the course of the disease, but other lower limb joints are often involved, especially the ankles and knees. Involvement of upper limb joints such as the wrists or elbows occurs less commonly. Acute gout is usually monoarticular and does not necessarily recur in the same joint. The best clinical account of acute gout is that of the English physician, Thomas Sydenham written in 1683, probably describing his own illness:

Its only forerunner is indigestion and crudity of the stomach . . . The day before the fit the appetite is unnaturally hearty. The victim goes to bed and

Table 18.9 Classification of Causes of Hyperuricemia and Hypouricemia

A. Primary hyperuricemia
  1. Increased purine production
     a. Idiopathic
     b. Enzyme abnormalities, e.g.:
        increased PP-ribose-P
        decreased HG-PRTase activity (Lesch-Nyhan syndrome)
  2. Idiopathic decreased renal uric acid clearance
B. Secondary hyperuricemia
  1. Increased purine catabolism
     a. Myeloproliferative and lymphoproliferative diseases
     b. Hemolytic anemias and hemoglobinopathies
     c. Psoriasis
     d. Cytotoxic drugs
  2. Decreased renal uric acid clearance
     a. All forms of chronic renal failure
     b. Sickle cell anemia
  3. Altered renal tubular handling of urate
     a. Drug-induced, e.g.,
        thiazide and other diuretics, low-dose salicylate
     b. Lactic-acidemia, e.g.:
        alcoholism, lactic acidosis, glucose-6-phosphatase deficiency
     c. Ketonemia, e.g.:
        diabetic ketoacidosis, starvation
C. Hypouricemia
  1. Increased uric acid excretion
     a. Reduced renal tubular urate resorption, e.g.:
        Fanconi syndrome, Wilson's disease
     b. Drug administration, e.g.:
        Probenecid and other uricosuric agents, allopurinol, radiocontrast media, high dose salicylates
  2. Decreased uric acid production
     a. Purine biosynthesis heritable enzyme deficiencies, e.g.:
        adenosine deaminase purine nucleoside phosphorylase, xanthine oxidase
     b. Acquired xanthine oxidase deficiency
     c. Acute intermittent porphyria

sleeps in good health. About 2 o'clock in the morning he is awakened by a severe pain in the great toe; more rarely in the heel, ankle or instep. The pain is like that of a dislocation and yet the parts feel as if cold water were poured over them. Then follow chills, shivers and a little fever . . . After a time this comes to its height, accommodating itself to the bones and ligament of the tarsus and metatarsus. Now it is a violent stretching and tearing of the ligaments, now it is a gnawing pain and now a pressure and tightening. So exquisite and lively meanwhile is the feeling of the part affected that it cannot bear the weight of the bedclothes . . . The night is passed in torture, sleeplessness . . . The tossing about of the body being as incessant as the pain of the tortured joint . . . As the fit goes off the foot itches intolerably, most between the toes; the cuticle scales off, and the feet desquamate as if ven-

omed . . . The disease being disposed of, the vigour and appetite of the patient return.

The veracity of this account of acute gout is such that it often seems that patients describing their attacks have read this passage. Most acute attacks of gout are self-limiting in duration, and subside within two to ten days. However, recurrent attacks of gout occur and after many episodes in the same joint, articular cartilage damage leads to secondary degenerative joint disease.

Chronic recurring gout is associated with the formation of deposits of urate as "tophi" in the proximity of joints, the Achilles tendon, the olecranon bursa, and, uncommonly, in the fibrocartilage of the outer helix of the ear. Aspiration of such a deposit provides crystals which may be readily identified by microscopy.

Mechanism of the Acute Attack of Gout

Most of the characteristic features of acute gouty attacks are explicable. Precipitating factors for acute episodes include dietary and alcoholic overindulgence, fasting, especially after surgery, and administration of drugs which alter purine and uric acid metabolism. The characteristic onset of attacks early in the morning waking the patient from sleep has been explained on the basis of increase in synovial fluid concentration above the limit of solubility. It is thought that small effusions accumulate in lower limb joints, notably the first metatarsophalangeal joint, during daytime ambulation. Recumbency at night permits resorption of water which passes more rapidly than does urate across synovium, which functions as a semipermeable membrane. The local increase in urate concentration leads to crystal formation and the sequence of events which follows favors further crystallization of urate.

Monosodium urate crystals have a strongly negative surface charge, which facilitates adsorption of IgG with the Fab portion preferentially oriented to the crystal surface. The Fc fragment is exposed and available to combine with receptors on neutrophil granulocytes and other phagocytic cells. Monosodium urate crystals are also able to interact with the complement system and have been shown to deplete total hemolytic complement activity in serum by adsorbing C1q and C4. Hageman factor also adsorbs to urate crystals and is activated by them, with sequential activation of plasmin and kinin precursors. Potent chemotactic factors are generated by neutrophils following crystal ingestion and also directly by activation of the complement system. Discharge of lysosomal enzymes decreases the pH in the joint cavity and this favors further urate crystallization. Additional crystal formation favors chemotaxis and a self-perpetuating vigorous inflammatory reaction ensues. The volume of inflammatory mediators liberated by the reaction is evident in the exquisite pain, marked local warmth, and acute swelling seen in the acute gouty attack.

Laboratory Findings

Hyperuricemia is usually present in patients during acute episodes of gout. Definitive diagnosis, however, requires the demonstration of urate crystals in synovial fluid aspirated from the affected joint. Joint fluid aspirated during attacks usually has a cell count in the range of $10,000/mm^3$ to $50,000/mm^3$, of which almost all are neutrophils. Phagocytosed urate crystals appear as long needle-shaped structures, often slightly larger than the ingesting cell. Although the shape and size of urate crystals is characteristic, further identification is required by examining the birefringence of crystals under polarized light in a suitable microscope. Two crossed polarizers are inserted in the optics of the microscope so that all unrefracted light is excluded. A first order red compensator is inserted, which changes the black background to red. When a crystal is seen, the microscope stage is located so that the long axis of the crystal lies parallel with the slow vibrations of the light. In these conditions monosodium urate crystals are bright yellow (negative birefringence) and they appear blue when the microscope stage is rotated through 90 degrees.

Investigation of patients seen between suspected acute attacks of gout can provide circumstantial evidence of the diagnosis. The finding of hyperuricemia may be accompanied by the finding of hyperuricosuria. Twenty-four hour urinary excretion of uric acid in excess of 600 mg when taking a purine-restricted diet is regarded as abnormal. Specific metabolic abnormalities causing hyperuricemia or hyperuricosuria are found in only a small proportion of patients with primary gout.

The etiology of primary gout remains obscure in the majority of patients. There may be a family history of the disease, but pedigree studies generally do not show clearly defined patterns of inheritance. Twenty percent of first-degree relatives of patients with primary gout have hyperuricemia but most do not have clinical gout. It is therefore concluded that primary gout has a polygenic basis. Metabolic studies with ^{14}C labelled urate precursors permit measurement of the body pool or urate. From these studies

it has been established that 90 percent of hyperuricemic patients with gout have relative underexcretion of uric acid and the remaining 10 percent have overproduction of urate. Investigation of gout requires exclusion of the secondary causes of gout. Coexistent diseases that have well-established associations with gout include obesity, diabetes mellitus, hypertension, and hypertriglyceridemia. Hyperuricemia has been proposed as a risk factor for coronary heart disease, but results in different studies have been at variance, especially when the serum urate concentrations were adjusted for effects of age, gender, and body mass.

Treatment

Effective treatment for acute gout has been available for more than 200 years. Colchicine, an extract of the plant Colchicum autumnale, is particulary effective. It is usually given in a dose of 0.6 mg taken orally at two hourly intervals until the arthritis improves or significant gastrointestinal side effects appear. Gastrointestinal side effects can be avoided by intravenous administration of colchicine 2 mg, followed by not more than 2 mg within the following 24 hours. This form of administration has the disadvantage of marked local reaction at the site of injection and risk of bone marrow toxicity if more than 5 mg is injected during the course of an acute attack. Indomethacin is effective in a dose of up to 50 mg four times daily. Phenylbutazone is similarly effective, but its half-life is longer than that of indomethacin and the attainment of suitable blood levels requires a high loading dose. Aspirin should be avoided in the treatment of acute gout because of its complex effects on renal handling of urate. Allopurinol is contraindicated in acute gout, but recurring acute gout indicates the necessity to consider prophylactic treatment with this agent. Recommendation of treatment, which should be continued for several years, requires full assessment of the patient. In patients with primary gout the urinary uric acid excretion should be estimated. For patients who excrete less than 700 mg in 24 hours, uricosuric agents such as probenecid or sulphinpyrazone are appropriate, and patients should be cautioned against taking aspirin. Allopurinol is the agent of choice in patients who are hypersecretors of uric acid or who have marked hyperuricemia, tophi, or evidence of uric acid renal calculi. During the first month or two of treatment with allopurinol there is a poorly understood tendency for acute attacks of gout to be induced and it is customary to administer indomethacin or colchicine with allopurinol during the first few weeks. Serum uric acid concentrations can usually be reduced to the region of 6 mg/dl with a dose of allopurinol in the range of 200 mg to 400 mg daily. Few side effects are experienced except for occasional development of skin rashes (especially in patients taking ampicillin). Prophylactic treatment of gout should be considered following recurrent acute attacks or in patients who have marked abnormality of uric acid metabolism at the time of their first attack. The frequency of acute attacks cannot be anticipated, and sufficient justification for long-term medication should be apparent both to the patient and the physician.

Dietary modification is generally not necessary in the modern management of gout. Low purine diets are inconvenient and less effective than pharmacological measures to reduce serum uric acid levels. Patients who find a particular dietary precipitant for their acute attacks should avoid that item. Excessive consumption of alcohol and administration of drugs which alter uric acid metabolism should be avoided.

Asymptomatic Hyperuricemia

In population surveys approximately 5 percent of males and a smaller number of females are found to be hyperuricemic, and these individuals are now being identified more frequently because of autoanalyzer screening. When causes of secondary hyperuricemia are excluded, there remains a significant number of individuals who have primary hyperuricemia. The major concern in asymptomatic hyperuricemia is that of renal damage, rather than the more readily treated problem of gout. In gouty subjects the risk of nephrolithiasis is around 20 percent when the urinary uric acid excretion is under 700 mg per day, but it rises to over 50 percent with a urine uric acid excretion over 1,100 mg per day. Allopurinol prophylaxis is beneficial in the prevention of uric acid and calcium oxalate calculi, which both occur in hyperuricosuric subjects. Treatment of asymptomatic hyperuricemia should be seriously considered in subjects who have a serum uric acid concentration above 9 mg/dl and either a urinary uric acid secretion greater than 700 mg per day, or a documented family history of gout.

Calcium Pyrophosphate Dihydrate Deposition Disease (Pseudogout)

Chondrocalcinosis is the radiographic appearance of calcification in articular cartilage. Following the observation that this finding was associated with an intermittent inflammatory arthritis, it was discovered that the acute arthritis was induced by crystal pyrophosphate dihydrate (CPPD). The features of the acute inflammatory episodes are reminiscent of acute gout, and the disease is sometimes referred to as "pseudogout."

Pathogenesis

Pyrophosphate is a by-product of many essential metabolic processes. It is produced in articular cartilage during the sulfation of glycosaminoglycans.

Pyrophosphate is of ubiquitous occurrence in many tissues and, for example, it is estimated that the normal daily synthesis of albumin generates up to 30 grams of pyrophosphate. Pyrophosphate is hydrolyzed to orthophosphate by intracellular pyrophosphatases, but will combine with calcium where the latter ion is available. Pyrophosphatases are inhibited by divalent cations, including calcium, iron, and copper. This may be relevant to the association of CPPD deposition disease with hyperparathyroidism, hemochromatosis, and Wilson's disease. The disease has also been described in association with the rare inherited syndrome of hypophosphatasia, which is accompanied by low serum alkaline phosphatase levels.

CPPD crystals are deposited in articular cartilage and when present in sufficient quantity are evident on radiographic examination as chondrocalcinosis.

Mechanism of the Acute Episode of Pseudogout

CPPD crystals may be somewhat less phlogistic than monosodium urate crystals. CPPD crystals are of low solubility and the initiating mechanism in attacks of pseudogout is probably shedding of crystals from deposits in articular cartilage, rather than crystallization from the fluid phase as occurs in gout. Phagocytosis of crystals leads to lysosomal discharge, reducing the local pH and favoring further shedding of crystals from articular cartilage matrix, as well as lysis of superficial cartilage matrix around CPPD crystals. Experimental observations have shown that CPPD crystals can directly activate the complement system and the chemotactic consequences of this activity in vivo would enchance the local inflammatory response. Acute attacks of pseudogout occur after surgery, especially parathyroidectomy, when rapid reduction of ionized plasma calcium is thought to increase the solubility of CPPD crystals, causing shrinkage and allowing embedded crystals to be shed from articular cartilage.

CPPD crystal deposition disease has been observed in diverse circumstances. Familial disease with dominant modes of inheritance has been reported in Czechoslavakian, Dutch, and Chilean pedigrees. Associated diseases include diabetes mellitus, hemochromatosis, Wilson's disease, hyperparathyroidism, Paget's disease of bone, and gout. Radiographic evidence of chondrocalcinosis increases with advancing age; in a survey of 58 persons with an average age of 83 years, 27 percent were found to have chondrocalcinosis on radiographic examination of the knees. The association with degenerative joint disease in the aged may be analgogous to the formation of calcification in atherosclerotic arteries.

Clinical Features

Symptomatic pseudogout is slightly more common in males than in females and is rare before middle life, except in individuals with associated metabolic disorders. The aphorism "the knee is to pseudogout as the big toe is to gout" indicates that large joints rather than small joints are usually involved in acute attacks. The acute inflammatory episodes are usually monoarticular, less dramatic than those of gout, and have a self-limiting duration from a few hours to several weeks. Acute attacks are sometimes preceded by surgery or severe medical illness such as stroke or myocardial infarction. As in gout, definitive diagnosis is achieved by the demonstration of crystals within cells and joint fluid during acute episodes. The crystals differ from those of monosodium urate in being smaller than the ingesting cells and they have a rhomboidal configuration. Under polarized light CPPD crystals show weak positive birefringence, appearing slightly blue when the long axis of the crystal is parallel with the slow vibrations of polarized light, and appear slightly yellow when the microscope stage is rotated through 90 degrees.

Circumstantial support for a diagnosis of pseudogout is obtained by the demonstration of chondrocalcinosis in a patient who describes episodes suggestive of the disease. Chondrocalcinosis is usually best seen in fibrocartilages and, in a patient with the appropriate history, radiographs should be taken of both knees to visualize the menisci, both wrists to visualize the triangular ligaments, and the pelvis to visualize the symphysis pubis.

Acute pseudogout is the most common manifestation of CPPD deposition disease, but other forms of chronic arthritis have been described. A syndrome resembling rheumatoid arthritis with multiple peripheral joint involvement and objective evidence of synovial thickening has been observed. Another pattern resembles degenerative joint disease affecting both large and small joints, with superimposed acute crystal-induced inflammatory episodes. Finally, CPPD deposition disease has been seen in some patients with gross destruction of large joints such as the knee or shoulder resembling the appearances of neuropathic joints, but in the absence of neurological abnormality.

Treatment

This group of diseases is less amenable than gout to pharmacological modification. Metabolic abnormality should be sought but is rarely found. Acute episodes of pseudogout respond to colchicine, but indomethacin is usually effective to the same degree. The same drugs should be administered on a prolonged basis with the aim of reducing subacute inflammatory activity.

Hydroxyapatite-Associated Arthropathy

Hydroxyapatite crystals have been demonstrated in joint fluids aspirated from patients who have a clinical picture of osteoarthritis with intermittent inflammatory episodes. These patients do not have radiographic signs of chondrocalcinosis or CPPD crystals in their joint fluids. Hydroxyapatite crystals are smaller than monosodium urate or CPPD crystals and require special visualization techniques. The crystals are barely visible on light microscopy using phase contrast methods but have been more reliably found by scanning electron microscopy and special crystallographic techniques such as energy dispersive analysis. Experimental observations in animals indicate that hydroxyapatite crystals are capable of inducing inflammatory responses in several varieties of tissue including synovium.

Deposits of hydroxyapatite are present in calcific tendonitis, the calcific deposits of scleroderma, and in a form of periarthritis observed in chronic renal failure patients undergoing regular dialysis.

RHEUMATOID ARTHRITIS

Rheumatoid arthritis is a common chronic disease with predominant articular manifestations frequently associated with nonarticular systemic complications. Typically the arthritis is progressive, symmetrical, and destructive of small peripheral joints and medium-sized limb joints. Involvement of the axial skeleton is uncommon except for joints of the cervical spine. The antiquity of rheumatoid arthritis has been questioned because detailed descriptions of the disease exist only from the middle of the 19th century. There are few references to the typical deformities caused by chronic rheumatoid arthritis in either medical or nonmedical literature before then. This is surprising because the deformities caused by progressive rheumatoid arthritis are striking; it is improbable that these would have escaped the notice of physicians or artists. The lack of descriptive or pictorial records has led to speculation that the disease may in some way be connected with environmental factors that appeared at the time of widespread industrialization. However, the disease has also been widely recorded in nonindustrialized countries and communities in the present century. The disease has been observed in most ethnic communities that have been examined. The overall prevalence in North America is estimated at 3.2 percent. Among persons below 35 years, the prevalence is estimated at 0.3 percent and rises to around 10 percent in persons aged 65 years and over. The prevalence is much below these ranges in Eskimo communities, and greater than average in some North American Indian communities.

Pathology of Articular Lesions

All synovial joints are liable to become involved in the synovitis of rheumatoid arthritis, and synovium in nonarticular sites such as tendon sheaths and bursae may become similarly involved. In the early stages the synovium becomes hyperemic and shows vascular congestion with fibrin formation on the synovial surface. Neutrophil granulocytes migrate into the joint, and the synovium becomes infiltrated with these cells and with lymphocytes. The lymphocytic infiltration appears diffusely throughout the synovium and also in small localized aggregates (lymphorrhages). As the disease progresses, increasing numbers of plasma cells appear in the synovium. The synovium becomes thickened by proliferation of fibroblasts and capillaries, and hypertrophied folds of tissue spread from the articular cartilage margins into the joint cavity. This encroaching *pannus* of hypertrophied and inflamed synovium and its products of inflammation begin to degrade articular cartilage. The erosive process commences at the articular cartilage margins, first entering subchondral bone and later eroding progressively into the deeper layers of cartilage. The joint capsule is first stretched by inflammatory synovial effusion

and, subsequently, products of the inflammatory reaction degrade the capsular collagen, leading to yet further joint capsule stretching and to subluxation or deformity of joints. Erosion of articular cartilage removes the cartilaginous spacing between adjacent bone, which further advances subluxation and deformity. Damage to articular cartilage also initiates changes of secondary osteoarthritis. In very advanced disease with massive destruction of articular cartilage, the mass of inflamed synovium undergoes metaplasia into fibrous tissue and eventually may even progress to the final stage of bony ankylosis. The pathological appearances of early rheumatoid synovitis resemble other forms of inflammatory synovitis and are not pathognomic of the disease. The most specific histological feature in rheumatoid arthritis is that seen in subcutaneous nodules present in established disease. There is a central zone of fibrinoid necrosis surrounded by palisades of microphages with an outer zone of chronic inflammatory granulation tissue, essentially comprised of lymphocytes. *Rheumatoid nodules* are found over extensor surfaces, especially the proximal ulna at the elbow, and seem to be situated at points of minor repeated trauma. It is uncertain whether rheumatoid nodules commence in small blood vessels or in some specific type of undifferentiated connective tissue.

Immunopathogenesis

A large body of evidence has accumulated which indicates that immunological processes mediate the synovitis of rheumatoid arthritis. The synovium becomes extensively infiltrated with lymphocytes and plasma cells. Lymphocyte characterization has shown that most of the cells in rheumatoid synovium are T-cells. Nevertheless, B-cells and plasma cells are present in large absolute numbers and local synthesis of IgG (and antiglobulins or rheumatoid factors) has been demonstrated. Indirect evidence of the importance of this infiltration has been obtained by experimental therapy with the procedure of thoracic duct drainage in which extensive depletion of the body pool of lymphocytes is followed by improvement in rheumatoid synovitis. Within the synovial fluid, immune complexes can be readily demonstrated together with depressed hemolytic complement activity. Immune complexes can also be demonstrated within synovial fluid cells. These inclusions may be visible in simple light microscopy ("ragocytes"). Immunofluorescent microscopy has permitted characterization of synovial fluid cell immune complexes, and these have been shown to contain IgG and IgM and complement components. The most characteristic serological finding in rheumatoid arthritis is the presence of antibodies with specificity for immunoglobulin (antiglobulins and rheumatoid factors). These antibodies are present in abundant quantities in rheumatoid synovial fluid and it has been estimated that at least 80 percent of the immunoglobulin produced by plasma cells in the rheumatoid synovium has antiglobulin activity. Further, these antibodies may be detected in synovial fluid of affected joints before they can be detected in blood.

The first step of major importance in the development of rheumatoid synovitis appears to be the intra-articular formation of immune complexes of immunoglobulin and antiglobulin. The complexes are phagocytosed by synovial Type A cells and by phagocytic cells in the synovial fluid. This initiates the sequence of inflammatory processes described in general terms earlier in this chapter. The consequences include complement activation, altered capillary permeability, chemotaxis of phagocytic cells, and the release of lysosomal enzymes. The lysosomal enzymes may have a special role in the perpetuation of rheumatoid arthritis. Some of the proteinases, notably cathespin D, have been shown to degrade IgG which, thus altered, then becomes a "foreign" antigen capable of inducing a further immune response. The secondary immune response induced in this way leads to further immune complex formation between the altered IgG and antibodies directed against that "foreign" molecule. Several varieties of antigen-antibody immune complexes have been demonstrated, or are theoretically possible, within the rheumatoid arthritic joint. These include: (1) normal IgG antigen with IgM as antibody, (2) normal IgG as antigen with IgG as antibody, (3) self-associating IgG and anti-IgG, (4) enzyme-altered IgG as antigen and IgG or IgM antibodies, (5) Type II collagen from degraded articular cartilage as antigen with antibodies to native or altered collagen, and (6) DNA and other nuclear debris from lysed cells as antigen with antinuclear antibodies. Immunochemical analysis of immune complexes in rheumatoid arthritis has shown their content to be almost entirely accounted for by immunoglobulin and other native proteins; there has been no consistent demonstration of viral or other infective agents in the complexes.

Etiology of Rheumatoid Arthritis

Although much is known regarding the immunopathogenesis of rheumatoid arthritis, the initiating etiology remains obscure:

1. Antiquity. Further investigation is necessary to establish whether rheumatoid arthritis is a disease of the modern era. If so, this would strongly support the possibility of environmental causation. Dietary factors are often blamed by patients with the disease, but no dietary trait or deficiency has been consistently found. Similarly, patients often attribute their disease to climatic vagaries. This seems to arise from variation in the intensity of the symptoms when there is change in the prevailing barometric pressure or humidity. Geographic studies give no credence to the possibility of climatic causation.

2. Heritable factors. Since rheumatoid arthritis is a common disease, familial aggregation of cases was attributed simply to chance in the past. However, more careful genetic studies show a small but significant heritable incidence. Analysis of pedigrees with several affected individuals indicates that the mode of inheritance is polygenic or multi-factorial (see Chapter 8). Observed differences in the prevalence of rheumatoid arthritis among different ethnic groups favors the possibility of heritable influence, but further studies are necessary to differentiate genetic and environmental causations.

Identical twin studies indicate an important genetic contribution in rheumatoid arthritis. The concordance rate for rheumatoid arthritis in monozygotic twins is around 30 percent, but only 9 percent of fraternal twins show concordance of rheumatoid arthritis. The histocompatability determinant HLA-DR4 has been reported in from 45 to 70 percent of series of patients with rheumatoid arthritis, but only in 15 to 40 percent of randomly ascertained control subjects in the same series of observations. The prevalence of DR4 rises to 90 percent in Felty's syndrome, a disorder seen almost exclusively in patients with very severe rheumatoid arthritis.

3. Infection. Many infective agents have been incriminated as possible causes of rheumatoid arthritis, including Streptococci, Mycobacteria, Diphtheroids, Mycoplasma, and many viruses, including the Epstein-Barr virus. None of these have been shown to have a clear causal relationship to rheumatoid arthritis, nor have these infections, when tested, been shown to be capable of reproducing the human disease in experimental animal models.

4. Antiglobulin induction. The striking immunopathological event of synthesis of antiglobulins in large quantities may be the central issue in the etiology of rheumatoid arthritis. This phenomenon implies loss of normal tolerance, or autoimmunity to immunoglobulin autoantigens. Other varieties of autoimmune disease have been associated with viral infection, aberrant cross-reaction with exogenous antigens of infective agents, drugs, and dietary

antigens, but it is uncertain to what extent these factors may apply in the etiology of rheumatoid arthritis. The antiglobulins formed in rheumatoid arthritis are predominantly directed against the Fc portion of the immunoglobulin molecule. In addition, their affinity is usually greater for non-human types of immunoglobulin, for example rabbit immunoglobulin, than for native human immunoglobulin. These observations have been interpreted to indicate that the stimulus to antiglobulin production is either from exogenous sources or from human immunoglobulin which has been attenuated.

Low titre antiglobulin production becomes more common with increasing age in both males and females and is found with increased frequency in asymptomatic first-degree relatives of patients with rheumatoid arthritis. Furthermore, prevalence studies of all age groups indicate that the overall frequency of positive rheumatoid factor tests is greater among individuals who do not have rheumatoid arthritis than those who do. Patients who have rheumatoid arthritis differ in that they usually have greater titres of rheumatoid factor antiglobulin activity in their sera. Finally, infusion of plasma containing high titres of rheumatoid factor activity into healthy volunteer subjects does not induce rheumatoid arthritis. Clearly, although the presence of antiglobulin rheumatoid factors must have great pathogenic significance in rheumatoid arthritis, this alone is insufficient to establish the disease process.

Clinical Features

Onset of symptoms of rheumatoid arthritis is unusual before the age of 12 years, but the disease may commence at any age, with the peak age of onset being in the fourth decade. There is a marked preponderance of female cases before 40 years, but beyond that age men are affected almost as frequently as women. There may be a premonitory illness with vague malaise and weight loss preceding the onset of joint symptoms. Early symptoms are pain and swelling in the metacarpophalangeal joints and pain in the metatarsophalangeal joints, with simultaneous or subsequent involvement of the proximal interphalangeal joints. Symmetry of symptomatic involvement is striking in most cases. Joint swelling may not be evident until some weeks or months after the onset of symptoms. Morning stiffness, or "morning gel," is a frequent and almost characteristic feature. After sleeping in a position of relative immobility, movement in the morning is painful and commonly referred to as "stiffness" by patients. The duration of morning stiffness is often useful as an indication of either advancing or decreasing disease activity. The rate of progression of disease activity throughout the peripheral joints may be highly variable. All of the peripheral synovial joints may become involved within a period of a few weeks in some patients, and in others there may be exacerbations and remissions of disease activity with cumulative joint damage following each exacerbation. Several patterns of clinical course may occur with a slowly progressive course being seen in approximately 50 percent of patients. Less than 10 percent become severely incapacitated by grossly destructive disease. In approximately 30 percent of patients the disease activity is intermittent with prolonged remissions between exacerbations. The course of the disease is relatively benign in the remainder of patients, with one or two episodes lasting a few weeks or a few months and no recurrence of disease. In the syndrome of "palindromic rheumatism," patients experience episodes of pain and swelling in peripheral joints which last two or three days and may recur at regular and frequent intervals over months or years; approximately 50 percent of patients with this presentation later proceed to typical sustained rheumatoid arthritis.

Progression of rheumatoid arthritis is generally in a centripetal distribution with small peripheral joint involvement being followed in frequency by wrist, knee, ankle, elbow, and shoulder disease. Hip involvement is uncommon. Any synovial joint or structure may become involved in advanced disease, including the cricoarytenoid joints of the larynx, the small joints of the inner ear, tendon sheaths, and bursae. Synovial effusion causes capsular stretching and laxity which is increased by the inflammatory destructive changes. Eventually there is bony erosion and distortion of the articular surface. The characteristic deformity of ulnar deviation or "drift" of the fingers at the metacarpophalangeal joints (Fig. 18.8), results from a combination of factors, including the normal alignment of the metacarpophalangeal joints, the tendency of the fingers to drop in an ulnar direction in the usual position of function, and from the bow-string effect caused by the pull of the long flexor and extensor tendons. With advancement of disease, the fingers may show a "swan-neck" deformity in which there is hyperextension of the proximal interphalangeal joints with flexion of the distal interphalangeal joints; or there may be a "buttonniere" deformity with reverse changes to that of the swan-neck configuration. In the latter deformity, the distal end of the proximal phalanx protrudes through the damaged extensor tendon sheath. Early involvement of the wrist causes tenderness over the ulnar

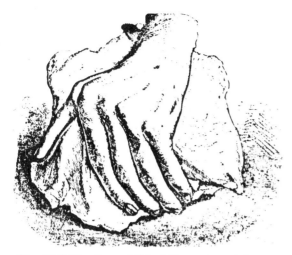

Fig. 18.8 The first published illustration of the typical hand deformity in rheumatoid arthritis, showing swelling and ulnar drift at the metacarpophalangeal joints. (From Garrod, AB: The Nature and Treatment of Gout and Rheumatic Gout. London, Walton and Maberly, 1859. Rheumatoid arthritis was first named and fully described in this monograph.

styloid process with later subluxation due to ligamentous damage commencing on the ulnar side of the wrist. Although symmetry of joint involvement is one of the most characteristic and diagnostically helpful features of rheumatoid arthritis, symmetry may become less apparent with advanced destructive disease. Lack of symmetry may arise from differential usage of joints and limbs, for example, in manual workers or from the effects of surgical intervention.

Joint deformity is the most obvious articular consequence of rheumatoid arthritis, and the cosmetic appearances of affected joints may cause distress to patients. Clearly, the extent of functional disability caused by swelling, distortion, or deformity of joints depends on the normal function of those joints. Disease in the small joints of the hands will impair fine movements such as writing or sewing, and disease in lower limb joints may greatly impair mobility. The metatarsophalangeal joints tend to be affected quite early in rheumatoid arthritis and transmission of body weight through the inflamed joints in normal walking may be extremely painful.

The erosive nature of rheumatoid arthritis has consequences beyond the immediate confines of joints. Rheumatoid synovitis of the knee may extend posteriorly to produce a popliteal, or Baker's cyst; rupture of the cyst with discharge of synovial fluid into the calf muscles may mimic acute deep venous thrombosis in the leg. In the neck, the atlantoaxial joint is at special risk from erosive damage causing destruction of both the odontoid peg and the dentate ligament. The consequent instability of the atlantoaxial joint predisposes to cervical cord impingement, long tract signs, and even quadriplegia. This is one of several forms of entrapment neuropathy consequent on rheumatoid synovitis; other examples include median nerve compression at the wrist giving rise to carpal tunnel syndrome, ulnar nerve compression at the elbow, superficial peroneal nerve pressure at the knee producing a drop-foot, and posterior tibial nerve compression in the foot giving rise to the tarsal tunnel syndrome.

Nonarticular manifestations of rheumatoid arthritis are frequent and occasionally become the dominant cause of morbidity.

Anemia occurs in the majority of patients and may become profound. Blood film smears show normochromic normocytic anemia typical of the anemia of chronic disorders. Bone marrow examination usually shows adequate iron stores and the defect appears to be one of iron utilization. The hematological picture may be complicated by drug effects, of which the most common is simple iron deficiency due to the gastrointestinal bleeding caused by prolonged ingestion of salicylates.

Rheumatoid nodule formation is the most characteristic of all the nonarticular manifestations of rheumatoid arthritis. Nodules typically occur in the subcutaneous tissues over extensor surfaces, and the most common site is over the olecranon. The sites of nodule formation may reflect areas of cutaneous pressure and in severely disabled patients confined to bed for long periods, nodules may be seen over the sacrum or occiput. Occasionally nodules appear within organs, where the pressure theory is unlikely to be applicable, such as in the lungs, the myocardium, in the sclera of the eye, and even within the cranium. Nodule formation is unusual in the first months of the disease and absence of nodules is unusual in patients with advanced erosive disease. Almost all patients with nodules have circulating antiglobulin rheumatoid factors, often in high titres.

A characteristic form of vasculitis involves small distal arteries in the digits causing typical "nail-fold" lesions which appear as small painful lesions at the nail edge. These infarcts heal, leaving the appearance of dark brown freckles around the finger nail. Cutaneous vasculitis may be associated with digital neuropathy or even mononeuritis multiplex because of vasa nervorum occlusion; this usually indicates severe disease and carries a poor prognosis. Chronic skin ulceration occurring over the lateral malleoli at the ankles is thought to have a vasculitic basis and may be seen as a feature of Felty's syndrome.

Felty's syndrome, comprising neutropenia, thrombocytopenia, and splenomegaly, occurs almost exclusively in patients who have severe advanced disease. The sera of most of these patients contain high titres of antiglobulin rheumatoid factors and antinuclear antibodies, some of which are granulocyte-specific.

Sjögren's syndrome typically occurs in association with extensive rheumatoid arthritis and is discussed further below. The keratoconjunctivitis sicca features of Sjögren's syndrome occur in approximately 20 percent of all patients with established arthritis. Other eye complications are rare. These include episcleritis, scleral thinning, giving a patchy blue appearance to the sclera, and scleromalacia perforans due to nodule formation in the globe.

Visceral complications of rheumatoid arthritis are usually encountered only in advanced disease, but occasionally may cause diagnostic confusion if seen with early disease. Pulmonary complications include pleural effusion, diffuse pulmonary fibrosis, and pulmonary nodule formation. The pleural effusions have the characteristics of exudates and the pleural fluid glucose is typically very low. In coal miners and others liable to coincident pneumoconiosis, extensive nodule formation and pulmonary fibrosis is seen (Caplan's syndrome). Pericardial effusion can be demonstrated by echocardiography in as many as 30 percent of patients with rheumatoid arthritis. However, symptomatic pericarditis is uncommon and, very rarely, pericarditis progresses to a constrictive syndrome. Nodular infiltration of the myocardium and heart valves have been described but are very rare. Evidence of mild biochemical liver dysfunction may occur occasionally in Felty's syndrome, but more commonly liver dysfunction in rheumatoid arthritis is due to the adverse effects of drugs. Renal amyloidosis is seen as part of a more generalized secondary amyloidosis and, for obscure reasons, is becoming very rare as a complication of rheumatoid arthritis. Analgesic nephropathy is a more frequent cause of renal insufficiency in patients with rheumatoid arthritis. Sustained high doses of salicylate do not appear to cause significant renal damage, but most patients with analgesic nephropathy have taken mixtures of analgesics, often as nonprescribed medication.

Diagnosis

The characteristic deformities of established erosive rheumatoid arthritis present no difficulty in diagnosis. However, early in the course of the disease, the symptoms and signs may be quite nonspecific. When considering the differential diagnosis, helpful symptoms include symmetry of involvement, the presence of actual swelling in addition to pain, and morning stiffness of peripheral joints. Typically, in early disease, careful examination will reveal synovitis in the second and third metacarpophalangeal joints and in the fourth and fifth metatarsophalangeal joints. The latter may be difficult to appreciate on clinical examination, but the presence of inflamed tissues can be detected by transverse compression of the metatarsal heads, giving rise to pain in the region of the lateral metatarsophalangeal joints.

Laboratory tests are useful in conforming the diagnosis of early rheumatoid arthritis and, to a lesser extent, assessing the established disease. The sedimentation rate is elevated in at least 90 percent of patients with established disease and, in general, the degree of elevation tends to correlate with the level of disease activity. The normochromic normocytic anemia of rheumatoid arthritis also tends to show a rough correlation with clinical disease severity. However, hemoglobin concentrations below 10 g/dl should raise suspicion of associated iron deficiency. Antiglobulin rheumatoid factors may not be detectable in the sera of patients during the first few months of symptoms but are detected by routine tests in at least 80 percent of patients who have had symptoms for more than six months. The proportion with positive tests rises to 95 percent in patients who have subcutaneous nodules and articular erosions. Negative tests in the presence of typical rheumatoid deformity suggests that the disease activity may be "burnt out" or that sero-negativity has been induced by treatment, for example, by gold salts or D-penicillamine. Synovial fluid aspirated from active joints has reduced viscosity and is usually turbid due to moderate pleocytosis. The total white blood cell count in synovial fluid is usually in the range of 5,000 to 15,000 cells/mm^3 of which 50 percent or more are polymorphonuclear leukocytes. Antinuclear antibodies are detected in up to 25 percent of patients with rheumatoid arthritis, the frequency of detection rising in patients with very long-standing disease and those with the complications of Felty's syndrome and Sjögren's syndrome. Serum complement activity is usually normal except in patients with severe vasculitis.

Synovial fluid complement activity and complement component concentrations are reduced in active disease, but estimation of these parameters has little clinical significance. DNA antibodies are not elevated except in a few patients with severe Felty's syndrome. Marked elevation of serum gamma globulin concentrations occurs in rheumatoid arthritis with

Sjögren's syndrome, but in most patients with rheumatoid arthritis protein electrophoresis is normal.

Radiographic abnormality other than soft tissue swelling cannot be detected until the disease has been active for several months. Periarticular osteopenia is the first radiographic sign and is most evident around small joints of the hands and feet. In late disease causing disability and immobility, more generalized loss of bone density is seen. The appearance of erosions is not inevitable in rheumatoid arthritis but when present indicates that the patient is more likely to develop an aggressive form of disease. Erosions appear first at the lateral margins of articular cartilage where the synovium is reflected. Cortical thinning is followed by subcortical bone erosion, which may eventually destroy the structure of the subchondral bone. Concurrently, the articular cartilage surface becomes eroded by the products of inflammation in the joint cavity and the radiolucent articular cartilage space seen between the bone ends becomes narrowed. When all joint space is lost and contiguous bone ends are in direct apposition, and changes of secondary degenerative joint disease including subchondral sclerosis begin to appear. In very advanced rheumatoid arthritis the articular anatomy is grossly distorted, and whole areas of bone may disappear on radiographic examination. The last stage, when the normal anatomy has been destroyed is progression to bony ankylosis with little remaining vestige of the original joint structure.

Treatment

In a disease so variable in its primary effects and complications as rheumatoid arthritis, it is essential to assess the severity, rate of progression, and complications when considering a treatment plan. The categories of management that should receive consideration in every patient are (1) education, (2) physical modes of therapy, (3) drug treatment of the immediate symptoms and remittive treatment for the underlying disease process, and (4) surgery.

Patient education is essential as part of the comprehensive treatment plan. Rheumatoid arthritis has an unfavorable public image and many patients have extreme anxiety about their prognosis. When the diagnosis has been established, the basic nature of the disease process and its chronicity should be carefully explained. Patients should be cautioned against fad diets, megavitamin therapy, and other dietary aberrations. It is explained that treatment is available for rheumatoid arthritis which modifies the course of the disease, but that a rapid "cure" cannot be provided. Reassurance should be given that only a small minority of patients become significantly disabled by the disease with modern forms of therapy. The necessity for prolonged medication should be explained and possible adverse effects mentioned so as to make it clear why laboratory monitoring may be necessary for complex types of treatment such as gold salts or D-penicillamine.

Since the functional consequences of rheumatoid arthritis impair movement, it is important to regard modes of physical management as being part of the treatment plan in the same way as the use of drugs should be part of an overall plan. The patient should be cautioned against both excessive immobility and excessive or unaccustomed physical exertion. During very active disease sore joints benefit symptomatically from splinting, but immobilization of the whole patient serves little purpose. Prolonged rest in bed during active phases aggravates "disuse atrophy" of muscles and often promotes the formation of joint contractures. So far as possible, the patient should continue with regular work and recreational activities. In excessively sedentary individuals a gentle exercise program should be encouraged. Swimming in warm water provides buoyancy and has a generally beneficial and soothing effect. In patients who have active wrist disease, rendering manual twisting and lifting tasks painful, wrist splints are a simple and usually effective device. Splinting of the neck by a collar may become essential in patients with atlantoaxial joint instability or other forms of destabilization of the cervical spine. Patients who have mild forms of these neck complications, not severe enough to warrant surgical stabilization, must wear their collars when travelling or in other activities which may jolt the neck. The application of warmth to actively diseased joints has a soothing effect and is especially helpful in patients with prolonged morning stiffness. A hot shower or bath after rising in the morning will usually shorten the period of morning stiffness. The use of wax bath dips for sore finger joints is traditional, but immersion of the hands in warm water generally achieves the same symptomatic benefit. Difficulties in activities of daily living should be evaluated, including such items as eating, dressing, grooming, proficiency in toiletry, and the activities involved in homemaking or earning a living. Simple modification of household utensils and work tools provided through an occupational therapy program can be effective in restoring both functional capacity and self-respect.

The basic principle to be followed in drug therapy of rheumatoid arthritis is that the simplest forms of treatment should be exploited first and the treatment regimen made more complex only according to the response to each preceding step and the rate of progression or severity of the patient's disease. Polypharmacy is usually necessary, but whenever possible the number of drugs being administered should be as small as possible. Aspirin is both analgesic and anti-inflammatory. The latter effect is achieved by high dosage which saturates hepatic pathways for salicylate metabolites and prolongs the plasma half-life of the drug. Total daily dosage in the range of 3 grams to 6 grams will give serum salicylate concentrations in the desirable range around 20 mg/dl. The optimum dose is usually a little below that which produces tinnitus. Enteric-coated tablets are preferable to plain tablets in the avoidance of gastrointestinal side effects. Nonsteroidal anti-inflammatory drugs may be used as an alternative to aspirin and, in certain circumstances, are used in conjunction with aspirin. Knowledge of the modes of action of aspirin and the various other anti-inflammatory drugs would suggest that little is to be gained by combinations of these agents. However, clinical practice demonstrates that further benefit may accrue when additional nonsteroidal anti-inflammatory agents are added to the treatment of patients with satisfactory serum salicylate levels. The most useful combination is that of aspirin with indomethacin. The latter drug given at bedtime in a dose of 50 mg to 100 mg as a slow-release tablet or as a suppository, will reduce night pain, disturbed sleep, and morning stiffness in most patients with rheumatoid arthritis. The combination of aspirin and naproxen has also been shown to produce more symptom relief than aspirin alone. Ibuprofen is useful in patients with gastric intolerance to aspirin, given in a total maximum daily dose of 2400 mg. Patients with mild disease may not require high dose aspirin treatment and medication with a phenylalkanoic acid derivative or indole derivative is often sufficient.

Oral corticosteroids should never be the initial drugs used in uncomplicated rheumatoid arthritis, however severe the symptoms. Corticosteroids are extremely effective in suppressing disease activity, but there is often a high price to be paid by the patient in late adverse effects including hypertension, osteoporosis, infection, cataracts, and other well-known consequences of prolonged steroid medication. Relatively early use of low dosage steroid treatment may be considered appropriate in elderly patients in whom symptomatic relief of symptoms is important and concern about remote side effects may be less. In younger patients, steroid treatment is appropriate only when conventional forms of remittive treatment have failed to be effective or have to be withdrawn because of adverse effects. It is customary to use these drugs in treating severe systemic complications including vasculitis, life-threatening Felty's syndrome, and pericarditis, although the value of such treatment in these circumstances remains uncertain. The usual commencing dose of prednisone is 5 mg to 10 mg daily with small increments, as necessary, if the clinical response is disappointing. It is inappropriate to commence with high doses with the intent of subsequent reduction because reduction of dose, unless it is extremely gradual, causes exacerbation of symptoms. Alternate day steroid treatment is used when necessary in severe childhood polyarthritis as a means of minimizing adverse effects and especially growth impairment; in adults, alternate day steroid therapy has not been shown to be safer than daily medication.

Gold salt treatment has been repeatedly shown to induce remission in some cases of rheumatoid arthritis. Between 40 and 60 percent of treated patients have major improvement, 20 to 40 percent have modest improvement and 10 to 20 percent of patients have no benefit or have to discontinue medication because of adverse effects. The best results are likely to be achieved if gold treatment is commenced before there is advanced joint destruction, but the potential side effects are such that other more conservative treatment should be fully exploited in the patient with early disease. Disease should have been present and active for at least four months and have been treated adequately with anti-inflammatory medication. Indications to commence gold at this stage include evidence of spread to joints not previously involved, severe continuing symptoms despite adequate anti-inflammatory medication, the appearance of subcutaneous rheumatoid nodules, and the radiographic appearance of erosions. Seronegative rheumatoid arthritis usually does not respond as well to gold (or D-penicillamine) as does typical seropositive disease. Gold should not be administered concurrently with D-penicillamine or immunosuppressive drugs. The compounds used are aqueous solutions of sodium aurothiomalate or thiosulphate or an oily suspension of aurothioglucose. An initial 10 mg dose is given as a test because some patients have idiosyncratic allergic reactions. If there is no reaction the subsequent dosage is 50 mg each week up to a total in the range of 1,000 mg. Provided that there have been no adverse effects, subsequent treatment beyond the total of 1,000 mg depends on the patient's progress. If there has been a good response with symptomatic improvement, objective improvement, a fall in sedimentation rate and rheumatoid factor titre, injections are continued at intervals of every two weeks for a further three or four months, followed by a monthly injection for at least a further year. Adverse effects include an itching eczematous skin rash, oral ulceration, bone marrow depression causing thrombocytopenia, leukopenia and aplastic anemia, proteinuria, nephrotic syndrome, chronic renal failure, and interstitial pneumonia. Because of the potential for serious bone marrow and renal side effects, each injection should be preceded by a complete blood count with platelet count, and urinalysis. Gold-induced skin rash is often accompanied by peripheral blood eosinophilia that may persist for several weeks or months following cessation of gold treatment.

D-penicillamine is capable of inducing remission in active rheumatoid arthritis; its remittive effect, like that of gold, takes three or more months to become apparent. D-penicillamine is not ulcerogenic but may cause nausea, anorexia, and disturbance of taste (dysgeusia). During the first few weeks of treatment with D-penicillamine, patients often experience a metallic taste, but this side effect usually resolves spontaneously. The serious potential adverse effects of D-penicillamine are similar to those of gold, namely, bone marrow depression and renal toxicity. Proteinuria develops in as many as 25 percent of patients and may proceed to an immune complex nephritis and nephrotic syndrome. Proteinuria exceeding 1 gram per 24 hours is an indication to discontinue treatment. Autoimmune phenomena have also been reported with prolonged D-penicillamine treatment, including myasthenia gravis, obliterative bronchiolitis, a lupus-like syndrome, and myositis. Penicillin allergy and previous adverse reactions to gold are not contraindications to treatment. The usual protocol for treatment is to commence with a dose of 250 mg daily increasing to 500 mg daily after three to four months of treatment if there is no evidence of improvement. Further increments in dosage to a maximum dose of 1,000 mg daily may be appropriate in the absence of a satisfactory response, having allowed sufficient time for improvement to occur. Symptomatic and objective improvement may not occur until after a full 12 months of treatment, but high-dose treatment should not be continued in the face of lack of response because of the significant risk of adverse affects. When remission is induced, the dose can usually be reduced by gradual decrements to 250 mg daily, without recurrence of disease activity. Because of the potential toxicity, it is necessary to have laboratory monitoring of therapy by means of complete blood count, including platelet counts, and urinalysis every two weeks for the first three months

of treatment and then monthly. Patients with rheumatoid arthritis seem to be especially susceptible to adverse effects with D-penicillamine treatment. The incidence of side effects is much greater in rheumatoid arthritis patients than in patients treated for Wilson's disease or cystinuria, who are able to tolerate doses up to 2,000 mg daily for many years without adverse effects.

Antimalarial drugs have remittive activity in rheumatoid arthritis through an unknown mechanism. The proportion of patients who derive benefit is less than the approximately two-thirds of patients treated with gold or with D-penicillamine. The major adverse effect is that of retinal toxicity and visual impairment. This risk is greater in dosage exceeding 3 mg per kilogram per day, and with chloroquine rather than with the preferred drug hydroxy-chloroquine.

Immunosuppressive drugs have only a minor role in the treatment of rheumatoid arthritis. Azathioprine and cyclophosphamide have been shown to have remittive effects comparable with the use of gold and D-penicillamine. However, the serious adverse effects of these drugs, especially bone marrow depression and increased susceptibility to infection, render the use of these agents appropriate only after inadequate response to the drugs previously discussed.

Intra-articular drug therapy of rheumatoid arthritis has a small but definite role. Intra-articular injection of microcrystalline steroid preparation can produce a significant, and sometimes lasting, reduction in synovitis in selected active joints in rheumatoid arthritis. The half-life of the injected steroid is around 24 hours, but the benefit may last for weeks or months, presumably by reducing the self-perpetuating cycle of inflammation within involved joints. This procedure is particularly useful when a small number of large joints show disproportionate activity and may obviate the need for vigorous systematic treatment. The microcrystalline nature of the depot preparations used may, however, induce inflammatory changes through a pseudocrystal arthropathy mechanism. For this reason, it is undesirable that intra-articular injections of steroid be given more frequently than once every four to six months in a particular joint. Also, in highly selected circumstances, the intraarticular injection of radioisotopes may have a beneficial effect. Colloidal preparations of radioisotope-labelled gold salts or yttrium silicate are taken up by phagocytic cells in the synovium and cause radiation-induced ablation of the synovium.

Several aspects of established rheumatoid arthritis

are amenable to surgical intervention. Joint replacement surgery is perhaps the most dramatic form of treatment and has been significantly refined during recent years. Prosthetic replacement of large joints, including the knees and hips, produces excellent relief of pain and usually moderate improvement in function. In general, the indications for replacement of joints are pain and loss of function associated with radiographic evidence of advanced loss of articular cartilage. Replacement of large joints is most successful in the knee and the hip. The small joints of the hand can be replaced by plastic prostheses, but often the patient has increased stiffness of the treated joints. The indications for joint replacement in the hands are to improve function and diminish pain, with the restoration of cosmetic appearance being of less importance.

Surgical repair of acutely ruptured tendons, due to rheumatoid tenosynovitis, should be done as soon as possible if adequate function is to be restored. Surgical fusion of unstable joints is functionally helpful with advanced wrist disease, and may be life-saving in patients with cervical instability and the risk of progressive spinal cord compression. Metatarsal head resection is a useful procedure in patients with advanced painful synovitis of the metatarsophalangeal joints. The role of surgical synovectomy is uncertain, the immediate results of surgical removal of hypertrophied synovial tissue are good, but the late effects may be those of devitalized joints with rapidly progressive degenerative joint disease. The procedure of surgical synovectomy is performed less often than was the case before joint replacement procedures became generally successful.

SERONEGATIVE ARTHROPATHIES

This group of inflammatory arthropathies was nosologically separated from rheumatoid arthritis by the discovery that the rheumatoid factor phenomenon associated with typical rheumatoid arthritis is absent in these diseases. The principal members of the group are ankylosing spondylitis, Reiter's syndrome, and psoriatic arthritis. Enteropathic arthritis and some forms of chronic arthritis of childhood are included because of their clinical, epidemiological, and genetic overlap with the principal members of the group. In recent years the group has been expanded to include forms of atypical seronegative arthritis that occur in individuals with the HLA-B27 phenotype.

The unifying features of the seronegative arthropathies include (1) involvement of the vertebral joints and the other joints of the axial skeleton; (2) a tendency to inflammation of ligaments and tendon insertions (enthesopathies); (3) a tendency to aggregation of cases within families, and also aggregation of different diseases of the group in different members of the same family; (4) absence of rheumatoid nodules and of IgM rheumatoid factor from serum; and (5) genetic association with the HLA-B27 phenotype. The clinical and genetic overlap between different members of the group of seronegative arthropathies is poorly understood and is often expressed in a diagram such as that in Figure 18.9.

Ankylosing Spondylitis

The chronic inflammatory process of ankylosing spondylitis usually commences in the sacroiliac joints and may extend in a variable manner to involve progressively higher levels of the spine. In its most extensive form, it may progress to bony ankylosis of the entire vertebral column. The duration of disease from initial symptoms to complete ankylosis may vary from as little as two to as many as 25 years. Large peripheral joints such as the hips and shoulders, may be the site of associated inflammatory disease, but, in contradistinction to rheumatoid arthritis, widespread systemic complications do not usually occur. The disease has been known for many centuries and has been associated with the names of Bechterew, Marie, and Strumpell. The old name "poker-back" aptly describes the advanced disease, but the term "rheumatoid spondylitis" is inappropriate, because this disease is not rheumatoid arthritis affecting the spine as was thought several decades ago. Since the discovery of the association of the disease with the HLA-B27 phenotype, it has become widely appreciated that minor incomplete forms of the disease are more common than the complete poker-back disease. In some individuals the disease produces no more than chronic low back pain associated with radiographic evidence of mild sacroiliitis. Family studies and studies of B27 individuals ascertained through blood donation programs have shown that some persons with radiographic evidence of the disease process may be asymptomatic. These recent studies suggest that mild disease is probably almost as frequent in females as in males, but extensive deforming ankylosing spondylitis is more common in males than in females with a sex ratio of the order of 5 to 1.

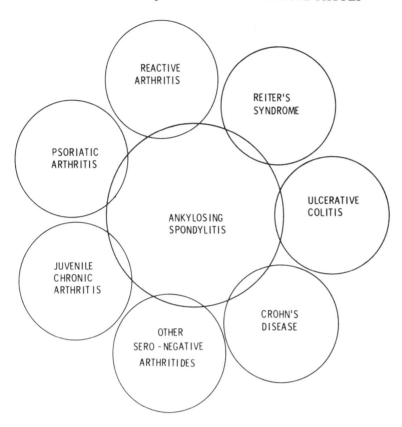

Figure 18.9 Concept of overlapping features in the seronegative arthropathies.

Pathology

The lower third of the sacroiliac joint has a synovial structure comparable with other synovial joints, and this tissue is the site of the initial inflammatory reaction. The major inflammatory reaction, however, in ankylosing spondylitis involves fibrocartilage, subchondral bone, periarticular periosteum, and the junctions of ligaments with bones. The nonsynovial synchondroses of the intervertebral joints and the major cartilaginous parts of the sacroiliac joints become involved in a chronic inflammatory process that may spread to the axial cartilaginous joints of the anterior chest wall and the symphysis pubis. An inflammatory infiltrate appears in these areas, mostly composed of lymphocytes and macrophages, which invade periosteum, fibrocartilage and connective tissue such as the annulus fibrosus of the intervertebral discs. Gradual metaplasia changes these tissues through a stage of fibrosis to ossification. This results in ankylosis of the spine, as the spinal ligaments lose their flexibility and slowly become transformed to bone. Synovial inflammation may be seen in some peripheral joints, but this is usually less marked than the synovitis of rheumatoid arthritis.

Etiology

Until recently it was believed that ankylosing spondylitis is inherited as an autosomal dominant trait with incomplete penetrance. The discovery that approximately 90 percent of patients with typical ankylosing spondylitis have the HLA-B27 phenotype led to a number of other important observations suggesting a multifactorial pattern of inheritance. Ankylosing spondylitis is some 20 times more common among individuals with inflammatory bowel disease than in the general population, but among patients who have the combination of ankylosing spondylitis and ulcerative colitis, only 70 percent have the HLA-B27 phenotype. Among the relatives of the 10 percent of patients who have typical ankylosing spondylitis but do not have the HLA-B27 phenotype, there may be found asymptomatic individuals who do have the B27 phenotype, or have inflammatory bowel disease, or psoriasis. Patients who have these associated diseases may develop spondylitis before or after the onset of their inflammatory bowel disease or psoriasis. These observations illustrate that the different disease processes do not have a simple causal relationship to B27. The male preponderance of cases of fully developed ankylosing spondylitis also indicates a multifactorial etiology. The HLA antigens are transmitted in a codominant manner, and gender-associated variation in antigenic expression has not been demonstrated for HLA-B27. Some other genetic or nongenetic factors must therefore influence the susceptibility to develop spondylitis or determine the pattern of disease evolution in susceptible individuals. It has been suggested that prostatitis in males might be a predisposing process, with spread of inflammation along the vertebral venous plexus. Although some males with ankylosing spondylitis do have a history of prostatitis and it has also been demonstrated that females with the disease may have chronic salpingitis, the majority of patients do not have discernible disease in their genital systems. Investigation of the fecal flora in spondylitics has yielded variable results, with excessive fecal carriage of Klebsiella strains being found in some series. The associations of spondylitis have given rise to a controversial hypothesis that the disease results from an aberrant immune response to surface components of certain gram-negative bacteria occurring in HLA-B27 individuals, or others with similar immune responsiveness.

Clinical Features

The onset of symptoms is usually before the age of 40 years and most commonly in the 15 to 25 year age range. Central low back pain most troublesome after sleep is the usual presentation. This may be episodic at first but later becomes more persistent. In 25 to 30 percent of patients the first symptom involves the peripheral joints with a painful hip, or pain and swelling of a knee or ankle. Presentation with peripheral joint involvement is more common in juvenile ankylosing spondylitis, and the diagnosis in these boys may become apparent only after several years have elapsed. The inflammatory process and disease symptoms may be present for many years, but symptoms of inflammatory activity are less common beyond 40 years of age. With rostral progression a characteristic postural abnormality develops with flattening of the lumbar lordosis, apparent accentuation of thoracic kyphosis and forward thrust of the head. In advanced disease the patient has a stooped posture with severe or complete limitation of all spinal movements. The most obvious abnormality to the casual observer is immobility of the head and inability to look upward; directional movement of gaze in walking or in conversation requires trunkal rotation. If the pathological process proceeds through inflammation to fibrosis and then finally bony ankylosis, the affected regions of the spine become painless.

The complications of ankylosing spondylitis are those caused by disease in the axial skeleton and also remote complications. Neurological abnormality occurs rarely and may mimic acute or chronic sciatica. A cauda equina syndrome involving the lower limbs with sphincter function disturbance has been described and has been attributed to associated arachnoiditis. Advanced ankylosis in the neck may rarely cause atlantoaxial subluxation and cord compression. Acute iritis is the most common of the nonskeletal accompaniments, occurring in up to 25 percent of patients. This is usually unilateral and may occur only once, or may be a recurring disorder, generally not following the clinical activity of the spondylitis. Cardiac lesions are rare (less than 5 percent), with inflammatory activity in the aorta and aortic valve ring leading to aortic regurgitation, and conduction tissue inflammation occasionally causing heart block. Severe disturbance of pulmonary function is also rare, but minor restrictive ventilatory abnormalities are frequent because of reduced costovertebral joint movement. Ventilation becomes dependent on diaphragm motion. Fibrosis of the lung apices has been described as a very rare complication of ankylosing spondylitis probably due to a low-grade interstitial penumonitis.

Physical Findings

The signs of early ankylosing spondylitis are subtle, and serial observation over months or years may be necessary before abnormalities are detected with certainty. In advanced disease, the diagnosis may be made from a considerable distance by the characteristic posture and gait. In early disease, the patient will usually point to the region of the sacroiliac joints as the site of discomfort. Percussion over the joints may cause pain and, in a few patients, maneuvers to stress the sacroiliac joints will also elicit pain. Slight flattening of the lumbar spinal lordosis is associated with paraspinal muscle spasm. Limited flexion of the lumbar spine is demonstrated by reduced distraction of marks made on the skin over a ten centimeter segment of the lumbar spine (Schober test). This is a more objective measure of reduced movement than measuring the distance from the finger tips to the floor on full forward flexion, which depends on the integrity of hip movement as well as that of the lumbar spine. Reduced chest expansion is often present because of costovertebral involvement before the patient has symptoms referred to the region of the thoracic spine. In advanced disease with increasing spinal flexion, progression can be measured by having the patient stand with his back to a wall, and the distance between the wall and the occiput is recorded (Forestier's fleche). Peripheral axial joint disease is most evident in the large joints with decrease in range of movement in the hips, pain and reduced range of motion in the shoulder, and recurring synovial effusions in the knees.

Laboratory Findings

The sedimentation rate is usually raised in early disease. There is usually a mild normocytic anemia in early disease. Biochemical investigations are normal with the exception of slight increase in the serum alkaline phosphatase concentration (perhaps due to active osteitis). Serum immunoglobulin concentrations IgA or IgG may be raised. The HLA-B27 phenotype is present in approximately 90 percent of patients, but its presence cannot confirm or refute a clinical diagnosis of ankylosing spondylitis because 10 percent of patients do not have that phenotype, and 80 percent or more of the population with the phenotype do not develop seronegative arthritis. If a patient with clinical features suspicious of ankylosing spondylitis has the HLA-B27 phenotype, this only provides circumstantial support for the diagnosis.

Radiology is the only definitive means of confirmation of the diagnosis of ankylosing spondylitis. Inflammatory sacroiliitis causes radiographic abnormality months to years after the onset of symptoms. The initial changes are in the lower two-thirds of the joint, and the changes are usually bilateral. Irregularity of the joint margin is followed by the appearance of subchondral sclerosis. Spread of the irregularity throughout both joints is followed by joint space narrowing and eventual loss of distinct joint margins as the sacroiliac joints become fused. Chondritis of the lumbar intervertebral discs is associated with adjacent osteitis and periostitis of the anterior margins of the vertebral bodies. This process tends to "square off" the anterior vertebral body margins, and the latter stages of the process are accompanied by the appearance of new bone formation at the margins of the annulus fibrosus and the formation of

syndesmophytes which bridge adjacent vertebral bodies. Ossification of the paraspinal ligaments may take place with the end result of bony bridging between vertebral bodies and the classical "bamboo spine" appearance. The radiographic changes reflect the clinical extent of disease and slowly spread up the spine until the whole length of the vertebral column becomes ankylosed. Radiographic recognition of advanced disease is a simple matter, but the diagnosis of early disease and the earliest changes in the sacroiliac joints is a more difficult matter. Radionuclide bone scanning has been used to detect minor degrees of sacroiliitis. This technique is valuable but has to be interpreted with caution; normal sacroiliac joints usually show more radionuclide uptake than adjacent areas. Late epiphyseal fusion of the sacroiliac joints gives a rather indistinct appearance to the joint margin until the late teens and often makes radiographic interpretation of these joints difficult at an age when the initial disease symptoms may be appearing.

Treatment

When the diagnosis of ankylosing spondylitis has been established, it is important to explain the chronic nature of the disease to the patient and the difficulty of predicting the extent of its eventual spread. Prognosis can be given with more confidence after observation of the rate of progression over a period of two or more years. Preservation of as much spinal mobility as possible is the most important aim of treatment. This requires careful education and physiotherapy to instruct the patient in maintenance of spinal extension and chest expansion. Prolonged rest and immobilization is contraindicated because of the danger of fusion in an excessively flexed position.

When large peripheral joints are affected, exercises designed to maintain the range of motion of those joints should be done. Occupations which involve sitting for prolonged periods are best avoided, because this tends to promote fusion in flexion, as does sleeping with more than one pillow. Anti-inflammatory medication is helpful in alleviating some or most of the associated pain of ankylosing spondylitis. High-dose salicylate treatment is usually effective. Phenylbutazone and indomethacin appear to be of particular symptomatic value in this disease, especially during acute exacerbations. The potential for serious bone marrow depression with long-term administration of phenylbutazone is such that its use is best avoided. Indomethacin is especially useful in a total dose of 50 to 150 mg daily. In many patients a single daily dose of indomethacin of 50 or 75 mg taken at night is sufficient to alleviate the more severe morning pain and stiffness of the disease. Administration of indomethacin or high-dose salicylate may be necessary over periods of months or years. In other patients, these drugs may be taken in high sustained doses for several weeks and then adequate relief of symptoms is maintained by low doses taken on a maintenance basis.

In the past, radiotherapy produced excellent relief of symptoms and appeared to slow, or wholly suppress, spread of the disease. Radiotherapy is no longer used in ankylosing spondylitis except in very severe disease where other therapeutic measures have been unsuccessful. Radiotherapy of the spine has been followed by the development of acute leukemia and aplastic anemia some years after irradiation in a significant number of patients. Surgical treatment has only a small place in the management of ankylosing spondylitis, but may be necessary to stabilize atlantoaxial subluxation.

Genetic counselling is occasionally requested; the risk that a patient who has ankylosing spondylitis will have a child likely to develop *severe* disease is probably not greater than 5 percent.

Reiter's Syndrome

Reiter's syndrome comprises the association of urethritis, or dysentry, with conjunctivitis and acute arthritis. Mucocutaneous lesions including balanitis, oral ulceration, and keratodermia blennorrhagica occur, usually in more severely affected patients. Acute disease with systemic illness and involvement of most of the tissues mentioned is relatively rare. However, incomplete forms of the syndrome are now known to be common, especially in males aged less than 40 years.

Pathology

The synovial pathology in Reiter's syndrome shows nonspecific abnormalities. Synovial biopsy in acute disease shows vascular congestion and infiltration with acute inflammatory cells. Following recurrent acute attacks or chronicity in the same joint, the synovial changes are similar to those of any chronic type of synovitis. Inflammation at sites of insertion of ligaments and tendons into bone (enthesopathy) may be prominent. The acute mucocutaneous lesions resemble sterile microabscesses; when these progress on the soles or palms to kera-

todermia blennorrhagica, the histological changes show a striking resemblance to those of psoriasis.

Etiology

The etiology of Reiter's syndrome is unknown, but the onset of disease appears closely allied to that of the reactive arthritides which follow infection with Salmonella, Yersinia, Campylobacter, and Shigella. The occurrence of Reiter's syndrome following urogenital inflammatory illness or acute diarrhea suggests, by analogy, that the disease process is stimulated by an infective agent, but infective agents have not been recovered from the joints or other inflammed tissues. Chlamydiae and Mycoplasmas have been isolated from the urogenital tract in only a minority of cases of acute Reiter's syndrome, but it is uncertain whether the majority of cases have had similar transient infection, or whether the disease is actually initiated by reaction to commensal organisms in the bowel or urogenital tract. The finding of the HLA-B27 phenotype in 75 to 85 percent of cases indicates an important immunogenetic component.

Clinical Features

Reiter's syndrome is predominantly a disease of young men, with a male to female ratio of at least 10 to 1, and acute disease is rare beyond 40 years. Following initial symptoms of diarrhea or urethritis lasting from one to several days, conjunctivitis, oral ulceration, circinate balanitis, and low grade fever occur, and these usually appear before the musculoskeletal symptoms. Almost any peripheral joint may be the site of arthritis in Reiter's syndrome, but most commonly the arthritis affects the larger joints of the lower limbs. It is unusual for more than four joints to be simultaneously symptomatic, and the distribution is nonsymmetrical. Affected joints show signs of very active synovitis with warmth, marked tenderness, and often large effusions. The presence of acute tendonitis, periostitis, and enthesopathic inflammation, especially around the ankle, is typical of Reiter's syndrome. Retrocalcaneal bursitis and inflammation of the insertion of the Achilles tendon are easily overlooked unless the ankle is examined from behind. The rash of keratodermia blennorrhagica is usually seen on the soles of the feet but sometimes occurs on the palms. These skin lesions resemble those of psoriasis but may show massive desquamation.

Most of the features of Reiter's syndrome resolve spontaneously during the course of a few weeks. Resolution usually includes the arthritis but this is the most variable and often the most persistent feature of the disease. A significant proportion of patients develop a chronic form of asymmetric arthritis as a remnant of the acute Reiter's syndrome. In less than 20 percent of patients this can persist for several months or even years, and may be associated with significant functional disability. Approximately 20 percent of patients with Reiter's syndrome develop sacroiliitis, sometimes as an acute manifestation of disease but more commonly as a chronic process recognized on radiographic examination.

Laboratory Findings

Laboratory investigation must be done to exclude pyogenic arthritis and gonococcal disease. The sedimentation rate is elevated and there is usually a mild neutrophil leukocytosis in the peripheral blood, Pyuria is common but culture of the urine, urethral, and cervical secretions is negative for Gonococci; and cultures of secretions, blood, and synovial fluid are sterile. The synovial fluid may resemble that in pyogenic arthritis with total white blood cell counts that may exceed 50,000/mm^3. HLA typing provides circumstantial support for the diagnosis of Reiter's syndrome if the patient is found to have the B27 phenotype.

There are no specific radiographic abnormalities in acute Reiter's syndrome. In subacute and chronic disease, periostitis may be seen and new bone formation may be evident at sites of enthesopathy, for example, in the formation of "plantar spurs." Sacroiliitis complicating Reiter's syndrome is radiographically indistinguishable from that seen in ankylosing spondylitis with the exception that the changes may be asymmetrical.

Treatment

The treatment of Reiter's syndrome is symptomatic. High-dose salicylate is usually effective, but indomethacin often gives superior symptomatic relief. It may be necessary to continue indomethacin 25 mg or 50 mg three times a day for several months.

Psoriatic Arthropathies

Arthritis occurs more frequently than would be expected by random occurrence among individuals with psoriasis, but the relationship is complex. Cutaneous psoriasis occurs in 1 to 2 percent of individuals in Caucasian populations. Six to 10 percent of individuals with psoriasis also have some form of arthritis, and as many as 7 percent of all patients who have chronic polyarthritis have some evidence of psoriasis. Several distinct patterns of joint disease have been described among patients with psoriasis, including:

1. Chronic arthritis predominantly involving distal interphalangeal joints
2. Extensive nonsymmetrical disease of small joints and large joints
3. Symmetrical disease resembling rheumatoid arthritis but without rheumatoid factors in serum
4. Monoarthritis or oligoarthritis
5. Spondylitis, with or without accompanying peripheral arthritis
6. Psoriasis with concomitant seropositive rheumatoid arthritis

The most common pattern is that of asymmetric involvement of several small and large joints, often with a tendency to exacerbations and remissions of disease activity. This pattern is seen in approximately 70 percent of patients with psoriatic arthritis. The more characteristic pattern with distal interphalangeal joint involvement accounts for approximately 15 percent of all patients with psoriatic arthritis. A severe deforming disease pattern, graphically described as arthritis mutilans occurs in fewer than 5 percent of all patients with psoriatic arthritis.

Pathology

The pathology of psoriatic arthritis is often indistinguishable from that of rheumatoid arthritis, but some characteristic features have been observed. Prominent thick-walled small arteries with perivascular infiltrates may be seen on synovial biopsy. Synovial fibrosis sometimes occurs in advanced disease.

Etiology

The etiology of psoriatic arthritis, like that of psoriasis, is obscure. The immunogenetic background is similar to that of the other seronegative arthropathies. The histocompatability antigens HLA B13, B17, B37, and Cw6 are all associated with psoriasis. Psoriatic arthritis is associated with the antigens A26, B27, B37, B38, and DR4. HLA-B27 occurs in 20 to 40 percent of patients with psoriatic spondylitis.

Clinical Features

Psoriatic arthritis may commence at almost any age between the first and seventh decades, but most commonly commences during the third decade. The sex ratio is close to unity. In the majority of patients there is not a clear relationship between the activity of the cutaneous disease and the activity of the arthritis. Simultaneous onset of skin and joint involvement is seen in about 10 percent of patients, but the onset of arthritis may be months or years following the onset of cutaneous disease. Occasionally joint disease appears before there are any cutaneous manifestations. The skin changes may be limited in extent, and in some instances the patient may not be aware that he or she has psoriasis. In such patients it is necessary to search carefully for evidence of psoriasis over the elbows, in the scalp, in the umbilicus, around the genitalia, and especially in the fingernails. Nail changes occur in 30 percent of all psoriatics but in as many as 80 percent of patients with psoriasis and arthritis. Either nail pitting or onycholysis may be the only cutaneous signs present to support a clinical suspicion of psoriatic arthritis. The nonarticular complications of rheumatoid arthritis do not occur in psoriatic arthritis. The presence of subcutaneous nodules suggests the concurrence of psoriasis and rheumatoid arthritis.

Laboratory Findings

There are no specific laboratory tests for psoriatic arthritis. During periods of active disease, nonspecific abnormalities include elevated sedimentation rate and normochromic anemia. Mild hyperuricemia occurs in patients with active skin disease and occasionally gives rise to diagnostic confusion in patients with acute psoriasis involving lower limb joints simulating acute gout. Synovial fluid analysis usually shows a moderate pleocytosis comparable with the findings in rheumatoid arthritis.

The radiographic features of psoriatic arthritis are distinct from those of rheumatoid arthritis. Juxta-articular osteoporosis is less prominent than in rheumatoid arthritis. Erosive changes tend to be asymmetrical and may be very aggressive. In the digital joints, whittling of bone ends leads to a typical "pencil in cup" deformity. In late psoriatic arthritis there is a greater tendency to ankylosis than is seen in rheumatoid arthritis. Psoriatic spondylitis may show some of the features seen in spondylitis associated with Reiter's disease, namely asymmetry of sacroiliac joint changes, erosive periostitis around the pelvis, and exuberant asymmetrical syndesmophyte formation bridging adjacent vertebrae.

Treatment

Treatment of psoriasis and treatment of associated arthritis should be regarded as separate management problems. Treatment of one does not usually affect the activity of the other. The remittive drugs used in rheumatoid arthritis are usually not effective in psoriatic arthritis except in those patients who have concomitant psoriasis and rheumatoid arthritis. Antimalarial agents are contraindicated in psoriatic arthritis because they may exacerbate the skin disorder.

The primary form of drug treatment is with antiinflammatory agents, of which high dose salicylate is the most important. Other nonsteroidal drugs are indicated in instances of adverse reaction to salicylate, in more severe cases of psoriatic arthritis, and sometimes in combination with salicylate. Oral steroid therapy is effective in very severe psoriatic arthritis, but the potential adverse effects and consequences of long-term steroid treatment are comparable with those encountered when rheumatoid arthritis is treated with systemic steroids. Immunosuppressive drugs are capable of suppressing both psoriasis and psoriatic arthritis but their use is reserved for severe progressive disease. Methotrexate is the most widely used immunosuppressive; its most important adverse effect is hepatic fibrosis.

Enteropathic Arthritis

Enteropathic arthritis refers to joint disease occurring in association with chronic inflammatory bowel disease, Whipple's disease, following intestinal bypass surgery, and following acute enteric infection. The last-mentioned association is discussed further in consideration of reactive arthritides.

Inflammatory Bowel Disease

Two distinct patterns of chronic seronegative arthritis occur in association with the chronic inflammatory bowel disease, ulcerative colitis and Crohn's disease: (1) an axial arthritis indistinguishable from ankylosing spondylitis, affecting the spine and large limb joints, and (2) peripheral arthritis in small or large joints. The relationship of chronic inflammatory bowel disease to ankylosing spondylitis is complex. Ankylosing spondylitis is approximately 20 times more common among patients with inflammatory bowel disease than in a random population sample, and both diseases are more common than would be expected among relatives of probands with one or other of the two types of disease. The symptomatic onset of ankylosing spondylitis may follow or precede the symptomatic onset of chronic inflammatory bowel disease. Further, the activity of the two processes is usually independent so that spondylitis may continue to progress with ulcerative colitis when the bowel disease is inactive or following colectomy. The relationship is made even more complex by the occurrence of mild forms of both diseases. Radiographic evidence of asymptomatic sacroiliitis is sometimes found in chronic inflammatory bowel disease and, conversely, endoscopic studies have suggested that mild asymptomatic inflammatory bowel disease may be present in a small proportion of patients with ankylosing spondylitis.

The HLA-B27 phenotype occurs in approximately 70 percent of patients who have ankylosing spondylitis and ulcerative colitis, and in approximately 50 percent of patients with Crohn's disease and ankylosing spondylitis. These data are open to differing genetic interpretation, but the simplest explanation is that genes which confer susceptibility to chronic inflammatory bowel disease also contribute to multifactoral susceptibility to develop ankylosing spondylitis. The clinical features of ankylosing spondylitis associated with chronic inflammatory bowel disease are similar to those of uncomplicated ankylosing spondylitis. Management is also similar except that drugs used in treatment of inflammatory bowel disease may secondarily benefit the spondylitis (the salicylate moiety of sulphasalazine, and oral steroids).

Peripheral arthritis occurs in approximately 10 percent of patients with ulcerative colitis and 20 percent of patients with Crohn's disease. Its activity follows that of the bowel disease more closely than occurs with associated axial disease. It tends to be present in those patients who have other extraintestinal complications such as erythema nodosum, aphthous stomatitis, and uveitis. Resolution of the colitis by medical treatment or by colectomy is usually followed by an improvement in the peripheral arthropathy. The distribution of joint involvement is usually nonsymmetrical and oligoarticular, sometimes showing a migratory pattern of involvement. Synovial fluid analysis shows a variable pleocytosis, with a predominance of neutrophils. The HLA-B27 phenotype is not encountered with increased frequency in this group of patients. Radiographic evidence of erosive joint disease is unusual. Treatment with salicylate or other anti-inflammatory drugs is usually effective. If the activity of the bowel disease merits the use of

steroid treatment, this will usually control the arthritis. The arthritis is of itself not an indication for the use of systemic steroid treatment.

Whipple's Disease

Whipple's disease is accompanied by joint symptoms in at least two-thirds of cases and in some patients rheumatic symptoms may precede gastrointestinal symptoms by several years. The arthritis tends to be episodic and transient with involvement of the larger limb joints such as the knees, ankles and wrists. The joint symptoms, as well as the intestinal symptoms, are improved by prolonged treatment with tetracycline.

Intestinal Bypass Arthropathy

Intestinal bypass surgery for the management of gross obesity has provided an interesting model of enteropathic arthritis. Following jejunocolic anastomosis, as many as 40 percent of patients develop peripheral polyarthritis comparable with the peripheral joint disease which occurs in some patients with chronic inflammatory bowel disease. The symptoms may appear at any time from a few weeks to many months following surgery. It is hypothesized that the surgical procedure gives rise to increased portal bacteremia, systemic bacteremia, formation of immune complexes containing bacterial components, and immune complex-induced synovitis. Intestinal bypass arthropathy responds to anti-inflammatory medication and regresses if the surgical procedure is reversed.

Reactive Arthritis

Reactive arthritis refers to arthritis occurring as an indirect consequence of infection. The arthritis in these circumstances may be caused by secondary products of the actual infection or as a secondary result of the host immune response to the infection, since organisms cannot be recovered from affected joints. These circumstances pertain to the acute arthritis of rheumatic fever, but usage of the term reactive arthritis generally refers to disorders in the group of seronegative arthropathies. Reiter's disease has many of the characteristics of a reactive arthritis, but the infective agent(s) is usually not apparent. Reactive arthritis is commonly associated with the enteric pathogens, *Yersinia enterocolitica, Shigella flex-*

neri, and Salmonella species. Yersinosis is common in Scandinavia where the primary presentation is that of a gastrointestinal illness with communicable acute diarrhea and an abdominal illness resembling acute appendicitis. A pattern of seronegative arthritis occurs in approximately 10 percent of individuals infected with Yersinia, and in some patients there are associated mucocutaneous lesions resembling those of Reiter's disease. The arthritis affects large or small joints in an asymmetrical pattern and persists for several weeks. Occasionally sacroiliitis follows Yersinia infection; this may proceed to ankylosing spondylitis and almost all such individuals have the HLA-B27 phenotype. Arthritis following Yersinia infection occurs less frequently in B27 negative individuals and in these persons the arthritis is of shorter duration and less liable to recurrence than is the case in B27 positive subjects.

Dysentery caused by Salmonella or Shigella species gives rise to oligoarthritis in a pattern resembling that of Reiter's disease in a minority of infected individuals. Follow-up studies of dysentery epidemics suggests that individuals with the HLA-B27 phenotype have a greatly increased risk of this particular complication. It has been estimated that 20 percent of HLA-B27 individuals infected in an outbreak of epidemic dysentery will develop joint symptoms. The arthritis begins one to eight weeks following infection and persists for periods varying from a few days to several months. Conjunctivitis, urethritis, and pharyngitis may be concomitants of arthritis in these patients.

B27-Associated Arthritis

Investigation of patients with unusual patterns of arthritis differing from the commonly recognized syndromes reveals a disproportionately high prevalence of the HLA-B27 phenotype. As many as 25 percent of patients considered to have "sero-negative rheumatoid arthritis" have this phenotype, a figure two or three times greater than would be expected on random sampling of most populations. The patterns of arthritis observed in this group include acute transient synovitis of large joints resembling the arthritis of Reiter's disease, and patterns of peripheral small and large joint disease analogous to the varieties of psoriatic arthritis, but in many patients precise categorization is not possible. Evolution and progression of the joint disease over months or years may permit diagnostic classification in a few patients, but often the diagnosis remains atypical seronegative arthritis.

ARTHRITIS DUE TO INFECTIVE AGENTS

Pyogenic Arthritis

Purulent joint infection is uncommon but potentially dangerous. It is uncommon because the enclosed joint space excludes infectious agents (and especially the larger agents such as bacteria or protozoa). It is dangerous because infection established within the enclosed joint space is not readily accessible to the humoral and cellular immune response mechanisms of the host.

Predisposition to joint infection occurs in joints previously damaged by disease and in individuals whose immune competence is impaired by pre-existent disease or by drugs. Joint infection is usually blood-borne except for rare instances of infection from perforating wounds or extension of osteomyelitis. The presence of multiplying bacteria within a joint rapidly activates the inflammatory processes described earlier in this chapter. Most joint infections are monoarticular; multiple joint infections are seen in immune-compromised individuals and portend a grave prognosis. Many microorganisms are capable of directly infecting joints, but different propensities are seen in different groups of subjects. Table 18.10 indicates commonly encountered varieties of bacterial infection and groups at particular risk.

Some bacteria have particular predilections to infect particular joints. Infections with gram-negative bacilli, including *Pseudomonas aeruginosa* and Klebsiella species, occur in abusers of intravenous drugs. In these individuals, infection often localizes to joints of the axial skeleton such as the sacroiliac joints, vertebral joints, and sternoclavicular joints. Joints damaged by rheumatoid arthritis are susceptible to infection, presumably because the intra-articular immune response has been compromised by the presence of immune complexes and depletion of complement and other immune effector systems. Secondary pyogenic infection should always be considered if a patient with rheumatoid arthritis complains that one joint has become more painful or swollen than other involved joints.

The symptoms of acute pyogenic arthritis are those of the classical inflammatory response, namely local heat, swelling, marked pain, and, in joints with a significant range of motion, loss of function. Small peripheral joints are infected less often than the large joints such as the hip or the knee. Involvement of two or more joints, or a migratory pattern is suggestive of gonococcal arthritis. General inquiry may disclose a history of preceding bacterial infection such as bacterial pharyngitis, urinary tract infection, or

Table 18.10 **Organisms and Predisposing Factors in Acute Pyogenic Arthritis**

Organisms	Frequency (%)	Risk Factors
Neisseria gonorrhoeae	40	Venereal infection
Staphylococcus aureus	35	Rheumatoid arthritis, diabetes, cirrhosis, debilitating illness
Streptococcus pyogenes, S. pneumoniae, S. viridans	10	As for *Staph aureus*
Gram-negative bacilli (*E. coli, Ps. aeruginosa,* Salmonella)	10	As for *Staph aureus,* IV drug abuse, myeloproliferative diseases
Hemophilus influenzae	5	Early childhood

skin infection. General symptoms of bacterial infection such as fever and chills may be present, but may not be evident in immunosuppressed or debilitated patients.

The physical findings are usually swelling, erythema, and marked local tenderness. Infection in joints of the axial skeleton and in the hip are not readily accessible to the examiner's hand and a high index of suspicion is necessary to achieve early diagnosis. The clinical features of gonococcal arthritis are discussed separately below.

Joint aspiration must be done whenever there is any suspicion of pyogenic arthritis. The joint fluid is turbid or frankly purulent. The total cell count may vary from as little as 3,000 cells/mm³ to more than 100,000 cells/mm³. There is usually an overwhelming predominance of neutrophils in the differential white cell count. Gram staining should be done immediately and the fluid innoculated for culture. Cultures should also be taken of possible primary sites of infection, including infected skin lesions. Blood cultures should be drawn, especially in debilitated patients. There is usually a peripheral blood leukocytosis but this may not be very impressive in debilitated or immunosuppressed patients.

Radiographic examination of infected joints does not show significant damage until several weeks have elapsed. Soft tissue swelling and widening of the joint space are occasionally observed in the early phase, with subsequent destruction of untreated joints. Radioisotope scanning methods are helpful when the diagnosis is in doubt, and in suspected infections of deeply situated joints such as the hip, sacroiliac and intervertebral joints.

General treatment measures should include analgesics and splinting of the involved limb. Antibiotic therapy should be commenced as soon as possible after specimens have been obtained for bacteriological investigation. The Gram stain findings usually indicate the group of antibiotics to be employed. Parenteral administration is indicated to achieve satisfactory blood levels. Intra-articular antibiotic administration is not necessary because of the increased synovial vascular permeability in pyogenic arthritis.

Infected joints should be aspirated repeatedly and the fluid analyzed and cultured to assess the benefit of treatment. Antibiotic treatment should continue for several weeks; parenteral antibiotic treatment is continued until the joint fluid is sterile. Surgical drainage should be considered immediately in cases of hip infection, if there is radiographic evidence of bone destruction at the time of presentation, and if medical management has been delayed, or has not produced improvement within seven days of initiating treatment. Pyogenic arthritis should be managed in consultation with an orthopaedic surgeon whenever this is possible.

Infection in prosthetic joints usually necessitates removal of the prosthesis for complete eradication of the infection. Patients with prosthetic joints should be managed in the same way as patients with prosthetic heart valves when being considered for dental, abdominal, or genitourinary surgery. Antibiotic management in these circumstances should be similar to that employed in the prophylaxis of bacterial endocarditis (see Chapter 7).

Gonococcal Arthritis

Infection with *Neisseria gonorrhoeae* is the most common form of bacterial arthritis in adults. Females appear to be more susceptible than males, particularly during menstruation. In males, arthritis usually follows urethritis within a week. There may be a period of migratory polyarthralgia followed by signs of arthritis in one or a small number of peripheral joints. The larger joints such as the knee are affected more often than small peripheral joints. Tenosynovitis is often a prominent feature in gonococcal disease. Characteristic skin lesions appear in approximately one-third of cases, usually appearing about the same time as the arthritis. The skin lesions appear as erythematous macules which develop a dark central vesicular core. Aspiration of synovial fluid from infected joints yields turbid fluid with a neutrophil pleocytosis. It is unusual to find gonococci on Gram staining of the synovial fluid because the number of organisms present is usually relatively small. The synovial fluid should be innoculated onto chocolate agar culture medium at the bedside. Positive culture results for gonococci are obtained in 60 percent of synovial fluids, 80 percent of urethral swabs and 25 percent of blood cultures. In appropriate circumstances, the pharynx and rectum should also be cultured. Treatment of gonococcal arthritis is with salicylate or nonsteroidal anti-inflammatory drugs, and antibiotics as outlined in Chapter 7.

Tuberculous Arthritis

Tuberculous arthritis has become uncommon in Western countries. Nevertheless, its incidence has remained at approximately 1 percent of all patients with tuberculosis. The majority of patients with tuberculous arthritis do not have active pulmonary disease. This and the tendency of tuberculosis to affect the deeply situated joints of the axial skeleton often leads to long delays in reaching the correct diagnosis. The intervertebral joints are most commonly affected, followed in frequency by the hip, the knee, wrist, and elbow. Tuberculous tenosynovitis sometimes occurs and, in the digits, produces a diffuse dactylitis. Factors predisposing to tuberculous arthritis include immunosuppressive treatment, diabetes and narcotic addiction. Tuberculous arthritis can supervene on rheumatoid arthritis, especially in patients treated with steroids or immunosuppressive drugs. Constitutional symptoms of weight loss, fever, and night sweats are not prominent unless there is associated pulmonary tuberculosis.

Synovial fluid analysis shows a moderate pleocytosis with a slight predominance of neutrophils and a low fluid glucose. Synovial biopsy sometimes reveals acid-fast bacilli or caseating granulomas, but synovial fluid and synovial tissue culture is usually necessary to establish the diagnosis. The tuberculin skin test is usually positive. The radiographic appearances of tuberculous arthritis show diffuse periarticular osteoporosis and bone destruction without very much reactive new bone formation. Treatment of tuberculous arthritis is discussed in Chapter 15.

Viral Arthritis

Many acute viral illnesses are accompanied by diffuse musculoskeletal complaints, but localized joint symptoms are infrequent and usually of brief duration. The importance of viral-induced arthritis pertains to the possibility that viruses may initiate chronic rheumatic diseases such as rheumatoid arthritis and systemic lupus erythematosus. The postulated mechanisms of virus-induced arthritis include: (1) direct viral invasion of joint tissues, (2) synovitis induced by deposition of circulating immune complexes containing viral antigen, and (3) the production of arthritogenic toxins. In most forms of viral arthritis, pain is more prominent than objective evidence of synovitis and there is no permanent articular damage.

Rubella Arthritis

Rubella infection, and vaccination with live rubella vaccines, are well-known but rather infrequent causes of polyarthritis. Females are affected more commonly than males and young adults are affected more frequently than children. Polyarthritis may precede the appearance of rash or may follow its appearance by a few days. Symmetrical polyarthritis affects the small joints of the fingers, the wrists, and the knees in a symmetrical manner and this may persist for one to three weeks. Wrist involvement has been associated with carpal tunnel syndrome in both the naturally occurring and vaccine-induced infection.

Hepatitis B Virus Arthritis

Hepatitis B virus causes polyarthralgia in 10 to 30 percent of patients with hepatitis. It occurs during the prodromal phase of the illness and usually subsides with the onset of clinical jaundice. The arthritis typically begins abruptly in small peripheral joints, especially in the fingers, being affected in a symmetrical pattern. Symptoms may persist for several days to several months, and the clinical appearance may resemble that of rheumatoid arthritis. Fifty percent of patients with arthritis have an associated rash with an urticarial or papular appearance. Circulating immune complexes have been detected in the sera of patients with hepatitis B associated arthritis. Synovial fluid analysis shows a neutrophil leukocytosis, and hepatitis B surface antigen has been found in synovial biopsy material.

Lyme Arthritis

Lyme arthritis was first identified in Lyme, Connecticut. The arthritis begins abruptly in one or two large joints and in some patients knee synovitis has persisted for more than a year. An erythematous papular rash often precedes the onset of arthritis and the progression of the skin lesions is reported to be typical of erythema chronicum migrans such as that caused by tick bites. It has been suggested that Lyme arthritis is caused by a spirochetal infection transmitted by arthropod vectors.

Arthritis In Childhood And Adolescence

Rheumatic Fever. The incidence of rheumatic fever has shown major decline in most developed countries. The disease remains common in socially disadvantaged groups and in nonindustrialized countries in conditions which favor endemic persistence of hemolytic streptococci. Acute rheumatic fever is most common between the ages of 5 and 15 years. Joint involvement becomes more common with increasing age and is usually the first symptomatic manifestation. Large joints are affected more often than small peripheral joints, and lower limb joints are affected slightly more often than upper limb joints. The arthritis characteristically shows a migratory pattern, with one or two joints being the site of active inflammation for a few days before migration to another joint. Each joint is usually affected only once, but in some patients the inflammatory process returns to the same joint two or three times. The other major features, laboratory findings and management are discussed in Chapter 16.

Juvenile Arthritis. The frequently used term "juvenile rheumatoid arthritis" is inappropriate for the majority of children and adolescents who have chronic forms of arthritis. Only a small minority of these patients have the form of rheumatoid arthritis seen in adults and the majority have other definable varieties of arthritis. Often the diagnosis is not evident until the child has been followed for many years, sometimes well into adulthood. Table 18.11 classifies the common forms of chronic arthritis of childhood.

Rheumatoid arthritis of the adult type with antiglobulin rheumatoid factors in serum is usually seen in children aged more than 10 years, and most of these patients are girls. The distribution of joint involvement, clinical features, and most of the complications are comparable with the adult form of disease. This "true" juvenile rheumatoid arthritis is best regarded as the adult disease occurring at an early age. The basic management and use of drugs is similar to that of the adult disease with the added requirement for very careful attention to prevention of deformities.

Table 18.11 **Arthritis of Childhood**

Disease	Frequency (%)
Seropositive rheumatoid arthritis	10
Juvenile ankylosing spondylitis	10
Other B27-associated arthritis	10
Still's disease	40
Oligoarticular or monoarticular disease	20
Other forms, including psoriatic arthritis, collagen vascular diseases, etc.	10

Juvenile ankylosing spondylitis is predominantly seen in boys. The presentation differs from the adult disease in that back pain is infrequent before the mid-teens. The usual presentation is with synovitis involving one of the large lower limb joints. This may persist or be present intermittently, with symptoms of back involvement appearing some years later. A family history of ankylosing spondylitis or one of the associated diseases is often helpful in reaching the correct diagnosis. HLA typing is of some value in the differential diagnosis of this condition in young persons. Radiographic evaluation of abnormality in the sacroiliac joints is very difficult until the epiphyses fuse after puberty. Radiography of the sacroiliac joint should be avoided in childhood because of the dose of radiation required and also because of the small likelihood of obtaining helpful information.

Other HLA-B27 associated forms of arthritis occur during childhood, mostly in boys. These may resemble acute Reiter's disease or may cause persistent synovitis or enthesopathy. HLA typing is useful in identifying susceptible individuals but the differentiation of this illness from juvenile ankylosing spondylitis is usually impossible without long-term follow-up.

Still's disease is characterised by chronic peripheral polyarthritis, often accompanied by systemic features, and represents the most common variety of childhood arthritis. It occurs in young adults as well as children. This disease is sometimes referred to as "juvenile rheumatoid arthritis" or "juvenile chronic polyarthritis," giving rise to confusion with other forms of childhood arthritis which are classified separately here. When the disease occurs after childhood it is usually referred to as "adult Still's disease." Approximately 50 percent of patients have systemic features, and these are often more prominent in older patients and in young adults. The polyarthritis affects the small peripheral phalangeal joints, as well as larger joints such as the knees and wrists. The involvement is usually symmetrical and slowly progressive. Joint swelling and mild deformities occur, but the extensive deformities of rheumatoid arthritis do not occur.

The systemic features of Still's disease include fever, hepatosplenomegaly, a characteristic skin rash, and iridocyclitis. The temperature chart differs from that of acute rheumatic fever in tending to return toward the baseline, with spikes of fever especially in the afternoon. The fever is less suppressible by salicylate than that of rheumatic fever. The skin rash resembles rubella but is often ephemeral, lasting only a few hours and most evident at the height of the fever. It is usually best seen on the trunk, buttocks, or thighs. The rash is of particular diagnostic value and may not be detected if these areas are not deliberately examined. Other features include pericarditis, generalized lymphadenopathy, and abdominal pain. Hepatitis without prominent arthralgia or arthritis may be the prominent presentation, especially in older children and young adults. Laboratory features of Still's disease include a marked elevation of sedimentation rate, striking leukocytosis, and thrombocytosis. Antiglobulin rheumatoid factors are not present in serum and antinuclear antibodies are not detected. Biochemical tests of liver function often show mild abnormality, especially in older patients.

Still's disease tends to run a self-limiting course lasting from a few weeks to several years. Most often the acute systemic type of disease runs a relatively short course, but activity in joints may persist for months or years. Treatment in mild cases is symptomatic, with salicylate being useful to treat arthritis symptoms. Severe disease, especially with marked systemic features may require corticosteroid treatment. Ophthalmic complications should receive prompt expert attention.

Oligoarticular and monarticular arthritis present great diagnostic difficulty at the time of presentation, when it is uncertain whether the symptoms represent the first manifestation of an extensive polyarticular disease. Some of these patients have a family history of seronegative arthritis and have the HLA-B27 phenotype. Other patients have a highly distinctive syndrome which appears to be confined to childhood. This affects one or two joints, usually in the lower limbs and generally occurs in young girls. It runs a self-limiting course and is notable for its frequent association with the presence of antinuclear antibodies and a propensity to develop chronic iridocyclitis. Fifty percent of these patients have antinuclear antibodies, but this figure rises to 90 percent in those who develop iridocyclitis. The eye involvement is sometimes asymptomatic and requires ophthalmic slit-lamp examination to detect its presence. This syndrome is associated with the HLA-DR5 phenotype. Unlike other forms of juvenile arthritis, this disease does not occur in adults.

ARTHRITIS IN SYSTEMIC DISEASES

Articular tissues are subject to involvement in many generalized and systemic diseases. The mechanisms of involvement are usually either immunological, affecting the synovium, or metabolic, causing deranged metabolism of articular cartilage.

Immunological Diseases

Serum Sickness

This process was initially described as an adverse reaction occurring seven to 14 days after administration of horse or other antisera. A similar reaction is now seen more commonly following exposure to nonserum allergens such as penicillin and other drugs. In experimental animal models of the disorder, arthritis occurs as a transient phenomenon, while immune complexes are circulating at the stage of approximate equivalence of antigen and antibody. The arthritis of human serum sickness mostly involves large joints such as the knees and wrists and causes pain, swelling, and effusion of a transient and often migratory nature. The condition is usually self-limiting but, if severe, a brief course of corticosteroid treatment may be necessary.

Erythema Nodosum

Erythema nodosum arthropathy represents a syndrome with numerous causes, although in many patients associated or underlying disease is not discovered. Arthralgia or arthritis is usually most notable at the ankles, but other large joints may be affected. Arthralgia and arthritis may precede or may accompany the erythema nodosum lesions on the lower legs. The syndrome usually runs a self-limiting course of two to six weeks' duration. Erythema nodosum is considered to be a hypersensitivity reaction to a variety of antigenic stimuli including:

1. Drugs, especially sulfonamides, penicillin and oral contraceptives
2. Infections, including Streptococcal lesions, tuberculosis, lymphogranuloma venereum, histoplasmosis, and psittacosis

3. Sarcoidosis
4. Chronic inflammatory bowel disease

Many patients with erythema nodosum and arthropathy have mild hilar adenopathy on chest radiographs but no other features of sarcoidosis; this may represent a mild and limited form of sarcoidosis.

Behcet's Disease

This rare disease comprises recurrent oral and genital ulceration with iritis, thrombophlebitis, central nervous system lesions, and arthritis. The arthropathy of Behcet's syndrome resembles the findings in inflammatory bowel disease with peripheral and axial forms. A mild peripheral polyarthritis occurs which rarely causes significant joint damage. The wrists, elbows, and knees are usually affected, rather than small peripheral joints. Sacroiliitis and spondylitis have been described complicating Behcet's disease.

Relapsing Polychondritis

This disorder causes recurring attacks of inflammation in several cartilaginous tissues, including articular cartilage. An immunological mechanism involving cell-mediated immunity to cartilage components has been suggested but has not been consistently substantiated. The arthropathy generally affects one or more large joints in the limbs or the intervertebral joints. Recurring episodes cause progressive articular destruction which may resemble low-grade rheumatoid arthritis.

Damage to cartilaginous tissue at other sites causes inflammatory lesions in the pinnae of the ears, collapse of the nasal cartilages and cartilaginous rings of the upper respiratory tract, and occasionally aortic insufficiency. The disease usually pursues a chronic relapsing course and the duration of the inflammatory exacerbations appears to be limited by the use of corticosteroids.

Familial Mediterranean Fever

This disease is most commonly seen in populations around the Mediterranean including Arabs, Jews, Turks, and Armenians. The disease causes periodic bouts of fever accompanied by acute abdominal pain, chest pain, and acute arthritis. Arthritis occurs in more than 70 percent of patients; larger joints such as the knees, elbows, and wrists are usually affected, and the involvement is commonly monoarticular or pauciarticular during each attack. The attacks may persist for two to six weeks during which time affected joints are swollen, tender, and often warm. Erosive damage is unusual in the limb joints. Sacroiliitis occurs in association with familial Mediterranean fever but does not often progress to ankylosing spondylitis. An immunological basis for the disease has been suggested by the circumstantial evidence of increased serum gammaglobulin levels and the association of the disease with amyloidosis. Long-term administration of colchicine appears to be an effective form of treatment in reducing the frequency and severity of attacks.

Amyloidosis

Involvement of joints has been described in both the primary varieties and in secondary amyloidosis complicating, for example, multiple myeloma. Amyloid infiltration occurs in synovium, articular cartilage, and periarticular tissues. The joints most frequently involved are shoulders, wrists, knees, and fingers. Shoulder involvement is particularly characteristic, giving rise to swelling which may be striking. Subcutaneous nodules comparable with rheumatoid nodules may be present, although antiglobulin rheumatoid factors are not usually detected. Synovial fluid analysis usually shows a modest pleocytosis, and amyloid deposits may be detected in the synovial fluid or in synovial membrane biopsies.

Metabolic and Endocrine Disorders

Alkaptonuria (Ochronosis)

This rare inborn error of metabolism results from deficiency of the enzyme homogentisic acid oxidase. This leads to accumulation of homogentisic acid, which is deposited in articular cartilage and fibrocartilage. The articular cartilage deposition in large joints, such as the knees, hips, and shoulders, impairs cartilage metabolism and leads to extensive degenerative joint disease. Deposits in the intervertebral discs lead to marked spondylosis, commencing in the lumbar region and spreading as far as the neck in many patients. Deposits in other tissues cause pigmentation of the ears and sclera and cardiac murmurs due to deposits in the mitral and aortic valve leaflets. This autosomal recessive disorder is of particular interest in illustrating the manner in which impaired articular cartilage metabolism predisposes to degenerative joint disease.

Hemochromatosis

Hemochromatosis produces a characteristic peripheral arthropathy, and the disease may first present with articular symptoms. Joints most frequently involved are the knees, metacarpophalangeal joints, and interphalangeal joints. Hemosiderin is deposited in synovial tissue and articular cartilage with resulting widespread chondrocalcinosis in the knees, wrists, intervertebral discs, symphysis pubis, and elsewhere.

Acromegaly

Musculoskeletal symptoms are very frequent in acromegaly, and include degenerative joint disease, backache, carpal tunnel syndrome, and proximal muscle weakness. The arthropathy involves small and large peripheral joints including the knees, shoulders, hips, and digital joints.

Hypothyroidism

Adult hypothyroidism commonly gives rise to musculoskeletal symptoms including arthritis, tenosynovitis, painful myopathy, and carpal tunnel syndrome. The arthropathy usually affects the knees, ankles, and metacarpophalangeal joints. Small effusions are found in affected joints with clinical signs suggesting hyperviscous synovial fluid. Synovial fluid analysis usually shows only a modest increase in total white cell count.

Miscellaneous Systemic Disease

Neuropathic (Charcot) Joints

Disruption of the proprioceptive signals from joints leads to a very destructive variety of degenerative joint disease. The mechanism is not entirely clear, but it appears that loss of joint sensation during movement decreases restraint of excessive joint movement by the surrounding musculature. Syphilitic tabes dorsalis is the classically associated disease and leads to gross destruction of knees, hips, ankles and joints of the lower spine. Diabetic neu-ropathy is now a more common cause, and typically the neuropathic joints are in the foot. Other associated neurological processes include lepromatous neuropathy, syringomyelia, paraplegia, and the hypertrophic neuropathy of Dejerine and Sottas. Radiographic examination of neuropathic joints shows gross abnormality with loss of joint space, marked osteophyte and subchondral cyst formation, and subluxation.

Hypertrophic Pulmonary Osteoarthropathy

Finger clubbing is usually present with hypertrophic osteoarthropathy but the reverse is not usually true. This condition is seen most commonly in patients with bronchogenic carcinoma (See Ch. 15). Swelling and pain occur most often in the wrists, ankles, and knees where there is both articular and periarticular swelling. Synovitis and synovial effusion is of moderate degree with the synovial cell counts usually being less than 2000/mm^3. Periarticular swelling and tenderness is accompanied by periostitis; radiographic examination shows periosteal new bone formation at the distal ends of the long bones of the forearm and leg.

Arthropathy in Bleeding Disorders

Hemophilia and the related bleeding diatheses are capable of causing extensive articular damage following recurrent acute hemarthroses which deposit iron in synovial phagocytes and in chondrocytes. Fortunately this has become a less serious problem because of the availability of cryoprecipitates rich in clotting factors. In hemophilia, acute hemarthrosis may occur spontaneously or following minor trauma and give rise to the rapid onset of pain, stiffness, limitation of movement and warmth in the affected joints. The knees, elbows, ankles, shoulders and wrists are most frequently involved. Repeated episodes cause synovial thickening, progressive loss of joint space and an accelerated form of degenerative joint disease. Periarticular osteoporosis due to prolonged immobilization may be striking but is uncommon now because of the availability of replacement therapy (see Chapter 4).

Sickle Cell Anemia

Severe polyarthralgia may occur during sickle cell crises as a consequence of infarction of synovium and adjacent tissue. Such patients usually also have bone infarction and periostitis causing diffuse limb pain. Swelling confined to joints is accompanied by synovial effusion which, on aspiration, may show a variable pleocytosis or evidence of hemarthrosis.

Hypermobility Syndrome

Hypermobility of joints due to ligamentous laxity is a well-recognized feature of the heritable disorders of connective tissue described earlier in this chapter. Lesser degrees of hypermobility are much more frequent than the rare heritable disorders. Such individuals become symptomatic in adolescence or early adult life complaining of nonspecific polyarthralgia, recurring effusions of large joints, such as the knee, and occasionally recurring subluxation of joints. Symptoms usually follow sports or other recreational activities, and there are no features suggesting inflammatory joint disease. Often there is a history of success in competitive gymnastics or in ballet consequent on the agility conferred by ligamentous laxity. Patients with marked hypermobility may be able to voluntarily sublux their glenohumeral joints or patellae. Examination shows ability to hyperextend the metacarpophalangeal joint beyond 90 degrees, hyperextend the elbows or knees and place the hands flat on the floor when keeping the knees extended. Hypermobility declines with aging, and the musculoskeletal symptoms associated with the hypermobility syndrome usually diminish after the second decade. However, chondrocalcinosis in middle-aged subjects has been associated with mild hypermobility, and it has been suggested that this may predispose to degenerative joint disease.

THE COLLAGEN VASCULAR DISEASES

The collagen vascular diseases are a group of disorders which, in their typical forms, represent distinctive syndromes but frequently merge in certain of their clinical and laboratory features. Many give rise to chronic systemic disease, and their variety of clinical presentations has long been a source of particular fascination to physicians in many branches of medicine. Immunological abnormalities are the basis of disease in joints, skin, and small blood vessels in solid organs. Abnormalities of humoral immune function and defects of cell-mediated immunity have been demonstrated in the majority of these illnesses.

The major diseases identified within the collagen-vascular disease group are: (1) systemic lupus erythematosus, (2) mixed connective tissue disease, (3) scleroderma (progressive systemic sclerosis), (4) Sjögren's syndrome, (5) the vasculitides, and (6) the inflammatory myositides. Each of these categories includes variants resembling the "parent" disease in clinical and laboratory features.

SYSTEMIC LUPUS ERYTHEMATOSUS

Lupus erythematosus was initially recognized as a cutaneous variant of lupus vulgaris late in the 19th century, and following the observations of Osler and others it was recognized that associated systemic disease could occur. A clinical picture of a rare and serious disease emerged, characterized by multisystem involvement, a striking facial rash, and early death from renal damage. It has become appreciated in recent years that the severe life-threatening form of the disease represents only the tip of an iceberg of a relatively common disease. When the "LE cell" phenomenon was discovered in 1948, it was thought to be specific for systemic lupus erythematosus (SLE) and the new technology permitted recognition of milder forms than hitherto recognized. With the development of the immunofluorescent method of detecting antinuclear antibodies in 1957, the frequency of diagnosis of mild cases increased again and it was appreciated that SLE is not a rare disease. The process of diagnosis was refined and expanded with the introduction of radioimmunoassay techniques for the measurement of DNA antibodies in the late 1960s. The present view of SLE is that of a disease that may produce a wide spectrum of activity and pathology and that does not affect vital organs in the majority of patients. It predominantly affects women in the reproductive age span and has a female to male ratio of the order of 9 to 1; in cases occurring in childhood and older age groups, the sex ratio is closer to equality. The prevalence rate varies in different groups studied with an average figure of 1 woman in 2,000 in the reproductive age span being affected. Ethnic and geographic variations have been observed, with the disease having increased prevalence in countries bordering the Mediterranean and the Carribean seas, and in American blacks.

Pathology

The two striking histopathological features of SLE are fibrinoid necrosis and hematoxylin bodies. Fibrinoid necrosis is seen as part of the vasculitic reaction in arterioles and capillaries and appears as homogeneous deposits which contain fibrinogen, complement, and gamma-globulin. The hematoxylin body is the tissue counterpart of the LE cell, and represents pyknosis of nuclei with resultant coalescence or phagocytosis. Renal involvement varies in severity from minimal histological findings to severe diffuse proliferative glomerulonephritis. Electron microscopy of the nephritic lesions shows electron-dense material on the endothelial aspect of the basement membrane with either a linear or lumpy-bumpy distribution. The deposits have been demonstrated to contain immunoglobulins with antibody specificity against DNA, complement, and fibrinogen. Analogous deposits can often be demonstrated at the dermoepidermal junction of skin by immunofluorescent methods. Fibrinoid deposition and perivascular fibrosis may be found in other organs affected, including serosal surfaces, synovium, and the spleen. Periarteriolar fibrosis in the spleen causes so-called onion skin lesions which are characteristic of SLE.

Etiology

The hallmark of SLE is the presence in serum of antinuclear antibodies, and especially antibodies to double-stranded DNA. Small quantities of DNA are present in the circulation in health but this does not give rise to the production of anti-DNA antibodies; in experimental circumstances, double-stranded DNA is not immunogenic unless it has been altered and denatured by, for example, ultraviolet irradiation or mild heating. In established disease, a wide range of antibodies may be present, including antibodies to single-stranded DNA, nuclear histones, RNA, cytoplasmic elements, immunoglobulins (rheumatoid factors), coagulation factors, and to the formed elements of blood, namely lymphocytes, granulocytes, red blood cells, and platelets. Organ-specific antibodies are present in some patients, including antineuronal antibodies and thyroid antibodies. Many of the histopathological features of the disease can be explained by the vascular deposition of circulating antigen-antibody immune complexes. Complement components are demonstrable in tissue lesions by immunofluorescent methods and serum concentrations of complement components tend to be depressed in active disease. Immune complexes concentrated in cryoprecipitates of SLE patients' sera have been analyzed for their antigen and antibody content; antinuclear antibodies and antibodies to

lymphocyte membranes have been consistently demonstrated by this technique. The lymphocyte specific antibodies are mostly active against T cells and this may have some relevance to the finding that suppressor T-cell activity and absolute numbers of these cells are both depressed in patients with active disease. The initiating cause of the many abnormalities of humoral and cellular immune function is uncertain but there has been particular interest in possible viral causes.

The great variation in susceptibility to organ-specific manifestations is not fully understood. Renal disease is associated with the presence of high avidity IgG anti-DNA antibodies, and it is thought that this may have a bearing on the type of immune complexes formed and the consequent deposition of antinuclear antibodies in the kidney. Cerebral disease has been associated with the presence of antineuronal antibodies and high concentrations of antilymphocyte antibodies.

Heritable etiological factors are suggested by the finding of occasional familial aggregations of cases, and also by the ethnic variation in disease prevalence. In studies of groups of patients the histocompatibility alloantigens HLA-B8, HLA-DR2, HLA-DR3 are found more frequently than in populations of control subjects. The predilection of the disease to affect females may have either a genetic or endocrine basis. In the New Zealand black and white (NZB/NZW) mouse model, castration of female animals delays the onset of the disease. The human disease is found with unexpected frequency in subjects who have Klinefelter's syndrome, which is suggestive that loci on the X chromosome have some importance in genesis of the disease. Patients with congential deficiency of some complement components including C2, C4, C5 and C8 are liable to develop a lupus-like disease. This association may be due to incomplete virus neutralization or deficiency in the ability to clear circulating immune complexes from the circulation.

A disease resembling SLE can be induced by prolonged administration of several drugs, most notably hydralazine and procainamide. Antibodies to nuclear histones are common in these patients, and it is believed that some drugs become bound by electrostatic forces to histones, giving rise to a haptenic immunogen. Chronic discoid lupus erythematosus occurs in patients with the systemic disease, but the relationship between the two processes is inconstant. Antinuclear antibodies and other immunological abnormalities are found in patients with chronic discoid lupus, but less than 1 patient in 20 who have the skin disease progresses to develop features of systemic disease.

Clinical Features

It is customary to say that the clinical manifestations of systemic lupus erythematosus are protean because almost every system and organ in the body may become involved. The course of SLE is characterized by a pattern of exacerbations and remissions. These dynamics must be taken into consideration when disease severity is being assessed, and it is preferable that treatment decisions be based on a period of observation rather than a single evaluation. The disease presents different faces to different medical subspecialities; in some patients hematological or renal complications are dominant, with other systems being only involved to a very small extent. Symptoms may be quite nonspecific and lead to inappropriate diagnosis of neuroticism. Nonspecific malaise, tiredness and low-grade fever are common. Occasionally the fever may reach 40°C during an exacerbation. Depression, irritability, headache, and the occurrence of vague pains in the joints, chest, or abdomen may be present for many months or even years before the correct diagnosis is appreciated. Table 18.12 ranks the major clinical manifestations of SLE derived from several large published series.

Musculoskeletal manifestations are very common. Synovitis is generally mild and is probably the result of deposition of circulating immune complexes in synovial tissue. Erosive arthritis and actual deformity other than mild periarticular swelling are uncommon, occurring in less than 5 percent of patients. The Jaccoud hand deformity is rare and causes hyperextension of the proximal interphalangeal joints with flexion of the distal interphalangeal joints. This is believed to be due to late fibrosis following tenosynovitis and capsular inflammation. The joint symptoms are usually mild, symmetrical, and predominently involve the small joints of the hands or feet, and less frequently the knees, wrists, and other joints. Avascular osteonecrosis is encountered in patients who have received immunosuppressive treatment but may occur without such treatment, perhaps as a result of vasculitis affecting small bone blood

Table 18.12 **Major Clinical Manifestations of Systemic Lupus Erythematosus**

Manifestation	Percentage Affected
Arthritis	87
Skin lesions	81
Renal disease	47
Pleurisy	44
Neuropsychiatric abnormality	44
Raynaud's phemenon	29
Pericarditis	28

vessels. The femoral head, tibial plateau, and humeral head are the areas most often affected. Nonspecific myalgia is common, but myositis causing weakness and functional disability is rare.

Cutaneous involvement is frequently found if sought carefully. Often patients may not be aware of having mild frontal alopecia or brittle frontal "lupus hairs" that are present in approximately 40 percent of patients. Alopecia areata is unusual except in patients who have extensive associated chronic discoid lupus erythematosus. Small areas of cutaneous vasculitis may be seen over the elbows, knees, and the knuckles. The well known butterfly-distribution rash over the face may show either a vasculitic appearance or that of chronic discoid lupus with follicular plugging. Exacerbation of skin lesions after prolonged or intense exposure to the sun may be a useful pointer to the diagnosis of SLE. Oral aphthous ulceration may be regarded as a cutaneous manifestation and occurs in approximately 20 percent of patients.

Lupus nephritis is the most important life-threatening complication of the disease. The extent of the nephritis may vary on biopsy appearance from minor mesangial hypertrophy or slight interstitial lymphocytic infiltration to glomerular destruction by focal glomerulonephritis, membranous disease, or diffuse proliferative glomerulonephritis. Diffuse proliferative glomerulonephritis carries the worst prognosis, with a median survival time in the range of 3 to 5 years. Concurrent necrotizing vasculitis associated with severe hypertension occurs in about 20 percent of patients with diffuse proliferative disease and carries a particularly poor prognosis. Features of the nephrotic syndrome may be present, but usually proteinuria is of a mild degree, not causing significant plasma protein depletion.

Neuropsychiatric abnormalities in SLE can mimic many other diseases, and, if the first or predominant clinical feature, may present great diagnostic difficulty. Minor personality changes, irritability, or depression may accompany general exacerbations of the disease. Generalized convulsions due to diffuse cerebritis are uncommon but localized cerebral disturbance may cause hemiparesis, cranial nerve palsy, and migrainous phenomena. Other neurological complications include aseptic meningitis, transverse myelitis, radiculopathies, and basal ganglia syndromes.

Pulmonary and cardiac involvement in SLE is most commonly evident through the mechanisms of serositis. Chest pain is common in SLE and is attributed to minor pleuritic changes. The pain is usually around the costal margin and intermittent. Diffuse pulmonary fibrosis causing respiratory insufficiency and large pleural effusions are relatively uncommon. Similarly, occasional mild pericarditis may occur but large pericardial effusions are rare. Verrucous endocarditis is a relatively frequent finding at necropsy but clinically evident valvular damage in SLE (Libman-Sacks syndrome) is rare. Infective endocarditis has been reported occurring on valves damaged by SLE.

Raynaud's phenomenon is usually mild in SLE, and severe symptoms may be an indication that the patient has mixed connective tissue disease. Prominent Raynaud's phenomenon may be observed in some patients with vasculitis, and an association with lupus nephritis has been suggested.

Hematological abnormality is usually not symptomatic except for purpura occurring with thrombocytopenia, or increased susceptibility to infection with leukopenia. The presence of coagulation factor antibodies, usually directed at Factors VII, IX and XII, rarely cause bleeding episodes. However, bleeding problems may occur in such patients following surgery or renal biopsy, especially in patients with active vasculitis.

Drug-induced lupus may closely resemble the idiopathic disease. Joint involvement, skin rashes, pleurisy, and pericarditis occur frequently. The occurrence of cerebral or renal involvement in a patient thought to have drug-induced lupus should give rise to suspicion that the patient has idiopathic SLE, or that these manifestations are consequences of the disease for which the incriminated drug has been prescribed.

Laboratory Findings

Diagnosis in early and mild cases requires careful clinical evaluation, and comprehensive laboratory investigation is frequently necessary to enable the diagnosis to be confirmed with reasonable confidence. Criteria for the classification of SLE have been designed by the American Rheumatism Association for epidemiological and other research purposes, and although more than 90 percent of cases of SLE meet these criteria, their use is not appropriate to confirm the diagnosis in an individual patient. Table 18.13 indicates some of the more common laboratory abnormalities in SLE.

Mild disturbance of a wide range of laboratory parameters is frequently found, but severe disturbances with clinical consequences are less common. For example, mild normochromic anemia, direct positive Coombs' test, mild leukopenia, and mild thrombocytopenia occur in more than 25 percent of pa-

Table 18.13 **Some Laboratory Findings in Systemic Lupus Erythematosus**

Laboratory Abnormality	Approximate % of SLE Patients
1. Hematologic	
Anemia	50
Hemolytic anemia	10
Positive Coomb's Test	25
Leukopenia, $< 4000/mm^3$	40
Lymphocyte antibodies	80
Thrombocytopenia, $< 100,000/mm^3$	25
2. Urinary	
Proteinuria, $> 3.5g/24$ hours	10–15
Urinary casts	10
3. Immunologic	
Reduced complement activity	30
Hypergammaglobulinemia	50
Antiglobulins	15
Antinuclear antibodies	
fluorescent ANA	99
double-stranded DNA	60–90
single-stranded DNA	90
histones (LE cell)	70
acid nucleoproteins	20–40
Coagulation factor antibodies	10
Positive test for syphilis	20

tients, but hemolytic anemia and thrombocytopenia sufficient to give rise to spontaneous bleeding are relatively rare. Patients who have a positive Coombs' test usually have immunoglobulin or complement on the surface of their red blood cells. Cold-reactive lymphocyte antibodies are present in the majority of patients with SLE, especially in those who have lymphopenia, but their presence does not have a clearcut correlation with overall disease activity. Proteinuria exceeding 3.5 g/24 hours and the presence of urinary casts indicates the presence of severe renal involvement but does not necessarily correlate well with the histological appearance if renal biopsy is performed.

Many immunological abnormalities may be demonstrable by routine laboratory tests in SLE. Diffuse mild hypergammaglobulinemia is usually present on protein electrophoresis. A small proportion of patients have selective IgA deficiency, and a very small number of patients have congenital deficiencies of complement components including C2 and C4. Much more commonly, however, reduced levels of complement components, notably C3 and C4, or reduced hemolytic complement activity indicates active disease. Complement levels often fall as the DNA antibodies levels rise concomitant with increased clinical activity of the disease. Antiglobulin rheumatoid factors are present in less than 20 percent of patients with SLE and the serum concentrations do not correlate with the extent or severity of articular involvement.

The presence of antinuclear antibodies is the most characteristic laboratory finding in SLE, and the diagnosis cannot be sustained if antinuclear antibodies are not present at some time during the course of the disease. Quantitative assays usually show varying levels of antinuclear antibody activity. The fluorescent antinuclear antibody test using a solid tissue substrate containing many different nuclear antigens is the most useful screening test, but it is not specific for SLE. The most specific routinely used test is for the presence of double-stranded DNA antibodies, which are usually measured by a radioimmunoassay method; the presence of such antibodies in high titre is virtually pathogonomic of SLE. The LE cell phenomenon can be demonstrated in approximately 70 percent of patients with idiopathic SLE and is dependent on IgG antibodies to histones. Specific histone antibodies are a frequent finding in the drug-induced SLE-like syndrome in which antibodies to double-stranded DNA are not detectable. Antibodies to acid extractable nuclear proteins are present in a minority of patients, but antibodies to one of these antigens, "Sm," shows very high specificity for SLE. False positivity for the routine serological test for syphilis is due to the presence of antibodies that react with cardiolipin. It should be noted that complement-fixation tests for syphilis and other types of similar tests may give spurious results because of the anticomplementary activity of immune complexes present in the sera of patients with SLE. Synovial fluid analysis of swollen joints usually shows only a modest pleocytosis and occasionally LE cells are observed.

Radiographic evaluation of symptomatic joints does not show any abnormality except in very rare instances of associated erosive disease. Chest radiographs may show small pleural effusion, mild elevation of the diaphragm, or small plate-like atelectases. Disturbances of pulmonary function on physiological testing, including mild defects in diffusing capacity, are somewhat more common than radiographic change.

Treatment

The tendency to exacerbation and remission implies that the patient's progress should be followed and treatment adjusted from time to time according to the clinical and laboratory findings. No form of treatment has been shown to eradicate or cure the disease, but treatment may have considerable supportive and symptomatic benefit. Prevention of exacerbations is only feasible in patients who have sun-related ultraviolet photosensitivity. These patients should avoid sunbathing and use barrier creams.

In many patients, arthralgia and arthritis are the most predominant symptoms, and symptomatic treatment with anti-inflammatory drugs alone is sufficient to control their illness. Salicylates and other nonsteroidal drugs are effective, but there appears to be an increased risk of hepatotoxicity in the use of salicylate in SLE.

Corticosteroids are the mainstay of treatment in SLE, and their use becomes necessary in patients who have hemolytic episodes, cerebral involvement, cardiac involvement, and in most patients with renal involvement. The value of steroids in treatment of these more serious and life-threatening complications is well established. However, there are major risks, and long-term administration of steroids seems to potentiate some disease consequences, such as impaired immune responsiveness and possibly vaculitis, so that steroid-treated patients are at special risk for the development of infections and avascular osteonecrosis.

The treatment of lupus nephritis is controversial. Less than 30 mg per day of prednisone does not appear to alter the course of severe diffuse proliferative glomerulonephritis. Larger doses of prednisone may be beneficial, but the risk of serious adverse effects may outweigh the possible benefit. Other modes of steroid treatment, including alternative day treatment and high-dose intraveneous pulsing, are of unproved value. Combinations of steroids with immunosuppressive drugs, including azathioprine, 6-mercaptopurine, and cyclophosphamide, have not shown definite advantage over steroid treatment alone. The value of renal biopsy in assessing the extent of lupus nephritis is also controversial. The extent of abnormality in the urinary sediment together with the extent of hematologic and immunologic abnormality may provide comparable information to that provided by renal biopsy. However, demonstration of severe diffuse proliferative glomerulonephritis by biopsy provides justification for aggressive immunosuppressive treatment. Hypertension associated with lupus nephritis may be treated in the usual manner, and the use of methyldopa and hydralazine is not contraindicated even though these drugs sometimes induce a lupus-syndrome.

Cerebral lupus is responsive to steroid medication, but this has to be administered with caution. High-dose steroid treatment may of itself induce psychosis and the differentiation of cerebritis due to lupus from steroid psychosis requires very careful clinical assessment. Laboratory and radiographic evaluation of cerebral lupus is notoriously difficult. Many forms of experimental treatment have been explored in systemic lupus erythematosus. These include repeated plasma exchange, and adsorption of DNA antibodies on special hemoperfusion columns. The value of these experimental forms of treatment has yet to be established.

Pregnancy in the course of systemic lupus erythematosus poses a common management problem. There is an increased risk of spontaneous abortion, but therapeutic abortion is not indicated except in patients who have severe renal disease or other life-threatening complications. Transient neonatal abnormality including thrombocytopenia and the presence of antinuclear antibodies in the neonate's serum are reported. Congenital heart block is a rare but well-documented complication of maternal lupus.

MIXED CONNECTIVE TISSUE DISEASE

The nomenclature of this illness causes confusion. Several of the collagen-vascular diseases have similar clinical presentations, and in a few patients differentiation between specific disease entities may be difficult. These patients are said to have "overlap" syndromes. Mixed connective tissue disease, however, is a specific disease entity that has features resembling systemic lupus erythematosus. scleroderma and polymyositis. The clinical features of mixed connective tissue disease occur in all three of these diseases but are present in a much greater proportion of patients with mixed connective tissue disease.

Table 18.14 illustrates comparative findings in SLE and mixed connective tissue disease. The clinical features of mixed connective tissue disease resemble mild SLE, but usually Raynaud's phenomenon is especially prominent. This may give rise to infarction of finger pulps and even digital gangrene, but more usually the fingers are diffusely swollen with a sausage-like appearance. After several years, the skin of the fingers becomes thickened and resembles the appearances in scleroderma. Arthralgia and arthritis are

usually mild and nondeforming. Proximal muscle weakness and myalgia are common. Dysphagia is usually not a major symptom, but esophageal motility abnormality has been demonstrated in 70 percent of patients with mixed connective tissue disease. Various forms of central nervous system abnormality occur but less frequently than in SLE. A syndrome resembling trigeminal neuralgia, sometimes accompanied by sensory loss has been reported as a particular neurological complication of mixed connective tissue disease. Renal disease is much less common than in SLE.

Early descriptions of the disease suggested that it was more likely to be steroid-responsive than SLE and the prognosis more favorable. Further experience has revealed that death may occur from renal disease, pulmonary arterial hypertensive disease, and infection.

Laboratory investigation shows a number of immunological abnormalities comparable to those found in SLE. Antibodies to ribonucleoprotein are often present in extremely high titre. DNA antibodies are usually also present but in lower concentrations than occur in SLE. Nonspecific findings include leukopenia and hypergammaglobulinemia. Serum concentrations of creatine phosphokinase and other muscle enzymes are moderately elevated in patients with prominent myositis.

Serological investigations by fluorescent antinuclear antibody (ANA) characterization often shows a speckled staining pattern. Investigation of the antinuclear antibodies has shown that their specificity is directed against antigens which can be extracted in aqueous solution from crude tissue homogenates (extractable nuclear antigens, or ENA). The principal antigen concerned is RNAse-sensitive and appears to be primarily of ribonucleoprotein origin. As in SLE, a variety of antinuclear antibodies may be present, but the emphasis in mixed connective tissue diseases is towards RNA rather than DNA-based antigens.

Treatment of mixed connective tissue disease is similar to that of the treatment of SLE. Mild cutaneous vasculitis and mild arthritis respond to salicylate and other anti-inflammatory agents. Patients with prominent Raynaud's phenomenon should not smoke cigarettes and should avoid excessive cold exposure. More severe disease and evidence of internal organ involvement is treated with corticosteroids. Arthritis, myositis, fever, rash, and other features of the disease usually respond well to small doses of prednisone. Scleroderma-like skin changes are reported to improve in some patients treated with steroids. As in SLE, long-term administration of high doses of steroids carries particular risk of adverse effects, including susceptibility to infections.

Table 18.14   **SLE Versus Mixed Connective Tissue Disease**

Finding	SLE	MCTD
Scleroderma changes	−	+ +
Raynaud's phenomenon	+	+ + +
Myositis	+	+
CNS disease	+ +	+
Renal disease	+ +	+
DNA antibodies	+ +	+
ENA antibodies	+	+ + +
Speckled ANF	+	+ +
Homogenous ANF	+	+

SCLERODERMA (PROGRESSIVE SYSTEMIC SCLEROSIS)

Although the major clinical manifestations of scleroderma are cutaneous, it is appropriate to consider the disease with the rheumatic and collagen-vascular disorders because of its noncutaneous associations. Scleroderma is a rare disease, with an annual estimated incidence of 12 cases per million population. There are several patterns of disease with variable extent. Progressive systemic sclerosis refers to scleroderma with internal organ involvement of a progressive nature.

Pathology

Skin biopsy appearances show marked thickening of the dermis with massive increase in the amount of collagen fibers in the reticular dermis and atrophy of skin appendages. Collections of lymphocytes (predominantly T cells) may be present. Small blood vessels show intimal proliferation that may progress to occlusion, hyalinization, and fibrosis. In late disease there is gross thickening of the dermis, atrophy of the epidermis, and increased melanin deposition in the basal epidermal layer. The serious and life-threatening complications of scleroderma arise from angiopathy in the renal and pulmonary vasculature. The renal intralobular arteries, interlobular arteries, and afferent glomerular arterioles show intimal proliferation, medial thinning, and adventitial collagen thickening. Pulmonary arteries tend to show similar intimal proliferation and medial hypertrophy.

Etiology

The etiology of scleroderma remains mysterious, but the clues to its cause, provided by the clinical associations of the syndrome and by experimental observations, suggest immunological mechanisms.

Clinical Findings

The generalized forms of scleroderma may commence at any time from the first decade of life to old age, but most commonly commence in females during the reproductive age. The onset of cutaneous symptoms is often preceded by the development of Raynaud's phenomenon, and in some instances this may have been present for 10 or more years without cutaneous change. Mild benign Raynaud's phenomenon is common in the general population, especially in females, but usually this will have been present from adolescence and be of mild degree. The abrupt onset of Raynaud's phenomenon after adolescence should be regarded with greater suspicion that it may represent the premonitory phase of scleroderma. Cutaneous disease sometimes commences with a relatively acute phase of generalized brawny edema of the extremities lasting from a few weeks to several months. This slowly regresses, and the typical thickened waxy-feeling skin change develops insidiously. The dorsal aspect of the digits are usually first involved (sclerodactyly). In progressing disease, the forearms, shins, and lower part of the face next become involved. With extensive progressing cutaneous scleroderma, there is spread to cause progressive joint contractures, cicatrization of the mouth and other body orifices, and cuirasse-like encasement of the trunk to the point that rib movement may be restricted. Synovitis is often present during the earlier phases of scleroderma and there may be a resemblance to rheumatoid arthritis. Later the skin overlying joints becomes tight and "hidebound," synovitis is less evident, and joint contractures develop. Synovitis in tendon sheaths may give rise to a distinctive type of leathery crepitus.

Usually the first symptomatic indication of systemic involvement is dysphagia, which may progress to the necessity for repeated bouginage. Sclerodermatous thickening of the lower gastrointestinal tract and impaired motility may cause malabsorption, constipation, and the symptoms of diverticular disease of the colon. Pulmonary involvement varies in severity from asymptomatic decrease in diffusion capacity to severe dyspnea caused by progressive pulmonary fibrosis. Symptoms of congestive heart failure can be caused by cor pulmonale consequent upon pulmonary fibrosis, or by progressive pulmonary arterial hypertension due to sclerodermatous pulmonary angiopathy. The most ominous complication of scleroderma is the appearance of renal involvement, manifested by hypertension and proteinuria. The hypertension is recalcitrant to conventional forms of antihypertensive treatment and pursues an accelerated course. The resultant renal reaction, accompanied by hyper-reninemia, causes hypertensive renal failure. Fewer than 10 percent of patients survive more than two years following the onset of renal disease in progressive systemic sclerosis.

The diagnosis of scleroderma is primarily based on clinical evaluation. Antinuclear antibodies are the most consistently demonstrable serological abnormality. Nonspecific elevations of sedimentation rate, immunoglobulin concentration, and antiglobulin concentrations may be present.

Treatment

Management of the more extensive and progressive forms of scleroderma is frustrating for the patient and for the physician. Progressive finger contractures associated with tightening of the skin require careful physiotherapy to prevent claw-hand deformities. Patients with prominent Raynaud's phenomenon should not smoke. Follow-up surveillance should include regular monitoring of blood pressure and urinalysis. Hypertension in progressive systemic sclerosis becomes increasingly difficult to manage with conventional antihypertensive drugs; Captopril has been reported to be the most effective agent in severe hypertension in scleroderma patients. Treatment of cutaneous manifestations has been attempted with numerous drugs, but it is difficult to establish their effectiveness because of difficulty in quantifying the extent of cutaneous disease, and also because spontaneous improvement or remission occurs in a number of patients. Among the drugs which have had some popularity are para-amino-benzoic acid and local application of dimethlyl sulphoxide. D-penicillamine has been shown to inhibit crosslink formation in collagen biosynthesis and appears of value in some patients with scleroderma if taken for months or years. Colchicine has also been used to inhibit the conversion of procollagen to collagen and may be useful in some patients. In general, however, no form of drug treatment has been shown to substantially impede or even reverse the cutaneous and internal organ involvement in progressive systemic sclerosis. Corticosteroid treatment has been very widely used, and sometimes combined with immunosuppressive cytostatic agents, but there is little evidence that this theoretically appropriate line of treatment is helpful.

CREST Syndrome

A relatively benign variant of scleroderma is nosologically separated as the CREST syndrome. This acronym indicates calcinosis, Raynaud's phenomenon, esophageal involvement, sclerodactyly, and telangiectasia. This syndrome differs markedly from progressive systemic sclerosis in representing an apparently benign end of the scleroderma spectrum. The course of this variant is measured in years or decades, and progression to life-threatening internal organ involvement is unusual. Raynaud's phenomenon is the primary feature and may have been present for many years before other features appear. Sclerodactyly develops very slowly and sclerodermatous skin changes may be apparent only in the digits and perhaps in the lower part of the face. Subcutaneous calcinosis appears after several years, comprising small deposits of hydroxyapatite in those areas affected by scleroderma. Esophageal motility abnormalities can be demonstrated by special investigation in many of these patients, although only a small proportion are symptomatic. Telangiectases, like calcinosis, are most likely to be found in those areas of skin showing sclerodermatous changes. They are most evident around the nail folds, fingertips and around the lips. Laboratory evidence that supports the view that the CREST syndrome should be regarded as a separate entity has been found by examination of the antinuclear antibody specificities; a high proportion of patients have antibodies with particular specificity for the centromere of dividing cells. Treatment of the CREST syndrome follows the same approach as described for scleroderma.

Eosinophilic Fasciitis

This recently described syndrome may be a benign variant of scleroderma. It is characterized by scleroderma-like skin changes, peripheral blood eosinophilia, lack of association with other collagen-vascular disease and absence of antinuclear antibodies. Although the disorder is called eosinophilic fasciitis, peripheral blood eosinophilia is a more constant feature of the syndrome than the presence of eosinophils in tissue infiltrates.

Oral steroid treatment of eosinophilic fasciitis usually results in softening of indurated skin, increased range of motion of joint contractures, and disappearance of peripheral blood eosinophilia. The natural history of the disease activity varies from periods of several months to one or more years, but the majority of patients have complete or near complete resolution of symptoms, and steroid treatment can slowly be withdrawn.

SJÖGREN'S SYNDROME

Sjögren's syndrome typically occurs with extensive rheumatoid arthritis, but this "keratoconjunctivitis sicca" syndrome occurs in association with collagen-vascular diseases such as SLE, or may occur in the absence of any associated articular or connective tissue disease. The lacrimal and salivary glands are the site of an inflammatory reaction, causing reduction in salivary and tear flow.

Pathology

The pathology of Sjögren's syndrome shows extensive lymphocytic and plasma cell infiltration of the salivary, lacrimal and other exocrine glands. The salivary glands may even resemble lymph nodes because of extensive infiltration with immunocytes. Inflammatory change has also been observed in proximity to glands in the respiratory tract, gastrointestinal tract, and the vagina.

Extensive humoral immune abnormality is indicated by elevation of serum immunoglobulin concentrations, sometimes to very high levels. Tissue specific autoantibodies directed against salivary gland duct epithelium have been demonstrated, but tissue and organ specific autoantibodies directed against many other tissues are also found in the sera of these patients. Antiglobulin rheumatoid factors are present in more than 90 percent of patients and these are also usually present at very high titre. Antinuclear antibodies are present in at least 70 percent of patients and anti-native DNA antibodies are present, usually in lower concentrations than found in SLE. Approximately 70 percent of patients have antibodies with specificity against an acid extractable nuclear antigen designated SS-B. Sjögren's syndrome is associated with the histocompatibility phenotypes HLA-B8 and DR3.

Sjögren's syndrome is also associated with renal tubular acidosis, hyperglobulinemic purpura, cryoglobulinemia, and a propensity to lymphoma formation.

Clinical Features

More than 90 percent of patients are female, with a mean age of 50 years. In the majority of patients, rheumatoid arthritis or collagen-vascular disease has been present for several years. Patients with rheumatoid arthritis who develop symptomatic Sjögren's syndrome usually have advanced erosive disease with nodule formation and high titres of antiglobulin rheumatoid factors. The usual first symptom is of dryness or grittiness in the eyes. Loss of the normal protective lubricating function of tears can progress to corneal ulceration and damage to the anterior chamber of the eye. Asymptomatic reduction in tear flow in rheumatoid arthritis is more common than

symptomatic keratoconjunctivitis sicca. Confirmation of keratoconjunctivitis requires opthalmic slit lamp examination.

Salivary insufficiency causes difficulty in mastication and swallowing. Patients drink increasing amounts of fluid to help swallow their meals, and dental caries may progress rapidly. Advanced Sjögren's syndrome causes dryness in the nose, pharynx, and larynx.

The physical findings are primarily those of the associated rheumatoid arthritis or collagen-vascular disease. Salivary gland enlargement, especially of the parotid glands is usually a late feature. Associated myositis may cause proximal weakness. Confirmation of the diagnosis of Sjögren's syndrome is primarily a clinical matter. Schirmer's test which measures wetting of absorbent paper, provides a rough indication of reduced tear flow. Salivary gland function can also be evaluated by scintigraphy and secretory sialography, but these techniques are usually not necessary in routine clinical practice. Biopsy of minor buccal salivary glands has been used as a simple and relatively innocuous means of obtaining a "tissue diagnosis."

Treatment

Treatment of Sjögren's syndrome is symptomatic. Artificial tears in the form of 0.5 percent methylcellulose instilled several times daily provide adequate replacement for deficient tear production. The oral aspects of the sicca syndrome require additional fluids with meals and regular dental attention.

VASCULITIS

Vasculitis is a frequent finding in the "collagen-vascular diseases," and in many this is the most important pathological feature. The inflammatory process underlying vasculitis in most of these diseases results from the deposition of circulating antigen-antibody immune complexes in the walls of blood vessels. This leads to activation of the complement system and local tissue destruction by recruitment of granulocytes with local release of lysosomal enzymes. (Type III immune response in the Gell and Coombs classification, see Chapter 6). This mechanism of tissue damage is well recognized in vasculitides affecting smaller arteries and capillaries, but the role of circulating immune complexes in vasculitides involving large and medium-sized arteries is less certain. In this latter group of disorders some evidence suggests a specific immune response directed against components of the arterial wall, and frequently in this subgroup a granulomatous infiltration of lymphocytes, plasma cells, and histiocytic giant cells may be found. A short classification of the vasculitides is shown in Table 18.15 with disorders listed by type of vessel involved and histological appearances.

Polyarteritis Nodosa

Polyarteritis nodosa is the prototype disease among the vasculitides. Arteritis is present in medium-sized and in some small muscular arteries that show fibrinoid change with neutrophil granulocyte infiltration and some fragmentation of the internal elastic lamina. Late lesions show obliteration and healing by fibrosis. Aneurysm formation occurs especially at points of bifurcation, giving the nodular abnormality implied in the name of the disease. These aneurysms are prone to rupture, causing hemorrhage in the gastrointestinal tract and elsewhere. The arteritis is widespread and has consequences in the skin, kidneys, lungs, heart, gastrointestinal tract, and peripheral nervous system.

The cause of polyarteritis nodosa is not apparent in the majority of patients. Analysis of serum cryoprecipitates has occasionally revealed hepatitis B antigen, and hepatitis B viral particles have been seen on electron microscopy of some cryoprecipitates. It is postulated that hepatitis B virus, or viral antigens, induce immune complex formation in individuals unable to completely clear the virus, and deposition of complexes gives rise to arteritis.

Clinical Features

The initial clinical features of polyarteritis nodosa are often vague and nonspecific, including weight loss, intermittent fever, myalgia, and arthralgia. In its typical presentation it is most often seen among middle-aged males, but atypical cases occur in females, and it has been reported in most age groups. Skin lesions are relatively infrequent in this form of vasculitis compared with other forms, but petechial or purpuric lesions may be seen. Renal involvement causes hypertension, proteinuria, and microscopic hematuria. Nodular swellings along the course of arteries at sites of aneurysm formation are only occasionally palpable but may be demonstrated by renal arteriography. Cardiac involvement may present with angina and congestive heart failure. Abdominal pain is a common symptom due to mesenteric involvement. The arterial supply to the gallbladder has a peculiar susceptibility to arteritis. Mononeuritis multiplex is one of the more frequent forms of neurological manifestations, occurring in some degree in 50 percent or more of patients. Pulmonary involvement causes asthma in some patients.

Laboratory findings in polyarteritis nodosa include neutrophil leukocytosis, sometimes to very high levels, moderate elevation of the sedimentation rate, thrombocytosis, and eosinophilia is present in approximately 20 percent of patients. Urinalysis may reveal proteinuria or hematuria. Tests for circulating immune complexes are positive in the majority of patients, and routine tests for hepatitis B surface antigen may be positive in 10 to 70 percent of patients. Chest radiographs may show transient pulmonary infiltrates. Celiac axis angiography has been found useful in patients with suspected polyarteritis nodosa

Table 18.15 **Simplified Classification of Vasculitic Syndromes**

Vasculitic Syndrome	Blood Vessels Involved
Takayasu's arteritis	Large arteries—aorta, cranial arteries
Giant cell arteritis	Cranial arteries and great vessels
Polyarteritis nodosa	Medium-sized muscular arteries
Wegener's granulomatosis	Medium-sized and small muscular arteries
Allergic granulomatosis (Churg-Strauss)	Small muscular arteries
Hypersensitivity vasculitides-including serum sickness, Henoch-Schonlein purpura, vasculitis associated with malignancy	Small arteries and arterioles
Vasculitis associated with rheumatic disease-including SLE, rheumatoid arthritis, mixed connective tissue disease, Sjogren's syndrome	Small arteries and arterioles
Miscellaneous vasculitis-including mucocutaneous lymph node syndrome (Kawasaki disease), thromboangiitis obliterans	Arterioles and venules
Leukocytoclastic vasculitis-associated with paraproteinemia, cryoglobulinemia; bacterial, viral, rickettsial and other infection; arthropod bites; drug and food allergic reactions; and malignant disease	Small arteries, arterioles, small veins, venules and post-capillary venules

who do not have prominent cutaneous or renal disease. This technique demonstrates aneurysm formation in branches of the celiac axis, including branches of the hepatic artery. Biopsy of cutaneous lesions when present is usually helpful. Biopsy of clinically affected organs is generally diagnostic; however, muscle biopsy is sometimes helpful in demonstrating arteritis in patients without clearly defined lesions in other organs.

Treatment

Corticosteroid treatment appears to prolong survival, but the rarity of the disease is such that controlled trials of different treatment regimens are difficult to perform. Immunosuppressive drugs including cyclophosphamide and azathioprine have also been used with apparent long-term benefit.

Wegener's Granulomatosis

Wegener's granulomatosis is a rare form of vasculitis involving the upper and lower respiratory tracts; often with associated glomerulonephritis. The process differs from polyarteritis nodosa by the presence of necrotizing granulomata and usual absence of aneurysm formation. Widespread vasculitis causes infarction in lungs, kidney, heart, spleen and other organs.

The clinical features of Wegener's granulomatosis include rhinorrhea, symptoms of sinusitis, and facial pain. Otitis media and hearing loss may occur. Skin lesions occur in various forms causing papules, nodules, and actual ulceration. Nonspecific arthralgia and arthritis affect approximately 50 percent of patients. Nephritis presents with hematuria, proteinuria or acute renal failure, and the suspicion of Wegener's granulomatosis is raised by the concurrence of upper respiratory tract and cutaneous lesions.

The chest radiograph may show solitary or multiple nodules, infiltrates, and cavitation. Normochromic anemia, raised sedimentation rate, and leukocytosis are found as nonspecific features. Eosinophilia is less common than in typical polyarteritis nodosa. Elevated serum concentrations of IgG and IgA are frequently found.

Wegener's granulomatosis is more responsive to combinations of corticosteroid and immunosuppressive treatment than to corticosteroids alone. The long-term survival in this disease has been greatly improved in recent years by treatment with cyclophosphamide in combination with prednisone.

Takayasu's Arteritis

This disease was initially described as a vascular ophthalmic disease in patients who had absent radial pulses (hence "pulseless disease"). The syndrome is characterized by an inflammatory reaction in the wall of the aorta and proximal parts of the major arteries. It is more common in Asia and Japan but has rarely been observed in most Western countries.

Histological examination of the affected great vessels shows a stenosing inflammatory reaction with intimal irregularity and fibrosis in the media. A granulomatous reaction with occasional giant cells is sometimes observed.

The patients are usually women in their late teens and early 20s. There is a generalized illness with fever, myalgia, and arthralgia. Partial obstruction of blood flow causes visual disturbance, upper limb claudication, and sometimes angina. Confirmation of the diagnosis is best provided by angiography. Takayasu's arteritis responds to steroid medication in many cases with disappearance of systemic symptoms and sometimes return of arterial pulses. Other forms of treatment, including anticoagulants and arterial surgery, have been employed with varying reported success.

Leukocytoclastic Vasculitis

The leukocytoclastic vasculitides are a group of disorders associated with several identifiable causes. The unifying feature is the pathological appearance of infiltration of necrotic blood vessel walls with neutrophil granulocytes and scattered nuclear debris (leukocytoclasis). The blood vessels involved are of small caliber and often involve postcapillary venules. Some of the disorders associated with leukocytoclastic vasculitis are listed in Table 18.15. Cutaneous lesions are the primary manifestation of the leukocytoclastic vasculitides. The characteristic skin lesion is purpura, often situated on the legs. Various forms of skin lesions may occur, however, including papular, ulcerative, urticarial, and necrotic lesions.

Henoch-Schönlein Purpura

Henoch-Schölein purpura is a vasculitic syndrome characteristically seen in children and young adults. The majority of patients with this disease have a mild illness requiring only general supportive measures. More severe disease with gastrointestinal or other bleeding and renal involvement are usually treated with high dose steroids (see Chapters 4 and 19).

Kawasaki Disease (Mucocutaneous Lymph Node Syndrome)

Kawasaki disease was initially observed in Japan but has been observed in children and young adults in many other countries. Features of the disease are fever, conjunctivitis, oral mucositis, erythema of the palms and soles, variable rash, and nonsuppurative cervical lymphadenopathy. Vasculitis occurs in conjunction with these features and has a particular predelection for the coronary arteries, which resembles the rare form of polyarteritis nodosa seen in children. The disease also resembles an acute childhood exanthem, and this has prompted speculation that it is caused by an infective agent.

Giant Cell Arteritis and Polymyalgia Rheumatica

Giant cell arteritis is also commonly known as temporal arteritis, or cranial arteritis. Although it is uncertain whether the symptoms of polymyalgia rheumatica are due to vasculitis in muscles, it is convenient to discuss this disease with giant cell arteritis because of the close relationship between the two. Both diseases are rare before the age of 55 years. Approximately 50 percent of patients with giant cell arteritis have symptoms typical of polymyalgia rheumatica. And approximately 10 to 20 percent of patients with polymyalgia rheumatica have symptoms of giant cell arteritis early in the course of their disease, and their illness may progress to typical giant cell arteritis.

The pathology of giant cell arteritis is that of an intense inflammatory reaction in the media and intima of medium-sized arteries with a high elastin content. The temporal and other superficial cranial arteries are most frequently involved, but the disease may also affect other large arteries. Microscopic examination shows fragmentation of the internal elastic lamina, intimal proliferation, and progression to occlusion of vessels. Within the arterial wall there is usually a granulomatous reaction with histiocytic giant cells, lymphocytes, and plasma cells.

The initial symptoms in both conditions are usually insidious and vague so that early recognition requires diagnostic vigilance when assessing older patients. Both conditions may be preceded by a phase of nonspecific fever, malaise, anorexia, weight loss,

and polyarthralgia. Polymyalgia rheumatica produces diffuse aching of shoulder girdle muscles, pelvic girdle muscles, and sometimes morning stiffness of muscles and joints. Giant cell arteritis causes temporal or occipital headache, scalp tenderness, diplopia, ptosis, and blurring of vision and may progress to transient or permanent blindness. Involvement of the arterial supply to the tongue and mastication muscles may give rise to "lingual claudication." Involvement of coronary arteries causes sudden onset of angina pectoris. There are no specific physical signs in uncomplicated polymyalgia rheumatica and objective muscle abnormality is unusual except for a few patients who have mild muscle tenderness. Giant cell arteritis may produce palpable thickening of affected arteries with progression to loss of temporal artery pulsation, scalp tenderness, and sometimes even scalp necrosis. Involvement of ophthalmic artery branches with consequent blindness is the most serious potential complication. This may occur within a few days of the onset of symptoms but may also occur many months after the initial polymyalgia symptoms.

Temporal artery biopsy is indicated whenever giant cell arteritis is suspected, and in cases of polymyalgia rheumatica where the diagnosis is in doubt. Temporal artery biopsy is abnormal in up to 90 percent of cases in giant cell arteritis, but may be normal due to patchy disease. Temporal artery biopsies done in uncomplicated polymyalgia rheumatica show abnormalities in from 20 to 40 percent of cases.

There are no specific blood tests for giant cell arteritis or polymyalgia rheumatica. The erthrocyte sedimentation rate usually shows marked elevation in both disorders. There may also be mild normochromic normocytic anemia, and mild disturbance of liver function tests but normal creatine kinase levels.

The natural history of giant cell arteritis and polymyalgia rheumatica is toward remission in a period of a few months to several years. Death early in the course of giant cell arteritis results from brainstem or other cerebral infarction, myocardial infarction, and ruptured aortic aneurysm. Late morbidity and mortality in both conditions are usually from adverse effects of steroid treatment. Progression to blindness can usually be averted by prompt diagnosis and steroid treatment. Visual involvement occasionally occurs during steroid treatment, but most cases with extensive visual loss are those in which the diagnosis was not made promptly. Treatment with prednisone will usually produce dramatic improvement in the muscle pain and stiffness within a few days, and this favorable response is often helpful in confirming the clinical diagnosis. An initial dose of prednisone of 15 mg daily to 30 mg daily is sufficient in polymyalgia rheumatica, with higher dosage being given for giant cell arteritis and for polymyalgia rheumatica in patients who may also have giant cell arteritis-associated symptoms. The steroid dosage is slowly reduced over a period of a few months, with the dose being titrated against the patient's symptoms and, to a lesser extent, the sedimentation rate. Some patients have symptomatic relapse on steroid withdrawal and it may be necessary to continue steroid treatment for two, three, or more years.

INFLAMMATORY MYOSITIS

Striated skeletal muscles are subject to a group of rare inflammatory diseases that have a number of features in common with the collagen-vascular disorders. These diseases occur in distinct form but may occur as components of multisystem collagen-vascular disease; inflammatory myositis is sometimes a major or prominent feature in systemic lupus erythematosus, scleroderma, mixed connective tissue disease, and Sjögren's syndrome. The inflammatory myositides are usually classified as follows:

Type 1—Adult polymyositis
Type 2—Adult dermatomyositis
Type 3—Polymyositis or dermatomyositis associated with malignancy
Type 4—Childhood myositis
Type 5—Myositis occurring in association with other rheumatic or collagen vascular disease

The gross histological appearances of muscle in each of the groups are similar and affect type I and type II fibers. An inflammatory cellular infiltrate is seen scattered throughout the muscle with associated degeneration and necrosis of muscle fibers, and occasional perivascular inflammatory infiltrates. In active disease, regeneration of muscle fibers may be evident. In long standing chronic disease interstitial fibrosis may be widespread, with calcinosis being a feature of advanced disease seen more often in childhood myositis than in adult disease.

Etiology

The association with collagen-vascular diseases suggests that there is an immune basis in most cases of inflammatory myositis. Experimental studies have shown the presence of lymphocytes capable of causing lysis of muscle fibers in tissue culture. A humoral immune process may be present: circulating immune complexes and cryoproteins are present in some patients and antinuclear antibodies are present in from 5 to 20 percent of patients. An antinuclear antibody with particular specificity, designated PM-1, is present in approximately 10 percent of patients. Viral particles have been observed in muscle biopsies in a small number of patients (usually children). The virus particles have usually resembled myxoviruses. Polymyositis and dermatomyositis are associated with internal malignancy in from 10 to 50 percent of patients. This association is seen more commonly than would be expected in matched random population samples, but the strength of the association has varied considerably in different series. The basis for the association of internal malignancy and myositis is not known, but some experimental observations have suggested that muscle fibers and some tumors may have cross-reacting surface antigens.

Polymyositis

The primary symptom is of muscle weakness that occurs in almost all patients and usually has a proximal distribution. This causes, for example, difficulty in climbing steps, and rising from a chair or combing hair. Involvement of neck flexor muscles causes difficulty in raising the head from a pillow. Symptomatic dysphagia occurs in only approximately 10 percent of patients, but esophageal abnormality can be demonstrated by radiographic means in approximately 30 percent of patients. Nonspecific arthralgia is sometimes present usually prior to the onset of muscle symptoms, and about one-third of patients have Raynaud's phenomenon. Visceral involvement is uncommon and most frequently involves the heart and lungs. Cardiac conduction defects, arrhythmia, congestive heart failure, and transient pneumonitis are infrequent causes of cardiorespiratory symptoms in myositic patients.

The physical signs of polymyositis are those of objective weakness in proximal muscle groups. In addition to weak muscles, the muscles may be tender and show evidence of wasting. In chronic polymyositis, muscle contracture causes further disability. The major laboratory abnormality is elevation of muscle enzymes, including creatine kinase and aldolase. The sedimentation rate may be normal or only slightly elevated. Serological findings include antinuclear antibodies and antiglobulin rheumatoid factors in less than 20 percent of patients. Electromyographic examination shows characteristic features.

Dermatomyositis

The clinical features of myositis in dermatomyositis are similar to those in polymyositis and may occur in association with a highly characterisitic rash. The skin may show a lilac discoloration of the eyelids (the heliotrope rash), an erythematous scaly rash involving the extensor surfaces of the joints, especially the fingers, the face, and the anterior upper chest (in a V-shaped pattern), and erythematous scaling patches (Gottron papules) over the metarcarpolphalangeal and proximal interphalangeal joints.

Treatment

Inflammatory myositis usually responds well to corticosteroid treatment. Prednisone, 20 to 30 mg daily, will usually produce symptomatic benefit. High doses of steroids may be necessary to induce improvement but should not be continued for long periods because a secondary steroid myopathy may cause symptoms similar to the inflammatory myositis. Improvement is evaluated by clinical assessment of muscle strength and by estimation of serum concentrations of muscle enzymes. In some patients, the muscle enzyme levels may remain high in the presence of clinical improvement in muscle strength. Patients whose myositis is recalcitrant to corticosteroid treatment often respond to cytotoxic drugs, including methotrexate and azathioprine. Approximately 75 percent of patients with inflammatory myositis respond to corticosteroid or cytotoxic drug therapy. The prognosis depends on the extent of inflammatory muscle damage at the time therapy is commenced.

The association of inflammatory myositis with malignancy indicates the necessity to look for possible occult neoplasia in middle-aged patients presenting with polymyositis or dermatomyositis. The association with malignancy appears to be stronger with dermatomyositis than with simple polymyositis. Associated malignancy most commonly involves the lungs, stomach, and ovary. Myositis may precede the appearance of overt malignancy by several years. If, therefore, initial examination for malignancy is negative, further examination should be undertaken at least once a year in patients whose myositis remains active following treatment.

RAYNAUD'S PHENOMENON

Raynaud's phenomenon is a frequent clinical feature in all of the collagen-vascular diseases. It should be regarded as a symptom-complex occurring in association with disease entities or as an isolated phenomenon, but not as a discrete disease. References to "Raynaud's disease" in earlier literature probably described patients with various collagen-vascular diseases now more clearly defined, for example mixed connective tissue disease and the varieties of vasculitis. Between 50 and 90 percent of patients with Raynaud's phenomenon do not have associated collagen-vascular or other disease, and these patients are said to have "primary Raynaud's phenomenon." The majority of such patients are female and their symptoms usually begin between the second and fourth decades. Suspicion of associated disease should arise in patients with an abrupt onset of symptoms, especially after the third decade, in males, and if the onset of symptoms is during the summer months.

Raynaud's phenomenon gives rise to intermittent and episodic ischemia of the digits. The fingers of both hands are usually affected and in more severe cases the toes, earlobes, and even the tip of the nose may be affected. The characteristic features in the fingers show a triphasic sequence of blanching, cyanosis, and erythema. The sequence is usually initiated by cold exposure or emotional episodes and is often painful during the later part of the sequence. After many years of Raynaud's phenomenon, the fingertips may show evidence of pulp atrophy, cutaneous ulceration, and paronychia. Raynaud's phenomenon is occasionally accompanied by dysphagia in the absence of features of scleroderma. Abnormal motility of the lower esophagus has also been demonstrated in patients with Raynaud's phenomenon in the absence of symptoms of esophageal dysfunction.

The pathogenesis of Raynaud's phenomenon is not clearly understood. The many associated conditions suggests that it represents the final common pathway of several possible mechanisms causing episodic vasospasm. Associated factors include blood hyperviscosity, inflammatory processes in the walls of small blood vessels, and extrinsic factors that may affect the vasomotor innervation. Raynaud's phenomenon is sometimes improved by cervical sympathectomy, and made worse by the administration of beta-blocking drugs, but the manner in which these procedures affect the phenomenon is uncertain.

The circumstances in which Raynaud's phenomenon is encountered are listed in Table 18.16.

Investigation and Management

Patients presenting with Raynaud's phenomenon as the major complaint should be carefully evaluated. If the history is not typical of Raynaud's phenome-

Table 18.16   Associations of Raynaud's Phenomenon

1. Primary Raynaud's phenomenon—50% to 90% of all individuals with Raynaud's phenomenon: no evidence of associated disease
2. Secondary Raynaud's phenomenon—associated with systemic disease or other identifiable cause:
    A. Collagen vascular diseases—scleroderma, progressive systemic sclerosis, CREST syndrome, mixed connective tissue disease, systemic lupus erythematosus, systemic vasculitis, polymyositis, and occasionally rheumatoid arthritis
    B. Central and peripheral vascular disease—cervical ribs and thoracic outlet syndrome giving rise to compression of the subclavian artery or of sympathetic fibres of the brachial plexus, arterial embolization, aneurysm and atherosclerotic disease
    C. Blood disorders—polycythemia, cryoglobulinemia, macroglobulinemia, and cold-agglutinin disease
    D. Toxins and drugs—ergot poisoning, prolonged contact with polyvinyl chloride, arsenic poisoning; methysergide, bleomycin and (?) beta blocking drugs
    E. Occupational and traumatic causes—e.g., pneumatic tool operators, typists, pianists, following prolonged cold exposure or frost bite

non, it may be useful to immerse the hand in cold water for a few minutes to see if the symptoms can be reproduced. If clinical examination and all investigations for the wide variety of associated conditions are negative, the patient is assumed to have primary Raynaud's phenomenon. Where the symptoms are severe or there is suspicion of associated disease, the hematological and serological investigation should be repeated at least annually.

The most effective forms of treatment for Raynaud's phenomenon are symptomatic, and drugs are usually of comparatively little benefit. Excessive cold-exposure should be avoided so far as possible, and gloves should always be worn in circumstances in which cold exposure is expected. Tobacco smoking should be discontinued. Some female patients appear to benefit from discontinuation of oral contraceptives, but the relationship is inconstant. Many different types of drugs have been used in Raynaud's phenomenon, but none show universal or consistent benefit. Most of the drugs employed have effects on sympathetic tone and include phenoxybenzamine, methyldopa, or papaverine. Surgical sympathectomy usually benefits the symptoms of Raynaud's phenomenon, but the improvement is usually temporary and the procedure is now rarely employed.

NONARTICULAR RHEUMATIC DISORDERS

Nonarticular rheumatic disorders are a major community health problem, even though the objective abnormality caused by these syndromes is usually trivial. The group of disorders is sometimes referred to as soft tissue, or nonarticular, rheumatism. The bland nomenclature of these conditions and their undramatic presentation belies their economic importance. Low back pain is a more important cause of lost industrial production that strikes in every industrialized country. The pathology of this group of diverse conditions is very poorly understood, since they are not fatal and rarely are serious enough to warrant biopsy or surgical investigation. Although several of the conditions have the suffix "itis," evidence for inflammatory pathology is generally absent. Most are symptom-complexes, and with the important exception of polymyalgia rheumatica, laboratory tests are characteristically normal. Very often careful history-taking will reveal an occupational or recreational activity which initiates the condition, and this gives a clue to the probable muscular basis of many of these disorders.

Soft tissue rheumatic disorders may mimic or precede more significant disease. Bursitis may be the initial manifestation of gout; nonspecific shoulder pain may be due to coronary artery disease; nonspecific low back pain may be due to bony metastasis of a malignancy, and so on.

FIBROSITIS SYNDROME

The fibrositis syndrome is a chronic painful disorder involving a characteristic group of body sites, and is not accompanied by abnormality on laboratory evaluation. The term *fibrositis* was introduced by the neurologist, Gowers, because it appeared that there was an inflammatory process in the fibers of symptomatic muscle regions. Clinical examination shows that the sites of tenderness are mostly in muscles, and hence the term *fibromyositis* is sometimes used. There may also be tenderness at the sites of muscle insertion such as the lateral humeral epicondyle, which gives origin to the wrist and finger extensors (tennis elbow sites). The fibrositis syndrome is usually seen as an isolated phenomenon with a somewhat lengthy self-limiting course. Occasionally, however, it may be a sequitur, or complication, of organic disease in the shoulder or cervical spine.

These instances give some insight into the etiology of this condition. Deep-seated pain from the neck or shoulder gives rise to painful spasm of the overlying muscles. It appears that sustained spasm causes some minor change in the affected muscle, which is of itself painful. This induces further protective muscle spasm, and so a self-perpetuating vicious circle of pain and spasm is established. Many patients with the fibrositis syndrome are tense or anxious, and in these individuals the fibrositis syndrome seems to represent a somatic reflection of psychological tenseness.

The sites of pain and tenderness are quite characteristic and their distribution constitutes a major feature of the fibrositis syndrome as a discrete entity. Often sites of localized tenderness can be elicited in the expected pattern, even though the patient was not aware of or complaining of symptoms in that particular region. Most typical is tenderness along the upper border of the trapezius muscles and the origins of the supraspinatus muscles close to the medial border of the scapula. Usually the findings are symmetrical, and occasionally areas of induration, or so-called fibrositic nodules, may be palpable. Other sites involved with tenderness include the region of the interspinous ligaments in the lower part of the neck, the lateral and medial epicondyles of the elbows, the region of the upper costochondral junctions at the origin of the pectoralis major muscles, the upper outer quadrants of the buttocks, and the medial joint line of the knee.

Muscle weakness is only associated with pain in use, and significant muscle wasting is not a feature of the fibrositis syndrome. No objective neurological abnormality is found. Some patients show mild hyperreflexia compatible with anxiety.

Anxiety in these patients is sometimes evident with a history of insomnia. Often patients with the fibrositis syndrome complain of more severe symptoms of pain and stiffness upon awakening, and it has been suggested that they do not become satisfactorily relaxed during sleep.

Laboratory investigation for inflammatory disease is uniformly negative in the fibrositis syndrome. The finding of a raised sedimentation rate should lead to consideration of polymyalgia rheumatica in elderly patients.

The fibrositis syndrome is usually self-limiting but may take many months to settle. A good occupational and recreational history should be taken to ascertain if any activity may be giving rise to overusage and initiating pain in symtomatic muscles. Physiotherapy, including range of motion exercises for symptomatic muscles with gentle application of heat, is often helpful. Treatment requires reassurance regarding the possibility of serious rheumatic disease. The possibility of anxiety should be carefully explored with the patient and its relationship to symptoms carefully explained. In some patients with symptomatic sleep disturbances a small dose of a benzodiazepine taken at night may modify the sleep pattern sufficiently to provide considerable relief of symptoms. Symptomatic treatment with small doses of analgesic or anti-inflammatory drugs is sometimes useful, but these drugs have only a minor role in this syndrome.

LOW BACK PAIN

Most patients complaining of low back pain have few, if any, abnormal physical signs to accompany their complaint. In the majority, no structural lesion can be demonstrated by radiographic examination. The anatomical structure of the lower part of the back is highly complex because of the necessity for agility and also the transmission of forces, which may reach the range of 3,000 kg exerted across the area of an intervertebral disc. The possible sources of pain in the low back are numerous, and include sensory nerve endings in apophyseal joint capsules, spinal ligaments, vertebral periosteum, muscles, tendons, and arterial walls. The posterior nerve roots and their branches may be the source of pain by direct pressure from prolapsed discs or osteophytes.

Paravertebral muscle spasm is one of the most common physical abnormalities found in patients with low back pain and appears to amplify and perpetuate pain arising in other structures. Pain arising in abdominal and pelvic viscera may be perceived as low back pain. Finally, the patient's psyche should be taken into account; many patients with persistent low back pain recalcitrant to the best therapeutic endeavours are found to have psychoneurotic, anxious, or frankly depressive traits.

A simple classification of causes of low back pain is listed below.

1. Traumatic, degenerative and mechanical causes, e.g., injury, abnormal posture, pregnancy, obesity, intervertebral disc disease, spondylolisthesis, degenerative joint disease

2. Intrinsic or metabolic bone disease, e.g., osteoporosis, osteomalacia, Paget's disease of bone

3. Infectious processes, e.g., (a) tuberculosis, vertebral and paravertebral abscess, brucellosis; (b) acute febrile illness

4. Inflammatory conditions, e.g., ankylosing spondylitis, sacroiliitis

5. Neoplasms, e.g., primary and metastatic malignancy, myeloma

6. Diseases of abdominal and pelvic organs, e.g., kidneys, uterus, pancreas, aortic aneurysm

7. Developmental abnormality, e.g., spinal stenosis, scoliosis

Intervertebral degenerative disc disease represents a special problem in the lumbar spine (and also in the cervical spine). Aging is associated with change in the annulus fibrosus and in the nucleus pulposus; the fibrillar structure of the annulus becomes coarse and fissuring appears, predisposing to nuclear herniation. These changes are comparable with the age changes described in articular cartilage affecting both collagen and proteoglycans. The gelatinous matrix of the nucleus pulposus is also subject to age changes with decreased proteoglycan size and increasing keratan sulfate content. The water content of the disc decreases with age.

Herniation of the nucleus pulposus through the annulus fibrosus is sometimes acute and caused by sudden mechanical stress. The symptoms include low back pain, with sciatica appropriate to the nerve root compressed by the herniated disc material. Typically the radiating pain is exacerbated by Valsalva maneuver procedures such as occur in coughing and defecation. The physical findings in this condition depend on the presence and extent of nerve root involvement. Evidence of neurological abnormality in the distribution of affected roots is of major diagnostic importance. Loss or impairment of sensation in lumbar or sacral segment(s) helps to define the level of disc prolapse. Impaired ability to raise a leg with the knee extended because of pain is highly suggestive of nerve root involvement. However, this finding may be due to hip disease, and sciatic stretch tests such as the Lasegue maneuver are necessary to confirm the sciatic origin of the pain. Midline disc herniation with involvement of sacral roots gives rise to bladder and rectal sphincter symptoms.

In the general examination of a patient with low back pain, it is important to note whether there is flattening of the normal lumbar lordosis, whether there is any lateral displacement of the spinous processes, indicating scoliosis, and whether there is associated asymmetry of the paravertebral musculature, indicating spasm. The area of pain should be palpated for areas of superficial myofascial tenderness, and percussed for areas of bone tenderness. The sacroiliac joints are deeply situated and covered with thick muscles so that considerable pressure is necessary to elicit tenderness in those joints.

SHOULDER PAIN

The shoulder has an extraordinary range of movement, which arises, in concert, at the glenohumeral joint, acromioclavicular joint, sternoclavicular joint, and scapulothoracic articulation. A patient complaining of pain in the shoulder may have something wrong with one of these joints, but it is necessary to recall that pain may be referred to the shoulder in cardiac abnormalities, from the diaphragm and from the cervical spine. In fact, the majority of patients complaining of shoulder pain do not have any abnormality of these structures but rather have a disorder involving the periarticular musculature and tendons.

The glenohumeral joint, like any other synovial joint, is subject to involvement in rheumatoid arthritis. It is also involved occasionally in ankylosing spondylitis and pseudogout, but involvement in generalized degenerative joint disease and in gout is uncommon. Neuropathic involvement of the shoulder joint occurs in syringomyelia.

Nonarticular causes of chronic shoulder pain involving the periarticular soft tissue include the following:

1. Rotator cuff lesions. Rotator cuff tears are usually of traumatic origin and have a sudden onset of symptoms. However, repeated occupational or recreational stress to the shoulder may weaken the supraspinatus, infraspinatus, and teres minor tendons that comprise the rotator cuff, and progress to actual rupture. Rotator cuff lesions cause inability or difficulty to abduct the arm but it can be held abducted if elevated to 90 degrees by the deltoid muscle.

2. Bicipital tendonitis and tenosynovitis cause anterior shoulder pain made worse by either internal rotation and/or abduction of the shoulder. Often the pain radiates along the bicipital groove and may be perceived mid-way between the shoulder and the elbow. This syndrome usually responds to injection of microcrystalline depot steroid around the biceps tendon.

3. Supraspinatus (calcific) tendonitis. The supraspinatus tendon and, to a lesser extent, the infraspinatus tendon are the site of degenerative and inflammatory lesions in middle-aged persons. Degeneration of the supraspinatus tendon is commonly followed by calcium deposition and this sometimes becomes symptomatic. Pain arising from the supraspinatus tendon region causes pain on movement, especially in abduction and forward flexion. An acute onset, or marked exacerbation, may occur if the deposit of hydroxyapatite discharges into

the subacromial bursa. Often patients with supraspinatus tendonitis have a "painful arc" in which maximum pain is experienced when the shoulder is abducted through an arc usually in the range of 70 to 100 degrees of abduction. Calcific supraspinatus tendonitis is one of the few lesions in which radiographic examination is useful in evaluation of the painful shoulder. Calcified deposits are seen in the suprasinatus and other tendons around the shoulder in approximately 3 percent of the general population, but the demonstration of such calcification in a patient with appropriate symptoms and signs is useful in confirming the clinical diagnosis. The symptoms of supraspinatus tendonitis often resolve spontaneously, but this may take several weeks or several months. Resolution can often be accelerated by physical modalities of treatment such as ultrasound, ice packs and short-wave diathermy. Local injection of steroid mixed with one to two ml of 1 percent local anesthetic may be helpful.

4. Bursitis. There are several bursae located around the shoulder, including the subacromial bursa and its lateral extension, the subdeltoid bursa, the subscapularis bursa, and bursae situated close to the insertions of several of the muscles around the shoulder. Subacromial bursal inflammation is the most frequent, and causes discomfort in abduction of the shoulder, often with a "painful arc" phenomenon. Local point tenderness may be evident on clinical examination. Treatment with physical modalities and injection of depot steroid is usually helpful, but anti-inflammatory medication may be necessary in addition to the other forms of treatment.

5. Frozen shoulder (adhesive capsulitis). The frozen shoulder syndrome occurs secondary to several local and remote causes. Fibrosis and tightening of the capsular and periarticular ligaments occurs, causing marked restriction of movement at the glenohumeral joint. It may follow trauma to the shoulder, or from any of the conditions previously described, causing chronic limitation of movement at the shoulder joint. The syndrome also occurs in association with coronary disease, stroke, following thoracotomy, and in association with disorders of the cervical spine. The physical findings are of diffuse tenderness and marked restriction of both active and passive movement at the shoulder. Treatment requires persistence with physiotherapy to mobilize the shoulder. Severe adhesive capsulitis may necessitate manipulation of the shoulder under general anesthesia. Analgesics and anti-inflammatory agents usually provide symptomatic relief, particularly during mobilization exercises.

6. Shoulder-hand syndrome (reflex neurovascular dystrophy). The shoulder-hand syndrome comprises the association of pain and limitation of movement at the shoulder together with pain, swelling, and stiffness involving the hand and fingers. The syndrome occurs in association with myocardial infarction, stroke, trauma to the neck and shoulder, spinal cord lesions, and administration of certain drugs, especially antituberculous drugs and barbiturates. In the later stages of this syndrome, the distal upper limb shows trophic skin changes and edema, and may be diffusely tender. The syndrome is bilateral in approximately one-fourth of cases. The pathogenesis is uncertain but it is believed to arise from a reflex sympathetic dystrophy comparable to causalgia. Radiographic examination of the hand in established cases often shows patchy or mottled osteoporosis. Treatment of the shoulder-hand syndrome is with analgesics and physical modalities, including local application of heat or cold. Severe shoulder-hand syndrome sometimes requires and responds to systemic steroid treatment given for a few weeks.

7. The fibrositis syndrome and polymyalgia rheumatica. These two syndromes have been previously described. They differ from most of the painful shoulder syndromes described above in that they usually produce bilateral shoulder pain. Polymyalgia rheumatica should always be suspected when an elderly patient complains of shoulder pain, especially if this is most marked on waking. The finding of an elevated sedimentation rate differentiates polymyalgia rheumatica from almost all of the other nonarthritic causes of painful shoulder.

REFERENCES

Disorders of Joints and Connective Tissues (Textbooks)

1. Katz, W.A., ed: Rheumatic Diseases—Diagnosis and Management. Philadelphia, J.B. Lippincott, 1977.
2. Kelley, W.M., Harris, E.D., Ruddy, S., Sledge, C.B., eds.: Textbook of Rheumatology. Philadelphia, WB Saunders, 1981.
3. McCarty, D.J., ed: Arthritis and Allied Conditions. 9th ed. Philadelphia, Lee and Febiger, 1979.

Specialized Reviews

4. Bitter, T., Calin, A., Hughes, G.V., eds: Symposium on Reiter's Syndrome. Annals of the Rheumatic Diseases, 38, supplement 1, 1979.

5. Cupps, T.R., Fauci, A.S.: The Vasculitides. Major Problems in Internal Medicine, XXI, Philadelphia, W.B. Saunders, 1981.
6. Hasselbacher, P., ed: The biology of the joint. Clinics in Rheumatic Diseases 7:3–87, 1981.
7. Lawrence, J.S.: Rheumatism in Populations. London, W. Heinemann, 1977.
8. Williams, R.C., Jr.: Rheumatoid Arthritis as a Systemic Disease. Philadelphia, W.B. Saunders, 1974.
9. Wright, V., Moll, J.M.H.: Sero-negative Polyarthritis. Amsterdam, North Holland, 1976.
10. New Directions for Research in Systemic Lupus Erythematosus. Arthritis and Rheumatism, 21, supplement 5, S1-S229, 1978.

19

Diseases of the Skin

Tom Enta, M.D.

The skin is so visible that patients expect every physician to make a diagnosis, prescribe an effective treatment and even a cure. With several thousands of skin disorders recorded, the non-dermatologist may find the correct diagnosis less than obvious. This chapter attempts to present principles which will provide some direction in the care of patients with skin diseases. A summary of structure and function of the skin is followed by an overview of important morphologic changes in disease. Three major areas of dermatology are emphasized: (1) serious skin diseases that require early recognition and treatment to prevent death, (2) common disorders which can be recognized by a few characteristic features, and (3) cutaneous changes that are associated with systemic diseases. These didactic approaches must be supplemented by practical experience in clinics and hospital wards.

STRUCTURE AND FUNCTION OF THE SKIN

STRUCTURE

Epidermis and Dermis

The skin consists of two layers, the epidermis and dermis. The epidermis is concerned with the production of keratin, which is constantly shed from the surface of the skin. It also contains the melanin-producing cell, the melanocyte. The dermis provides strength through its fibrous elements and contains other vital structures (Fig. 19.1).

The epidermis is made up of a stratified cellular layer, held together by intracellular processes, known as desmosomes (Fig. 19.2). The basal cells divide repetitively and move to the surface. They are initially cuboidal but become flat and anuclear as they move to the surface. The maturing cells produce a fibrillar protein, keratin, which gives the outermost layer, the stratum corneum, its toughness. Migration of the cells from the basal area to the surface takes approximately 28 days. The melanocytes, scattered between the basal cells, produce melanin from phenylalanine and pass the pigment to the keratinocytes by injection through their dendritic processes. The epidermis is firmly attached to the dermis by desmosomes that anchor into the basal lamina, which in turn is attached to the dermis through fibrils resembling collagen.

The dermis is a highly organized structure. Its main component is collagen fibers, which may vary in thickness depending on age, sex, or site; the thickest area is on the back and the thinnest is on the eyelids. The collagen fibers, secreted by fibroblasts, are arranged in a three-dimensional pattern, apparently organized to withstand stress. Elastic fibers, which are finer and take up much less volume are associated with the collagen; these fibers are embedded in a ground substance containing mucopolysaccharides. Other cells in the dermis include mast cells and histiocytes. The dermis also contains nerve endings, blood vessels, and appendages.

Free nerve endings occur most frequently around hair follicles. The specialized nerve endings, such as Pacinian and Meissner's corpuscles, and Merkel's disc, occur in non-hairy areas and along mucocutaneous junctions. Temperature, touch, and pain are transmitted through the free nerve endings. The Pacinian corpuscle is involved in pressure sensation.

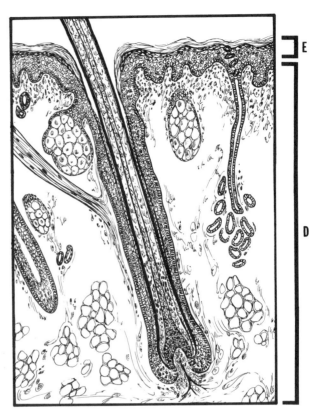

Fig. 19.1 The skins 2 layers: epidermis (E), dermis (D). The apparently loosely structured dermis is highly organized with a structured network of collagen and elastin, blood vessels, glands and several specialized cells.

Skin Vasculature

The skin vessels are found in the dermis and consist of vessels that lie in the reticular dermis, and the vital microcirculation in the papillary zone. The arterioles and venules lie horizontally in the subpapillary zone. A fine ascending capillary comes off the arteriole and courses into the papillary area, makes a loop and then descends down and joins the postcapillary venules. Lymphatic vessels, present in great abundance in the skin, begin in the papillary area and extend downward in a network to form larger vessels. Their role is to remove protein, water, and minerals from the extracellular space of the dermis.

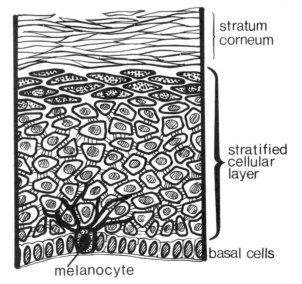

Fig. 19.2 The epidermis with three layers and a melanocyte. See text for details.

Hair

Hairs are present everywhere except on the palms and soles. There are some five million hairs; the scalp contains one hundred thousand. Hair follicles remain constant in number after birth, although the number of hairs is modified throughout life, showing a decline after middle age. The hair grows from a root consisting of specialized epidermal cells surrounding a core of dermal tissue (Fig. 19.3). The cells of the root contain melanocytes that provide color to the hair. Many of the characteristics, including growth, of hair are genetically controlled. The length of the hair is dependent on the follicular growth phase, which lasts for three to four years (anagen) (Fig. 19.4). At this time, the follicle rapidly involutes (catagen) and the hair is left resting with its root in the upper dermis. This resting hair, called club hair, falls out in two to three months (telogen). Usually a new hair develops in a new follicle in the vicinity of the old as the resting hair is shed. In early infancy, the

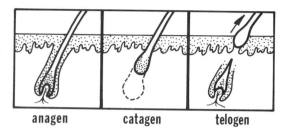

Fig. 19.4 The three growth phases of a hair, see text for description.

hair follicles of the scalp are in the same growth phase so that hair loss and growth tend to be synchronous. Later in childhood, and in the adult, hair follicles grow independently and the growth and shedding are now asynchronous, with 80 percent or more of the hairs being in the growth phase. After acute disease such as pneumonia or after surgery or pregnancy, a greater number of hairs tend to rest together and this leads to a transient hair loss known as telogen effluvium.

Nails

The nails, hard laminated keratin plates at the dorsal ends of the digits, grow approximately 0.1 mm per day. The nail plate develops from the nail matrix, a special group of epidermal cells that grows downward into the skin. The end of the matrix is the lunula, marked by the pale, opaque semilunar portion at the proximal end of the nail. Much of the nail plate is produced by the matrix in a process of keratinization similar to hair or epidermis, although a small contribution comes from the keratin of the underlying nail bed. The nail plate, nail bed, and the nail folds may be involved in disease processes.

Sebaceous Glands

These lobulated oil glands empty into the associated hair follicles. They are found in great numbers on the scalp, face, upper parts of the chest, and back. Their secretions consist of a mixture of fatty acids, triglycerides, squalene, wax esters, and cholesterol. They are under endocrine control, with their greatest activity beginning at puberty and then declining over many years.

Apocrine Glands

Apocrine sweat glands are found in the axillae and anogenital areas. The apocrine glands open to the skin or into the hair follicles and are structured like

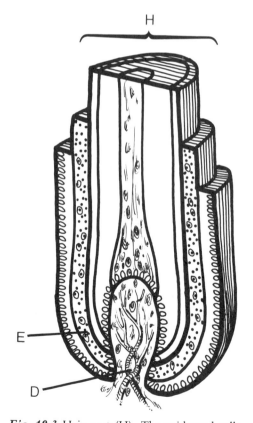

Fig. 19.3 Hair root (H). The epidermal cells (E) surround the hair follicle and a pouch of dermal tissue (D) forms at the base of the nerve root. See also Fig. 19.1 and the text.

the eccrine glands. The secretions are odorless but become foul smelling as a result of bacterial action.

Eccrine Sweat Glands

Eccrine sweat glands cover most of the body. They consist of a secretory coil in the deep dermis that passes upward to the epidermis through a straight duct, which coils in a spiral fashion as it passes through the stratum corneum. The glands are innervated by sympathetic fibers but are cholinergically mediated. Sweat plays an important role in electrolyte transport and thermoregulation. Sweating under emotional stress (psychogenic sweating) is confined to such areas as the palms, soles, face, and axillae, while sweating under stimulus of temperature (thermal sweating) is more generalized.

Smooth Muscle

The dermis contains narrow bands of smooth muscle that attach to the hair follicle at one end and the dermal collagen at the other (arrector pili). Contraction of the muscle leads to the "goose pimple" effect of the skin. There are larger accumulations of smooth muscle around the nipple and scrotum.

FUNCTION

The skin plays a major role in protection against a hostile environment and allows man to adapt to a wide variation of environmental conditions. Its tough dermal collagen fibers equip the skin to resist mechanical injury, while the stratified and keratinized epidermis is impervious to microorganisms, chemicals, or even body fluids. Pigmentation in the epidermis establishes resistance to ultraviolet injury.

Skin plays a vital role in temperature control. The reduction of skin blood flow on exposure to cold reduces body heat loss. Increase in blood flow to the skin in response to heat, and the evaporation of sweat from the eccrine sweat glands, increases heat loss and enables man to remain cool in a hot environment, or to defervesce after a fever.

The production of vitamin D_3 in the epidermis is an important function in the absence of dietary vitamin D. The provitamin is converted by short ultraviolet light to vitamin D_3, which is removed from the skin and transported to the liver through the bloodstream.

The skin is a sensitive organ of sensation, responding to hot, cold, pain, and touch. This plays an es-

sential protective function, as well as a vital role in social and sexual communication.

THE BASIS OF DERMATOLOGIC DIAGNOSIS

EXAMINATION

The traditional approach to a medical problem is to take a careful history followed by a thorough examination. In dermatology it is often advantageous to see the lesion and then ask questions. The color and characteristic morphologic changes are often sufficient to suggest the diagnosis. The questions in the history can then be asked to pursue the suspected diagnosis.

The color of normal skin results from the reflection of light from components of the epidermis such as melanin, carotenoids, and components of the dermis (connective tissue and blood vessels). The normal skin is pink-white in color in a lightly pigmented individual. Temporary changes in color from red (erythema) to blue (cyanosis) result from the amounts and proportions of oxyhemoglobin and reduced hemoglobin. The longer-lasting color changes of the skin referred to as hyper- or hypo-pigmentation result from the presence of melanin and at times hemosiderin in the epidermal keratinocytes and the dermal macrophages. An example is hyperpigmentation, seen at the ankle in stasis dermatitis. The most obvious absence of pigment is vitiligo.

Characteristics of Skin Lesions

The skin involved in disease presents with a variety of visible and palpable changes (Fig. 19.5). Descriptive terms help to characterize the lesions:

Papule—the simplest change in the skin, a small (1–3 mm) bump or elevation.
Macule—an area of color change on the surface of the skin, of varying size, usually with no elevation.
Nodule—a solid palpable mass in the skin.
Tumor—often used interchangeably with nodule, usually refers to a larger mass.
Plaque—an elevated macule resulting from a confluence of papules or abnormal thickening of some layers of the skin.
Wheal—a raised macule usually round in configuration, with the bulk of the swelling consisting of extracellular fluid. It is evanescent.
Vesicle—a small blister.

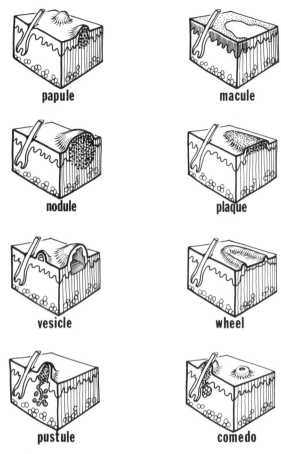

Fig. 19.5 Typical visible or palpable abnormalities of skin. See text for definition of each lesion.

Bulla—a larger blister. Vesicles and bullae may arise within the epidermis, at the dermoepidermal junction, or subepidermally.

Pustule—a distinct type of papule made up of pus.

Comedo—a papule, associated with a sebaceus gland in which the opening pore is obstructed by dark keratinous material (blackhead).

Purpura—the dark bluish discoloration of the skin resulting from extravasated red blood cells.

Petechia—multiple, punctate, purplish-brown accumulations of red blood cells.

Ecchymosis—well-demarcated blue or purplish-brown discoloration due to collections of blood in the dermis and subcutaneous tissues.

Telangiectasis—visible, dilated capillaries which may develop with age or during pregnancy, in systemic disorders, including cirrhosis, and certain collagen vascular diseases.

Skin lesions are commonly accompanied by secondary changes that result from breakdown of the primary lesion, for example infection of a vesicle, or scratching and rubbing of a wheal.

Acutely inflamed skin often weeps or oozes exudate, particularly after denuding or erosion as a result of scratching. The exudate will dry, producing *crusts*. Inflammation of the skin leads to increased keratinization of the epidermis with subsequent desquamation or *scaling* from the surface. Inflammatory lesions at the angles of the orifices and at the folds with loose skin may form *fissures*. Involvement of epidermis and dermis leads to loss of the surface resulting in *ulcers*. As lesions heal, they may form *scars* that may be atrophic and appear depressed or hypertrophic as a result of proliferation of collagen. *Lichenification* is the palpable thickening of the skin, usually as a result of long standing rubbing and scratching.

The surface configuration may direct our thinking toward a diagnosis. The annular or ring-like pattern is characteristic of the fungal infection in tinea corporis or granuloma annulare. Linear lesions are characteristic of scratch or injury lines. Concentric circles referred to as iris, target, or bull's eye lesions are found in erythema multiforme. Some lesions like those of herpes simplex or herpes zoster appear in grape-like clusters, or may involve a band of skin, often following a dermatome.

Many skin conditions appear at characteristic sites. Psoriasis is often found on the elbows and knees, but the reason for this localization is unknown. In some, there is an explanation for the sites of predilection; sun sensitive dermatosis appear on the exposed areas, candidiasis is found in the axillae and groins since the causative organism thrives in warm moist areas.

HISTORY

The appearance of the skin change is the guide to questioning. The history is essential in allergic contact dermatitis, drug-related eruptions, or occupational dermatitis. Functional inquiry regarding body systems will help to determine whether a skin change is part of a systemic disorder (see section below entitled Cutaneous Manifestations of Systemic Diseases). A family history is essential in genetic disorders. A few appropriate questions will yield vital information regarding the onset of the condition, the nature of the topical or systemic therapy, and response to past medications and surgical procedures.

LABORATORY INVESTIGATIONS

Many patients require no specific laboratory investigation. Where the eruption is part of a systemic disease, appropriate blood work, urinalysis, and radiological examinations are undertaken. The use of an adequate light microscope is essential. In suspected fungus infection, examination of hair, scales, and nails, using potassium hydroxide solution to reduce the obscuring keratin, may be diagnostic. An ultraviolet lamp (Wood's lamp) is useful in fungus infection of the scalp and tinea versicolor, revealing a blue-green fluorescence. Cultures for fungi may be helpful but take several weeks. In viral infections such as herpes simplex, chicken pox, and zoster, a smear of the vesicular contents stained with Wright's or Giemsa's stain (Tzank smear) reveals the typical giant cells under the light microscope. A Gram stain of exudates and pus from abscesses will identify the nature of the infection. A Scotch tape smear taken from the perianal skin will reveal the ova of pinworms.

Skin biopsy is a relatively simple procedure that should be used selectively. The skin biopsy may be a superficial shave using a scalpel, a punch biopsy, or an incisional or excisional biopsy. Appropriate stains and examination by light microscopy, electron microscopy, or immunofluorescence may permit definitive diagnosis. The specific diagnostic approaches are discussed in relation to each condition.

POTENTIALLY LETHAL SKIN DISORDERS

Every physician should be able to recognize potentially life threatening skin conditions, which are fortunately few in number.

TOXIC EPIDERMAL NECROLYSIS AND THE STAPHYLOCOCCAL SCALDED SKIN SYNDROME

These two conditions are characterized by marked erythema of the skin, followed by large flaccid blisters and shedding of inflamed necrotic epidermis (Fig. 19.6). In toxic epidermal necrolysis (TEN), the raw, oozing, painful surfaces appear like a burn. Death has occurred in 20 percent or more of the cases. The major cause is drugs such as phenylbutazone, sulphonamides, and hydantoin. Treatment consists of stopping the causal drug, administration of systemic corticosteroids, and symptomatic treatment of the denuded skin.

In the staphylococcal scalded skin syndrome (SSS) the presentation is usually somewhat different from TEN. The eyelids, neck, and axillae become involved first. The cause in a child is infection of the conjunctiva and skin with staphylococcus. The condition is histologically distinct from TEN. The

course is self limiting and death is unusual, but treatment with the appropriate antibiotic hastens the cure.

ERYTHEMA MULTIFORME

Erythema multiforme is characterized by recurrent attacks of red papules, target lesions, and in severe forms, large bullae of the skin. The most severe bullous form known as *Stevens-Johnson syndrome* is characterized by sudden onset of lesions involving many areas of the skin, as well as mucous membranes of the eyes, mouth, genitalia, and pharyngeal and bronchial mucosa (Fig. 19.7). The disease is usually associated with marked constitutional symptoms and high fever. The mucous membranes show extensive bullous formation followed by erosions. Involvement of the bronchi and lungs is manifested by cough, dyspnea, and secondary infection. Purulent conjunctivitis may be complicated by corneal ulcerations and anterior uveitis. Oral lesions make food intake very painful. Renal and cardiac involvement may occur. The mortality rate of untreated cases has been as high as 15 percent. The Stevens-Johnson syndrome results from a hypersensitivity to drugs, or viral or mycoplasma infections. In the severe bullous form, treatment requires high doses of a corticosteroid (prednisone 60 to 80 mg daily) and supportive measures including fluids and systemic antibiotics.

PEMPHIGUS VULGARIS

Pemphigus vulgaris is probably the most lethal of the various blistering disorders. It is found in both sexes and at all ages, but generally occurs in the 40 to 60 year age group. Prior to the use of corticosteroids, death was the most likely outcome. The blisters form in the suprabasalar region of epidermis as a result of loss of epidermal cell adhesion, associated with an immune reaction directed at the intercellular substance. An unexplained specific IgG antibody is found in the serum and between the epidermal cells. The disease often starts slowly, with lesions localized in the mouth or on some part of the skin. The large blisters break, leaving poorly healing erosions in the mouth and on the skin. A blister extends when it is pressed due to acantholysis, and the epidermis will separate when rubbed, touched, or pinched (Nikolsy sign). Secondary infection is common.

The diagnosis is suggested by the involvement of the mouth and the presence of rapidly breaking bullae. Skin biopsy examined with light microscopy and with immunofluorescence will confirm the diagnosis. Treatment requires a high daily dose of prednisone (100 – 150 mg daily) and immunosuppressive

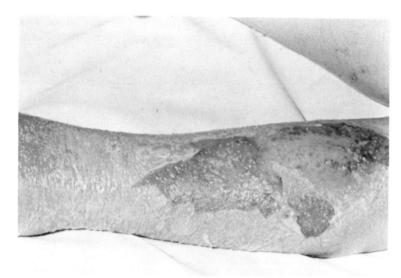

Fig. 19.6 Toxic epidermal necrolysis with extensive epidermal loss

drugs such as azathioprine. The disease can generally be controlled. Death, when it occurs, is then related to drug toxicity.

MALIGNANT TUMORS OF THE SKIN

Malignant Melanoma

This tumor arising from epidermal melanocytes or the junctional component of a nevus has a great potential for metastasizing widely. The lesions are found on any part of the body and appear to have a clear relationship to long-standing sun exposure. It occurs most commonly in fair-complexioned persons. While it accounts for only 3 percent of malignant skin tumors, it is responsible for two-thirds of deaths due to skin malignancies. The rate of growth, clinical course, and response to treatment are remarkably variable. There are at least three distinctive forms of melanomas.

Superficial spreading melanoma (SSM) appears as a pigmented lesion in which there is a color variation with shades of black, purple, brown, red and an area of white. The border appears to extend outward and takes on an irregular contour. The surface changes from being flat and smooth to irregular and will eventually show ulceration. SSM grows laterally for several years, but will eventually show vertical penetration (Fig. 19.8).

Nodular melanoma appears as a black or dark dome-shaped lesion, usually with a smooth surface. This form of melanoma has greater metastatic potential, since it quickly penetrates the dermis and invades un-

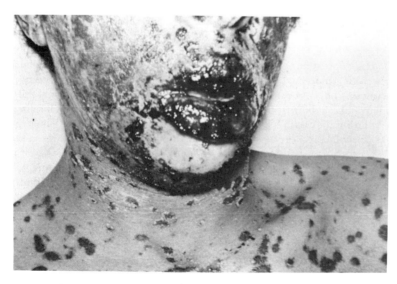

Fig. 19.7 Stevens-Johnson Syndrome with extensive involvement of skin, oral and pharyngeal mucosa

derlying tissues. A large clear cell is characteristically seen in the biopsy. When malignant cells remain at the epidermodermal junction it is classified as level one; when cells reach the papillary dermis, level two; when cells penetrate the reticular dermis, level three; and those that penetrate the lower reaches of the dermis and beyond, levels four and five. Prognosis is related to the depth of penetration and the thickness of the tumor.

The *melanotic freckle* of Hutchison (Lentigo Maligna) is a much more benign lesion. This begins as a freckle in the elderly and over many years enlarges. The area eventually becomes melanomatous but behaves much like a basal cell carcinoma, rarely metastasizing.

The primary treatment of melanomas is surgical, and the ultimate prognosis and survival rate depend on the complete excision of lesions with the least penetration. Chemotherapy and immunotherapy are under active investigation and show promise for certain tumors.

Invasive Squamous Cell Carcinoma

Squamous cell carcinoma results from environmental factors including sunlight, x-rays, gamma rays and derivatives of tar and oil. Squamous cell carcinoma also develops in chronic scars, ulcers, and inflammatory sinuses. A squamous cell carcinoma usually appears as a flat scaly lesion with a base of mild erythema. At this stage only a biopsy will differentiate this from an actinic keratosis. As the carcinoma develops, the lesion becomes elevated, firm,

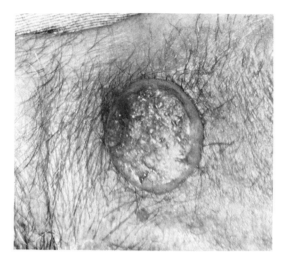

Fig. 19.9 Squamous cell carcinoma

bleeds easily, crusts, and fails to heal (Fig. 19.9). Squamous cell carcinoma is seen commonly on the pinnae of the ears, the backs of the hands, on the lower lip, and at sites of chronic irritation. Metastasis from a squamous cell carcinoma arising in an actinic keratosis is very low, while those arising in areas of radiation dermatitis, scars, and inflammatory ulcers metastasize frequently. Early treatment by excision, electrosurgery, and radiation therapy effectively reduce the mortality of invasive squamous cell carcinoma.

Cutaneous Metastasis

Cutaneous metastases generally appear as firm, flesh-colored or purple nodules or papules, generally in the dermis or subcutaneous tissues. These are readily biopsied and their histology may indicate the probable site of the primary tumor. This extent of metastases indicates a grave prognosis unless the tumor is sensitive to chemotherapy or radiation therapy.

COMMON SKIN DISORDERS

BLISTERING DISORDERS

Several skin disorders present with blisters as the dominant clinical feature. The potentially lethal disorders are pemphigus vulgaris, TEN and Erythema Multiforme, discussed in the preceding section. Milder conditions are outlined below.

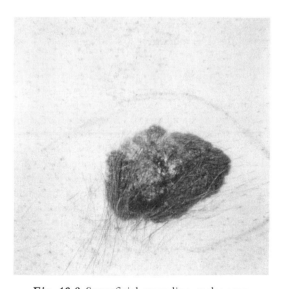

Fig. 19.8 Superficial spreading melanoma

Pemphigoid

Pemphigoid, a milder variant than pemphigus vulgaris, is seen in the elderly and associated with antibody (IgG) directed at the epidermodermal junction. The blisters are often preceded by pruritis and urticaria. They are usually large, numerous, and found on the chest and abdomen. The mouth may be involved. The blister ultimately ruptures, leaving an ulceration that heals slowly. A distinctive mucous membrane form may attack the mouth, rectum, vagina, and eyes, leading to fibrous scarring. The treatment consists of systemic corticosteroids and immunosuppressive drugs.

Dermatitis Herpetiformis

This blistering condition of unknown cause occurs about twice as frequently in men and appears at any age, though it is more common in the third to fifth decades. The outstanding features include intense burning or itching, eruptions of red papules, urticarial lesions, and at times grouped vesicles on the elbows, knees, upper back, and buttocks. The eruptions usually continue for years. The disease is associated with distinctive deposition of IgA at the epidermodermal junction. About 80 percent of the patients have coeliec disease, though the exact relationship is uncertain. The disease responds fairly well to diaminodiphonyl sulfone.

Sunburn

Acute skin lesions ranging from erythema to induration and vesiculation may result from sun exposure. Persons with little skin pigmentation and fair hair are more vulnerable than the deeply pigmented. The intensity and duration of exposure are also important factors.

Several factors predispose to this form of ultraviolet light injury: albinism, because there is lack of pigment shielding; xeroderma pigmentosa, due to defects in skin repair mechanisms; and porphyria, due to development of toxic metabolites. Photosensitivity is also seen as a result of a wide range of medications (see Cutaneous Reactions to Drugs) and in diseases such as lupus erythematosus.

The best preventive measure consists of shading from sunlight; a variety of sunscreen lotions provide substantial screening for ultraviolet rays.

Premature skin aging and skin carcinomas occur as a result of excessive and recurrent sun exposure.

ECZEMATOUS GROUP

Seborrheic Dermatitis

This is a common disorder, affecting individuals from the cradle to the grave. It consists of simple scaling on a mild to moderate erythematous base located in the hirsute areas of the body. It is found on the scalp, particularly in infants as adherent scaling (cradle cap), postauricular area, external ear canals (otitis externa), eyelids (marginal blepharitis), nasolabial areas of the face, central areas of the chest, back, axillae, and groin. In infants, it may be widespread, looking not unlike psoriasis and causing considerable diaper dermatitis. The cause of this subacute inflammatory process of the pilosebaceus unit is unknown, although it is localized to areas with a high density of sebaceus glands. Curiously, it occurs in some adults who are confined in the intensive coronary units following a myocardial infarction, or on neurological units in patients who have had a stroke or suffer from Parkinsonism. Perhaps these individuals who cannot carry on a normal hygienic routine of face and body washing suffer from the irritating effects of the sebaceus material. The course of seborrheic dermatitis is variable; in infants it disappears in a year or more; in adults it is recurrent, diminishing in the summer but returning in the winter. Ultraviolet light has beneficial effects, as does regular washing with soap and shampooing of the scalp. The condition is well controlled with solutions and creams of topical corticosteroids including hydrocortisone.

Nummular Dermatitis

This is a common eczematous eruption with multiple coin-sized lesions, particularly on the extremities. The lesions begin as papules that rapidly enlarge to 2 to 3 cm in diameter and show fine vesiculation on the surface. These lesions are extremely pruritic and often associated with dyshidrosis of the hands and feet. Some individuals with atopic dermatitis develop lesions with a nummular pattern, but true nummular dermatitis is a distinctive entity. The cause is unknown and the course is unpredictable. The histologic appearance consists of a perivascular lymphocytic infiltration of the dermis and spongiosis of the epidermis. It responds reasonably well to topical corticosteroids but on occasion requires systemic corticosteroids.

Dyshidrosis

This is one of the more common and most troublesome vesicular eruptions of the hands and feet. Small vesicles containing clear fluid, often seen at the sides of the fingers and on the palms, are rapidly followed by inflammation of the skin with swelling, redness, desquamation, and fissuring. At times the vesicles become pustular and a true secondary infection may take place. Dyshidrosis can begin in childhood, although generally it occurs in adults. It is tempting to assume that the vesicles represent obstructed eccrine sweat glands, but this does not appear to be the case and the cause remains an enigma. The histological changes consist of nonspecific inflammation with intraepidermal vesicles. The usual course is one of numerous recurrences requiring topical or occasionally oral corticosteroids, and appropriate antibiotics.

Prurigo and Lichen Simplex Chronicus

In the temperate zones with cold winters, prurigo hemalis is common. This is characterized by extreme drying of epidermis (xerosis), with noticeable desquamation. It is often accompanied by cracking of the surface down to the basal layers of epidermis. This leads to mild inflammation and considerable itching. This so-called *eczema cracquele* responds well to measures designed to preserve skin moisture, such as less frequent bathing and bathing followed with an emollient, or an emollient containing mild strength corticosteroid.

Lichen Simplex Chronicus has replaced the older term of *localized neurodermatitis*. This is characterized by palpably thickened plaques, usually accompanied by hypo- and hyperpigmentation. The acanthosis or thickening of the epidermis is induced by repeated scratching and rubbing. In some patients the thickening may be nodular (prurigo nodularis). Treatment requires persistent application of topical corticosteroids, sometimes aided by polyethylene film cover, or occasionally intralesional corticosteroid injections.

Pityriasis Alba

This common affliction of children and young adults is characterized initially by mild erythematous patches on the face and outer aspects of the upper extremities. The mild inflammation is replaced by circular hypopigmented patches, at times confused with vitiligo. Other than its annoying cosmetic effect, it is usually asymptomatic. The cause is unknown. Treatment may be undertaken with topical corticosteroid on the eczematous areas or exposure to sunlight to aid in repigmentation of the spots.

Stasis Dermatitis

Stasis dermatitis occurs after the third decade and is a result of poor venous return from the lower extremities in patients with varicose veins, valvular incompetence, thrombophlelitis of the leg and pelvic veins, or in association with increased abdominal pressure due to ascites, pregnancy, or obesity. The poor venous return leads to chronic edema of the lower extremity.

The dermatitis consists of hyperpigmentation of the lower third of the leg, particularly around the ankle areas, as a result of extravasation of red blood cells into the dermis through ruptured capillaries. The vitality of the skin of this area is jeopardized, leading to eczematous changes with scaling, itching, and exudation, often complicated by secondary cellulitis. Some patients with severe stasis dermatitis develop a papulomacular eruption on distant parts of the body. This autoeczematous reaction is thought to be secondary to some form of autoimmunity. The final stage of the dermatitis is ulceration (stasis ulcers) of the skin, most commonly just above the level of the maleoli. Treatment requires assessment of the venous problems and treatment of underlying disease (see Chapter 4, Postphlebitic Syndrome). The limb must be elevated frequently and for prolonged periods to improve venous return. Fitted, pressure gradient support stockings may help control edema. Topical corticosteroid often reduces the eczematous changes. Appropriate systemic antibiotics and bland topical preparations are valuable in healing superficial lesions.

A peculiar white scarring process (atrophie blanche) is seen at times in association with stasis dermatitis and thrombophlebitis. It is not common but is distinctive in that the healing process is characterized by white atrophic plaques and fine telangiectasis in the area.

Contact Dermatitis

Contact dermatitis is a result of the innumerable naturally existing agents and synthetic chemicals that can cause skin lesions as a result of direct exposure. The simplest form, *irritant dermatitis*, occurs when an irritant material creates a dermatitis at the site of direct skin contact. This may occur in any person as a result of a sufficiently irritative material, such as acids and alkali. No immune mechanism is involved, and treatment is obvious. In *allergic contact dermatitis*, the eruption develops at the site of contact to a topical allergen in a previously sensitized individual. The development of sensitivity depends on the potency of the sensitizer (or agent with similar chemical characteristics), frequency of contact, and the individual susceptibility.

Since the eruption occurs at the site of contact, the diagnosis and the agent involved can be suspected (e.g., ear lobe dermatitis from earrings, eyelid dermatitis from eye makeup). The diagnosis is made by patch testing with the agent or the appropriate chemical at the proper concentration. The test patch is applied to the skin of the arm or back under occlusion and examined at 48 to 96 hours for evidence of eczematization at the site. Allergic contact dermatitis is treated by discovering and removing the causative agent and treating the eczematous area with cold compresses in the acute phase and later with topical corticosteroid.

Atopic Dermatitis

This is a fairly common disorder with genetic predisposition that often occurs in patients with hay fever and asthma. The eruption commonly occurs in early childhood and may disappear by school age, though in some it can continue to be troublesome throughout life. These patients appear to be worse in winter, because of increased drying of the epidermis. The eruption is very pruritic, involving the flexural areas of the neck and extremities. These patients show white dermographism rather than the normal triple response when the skin is stroked. It is generally accepted that an atopic individual does not have an increased propensity to contact allergic dermatitis. The diagnosis is clear in patients with chronic flexural dermatitis beginning in early childhood with a family background of asthma, hay fever and eczema.

There are several distinctive immune changes. These patients develop increased levels of reaginic antibogy (IgE) that appear to correspond to severity of the eruption. The eczematous response in the skin shows a lymphocytic reaction that reflects delayed hypersensitivity. There appears to be some impairment of cellular immunity, and the skin of atopic individuals becomes infected easily.

The management of atopic dermatitis requires understanding and patience on the part of the patient and parents. Topical corticosteroids are a godsend,

but, in view of the chronic disease, a balance must be struck to use the lowest concentration of steroid to keep the condition under reasonable control. Where infection is suspected, systemic antibiotics are indicated. The role of topical antibiotics has been controversial but in recent times they have been considered helpful. Pruritis is treated with oral antihistamine (H_2 antagonists).

Pityriasis Rosea

This common seasonal eruption is characterized by presence of a herald patch followed in a few days by numerous smaller similar macules showing fine adherent scaling at the periphery. The herald patch is usually on the trunk and often mistaken for tinea corporis. The process lasts 5 to 6 weeks, leaving no residual change. The present accepted etiology is viral; no treatment is indicated.

Psoriasis

This is an extremely common disorder genetically inherited as a dominant trait. The main diagnostic features of the disease are the presence of red papules and macules topped by silvery scaling found characteristically on the scalp, the extensor surface of the extremities and the intertriginous areas. The disease occurs in about 2 percent of the population, affecting both sexes and individuals of all ages. There is a tendency for psoriasis to appear before the age of 30.

The psoriatic patch results from a rapid epidermatization in which the transit time of a cell produced by division from the basal cell progresses upward, reaching the surface in 3 to 4 days compared to a skin transit time of 28 to 30 days. The histologic picture is characterized by increase in rete ridges of epidermis with corresponding elongation of dermal papillae, increased blood supply, marked retention of nuclei of the keratinizing cells (parakeratosis), and collections of pyknotic nuclei of neutrophils in the epidermis forming Munro abscesses. Psoriasis has a variety of clinical presentations. In the young, particularly after an infection, the psoriasis appears as numerous red papules and small macules, usually with scaling. This *guttate form*, confined to covered areas of the body, tends to last for several months and disappear only to return at a later date. It will show the characteristic silvery scaling. A *pustular form* appears as pustules on the palms and soles and at times in crops of small sterile pustules involving larger areas of the body with considerable toxic reaction. Psoriasis can become extensive, with considerable exfoliation and erythema secondary to a drug eruption, after the application of irritating topical agents or after the withdrawal of systemic corticosteroids (psoriatic erythroderma). The nails are often involved, the initial change being pitting of the surface. There will be an increase in the free edge of the nail, with brown discoloration proximal to the free edge, and marked accumulation of subungual keratin.

Patients with psoriasis have a high association with certain HLA types; particularly patients with arthropathy (see Chapter 18).

The treatment of psoriasis consists of:

1. Corticosteroids, either as topical agents or injected intralesionally
2. Coal tar and dithranol paste topically
3. Coal tar, dithranol, and ultraviolet B light
4. Cytotoxic and immunosuppressive drugs (methotrexate is usually used) on a cyclic basis
5. Phototherapy utilizing ultraviolet A light and oral 8-methoxy-psoralen
6. Others: oral retenoids, plasmapheresis and peritoneal dialysis are experimental.

Lichen Planus

This disease appears as flat topped violaceus papules on the wrists and shins with white lace-like lesions on the oral and genital mucosa. In some areas, lichen planus will appear as hypertrophic plaque or annular lesions. Two distinctive forms include the idiopathic variety that appears spontaneously and lichen planus-like drug eruption. This lichenoid eruption may occur following the use of antimalarials, antibiotics, or after topical sensitization to chemicals in color photography. A lichenoid eruption has been seen in the chronic phase of graft-versus-host reaction.

The histological changes are characteristic with a dense band-like infiltration of lymphocytes of the upper dermis hugging the epidermis. There is often destruction of the basal area giving a sawtooth appearance to the epidermodermal junction. The disease may affect the nails and the scalp. The treatment usually consists of topical, intralesional, or oral corticosteroids.

Acne Vulgaris

Acne is seen in adolescents and is characterized by opened (blackhead) and closed (whitehead) comedones, inflammatory papules and pustules in the se-

baceous areas with a tendency to heal with pitted scarring. Sebaceous glands become active and larger, beginning in the second decade of life. Acne results from obstruction of the pilosebaceous duct at the infundibular portion of this unit. The blocking effect is created by adrenal hormone effects. The obstruction leads to an excessive accumulation of sebum. With colonization by saprophytic *Corynebacterium acnes*, the sebum content becomes markedly acidified, leading to inflammatory changes. Acne may only last for several years or continue into the twenties or even into middle age.

Acne may be seen shortly after birth and last several months. This neonatal acne is related to circulating maternal hormones. Certain drugs induce acne, including iodides, corticosteroids, and androgens. A number of topically applied agents promote acne secondary to follicular plugging.

The wide range of remedies available indicates that no given medication is suitable for all. Currently, topical benzol peroxide and broad-spectrum antibiotics appear moderately successful. Oral tetracycline and other antibiotics have been extensively used with unpredictable results. Acne surgery, extracting the comedone, and injection of the inflamed cysts with intralesional corticosteroids is used with good results.

Hidradenitis suppurativa is a chronic inflammatory process affecting the axillary and anogenital regions. A large painful boil or abscess may form suddenly. Though it was considered to be an inflammatory process of apocrine glands, it may be of sebaceous origin as well. Effective therapy requires surgical excision of the glands.

Rosacea

This disease affects individuals in the middle years. It is characterized by transient facial erythema initially followed by inflammatory papules and pustules, particularly of the nose and adjacent areas. With the progress of the disease, the erythema becomes marked and there is hypertrophy, particularly of the nose, known as rhinophyma. This disease responds slowly to oral tetracycline.

CUTANEOUS REACTIONS TO DRUGS

Table 19.1 outlines a classification of cutaneous lesions and the drugs that are commonly responsible. In most instances the precise mechanism is unknown, but disordered immunity is commonly demonstrable. The best therapy is withdrawal of the drug, care-

Table 19.1   **Cutaneous Reactions to Drugs**

Reactions	Drugs

Severe reactions
    Exfoliative dermatitis
    Toxic epidermal necrolysis
    Stevens-Johnson syndrome
    Systemic lupus erythematosis
	Penicillin, sulfonamides, barbiturates, hydantoins, phenylbutazone, phenolphthalein, hydralazine, many others

Contact dermatitis	Antihistamines, arsenicals, bacitracin, chloramphonicol, sulfonamides, many others
Acne	Corticosteroids, androgenic steroids, bromides, iodides, oral contraceptives
Erythema nodosum	Penicillin, sulfonamides, phenacetin, salicylates, barbiturates, thiazide diuretics, oral contraceptives
Rashes and urticaria	Penicillins, allopurinol, barbiturates, thiazides, gold salts, hydantoins, salicylates, opiates, quinidine, many others
Hyperpigmentation	Busulfan, 6-mercaptopurine, phenothiazines, corticosteroids, ACTH, vitamin A, chloroquin, Gold (chrysiasis), Silver (argyria)
Alopecia	Cytotoxic agents, heparin, clofibrate, chloroquin, oral contraceptives, many others
Hirsutism	Androgens, oral contraceptives, corticosteroids, hydantoins, diazoxide, minoxidil
Photo dermatitis	Griseofulvin, sulfonamides, sulfonureas, demeclocycline, thiazides, many others
Necrotizing vasculitis	Anticoagulants, barbiturates, sulfonamides, penicillin

ful search for medication mixtures that may contain an offending drug, and, in severe reactions, systemic corticosteroid therapy. While certain drugs are more likely to induce certain reactions, all drugs must be considered the potential cause of cutaneous abnormalities in a given patient.

VASCULAR REACTIONS

Urticaria

Urticaria or hives is a common disorder characterized by transient pruritic wheals. The wheal results from escape of fluid and at times red blood cells into the dermis from dilated capillaries. The vascular leakage is created by mediators of which histamine is the most important. In some forms, IgE antibodies are thought to be involved. In serum sickness, a complex of antigens and antibody (usually IgG) precipitate out in the skin, kidney, and blood vessels leading to the urticaria.

Acute urticaria develops with wheals of varying size, some with polycyclic configuration. There may be swelling of the eyelids, lips, synovial tissue, and at times the laryngeal membranes. The urticarial reaction is transient, disappearing with no residual change, but new wheals may appear. Often a drug, food, or infection appears to play a role. In chronic urticaria, the wheals appear more or less continuously for two or more years. Despite considerable laboratory investigation, elimination of medication, and restricted diet, the cause may not be found. Treatment generally consists of oral antihistamines.

Urticaria pigmentosa is a condition which generally occurs in children, characterized by excessive cutaneous mast cell infiltration. These patients have small, discrete to reddish-brown, pigmented macules that become hive-like on stroking, as a result of release of histamine. Rarely systemic mast cell disease occurs, particularly in adults, and may result in nodular mast cell tumors of multiple organs.

Dermographism

On occasion, an individual will develop pruritic urticaria at sites of pressure or scratching. The cause is unknown.

Purpura

Bleeding into tissues causes bluish discoloration of the overlying skin. Resolution occurs during subsequent days to weeks with color changes through brown, green, yellow, and then delayed clearance of a brownish pigmentation.

Underlying causes are discussed in Chapter 4 under Bleeding Disorders.

Vasculitis

This includes a group of reactions resulting from an inflammatory response of the blood vessels. The skin lesions range from erythematous plaques to combined lesions including necrosis and ulceration.

Secondary changes due to scratching may be the dominant visible feature.

Leucocytoclastic Angiitis

This is characterized by purpura in which vascular damage results from immune-complex deposition in vessel walls with subsequent leukocyte infiltration and destruction. This process is probably involved in vasculitis due to infections, drugs, collagen-vascular diseases, and lymphoreticular disorders. *Henoch-Schöenlein purpura* is a variant seen in children, characterized by purpura of the extremities with associated involvement of the bowel, joints, and kidneys (see Chapter 4 and Chapter 19).

Erythema multiforme, described above, is thought to be an immune response within the vessel walls.

Vasculitis with Nodules

Erythematous, hot, tender nodules may develop with involvement of the lower dermis and panniculus due to an intensive vascular inflammation. In erythema nodosum, well demarcated, painful swelling of the shins will slowly resolve over 3 to 4 weeks. This immune response may occur with streptococcal infections of the upper respiratory tract, sarcoidosis, tuberculosis, fungus, viral infections, or use of certain drugs. It may also occur in granulomatous bowel diseases such as ulcerative colitis.

INFECTIONS

Bacterial Infections

The skin is colonized by many harmless bacteria. Their numbers vary from time to time and from site to site. Occasionally, due to imbalance of numbers or injury to the skin, a given organism grows excessively or a pathogenic organism establishes infection.

Impetigo

This is a common superficial infection of children caused by staphylococci, streptococci, or both. The lesions show adherent honey-colored crusting and oozing. Primary skin disorders that are pruritic often become infected secondarily. There is always danger of bacteremia. Persistent impetigo may predispose to acute glomerulonephritis. A dramatic form of staphylococcal infection in children is the scalded skin syndrome (discussed above). Treatment consists of good skin hygiene and appropriate systemic antibiotics.

Furuncles and Carbuncles

Infection of the pilosebaceous unit caused by pathogenic staphylococci results in a furuncle (boil). The lesion begins as a tender red papule that becomes painful and swollen with a fluctuant centre. Rupture may occur with discharge of pus. A carbuncle is a larger lesion involving multiple follicles. Large or progressive lesions may require surgical drainage. When surrounding cellulitis develops, systemic antibiotics are indicated.

Ecthyma is an infection of skin that extends deeper than the epidermis, often to the depth of the subcutaneous fat. It appears as a punched-out ulcer. This occurs in children and in poorly nourished elderly patients.

Cellulitis and Erysipelas

Cellulitis or erysipelas is characterized by a well-demarkated, somewhat tender erythematous swelling of the skin due to group A streptococci. In elderly patients the tissues of the face, including the nose, cheeks, and adjacent eyelids, may be involved. The skin of the involved area is warm and tense; the swelling spreads during hours of observation; and vesicles or bullae may develop at some point. Constitutional features include malaise and fever. The peripheral blood cell count may be elevated. Septicemia is a major hazard. Generally it is not possible to isolate the organism. Systemic penicillin is the drug of choice. A swelling resembling erysipelas occurs on the hands and forearm of workers handling animals, fish, or birds. This is an infection with *Erysipelothrix rhusiopathiae* and is known as erysipeloid.

Tuberculosis

Skin lesions rarely result from Mycobacterium tuberculosis in North America. Cutaneous lesions due to atypical mycobacterial infection are more common (e.g. the swimming pool granuloma that may present as nodules or chronic indolent discharging lesions). Biopsy reveals the granuloma with giant cells. Appropriate tissue cultures should grow the organism.

Leprosy

Leprosy was long considered to be a tropical and subtropical disorder but is now appearing in many temperate zones as a result of worldwide travel. This severe, disabling disease affects up to 2 percent of the people in some third-world countries. The causative agent, *Mycobacterium leprae,* has a predilection for the skin, peripheral nerves, and the mucosa of the upper respiratory tract. This organism is transferred by close contact, but due to slow growth the first lesions appear after a number of years. The early lesion is a hypopigmented macule, termed indeterminate leprosy. In patients with high resistance, further skin lesions are limited and appear as slightly infiltrated hypopigmented anesthetic macules. This is the *tuberculoid* form. Patients with poor resistance to the Mycobacterium will develop *lepromatous leprosy* with numerous patches, as well as diffuse infiltrations. Some will develop a mixture of lesions that are clinically and histologically a combination of tuberculoid and lepromatous type (dimorphous leprosy). The peripheral neuropathy is responsible for anesthesia, leading to severe, traumatic destructive changes of involved tissues. Response to treatment is favorable, and both forms of leprosy respond well to sulfones and rifampicin, provided drug therapy can be maintained through many years. Problems of drug resistance of the organism and compliance of the patients seriously influence therapeutic outcome.

Syphilis

With the advent of diagnostic serological tests and curative antibiotics, devastating late syphilis appears to be rare. However, recent trends to more varied sexual practices are associated with an increasing rate of syphilis infections.

The natural course of syphilis can be divided into four phases. In general, the primary and secondary stages present with skin lesions. The primary stage is characterized by the chancre, a shallow painless ulcer at the point of infection, occuring 1 to 5 weeks after contact. This chancre is generally on the genital mucosa, though extragenital chancres are seen surprisingly often. The most useful diagnostic aid in the early stage is the darkfield examination or phase-contrast microscopy, since the chancre contains numerous motile organisms, *Treponema pallidum.* After 3 to 4 weeks, the chancre will disappear spontaneously, although this occurs more quickly with antibiotic therapy. As the chancre disappears, in the untreated case, the secondary phase presents with a variety of skin lesions. The most characteristic lesion is a red maculopapular eruption, localized or widespread, with fine peripheral scaling. Palmar and plantar macules are pathognomonic for secondary syphilis. Syphilis, the great mimicker, is often confused with other eruptions such as pityriasis rosea, drug eruptions, guttate psoriasis, viral infections, and even acne vulgaris. For a discussion of systemic manifestations, diagnostic serology, and treatment, see Chapter 7.

Gonorrhea

Gonococcal infections are increasing in number despite our educational and therapeutic efforts. The majority of gonococcal infections are urethral or internal. On occasion, an enlarged infected Bartholin cyst may present as swelling in the lateral margin of the vaginal introitus. The cutaneous form of gonococcal infection, though rare, is part of disseminated gonococcemia and appears as a few purpuric macules on the distal extremities. It affects women more often than men (10:1) and generally follows the menses. There is often an associated arthropathy. The clinical picture is diagnostic. Culture from the cutaneous lesions is usually negative. For detailed discussion of gonococcal disease, see Chapter 7.

Superficial Fungal Infections (Tinea)

Fungal infections of the skin are caused by organisms that are transmitted from other humans (anthopophilic), animals (zoophilic), and from the environment (geophilic). The clinical classification is based on the site of involvement.

Tinea Pedis

Tinea of the feet (athlete's foot) is the most common fungus infection. It may appear as a dry scaly pruritic involvement of one or both feet and commonly involves only one hand. The causative agent is *Trichophyton rubrum.* A second more inflammatory form of athletes foot appears as pruritic and painful blisters, caused by *Trichophyton mentagrophytes.*

Tinea Cruris

This relatively common infection appears as a red extending macule with an active border on the inner aspects of the upper thigh. The causative agents are

Epidermophyton floccosum and *Trichophyton mentagrophytes.*

Tinea Corporis

This is the classical ringworm with an active red scaly border and central clearing (Fig. 19.10). This is most often caused by *Trichophyton mentagrophytes, Microsporum canis,* or *Trichophyton verrucosum.* Those that are caused from animal sources tend to be highly inflamed and produce a carbuncle-like lesion known as a kerion.

Tinea capitis has been caused by a variety of agents such as *Microsporum audouini, Microsporum canis, Trichophyton schoenleini,* and *Trichophyton mentagrophytes.* It is the form that fluoresces under Woods' lamp as a blue-green color.

Tinea of Nails

This appears as yellow-white involvement of the nail plate, usually extending from the free edge proximally. Diagnosis of tinea is made on clinical grounds. Skin scrapings examined microscopically with potassium hydroxide solution (20 percent) will reveal the telltale mycelia or hyphae of the dermatophyte.

Tinea Versicolor

This benign lesion is not considered a true dermatomycosis. It is commonly found on the chest, back, and adjacent areas of the arms, appearing as hypopigmented macules with fine scaling on the surface. It tends to be brown in winter and whiter in summer, sometimes mistaken for vitiligo. The causative agent, *Malassezia furfur,* can be identified in skin scrapings under the microscope, but cannot be cultured on routine mycological media.

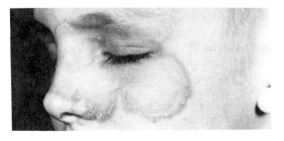

Fig. 19.10 Tinea corporis with characteristic border

Candidiasis

Candida albicans is an opportunistic agent that often grows well in moist intertriginous areas. In infants it is often found on the skin in diaper dermatitis. Women with excessive perspiration and large pendulous breasts may develop infection in the skin folds. It is found in the vagina and oral mucous membranes in patients taking birth control pills, broad spectrum antibiotics, patients with diabetes mellitus, and patients receiving corticosteroids. In the mouth, whitish-gray plaques of organisms may be scraped, leaving a friable, erythematous base, sometimes with serrated edges (thrush). Eating and swallowing may be painful.

Treatment of Cutaneous Fungal Infection

The treatment of fungal skin infections usually depends on topical agents, which are reasonably effective. For nail involvement, griseofulvin and ketoconozol may be necessary.

Viral Infections

Warts (Verruca)

Warts are very common, accounting for about 10 percent of all dermatologic diagnosis. This viral disease can be found anywhere on the skin as well as on the mucous membrane. The common wart is found on the extremities, usually the hands. Plantar warts may appear as calluses, since pressure on the surface creates a wart that is predominantly below the surface. Condyloma accuminata are cauliflower-like warts on the moist areas of genital organs, perianal skin, and mouth. At least 6 serological types of viral agents have been implicated as causing warts.

Warts often regress spontaneously, and for very young children the best treatment appears to be "tincture of time." In older children and adults, a variety of destructive methods such as topical liquid nitrogen, electrofulguration, excision, topical acid, keratolytic agents, and intralesional bleomycin all have been used with varying degrees of success.

Molluscum Contagiosum

This is a relatively common viral infection characterized by translucent dome-shaped papules measuring 2 to 3 mm. They have a central umbilication, which covers an accumulation of viral particles in the epidermal cells (molluscum body). They are common in the genital and flexural areas. The most effective treatment is incision and extraction using a Schamberg comedone extractor. Young children will not tolerate this procedure and do require a general anesthetic for removal.

Herpes Simplex Labialis and Genitalis

Herpes simplex labialis (Type I) is the formal term for what everyone knows as cold sores. Most individuals who have recurrent labial herpes are infected in early childhood. The lesion appears as a cluster of tiny vesicles usually at the mucocutaneous margin of the lip. A short prodromal period characterized by itching precedes the appearance of the vesicles. The vesicles break in 3 to 4 days, become crusted and heal in 10 to 12 days. In some individuals, herpes simplex may be found elsewhere, such as on the tip of the finger or back of the neck. The major complications are involvement of the cornea of the eye and, on rare occasions, generalized infection in immunosuppressed individuals or those with atopic dermatitis (Kaposi's varicelliform eruption).

Herpes genitalis (Type II) is transmitted sexually and vesicles are found on the genitals or adjacent areas. This is discussed under Sexually Transmitted Diseases, Chapter 7.

In herpes labialis, recurrence of lesions is often associated with some insult to the skin, such as considerable sunlight, or a febrile illness, such as influenza or pneumonia. It is thought that the herpesvirus lodges in the nucleus of the cutaneous nerve root supplying the skin, but leaves the nucleus and migrates to the epidermal cells during times of clinical infection.

The diagnosis is easily confirmed. Examination of the contents of the blister, stained with Wright stain (Tzank smear) reveals large multinucleated neutrophils. Viral cultures and electron microscopy (for inclusion bodies) also aid in the diagnosis. Idouridine and acyclovir may be useful in treating severe infections.

Herpes Zoster

These skin lesions are characterized by grouped red papules that become vesicular and then pustular, distributed in a continuous or interrupted fashion along the course of one or two dermatomes. These skin lesions are often preceded by pain and dysesthesia for 3 to 5 days. Lymph nodes draining the area become tender and enlarged. The lesions usually disappear, leaving some minor hypopigmented change, after 3 to 4 weeks; the pain usually subsides as the eruption appears. Seventy to 75 percent occur in the thoracic and neck areas, and the opthalmic area is involved in approximately 15 percent. In some patients, diffuse vesicles may accompany the dermatomal zoster. In elderly individuals the eruption may become necrotic with delayed healing, considerable scarring, and persistent pain. Zoster occasionally involves motor nerve roots and visceral nerves. Opthalmic zoster is dreaded, since complications of corneal ulcers and infection occur in 50 percent of cases. Patients with lymphoma may develop severe, progressive zoster.

Varicella and zoster are caused by the same virus. It is felt that varicella is the primary infection with herpes varicella virus, and zoster results from the activation of a latent infection in a partially immune host.

In varicella and zoster the cells of the malpighian layer show ballooning of the cytoplasm and multinuclear giant cells are found in the vesicles on Wright stains.

Treatment with analgesic and local therapy is sufficient in the mild attack. Patients with severe pain may derive symptomatic improvement from high dose corticosteroid treatment (e.g., 60–80 mg Prednisone per day). Intralesional corticosteroid (triamcinolone 2 mg/cc) has been advocated, injecting directly into the area of pain.

Scabies and Lice Infections

Scabies occurs at all ages, and is a result of the itchmite, *Sarcoptes scabei*. Intense pruritis on the hands, wrists, and genital organs occurs, particularly at night. Similar symptoms are common in friends and family. The skin lesion appears as a 2 to 3 mm scratch-like mark with a tiny black dot at the end. This is the burrow of the gravid female mite and is best seen on the hands, feet, and the glans penis. The female mite is the black dot, and can be extracted using a magnifying lens and a pointed scalpel blade and then identified under the microscope.

Lice infestations appear as mild itching of the scalp, body, or pubic areas. Examination of the hairs reveal the eggs (nits) attached firmly to the hair shafts. A careful search will reveal the cigar-like head louse (*Pediculus humanis*) or the crab louse (*Phthirus pubis*) tightly clinging to the hairs. On occasion, crab lice can be seen clinging onto the eyelashes.

Both scabies and lice are rapidly removed by the use of topical gamma benzene hexachloride. In scabies, patients will find their intense itching reduced with the first application, but some degree of itching may continue for days, requiring the use of oral antihistamines and topical corticosteroids.

HAIR DISORDERS

Hair has limited functional value in the human; however, careful study of the amount, distribution, and quality of the hair may be helpful in diagnosis of systemic disease. More frequently patients come because of cosmetic concerns.

Alopecia

Alopecia Areata

This is a relatively common disorder affecting older children and adults of all ages. One or more discrete, circular patches or hair loss occur without any visible damage to the skin. These occur on the scalp or any other part of the body. Close examination may reveal short hairs with expanded tips and tapering above the tip (exclamation mark hairs).

There is a tendency for the hair to regrow, usually within a year. The hairs may be white initially, but the pigment slowly returns. Children who develop alopecia areata tend to have recurrent bouts. Where hair is lost from the peripheral zones of the scalp, the regrowth is often slow and incomplete. The disorder may be associated with other conditions such as thyroiditis, pernicious anemia, vitiligo, and diabetes mellitus. Hair may be totally lost from the scalp (alopecia totalis) and occasionally the whole body is affected (alopecia universalis).

Treatment should be withheld for 4 to 6 months after the loss of the patches. If regrowth does not occur spontaneously, the most effective treatment is intralesional injection with corticosteroids (triamcinolone).

Androgenic–Male Pattern Baldness

This is the most common form of hair loss in men. The disorder is transmitted as a dominant trait and requires the presence of an adequate concentration of androgen. In those who will develop male pattern baldness, early loss may be seen in the late teens as bilateral temporal recession. The crown will thin and with time the receding temporal areas will join the crown portion to produce a single large area of alopecia, with hair only on the sides and occiput. Despite claims, hair lost in this way cannot be regrown. Autotransplantation of hair from the sides and back of the scalp to the central portion produces reasonable cosmetic effects in some individuals.

Telogen Effluvium

Worrisome, diffuse hair loss may occur primarily in women, due to large numbers of hair in the decline or resting phase of growth. The patient suddenly notices a greater than normal number of hairs on her pillow or coming out with combing and brushing. The examiner will find a mild diffuse loss with no localization.

This tends to occur following such common events as parturition, acute febrile illness, surgery, or prolonged emotional stress because greater number of hairs come into synchrony in the catagen and telogen phases (see Structure and Function of the Skin, Hair; above). This causes many more hairs to be shed 2 to 3 months later as new hairs begin to grow (anagen phase). In the absence of alopecia areata and other forms of alopecia, patients with antecedent history of a stressful event permit this diagnosis. Treatment is restricted to explanation and reassurance.

Diffuse Alopecia in Women

This is the diffuse scalp hair loss in women beginning in the third or fourth decade. There is no specific explanation for this process although it probably represents a decline in the number of active follicles associated with aging. In some, it appears to be part of telogen effluvium after pregnancies, in which the hair loss was not fully regained. Hypothyroidism and iron deficiency should be considered. The condition progresses slowly and effective treatment is not available.

Alopecia and Drugs

Alopecia occurs temporarily with radiation and cytotoxic drugs. These affect the anagen hairs. Anticoagulants may produce diffuse alopecia after several weeks to months.

Hirsutism

Excessive hair in areas that normally are considered hairless is particularly undesirable in women. Some women have what they would consider more hair than normal on their faces. This may be a normal familial or racial trait.

In some women, hirsutism is a result of adrenal adrogenic stimulation. These individuals show systemic virulism. In many, however, there is no evidence of virulism, but simply excessive facial hair. The mechanism may be increased androgen production or increased response of hair follicles to the hormone. Patients with hirsutism and virilization should be thoroughly evaluated to assess the possibility of adrenal or ovarian tumors (see Chapter 13).

Drugs such as minoxidil, corticosteroids, phenytoin and diazoxide have been associated with hirsutism. Topical treatment includes plucking out darker and firmer hair, or frequent shaving. Destruction of the hair follicles by electrolysis is more permanent but extremely costly. Cyclic estrogen-progesterone therapy, cimetidine, and spironolactone have all been used for management of severe hirsutism.

NAIL DISORDERS

Nails are affected in many primary cutaneous diseases that are usually distinguishable from those associated with a systemic disorder.

Transverse Lamellar Nail Dystrophy

The nail consists of shingle-like cells glued together into a many-layered plate. Although the nail is markedly impervious to water, with repeated immersion of the hands in water and detergent the layers of the nail cells will separate, producing transverse splitting. This is an occupational hazard of housewives and dishwashers.

Dystrophica Mediana Canaliformis

A central longitudinal split of the nail plate of the thumb occurs uncommonly. An abnormality deep to the posterior nail fold, in contact with the nail matrix effectively hinders the nail growth at this point.

TUMORS

Common Benign Tumors

Nevus

This is the most common benign tumor of the skin. It arises from melanocytes as a flat junctional nevus, or elevated as the classical dark or flesh-colored dermal or compound nevus. Nevi appear at an early age, reach their greatest number at puberty, and may continue to appear at any age. The halo nevus is surrounded by a halo of vitiligo. Leukoderma engulfs the nevus, and eventually the tumor disappears as well. In the dark, uniformly colored blue nevus melanocytes extend deep in the dermis. In children an active brown-red compound nevus often seen in the face is known as a juvenile melanoma. The importance is that the nevus is benign, despite the melanoma-like histologic appearance of the cells (see malignant melanoma, above).

The large congenital nevus known as the giant hairy nevus may involve portions of the trunk, arm, or leg. It may be grotesque in appearance, and has considerable potential risk of developing melanocarcinoma. It must be followed regularly and any site showing change must be biopsied.

Lentigo is the common pigmented macular lesion seen in the aged in areas exposed to the sun. Often referred to as a liver spot, this results from the elongation of rete ridges of the epidermis and increased concentration of melanocytes.

Skin Tags

These are the flesh colored or pigmented pedunculated soft tumors about the neck, eyelids, and axillae, where rubbing is common. They are made up of a flattened epidermis surrounding a small amount of loose connective tissue. These are easily removed by snipping with a sterile pair of scissors.

Seborrheic Keratosis

This verrucous, waxy tumor is extremely common on the upper body of the elderly. Histologically the lesion shows an overgrowth of basal cells with numerous islands of keratin. A papular form found in dark skinned individuals at an earlier age is labelled dermatosis papulosa nigra. These are treated if necessary by curettage and light electrodesiccation.

Hemangiomata

Tumors derived from blood vessels occur in several forms. The *capillary hemangioma* appears as a bright red macule shortly after birth. This port-wine stain or nevus flammeus remains throughout life. It may be part of the Sturge-Weber syndrome in which the hemangioma appears on the face.

The *strawberry hemangioma* is a large lobulated tumor that appears early and tends to increase in size for the first year of life; many then regress spontaneously. The large hemangiomas may create difficulties when they occur around the eyes, mouth, or in the pharyngeal area.

Cavernous hemangiomas are the deeper colored vascular tumors that lie in the subcutaneous tissues. Arteriovenous fistulae may be associated with cutaneous telangiectasis (Osler-Weber-Rendu Syndrome).

Premalignant and Malignant Tumors

Actinic Keratosis

The elderly Caucasian who has spent considerable time in the sun will develop many actinic keratosis in the sun-exposed areas. An actinic keratosis appears as a scaling lesion on an erythematous base without much elevation, most prominent on the face, the rim of the ear pinna, and on the dorsum of the hands. The lesion is slightly tender. The epidermal cells in this lesion show dyskeratosis with cellular atypia and abnormal keratinization. In some actinic keratosis, the abnormal keratin will remain adherent to form a cutaneous horn. Solar keratosis may develop into squamous cell carcinoma, which tends not to metastasize.

Leukoplakia is a white, slightly elevated lesion on the lip or other mucous membrane. Histologically, the changes are much like actinic keratosis. This may progress to squamous cell carcinoma; those that develop from oral or vulvular leukoplakia have a much greater tendency to metastasize.

A slowly enlarging erythematous patch on any part of the body should raise the possibility of Bowen's disease. This lesion does not have the pearly border seen with basal cell carcinoma. This persistent lesion may become invasive after many years and may develop distant metastasis. Histologically, it is an intraepidermal squamous cell carcinoma.

A similar lesion to Bowen's disease may be found on the glans penis. It appears as a persistent red velvety area with slight elevation and ulceration.

These premalignant and malignant lesions are easily biopsied and treated by electrodessication, excisional surgery, cryotherapy, or topical 5-fluorouracil cream.

Basal Cell Carcinoma

This tumor accounts for more than 70 percent of malignancies of the skin. It arises from the basal cells of the epidermis, grows at or near the site of origin, and rarely metastasizes. Approximately 90 percent of

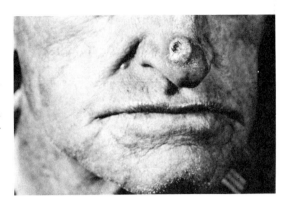

Fig. 19.11 Basal cell carcinoma

basal cell carcinomas appear on the sun-exposed areas, particularly the face and neck. Males are affected more often than females in a ratio of 4:1. They generally occur after age 40 but may appear at a younger age group in fair-skinned individuals. They occur in the teens and twenties in those who have the basal cell nevoid syndrome and xeroderma pigmentosa.

Basal cell carcinoma may appear in several clinical forms. The most common is the pearly elevated nodule with the surface marked by fine telangiectasis. When ulceration occurs (rodent ulcer), the border will show the characteristic pearly rolled edges (Fig. 19.11). Occasionally the tumor may show a blister, resulting from necrosis of cells within the tumor. Some basal cell carcinomas have considerable black pigmentation, suggesting a possible melanoma. A rare type of basal cell carcinoma, the morphea type, appears as a firm white macule, usually on the face.

This tumor grows slowly, and can be cured by a variety of methods: excision, curettage and electrodessication, Moh's chemoexcision, cryotherapy, and radiotherapy.

CUTANEOUS MANIFESTATIONS OF SYSTEMIC DISEASE

CUTANEOUS SIGNS OF ENDOCRINE DISORDERS

Pituitary and Adrenal Disease

Acromegaly

Hypertrophy of skin results from excessive secretion of growth hormone. The skin is diffusely thickened and may be furrowed (cutis gyrata) on the forehead and scalp, with hyperactivity of sebaceous and sweat glands. Moderate pigmentation and hirsutism may develop.

Adrenal Hypersecretion

Hypercortisolism resulting from excess of adrenal glucocorticoids may occur in patients with adrenal tumors, secondary to excessive pituitary ACTH, or due to drugs. The skin changes include acne, hirsutism, increased pigmentation, purple striae, and the characteristic "moon face" and "buffalo hump" due to preauricular and suboccipital fat pads. Excess production of adrenal androgens (generally due to tumors) will lead to hirsutism, male pattern baldness, seborrhea and acne, and increased pigmentation.

Adrenal Hyposecretion

In adrenal failure, diffuse hyperpigmentation results from increased production of melanin, with accentuation at sun-exposed sites and areas of friction. Mechanisms for the melanocyte stimulation probably result from failure of feedback inhibition of the pituitary gland (see Chapter 13).

Thyroid Disorders

Hyperthyroidism

The skin tends to be warm, smooth, and vasodilated. The hair is fine, and alopecia areata is more common than in normal subjects. Onycholysis, the separation of the nail plate from the nail bed, occurs commonly.

A curious cutaneous feature of thyrotoxicosis follows treatment by surgery or radioactive iodine. Waxy plaques with prominent follicular orifices develop on the shin, showing the changes of peau-de-orange. This results from deposition of acid mucopolysaccaride in the dermis.

Hypothyroidism

Myxedematous patients have pale skin that is coarse and puffy. The hair is coarse and sparse on the scalp and brows. The skin takes on a whitish-yellow color related to a number of factors; decrease in melanin, anemia, vasoconstriction and increased carotene.

The Parathyroids

Hyperparathyroidism

In hyperparathyroidism secondary to renal disease, itching is common, and reports indicate relief after parathyroidectomy. Cutaneous calcification has also been associated with secondary hyperparathyroidism.

Hypoparathyroidism

Hypoparathyroidism produces skin that is rough and scaly; the hair is sparce and nails are broken and brittle. In idiopathic hypoparathyroidism, widespread mucocutaneous candidiasis may occur.

Diabetes Mellitus

The skin is involved in a variety of ways in diabetes mellitus. In some patients the skin lesions may be the presenting feature.

Necrobiosis Lipoidica

This yellow atrophic plaque on the shins develops at all ages and is more common in women. The lesion progresses with degeneration of collagen and atrophy and at times ulceration of the surface. It is intimately related to diabetes, although it has occured in the absence of diabetes. Adequate control of diabetes does not seem to alter the course. Treatment is with topical corticosteroids or intralesional corticosteroid injections.

Granuloma Annulare

The association of granuloma annulare with diabetes is not as definite as necrobiosis lipoidica. Granuloma annulare occurs on the hands, fingers, ankles, and feet and may persist for a number of months, slowly increasing in size. This lesion in its early phase often resembles necrobiosis, both clinically and histologically. However, it does not show the epidermal atrophy and the lipid accumulation of necrobiosis.

Dermopathy Diabeticorum

Pigmented atrophic macules appear on the shins, looking like a posttraumatic scar. This is thought to result from the microangiopathy seen in diabetics.

Skin Infection

Bacterial infections were once a major problem but are less common with the use of antibiotics and greater attention to infection. Candidiasis is particularly common in the intertriginous areas as well as in the anogenital regions. Chronic dermatophyte infection is also common.

Neuropathy

The feet often will be involved with paresthesia and impairment of sensation, leading to trauma with callus formation and poor tissue resistance. The area under the metatarsal head may ulcerate, taking months to heal (malperforans).

Eruptive Xanthoma

The poorly controlled diabetic may develop yellow-pink papules on the extensor surfaces, which result from increased serum triglycerides.

Ischemia

With atherosclerosis and reduced cutaneous circulation, the lower extremities will show gangrene of the toes and feet and ischemic ulceration.

Pruritus

This is common and at times troublesome, but generally there are no visible changes to account for the itching.

METABOLIC DISORDERS

The Porphyrias

Abnormal porphyrin synthesis leads to syndromes that involve the skin, because the metabolites produced in excess are very photoactive. The two forms of porphyria that prominently affect the skin are porphyria cutanea tarda and erythropoietic protoporphyria. The photoactivation of porphyria in the skin is at a wavelength of 400 nm.

Porphyria Cutanea Tarda

This form of porphyria is common and is provoked by excessive alcohol intake, use of contraceptive pills, and toxic liver disease. The patient appears with pigmentation of the sun-exposed areas. The skin of the hands "peels" with minor trauma. Often tense blisters will appear on the back of the hands. As damaged areas heal, they produce white inclusion papules (milia). Excessive hair is most noticeable in women. A number of patients show sclerodermoid

thickening around the neck and upper chest. The clinical features are diagnostic. The skin biopsy is characteristic as is the urinary uroporphyrin excretion.

Erythropoietic Protoporphyria

This rarer form of porphyria appears in young children and results in considerable itching, erythema, and urticaria, leading to crusted vesicular lesions of sun-exposed areas. These changes cause scarring on the nose, face, and the backs of the hands.

The diagnosis is confirmed by the presence of increased blood and fecal protoporphyrin. Oral B-carotene appears to reduce the photoreaction considerably.

Lipid Metabolism

The skin manifestations of disordered lipid metabolism are characterized by yellow papules, nodules, and plaques distributed symmetrically (xanthoma). They occur on eyelids, palms, neck, and trunk. The eyelid lesions, xanthelasma, are associated with hypercholesterolemia 50 percent of the time. *Plane xanthoma* are features of Type II, III, and IV hyperlipidemia. *Tuberous xanthoma* occur on the extensor aspects of joints and on the buttocks. They are a feature of Type II and III hyperlipidemia.

Tendinous xanthoma occur mainly on the extensor tendons and occur in Type II and Type III hyperlipidemia (see Chapter 2).

Angiokeratoma Corporis Diffusum (Anderson-Fabry Disease)

This rare systemic lipid storage disease is transmitted as an X-linked recessive trait. Petechiae-like lesions begin on the lower part of the body starting before puberty and appear in great numbers as time passes. Those affected have low-grade pain, particularly of the legs. These patients succumb before the age of 40 with cardiac and renal failure. The lipid may be found in the urine. Biopsy of a lesion will show the characteristic lipid involvement of blood vessel wall.

Nutritional Disorders

A careful dietary history is important in patients with generalized dryness, hyperkeratosis, mucous membrane inflammation, or oral fissures. Generalized protein-calorie deficiency, excess intake of vitamin A, and deficiency of niacin commonly result in skin lesions. Vitamin C deficiency (scurvy) may present with perifollicular swelling and petechiae.

COLLAGEN-VASCULAR DISEASES

These conditions are described in detail in Chapter 18; only the cutaneous features are covered here.

Lupus Erythematosus

This may be purely cutaneous or systemic, with involvement of many organs.

Discoid lupus erythematosus (DLE) begins in the fourth decade and appears as discrete erythematous scaly patches on the scalp, face, neck, and arms. Often they will appear after sun exposure. The lesions tend to persist for some time, finally healing with atrophic hypopigmented scars. The lesions are diagnostic histologically. These lesions often respond to topical or intralesional corticosteroids.

Systemic lupus erythematosus (SLE) shows lesions similar to DLE, but they may be more extensive. There may be diffuse hair loss. Telangiectasis are common on the fingers, palms, and feet. Urticaria, an early sign, may be found in 10 percent of patients. Ulceration, lividoreticularis, and purpura are also seen.

Dermatomyositis

The characteristic sign of dermatomyositis is the erythematous change of the face and particularly the eyelids, resembling an allergic contact dermatitis. This erythema is also found over the knuckles, elbows, and knees. The cutaneous lesions may resemble other collagen diseases.

Scleroderma

This disorder includes purely cutaneous forms and the serious systemic sclerosis.

Localized Forms

Morphea is a discrete patch initially characterized by hyperpigmentation; the central areas become hypopigmented and firm, but the edge shows a cyanotic or purple hue. The lesion slowly resolves over several years. In the diffuse form, many patches of morphea occur on the chest and trunk. The usual course is one of extensive involvement with slow recovery over many years. Linear morphea presents as a linear sclerodermatous patch usually on the extremities. It may involve the underlying connective tissue, muscles, and long bone. The skin will contract and become firm, producing a linear depressed scar. When it involves the face it may extend beyond the hairline into the scalp and to the eyebrows. At times there may be facial atrophy as well. It tends to slowly resolve over many years.

Systemic Sclerosis

Progressive systemic sclerosis is a generalized disease involving most organs with atrophy and fibrosis of the connective tissue. Raynaud's phenomenon often precedes other features for many years. The skin becomes thickened and firm. The skin over the fingers and hands appears and feels tight and bound down. Many areas including the face, chest, and upper and lower extremities become involved. The skin often becomes diffusely pigmented, with widespread telangiectasis. Calcification develops in many areas of skin.

CUTANEOUS SIGNS OF INTERNAL MALIGNANCIES

There are two major ways in which skin changes are associated with internal malignancies: (1) direct invasion or metastasis, discussed under Malignant Tumors, above, and (2) skin changes without metastasis.

Skin Changes without Metastasis

Humoral Syndromes

A number of nonendocrine tumors secrete humoral agents that mimic endocrine disease. Oat cell carcinoma of the lung may produce hyperadrenal cortisolism with pigmentation. The most dramatic endocrine syndrome is related to carcinoid tumors. Patients develop bright red-purple flushing of the face and neck that is transient initially but becomes more permanent with repeated attacks. Widespread telangiectasis develops. The vascular response, symptoms of wheezing and diarrhea are a result of secretion of serotonin and bradykinin from the tumor. The intestine, appendix, or bronchus are usual primary sites.

Inflammatory Changes

Generalized pruritus or itching is uncommon but occurs with lymphoma, particularly Hodgkins type. Scaling of a generalized nature much like ichthyosis is most commonly seen with lymphomas. A generalized erythroderma is the hallmark of Sezary's syndrome due to lymphoma. Plaque-like infiltrations with erythema are common in leukemia and lymphoma. Dermatomyositis in the adult is often associated with carcinoma; the lungs, breast, and gastrointestinal tract are the most common primary sites.

Figurate erythema and erythema multiforme are uncommon presentations, found with breast, lung, and cervical carcinoma.

Acanthosis Nigricans

This is characterized by velvety hyperpigmentation of skin folds in the axillae and perineal areas (Fig. 19.12). It is commonly associated with adenocarcinoma.

MISCELLANEOUS SYSTEMIC DISORDERS

Pseudoxanthoma Elasticum

This is a genetic disorder in which there is destruction and calcification of elastic tissue throughout the body. Yellow papules, like the skin of a "plucked chicken," occur in the flexures of the neck, axillae, and anticubital areas, and the skin becomes lax. The disease has its greatest impact on elastic tissue of the blood vessels, leading to rupture and bleeding. Opthalmoscopic examination may demonstrate the angioid streaks of Bruchs membrane of the retina, which lead to considerable decline in visual accuity. No effective treatment is available.

Skin Manifestations of Gastrointestinal Disorders

Diseases of Stomach

Pernicious anemia may be associated with vitiligo. Pigmentation of the lips and other parts of skin may be associated with gastric polyposis in the Peutz-Jegher syndrome. Gastric carcinoma may be associated with acanthosis nigricans (See Cutaneous Signs of Internal Malignancy).

Diseases of Bowel

Malabsorption may be associated with cutaneous changes. Dermatitis herpetiformis often occurs in patients with spruelike changes of the small bowel. Other changes in patients with malabsorption include dry scaly skin, pigmentation, and eczematization; in acrodermatitis enteropathica, there is poor absorption of zinc. This is associated with the presence of perioral eruption and alopecia. This condition is reversed by zinc administration.

In regional ileitis, there may be abdominal fistulae and rectal abscesses. In ulcerative colitis, skin lesions appear as a large ulcer with vegetating border (pyoderma gangrenosum), multiple pustules on the skin (pyostomatitis vegetans), erythematous tender nod-

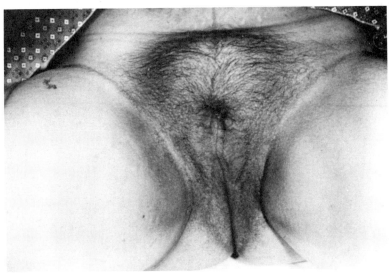

Fig. 19.12 Acanthosis Nigricans

ules usually on the shins (erythema nodosum), and apthous ulcers of the mouth.

In *dermatogenic enteropathy*, malabsorption develops as a result of moderate to severe skin disease such as psoriasis or eczema. The jejunal biopsy is normal and the steatorrhea does not respond to a gluten-free diet. The degree of malabsorption correlates with the degree of skin involvement and disappears with clearing of the erythroderma. The mechanism of dermatogenic enteropathy has not been elucidated.

Liver Disease

The presence of bile pigments in liver disease, caused by a variety of disorders, leads to jaundice. There may be diffuse pigmentation associated with biliary cirrhosis and hemochromatosis. Spider hemangiomata are common in women and children, but appear in greater numbers in pregnancy and cirrhosis. Palmar erythema is also prominent in liver disease. Purpura and bruising may result from vitamin K deficiency and thrombocytopenia.

The nails may become white with absence of lunula and clubbing may develop. The hair may be fine and sparse.

Pruritus is often present in advanced liver disease and is more marked when there is cholestasis.

Renal Disease

Renal failure may lead to itching, particularly in severe renal failure. The itching may be relieved by dialysis or those patients with secondary hyperparathyroidism may require a parathyroidectomy. The skin may be dry, pale, and often hyperpigmented. Rarely, uremic frosting due to white urea crystals is seen on the skin.

Pulmonary Disease

Pulmonary sarcoidosis and infections such as psittacosis, histoplasmosis, and coccidiomycosis may present with erythema nodosum. Subcutaneous nodules consisting of characteristic granulomas may be present in sarcoidosis. Many pulmonary diseases including bronchiectasis, interstitial fibrosis, and carcinoma may present with clubbing. Hypoxemia is seen as cyanosis and chronic hypoxemia with polycythemia results in a ruddy complexion or plethora.

Diseases of Nervous System

Neurofibromatosis (von Recklinghausen's disease) is a systemic, dominantly inherited disorder affecting skin, bones, and subcutaneous tissues. Soft, flesh-colored, pedunculated tumors arise along nerve sheaths anywhere in the body. They may be sessile, doughy, and easily invaginated. Pigmented macular lesions (café-au-lait spots) are frequently present with axillary freckles. Associated clinical features include kyphoscoliosis, evidence of mass effect in cranial nerves or organs such as the lung, and an increased incidence of pheochromocytoma.

Ataxia telangiectasia is a neurocutaneous order recognized by telangiectasis of the malar eminences, bulbar conjunctiva, head and neck, associated with cerebellar ataxia. Unexplained immune deficiencies including IgA and IgE deficiencies are common.

REFERENCES

1. Braverman, I.M.: Skin Signs of Systemic Disease. Philadelphia, W.B. Saunders, 1970.
2. Cronin, E.: Contact Dermatitis. London, Churchill Livingstone, 1980.
3. Fitzpatrick, T., Eisen, A., Wolff, K., et al: Dermatology in General Medicine. New York, McGraw-Hill, 1979.
4. Kimmig, J., Janner, M.: Color Atlas of Dermatology. Philadelphia, W.B. Saunders, 1966.
5. Lever, W.F., Schaumberg-Lever, G.: Histopathology of Skin. 5th ed. Philadelphia, J.B. Lippincott, 1975.
6. Rook, A.; Wilkinson, D.S., Ebling, F.J.G.: Textbook of Dermatology. Oxford, Blackwell Scientific Publication, 1979.
7. Shuster, S.: Dermatology in Internal Medicine. Oxford, Oxford Universal Press, 1978.
8. Wisdom, A.: Color Atlas of Venereology. Chicago, Year Book Medical Publication, 1973.

APPENDIX:
COMMON LABORATORY VALUES

Abbreviations: B-Blood, S-Serum, P-Plasma, U-Urine, Sf-Spinal fluid, d-day, h-hour, C°-Celsius degrees, dl-decilitre (100 ml), L-Litre, g-gram, μ-micro, n-nano, p-pica, mol-mole, Eq-equivalents.

Electrolytes	Common Lab Units	International Units
Calcium (S) Male	8.8–10.3 mg/dl	2.20–2.58 mmol/L
Female <50 yrs	8.8–10.0 mg/dl	2.20–2.50 mmol/L
Female >50 yrs	8.8–10.2 mg/dl	2.20–2.56 mmol/L
Calcium (S) ionized	2.00–2.30 mEq/L	1.00–1.15 mmol/L
Calcium (U) normal diet	<250 mg/24h	<6.2 mmol/d
Carbon dioxide content (B,P,S)	22–28 mEq/L	22–28 mmol/L
Chloride (S)	95–105 mEq/L	95–105 mmol/L
Magnesium (S)	1.8–3.0 mg/dl	0.80–1.20 mmol/L
	1.6–2.4 mEq/L	
Phosphate (S)	2.5–5.0 mg/dl	0.80–1.60 mmol/L
Potassium (S)	3.5–5.0 mEq/L	3.5–5.0 mmol/L
Potassium (U) diet dependant	25–100 mEq/24h	25–100 mmol/d
Sodium (S)	135–147 mEq/L	135–147 mmol/L
Sodium (U) diet dependant	mEq/24h	mmol/d

Enzymes:	Common Lab Units	International Units
Alanine amino transferase (S) ALAT	0–35 U/L	0–35 U/L
Aldolase (S)	0–6 U/L	0–6 U/L
Amylase		
Enzymatic	0–130 U/L	0–130 U/L
Somogyi	50–150 Somogyi units/dl	100–300 U/L
Aspartate amino transferase (S) ASAT	0–35 U/L	0–35 U/L
Cholinesterase (S)	620–1370 U/L	620–1370 U/L
Creatine kinase (S) CK	0–130 U/L	0–130 U/L
Creatine kinase isoenzymes – MB fraction	>5 in myocardial infarction	>0.05
Gamma-glutamyl transferase (S) GGT	0–30 U/L	0–30 U/L
Lactate dehydrogenase (S)	50–150 U/L	50–150 U/L
Lipase (S)	0–160 U/L	0–160 U/L
Phosphatase, acid (P)	0–3 King-Armstrong units/dl	0–55 U/L
Phosphatase, alkaline (S)	30–120 U/L Bodansky units/dl	30–120 U/L

Blood Cells	Common Lab Units	International Units
See Chapter 17, Table 17-1		

Blood Proteins	Common Lab Units	International Units
Albumin (S)	4.0–6.0 g/dl	40–60 g/L
Alpha₁ antitrypsin (S)	150–350 mg/dl	1.5–3.5 g/L
Complement, C3 (S)	70–160 mg/dl	0.7–1.6 g/L
Electrophoresis, protein (S)		
Albumin	3.6–5.2 g/dl	36–52 g/L
Alpha 1	0.1–0.4 g/dl	1–4 g/L
Alpha 2	0.4–1.0 g/dl	4–10 g/L
Beta	0.5–1.2 g/dl	5–12 g/L
Gamma	0.6–1.6 g/dl	6–16 g/L
Haptoglobin (S)	50–220 mg/dl	0.50–2.20 g/L
Hemoglobin (B)		
Male	14.0–18.0 g/dl	140–180 g/L
Female	11.5–15.5 g/dl	115–155 g/L
Immunoglobulins (S)		
IgG	500–1200 mg/dl	5.00–12.00 g/L
IgA	50–350 mg/dl	0.50–3.50 g/L
IgM	30–230 mg/dl	0.30–2.30 g/L
IgD	<6 mg/dl	<60 mg/L
IgE 10–20 yrs	25–1200 ng/ml	25–1200 μg/L
20–70 yrs	20–1000 ng/ml	20–1000 μg/L
Protein, total (S)	6–8 g/dl	60–80 g/L
(Sf)	<40 mg/dl	<0.40 g/L
(U)	<150 mg/24h	<0.15 g/d

Blood Lipids:	Common Lab Units	International Units
Cholesterol (P) <30 yrs	<200 mg/dl	<5.20 mmol/L
>50 yrs	<265 mg/dl	<6.85 mmol/L
Lipids, total (P)	400–850 mg/dl	4.0–8.5 g/L
Lipoproteins (P)		
Low density–LDL	50–190 mg/dl	1.30–4.90 mmol/L
High density–HDL		
Male	30–70 mg/dl	0.80–1.80 mmol/L
Female	30–90 mg/dl	0.80–2.35 mmol/L
Triglycerides (P)	<160 mg/dl	<1.80 mmol/L

Hormones:	Common Lab Units	International Units
Aldosterone (S)		
Normal salt diet	8.1–15.5 ng/dl	220–430 pmol/L
Restricted salt diet	20.8–44.4 ng/dl	580–1240 pmol/L
Cortisol (S)		
0800 h	4–19 µg/dl	110–520 nmol/L
1600 h	2–15 µg/dl	50–410 nmol/L
2400 h	<5µg/dl	<140 nmol/L
Cortisol (U)	10–110 µg/24 h	30–300 nmol/d
Epinephrine (P)	31–95 (At rest for 15 minutes)	170–520 pmol/L
(U)	<10 µg/24h	<55 nmol/d
Estriol (U)		
Onset of menstruation	4–25 µg/24h	15–85 nmol/d
Ovulation peak	28–99 µg/24h	95–345 nmol/d
Luteal peak	22–105 µg/24h	75–365 nmol/d
Menopausal women	1.4–19.6 µg/24h	5–70 nmol/d
Male	5–18 µg/24h	15–60 nmol/d
Estrogens (S)		
Female	20–300 pg/ml	70–1100 pmol/L
Peak Production	200–800 pg/ml	750–2900 pmol/L
Male	<50 pg/ml	<180 pmol/L
Follicle Stimulating Hormone (P)–FSH		
Female	2.0–15.0 mIu/ml	2–15 IU/L
Peak production	20–50 mIu/ml	20–50 IU/L
Male	1.0–10.0 mIu/ml	1–10 IU/L
Follicle Stimulating Hormone (U)–FSH		
Midcycle, peak	8–40 Iu/24h	8–40 IU/d
Menopausal women	35–100 Iu/24h	35–100 IU/d
Male	2–15 Iu/24h	2–15 IU/d
Gastrin (S)	0–180 pg/ml	0–180 ng/L
Glucagon	50–100 pg/ml	50–100 ng/L
Growth Hormone (P,S)		
Male, fasting	0–5 ng/ml	0–5 µg/L
Female, fasting	0–10 ng/ml	0–10 µg/L
Insulin (P,S)	5–20 µU/ml	35–145 pmol/L
	5–20 mU/L	
	0.20–0.84 µg/L	
Pregnanediol (U)		
Normal	1.0–6.0 mg/24h	3.0–18.5 µmol/d
Pregnancy	depends on gestation	
Pregnanetriol (U)	0.5–2.0 mg/24h	1.5–6.0 µmol/d
Progesterone		
Follicular phase	<2 ng/ml	<6 nmol/L
Luteal phase	2–20 ng/ml	6–64 nmol/L
Prolactin (P)	<20 ng/ml	<20 µg/L
Steroids (U)		
Hydroxycorticosteroids		
Female	2–8 mg/24h	5–25 µmol/d
Male	3–10 mg/24h	10–30 µmol/d
17 Ketogenic steroids		
Female	7–12 mg/24h	25–40 µmol/d
Male	9–17 mg/24h	30–60 µmol/d
17 Ketosteroids		
Female	6–17 mg/24h	20–60 µmol/d
Male	6–20 mg/24h	20–70 µmol/d
Testosterone (P)		
Femal	<0.6 ng/ml	<2.0 nmol/L
Male	4.0–8.0 ng/ml	14.0–28.0 nmol/L
Thyroid Stimulating Hormone (S)–TSH	2–11 µU/ml	2–11 mU/L
Thyroxine (S)–T_4	4–11 µg/dl	51–142 nmol/L
Thyroxine binding globulin (S)–TBG	12–28 µg/dl	150–360 nmol/L
Triiodothyronine (S)–T_3	75–220 ng/dl	1.2–3.4 nmol/L
T_3 Uptake (S)	25–35%	0.25–0.35

Misc. Chemistry:	Common Lab Units	International Units
Bilirubin, total (S)	0.1–1.0 mg/dl	2–18 μmol/L
Conjugated	0–0.2 mg/dl	0–4 μmol/L
Copper (S)	70–140 μg/dl	11.0–22.0 μmol/L
(U)	<40 μg/24h	<0.6 μmol/d
Creatinine (S)	0.6–1.2 mg/dl	50–110 μmol/L
(U)	variable g/24h	variable mmol/d
Fecal fat (F)	2.0–6.0 g/24h	7–21mmol/d
Ferritin (S)	18–300 ng/ml	18–300 μg/L
Folate (S)	2–10 μg/dl	4–22 nmol/L
Gases, arterial (B)		
pO_2	75–105 mmHg (= Torr)	10.0–14.0 kPa
pCO_2	33–44 mmHg (= Torr)	4.4–5.9 kPa
Glucose (P)	70–110 mg/dl	3.9–6.1 mmol/L
(Sf)	50–80 mg/dl	2.8–4.4 mmol/L
5-Hydroxyindoleacetate (U)	2–8 mg/24h	10–40 μmol/d
Iron (S) Male	80–180 μg/dl	14–32 μmol/L
Female	60–160 μg/dl	11–29 μmol/L
Iron binding capacity (S)	250–460 μg/dl	45–82 μmol/L
Lactic Acid (P)	0.5–2.0 mEq/L	0.5–2.0 mmol/L
	5–20 mg/dl	
Metanephrines (U)	0–2.0 mg/24h	0–11.0 μmol/d
Osmolality (P)	280–300 mOsm/kg	280–300 mmol/kg
(U)	50–1200 mOsm/kg	50–1200 mmol/kg
Porphobilinogen (U)	0–2 mg/24h	0–8.8 μmol/d
Porphyrins		
Coproporphyrin (U)	45–180 μg/24h	68–276 nmol/d
Protoporphyrin (Erc)	15–50 μg/dl	0.28–0.90 μmol/L
Uroporphyrin (U)	5–20 μg/24h	6–24 nmol/d
Renin (P)		
Normal sodium diet	1.1–4.1 ng/ml/h	$0.30–114 \ ng \cdot L^{-1} \cdot S^{-1}$
Restricted sodium diet	6.2–12.4 ng/ml/h	$1.72–3.44 \ ng \cdot L^{-1} \cdot S^{-1}$
Uric Acid (S)	2.0–6.0 mg/dl	120–360 μmol/L
Urobilinogen (U)	0–4.0 mg/24h	0.0–6.8 μmol/d
Vanilylmandelic acid (U)–VMA (4-hydroxy-3-methoxy mandelic acid)	<6.8 mg/24h	<35 μmol/d
Vitamin B_{12} (P,S)	200–1000 pg/ml ng/dl	150–750 pmol/L

Drugs and Poisons:	Common Lab Units	International Units
Acetominophen (P)		
Therapeutic	0.2–0.6 mg/dl	13–40 μmol/L
Toxic	>5.0 mg/dl	>300 μmol/L
Amitriptyline (S)		
Therapeutic	50–200 ng/ml	180–720 nmol/L
Barbiturate (S)		
Overdose	Depends on composition of mixture	
Therapeutic phenobarbital	2–5 mg/dl	85–215 μmol/L
Diazepam (P)		
Therapeutic	0.1–0.25 mg/L	350–900 nmol/L
Toxic	>1.0 mg/L	>3510 nmol/L
Digoxin (P)		
Therapeutic	0.5–2.2 ng/ml	0.6–2.8 nmol/L
	0.5–2.2 μg/L	0.6–2.8 nmol/L
Diphenylhydantoin (P)		
Therapeutic	10–20 mg/L	40–80 μmol/L
Ethanol (P)		
Legal limit, driving	<80 mg/dl	<17 mmol/L
Toxic	>100 mg/dl	>22 mmol/L
Ethchlorvynol		
Therapeutic	<40 mg/L	<280 μmol/L
Glutethimide (P)		
Therapeutic	<10 mg/L	<46 μmol/L
Toxic	>20 mg/L	>92 μmol/L
Imipramine (P)		
Therapeutic	50–200 ng/ml	180–170 nmol/L
Isoniazid (P)		
Therapeutic	<2.0 mg/L	<15 μmol/L
Toxic	>3.0 mg/L	>22 μmol/L
Lead (B) Toxic	>60 μg/dl	>2.90 μmol/L
(U) Toxic	>80 μg/24h	>0.40 μmol/d
Lithium (S) Therapeutic	0.50–1.50 mEq/L	0.50–1.50 mmol/L
Primidone (P)		
Therapeutic	6–10 mg/L	25–45 μmol/L
Toxic	>10 mg/L	>46 μmol/L
Procainamide (P)		
Therapeutic	4.0–8.0 mg/L	17–34 μmol/L
Toxic	>12 mg/L	>50 μmol/L
Propranolol (P)		
Therapeutic	50–200 ng/ml	190–770 nmol/L
Quinidine (P)		
Therapeutic	1.5–3.0 mg/L	4.6–9.2 μmol/L
Toxic	>6.0 mg/L	>18.5 μmol/L
Salicylate (S)		
Toxic	>20 mg/dl	>1.45 mmol/L
Theophylline (P)		
Therapeutic	10.0–20.0 mg/L	55–110 μmol/L
Warfarin (P)		
Therapeutic	1.0–3.0 mg/L	3.3–9.8 μmol/L

Index

Illustrations are indicated with an "f" after page number, tables are indicated with a "t" after page number.